THE LYMPHOMAS

Second Edition

THE LYMPHOMAS

Second Edition

Editors

George P. Canellos, M.D., F.R.C.P., Dr.S (Hon.)
William Rosenberg Professor of Medicine
Harvard Medical School
Department of Medical Oncology
Dana-Farber Cancer Institute
Boston, Massachusetts

T. Andrew Lister, M.D., F.R.C.P., F.R.C.Path.
Professor of Medical Oncology
Cancer Research UK Medical Oncology Unit
St. Bartholomew's Hospital
London, United Kingdom

Bryan D. Young, Ph.D.
Professor of Molecular Oncology
Cancer Research UK Medical Oncology Unit
St. Bartholomew's Hospital Medical School
London, United Kingdom

SAUNDERS
ELSEVIER

SAUNDERS
ELSEVIER

1600 John F. Kennedy Blvd.
Suite 1800
Philadelphia, PA 19103-2899

THE LYMPHOMAS, SECOND EDITION

ISBN-13: 978-0-7216-0081-9
ISBN-10: 0-7216-0081-6

Library of Congress Cataloging-in-Publication Data
The lymphomas / [edited by] George Canellos, T. Andrew Lister, Bryan Young.—2nd ed.
p. ; cm.
Includes bibliographical references and index.
ISBN 0-7216-0081-6
1. Lymphomas. I. Canellos, Geogre P. (George Peter), 1934 II. Lister, T. A. (Thomas Andrew) III. Young, G. Bryan (Gordon Bryan)
[DNLM: 1. Lymphoma WH 525 L9852 2006]
RC280.L9L953 2006
616.99'446—dc22

2005056129

Acquisitions Editor: Dolores Meloni
Developmental Editor: Kristina Oberle
Project Manager: David Saltzberg

Printed in China

Last digit is the print number: 9 8 7 6 5 4 3 2 1

To the memory of our
colleague, Dr. Stanley Korsmeyer.

Preface

Research in the field of malignant lymphoma has moved faster than any other component of medical oncology. The second edition of *The Lymphomas* is an attempt to bring the changing basic science and clinical information up-to-date and to conform with the new understanding of the biological features and natural history of the various malignant lymphomas. Since the last edition, there has been a comprehensive review by the World Health Organization resulting in a classification scheme that embodied some of the principles of the REAL [revised European American lymphoma] classification as well as a consensus among pathologists and clinicians regarding the appropriateness of the various subdivisions of Hodgkin lymphoma and non-Hodgkin's lymphoma. New contributors who are active in their various fields of specialization have been brought into the second edition, bringing a new vitality to this edition. A molecular biologic basis of the cytogenetic translocations that characterize the various forms of lymphoma has been completely updated. The immunophenotypic as well as molecular genetic abnormalities are described, which may lend themselves to the targeted therapy. To that end, the section on biological therapy has been completely rewritten with a comprehensive consideration of all of the new information available on the biological therapy of lymphoma. The major subdivisions within the WHO classification have been separated and discussed individually. As in the previous edition, the therapeutic modalities—such as chemotherapy, radiation therapy, and bone marrow transplantation—are updated in separate chapters.

The pace of biological discovery is very quick leading to a host of new agents targeted to cell surface markers as well as unique molecular abnormalities. Microarray technology has begun to define the various lymphomas according to molecular genetic signatures which correlate with natural history. In addition, this technique may define specific abnormalities against which targeted therapies could be developed. The basic scientific sections have a new editor in Dr. Bryan Young, who has been an active investigator in the field. This second edition is an attempt to offer the reader a comprehensive view of the basic and clinical science in the field with recommendations as to therapeutic approaches. It is assumed that this field will continue to change as new therapeutic tactics emerge.

The editors wish to thank all of the contributors, their administrative assistants and secretaries for their dedicated efforts with this Second Edition. The editors gratefully acknowledge the inspiration of their mentors in the field of lymphoma therapy, some of whom have passed on, including Professor G. Hamilton Fairley, Professor Timothy McElwain, Drs. Paul Carbone and John Ultmann.

George P. Canellos
T. Andrew Lister
Bryan D. Young

Contributors

Ranjana Advani, M.D.
Assistant Professor of Medicine, Department of Medicine and Oncology, Stanford University, Stanford, California, USA

James O. Armitage, M.D.
Joe Shapiro Professor of Medicine, Department of Internal Medicine, University of Nebraska Medical Center, Omaha, Nebraska, USA

Francesco Bertoni, M.D.
Honorary Senior Lecturer, Barts and The London, London, United Kingdom; Head of the Functional Genomics Unit, Laboratory of Experimental Oncology, Oncology Institute of Southern Switzerland, Bellinzona, Switzerland

Magnus Björkholm, M.D., Ph.D.
Department of Medicine, Division of Hematology, Karolinska Hospital, Stockholm, Sweden

Kristie A. Blum, M.D.
Assistant Professor of Medicine, Division of Hematology and Oncology, The Ohio State University, The Arthur G. James Comprehensive Cancer Center, Columbus, Ohio, USA

Jennifer R. Brown, M.D., Ph.D.
Instructor in Medicine, Harvard Medical School, Department of Medical Oncology, Dana-Farber Cancer Institute, Department of Medicine, Brigham & Women's Hospital, Boston, Massachusetts, USA

John C. Byrd, M.D.
Division of Medicinal Chemistry, Department of Pharmacy, The Ohio State University Columbus, Ohio, USA

Elias Campo, M.D. Ph.D.
Professor of Pathology, Chief, Department of Pathology and Hematopathology Unit, Hospital Clinic, University of Barcelona, Barcelona, Spain

George P. Canellos, M.D., F.R.C.P., DR.S (Hon.)
William Rosenberg Professor of Medicine, Harvard Medical School, Department of Medical Oncology, Dana-Farber Cancer Institute, Boston, Massachusetts, USA

Franco Cavalli, M.D., F.R.C.P.
Professor of Medicine, University of Bern, Switzerland, Director of the Oncology Institute of Southern Switzerland, Ospedale San Giovanni, Bellinzona, Switzerland

Bruce D. Cheson, M.D.
Head of Hematology, Georgetown University Hospital, Washington, DC, USA

Bertrand Coiffier, M.D.
Hospices Civils de Lyon & Université Claude Bernard, Lyon, France; Hematology Department, Pierre Benite, France

Joseph M. Connors, M.D., F.R.C.P.C.
British Columbia Cancer Agency, Vancouver, BC, Canada

Andrew Davies, B.Sc., B.M., M.R.C.P.
Clinical Research Fellow and Honorary Lecturer, Department of Medical Oncology, Institute of Cancer and the CR-UK Clinical Centre, Barts and the London, Queen Mary's School of Medicine and Dentistry, London, United Kingdom

Martin Dreyling, M.D., Ph.D.
University Hospital Grosshadern, Department of Internal Medicine III, Ludwig-Maximilians-University, Munich, Germany

Andrew L. Feldman, M.D.
Clinical Fellow, Laboratory of Pathology, National Cancer Institute, National Institutes of Health, Bethesda, Maryland, USA

Howard A. Fine, M.D.
Chief of the Neuro-Oncology Branch, National Cancer Institute, National Institutes of Neurological Disorders and Stroke, National Institutes of Health, Bethesda, Maryland, USA

Richard I. Fisher, M.D.
Samuel E. Durand Professor of Medicine, Director, James P. Wilmot Cancer Center, Director, Hematology-Oncology Division, Director of Cancer Services, Strong Health, University of Rochester School of Medicine, Rochester, New York, USA

Jonathan W. Friedberg, M.D.
Assistant Professor of Medicine and Oncology, University of Rochester School of Medicine, James P. Wilmot Cancer Center, Rochester, New York, USA

John G. Gribben, M.D.
Cancer Research UK Medical Oncology Unit, St. Bartholomew's Hospital, Barts and the London School of Medicine and Dentistry, London, United Kingdom

Wolfgang Hiddemann, M.D., Ph.D.
University Hospital Grosshadern, Department of Internal Medicine III, Ludwig-Maximilians-University, Munich, Germany

Richard T. Hoppe, M.D.
Henry S. Kaplan-Harry Lebeson Professor of Cancer Biology, Department of Radiation Oncology, Stanford University School of Medicine, Stanford, California, USA

Doug Horsman, M.D.
Director, Cancer Genetics Laboratory, British Columbia Cancer Agency, Vancouver, British Columbia, Canada

Roland Hustinx, M.D., Ph.D.
Centre Hospitalier Universitaire Sart Tilman, University of Liège, Belgium

Naoko Ishibe, Sc.D.
Nuclear Medicine, Centre Hospitalier Universitaire Sart Tilman, Belgium

Elaine S. Jaffe, M.D.
Chief, Hematopathology Section, Acting Chief, Laboratory of Pathology, National Cancer Institute, National Institutes of Health, Bethesda, Maryland, USA

Guy Jerusalem, M.D., Ph.D.
Medical Oncology, Centre Hospitalier Universitaire Sart Tilman, University of Liège, Belgium

Youn H. Kim, M.D.
Professor of Dermatology, Director, Multidisciplinary Cutaneous Lymphoma Clinic, Department of Dermatology, Stanford University School of Medicine, Stanford, California, USA

Anton W. Langerak, Ph.D.
Department of Immunology, Erasmus MC, University Medical Center Rotterdam, Rotterdam, The Netherlands

Rifca Le Dieu, M.B.B.S.
Clinical Research Fellow, Cancer Research UK Medical Oncology Unit, St. Bartholomew's Hospital, Barts and the London School of Medicine and Dentistry, London, United Kingdom

Georg Lenz, M.D.
Fellow, Metabolism Branch, National Cancer Institute, National Institutes of Health, Bethesda, Maryland, USA

Alexandra M. Levine, M.D.
Keck School of Medicine, University of Southern California, Los Angeles, California, USA

Raymond Liang, M.D., F.R.C.P., F.R.A.C.P.
S.H. Ho Chair Professor in Haematology and Oncology, Department of Medicine, University of Hong Kong, Hong Kong

T. Andrew Lister, M.D., F.R.C.P., F.R.C.Path.
Professor of Medical Oncology, Centre for Medical Oncology, Institute of Cancer and the CR-UK Clinical Centre, Barts and the London, Queen Mary's School of Medicine and Dentistry, London, United Kingdom

Jay S. Loeffler, M.D.
Herman and Joan Suit Professor of Radiation Oncology, Harvard Medical School, Chair, Department of Radiation Oncology, Massachusetts General Hospital, Boston, Massachusetts, USA

Gerard Lozanski, M.D.
Department of Pathology, Ohio State University, Columbus, Ohio, USA

Masao Matsuoka, M.D., Ph.D.
Institute for Virus Research, Kyoto University, Kyoto, Japan

Silvia Montoto, M.D.
Senior Lecturer, Centre for Medical Oncology, Institute of Cancer and the CR-UK Clinical Centre, Barts and the London, Queen Mary's School of Medicine and Dentistry, London, United Kingdom

Emili Montserrat, M.D., Ph.D.
Professor of Medicine, Director, Institute of Hematology and Oncology Hospital Clínic, University of Barcelona, Barcelona, Spain

Andrea K. Ng, M.D., M.P.H.
Assistant Professor of Radiation Oncology, Harvard Medical School, Brigham and Women's Hospital, Boston, Massachusetts, USA

Vassaliki I. Pappa, M.D.
Second Department of Internal Medicine, Propaedeutic, University of Athens, Attikon University General Hospital, Athens, Greece

Stefania Pittaluga, M.D., Ph.D.
Staff Clinician, Laboratory of Pathology, National Cancer Institute, National Institutes of Health, Bethesda, Maryland, USA

Rodney H. Reznek, M.B., Ch.B., F.R.C.P., F.R.C.R.
Professor of Diagnostic Imaging and Consultant Radiologist, Cancer Imaging, St. Bartholomew's Hospital, London, United Kingdom

Ama Z. Rohatiner, M.D., F.R.C.P.
Professor of Hemato-Oncology, Centre for Medical Oncology, Institute of Cancer and the CR-UK Clinical Centre, Barts and the London, Queen Mary's School of Medicine and Dentistry, London, United Kingdom

Vaskar Saha, M.D.
Cancer Research UK Children's Cancer Group, Department of Paediatric Haematology and Oncology, Institute of Cancer, Barts and The London School of

Medicine and Dentistry, Queen Mary University of London, London, United Kingdom

A. Shankar, M.D.
Cancer Research UK Children's Cancer Group, Department of Paediatric Haematology and Oncology, Institute of Cancer, Barts and The London School of Medicine and Dentistry, Queen Mary University of London, London, United Kingdom

Tamara N. Shenkier, M.D., F.R.C.P.C.
Medical Onoclogist, British Columbia Cancer Agency, Clinical Assistant Professor of Medicine, University of British Columbia, Vancouver, BC, Canada

Arthur T. Skarin, M.D., F.A.C.P., F.C.C.P.
Associate Professor of Medicine, Harvard Medical School, Department of Medical Oncology, Dana-Farber Cancer Institute, Department of Medicine, Brigham & Women's Hospital, Boston, Maryland, USA

Louis M. Staudt, M.D., Ph.D.
Chief, Lymphoid Malignancies Section, Metabolism Branch, Center for Cancer Research, National Cancer Institute, National Institutes of Health, Bethesda, Maryland, USA

John W. Sweetenham, M.D.
Professor of Medicine, Hematology and Oncology, Cleveland Clinic Foundation, Cleveland, Ohio, USA

Lode J. Swinnen, M.D.
Division of Hematological Malignancy, Department of Oncology, Johns Hopkins Cancer Center, Baltimore, Maryland, USA

Tomasz Szczepański, M.D., Ph.D.
Silesian School of Medicine, Department of Pediatric Hematology and Oncology, Zabrze, Poland

Catherine Traullé, M.D.
Hospices Civils de Lyon, Hematology Department, Centre Hospitalier Lyon-Sud, Pierre Benite, France

Margaret Tucker, M.D.
Director, Human Genetics Program, Genetic Epidemiology Branch, Division of Cancer Epidemiology and Genetics, National Cancer Institute, National Institutes of Health, Rockville, Maryland, USA

Vincent H.J. van der Velden, Ph.D.
Department of Immunology, Erasmus MC, University Medical Center Rotterdam, Rotterdam, The Netherlands

Jacques J.M. van Dongen, M.D., Ph.D.
Department of Immunology, Erasmus MC, University Medical Center Rotterdam, Rotterdam, The Netherlands

Sarah J. Vinnicombe, B.Sc.(Hons.), M.R.C.P., F.R.C.R.
Department of Diagnostic Imaging, St Bartholomew's Hospital, London, United Kingdom

Rein Willemze, M.D.
Leiden University Medical Center, Department of Dermatology, Leiden, The Netherlands

Wyndham H. Wilson, M.D., Ph.D.
Senior Investigator and Chief, Lymphoma Therapeutics Section, Metabolism Branch, Center for Cancer Research, National Cancer Institute, National Institutes of Health, Bethesda, Maryland, USA

Joachim Yahalom, M.D.
Co-chair, Lymphoma Disease Management Team, Attending, Department of Radiation Oncology, Member, Memorial Sloan-Kettering Cancer Center, Professor of Radiation Oncology in Medicine, Weill Medical College of Cornell University, New York, New York, USA

Bryan D. Young, Ph.D.
Professor of Molecular Oncology, Cancer Research UK Medical Oncology Unit, St. Bartholomew's Hospital Medical School, London, United Kingdom

Andrew Zelenetz, M.D., Ph.D.
Chief, Lymphoma Service, Head, Laboratory of Hemato-Oncology, Memorial Sloan-Kettering Cancer Center, New York, New York, USA

Pier Luigi Zinzani, M.D., Ph.D.
Institute of Hematology and Medical Oncology "Seràgnoli", University of Bologna, Bologna, Italy

Emanuele Zucca, M.D.
Privatdozent of Oncology/Haematology, University of Bern, Switzerland, Head of the Lymphoma Unit, Oncology Institute of Southern Switzerland, Ospedale San Giovanni Bellinzona, Switzerland

Contents

Color Plate Section

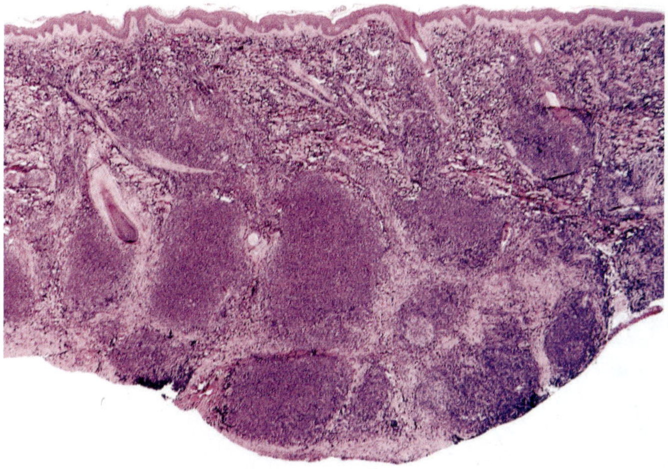

A

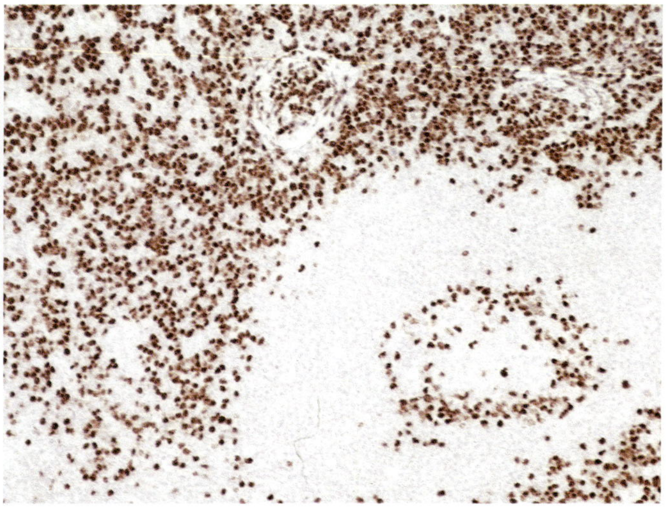

B

Figure 1–1. Precursor B-lymphoblastic leukemia/lymphoma. **A:** This scalp lesion was the initial presenting site of disease in this 10-year-old female. The tumor infiltrates the reticular dermis, but leaves a Grenz zone beneath the epidermis. **B:** Lymphoblasts demonstrate nuclear staining for terminal deoxynucleotidyl transferase (TdT). This example of lymph node involvement shows diffuse paracortical involvement with relative sparing of germinal centers **(lower right).**

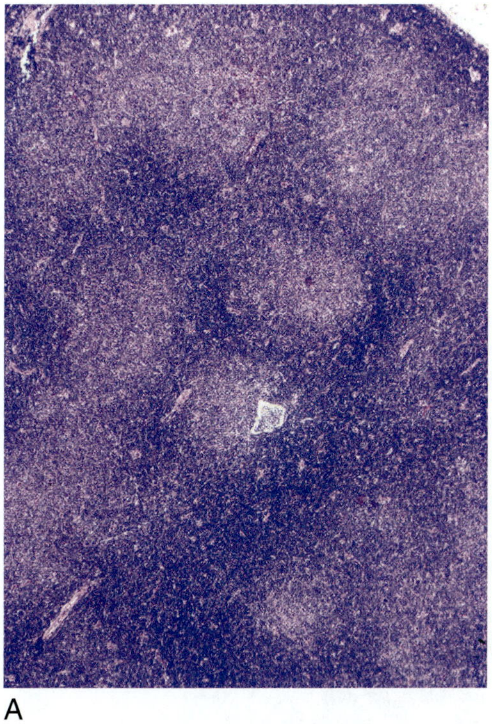

A

Figure 1–2. CLL/SLL, lymph node. **A:** The lymph node shows diffuse architectural effacement with a pseudofollicular pattern, seen as pale areas representing proliferation or growth centers.

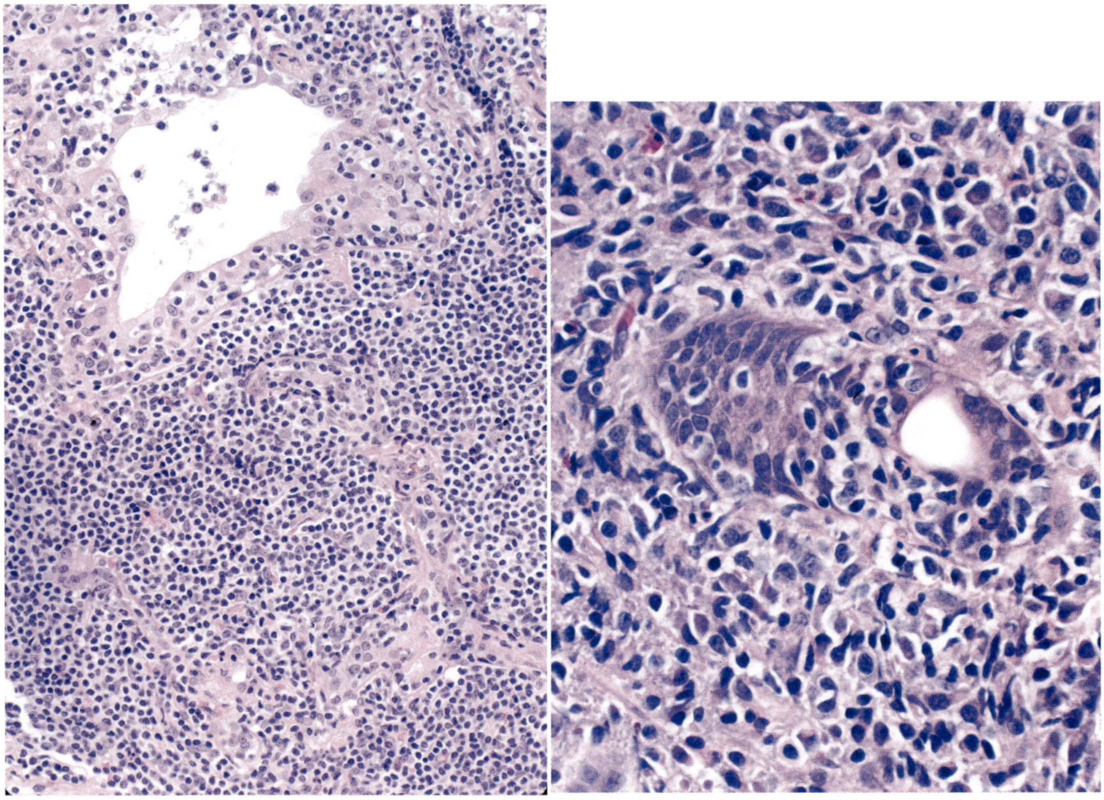

A B

Figure 1–4. MALT lymphoma. **A:** In this lung lesion, monocytoid-appearing cells with pale cytoplasm infiltrate and surround the bronchial epithelium. **B:** Lymphoepithelial lesion in a case of gastric MALT lymphoma, showing lymphoma cells invading an epithelial gland.

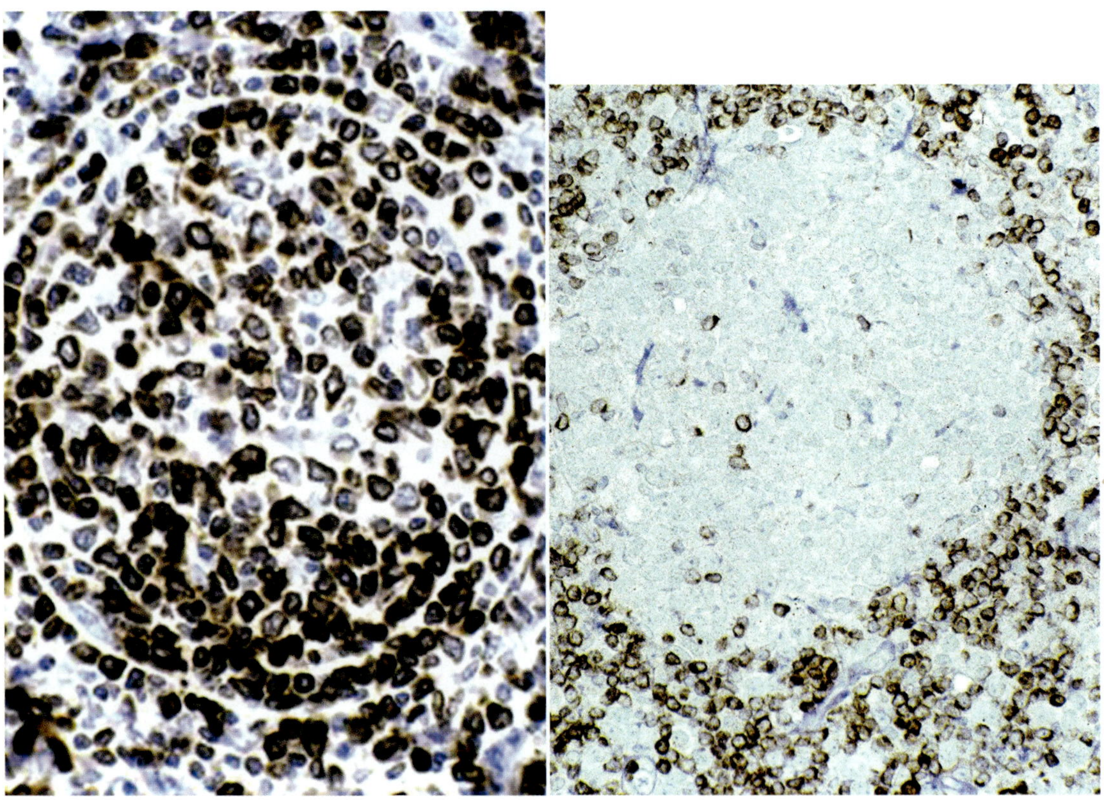

B C

Figure 1–5. Follicular lymphoma, lymph node. **B:** The t(14;18) translocation leads to overexpression of Bcl-2 protein in the neoplastic follicles of follicular lymphoma (dark cytoplasmic staining). **C:** Bcl-2 protein is not expressed in reactive, non-neoplastic germinal center B cells. The positive cells seen represent reactive T cells.

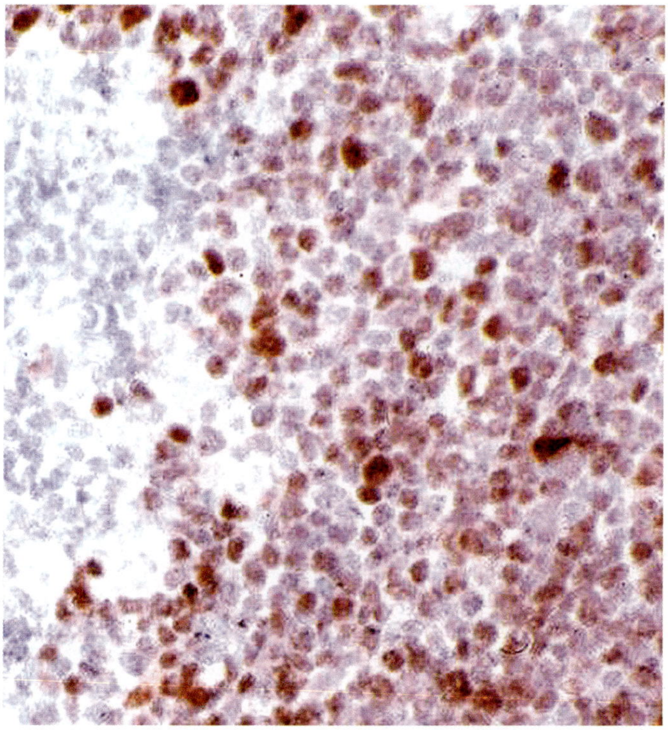

Figure 1–6. Mantle cell lymphoma, lymph node. A monotonous lymphoid infiltrate highlighted by nuclear staining for cyclin D1 maintains its mantle zone pattern, surrounding a non-neoplastic germinal center (negative staining, **left**).

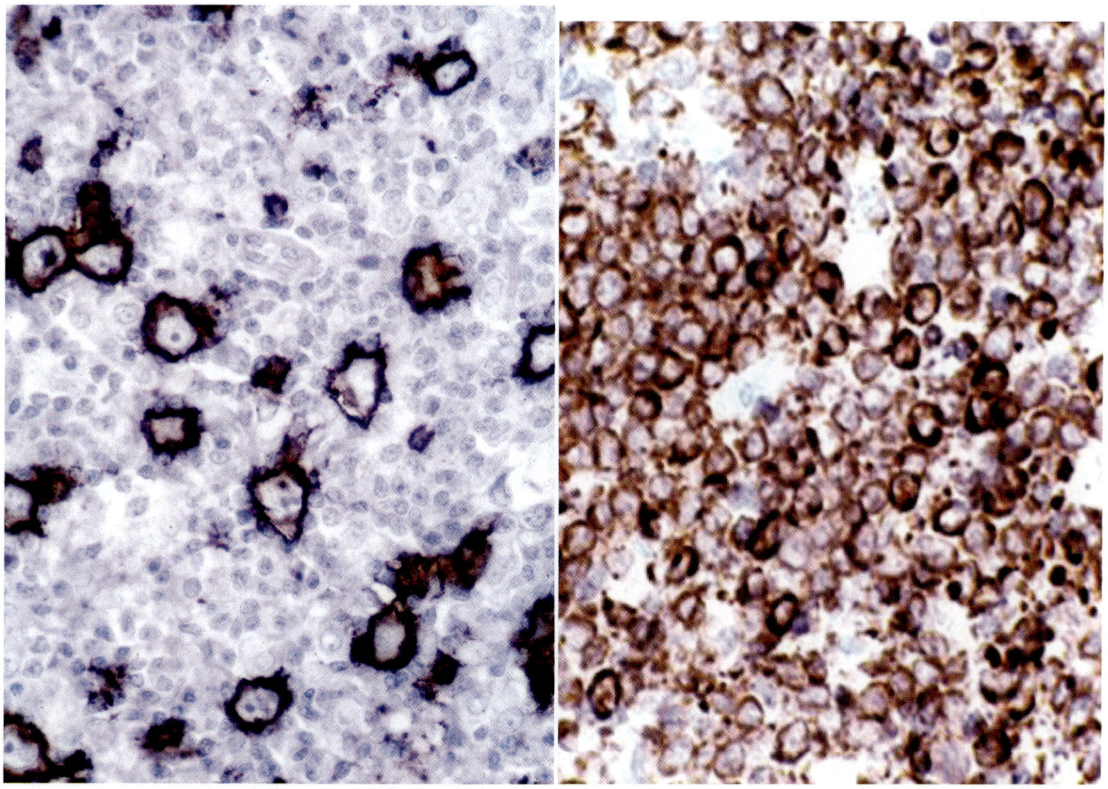

B C

Figure 1–7. Diffuse large B-cell lymphoma. **B:** In the T-cell/histiocyte-rich variant of DLBCL, a background of small non-neoplastic T cells surrounds the large neoplastic B lymphocytes, which are highlighted by immunostaining for CD20. **C:** A case of DLBCL demonstrating Bcl-2 protein expression (dark cytoplasmic staining), a finding generally associated with adverse outcome.

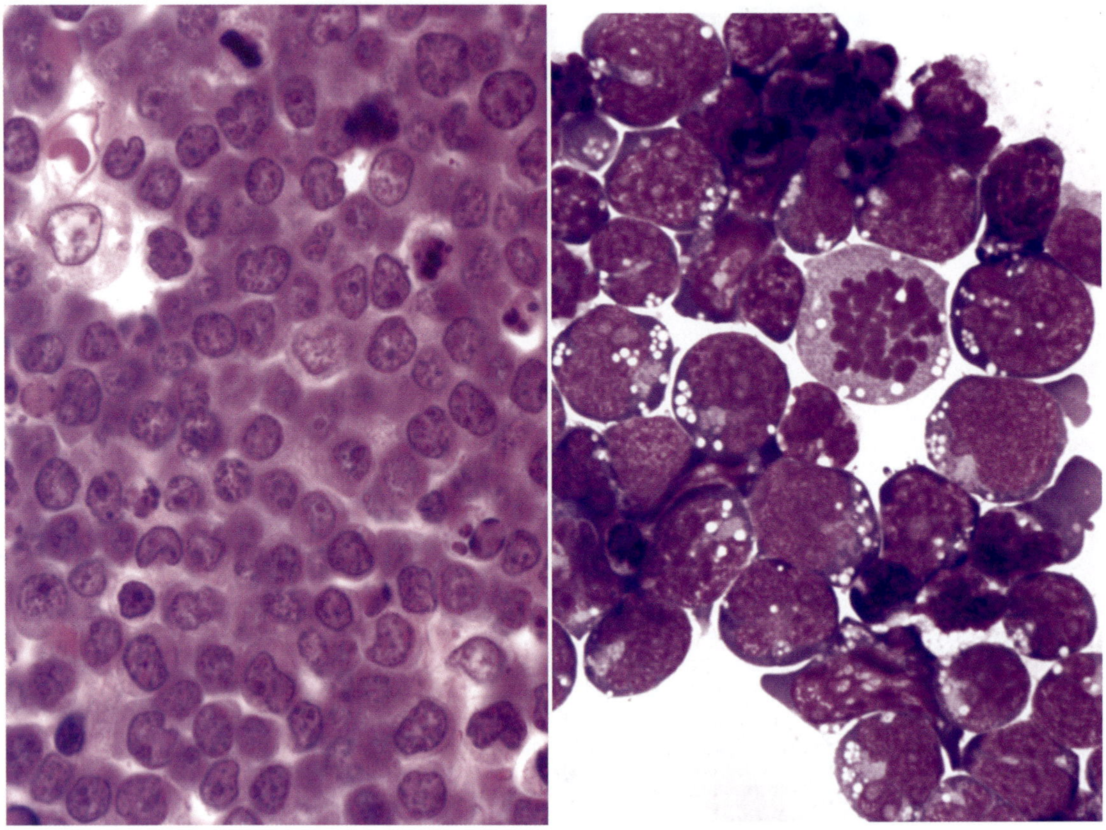

A B

Figure 1–8. Burkitt's lymphoma. **A:** The cells are uniform, round to oval, with multiple small basophilic nucleoli. The nuclear size is similar to that of the "starry sky" histiocyte in the **upper left.** Mitotic activity is present. **B:** A touch preparation demonstrates lipid vacuoles in the deeply basophilic cytoplasm.

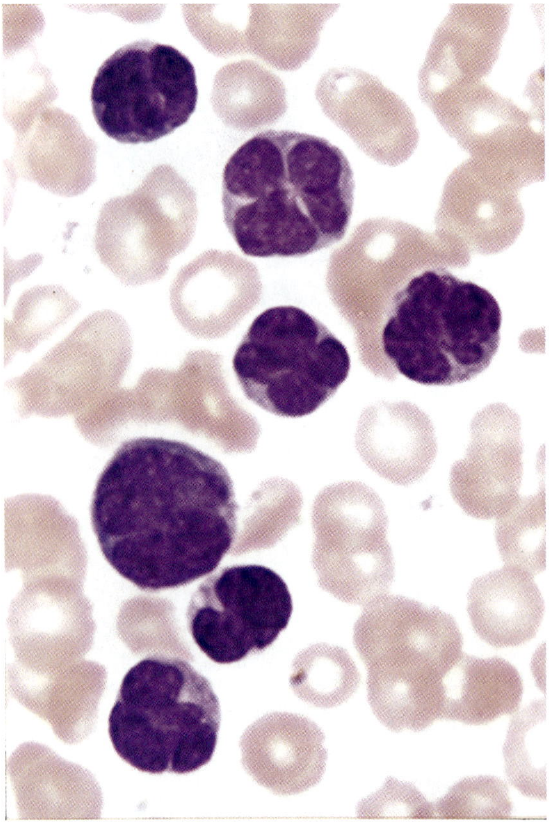

Figure 1–10. Adult T-cell leukemia/lymphoma. Markedly polylobated ("flower") cells circulate in the peripheral blood.

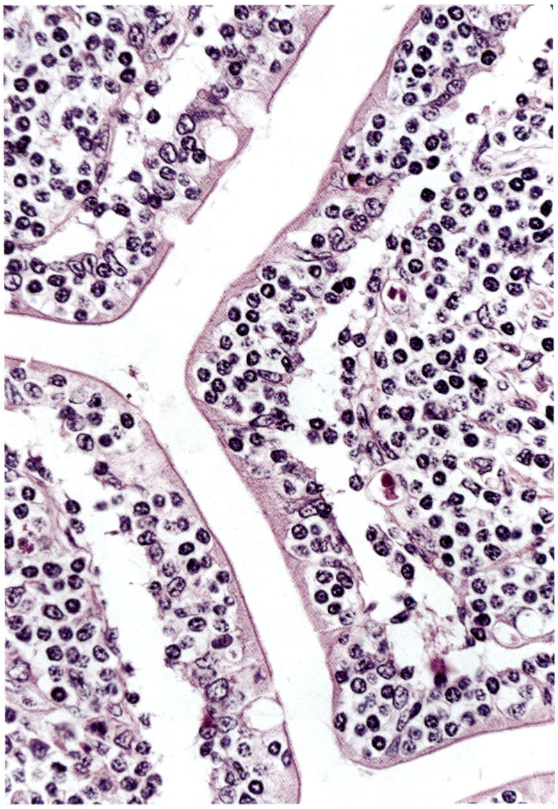

Figure 1–12. Enteropathy-type T-cell lymphoma. Atypical lymphocytes with pale cytoplasm infiltrate the epithelial mucosa and lamina propria of small intestinal villi.

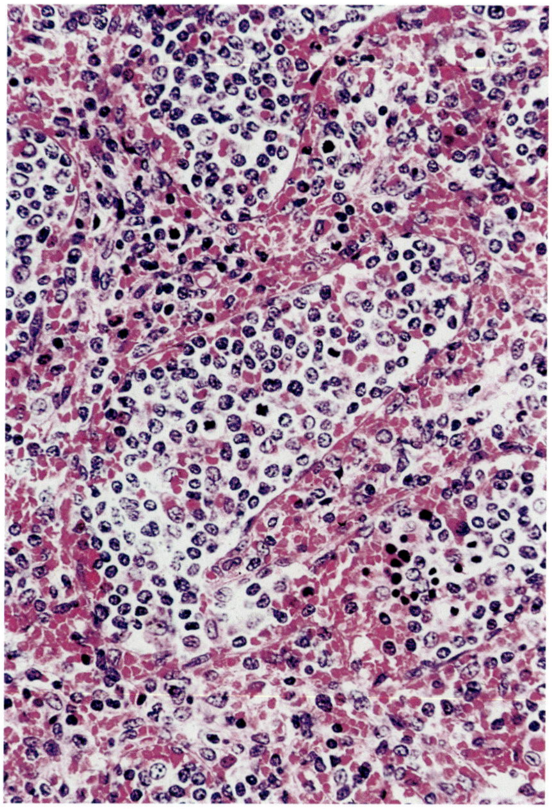

Figure 1–13. Hepatosplenic T-cell lymphoma. This liver biopsy shows a monotonous population of medium-sized cells with pale cytoplasm distending the hepatic sinusoids.

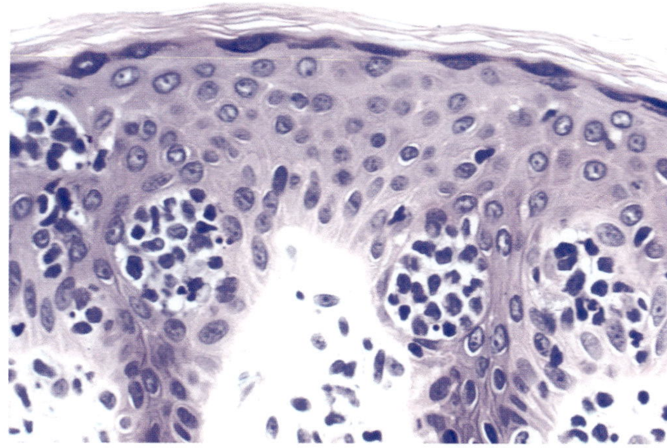

Figure 1–15. Mycosis fungoides. This skin biopsy shows neoplastic lymphocytes with convoluted nuclei forming Pautrier microabscesses within the epidermis.

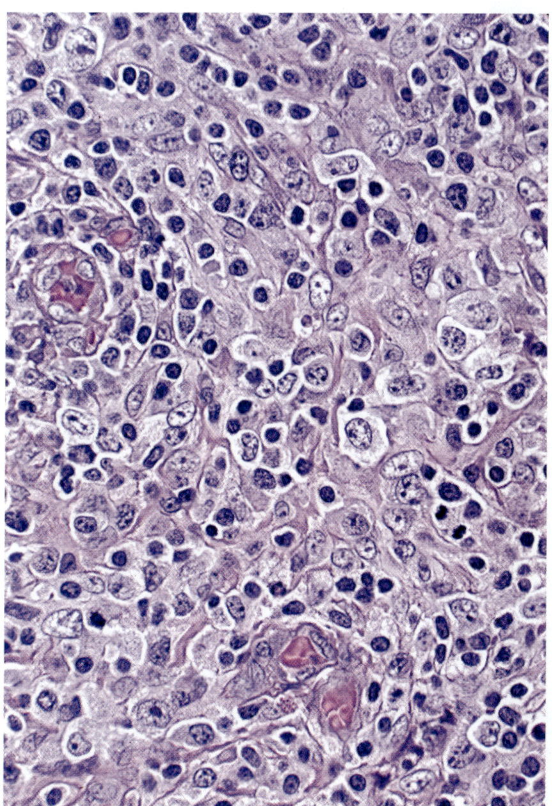

Figure 1–16. Angioimmunoblastic T-cell lymphoma. There is an infiltrate of atypical lymphoid cells with pale cytoplasm in a mixed inflammatory background, and prominent post-capillary venules with plump endothelial cells.

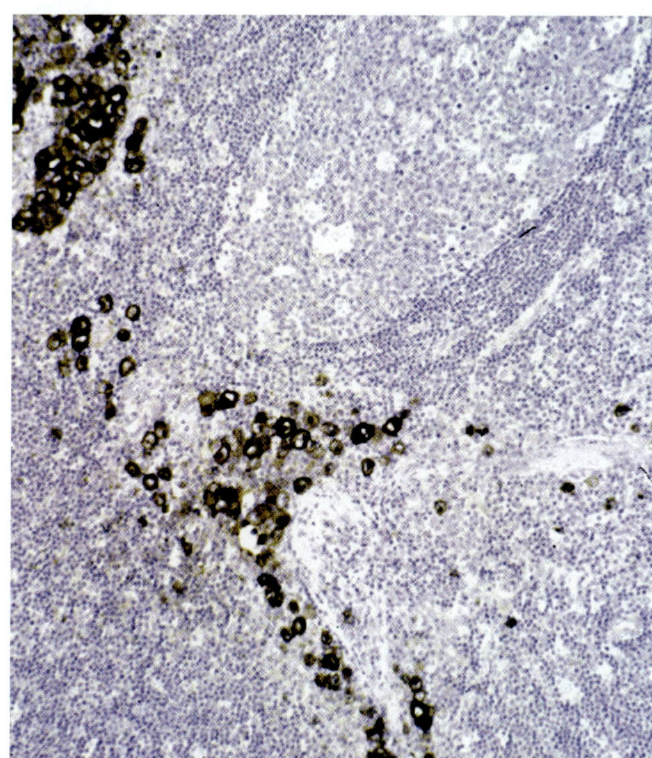

B

Figure 1–18. Systemic anaplastic large cell lymphoma (ALCL). **B:** The malignant cells are strongly positive for CD30 by immunohistochemistry.

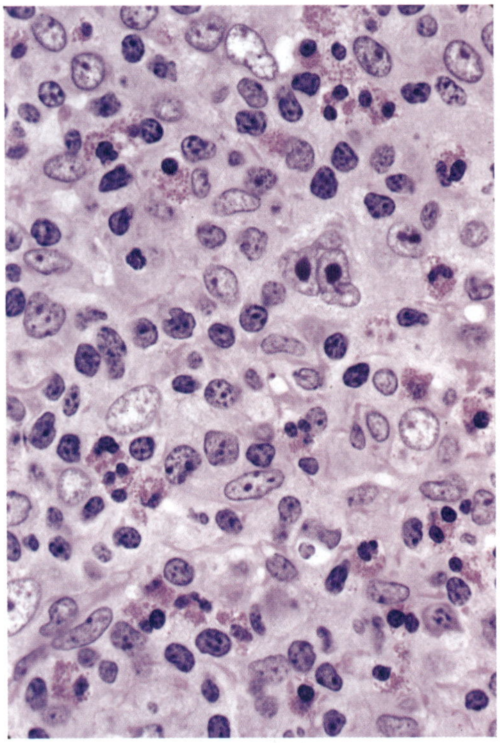

B

Figure 1–19. Hodgkin's lymphoma. **B:** Mixed-cellularity Hodgkin's lymphoma, showing classic Reed–Sternberg cells admixed with lymphocytes, plasma cells, and eosinophils.

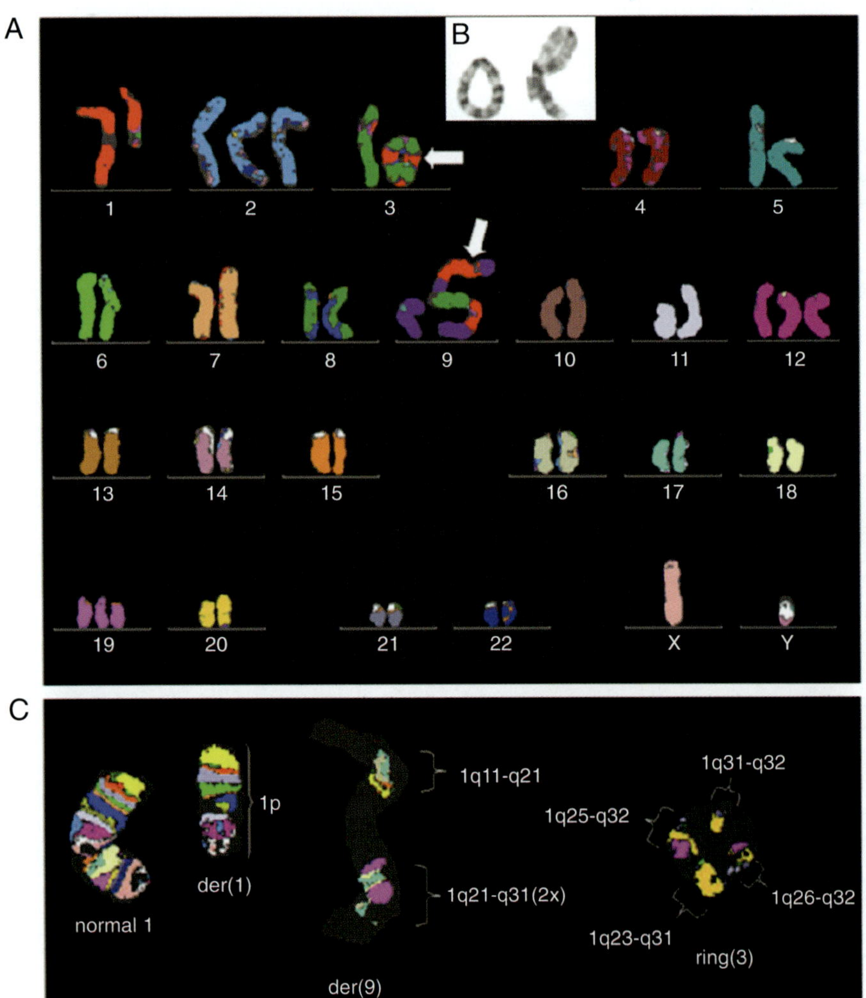

Figure 2–3. Multicolor karyotype (MFISH) of a representative case of diffuse, large B-cell lymphoma. **A:** The karyotype reveals a deletion of the q arm of chromosome 1, trisomy for chromosomes 2, 12, and 19, and two complex rearrangements *(white arrows)* representing a large-ring chromosome 3 composed of alternating segments of material from chromosome 1 and chromosome 3, and a large derivative chromosome 9 composed of alternating segments of material from chromosomes 1, 3, and 9. **B:** G-banded image of ring (3) and der (9). **C:** Multicolor banding pattern of the chromosome 1 segments of der (1), der (9), and ring (3). Normal chromosome 1 is shown on the left.

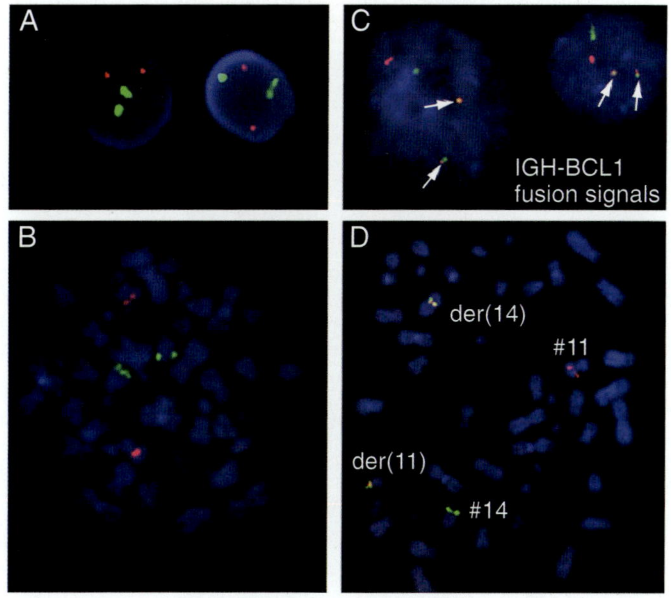

Figure 2–4. Locus-specific FISH images of a representative case of mantle cell lymphoma obtained with a commercial Vysis LSI IGH/BCL1 dual-color, dual-fusion translocation probe. The normal pattern of two BCL1 (red) and two IGH (green) signals are evident in **(A),** an interphase nucleus, and **(B),** a metaphase. An abnormal pattern of one BCL1 signal (red), one IGH signal (green), and two IGH-BCL1 fusion signals are evident in **(C),** an interphase nucleus (fusion signals indicated by *white arrows*), and **(D),** in a metaphase containing the t(11;14) of MCL (normal and derivative chromosomes indicated with *white lettering*).

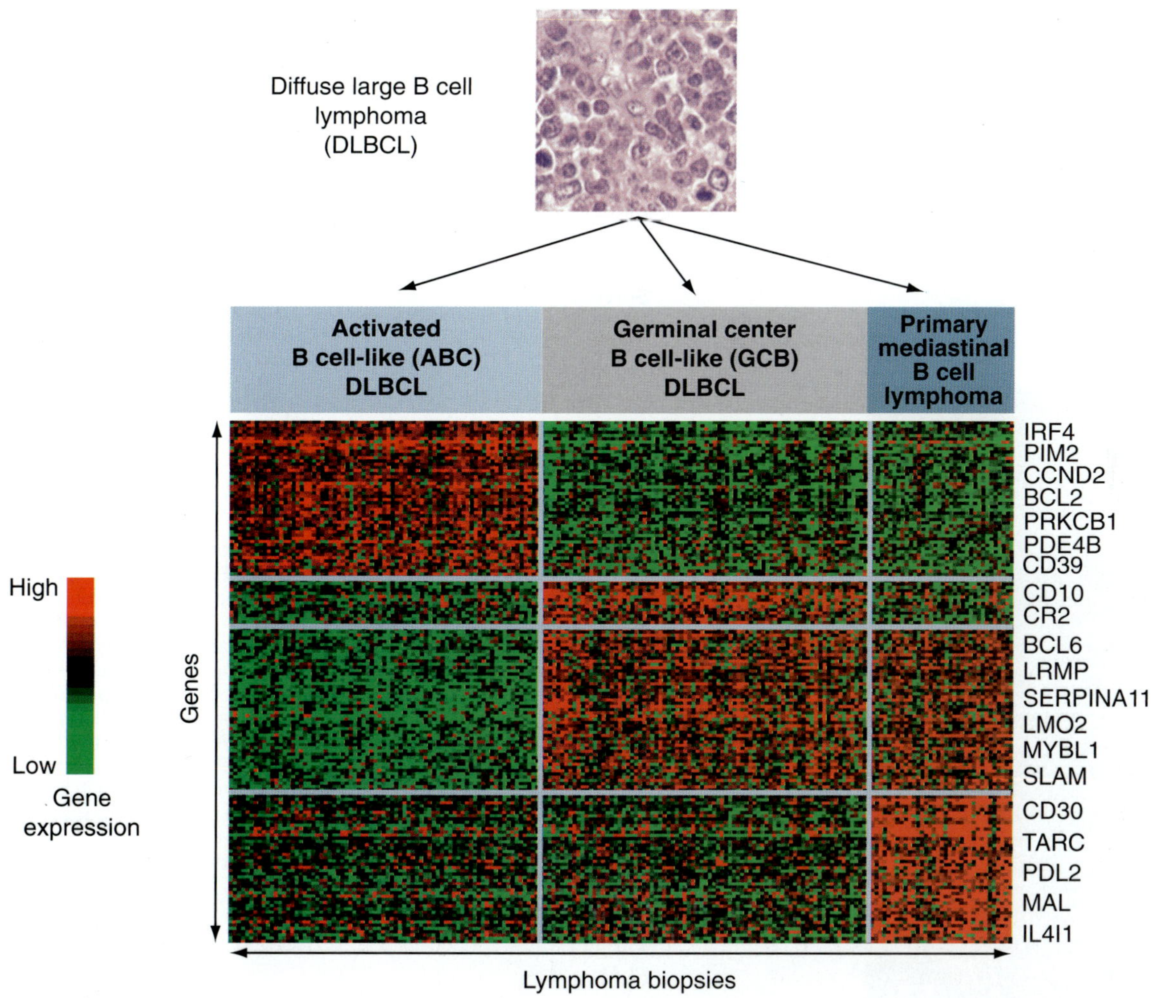

Figure 5–1. Definition of molecularly and clinically distinct subgroups of diffuse large B-cell lymphoma (DLBCL) by gene expression profiling. Gene expression differences between germinal center B-cell–like (GCB) DLBCL, activated B-cell–like DLBCL, and primary mediastinal B-cell lymphoma (PMBL). Each row represents gene expression data from an individual biopsy sample, and each column represents a single gene on the DNA microarray. Relative gene expression is indicated according to the color bar shown at the left. Representative genes that distinguish the DLBCL subgroups are indicated. Not shown are ~18% of DLBCLs that do not fit any of the three gene expression subgroups well.

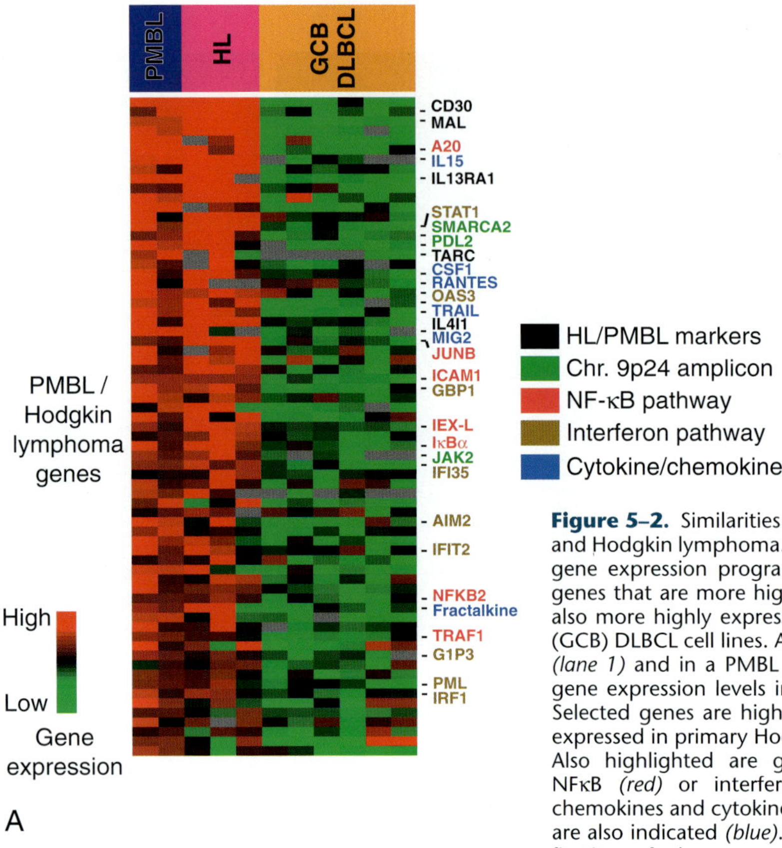

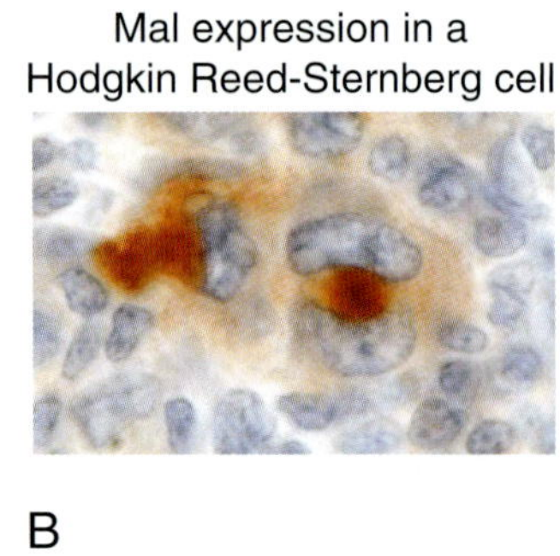

Figure 5–2. Similarities between primary mediastinal B-cell lymphoma (PMBL) and Hodgkin lymphoma. **A:** PMBL and Hodgkin's lymphoma (HL) share a broad gene expression program. The 69 genes depicted are all PMBL "signature" genes that are more highly expressed in PMBL than in other DLBCLs, and are also more highly expressed in HL cell lines than in germinal center B-cell–like (GCB) DLBCL cell lines. Average gene expression levels in primary PMBL tumors *(lane 1)* and in a PMBL cell line, K1106 *(lane 2)*, are shown. Also shown are gene expression levels in three HL cell lines and in six GCB DLBCL cell lines. Selected genes are highlighted that have been shown to be characteristically expressed in primary Hodgkin's Reed–Sternberg cells and/or PMBL cells *(black)*. Also highlighted are genes that are activated by signaling through the NFκB *(red)* or interferon *(brown)* pathways. Numerous genes encoding chemokines and cytokines, many of which are activated by the NF-κB pathway, are also indicated *(blue)*. PMBL and HL tumors frequently harbor a gain/amplification of chromosome region 9p24, which contains several genes that are characteristically expressed in both lymphoma types *(green)*. **B:** Detection of Mal protein expression in a primary Hodgkin's Reed–Sternberg cell by immunohistochemistry.

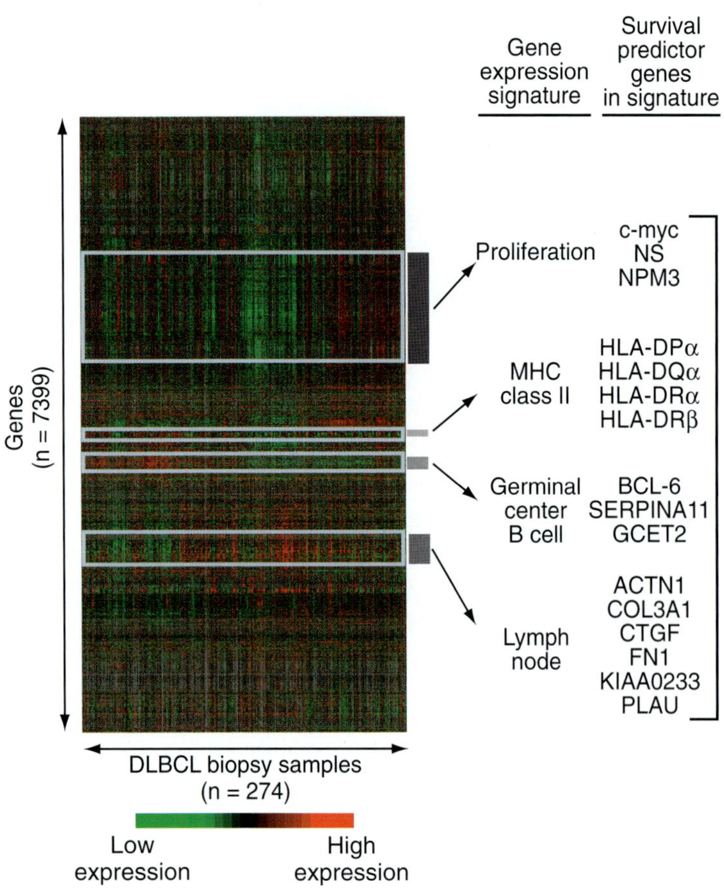

Figure 5–4. A gene expression–based predictor of survival following chemotherapy for DLBCL. Hierarchical clustering of the gene expression data reveals gene expression signatures containing survival predictor genes. A hierarchical clustering algorithm was used to organize genes based on their expression across 274 DLBCL biopsy samples. Four gene expression signatures are indicated, each of which is composed of coordinately expressed genes that reflect a specific biological aspect of the tumors (see text for details). A supervised method was used to discover genes whose expression patterns were correlated with the length of survival, and the majority of these "survival predictor genes" belonged to one of the four indicated gene expression signatures.[10] Shown are 16 representative survival predictor genes from these four signatures that were used to create a multivariate model of survival.

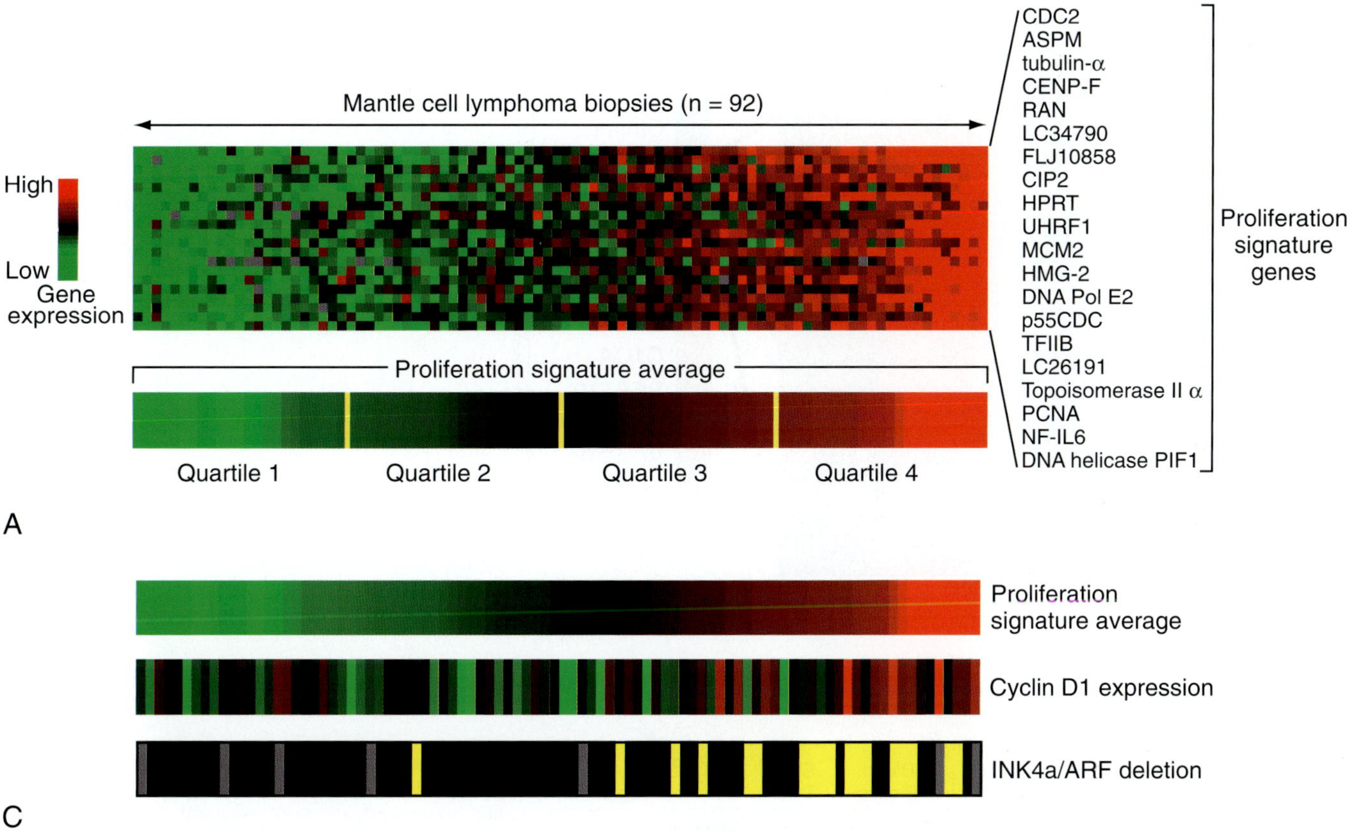

Figure 5–5. The length of survival in mantle cell lymphoma is predicted by gene expression in the tumor at diagnosis. **A:** Development of a gene expression–based survival predictor for mantle cell lymphoma. A supervised method was used to identify genes whose expression patterns were correlated with length of survival following diagnosis of mantle cell lymphoma. The majority of these genes belong to the proliferation gene expression signature, which includes genes that are more highly expressed in proliferating than in quiescent cells. The expression levels of the 20 proliferation signature genes shown were averaged to create a proliferation signature average for each of 92 mantle cell lymphoma patients. Patients were divided into four equal quartiles based on the proliferation signature average. **C:** The proliferation signature average is a quantitative character of multiple oncogenic events that influence the proliferation rate. A higher expression level of the cyclin D1 mRNA coding region is observed in many tumors with high proliferation signature averages (see text for details). Tumors with deletion of the INK4a/ARF locus encoding p16 and p14ARF are indicated in yellow, and are more commonly observed in tumors with a high proliferation signature average. (Data are adapted from Figs. 2A and B, 4A, and 5A in Rosenwald A, Wright G, Wiestner A, et al. The proliferation gene expression signature is a quantitative integrator of oncogenic events that predicts survival in mantle cell lymphoma. Cancer Cell 2003;3:185–97, with permission.)

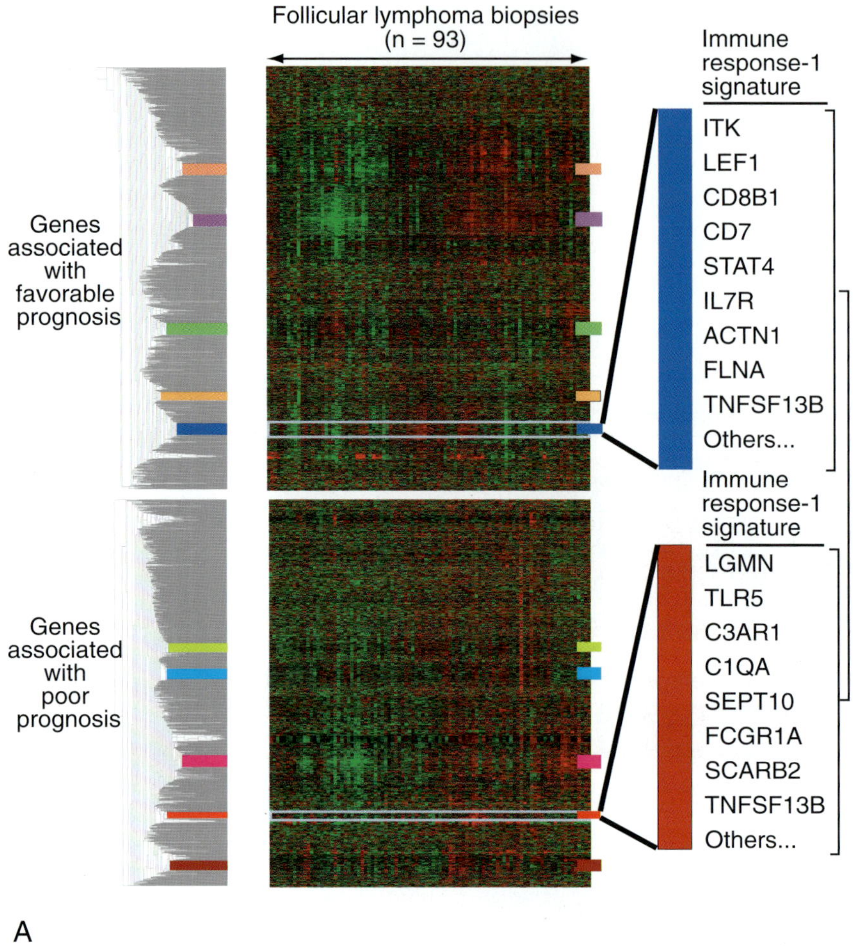

Figure 5–6. A gene expression–based survival model in follicular lymphoma. **A:** Identification of gene expression signatures associated with good or poor prognosis in follicular lymphoma. Genes with expression patterns that correlated with long survival **(top panel)** or short survival **(bottom panel)** following diagnosis were organized by hierarchical clustering across 93 follicular lymphoma biopsy samples. Ten gene expression signatures were identified *(colored bars)*, two of which were used to create an optimal model of survival.[67] Representative genes in these two signatures, termed immune response-1 and immune response-2, are shown.

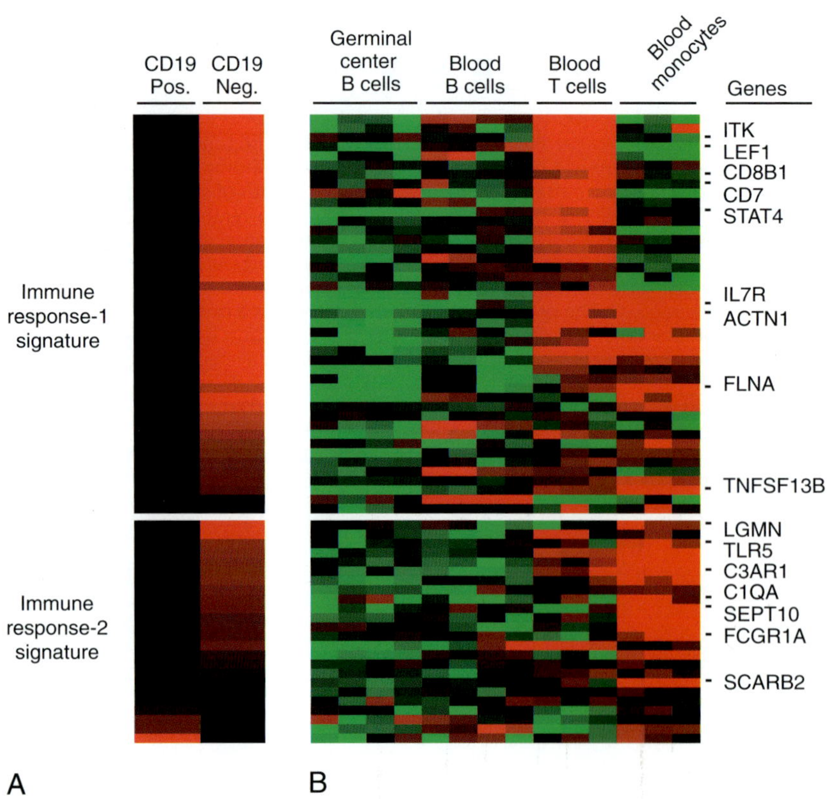

Figure 5–7. Genes with expression patterns that predict the length of survival in follicular lymphoma are expressed in nonmalignant tumor–infiltrating immune cells. **A:** Expression of genes in the immune response-1 and immune response-2 signatures in malignant and nonmalignant cell populations isolated from follicular lymphoma biopsy samples. Magnetic cell sorting was used to isolate CD19-positive malignant cells and CD19-negative nonmalignant cells from follicular lymphoma biopsies. The majority of genes in both the immune response-1 and immune response-2 signatures are more highly expressed *(red)* in the nonmalignant cell fraction. **B:** Expression of the immune response-1 and immune response-2 signature genes in various normal subpopulations of immune cells. Tonsilar germinal center B cells and blood B cells, T cells, and monocytes were analyzed by gene expression profiling. Most genes belonging to the immune response-1 signature are highly expressed in blood T cells or monocytes, whereas the majority of genes in the immune response-2 signature are most highly expressed in monocytes. Neither gene expression signature is highly expressed in germinal center B cells, the cell of origin for follicular lymphoma. (Data are adapted from Figs. 2A and 3B in Dave SS, Wright G, Tan B, et al. A molecular predictor of survival following diagnosis of follicular lymphoma based on the profile of non-malignant tumor-infiltrating immune cells. N Engl J Med 2003;351:2159–69, with permission.)

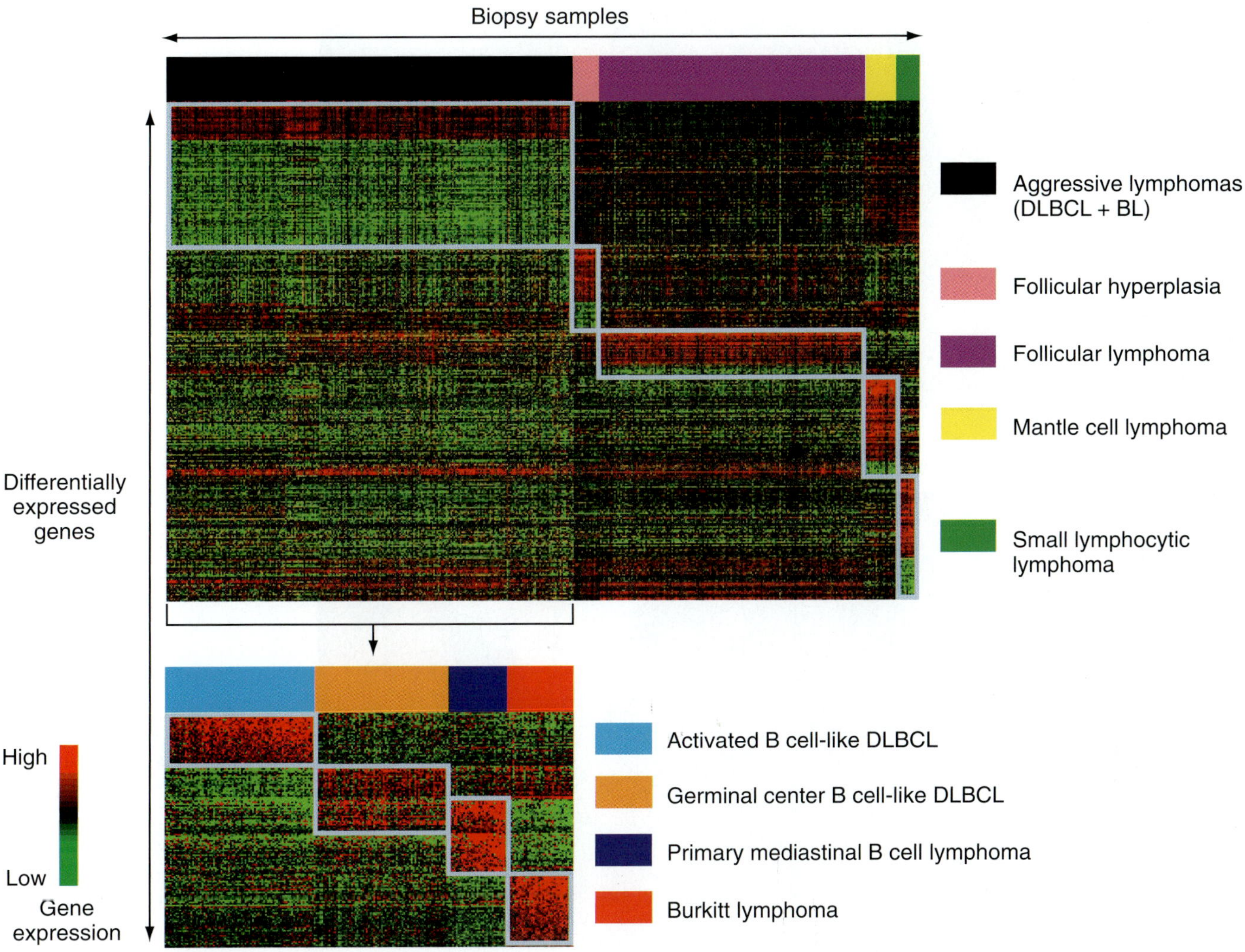

Figure 5–8. Molecular diagnosis of lymphomas by gene expression profiling. Gene expression of several hundred genes can be used to reliably assign a biopsy specimen to a lymphoma type.[84] The first step of the algorithm separates aggressive lymphomas (DLBCL), Burkitt's lymphoma (BL), and other common lymphoma types from one another **(top panel).** The second step distinguishes BL from the three DLBCL subgroups **(bottom panel).** A custom DNA microarray can be used to make these distinctions, and to provide prognostic information for patients with DLBCL, mantle cell lymphoma, and follicular lymphoma.

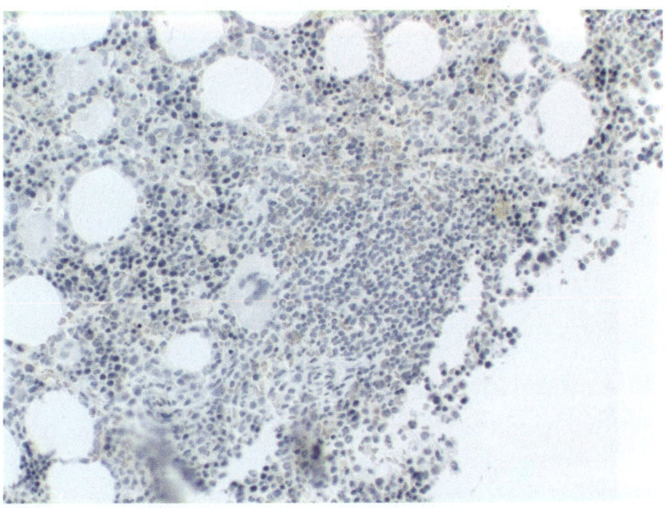

C

Figure 8–2. C: Positive staining with anti-CD3. The above pattern demonstrates the reactive nature of the nodule.

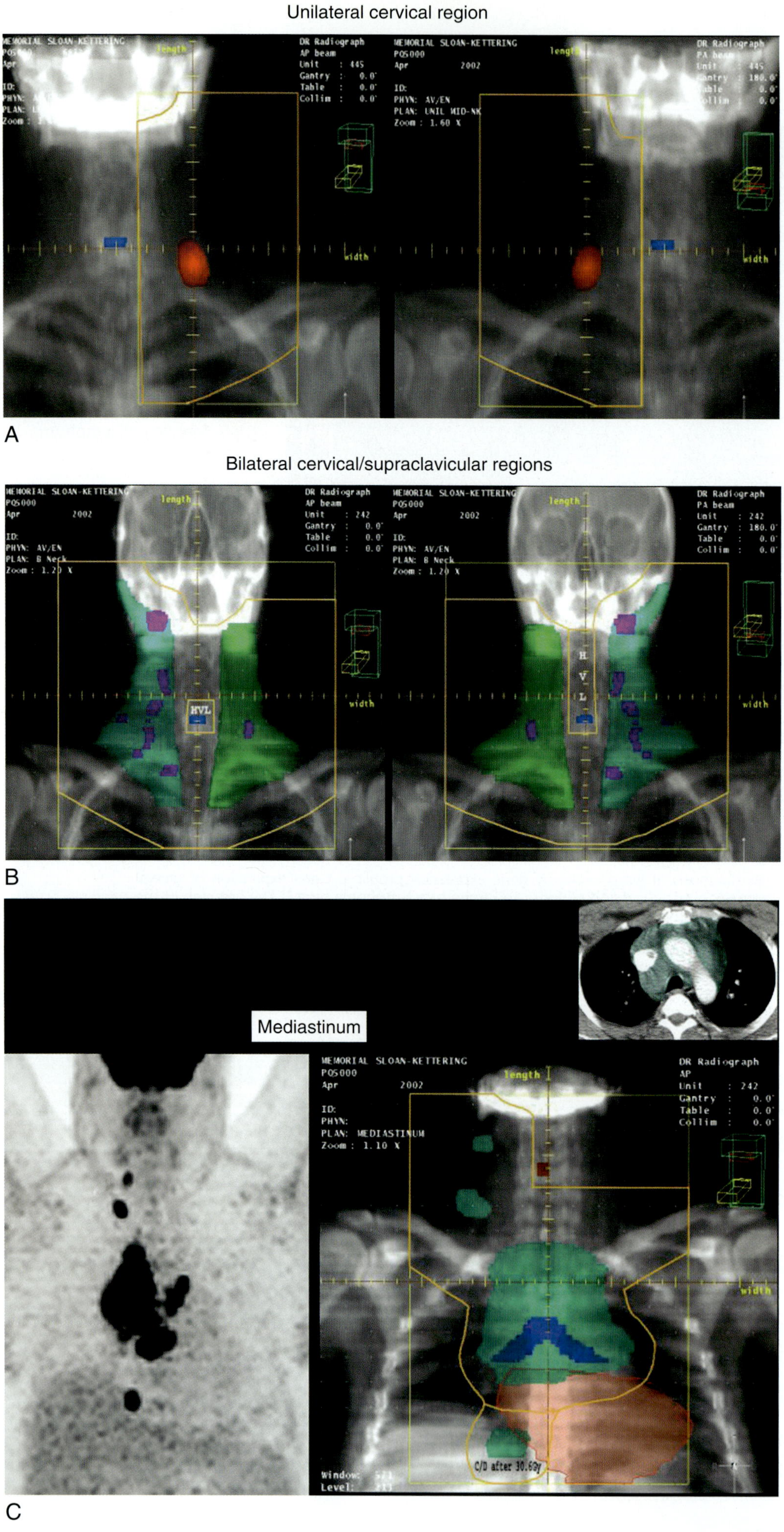

Figure 12–1. Involved field radiotherapy. **A:** Stage I HL involving the right neck. **B:** Stage II HL involving the right neck and the left lower neck. **C:** Stage IIX HL with involvement of the right neck, bulky mediastinum, right hilum, and right cardiophrenic area.

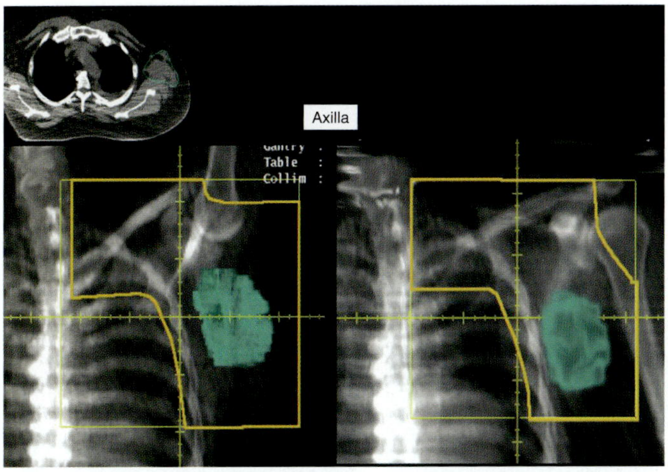

Figure 12–2. Regional field radiotherapy. Stage I HL involving the left axilla.

CT-MR fusion
for target localization

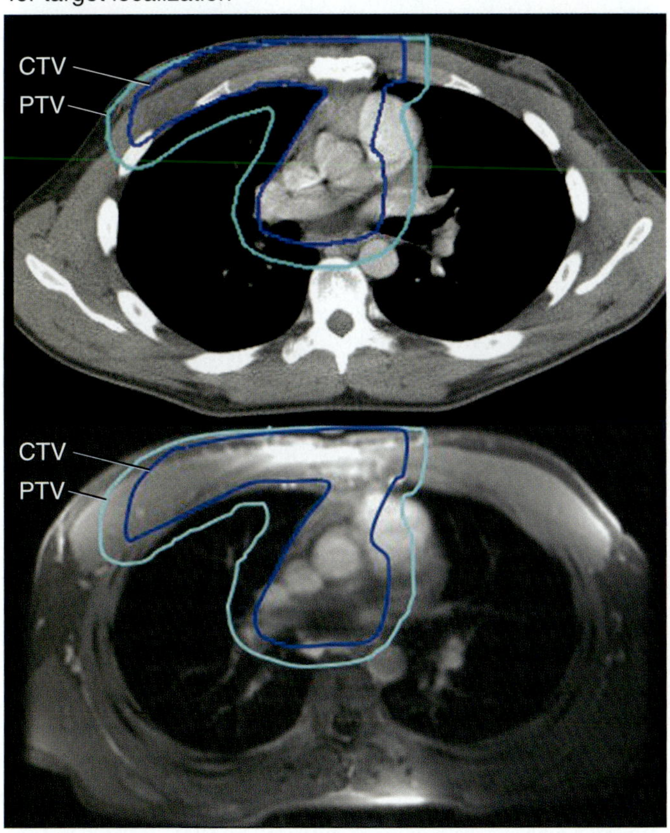

A

Figure 12–6. **A:** Intensity-modulated radiation therapy for extensive HL involving the mediastinum and the chest wall.

Case:
TLI – mantle

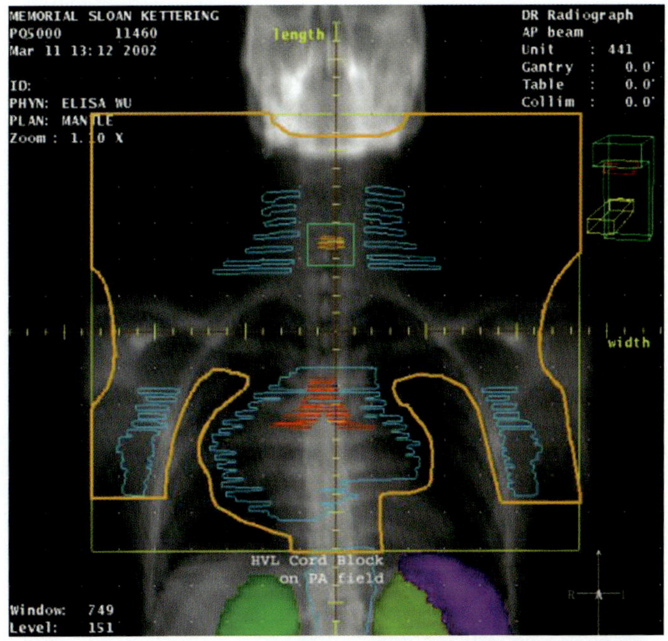

A

Case:
TLI – inverted Y

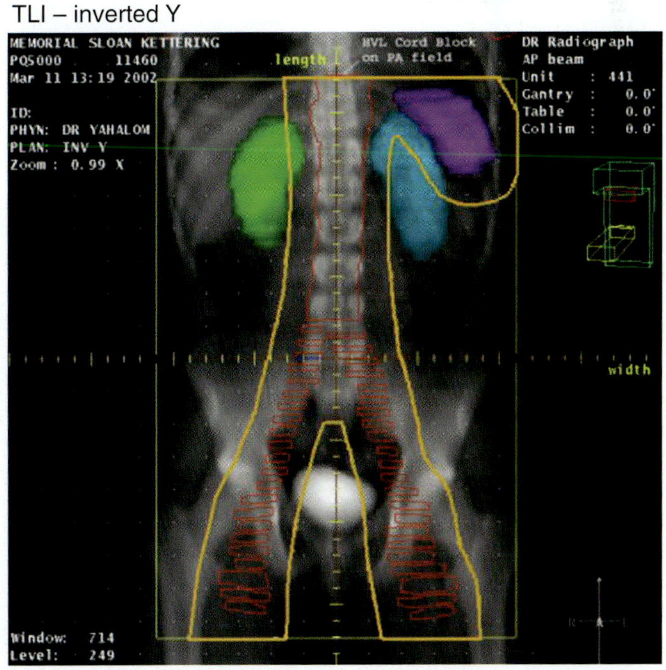

B

Figure 12–3. Extended field. **A:** Mantle field. **B:** Inverted Y.

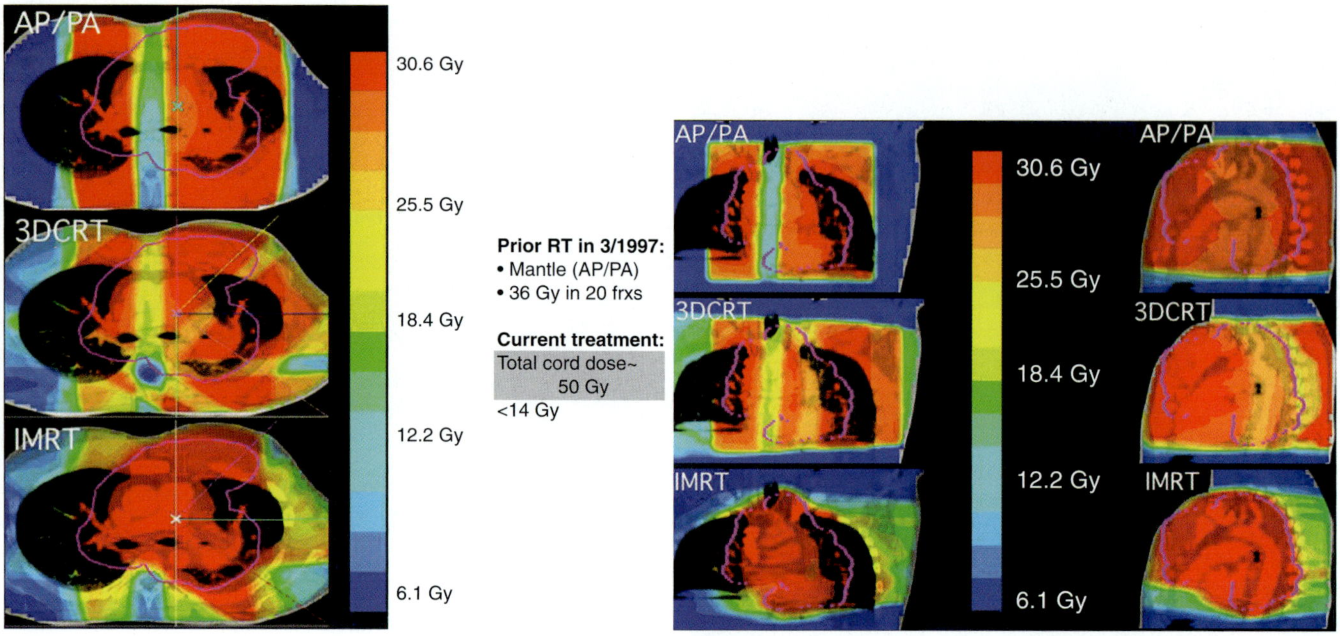

D E

Figure 12–7. (D and E): Reirradiation of a relapsed mediastinal mass using intensity-modulated radiation therapy to avoid the spinal cord.

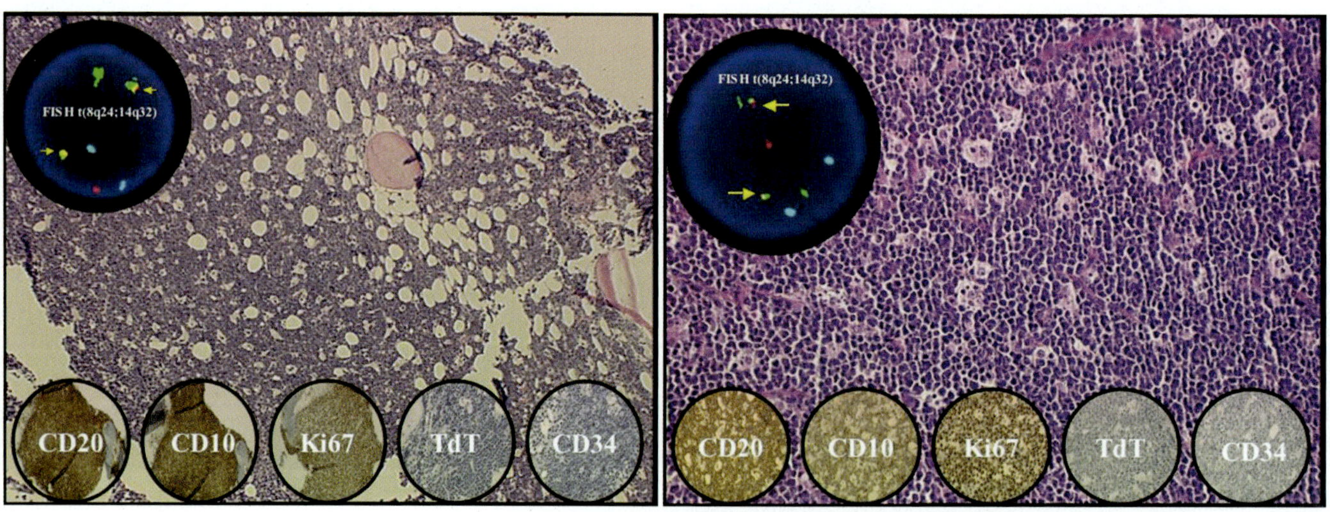

A B

Figure 16–1. Typical morphology of bone marrow with involvement by Burkitt's lymphoma. **(A,B)** Characteristic immunophenotype illustrated by immunohistochemistry: CD20+, CD10+, Ki67+ (100%), TdT– and CD34–. Classical translocation involving cMYC and immunoglobulin heavy-chain genes is illustrated by FISH analysis with probes for 14q32 (IgH), *green;* 8q24 (MYC), *red;* and chromosome 8 centromere probe, *aqua.* Fusion product t(8q24; 14q32) in *yellow* (indicated by *arrows*).

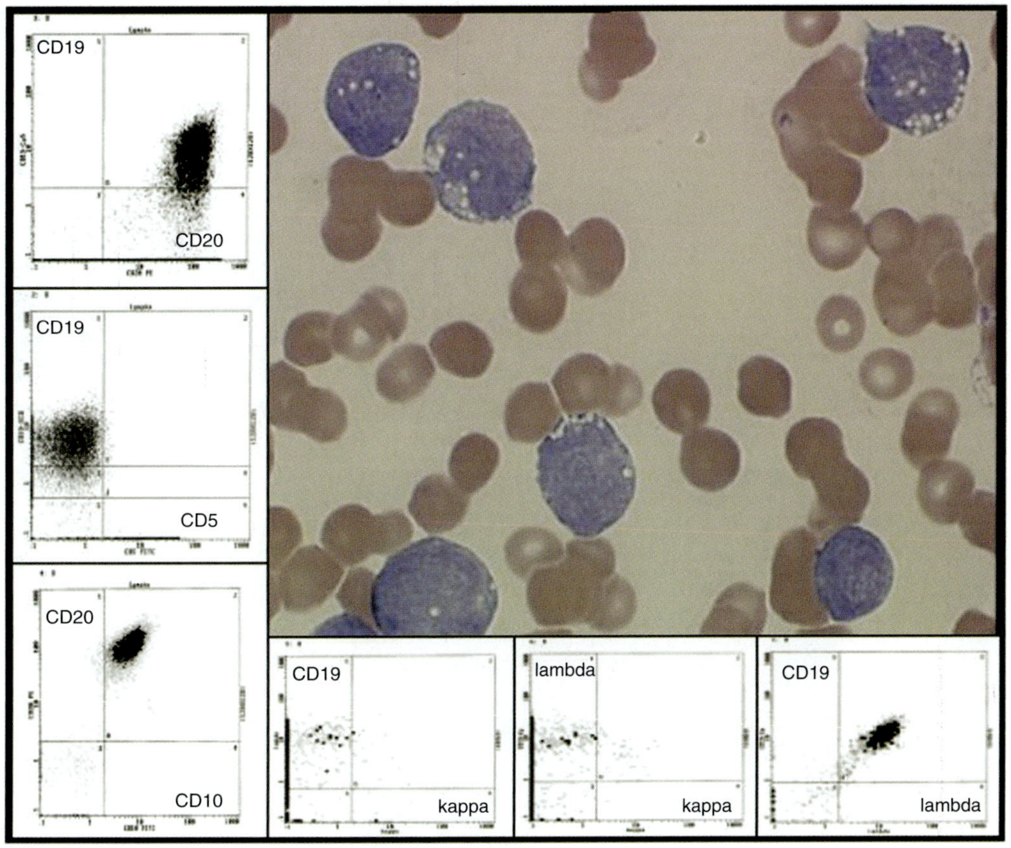

Figure 16–2. Typical morphology of Burkitt's leukemia. Characteristic immunophenotype is illustrated by flow cytometric analysis: CD10+, CD19+, CD20+ (bright), surface immunoglobulin light-chain lambda restricted (bright), and CD5–.

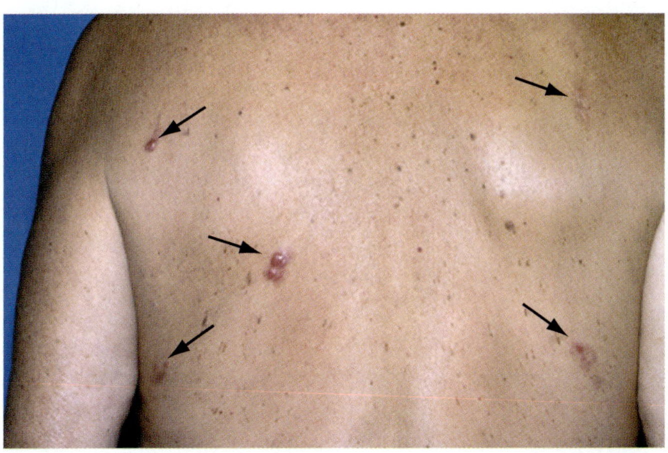

Figure 24–1. Primary cutaneous marginal zone B-cell lymphoma. Typical clinical presentation with multiple nodules on the back.

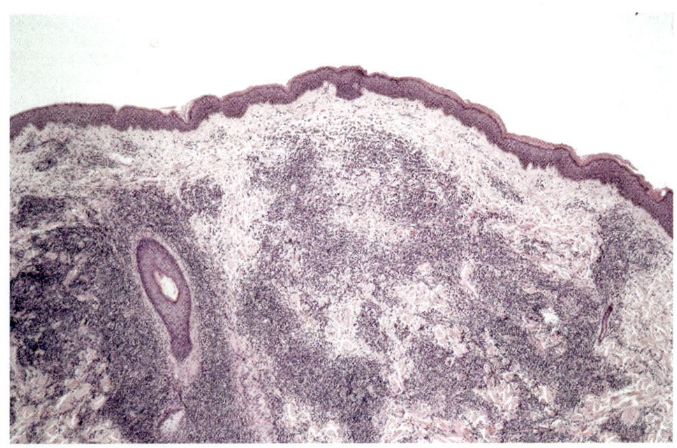

A

Figure 24–2. Primary cutaneous marginal zone B-cell lymphoma. **A:** Patchy infiltrates throughout the dermis.

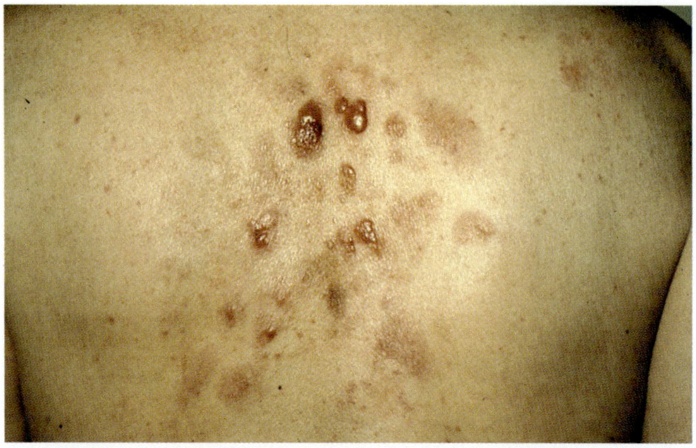

A

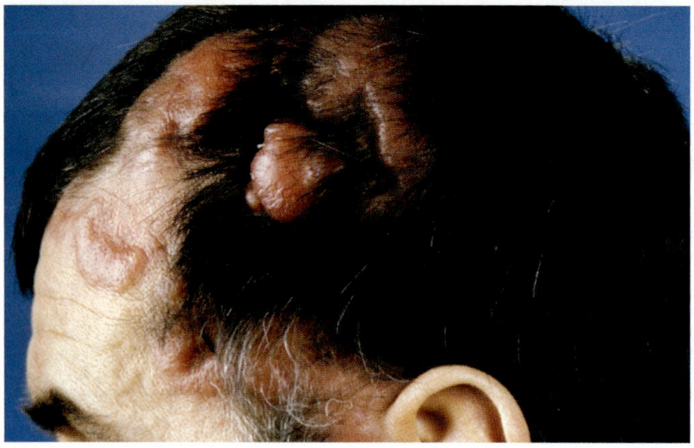

B

Figure 24–3. Primary cutaneous follicle center lymphoma. Characteristic clinical presentation with localized skin lesions **(A)** on the back (Crosti's lymphoma) and **(B)** on the scalp.

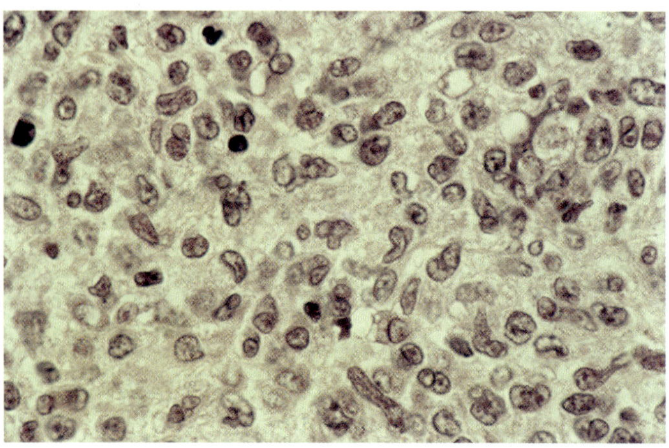

A

Figure 24–4. Primary cutaneous follicle center lymphoma. **A:** Histology of a skin tumor showing a diffuse infiltrate of large centrocytes (large cleaved cells) including many cells with multilobated nuclei.

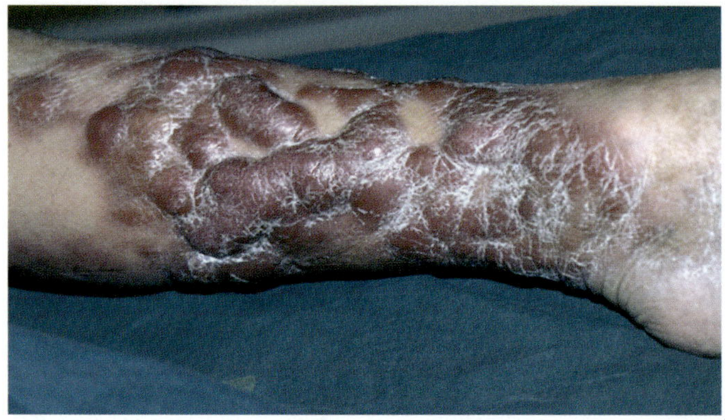

Figure 24–5. Primary cutaneous large B-cell lymphoma, leg type.

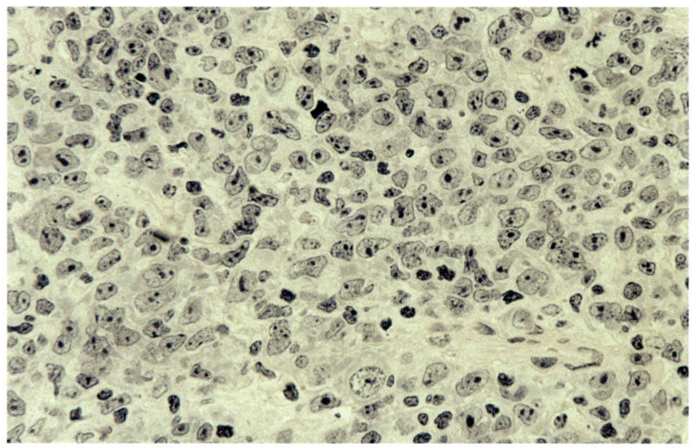

A

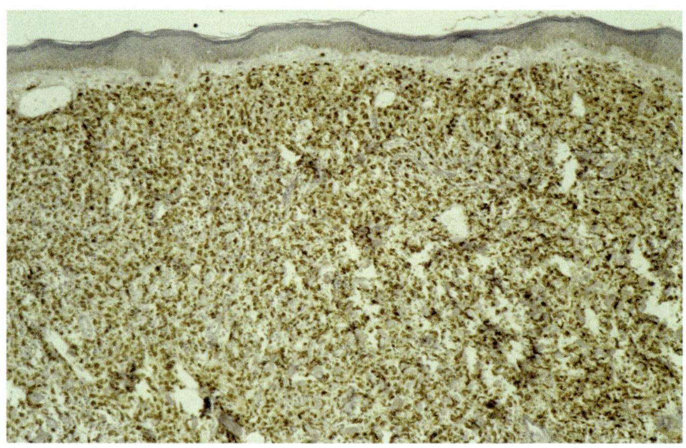

B

Figure 24–6. Primary cutaneous large B-cell lymphoma, leg type. **A:** diffuse proliferation of centroblasts and immunoblasts. **B:** Tumor cells show strong reactivity for bcl-2.

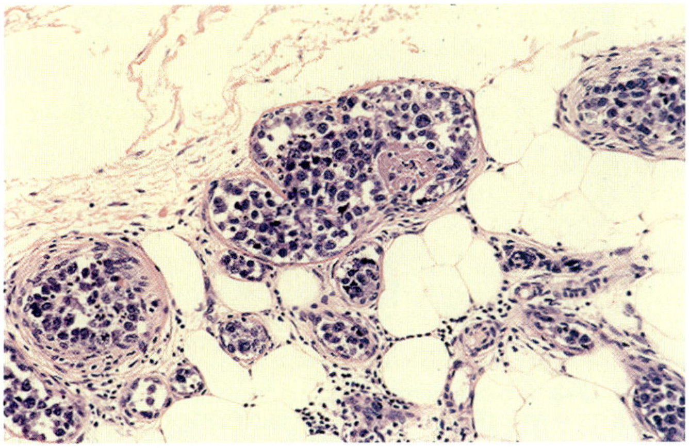

B

Figure 24–7. Primary cutaneous intravascular large B-cell lymphoma. **B:** Intravascular population of large neoplastic B cells.

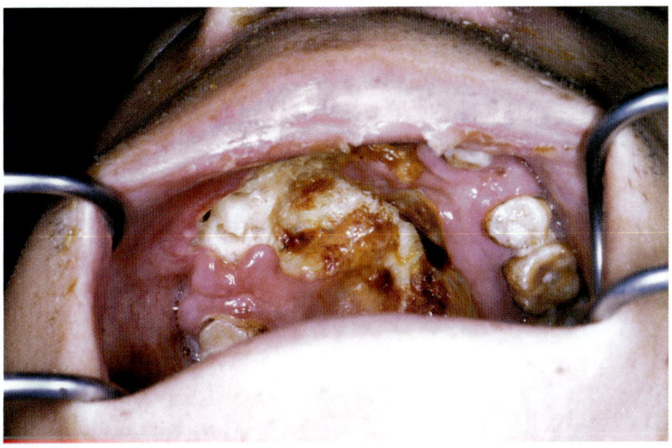

Figure 27–1. Primary nasal NK-cell lymphoma infiltrating hard palate.

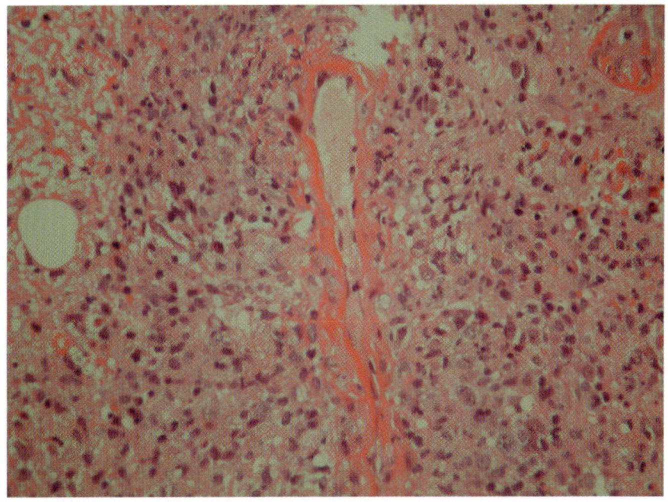

Figure 27–3. Nasal NK-cell lymphoma showing angiocentricity.

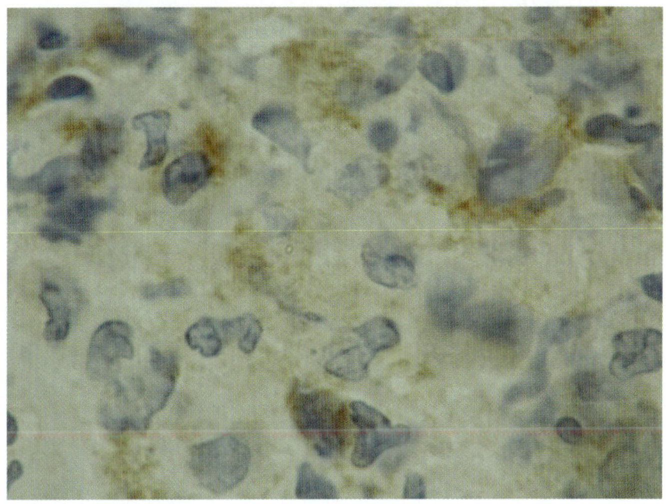

Figure 27–4. Nasal NK-cell lymphoma showing positive CD56 immunostaining.

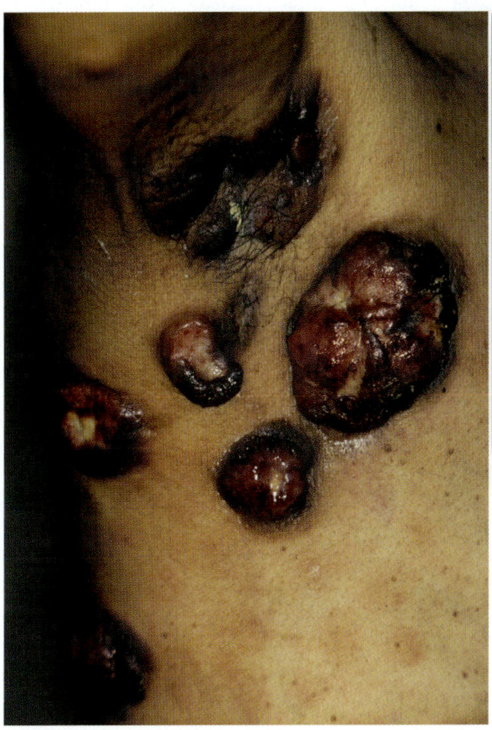

A

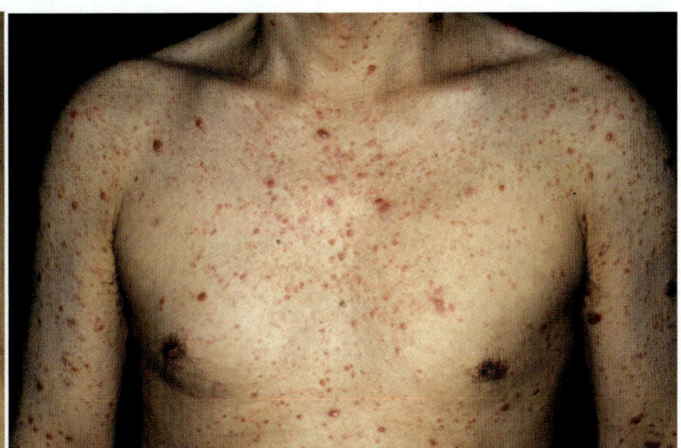

B

Figure 29–4. Skin lesions in ATL patients. Skin lesions observed in ATL patients are variable. Tumor formation is common among skin involvement in ATL patients **(A).** Papule is also observed in a patient with acute ATL **(B).**

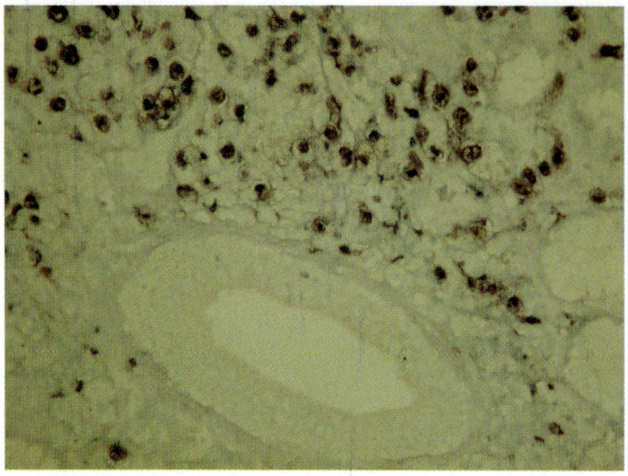

Figure 27–5. Nasal NK-cell lymphoma showing positive EBER staining on in situ hybridization.

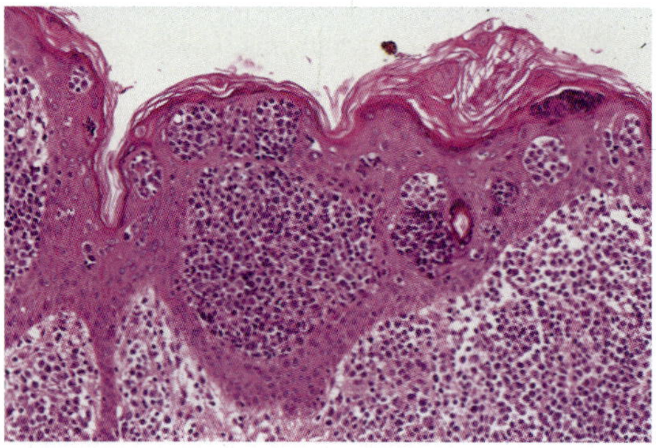

Figure 29–5. Skin involvement of ATL. ATL cells infiltrate into epidermis and form Pautrier's microabscesses.

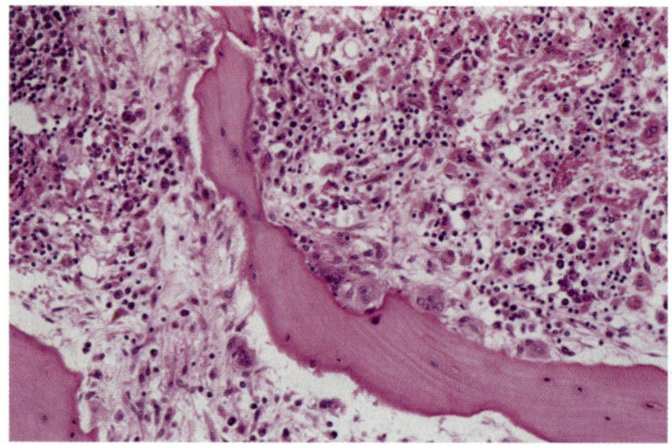

Figure 29–8. Increased osteoclasts in a hypercalcemic ATL patient. In a hypercalcemic patient, the number of osteoclast increased in the bone, which accelerated bone resorption.

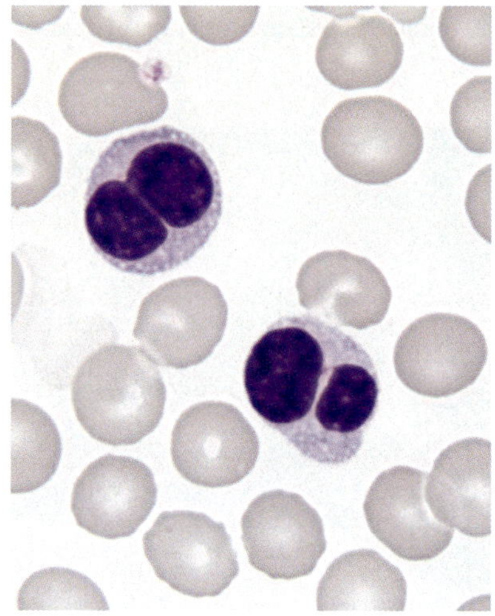

B

Figure 29–9. Cell morphology of ATL cells. ATL cells from an acute ATL **(B)** are shown.

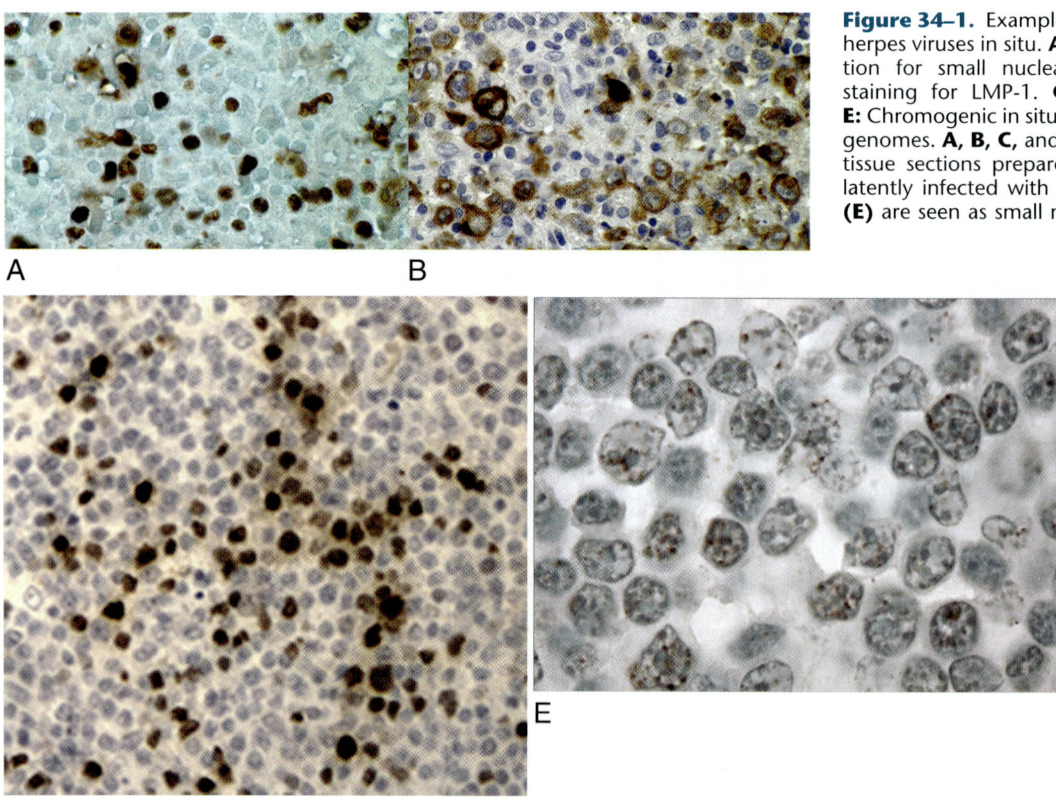

A B C E

Figure 34–1. Examples of detection of EBV and related herpes viruses in situ. **A:** Chromogenic in situ hybridization for small nuclear RNAs (EBERs). **B:** Immunostaining for LMP-1. **C:** Immunostaining for EBNA2. **E:** Chromogenic in situ hybridization for the human EBV genomes. **A, B, C,** and **E** represent stains performed on tissue sections prepared from human PTLDs that are latently infected with EBV. Individual EBV genomes in **(E)** are seen as small nuclear dots.

1 Pathophysiology

1

Classification and Histopathology of the Lymphomas

Andrew L. Feldman, M.D.
Stefania Pittaluga, M.D., Ph.D.
Elaine S. Jaffe, M.D.

The classification of the malignant lymphomas has undergone significant reappraisal over the past 50 years. These changes have resulted from insights gained through the application of immunologic and molecular techniques, as well a better understanding of the clinical aspects of lymphoma through advances in diagnosis, staging, and treatment. At one time lymphomas were seen as no more than four or so generic types: lymphosarcoma, reticulum cell sarcoma, giant follicle lymphoma, and Hodgkin's lymphoma (Hodgkin's disease). Currently, more than 40 distinct entities are recognized in the World Health Organization (WHO) classification (Table 1–1).[1] Each variant can be distinguished using a combination of morphologic, immunophenotypic, and genotypic analyses, and each is associated with characteristic clinical behavior, pattern of spread, and response to therapy.

CLASSIFICATION OF THE NON-HODGKIN'S LYMPHOMAS

The Rappaport classification, first introduced in 1956,[2] divided lymphomas according to pattern (nodular or diffuse), and then according to cell type, based on the degree to which the lymphoid cells morphologically resembled either normal lymphocytes or histiocytes.[3] Advances in immunology in the 1970s made it apparent that this approach was flawed and that the cells termed "histiocytic" were for the most part transformed lymphocytes. In addition, the recognition of T cells, B cells, and various other subsets made it possible to see lymphomas in functional terms, each deriving from a unique cell type. Both the Kiel classification, proposed by Karl Lennert and colleagues,[4] and the Lukes–Collins scheme[5] were immunologically based, although at the time immunologic techniques were still in their infancy, and monoclonal antibodies as a diagnostic tool were not yet available.

In the 1970s, six different classifications had been proposed, and at least four were in use: the Rappaport and Lukes–Collins schemes in the United States, the Kiel classification in Europe, and the classification system of the British National Lymphoma Investigation (BNLI)[6] in Great Britain. Although several meetings attended by both pathologists and clinicians were held in an attempt to reach consensus (in London, Florence, and Airlie, Virginia) no agreement could be reached.

The National Cancer Institute (NCI) responded by sponsoring a study to test each of the classification schemes using a database containing clinical data from approximately 1200 cases of lymphoma treated on prospective clinical trials from four different institutions.[7] The NCI study indicated that each of the schemes could segregate the tumors into broad groups of low, intermediate, and high clinical grade, as determined by survival in the test group of cases. No one scheme appeared superior to any other. Moreover, the study demonstrated both a relatively high lack of reproducibility by individual pathologists (0.53 to 0.93) when confronted by the same slides on a second review, as well as a low rate of concordance among the various pathologists (0.21 to 0.65) in trying to reproduce diagnoses within a given scheme. It should be noted that the pathologists were restricted to only routine hematoxylin- and eosin-stained sections and limited clinical information (age, sex, and anatomic site). Nevertheless, the clinicians involved in this study reached the conclusion that "clinical outcome" was a reasonable basis for a lymphoma classification scheme, since agreement could not be achieved regarding the individual pathologic entities.

The participants proposed the Working Formulation (WF) for the non-Hodgkin's lymphomas (NHLs) based on the clinical and pathologic findings. The original intent was to have the WF serve as a common language to translate among classifications, and not to serve as a free-standing classification scheme. However, because it was a convenient guide to therapy, it quickly became popular among clinicians and was adopted for use in many centers in the United States for clinical trials. In reality, the WF was in essence the Rappaport scheme. It substituted the term "large cell" for "histiocytic," and divided the "histiocytic" lymphomas of the Rappaport scheme into two subgroups: large cell and large-cell immunoblastic. This separation split the "histiocytic" lymphomas among the intermediate and high-grade categories, a division that has been controversial and not supported by subsequent analyses.

Another more basic flaw in the WF was that it was a classification based on treatment outcome, not the recognition of individual disease entities or cell of origin for a malignant neoplasm. This conceptual approach is a significant deviation from the way in which classification systems have been developed for other organ systems. It lumps diseases that share a similar cell size and survival into single categories, and splits diseases with variations in cytologic composition and clinical grade into separate categories. It is apparent that major differences exist in the incidence of subtypes of lymphoma (and other cancers) in different geographic regions and among different racial and ethnic populations. In order to pursue these epidemiologic differences, standardized

Table 1–1. World Health Organization (WHO) Classification of Lymphoid Tumors

B-CELL NEOPLASMS
Precursor B-cell neoplasm
Precursor B-lymphoblastic leukemia/lymphoma
Mature B-cell neoplasms
Chronic lymphocytic leukemia/small lymphocytic lymphoma
B-cell prolymphocytic leukemia
Lymphoplasmacytic lymphoma/Waldenström macroglobulinemia
Splenic marginal zone lymphoma
Hairy cell leukemia
Plasma cell neoplasms: plasma cell myeloma, plasmacytoma, monoclonal immunoglobulin deposition diseases, heavy-chain diseases
Extranodal marginal zone B-cell lymphoma (MALT lymphoma)
Nodal marginal zone B-cell lymphoma
Follicular lymphoma
Mantle cell lymphoma
Diffuse large B-cell lymphoma
Large B-cell lymphoma subtypes: mediastinal (thymic), intravascular, primary effusion lymphoma; plasmablastic, ALK+ large B-cell lymphoma
Burkitt's lymphoma/leukemia
Lymphomatoid granulomatosis
T-CELL NEOPLASMS
Precursor T-cell neoplasm
Precursor T-lymphoblastic leukemia/lymphoma
Mature T-cell and NK-cell neoplasms
T-cell prolymphocytic leukemia
T-cell large granular lymphocytic leukemia
Aggressive NK-cell leukemia
Adult T-cell leukemia/lymphoma
Extranodal NK/T-cell lymphoma, nasal type
Enteropathy-type T-cell lymphoma
Hepatosplenic T-cell lymphoma
Subcutaneous panniculitis-like T-cell lymphoma
Blastic NK-cell lymphoma
Mycosis fungoides/Sézary syndrome
Primary cutaneous CD30-positive T-cell lymphoproliferative disorders: primary cutaneous anaplastic large cell lymphoma, lymphomatoid papulosis, borderline lesions
Angioimmunoblastic T-cell lymphoma
Peripheral T-cell lymphoma, unspecified
Systemic anaplastic large cell lymphoma
HODGKIN'S LYMPHOMA (HODGKIN'S DISEASE)
Nodular Lymphocyte Predominant Hodgkin's Lymphoma
Classic Hodgkin's Lymphoma
Nodular sclerosis Hodgkin's lymphoma
Mixed cellularity Hodgkin's lymphoma
Lymphocyte-rich classic Hodgkin's lymphoma
Lymphocyte depleted Hodgkin's lymphoma

classifications of disease should be employed on a worldwide basis. More important, precise identification of disease entities is required to gain insight into pathogenesis. The WF, while a useful scheme for the oncologist in providing clinical groupings as a guide to therapy, did not for the most part delineate disease entities. In recent years there have been many advances in understanding the pathogenesis of lymphoma (Table 1–2). Most of the currently recognized disease entities, other than follicular lymphoma and Burkitt's lymphoma, were not identified in the WF. Therefore, clinical and epidemiologic studies employing the WF were limited in their ability to identify differences in the clinical behavior and incidence of individual lymphoma subtypes, and hampered further studies of lymphoma biology.

Of the classifications originally tested in the NCI study,[7] only the Kiel classification remained in widespread use, mainly in Europe and Asia. Several revisions were published, adding some of the more newly described entities, such as anaplastic large cell lymphoma (ALCL). However, several aspects of the Kiel scheme were not accepted universally. For example, it was intended for nodal lymphomas only, and did not delineate distinct disease entities arising in extranodal sites. Additionally, the absence of grading criteria for follicular lymphoma (FL) made it unpopular in the United States, where FL is the most common lymphoma subtype, accounting for about 40% of NHLs.

In 1994, the International Lymphoma Study Group (ILSG) proposed the revised European–American classification of lymphoid neoplasms (REAL),[8] which classified disease entities according to cell of origin, principally T cell or B cell, and stage of differentiation when known. The major differences between the REAL classification and prior classification schemes were the focus on the definition of "real" entities incorporating all available data, and the recognition that the complexity of the field necessitated a broad consensus rather than different classifications proposed by individual pathologists. Each variant in the REAL classification was associated with a distinct combination of morphologic, immunophenotypic, and genotypic features, as well as characteristic etiologic, epidemiologic, and clinical characteristics. In addition, the REAL classification emphasized the distinction between histologic grade and clinical behavior, and suggested the application of histologic grading schemes within individual diseases. The classification also noted the importance of site (e.g., nodal vs. extranodal) in predicting the biologic behavior of many lymphomas. The validity, applicability, and reproducibility of the REAL classification were evaluated in an international study undertaken by a group of expert pathologists, taking into account the contributions of immunophenotype and clinical data in lymphoma diagnosis.[9] The study concluded that the REAL classification improved diagnostic accuracy and decreased interobserver variation. The classification also was enhanced by the incorporation of immunophenotype (which was particularly critical in the evaluation of certain diseases such as peripheral T-cell lymphoma[10]) and clinical factors (such as the International Prognostic Index [IPI][11]).

On the basis of these data, WHO adopted the general approach of the REAL classification and organized a Clinical Advisory Committee (CAC) composed of expert hematologists and oncologists to advise the pathologists and ensure that the resulting classification scheme was clinically useful.[12] In addition to modifications proposed by the CAC, the WHO classification incorporated new data published since the development of the REAL classification, and proposed some minor changes in terminology.[1] The WHO classification recognizes three main categories of lymphoid neoplasms: B-cell neoplasms, T- and NK-cell neoplasms,

Table 1–2. Pathogenic Insights Based on Disease-Oriented Approach to Lymphoma Classification

Disease	Pathogenesis/Co-factor	Epidemiology
Burkitt's lymphoma	EBV, malaria, immunodeficiency, *c-Myc*	Endemic vs. sporadic in North America
Adult T-cell leukemia/lymphoma	HTLV-1	SW Japan, Caribbean
Primary effusion lymphoma	KSHV/HHV-8	HIV, Mediterranean
MALT lymphomas	*Helicobacter, MALT1/MLT*	Feltre, Italy
Extranodal NK/T-cell lymphoma, nasal type	EBV, genetics	Asia, Central and South America
Follicular lymphoma	*Bcl-2*	United States, Western Europe
Mantle cell lymphoma	*Cyclin D1*	Southern Europe
Anaplastic large cell lymphoma	*ALK*	Unknown

and Hodgkin's lymphoma (HL). Many distinct lymphoma entities have ranges in both histologic grade and clinical aggressiveness. This point is exemplified by follicular lymphoma (FL), which is recognized as a single disease entity with a common molecular pathogenesis in the majority of cases. However, variations in cytologic grade are a valid basis for stratifying patients for therapy. Thus, grading schemes and other prognostic factors for FL and other disease entities are incorporated in the WHO classification.

While the classification of Hodgkin's lymphoma has undergone relatively few revisions since the institution of the Rye modification of the Lukes–Butler scheme, it has become apparent that the cell of origin of HL is lymphoid. Moreover, a sharp distinction between HL and NHL often is not possible. Instances of composite HL/NHL and sequential HL/NHL further indicate a close relationship.[13] Therefore, while for clinical purposes we segregate HL and NHL, conceptually it is appropriate for both to be included in any classification scheme of lymphomas. The WHO classification thus includes all lymphoid neoplasms. However, for the purposes of this chapter those entities other than the malignant lymphomas will be touched on only briefly, or not discussed.

The WHO classification is a significant achievement in that it represents a new level of cooperation, communication, and consensus among pathologists, hematologists, and oncologists. Furthermore, it is recognized that any classification system is an evolving process. For example, the WHO classification notes the ability of gene expression profiling using cDNA microarrays to identify discrete subsets of diffuse large B-cell lymphoma (DLBCL), which have major prognostic significance independent of IPI score.[14] New data resulting from ongoing technologic advances in the fields of genomics[15] and proteomics[16] provide novel diagnostic tools to refine this classification. Thus, the continued cooperation of the major hematopathology societies with multidisciplinary input and periodic review and revision to incorporate new findings can be expected to maintain a classification that not only will be widely accepted but will also be capable of withstanding the test of time.

B-CELL NEOPLASMS

Precursor B-Lymphoblastic Leukemia/Lymphoma (B-ALL/B-LBL)

WF: malignant lymphoma, lymphoblastic
Kiel: lymphoblastic, B-cell type
REAL: precursor B-lymphoblastic leukemia/lymphoma

While most cases of B-ALL/B-LBL present as leukemia, lymphomatous presentation occurs in approximately 5% to 10% of patients.[17,18] Frequent sites of involvement include lymph nodes, skin, and bone. Skin lesions in children frequently present in the head and neck region, including the scalp (Fig. 1–1A).[17,19] Progression to leukemia will occur in the majority of cases if a complete remission is not achieved. B-LBL is most common in children and young adults, and is considered the solid tumor equivalent of common acute lymphoblastic leukemia and pre-B-cell acute lymphoblastic leukemia.

Cytologically, B-LBL is composed of lymphoblasts that are usually somewhat larger than a small lymphocyte, but smaller than the cells of diffuse large B-cell lymphoma.[20] The cells have finely stippled chromatin with very sparse cytoplasm and inconspicuous nucleoli. The nuclei may be round or convoluted; however, the presence or absence of nuclear convolutions is not useful in predicting immunophenotype in lymphoblastic malignancies. Mitotic figures are frequent, in keeping with the high-grade nature of this neoplasm.

The differential diagnosis of B-LBL includes the blastic variant of mantle cell lymphoma (MCL).[21] The cells of MCL usually have more abundant cytoplasm and some evidence of chromatin clumping. The clinical presentation is useful in that MCL is much more common in adults. Immunophenotypic studies aid in the differential diagnosis. The lymphoblasts of B-LBL express terminal deoxynucleotidyl transferase (TdT; Fig. 1–1B), unlike the mature B-cell phenotype of the blastic variant of MCL. B-LBL does not normally express immunoglobulin, although B-cell markers expressed at the time of heavy chain gene rearrangement, such as CD19 and CD79a, will be present.[22] CD20, acquired at the time of light chain gene rearrangement, is expressed in approximately 50% of cases.[23] Immunostaining for the B-cell-specific transcription factor Pax-5 has been advocated as a more sensitive and specific marker of B-cell lineage, and may be particularly useful when CD20 is negative.[24] Documenting expression of the transcription factors PU.1 and Oct-2 (along with its coactivator BOB.1) may be additionally helpful in this regard.[25,26] It should be noted that both pre-T and pre-B LBL may be negative for leukocyte common antigen (LCA, CD45), and are positive for CD99 (MIC-2 gene product) in a high proportion of cases. Because CD99 is expressed in Ewing's sarcoma, a non-lymphoid malignancy of children and young adults, an extensive immunohistochemical panel is required for accurate diagnosis in some cases.[27] The classification of lymphoblastic leukemias/lymphomas is likely to attain even

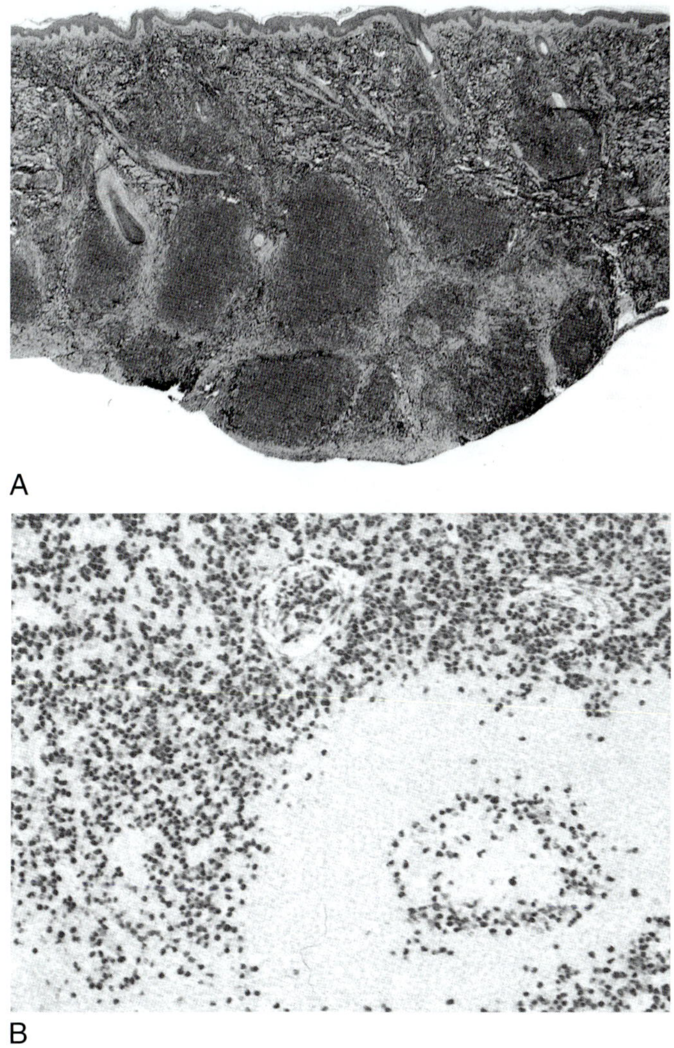

Figure 1–1. Precursor B-lymphoblastic leukemia/lymphoma. A: This scalp lesion was the initial presenting site of disease in this 10-year-old female. The tumor infiltrates the reticular dermis, but leaves a Grenz zone beneath the epidermis. B: Lymphoblasts demonstrate nuclear staining for terminal deoxynucleotidyl transferase (TdT). This example of lymph node involvement shows diffuse paracortical involvement with relative sparing of germinal centers (**lower right**). (See color insert.)

greater accuracy and prognostic value through the application of recently described gene expression profiling approaches.[28]

Chronic Lymphocytic Leukemia/Small Lymphocytic Lymphoma (CLL/SLL)

WF: small lymphocytic, consistent with CLL
Kiel: CLL; immunocytoma, lymphoplasmacytoid type
REAL: B-cell CLL

CLL/SLL usually presents in adults with generalized lymphadenopathy, frequent bone marrow and peripheral blood involvement, and often hepatosplenomegaly. Presentation as leukemia (CLL) is more common than as lymphoma (SLL). Even in patients with a lymphomatous presentation, careful examination of the peripheral blood may disclose a circulating monoclonal B-cell component. Nevertheless, there are some patients who will present with generalized lymphadenopathy, and while progression to leukemia is frequent, it does not necessarily occur in all cases.[29]

Histologically, the lymph nodes involved by CLL/SLL show diffuse architectural effacement (Fig. 1–2A), although occasional residual naked germinal centers may be present. In this regard, the process may simulate mantle cell lymphoma, but usually can be readily distinguished from MCL on cytologic grounds. While the predominant cell is a small lymphocyte with clumped nuclear chromatin, varied nuclear morphology usually is seen. Pseudofollicular growth centers or proliferation centers are present in the majority of cases,[30] and contain a spectrum of cells ranging from small lymphocytes to larger prolymphocytes and paraimmunoblasts (Fig. 1–2B). The prolymphocytes and paraimmunoblasts have somewhat more dispersed chromatin and usually have centrally placed, prominent nucleoli. There is a moderate amount of amphophilic cytoplasm. Paraimmunoblasts are larger than prolymphocytes but are similar in other respects.

In some cases the small lymphoid cells may show nuclear irregularity, providing an additional source of confusion with mantle cell lymphoma. However, the presence of pseudofollicles and paraimmunoblasts argues strongly in favor of a diagnosis of CLL/SLL over MCL. It has been shown that cases with cleaved nuclear morphology and pseudofollicles exhibit the indolent clinical behavior of CLL/SLL rather than the more aggressive clinical course of MCL.[31,32] Immunophenotypic studies are helpful in this differential diagnosis. CLL/SLL is characterized by CD5+, CD23+ B cells expressing dim CD20 and usually dim surface immunoglobulin (sIg).[33,34] The absence of cyclin D1 staining can help rule out MCL, which also is usually CD23$^-$ (Table 1–3).[35] CLL and SLL have been shown to be heterogeneous with respect to somatic mutation of the VH genes,[36–38] thus cells can be at a pre- or post-germinal center stage of differentiation. Immunohistochemical staining for ZAP-70 can distinguish mutated from unmutated cases and may be clinically useful as a surrogate marker for mutation status, with ZAP-70 expression correlating with unmutated status and poor prognosis.[39–41] CD38 also has been proposed as a surrogate marker for mutation status,[42,43] although assigning appropriate cut-offs for CD38 expression has been controversial. Cytogenetic findings also correlate with mutation status and outcome. Trisomy 12, 11q deletion, and 17p deletion have been reported in 10% to 20% of cases, and are associated with unmutated VH genes and poor prognosis.[38,42,44]

The proliferative rate in CLL/SLL varies. However, grading schemes with clinical relevance have not been validated. The proliferating cells generally resemble prolymphocytes. Prolymphocytic transformation may occur, ultimately leading to an aggressive large B-cell lymphoma, the so-called Richter's syndrome.[45] However, some large B-cell malignancies occurring in patients with CLL/SLL appear to be secondary, derived from a separate B-cell clone.

A Hodgkin's-like transformation also has been described in CLL/SLL. This transformation can take one of two forms. In some cases Reed–Sternberg (RS) cells and mononuclear variants are seen in a background of small round B-lymphocytes demonstrating the features of CLL/SLL.[46] The

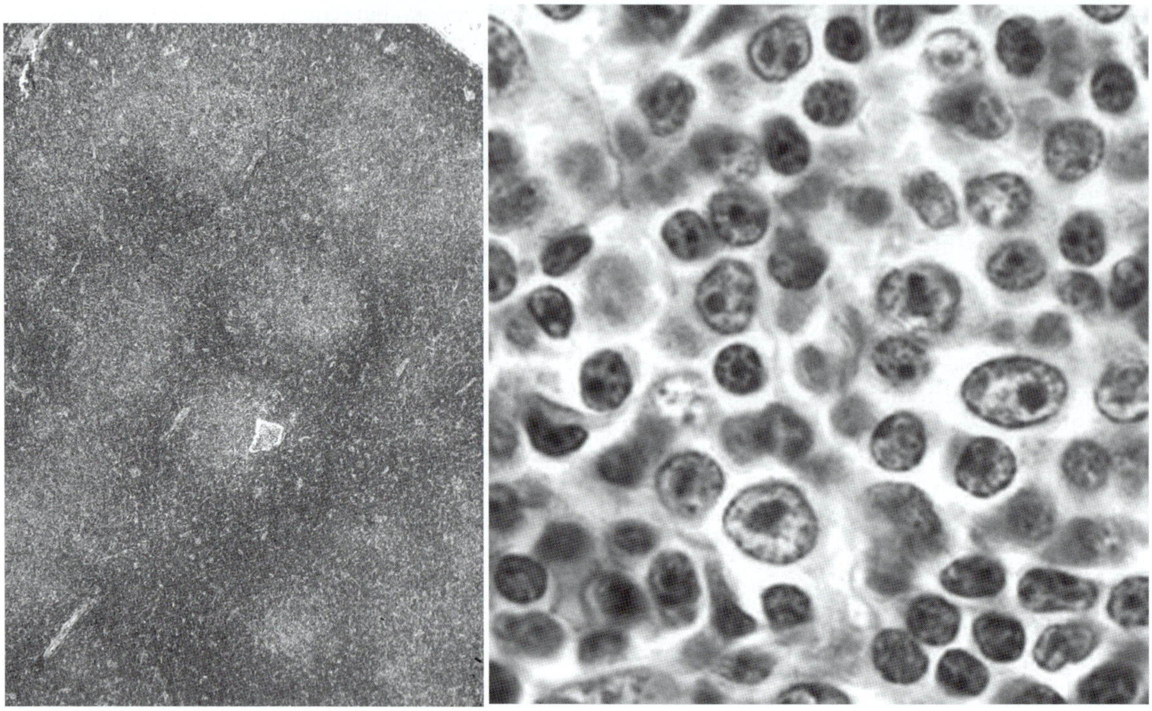

A B

Figure 1–2. CLL/SLL, lymph node. **A:** The lymph node shows diffuse architectural effacement with a pseudofollicular pattern, seen as pale areas representing proliferation or growth centers. (See color insert.) **B:** These growth centers appear pale due to the presence of larger lymphoid cells (prolymphocytes and paraimmunoblasts) in addition to small lymphocytes with clumped chromatin.

process lacks the rich inflammatory background of eosinophils, plasma cells, and histiocytes characteristic of Hodgkin's lymphoma. However, patients with this type of Hodgkin's transformation appear to progress to a process that is more typical of HL, with loss of the B-cell small lymphocytic component. In other instances, classic Hodgkin's lymphoma of the mixed cellularity or nodular sclerosis subtype may be seen in patients with a history of CLL/SLL.[47] Studies have implicated Epstein–Barr virus (EBV) in the HL type of Richter's transformation.[48] The Reed–Sternberg cells and variants are EBV+, and the implication is that they are derived from the underlying B-cell clone.

In some cases of CLL/SLL, limited plasmacytoid differentiation may occur.[49] The cytology resembles that of CLL/SLL, but the cells contain moderate amounts of cytoplasmic immunoglobulin, and a small monoclonal immunoglobulin spike may be detected in the serum. These cases conform to the lymphoplasmacytoid subtype of immunocytoma in the Kiel classification.[50] Such cases retain the immunophenotype of classic CLL/SLL and are regarded as a variant of CLL/SLL in the WHO classification.[51]

Lymphoplasmacytic Lymphoma (LPL)

WF: small lymphocytic, plasmacytoid
Kiel: immunocytoma, lymphoplasmacytic type
REAL: lymphoplasmacytoid lymphoma/immunocytoma

This tumor conforms in most cases to the clinical picture of Waldenström macroglobulinemia (WM), a disease of adult life that usually presents with generalized lym-

Table 1–3. Differential Diagnosis of "Small" B-Cell Lymphomas

Disease	CD5	CD10	CD23	CD43	Cyclin D1	Ig class
FL	−	+	+/−	−	−	IgM, IgG
MCL	+	−	−	+	+	IgM/IgD
CLL/SLL	+	−	+	+	−	IgM/IgD
LPL	−	−	−	+/−	−	IgM (c)
MALT	−	−	−	+/−	−	IgM (c, s)
SMZL	−	−	−	−	−	IgM/IgD
HCL	−	−	−	−	−/+	IgG

FL, follicular lymphoma; MCL, mantle cell lymphoma; CLL/SLL, chronic lymphocytic leukemia/small lymphocytic lymphoma; LPL, lymphoplasmacytic lymphoma; MALT, marginal zone lymphoma of MALT type; SMZL, splenic marginal zone lymphoma; HCL, hairy cell leukemia; Ig class, most commonly expressed heavy chain classes; c, cytoplasmic Ig; s, surface Ig.

phadenopathy, vague constitutional symptoms, anemia, and splenomegaly. Autoimmune hemolytic anemia is a common complication. IgM monoclonal gammopathy may be associated with increased serum viscosity leading to neurologic and vascular complications.[33,52–54] However, this phenomenon also is observed in other lymphomas. Peripheral blood involvement with an absolute lymphocytosis is less common in LPL than in CLL/SLL.

The neoplastic cells in LPL show evidence of plasmacytic differentiation (Fig. 1–3).[54] They have been referred to as "lymphoplasmacytoid" because, while the cytoplasm assumes a distinctly plasmacytic appearance with amphophilic cytoplasm and a perinuclear hof, the nucleus retains the condensed nuclear chromatin characteristic of a lymphocyte. LPL may show considerable morphologic heterogeneity.[55] Usually, a spectrum of plasmacytoid differentiation is seen, with the most plasmacytoid-appearing cells found in a perivascular and perisinusoidal distribution. Dutcher bodies are another characteristic cytologic feature of LPL. An interesting architectural feature of LPL is the tendency for lymphoid sinuses to be preserved, and even congested and distended. This apparent preservation of nodal architecture may cause problems in diagnosis. However, careful examination will usually reveal absence of follicles and paracortical regions, indicating architectural effacement by the lymphoid neoplasm.

By immunohistochemistry, cells showing plasmacytoid differentiation demonstrate expression of surface and cytoplasmic (some cells) immunoglobulin, usually of the IgM type (occasionally G, rarely A, and typically not D). The tumor expresses B-cell–associated antigens (CD19, 20, 22, 79a) but lacks CD5 and CD10. CD25 or CD11c may be faintly positive in some cases.[33,50,53,54] Lack of CD5 and presence of cytoplasmic immunoglobulin (cIg) are useful in distinction from CLL/SLL. The immunophenotype suggests a late stage in B-cell differentiation, just prior to the plasma cell stage; the postulated normal counterpart is thought to be a post-follicular medullary cord B cell,[33,56] based in part on the presence of somatic mutations in the Ig heavy and light chain variable region genes.[57] A recurrent chromosomal abnormality, t(9;14)(p13;q32), has been detected in approximately 50% of patients with LPL, especially those with WM.[58] This translocation involves the Pax-5 gene, which encodes a B-cell–specific transcription factor involved in the control of B-cell differentiation and proliferation.[59]

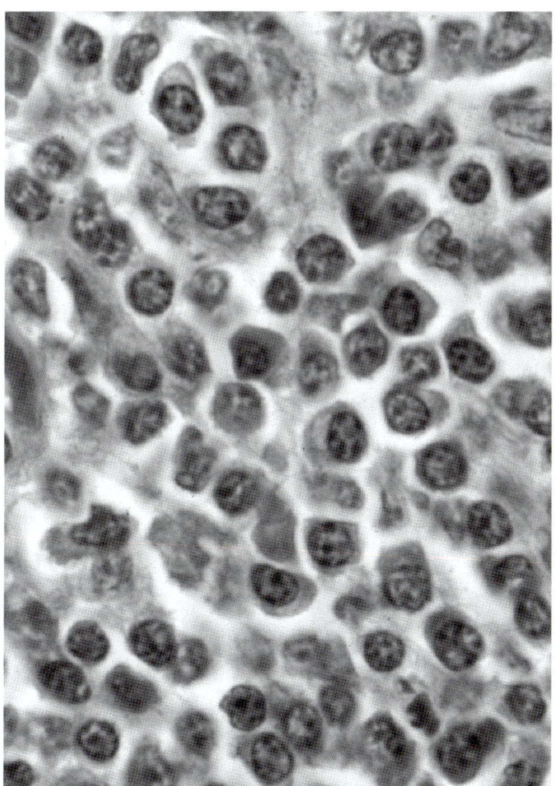

Figure 1–3. Lymphoplasmacytic lymphoma, lymph node. A spectrum of cell types is present, including small lymphocytes, plasmacytoid cells, and plasma cells with eccentric nuclei and amphophilic cytoplasm.

Splenic Marginal Zone Lymphoma (SMZL)

WF: small lymphocytic, small lymphocytic plasmacytoid
Kiel: not listed
REAL: splenic marginal zone lymphoma (provisional category)

SMZL presents in adults and is slightly more frequent in females than males.[60] The clinical presentation is splenomegaly, usually without peripheral lymphadenopathy. The majority of patients have bone marrow involvement, but there is usually only a modest lymphocytosis, with elevations in the lymphocyte count that are usually less than those seen in CLL. Some evidence of plasmacytoid differentiation may be seen, and patients may have a small M component. The abundant pale cytoplasm evident in tissue sections may also be seen in peripheral blood smears. The cytologic features may be mistaken for hairy cell leukemia. The disorder described as splenic lymphoma with villous lymphocytes (SLVL) appears equivalent to splenic marginal zone lymphoma.[61,62] The course is indolent, and splenectomy may be followed by prolonged remission.[63]

Histologically, the spleen shows expansion of the white pulp, but usually some infiltration of the red pulp is present as well.[64–67] In early cases, preferential involvement of the marginal zone may be seen, with residual mantle cells present.[68] Subsequently, a characteristic biphasic pattern in the neoplastic white pulp can be seen,[62] in which a peripheral zone of larger cells resembling marginal zone cells surrounds a central zone of small lymphocytes, with effacement of the normal mantle. Progression to DLBCL, often involving the spleen, can be seen.[69] Involvement of the bone marrow by SMZL is characterized by large, ill-defined, nonparatrabecular aggregates, with the neoplastic cells typically infiltrating bone marrow sinusoids.[65] Splenic hilar lymph nodes usually show diffuse infiltration, often with preservation of lymph node sinuses.

Immunophenotypic studies are useful in distinguishing SMZL from CLL/SLL involving the spleen. Whereas typical CLL/SLL is CD5+, SMZL usually is CD5–.[64] Careful attention to the cytologic features in these cases indicates that the cells have somewhat more abundant cytoplasm than those of typical CLL/SLL and resemble lymphocytes of the normal splenic marginal zone. The nuclei are usually predominantly round but may be slightly irregular. They have a moderate amount of pale cytoplasm. The phenotype of these cells resembles other MZLs; however, IgD expression is more frequently present.[65] Up to 40% of cases of SMZL show allelic loss of chromosome region 7q31-32.[70,71]

Plasmacytoma/Plasma Cell Myeloma

WF: extramedullary plasmacytoma
Kiel: plasmacytic lymphoma
REAL: plasmacytoma/myeloma

Plasmacytomas are rare in lymph nodes but occur with some frequency in extranodal sites. Patients with localized plasmacytomas involving lymph nodes or other organs are at risk to develop systemic disease, that is, plasma cell myeloma. The majority of localized plasmacytomas are well differentiated, clinically low grade, and morphologically composed of normal-appearing plasma cells.[72]

Some plasma cell malignancies are composed of immature cells with prominent central nucleoli and abundant deeply amphophilic cytoplasm.[73] Marked nuclear irregularity may be seen in rare cases.[74] This morphologic appearance has been termed "anaplastic myeloma." Patients with this high-grade histology are at greater risk to develop disease outside the bone marrow (e.g., lymph nodes, spleen, and liver). In addition, anaplastic myeloma may be difficult to distinguish from DLBCL exhibiting plasmacytoid differentiation, or so-called plasmablastic lymphoma.[75] The clinical behavior of these high-grade malignancies is more similar to aggressive lymphoma than typical multiple myeloma.

Immunophenotypically, plasma cell myelomas and plasmacytomas characteristically express monoclonal cytoplasmic Ig but lack surface Ig.[76] IgG is the most common Ig class, followed by IgA, and rarely IgD, IgE, or IgM. In 15% of cases only light chain is expressed (Bence–Jones myeloma). Most cases are negative for CD19 and CD20, but positive for CD38 and CD138 (syndecan-1).[77] CD79a is positive in approximately 50% of cases of multiple myeloma.[78] Additional markers that may be present include CD10[79] and CD56.[80] Cytogenetic abnormalities in patients with myeloma typically are complex, with abnormalities of chromosome 13 being among the most common findings.[81] Some patients demonstrate a t(11;14) translocation juxtaposing the cyclin D1 gene and the immunoglobulin heavy chain locus, and nuclear cyclin D1 protein can be detected immunohistochemically.[82] Cyclin D1 gene overexpression appears associated with improved outcome,[83] and ongoing gene microarray studies show promise in identifying new prognostic groups among patients with myeloma and identifying potential therapeutic targets.[84,85]

Extranodal Marginal Zone B-Cell Lymphoma of Mucosa-Associated Lymphoid Tissue (MALT Lymphoma)

WF: small lymphocytic, lymphoplasmacytoid, diffuse small cleaved cell
Kiel: immunocytoma
REAL: extranodal low-grade B-cell lymphoma of MALT

Most lymphomas of marginal zone derivation present in extranodal sites and have the histopathologic and clinical features identified by Isaacson and Wright as part of the spectrum of MALT lymphomas.[86,87] MALT lymphomas are characterized by a heterogeneous cellular composition that includes marginal zone or centrocyte-like cells, monocytoid B cells, small lymphocytes, and plasma cells (Fig. 1–4). In most cases, large transformed cells are infrequent. Reactive germinal centers are nearly always present. Therefore, it is not surprising that based on the heterogeneous cellular composition and presence of reactive follicles, most MALT lymphomas were diagnosed in the past as pseudolymphomas or atypical hyperplasias. However, recent studies have shown the majority to be composed of monoclonal B cells. The follicles usually contain reactive germinal centers, but the germinal centers may become colonized by neoplastic cells. When follicular colonization occurs, the process may simulate follicular lymphoma.[88] The plasma cells are usually found in the subepithelial zones and are monoclonal in up to 50% of cases.

MALT lymphomas have been described in nearly every anatomic site but are most frequent in the stomach, lung, thyroid, salivary gland, and lacrimal gland.[56,89] Other less common sites of involvement include the orbit, breast, conjunctiva, bladder, kidney, and thymus gland.[90] Most patients present with localized disease, although regional lymph node involvement is common in gastric and salivary gland MALT lymphoma. The involved lymph nodes in those cases resemble monocytoid B-cell lymphoma, and it now is recognized that monocytoid B-cell lymphoma is the nodal equivalent of MALT lymphoma.[91–95] Widespread nodal involvement is infrequent, as is bone marrow involvement. The clinical course is usually quite indolent, and many patients are asymptomatic. MALT lymphomas tend to relapse in other MALT-associated sites. For example, a patient with a salivary gland lymphoma may relapse with lacrimal gland involvement or conjunctival disease.[56]

MALT lymphomas of the salivary gland are usually associated with Sjögren syndrome and a history of autoimmune disease. Similarly, MALT lymphomas of the thyroid are associated with Hashimoto's thyroiditis. Helicobacter gastritis is frequent in patients with gastric MALT lymphomas, and it has been suggested that antigen stimulation is critical to both the development of MALT lymphoma and the maintenance of the neoplastic state.[96] Indeed, antibiotic therapy and eradication of *Helicobacter pylori* has led to the spontaneous remission of gastric MALT lymphoma in some cases.[97] Antibiotic treatment is currently advocated as first-line therapy, although the therapy of MALT lymphomas is still controversial. Isolated lesions readily amenable to surgical excision should be removed. Systemic chemotherapy may be warranted for more widespread disease, and local radiation therapy may play a role in the control of localized tumor masses, especially for gastric and orbital MALT lymphomas.

Immunophenotype is helpful in distinguishing MALT lymphomas from cytologically similar lymphomas such as CLL/SLL and MCL. MALT lymphomas are positive for B-cell associated antigens (CD19, CD20, and CD22), but typically are negative for CD5, in contrast to most systemic small lymphocytic malignancies. The absence of cyclin D1 expression is useful in ruling out MCL, especially in intestinal disease. Rare cases of MALT lymphoma

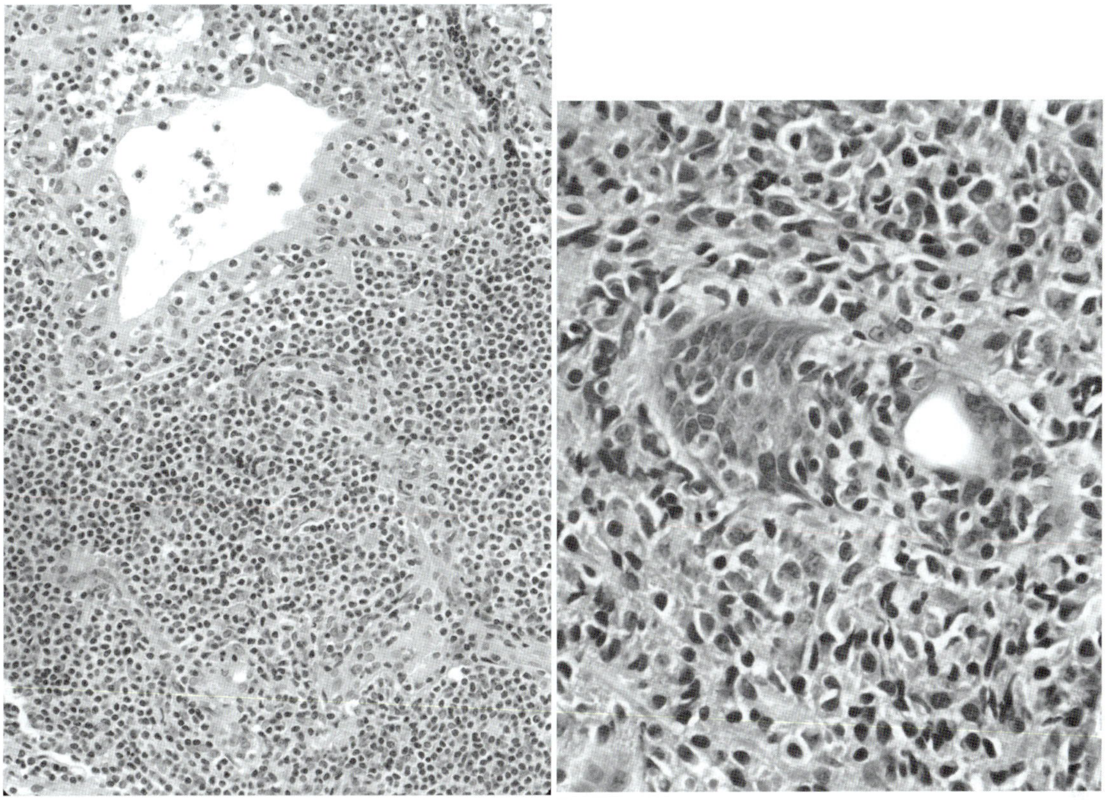

A B

Figure 1–4. MALT lymphoma. **A:** In this lung lesion, monocytoid-appearing cells with pale cytoplasm infiltrate and surround the bronchial epithelium. **B:** Lymphoepithelial lesion in a case of gastric MALT lymphoma, showing lymphoma cells invading an epithelial gland. (See color insert.)

have been reported to be CD5+, and in some but not all instances this has been associated with more aggressive disease.[98–100]

The t(11;18) translocation has been observed in 50% of extranodal MALT lymphomas.[101–104] The genes involved are *API2*, encoding an inhibitor of apoptosis, and the *MALT1/MLT* gene on 18q21 (function unknown).[105] The fusion protein may confer a survival advantage to the neoplastic cells through an anti-apoptotic effect.[105] The t(1;14) translocation involving the *Bcl-10* gene is more infrequent;[106] Bcl-10 protein overexpression may be seen in MALT lymphomas with or without the t(1;14).[107,108] Both translocations are felt to activate the NF-κB pathway.[109,110] Additionally, another translocation recently was identified involving the MALT1 gene and the immunoglobulin heavy chain gene. This translocation, t(14;18)(q32;q21), appears to be absent in gastric MALT lymphoma, but may be more common in MALT lymphomas presenting in the ocular adnexae, liver, and skin.[111]

The putative cell of origin of MALT lymphoma is a postgerminal center memory B cell.[112,113] As noted above, most MALT lymphomas are clinically low grade and contain a paucity of large transformed cells. Increased numbers of transformed cells may occur, although the clinical significance of this is uncertain.[114] The t(11;18) translocation is associated exclusively with low-grade extranodal MALT, and is not detected in cases with simultaneous low- and high-grade tumors, or in "primary" extranodal large cell lymphomas. Thus, it is unlikely that these primary extranodal large B-cell lymphomas are in fact related to low-grade MALT,[104,115–117] and the WHO Clinical Advisory Committee recommended against the use of the ambiguous term "high-grade MALT" for primary extranodal large cell lymphomas arising in MALT sites.[118]

Nodal Marginal Zone B-Cell Lymphoma (NMZL)

WF: small lymphocytic, plasmacytoid; follicular or diffuse small cleaved cell; follicular or diffuse mixed small and large cell
Kiel: monocytoid B cell
REAL: nodal marginal zone B-cell lymphoma with monocytoid B cells (provisional)

The existence of primary NMZL has been controversial, with many cases representing secondary involvement of lymph nodes by extranodal MALT lymphomas.[95,119,120] The existence of the primary extranodal disease may not be immediately apparent. Furthermore, relapses in nodal sites may occur many years after primary diagnosis. Nevertheless, there are several recent, well-documented reports of primary nodal lymphomas with features of MZL.[121,122] These patients often have bone marrow involvement, and tend to have a more aggressive clinical course than patients with extranodal MALT lymphomas.[120–122]

The neoplastic proliferation is polymorphous and composed of monocytoid B cells, plasmacytoid cells, and interspersed large blast-like cells. There is an expansion of the marginal zone area, often with preservation of the nodal architecture. The mantle zone may be intact, attenuated, or effaced.[95] The immunophenotype is similar to other MZLs, that is, CD20+, CD5–, and CD10–, with variable IgD expression (weak to negative). Some NMZLs have a morphology and immunophenotype similar to that of splenic MZL, and are IgD positive.[95] Because there are no precise immunophenotypic or genotypic markers of NMZL, the diagnosis sometimes is one of exclusion. A continuing problem is the differential diagnosis with LPL, which has overlapping morphologic and immunophenotypic features.[55] The presence of marked plasmacytic differentiation with prominent Dutcher bodies favors LPL. Clinical correlation is important in this distinction.

A morphologically similar but biologically distinct phenomenon is monocytoid B-cell differentiation in a primary nodal lymphoma. Monocytoid B lymphocytes have been described in many low-grade lymphomas, most commonly follicular lymphoma (FL, see next section).[123] The monocytoid B-cell component appears to occupy the marginal zone. Nevertheless, the immunophenotype and genotype of the neoplastic cells is that of FL. Monocytoid differentiation is an interesting morphologic variant, but does not yet have proven clinical or biologic significance. One study suggested that cases of FL with monocytoid B cells have a more aggressive clinical course,[124] but these results have not yet been confirmed.

Follicular Lymphoma (FL)

WF: follicular, small cleaved, mixed small cleaved and large cell, large cell
Kiel: centroblastic/centrocytic follicular, follicular centroblastic
REAL: follicle center lymphoma

FL is the most common subtype of non-Hodgkin's lymphoma in the United States and accounts for approximately 40% of all newly diagnosed cases. It has a peak incidence in the 5th and 6th decades and is rare under age 20. Men and women are equally affected. FL is less common in black and Asian populations. Most patients have Stage 3 or 4 disease at diagnosis, with generalized lymphadenopathy.[7] Staging evaluation will usually detect bone marrow involvement. Approximately 10% of patients have circulating malignant cells.[125] However, careful immunophenotypic or molecular analyses may disclose peripheral blood involvement in a higher proportion of patients.[126]

The natural history of the disease is associated with histologic progression of both pattern and cell type. A heterogeneous cytologic composition is one of the hallmarks of FL. Usually, all of the follicle center cells are represented, but in varying proportions.[4] It should be stressed that the variation in cytologic grade is a continuum (Fig. 1–5A), and therefore precise morphologic criteria for subclassification are difficult to establish. Most studies have shown that subclassification of follicular lymphoma is difficult to reproduce among groups of pathologists. The WHO classification includes three major grades: Grade 1 (0 to 5 centroblasts/high power field [hpf]); Grade 2 (6 to 15 centroblasts/hpf); and Grade 3 (>15 centroblasts/hpf), based on the method of Mann and Berard.[127] In addition, Grade 3 FL is further subdivided into Grade 3a (>15 centroblasts/hpf, but centrocytes still present) and Grade 3b (solid sheets of centroblasts). Recent studies indicate that FL Grade 3b may be more closely related biologically to DLBCL.[128,129] These data might provide a biological explanation for the greater curability of Grade 3 FL with aggressive therapy,[130] although some studies have not found support for this hypothesis.[131] Differences in diagnostic criteria might account for some of this apparent discrepancy.[132]

The majority of FLs (approximately 85%) are associated with a t(14;18) involving rearrangement of the Bcl-2 gene.[133] This translocation results in constitutive expression of Bcl-2 protein, which inhibits apoptosis in lymphoid cells (Fig. 1–5, B and C).[134] By avoiding apoptosis, FL cells accumulate and are at risk to undergo secondary mutations associated with histologic progression. The proportion of FLs expressing Bcl-2 protein varies with histologic grade, and is lowest in Grade 3 FL.[135] Recent data using protein microarrays have shown distinct alterations in the apoptotic pathways of Bcl-2-negative FLs, suggesting that this subset may have a different pathogenesis.[136] It has been postulated that the Bcl-2/JH translocation occurs during immunoglobulin gene rearrangement in the bone marrow at the pre–B-cell stage of development. This hypothesis might explain the difficulty in eradicating the neoplastic clone with chemotherapy. However, more recent studies have suggested that the translocation might occur in a mature B cell within the germinal center.[137,138] In some instances, FL may be restricted to isolated germinal centers within a lymph node, termed in situ localization of FL.[138] This pattern may be seen in conjunction with conventional FL at other sites, or may be the only manifestation of disease in some patients. The risk for progression in this latter group is not fully established.

The neoplastic cells of FL have a mature B-cell phenotype, with expression of the B-cell antigens CD19, CD20, and CD22. Surface Ig is positive, most commonly showing expression of IgM, but IgG or IgA can be seen in many cases. CD10 is positive, but CD5 is negative.[139] The presence of CD10+ cells in the interfollicular region can be a diagnostic clue, as this pattern is not seen in normal lymph nodes.[140] As evidence of the germinal center origin of FL, Bcl-6 is nearly always expressed.[141] FL was one of the first examples in which immunophenotype provided evidence for the normal lymphoid equivalent from which a lymphoma was derived,[139,142,143] in this case being the neoplastic counterpart of reactive germinal center cells.[144] As in their normal counterpart, intraclonal heterogeneity with a high number of somatic mutations and ongoing mutations of the Ig genes has been detected in FL cells.[145]

Most cases of FL present in lymph nodes. A subset of cases with the morphologic features of FL may present in skin.[146] Clinically, these tumors usually are localized and infrequently are associated with lymph node involvement. They have an excellent prognosis, and complete remissions may be obtained with either surgical excision or local radiation therapy.[147,148] Interestingly, cutaneous FL frequently lacks the Bcl-2 translocation associated with nodal FL. FL generally is rare in children; the nasopharyngeal and palatine tonsils and gastrointestinal tract are among the most common sites.[149] Pediatric FL also may present as an isolated testicular mass.[150] In contrast to FLs in adults, these tumors are usually Bcl-2 protein negative and lack Bcl-2 gene rearrangements. They typically are Grade 3, with a predominance of centroblasts and a high mitotic rate. FL in

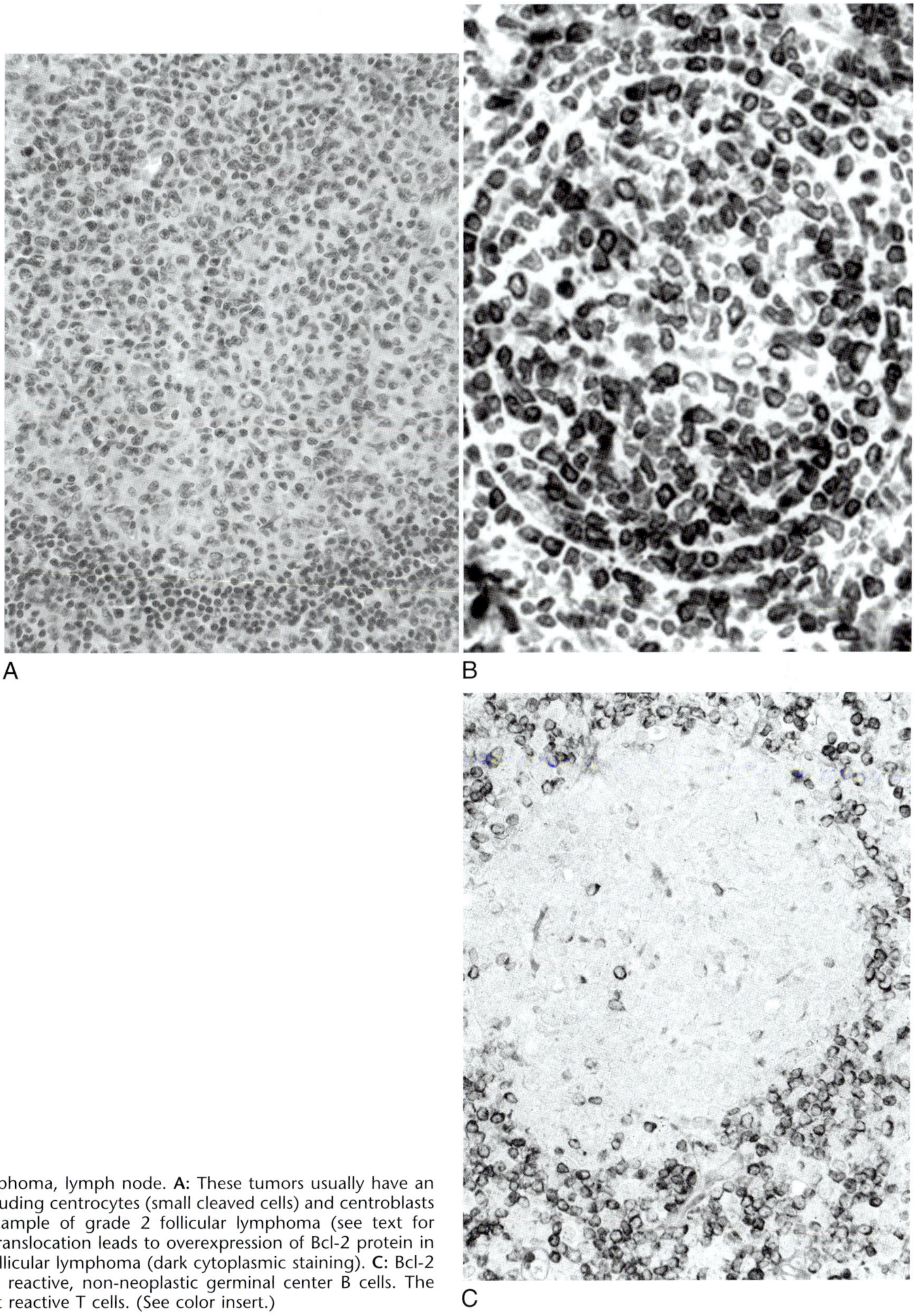

Figure 1–5. Follicular lymphoma, lymph node. **A:** These tumors usually have an admixture of cell types, including centrocytes (small cleaved cells) and centroblasts (large cells). This is an example of grade 2 follicular lymphoma (see text for grading). **B:** The t(14;18) translocation leads to overexpression of Bcl-2 protein in the neoplastic follicles of follicular lymphoma (dark cytoplasmic staining). **C:** Bcl-2 protein is not expressed in reactive, non-neoplastic germinal center B cells. The positive cells seen represent reactive T cells. (See color insert.)

the pediatric age group probably is a biologically distinct disease.

Mantle Cell Lymphoma (MCL)

WF: diffuse or follicular, small cleaved cell (rarely diffuse large cleaved cell)
Kiel: centrocytic lymphoma
REAL: mantle cell lymphoma

MCL is a distinct clinical pathologic entity that has been more precisely defined in recent years through the integration of immunophenotypic, molecular genetic, and clinicopathologic studies.[151,152] Early on it was noted that this tumor tended to surround residual naked germinal centers, and a derivation from the follicular lymphoid cuff was postulated.[153] Tumors with a very conspicuous mantle zone pattern of growth were also termed "mantle zone lymphoma."[154]

MCL occurs in adults (median age, 62), with a high male-to-female ratio. Most patients present with Stage 3 or 4 disease at diagnosis.[155–158] Common sites of involvement include the lymph nodes, spleen, bone marrow, and lymphoid tissue of Waldeyer's ring. Gastrointestinal tract involvement is frequent, and is associated with the picture of lymphomatous polyposis.[159] Like other low-grade lymphomas, this tumor appears to be incurable with available treatment. However, the median survival is shorter than for most other low-grade lymphomas and is in the range of 3 to 5 years. The median survival of the blastic variant is less than 3 years.[21]

The hallmark of MCL is a very monotonous cytologic composition. Within a given case the cells are usually of comparable size and share similar cytologic features. In the typical case, the cells are slightly larger than a normal lymphocyte with finely clumped chromatin, scant cytoplasm, and inconspicuous nucleoli. The nuclear contour is usually irregular or cleaved. Transformed cells resembling centroblasts or immunoblasts are essentially absent, providing an important distinction from follicular lymphoma. In addition, transformation to DLBCL, a common event in many other low-grade lymphomas, is not seen. Approximately 25% of cases of MCL have cells with large nuclei, more dispersed chromatin, and a higher proliferation fraction. This cytologic variant has been termed the blastic variant, because of the resemblance of the cells to lymphoblasts.[21] "Blastoid" MCLs include the classic blastic variant and a pleomorphic variant, and are associated with a more aggressive clinical course.[160–162] A high mitotic rate consistently has been found to be an adverse prognostic indicator.[163,164] Additionally, a proliferation signature identified by gene-expression profiling of MCLs recently was shown to correlate with survival.[165]

The immunophenotype of MCL is distinctive, and is characterized by expression of IgM/IgD and CD5, but lack of CD10 and CD23. The postulated normal counterpart is the CD5+, IgM/IgD+ "virgin" B cell that can be found in the peripheral blood and in the mantle zones of reactive germinal centers. In addition, the chromosomal translocation t(11;14) involving cyclin D1 located at the Bcl-1/Prad-1 locus is associated with MCL, but is absent in most other B-cell malignancies.[152,166] Virtually all cases of MCL express cyclin D1 (Fig. 1–6), including those rare cases lacking CD5 expression.[167–169] Alterations of other cell cycle regulatory molecules, including RB, p53, p16, and p27, have been described in the more aggressive forms of MCL.[170–175]

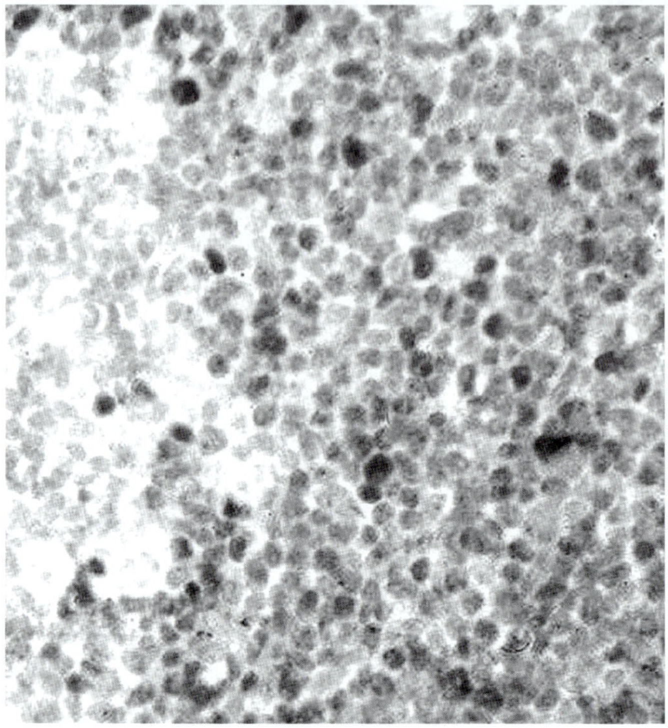

Figure 1–6. Mantle cell lymphoma, lymph node. A monotonous lymphoid infiltrate highlighted by nuclear staining for cyclin D1 maintains its mantle zone pattern, surrounding a non-neoplastic germinal center (negative staining, **left**). (See color insert.)

Diffuse Large B-Cell Lymphoma (DLBCL)

WF: diffuse mixed small and large cell, diffuse large cell, large cell immunoblastic
Kiel: centroblastic, immunoblastic, large cell anaplastic (B cell)
REAL: diffuse large B-cell lymphoma

DLBCL is one of the more common subtypes of non-Hodgkin's lymphoma, representing up to 40% of cases. It has an aggressive natural history but responds well to chemotherapy. The complete remission rate with modern regimens is 75% to 80%, with long-term disease-free survival approaching 50% or more in most series.[176] DLBCL may present in lymph nodes or in extranodal sites, including bone, skin, thyroid, gastrointestinal tract, and lung.

Because there is variation in the responsiveness to chemotherapy, and because DLBCL is one of the more common lymphomas, there has been great interest over the years in identifying morphologic or immunophenotypic features that might be prognostically important. In most studies, tumors composed of centroblasts have a better prognosis than those composed predominantly of immunoblasts.[7,177,178] Although this finding has not been consistently reproducible, the centroblastic variant often is seen in DLBCLs with a germinal center–like B-cell (GCB) gene-expression profile, a signature associated with a relatively favorable outcome (see below).[14]

DLBCLs are composed of large, transformed lymphoid cells with nuclei at least twice the size of a small lymphocyte. The nuclei generally have vesicular chromatin, prominent nucleoli, and basophilic cytoplasm, resembling the centroblasts of the normal germinal center (Fig. 1–7A). Marked variation in the nuclear contour may be seen, and the cells may be polylobated or cleaved.[179] In the immunoblastic variant of DLBCL, the majority of cells (>90%) have prominent central nucleoli and abundant, deeply staining cytoplasm, characteristic of immunoblasts.[52]

The T-cell/histiocyte-rich morphologic variant of DLBCL contains abundant non-neoplastic T lymphocytes with or

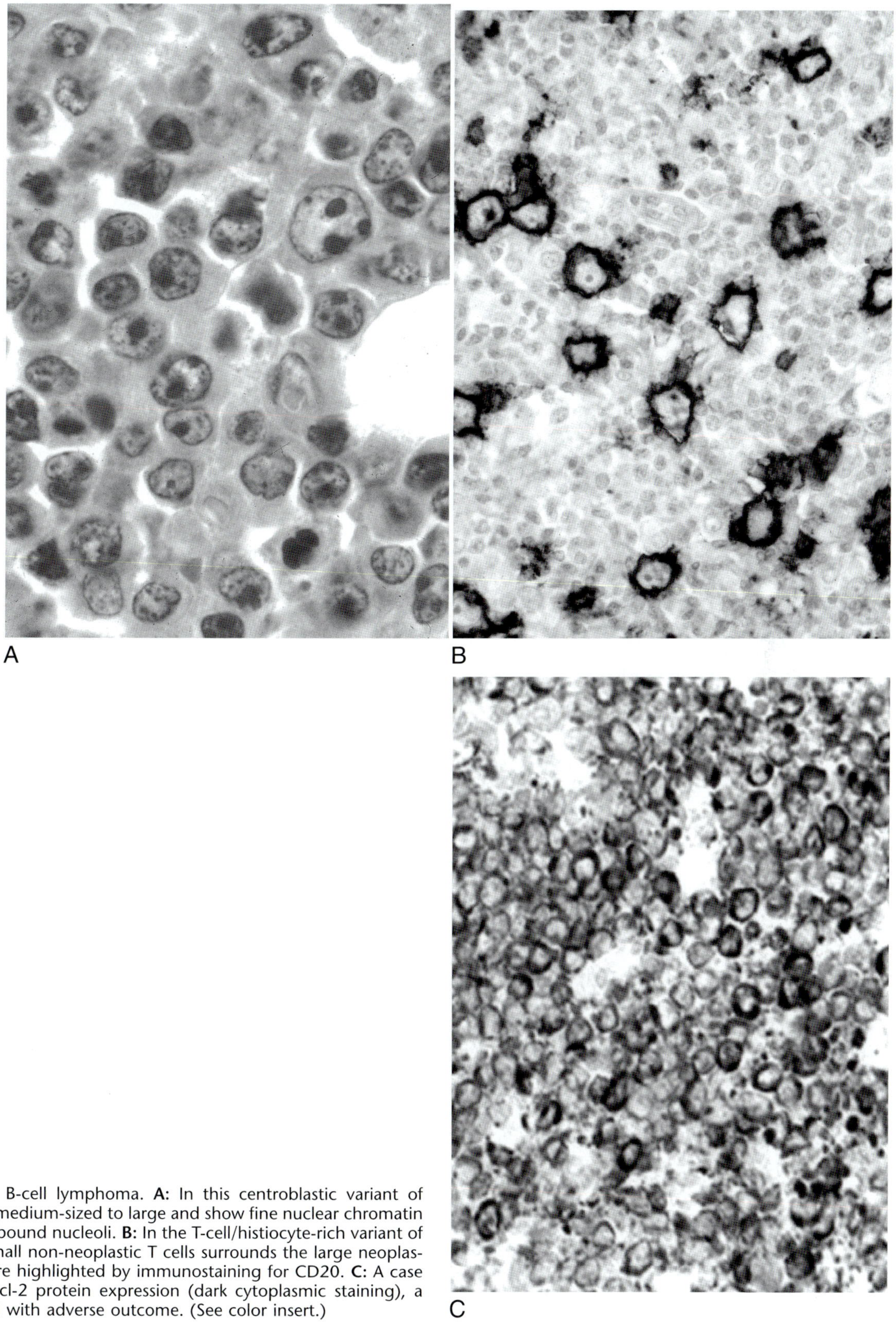

Figure 1–7. Diffuse large B-cell lymphoma. **A:** In this centroblastic variant of DLBCL, the tumor cells are medium-sized to large and show fine nuclear chromatin and prominent membrane-bound nucleoli. **B:** In the T-cell/histiocyte-rich variant of DLBCL, a background of small non-neoplastic T cells surrounds the large neoplastic B lymphocytes, which are highlighted by immunostaining for CD20. **C:** A case of DLBCL demonstrating Bcl-2 protein expression (dark cytoplasmic staining), a finding generally associated with adverse outcome. (See color insert.)

without histiocytes, and less than 10% large neoplastic B cells (Fig. 1–7B). It has been associated with aggressive clinical behavior, and often presents with advanced stage and bone marrow involvement.[180–183] Histologically, it may resemble classical Hodgkin's disease or even peripheral T-cell lymphoma.[184–186] Some cases appear related to nodular lymphocyte predominant Hodgkin's disease (NLPHD), with the neoplastic cells having a popcorn-like morphology and expressing epithelial membrane antigen (EMA).[184]

DLBCLs consistently express B-cell markers, especially CD20. Surface and/or cytoplasmic Ig may be demonstrated. A subset of cases express CD5 or CD10. Numerous studies have addressed the possible prognostic significance of immunophenotypic markers. Some data suggest that high growth fraction is an adverse prognostic marker;[187] however, other studies have reached the opposite conclusion, suggesting that lymphomas with a high growth fraction may be more sensitive to chemotherapy.[188] The prognostic significance of Bcl-2 protein expression and Bcl-2 gene rearrangement in DLBCL is controversial. However, in several studies the expression of Bcl-2 protein (irrespective of the presence of t(14;18)) has been associated with reduced disease-free survival (Fig. 1–7C).[188–190] This finding may be related to the anti-apoptotic effect of Bcl-2, abrogating apoptosis induced by chemotherapy. However, recent data suggest that Bcl-2-associated resistance to chemotherapy can be overcome using Rituximab in elderly patients with DLBCL.[191] The presence of Bcl-6 gene rearrangement in DLBCL, described mainly in cases with extranodal involvement, has been associated with a better prognosis[192]; however, these data have not been confirmed in other studies.

As mentioned above, cDNA microarray analysis of DLBCLs has demonstrated at least two major patterns of gene expression, the germinal center B cell (GCB) signature and the activated B-cell (ABC) signature.[14] The ABC signature was associated with shortened overall survival; furthermore, the gene expression profile was a predictor of outcome independent of the International Prognostic Index (IPI). Further studies demonstrated a third (Type 3) gene expression signature, which is more heterogeneous than the ABC and GCB groups, but appears to correlate with poor outcome, similar to DLBCLs with an ABC signature.[193] The cDNA microarray–based classification of DLBCLs has been validated by an immunohistochemical approach using tissue microarrays.[194] This study used immunohistochemistry to identify surrogate markers of the gene expression profile. The co-expression of Bcl-6 and CD10 with negative staining for MUM-1 correlated with a good prognosis.

Distinct Subtypes of Diffuse Large B-Cell Lymphoma

Mediastinal (Thymic) Large B-Cell Lymphoma

WF: large cell, large cell immunoblastic
Kiel: discussed as "rare and ambiguous subtype"
REAL: primary mediastinal (thymic) large B-cell lymphoma

This lymphoma has emerged in recent years as a distinct clinicopathologic entity.[195–197] Cytologically, it resembles many other large B-cell lymphomas and is composed of large transformed cells that can resemble centroblasts or even immunoblasts. A constant feature is relatively abundant pale cytoplasm, often with distinct cytoplasmic membranes.[196] Many cases have fine compartmentalizing sclerosis, which may even lead to misdiagnosis as an epithelial tumor, such as thymoma. The tumor appears to be derived from medullary B cells within the thymus gland.[195,198,199] The neoplastic cells express CD20 and CD79a, but not surface Ig.[199] CD30 frequently is positive, though often weak.[200,201] In some cases, the distinction from nodular sclerosis Hodgkin's lymphoma (NSHL) can be difficult (so-called "grey-zone" lymphomas).[202] Positive immunohistochemical staining for Pax-5, BOB.1, Oct-2, and PU.1 in mediastinal large B-cell lymphomas may help in the differential diagnosis.[201,203] Mediastinal large B-cell lymphomas also appear to lack the "crippling" immunoglobulin gene mutations seen in some cases of HL.[201,204] However, mediastinal large B-cell lymphoma may occur as a secondary malignancy following NSHL, supporting the possibility of a biologic relationship between these two entities.[205,206] Recently, gene expression profiling studies have found that mediastinal large B-cell lymphoma bears a distinct molecular signature that differs from that of other DLBCLs, and shares features of classic Hodgkin's lymphoma (CHL).[207,208]

Clinically, mediastinal large B-cell lymphoma is much more common in females than males.[209] It is common in adolescents and young adults with a median age at presentation in the fourth decade. The clinical presentation is that of a rapidly growing anterior mediastinal mass, frequently with superior vena cava syndrome and/or airway obstruction. Nodal involvement is uncommon at presentation and also at relapse. Frequent extranodal sites of involvement, particularly at relapse, include the liver, kidneys, adrenal glands, ovaries, gastrointestinal tract, and central nervous system. Early studies suggested that the tumor was associated with an unusually aggressive clinical course and poor response to conventional chemotherapy. This may have been due to inadequate therapy, since the tumor usually presents with Stage I or II disease, and more recent studies have reported cure rates similar to those seen for other large B-cell lymphomas after combined chemotherapy and irradiation.[210]

Intravascular Large B-Cell Lymphoma

Kiel: angio-endotheliotropic (intravascular) lymphoma
REAL: diffuse large B-cell lymphoma

Intravascular large B-cell lymphoma is a rare form of DLBCL characterized by the presence of lymphoma cells only in the lumens of small vessels, particularly capillaries.[211] The neoplasm is composed of a disseminated intravascular proliferation of large lymphoid cells of B-cell phenotype. The tumor cells have vesicular nuclei and prominent nucleoli, resembling centroblasts or immunoblasts. Lymph node involvement is rare: The tumor presents in extranodal sites and is most readily diagnosed in the skin.[212] Neurologic symptoms associated with plugging of small vessels in the central nervous system are common. The disease often is not diagnosed until autopsy, because of the varied symptomatology and lack of definitive radiologic or clinical evidence of disease.

Primary Effusion Lymphoma (PEL)

PEL is a novel lymphoproliferative disorder associated with human herpesvirus 8 (HHV-8) infection.[213] Most PELs develop in HIV-seropositive individuals and the neoplastic cells usually are coinfected with Epstein–Barr virus (EBV). Most patients are young to middle-aged homosexual males.[214] The disease also occurs in areas with high seroprevalence for HHV-8 infection, such as the Mediterranean, usually in elderly males.[215] Many affected patients also have a history of Kaposi sarcoma, and less commonly multicentric Castleman's disease.[216] The most common sites of involvement are the pleural, pericardial, and peritoneal cavities. Some cases may present with tumor masses involving the gastrointestinal tract, soft tissue, or other extranodal sites.[217]

The neoplastic cells usually exhibit plasmablastic or immunoblastic morphology, with some cells having a more anaplastic morphology. The cytoplasm is very abundant and deeply basophilic. The disease should be distinguished from pyothorax-associated DLBCL, which usually presents with a pleural mass lesion, and is EBV-positive but HHV-8-negative. The cells of PEL often have a "null-cell" phenotype, with loss of B-cell surface markers, in keeping with a late B-cell stage of differentiation. However, sIg and cIg often are absent. Markers of activation and plasma cell differentiation, such as CD30, CD38, and CD138, usually can be demonstrated.[218] Aberrant cytoplasmic CD3 expression has been reported.[219] Because of the markedly aberrant phenotype, it often is difficult to assign a lineage using immunophenotyping. Genotypic studies typically show IgH gene rearrangement,[220] but aberrant rearrangement of T-cell receptor genes also has been reported.[221] The nuclei of the neoplastic cells are positive by immunohistochemistry for the HHV-8/KSHV-associated latent nuclear antigen-1 (LNA-1/ORF-73),[222] which is a useful diagnostic test.

Plasmablastic Lymphoma (PBL)

The plasmablastic variant of DLBCL represents more than a single entity.[75] The term is most commonly associated with plasmablastic lymphomas of the oral cavity, usually diagnosed in the setting of HIV infection.[223] Most cases are EBV-positive. The tumor cells have immunoblastic or plasmablastic features, but do not show evidence of ongoing plasmacytic differentiation. Other rare examples of PBL may complicate multicentric Castleman's disease and contain HHV-8.[224] Although these lymphomas are indistinguishable from some examples of immunoblastic lymphoma on morphologic grounds, the lymphoma cells are negative for CD20 and CD45, but express plasma cell markers such as CD138.[225] Still another type of PBL is ALK-positive large B-cell lymphoma.[226] This lymphoma expresses the ALK tyrosine kinase usually expressed in T-cell–derived, anaplastic large cell lymphoma (ALCL). The mechanism of overexpression is complex, and most cases express full-length ALK, although translocations involving the ALK gene and other partners such as clathrin and nucleophosmin recently have been described.[227,228] The tumor presents with aggressive disease in adults, and shows a male predominance. Sinusoidal invasion frequently is present in lymph nodes.

Burkitt's Lymphoma

WF: small non-cleaved cell, Burkitt's type
Kiel: Burkitt's lymphoma
REAL: Burkitt's lymphoma

Burkitt's lymphoma (BL) is most common in children and accounts for up to one-third of all pediatric lymphomas in the United States.[229] It is the most rapidly growing of all lymphomas, with 100% of the cells in cell cycle at any time. It usually presents in extranodal sites. In nonendemic regions, such as the United States, frequent sites of presentation are the ileocecal region, ovaries, kidneys, or breasts. Jaw presentations, as well as involvement of other facial bones, are common in African or endemic cases, and are seen occasionally in nonendemic regions. Some cases present as acute leukemia with diffuse bone marrow infiltration and circulating Burkitt tumor cells (formerly known as L3-ALL in the FAB classification). Even in patients with typical extranodal disease, bone marrow involvement is a poor prognostic sign.

BL is one of the more common tumors associated with HIV infection.[230] It can present at any time during the clinical course. In some patients with HIV infection, Burkitt's lymphoma may be the initial AIDS-defining illness. The pathogenesis of BL is related to translocations involving the c-Myc oncogene, which are seen in virtually 100% of cases.[231,232] Most cases involve the immunoglobulin heavy-chain gene on chromosome 14. Less commonly the light-chain genes on chromosomes 2 and 22 are involved in the translocation. African BL occurs in regions endemic for malaria, and it has been postulated that immunosuppression associated with malarial infection places patients at increased risk for Burkitt's lymphoma.[133] In this regard, the pathogenesis appears similar to that seen with HIV infection.

EBV is closely linked to Burkitt's lymphoma in endemic regions but is less frequently seen (15% to 20%) in European and North American cases.[229] Burkitt's lymphoma is more often EBV-positive (50% to 70% of cases) in regions characterized by low socioeconomic status and EBV infection at an early age.[233] These data support the hypothesis that EBV is a co-factor for the development of BL. Differences in the proportion of cases associated with the two EBV strains (Types 1 and 2) also have been shown in sporadic and endemic EBV-positive BL.[234]

Cytologically, BL is monomorphic, consisting of medium-sized cells with round nuclei, moderately clumped chromatin, and multiple (2 to 5) basophilic nucleoli (Fig. 1–8A). The cytoplasm is deeply basophilic and moderately abundant. The cells contain cytoplasmic lipid vacuoles, which are probably a manifestation of the high rate of proliferation and high rate of spontaneous cell death. Lipid vacuoles are usually evident on imprints or smears but not in tissue sections (Fig. 1–8B). The "starry sky" pattern characteristic of BL is a manifestation of the numerous benign macrophages that have ingested karyorrhectic or apoptotic tumor cells. BL has a mature B-cell phenotype. The neoplastic cells express CD19, CD20, CD22, CD79a, and monoclonal surface Ig, nearly always IgM. CD10 and Bcl-6 are positive in nearly all cases, while CD5, CD23, and Bcl-2 are consistently negative.[235]

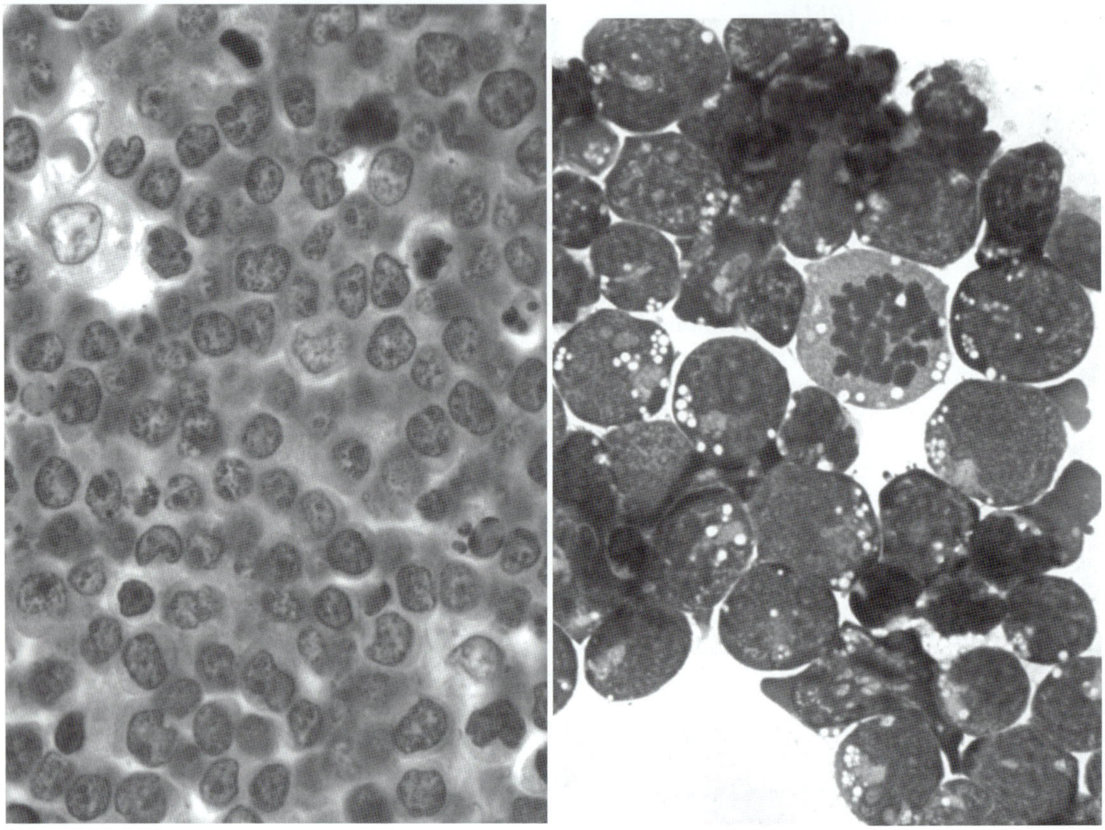

A B

Figure 1–8. Burkitt's lymphoma. **A:** The cells are uniform, round to oval, with multiple small basophilic nucleoli. The nuclear size is similar to that of the "starry sky" histiocyte in the **upper left**. Mitotic activity is present. **B:** A touch preparation demonstrates lipid vacuoles in the deeply basophilic cytoplasm. (See color insert.)

The WHO classification includes three clinical variants of BL that are associated with different clinical settings: endemic BL, sporadic BL, and AIDS-associated BL. In addition, three morphologic variants are defined: classic BL, atypical BL, and BL with plasmacytoid differentiation. The last variant is most often seen in association with HIV infection,[236] whereas the other two variants can be encountered in both endemic and sporadic clinical settings. The distinction of BL from morphologically similar aggressive B-cell lymphomas has been problematic for pathologists and clinicians. The category of small non-cleaved cell lymphoma, non-Burkitt, in the WF was biologically and clinically heterogeneous. In addition, the c-Myc translocation as a secondary event is not associated with identical clinical consequences.

The atypical variant of BL is composed of medium-sized Burkitt cells and shows other features of BL (high degree of apoptosis, high mitotic index). However, in contrast to classic BL, the cells show greater pleomorphism in nuclear size and shape. Nucleoli are more prominent and fewer in number. The diagnosis requires a growth fraction of 100% and the appropriate immunophenotype for BL. Because of imprecision in the cytologic features, molecular studies to identify a c-Myc translocation are highly desirable, if not required, for diagnosis. This designation should not be utilized for cases of DLBCL composed of medium-sized cells. It also differs from the provisional category of "Burkitt-like lymphoma" in the REAL classification, which was admittedly heterogeneous, including cases of both atypical BL and DLBCL.

While the c-Myc translocation is the hallmark of BL, it may occur as a secondary event in other lymphomas, including follicular lymphoma, mantle cell lymphoma, and DLBCL.[237,238] In follicular lymphoma, secondary c-Myc translocations have been associated with high-grade transformations showing Burkitt-like or lymphoblastic cytology.[239] Mantle cell lymphomas with c-Myc deregulation are aggressive or blastic in appearance.[240]

Lymphomatoid Granulomatosis (LYG)

LYG is an angiocentric lymphoproliferative disease that exhibits many similarities both clinically and pathologically to extranodal NK/T-cell lymphoma, nasal type, from which it must be distinguished.[241,242] Only recently, both diseases were considered part of the same spectrum of angiocentric immunoproliferative lesions. However, recent data indicate that LYG is an EBV-positive B-cell proliferation associated with an exuberant T-cell reaction.[243] LYG also presents in extranodal sites, but the most common site of involvement is the lung.[244] The kidney and central nervous system also are frequently involved, as are skin and subcutaneous tissue. Morphologically, LYG is an angiocentric, angiodestructive lesion, typically showing lymphocytic vasculitis with areas of necrosis, mediated in part by EBV-induced chemokine production (Fig. 1–9).[245] The lesion is charac-

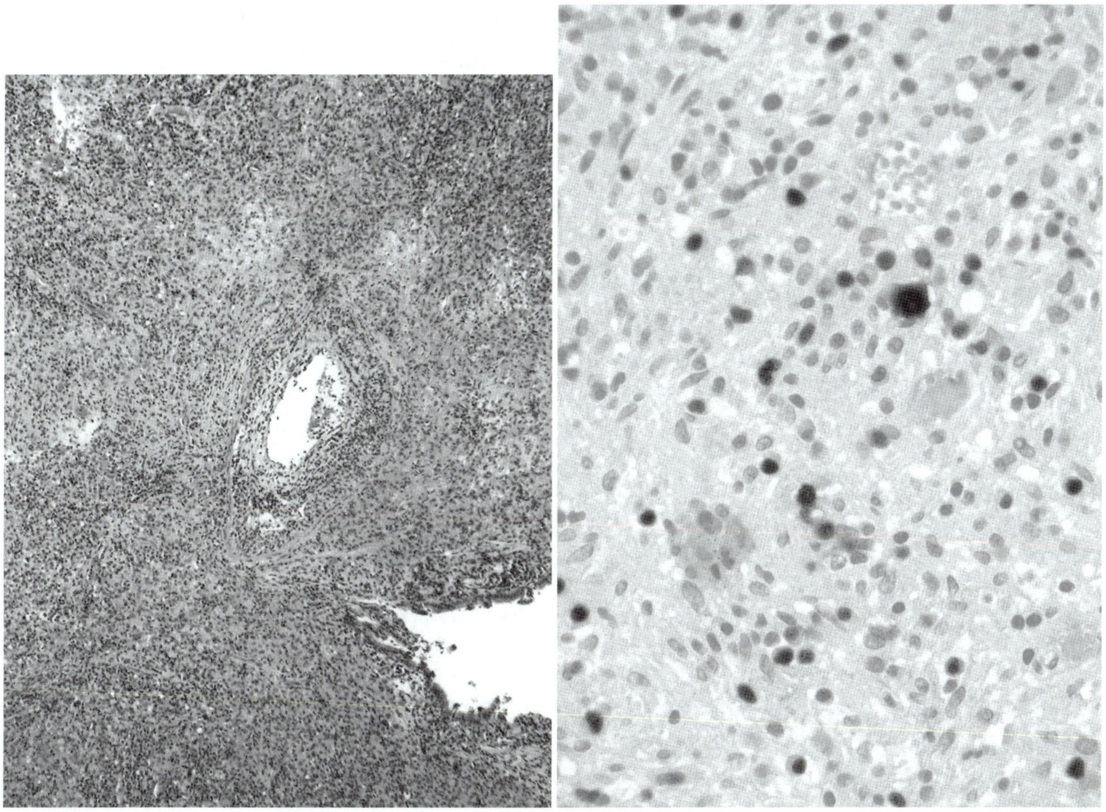

A B

Figure 1–9. Lymphomatoid granulomatosis, lung. **A:** The angiocentric, angiodestructive nature of the polymorphous lymphoid infiltrate is shown in the center of the field. **B:** The mixed inflammatory background contains relatively sparse atypical EBV-positive B cells, highlighted by in situ hybridization (*dark nuclear staining*).

terized by a relatively small number of EBV-positive B cells, usually demonstrating atypia, superimposed on a mixed inflammatory background of small lymphocytes, plasma cells, immunoblasts, and histiocytes.[243,246] Most of the background lymphocytes are CD3+ T cells (CD4>CD8). The EBV-positive B cells express CD20, with variable expression of CD79a and CD30. CD15 is negative. These cells can be highlighted using in situ hybridization for EBV sequences using the EBER1/2 probe. The frequency of positive cells can be used to assist in grading, with Grade I lesions having less than 5 EBV-positive cells per hpf, Grade II lesions having 5 to 20 per hpf, and Grade III lesions having numerous such cells and corresponding to frank malignant lymphoma.[247] Clonal immunoglobulin gene rearrangements can be demonstrated in most Grade II and III lesions. Grade I and II lesions may respond to interferon-alpha 2b,[247] whereas Grade III lesions are considered a subtype of DLBCL and may respond to aggressive chemotherapy.[242]

T-CELL AND NK-CELL LYMPHOMAS

Overview of T-Cell and NK-Cell Neoplasm Classification

While the definition of precursor T-cell or lymphoblastic neoplasms is straightforward, the classification of peripheral T-cell lymphomas has been controversial. Most previously published classification schemes for the malignant lymphomas published in the United States or Europe have been based on B-cell malignancies, as these are far more common than their T-cell counterparts. The classification of T-cell and NK-cell neoplasms proposed by the WHO emphasizes a multiparameter approach, integrating morphologic, immunophenotypic, genetic, and clinical features. Clinical features are of particular importance in the subclassification of these tumors, in part due to the lack of specificity of other parameters. T-cell lymphomas show great morphologic diversity, and a spectrum of histologic appearances can be seen within individual disease entities. The cellular composition can range from small cells with minimal atypia to large cells with anaplastic features. Such a spectrum is seen in anaplastic large cell lymphoma, adult T-cell leukemia/lymphoma, and extranodal NK/T-cell lymphoma, nasal type, as selected examples. Moreover, there is morphologic overlap between disease entities. Many of the extranodal cytotoxic T-cell and NK-cell lymphomas share similar appearances, including prominent apoptosis, necrosis, and angioinvasion.[248]

In contrast to B-cell lymphomas, specific immunophenotypic profiles are not associated with most T-cell lymphoma subtypes. While certain antigens are commonly associated with specific disease entities, these associations are not entirely disease-specific. For example, CD30 expression is a universal feature of anaplastic large cell lymphoma, but also can be expressed, usually to a lesser degree, in other T- and B-cell lymphomas. CD30 is, of course, also positive in classic Hodgkin's lymphoma. Similarly, while CD56 expression is a characteristic feature of extranodal NK/T-cell lymphomas, it can be seen in other T-cell lymphomas, and even malignant plasma cell neoplasms.[80,249,250]

Presently, specific genetic features have not been identified for many of the T-cell and NK-cell neoplasms. One exception is anaplastic large cell lymphoma, which is associated with the t(2;5) and other variant translocations.[251] However, the molecular pathogenesis of most T-cell and NK-cell neoplasms remains to be defined. The lack of specific genetic and immunophenotypic markers increases the importance of clinical features for the mature T-cell lymphomas.

Precursor T-Lymphoblastic Leukemia/Lymphoblastic Lymphoma (T-ALL/T-LBL)

WF: lymphoblastic
Kiel: T lymphoblastic

Most T-LBLs are cytologically indistinguishable from their B-cell counterparts. The cells usually are convoluted, but non-convoluted forms also exist.[20,252] The cells have finely distributed chromatin, inconspicuous nucleoli, and sparse, pale cytoplasm. Eighty-five percent of patients with lymphoblastic lymphoma have a tumor of precursor T-cell phenotype. This is a disease of adolescents and young adults, with an increased male-to-female ratio. Fifty percent to 80% of patients present with an anterior mediastinal mass, usually with involvement of the thymus gland. T-LBL is a high-grade lymphoma, and rapid growth may be associated with airway obstruction. Bone marrow involvement is common, and progression to a leukemic picture will occur in the absence of effective therapy. The tumor also has a high frequency of central nervous system (CNS) involvement, a poor prognostic sign. T-LBL is closely related to T-ALL, although the lymphomatous forms usually exhibit a more mature T-cell phenotype.[253] Translocations involving T-cell receptor loci have been detected in T-ALL/LBL, leading to dysregulation of various genes, such as TAL1[254] and HOX11.[255] These oncogenes also can be activated in the absence of chromosomal abnormalities, and gene expression profiling has helped to characterize the transforming events in T-ALL and identify new prognostic groups.[256]

In lymph nodes, T-LBL shows a diffuse leukemic pattern of infiltration. There is very little stromal reaction, and the cells diffusely infiltrate the lymph node parenchyma. Streaming of cells in the medullary cords may be prominent, especially around vascular structures. Some residual follicles may be present, but ultimately architectural effacement is the rule. A starry sky pattern is seen in approximately one-third of cases. Mitotic figures are readily observed. Histologically, it is not possible to differentiate T-LBL from B-LBL; however, immunophenotypic studies can usually identify the cell of origin. The lymphoblasts in T-LBL express TdT and show variable positivity for T-cell markers, most commonly CD7 and cytoplasmic CD3. Of these, CD3 is considered lineage-specific. CD4 and CD8 are frequently co-expressed.

T-Cell Prolymphocytic Leukemia (T-PLL)

WF: small lymphocytic, consistent with CLL, diffuse small cleaved cell, unclassified
Kiel: T-cell CLL/PLL
REAL: T-cell prolymphocytic leukemia/T-cell chronic lymphocytic leukemia

T-PLL presents with leukemia, with or without lymphadenopathy, and usually with markedly elevated white blood cell counts.[257,258] Instances of primary lymph node involvement are exceedingly rare. The lymph node involvement is diffuse and primarily paracortical, with sparing of the follicles. The cellular infiltrate is usually more monotonous than that of CLL/SLL and lacks pseudofollicular proliferation centers. Involvement of the spleen is associated with diffuse red pulp infiltration. Hepatomegaly is frequently present. Clinically, T-PLL is much more aggressive than CLL/SLL. In most cases, some cytologic atypia is present, so that the cells do not resemble small, round normal-appearing lymphocytes. The immunophenotype is that of T prolymphocytes, which are TdT and CD1a negative, and CD2, CD3, and CD7 positive. In 25% of cases, CD4 and CD8 are co-expressed; 60% express CD4 only, while 15% express CD8 only.[257]

T-Cell Large Granular Lymphocyte Leukemia (T-LGL)

WF: small lymphocytic, consistent with CLL
Kiel: T-CLL
REAL: large granular lymphocyte leukemia, T-cell type

This disorder is not generally considered with the malignant lymphomas, and will be discussed only briefly. The cells have more abundant pale cytoplasm than those of T-PLL. In smear preparations azurophil granules are readily identified. Most cases of T-LGL have been shown to be clonal, based on analysis of T-cell receptor gene rearrangement.[259] In addition to peripheral blood involvement, the cells infiltrate the marrow, splenic red pulp, and liver. Lymphadenopathy is uncommon, and the clinical course is indolent. The neoplastic cells have a mature T-cell immunophenotype[260] and consistently express CD3. Most commonly (80%) the cells are T-cell receptor (TCR) $\alpha\beta$+, CD4−, and CD8+, but rare variants exist. Cases resembling T-LGL but exhibiting an NK-cell immunophenotype are grouped with the NK disorders in the WHO classification.

Adult T-Cell Leukemia/Lymphoma (ATLL)

WF: diffuse small cleaved, diffuse mixed small and large cell, large cell, large cell immunoblastic, small non-cleaved non-Burkitt
Kiel: pleomorphic small cell, medium sized and large cell, immunoblastic (HTLV-1 positive)
REAL: adult T-cell leukemia/lymphoma

Adult T-cell leukemia/lymphoma (ATLL) is a distinct clinicopathologic entity originally described in southwestern

Japan, which is associated with the retrovirus HTLV-1.[261,262] HTLV-1 is found clonally integrated in the T cells of this lymphoma. HTLV-1 is also endemic in the Caribbean, where clusters of ATLL have been described, predominantly among blacks.[263,264] It is seen with lesser frequency in blacks in the southeastern United States.[265] The median age of affected individuals is 45 years. Patients in the Caribbean tend to be slightly younger than those in Japan.[266] Patients may present with leukemia or with generalized lymphadenopathy. The leukemic form predominates in Japan, whereas lymphomatous presentations are more common in the Western hemisphere. Other clinical findings include lymphadenopathy, hepatosplenomegaly, lytic bone lesions, and hypercalcemia.[267] The acute form of the disease is associated with a poor prognosis and a median survival of less than 2 years.[265] Complete remissions may be obtained, but the relapse rate is nearly 100%.

Chronic and smoldering forms of the disease are seen less commonly.[268] These are associated with a much more indolent clinical course. There is usually minimal lymphadenopathy. The predominant clinical manifestation is skin rash, with only small numbers of atypical cells in the peripheral blood. In the chronic and smoldering forms, HTLV-1 virus also is found integrated within the atypical lymphoid cells.

The cytologic spectrum of ATLL is extremely diverse. The cells may be small with condensed nuclear chromatin and a markedly polylobated nuclear appearance (Fig. 1–10).[265,269] Larger cells with dispersed chromatin and small nucleoli may be admixed and predominate in some cases. RS-like cells can be seen, simulating Hodgkin's lymphoma.[270] The RS-like cells represent EBV-infected B cells, expanded secondary to underlying immunodeficiency.[271] In the smoldering form of ATLL, the cells often are small and show minimal cytologic atypia, and may resemble the cells of SLL. The larger cells usually show abundant cytoplasmic basophilia. Skin involvement is seen in approximately two-thirds of patients, and the cutaneous infiltrates often show prominent epidermotropism, simulating mycosis fungoides. Immunophenotypically, the neoplastic cells are positive for T-cell–associated antigens such as CD2, CD3, and CD5, but typically are CD7−. Most cases are CD4+/CD8−. Nearly all cases are CD25+.

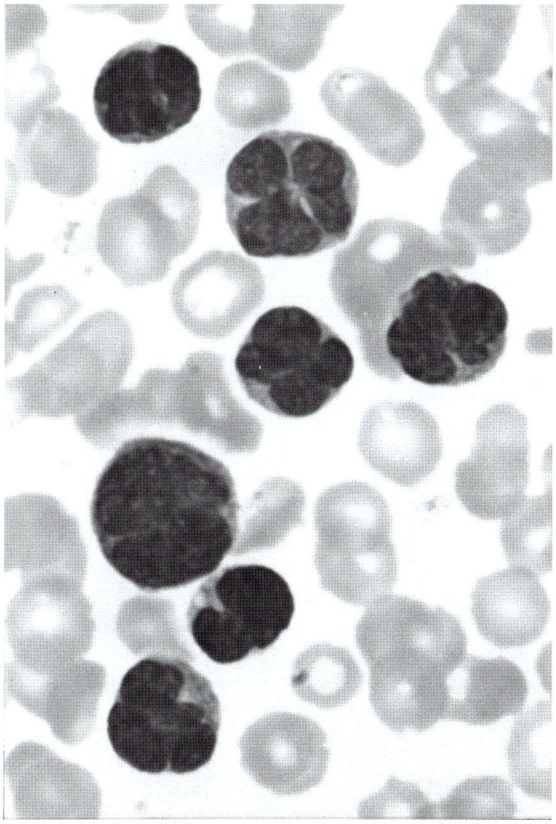

Figure 1–10. Adult T-cell leukemia/lymphoma. Markedly polylobated ("flower") cells circulate in the peripheral blood. (See color insert.)

Extranodal NK/T-Cell Lymphoma, Nasal Type

WF: diffuse small cleaved, mixed small and large cell, large cell immunoblastic
Kiel: pleomorphic small cell, medium and large cell (HTLV-1 negative)
REAL: angiocentric T-cell lymphoma

Extranodal NK/T-cell lymphoma, nasal type, is a distinct clinicopathologic entity highly associated with EBV.[272,273] It affects adults (median age, 50), and the most common clinical presentation is with a destructive nasal or midline facial tumor. Palatal destruction, orbital swelling, and edema may be prominent.[274] NK/T-cell lymphomas have been reported in other extranodal sites, including skin, soft tissue, testis, upper respiratory tract, and gastrointestinal tract. Aggressive NK-cell leukemia/lymphoma is a closely related disorder.[275] The clinical course usually is highly aggressive with a slightly improved median survival in patients with localized disease. However, the outcome remains poor with current chemotherapy. Radiation therapy may be effective in localized disease. A hemophagocytic syndrome is a common clinical complication, and adversely affects survival in extranodal NK/T-cell lymphoma, nasal type.[276] It is likely that EBV plays a role in the pathogenesis of the hemophagocytic syndrome. Extranodal NK/T-cell lymphoma, nasal type, is much more common in Asians than in individuals of European background. Clusters of the disease also have been reported in Central and South America in individuals of Native American heritage, suggesting that ethnic background may play a role in the pathogenesis of these lymphomas.[277]

Extranodal NK/T-cell lymphomas demonstrate a broad cytologic spectrum. The atypical cells may be small or medium in size. Large, atypical, hyperchromatic cells may be admixed or may predominate. If small cells are in the majority, the disease may be difficult to distinguish from an inflammatory or infectious process. In early stages, there also may be a prominent admixture of inflammatory cells, further causing difficulty in diagnosis.[242]

Although the cells express some T-cell–associated antigens, most commonly CD2, other T-cell markers such as surface CD3 are usually absent.[278] The cells express cytoplasmic CD3ε, and are usually CD56+. Cytotoxic markers such as granzyme B and TIA-1 are present. Molecular studies are negative for T-cell receptor gene rearrange-

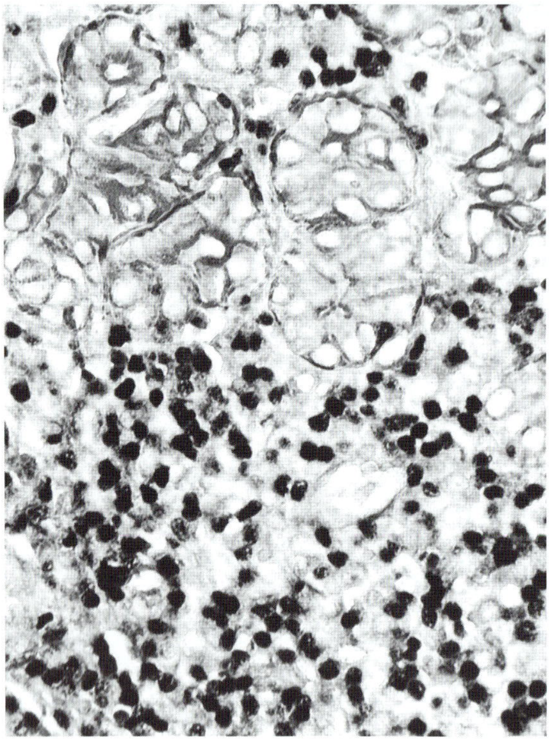

Figure 1–11. Extranodal NK/T-cell lymphoma, nasal type. The tumor cells are diffusely positive for EBV-encoded RNA by in situ hybridization (*dark nuclear staining*), whereas epithelial glands are negative for EBV and are stained for keratin (**top**).

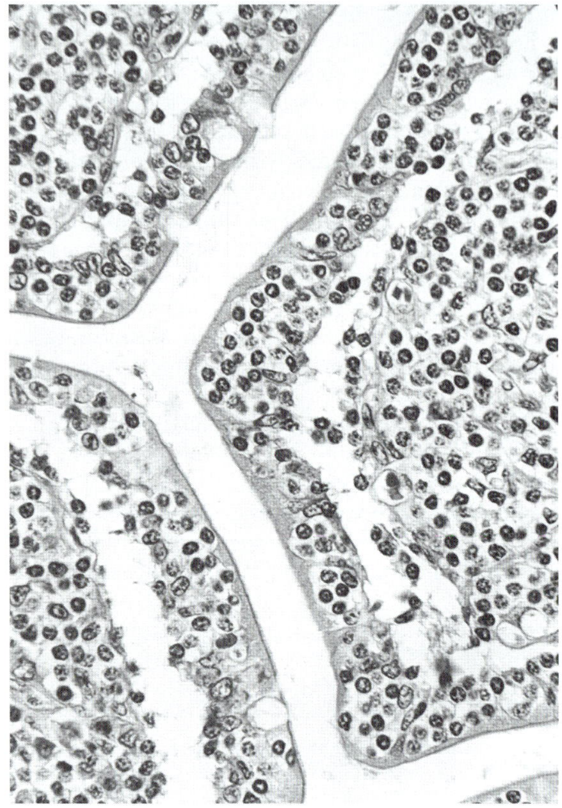

Figure 1–12. Enteropathy-type T-cell lymphoma. Atypical lymphocytes with pale cytoplasm infiltrate the epithelial mucosa and lamina propria of small intestinal villi. (See color insert.)

ment, despite the demonstration of clonality by other methods.[278–280] Because virtually all cases of extranodal NK/T-cell lymphoma, nasal type, are positive for EBV, in situ hybridization studies with probes to EBV-encoded small nuclear RNA (EBER 1/2) may be very helpful in diagnosis and can detect even small numbers of neoplastic cells (Fig. 1–11).[278,281]

Enteropathy-Type T-Cell Lymphoma (ETL)

WF: diffuse small cleaved, diffuse mixed small and large cell, diffuse large cell immunoblastic
Kiel: pleomorphic small, medium, and large
REAL: intestinal T-cell lymphoma (with and without enteropathy)

ETL was originally termed malignant histiocytosis of the intestine; however, the demonstration of clonal T-cell receptor gene rearrangement indicated that it was a T-cell lymphoma.[282,283] The small bowel usually shows ulceration, frequently with perforation. A mass may or may not be present. The infiltrate shows a varying cytologic composition with an admixture of small, medium, and larger atypical lymphoid cells (Fig. 1–12). Anaplastic cells strongly positive for CD30 may be present. The neoplastic cells are CD3+, CD7+ T cells, which are negative for CD4, often show loss of CD8,[284] and express the homing receptor CD103 (HML-1).[285] The cells express cytotoxic molecules, a feature shared by nearly all extranodal T-cell lymphomas, and appear to be part of the innate immune system.[286] EBV generally is negative. EBV has been detected in some intestinal NK/T-cell lymphomas in certain geographic regions, such as Mexico and Asia, but whether these lymphomas are true ETLs or in fact extranodal NK/T-cell lymphomas involving the intestine remains to be determined.[287,288] The gastrointestinal tract is a common site of secondary involvement by extranodal NK/T-cell lymphoma, nasal type (see above).[289]

This disease occurs mostly in adults with either overt or clinically silent gluten-sensitive enteropathy, including those with refractory celiac disease.[290,291] Most patients have the HLA DQA1*0501, DQB1*0201 genotype.[292] The adjacent small bowel usually shows evidence of villous atrophy.[293] Although celiac disease usually is associated with an increase in intraepithelial $\gamma\delta$ T cells, the cells of ETL are usually of $\alpha\beta$ origin.[294] TCR-β and -γ genes are clonally rearranged. Similar clonal rearrangements may be found in the adjacent intestine, suggesting that the associated increase in intraepithelial T cells constitutes a neoplastic or preneoplastic population.[295] The most common genetic aberration is amplification at the 9q34 locus, seen in 40% of patients with informative genotypes.[296] Patients usually present with abdominal symptoms such as pain, small bowel perforation, and associated peritonitis. The clinical course is aggressive, and most patients have multifocal intestinal disease.

Hepatosplenic T-Cell Lymphoma

WF: diffuse small cleaved cell, unclassified
Kiel: pleomorphic small cell, medium size cell (HTLV-1 negative)
REAL: hepatosplenic $\gamma\delta$ T-cell lymphoma

Hepatosplenic T-cell lymphoma presents with marked hepatosplenomegaly in the absence of lymphadenopathy.[297,298] The majority of cases are of γδ T-cell origin.[299,300] Most patients are male, with a peak incidence in young adulthood. Although patients may respond initially to chemotherapy, relapse has been seen in the majority of cases, and the median survival is less than 3 years. Rare long-term survival has been seen following allogeneic bone marrow transplantation.[300] The cells of hepatosplenic T-cell lymphoma are usually moderate in size, with a rim of pale cytoplasm (Fig. 1–13). The nuclear chromatin is loosely condensed with small, inconspicuous nucleoli. The liver and spleen show marked sinusoidal infiltration, with sparing of both portal triads and white pulp, respectively. Abnormal cells are usually present in the sinusoids of the bone marrow but may be difficult to identify without immunohistochemical stains. The neoplastic cells have a phenotype that resembles that of normal resting γδ T cells. They often are negative for both CD4 and CD8, although CD8 may be expressed in some cases. They are positive for CD3 and TCRγ, but negative for βF1. CD56 often is positive.[298,300] A small percentage of cases appear to be of αβ origin.[301–303] The neoplastic cells express markers associated with cytotoxic T cells, such as TIA-1. However, perforin and granzyme B are usually negative, suggesting that these cells are not activated.[300,304] Isochromosome 7q is a consistent cytogenetic abnormality, and often is seen in association with trisomy 8.[305–307]

While hepatosplenic T-cell lymphoma is a tumor of inactive or immature γδ T cells, other forms of γδ T-cell lymphoma exist. For example, a γδ phenotype can be seen in cases of Pre-T LBL/ALL,[308] and tumors of activated γδ T cells arise in a variety of mucocutaneous sites (see next section).

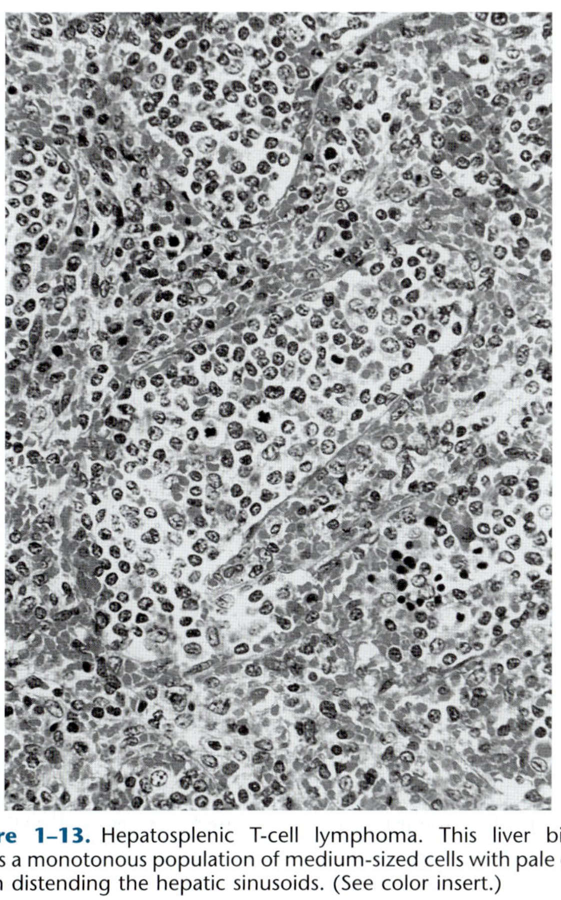

Figure 1–13. Hepatosplenic T-cell lymphoma. This liver biopsy shows a monotonous population of medium-sized cells with pale cytoplasm distending the hepatic sinusoids. (See color insert.)

Subcutaneous Panniculitis-Like T-Cell Lymphoma (SPTCL)

WF: diffuse mixed small and large cell, large cell immunoblastic, small cleaved cell
Kiel: pleomorphic medium mixed and large cell (HTLV-1 negative)
REAL: subcutaneous panniculitic T-cell lymphoma

SPTCL is sufficiently distinct to warrant separation from other forms of peripheral T-cell lymphoma.[309] The disease usually presents with subcutaneous nodules, primarily affecting the extremities and trunk. The nodules range in size from 0.5 cm to several centimeters in diameter. Larger nodules may become necrotic. In its early stages, the infiltrate may appear deceptively benign, and lesions are often misdiagnosed as panniculitis.[309,310] However, histologic progression usually occurs, and subsequent biopsies show more pronounced cytologic atypia, permitting the diagnosis of malignant lymphoma.

The cytologic composition of subcutaneous panniculitic T-cell lymphoma may vary. The lesions may contain a predominance of small to medium-sized lymphoid cells with clear cytoplasm, or larger cells with hyperchromatic nuclei (Fig. 1–14). Admixed reactive histiocytes often are present, particularly in areas of fat infiltration and destruction. The histiocytes frequently are vacuolated, due to ingested lipid material. Vascular invasion may be seen in some cases, and necrosis and karyorrhexis are common.

The neoplastic cells are CD8+ T cells, which also are positive for the cytotoxic proteins perforin, granzyme B, and TIA-1.[250] These proteins may be responsible for the cellular destruction seen in these tumors. Most cases are of αβ T-cell origin, but up to 25% of cases are of γδ T-cell origin and demonstrate more aggressive clinical behavior (see below).[250,311,312] The cells are EBV-negative, but show clonal rearrangement of T-cell receptor genes.

A hemophagocytic syndrome is a frequent complication of subcutaneous panniculitic T-cell lymphoma.[309] Patients present with fever, pancytopenia, and hepatosplenomegaly. This complication is most readily diagnosed in bone marrow aspirate smears, where histiocytes containing phagocytosed erythrocytes, platelets, and other blood elements may be observed. The hemophagocytic syndrome usually precipitates a fulminant downhill clinical course. However, if therapy for the underlying lymphoma is instituted and is successful, the hemophagocytic syndrome may remit. The cause of the hemophagocytic syndrome appears related to cytokine production by the malignant cells. Interferon gamma, granulocyte–monocyte colony-stimulating factor, and MIP-1α have been identified.[310,313] Dissemination to lymph nodes and other organs is uncommon and usually occurs late in the clinical course.

Mucocutaneous γδ T-Cell Lymphomas

The mucocutaneous γδ T-cell lymphomas previously were not identified as a distinct subtype of lymphoid neoplasm. However, recent data demonstrating their aggres-

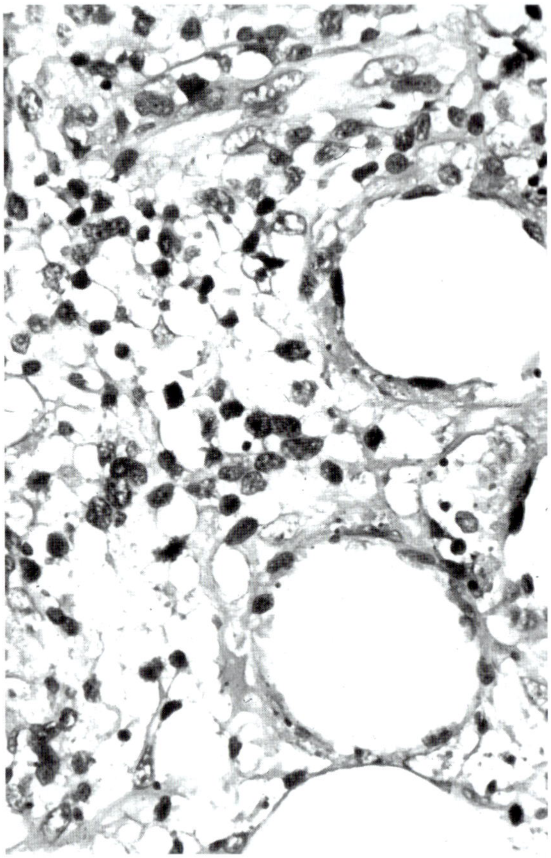

Figure 1–14. Subcutaneous panniculitis-like T-cell lymphoma. The subcutaneous adipose shows a lace-like infiltrate of neoplastic lymphoid cells and admixed histiocytes, with foci of necrosis and karyorrhexis.

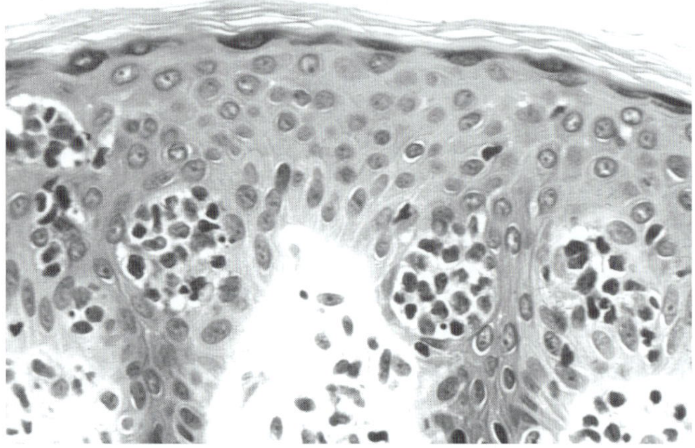

Figure 1–15. Mycosis fungoides. This skin biopsy shows neoplastic lymphocytes with convoluted nuclei forming Pautrier microabscesses within the epidermis. (See color insert.)

sive clinical course suggest that this entity merits special consideration.[312,314] Non-hepatosplenic lymphomas of γδ T-cell origin may involve the skin, nasal cavity, or mucosal surfaces of the gastrointestinal or respiratory tract.[314] Cutaneous γδ T-cell lymphomas involving the subcutaneous fat (panniculitis-like) appear to have a poorer prognosis than those with dermal involvement and/or epidermotropism.[312] Mucocutaneous γδ T-cell lymphomas frequently are double negative for CD4 and CD8, and demonstrate an activated cytotoxic T-cell phenotype with expression of perforin, TIA-1, granzyme B, and granzyme M.[248,286,314] EBV sequences have been detected in some lesions, and an association with chronic antigen exposure and/or immunodeficiency has been noted.[314] These findings suggest a relationship between these lymphomas and the proposed role of γδ T cells in epithelial immune surveillance.[314,315]

Mycosis Fungoides/Sézary Syndrome (MF/SS)

WF: mycosis fungoides
Kiel: small cell, cerebriform
REAL: mycosis fungoides/Sézary syndrome

MF/SS by definition presents with cutaneous disease. Skin involvement may be manifested as multiple cutaneous plaques or nodules, or with generalized erythroderma. Lymphadenopathy is usually not present at presentation and, when identified, is associated with a poor prognosis.[316] In early stages, enlarged lymph nodes may show only dermatopathic changes (Category I).[317] If malignant cells are present in significant numbers and are associated with architectural effacement (Category II or III), the prognosis is significantly worse.[1]

Cytologically, the small cells of MF/SS demonstrate cerebriform nuclei with clumped chromatin, inconspicuous nucleoli, and sparse cytoplasm. The larger cells may be hyperchromatic or may have more vesicular nuclei with prominent nucleoli. Nuclear pleomorphism usually is evident in the large cells, and RS-like cells may be seen, especially in advanced lesions. Epidermotropism is usually a prominent feature of the cutaneous infiltrates (Fig. 1–15). The typical immunophenotype is CD2+, CD3+, CD5+, CD4+, and CD8–. The absence of CD7 expression is a constant feature, but also may be seen in reactive conditions, and therefore is of limited diagnostic value.[318] Aberrant expression of other T-cell antigens may be observed, but mainly occurs in advanced (tumor) stages.

T-cell receptor genes are clonally rearranged in most cases. The identification of clonality is clinically useful but not entirely specific, since benign cutaneous infiltrates also may be clonal by PCR.[319] Inactivation of p16 and PTEN has been identified in some cases, and may be associated with disease progression.[320–322] Although Sézary syndrome is much more aggressive, the presence of common genetic pathways supports a close relationship between MF and SS.[323] Some studies have identified retroviral sequences related to HTLV-I, but association of the disease with a specific retroviral agent is controversial.[324]

Primary Cutaneous CD30-Positive T-Cell Lymphoproliferative Disorders

Kiel: anaplastic large cell
WF: various, including diffuse large cell, immunoblastic
REAL: primary cutaneous anaplastic large cell (CD30+) lymphoma

Lymphomatoid papulosis and primary cutaneous anaplastic large cell lymphoma (C-ALCL) are part of the spectrum of CD30-positive cutaneous lymphoproliferative diseases, which also includes a category of borderline lesions with overlapping clinicopathologic features.[325–329] C-ALCL differs clinically, immunophenotypically, and molecularly from systemic ALCL.[325–328] Small lesions are likely to regress. Patients with large tumor masses may develop disseminated disease with lymph node involvement. However, C-ALCL is a more indolent disease than other cutaneous T-cell lymphomas. Most patients with primary C-ALCL have multiple skin lesions. Because the skin nodules may show spontaneous regression, a period of observation usually is warranted before instituting chemotherapy.[330] C-ALCL is CD30+ but ALK negative, and usually is negative for EMA. It also lacks the t(2;5) translocation.[325,327]

Angioimmunoblastic T-Cell Lymphoma (AILT)

WF: diffuse mixed small and large cell, large cell immunoblastic, AILD
Kiel: angioimmunoblastic
REAL: angioimmunoblastic T-cell lymphoma

AILT initially was thought to represent an abnormal immune reaction or form of atypical lymphoid hyperplasia with a high risk of progression to malignant lymphoma.[331] Because the majority of cases show clonal rearrangements of T-cell receptor genes, it is now regarded as a variant of T-cell lymphoma.[332] The median survival generally is less than 5 years; thus, designation as a lymphoma also is warranted on clinical grounds.[333]

The nodal architecture generally is effaced, but peripheral sinuses often are open and even dilated. The abnormal infiltrate usually extends beyond the capsule into the surrounding tissue. Hyperplastic germinal centers are absent. However, there may be regressed follicles containing a proliferation of dendritic cells and blood vessels. At low power there usually is a striking proliferation of post-capillary venules with prominent arborization, and the cellularity of the lymph node often appears reduced or depleted. Clusters of lymphoid cells with clear cytoplasm may be seen. The neoplastic cells are admixed with a polymorphous cellular background containing small, normal-appearing lymphocytes, basophilic immunoblasts, plasma cells, and histiocytes, with or without eosinophils (Fig. 1–16). The abnormal cells usually are CD4+ T cells that show expression of CD10 and sometimes Bcl-6.[334] A helpful diagnostic feature is the presence of numerous CD21+ dendritic reticulum cells, which are especially prominent around post-capillary venules.[335] EBV-positive large B-cell blasts are nearly always present in the background.[336,337] The EBV-positive cells may have an RS-like appearance, simulating Hodgkin's lymphoma.[338]

AILT presents in adults. Most patients have generalized lymphadenopathy and prominent systemic symptoms with fever, weight loss, and skin rash. There usually is a polyclonal hypergammaglobulinemia.

Peripheral T-Cell Lymphoma, Unspecified (PTCL)

WF: diffuse small cleaved, diffuse mixed small and large cell, large cell immunoblastic

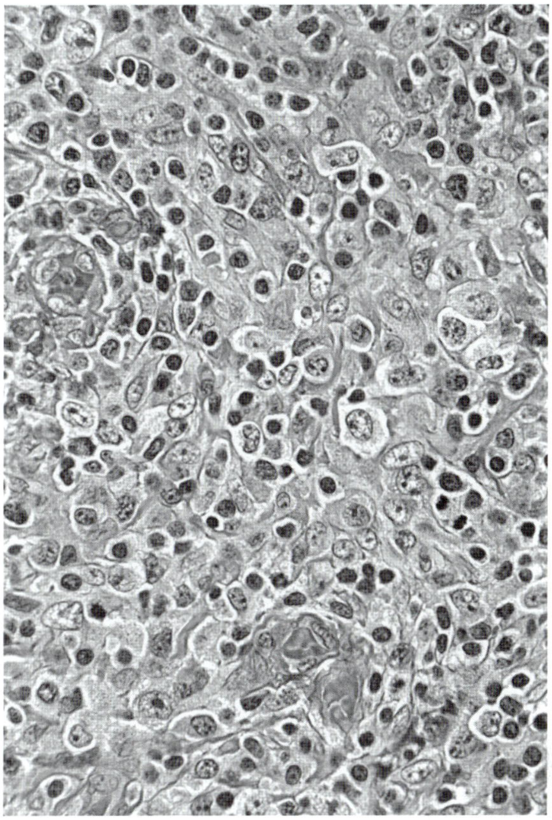

Figure 1–16. Angioimmunoblastic T-cell lymphoma. There is an infiltrate of atypical lymphoid cells with pale cytoplasm in a mixed inflammatory background, and prominent post-capillary venules with plump endothelial cells. (See color insert.)

Kiel: T-zone lymphoma; lymphoepithelioid cell lymphoma; pleomorphic small, medium, and large cell (HTLV-1 negative); immunoblastic (HTLV-1 negative)
REAL: peripheral T-cell lymphoma, unspecified (provisional cytologic categories: large cell, medium-sized cell, mixed large/medium-sized cell)

PTCL is a diagnosis of exclusion and admittedly is a heterogeneous category. Most cases are nodal in origin and characterized by a heterogeneous cellular composition. There is usually a mixture of small and large atypical lymphoid cells, frequently in an inflammatory background consisting of eosinophils, plasma cells, and histiocytes (Fig. 1–17). If epithelioid histiocytes are numerous and clustered, the neoplasm fulfills the criteria for the lymphoepithelioid cell variant of PTCL (Lennert lymphoma).[339,340] The T-zone variant is composed of small to medium-sized cells that preferentially involve the paracortical regions of the lymph node.[341,342]

Clinically, PTCL most often presents in adults. Most patients exhibit generalized lymphadenopathy, hepatosplenomegaly, and frequently bone marrow involvement. Constitutional symptoms, including fever and night sweats, are common, as is pruritus. The clinical course is aggressive, although complete remissions may be obtained with combination chemotherapy.[343–345] However, the relapse rate is higher for PTCL than for aggressive B-cell lymphomas, including DLBCL.[343]

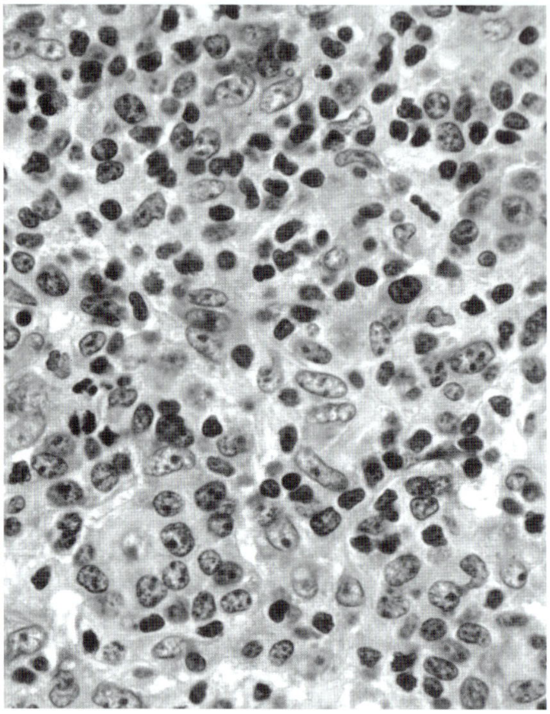

Figure 1–17. Peripheral T-cell lymphoma, unspecified. This case shows a range of small to medium-sized atypical lymphocytes with irregular nuclear outlines in a background of mixed inflammatory cells.

PCTL, as defined in the WHO classification, remains heterogeneous. It is likely that individual clinicopathologic entities will be delineated in the future from this broad group of malignancies. Thus far, immunophenotypic criteria have not been helpful in delineating subtypes. Most cases have a mature T-cell phenotype, and express one of the major subset antigens (CD4 more commonly than CD8). These are not clonal markers, and antigen expression can change over time. Loss of one of the pan-T-cell antigens (CD2, CD3, CD5, or CD7) is seen in 75% of cases, with CD7 most frequently being absent.[346]

Systemic Anaplastic Large Cell Lymphoma (ALCL)

WF: large cell, large cell immunoblastic
Kiel: ALCL (Ki-1+ T cell)
REAL: anaplastic large cell lymphoma

ALCL is characterized by pleomorphic or monomorphic cells that have a propensity to invade lymphoid sinuses.[347] A constant feature is the presence of cells with lobulated and indented nuclei, so-called "hallmark" cells (Fig. 1–18A).[348,349] Nucleoli are present but tend not to be prominent and frequently are basophilic. In some cases the nuclei may be round. The cytoplasm usually is abundant and amphophilic, and there are distinct cytoplasmic borders. A prominent Golgi region usually is apparent. Because of the sinusoidal location of the tumor cells, and their lobulated nuclear appearance, this disease previously was interpreted as a variant of malignant histiocytosis. Misdiagnosis as metastatic carcinoma or melanoma also is common.

Recently, histologic variants of ALCL have been described. In the lymphohistiocytic variant, there is an admixture of histiocytes, which may lead to misdiagnosis as an inflammatory condition.[350] In the small-cell variant, the cells are small to medium in size with abundant cytoplasm.[351] Hallmark cells are always present, although often localized around blood vessels.[349]

A consistent feature of ALCL is the expression of the CD30 antigen, which is a hallmark of this disease (Fig. 1–18B).[352] The older terminology of Ki-1+ lymphoma is not favored because CD30 expression is not specific for ALCL and also is seen in other conditions, including classic Hodgkin's lymphoma (Table 1–4).[353,354] The neoplastic cells of ALCL exhibit an aberrant immunophenotype, with loss of many of the T-cell–associated antigens. Both CD3 and CD5 are negative in more than 50% of cases. CD2 and CD4 often are positive. CD8 usually is negative. ALCL cells, despite the CD4+/CD8– phenotype, exhibit positivity for the cytotoxic associated antigens TIA-1, granzyme B, and perforin.[355] The prominent Golgi region usually shows intense staining for CD30 and EMA.[356] In most cases, molecular studies demonstrate clonal T-cell receptor gene rearrangement, confirming a T-cell origin.

Systemic ALCL is associated with a characteristic chromosomal translocation, t(2;5)(p23;q35), involving the ALK (2p23) and NPM (5q35) genes.[357] A number of variant translocations have been identified that involve partners other than NPM. All lead to an overexpression of ALK protein, although the cellular distribution of ALK varies according to the gene partner (Fig. 1–18C).[358,359]

ALCL is most common in children and young adults. A bimodal age distribution has been reported; however, the t(2;5) and ALK protein expression are lacking in most elderly patients, suggesting that these cases may be part of a different clinicopathologic entity.[360] ALCL shows a

Table 1–4. Differential Diagnosis of Systemic Anaplastic Large Cell Lymphoma

Disease	CD30	CD15	LCA	CD3	TIA-1	EMA	Clu	ALK	CD20
ALCL	+	–	+	–/+	+	+	+	+	–
CHL	+	+	–	–	–	–	–	–	–/+
NLPHL	–	–	+	–	–	+/–	–	–	+
PTCL	–/+	–	+	+	–/+	–	–	–	–
DLBCL	–/+	–	+	–	–	+/–	–	–	+

ALCL, anaplastic large cell lymphoma; CHL, classic Hodgkin's lymphoma; NLPHL, nodular lymphocyte predominant HL; PTCL, peripheral T-cell lymphoma, unspecified; DLBCL, diffuse large B-cell lymphoma (includes T-cell/histiocyte-rich large B-cell lymphoma).

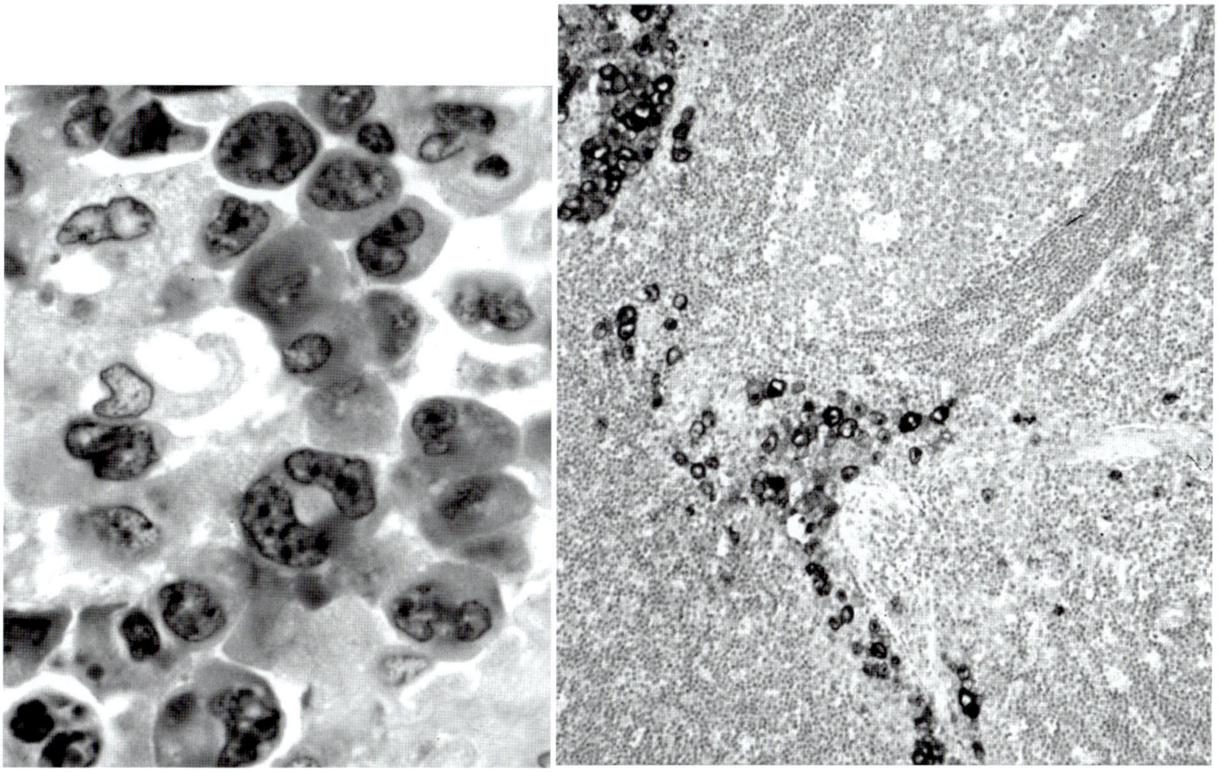

A B

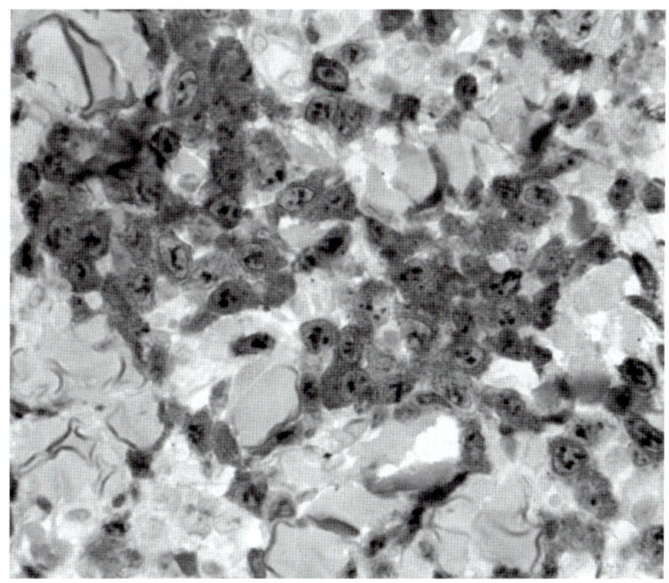

C

Figure 1–18. Systemic anaplastic large cell lymphoma (ALCL). **A:** Large "hallmark" cells are pleomorphic, with eccentric kidney-shaped nuclei. **B:** The malignant cells are strongly positive for CD30 by immunohistochemistry. (See color insert.) **C:** This case contained the *NPM/ALK* translocation, leading to both nuclear and cytoplasmic ALK protein immunoreactivity.

marked male predominance. Patients usually present with nodal disease, often with involvement of extranodal sites as well, including skin, bone, and soft tissue. About 75% of cases present with advanced stage and systemic symptoms.[361] Although these lymphomas have an aggressive natural clinical history, they respond well to chemotherapy; overall survival and disease-free survival are significantly better among ALK+ cases than among ALK- cases.[361,362] Recent studies suggest that the International Prognostic Index (IPI) is prognostically useful, in contrast with early reports.[361,362] Whether ALK-negative ALCL should be considered a separate disease remains controversial, but at present the WHO classification recommends that if ALK is negative, this finding should be designated in the diagnostic report.[348]

HODGKIN'S LYMPHOMA

The modern classification of Hodgkin's lymphoma (HL) is based on the Lukes–Butler classification scheme.[363] The original Lukes–Butler scheme contained six histologic subtypes (Table 1–5), which were reduced to four at the Rye

Table 1–5. Classification of Hodgkin's Lymphoma (HL)

Lukes–Butler	Rye Modification	ILSG Scheme	WHO Classification
Lymphocytic and/or histiocytic	Lymphocytic predominance	Lymphocyte predominance, nodular +/– diffuse	Nodular lymphocyte predominant HL
Nodular diffuse		Lymphocyte rich, classic HL	Lymphocyte-rich classic HL
Nodular sclerosis	Nodular sclerosis	Nodular sclerosis	Nodular sclerosis
Mixed cellularity	Mixed cellularity	Mixed cellularity	Mixed cellularity
Diffuse fibrosis	Lymphocytic depletion	Lymphocytic depletion	Lymphocyte depleted
Reticular			

Conference.[364] It should be noted that in the WHO classification the term *Hodgkin's lymphoma* is favored over *Hodgkin's disease*, since the Reed–Sternberg (RS) cell now is known to be of lymphoid origin. The WHO classification subclassifies HL into two disease entities based on recent clinical and biologic data. These two subtypes, *nodular lymphocyte predominant Hodgkin's lymphoma (NLPHL)* and *classic Hodgkin's lymphoma (CHL)*, are distinct in their clinical presentation, behavior, morphology, immunophenotype, and molecular characteristics. NLPHL and CHL share the somewhat unique feature among the malignant lymphomas that RS cells and variants, the malignant cells, constitute the minority of cells present in the tumor mass. These are associated with a rich inflammatory background containing lymphocytes, eosinophils, neutrophils, histiocytes, and plasma cells in varying proportions.

Nodular Lymphocyte Predominant Hodgkin's Lymphoma (NLPHL)

Lukes–Butler: lymphocytic and/or histiocytic (L&H) predominance
REAL: nodular lymphocyte predominance

This subtype of HL has undergone significant reappraisal in recent years. As currently defined, NLPHL represents approximately 5% of all cases of HL. It is more common in males than females, and presents in young adults with a median peak incidence in the 4th and 5th decades. Patients typically present with localized peripheral lymphadenopathy (Stage I or II), generally involving axillary, cervical, or inguinal lymph nodes. In contrast to other forms of HL, mediastinal lymphadenopathy is rare.

NLPHL typically has a nodular, or nodular and diffuse, growth pattern. A predominantly diffuse pattern is uncommon. Classic RS cells are not seen or are exceedingly rare. The neoplastic cells are referred to as L&H cells or "popcorn" cells (Fig. 1–19A). These have a lobulated nuclear contour, dispersed chromatin, and inconspicuous nucleoli. They generally cluster within nodules in association with lymphocytes and histiocytes. L&H cells typically are positive for CD20, CD79a, Bcl-6, and CD45; they generally are negative for CD15 and negative or weakly positive for CD30. EMA is positive in about half of cases. PU.1, Oct-2, and BOB.1 are expressed, unlike CHL.[365,366] The nodules characteristically show expanded meshworks of CD21+ follicular dendritic cells with numerous small B cells and CD57+ T cells. T cells are more numerous in the diffuse areas, and tend to increase over time in the nodular areas as well.[367]

NLPHL has a very indolent clinical course but a paradoxically high relapse rate. However, relapses are not necessarily associated with clinical progression, and survival remains excellent, even in patients with recurrent disease. Progression to a large-cell lymphoma of B-cell phenotype occurs in a small proportion of cases.[368] These large-cell lymphomas occasionally disseminate and pursue an aggressive clinical course. The differential diagnosis between NLPHL and T-cell/histiocyte–rich DLBCL can be difficult, although differences in the non-neoplastic background cells and expression of PU.1 by NLPHL can help in this distinction.[366,369] Nevertheless, both diseases can occur as composite lymphomas or sequentially in the same patient, and current data suggest a biologic relationship between them.[180,369,370]

Classic Hodgkin's Lymphoma (CHL)

CHL comprises 95% of all cases of HL and demonstrates a bimodal age distribution, with a first peak at age 15 to 35 and a second peak later in life. In 75% of cases, it involves the cervical lymph nodes, followed by nodes in the mediastinal, axillary, and para-aortic regions. Splenic involvement occurs in approximately 20% of cases, and the bone marrow is involved in around 5%; however, primary extranodal involvement is rare. The RS cells and variants are nearly always positive for CD30, and usually positive for CD15. CD20 may be expressed on a minority of RS cells. EMA expression is rare. In contrast to the L&H cells of NLPHL, the RS cells of CHL typically lack expression of PU.1, Oct-2, and BOB.1, which are critical in immunoglobulin transcription.[365,366,371,372] Despite defective Ig transcription, RS cells demonstrate clonal Ig gene rearrangement in nearly all cases, and recent analyses of somatic mutations in *VH* genes have suggested that the RS cell of CHL is of germinal center origin.[372,373]

Nodular Sclerosis Hodgkin's Lymphoma (NSHL)

NSHL is the most common subtype of HL, accounting for approximately 75% of cases in the United States.[363] This is the only subtype without a male predominance (male : female ratio approximately 1 : 1). It tends to occur in young adults, usually under age 50 years. Anterior mediastinal involvement is exceedingly common, with subsequent involvement of cervical and supraclavicular lymph nodes, upper abdominal lymph nodes, and spleen. Most patients present with Stage II disease. Bulky mediastinal

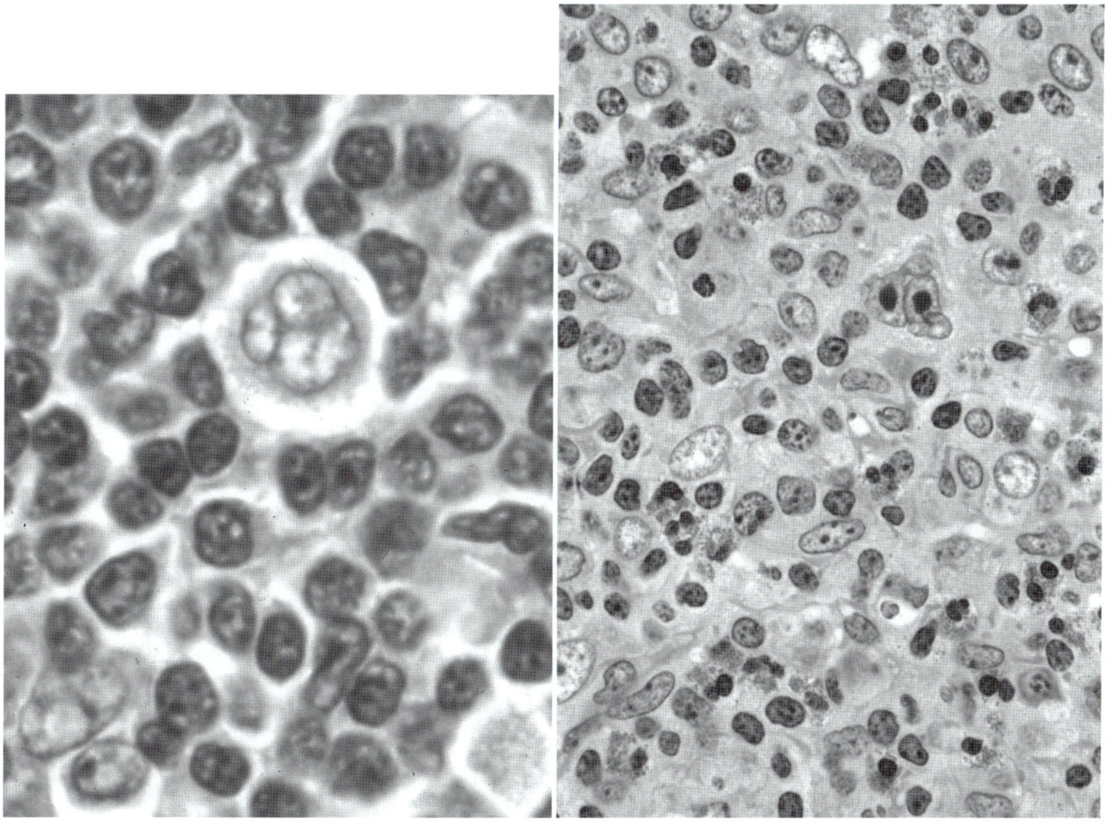

A B

Figure 1–19. Hodgkin's lymphoma. **A:** Nodular lymphocyte predominant Hodgkin's lymphoma, showing a "popcorn" or lymphocytic and/or histiocytic cell with its lobated nucleus in a background of small lymphocytes and an occasional histiocyte. **B:** Mixed-cellularity Hodgkin's lymphoma, showing classic Reed–Sternberg cells admixed with lymphocytes, plasma cells, and eosinophils. (See color insert.)

masses may occur and are a poor prognostic sign. The disease also may extend directly into the adjacent lung.

The diagnosis of NSHL requires the presence of (1) a nodular growth pattern, (2) broad bands of fibrosis, and (3) a characteristic variant of the RS cell known as the lacunar cell. The lacunar cell has abundant clear cytoplasm with a sharply demarcated cell membrane. In formalin-fixed tissue a characteristic artifact often occurs; the cytoplasm of the cell retracts, leaving a clear space or lacunus. The lacunar cell may be mononuclear, hyperlobated, or multinucleated. The nucleoli of lacunar cells generally are smaller than those seen in classic RS cells. In the cellular phase of NSHL, tissue sections show a nodular growth pattern with lacunar cells, but with absent or minimal fibrous bands. This finding represents a phase in the development of NSHL and is not associated with unique clinical features. A syncytial variant of NSHL has been described, in which prominent aggregates of lacunar cells are seen, often with frequent eosinophils.

The BNLI has developed a grading system for NSHL, based on the frequency of malignant cells. In Grade 1 lesions, at least 75% of the nodules contain scattered RS cells, whereas in Grade 2 lesions, at least 25% of the nodules contain numerous malignant cells which sheet out, often surrounding areas of necrosis.[374,375] BNLI Grade 2 lesions, corresponding to the previous designation of lymphocyte-depleted NSHL, are associated with a more aggressive clinical course.

Mixed Cellularity Hodgkin's Lymphoma (MCHL)

MCHL, although originally considered a diagnosis of exclusion in the Lukes–Butler scheme, is considered a defined subtype of CHL in the WHO classification. RS cells are of the classic type with prominent inclusion-like nucleoli. Lacunar cells are inconspicuous, and nodular fibrosing sclerosis is absent. MCHL usually is associated with diffuse architectural effacement, but many cases show an interfollicular pattern of involvement, with residual hyperplastic follicles. MCHL contains a rich inflammatory background with numerous eosinophils, plasma cells, and histiocytes (Fig. 1–19B).

MCHL is more common in males than females.[364] It frequently is associated with disseminated disease at presentation,[376] and B symptoms are common.[377] It is one of the variants of Hodgkin's lymphoma, along with lymphocyte-depleted HL (see next section), that are seen in association with HIV infection. MCHL is the subtype of HL most often positive for EBV sequences.[378,379]

Lymphocyte-Rich Classic Hodgkin's Lymphoma (LRCHL)

LRCHL is characterized by a background of abundant small lymphocytes. Eosinophils and neutrophils are rare or absent. The tumor contains infrequent RS cells, but the RS cells have the classic morphology and immunophenotype. They occasionally may resemble L&H or lacunar cells. The most common growth pattern is nodular, though a diffuse pattern rarely may be seen.[367,380] Immunostaining shows the nodules to contain predominantly small CD20+ B cells. CD21 staining highlights follicular dendritic cell meshworks within expanded mantle zones. Regressed germinal centers also may be present, although the RS cells typically are located at the periphery of the mantles rather than in the germinal centers.

LRCHL is more common in males and presents at a somewhat higher median age than other subtypes of HL. Most patients present with Stage I or II disease, and B symptoms are rare. Survival appears slightly better compared to that of patients with other types of CHL.[367,381]

Lymphocyte-Depleted Hodgkin's Lymphoma (LDHL)

LDHL is the most uncommon subtype of HL, accounting for less than 5% of cases.[374] It is more common in males than females. Most patients present with advanced-stage disease and B symptoms. Historically, many cases of high-grade non-Hodgkin's lymphoma were misdiagnosed as LDHL.[374] With improvements in diagnostic criteria, including immunohistochemical techniques, LDHL is diagnosed with much less frequency. Although it still is considered an aggressive form of HL, complete remissions can be obtained. The exceedingly poor prognosis historically associated with LDHL was most likely the result of the misdiagnosis of aggressive non-Hodgkin's lymphomas as HL.

LDHL has variable morphology, but consistently shows a relative predominance of RS cells and variants, with depletion of non-neoplastic lymphocytes. In some cases, the presence of pleomorphic RS cells produces a sarcomatous appearance. The immunophenotype of the RS cells is the same as in other subtypes of CHL. EBV infection often can be demonstrated when LDHD occurs in HIV+ patients.[382]

Second Hematologic Malignancies Following Hodgkin's Lymphoma

Among the second malignancies following treatment for HL, acute non-lymphocytic leukemias and non-Hodgkin's lymphomas are the most common.[383] Acute leukemias occur usually 2 to 5 years after initial therapy but can be seen as late as 12 years. Patients receiving both radiation and chemotherapy are at increased risk. NHL occurs later, most often 10 or more years after the diagnosis of HL. The risk is relatively small (<2% of cases of CHL).[384] In most cases, the NHL is a DLBCL or Burkitt-like lymphoma, often presenting as an abdominal mass with involvement of the gastrointestinal tract. Rare cases of T-cell lymphoma have been described.[384] It has been postulated that these tumors might be secondary to the immunodeficiency of HL, possibly aggravated by additional immunosuppressive therapy.[206] Although a role for EBV has been proposed, less than 20% of these tumors are EBV-positive.[385]

Large B-cell lymphomas also occur in patients with NLPHL. In large series, this phenomenon occurs in less than 5% of cases.[368] These tumors may represent clonal progression of the original malignancy, since composite NLPHL/large-cell lymphomas are observed with some frequency.[386] In both tumors the cells express a B-cell phenotype, and a clonal relationship has been demonstrated in a small number of cases.[387,388] Large-cell lymphomas in patients with NLPHL often do not pursue an aggressive clinical course, especially if detected simultaneously with NLPHL.[368,386]

References

1. Jaffe ES, Harris NL, Stein H, et al. Pathology and Genetics of Tumours of Haematopoietic and Lymphoid Tissues. Lyon, France: IARC Press. 2001.
2. Rappaport H, Winter W, and Hicks E. Follicular lymphoma. A re-evaluation of its position in the scheme of malignant lymphoma, based on a survey of 253 cases. Cancer 1956;9:792–821.
3. Rappaport H. Tumors of the Hematopoietic System. Atlas of Tumor Pathology. Series I edition. Washington, DC: Armed Forces Institute of Pathology, 1966.
4. Lennert K, Mohri N, Stein H, et al. The histopathology of malignant lymphoma. Br J Haematol 1975;31(suppl): 193–203.
5. Lukes R and Collins R. Immunologic characterization of human malignant lymphomas. Cancer 1974;34:1488–1503.
6. Bennett MH, Farrer–Brown G, Henry K, et al. Classification of non-Hodgkin's lymphomas. Lancet 1974;2:405–6.
7. Bennett MH, Farrer–Brown G, Henry K, et al. Non-Hodgkin's lymphoma pathologic classification project. National Cancer Institute–sponsored study of classifications of non-Hodgkin's lymphomas: summary and description of a working formulation for clinical usage. Cancer 1982;49:2112–35.
8. Harris NL, Jaffe ES, Stein H, et al. A revised European–American classification of lymphoid neoplasms: a proposal from the International Lymphoma Study Group. Blood 1994;84:1361–92.
9. Harris NL, Jaffe ES, Stein H, et al. The Non-Hodgkin's Lymphoma Classification Project: a clinical evaluation of the International Lymphoma Study Group classification of non-Hodgkin's lymphoma. Blood 1997;89:3909–18.
10. Gisselbrecht C, Gaulard P, Lepage E, et al. Prognostic significance of T-cell phenotype in aggressive non-Hodgkin's lymphomas. Groupe d'Etudes des Lymphomes de l'Adulte (GELA). Blood 1998;92:76–82.
11. Shipp MA. Prognostic factors in aggressive non-Hodgkin's lymphoma: who has "high risk" disease? Blood 1994;83: 1165–73.
12. Harris NL, Jaffe ES, Diebold J, et al. World Health Organization classification of neoplastic diseases of the hematopoietic and lymphoid tissues: report of the Clinical Advisory Committee meeting, Airlie House, Virginia, November 1997. J Clin Oncol 1999;17:3835–49.
13. Jaffe ES, Zarate OA, and Medeiros LJ. The interrelationship of Hodgkin's disease and non-Hodgkin's lymphomas—lessons learned from composite and sequential malignancies. Semin Diagn Pathol 1992;9:297–303.
14. Alizadeh AA, Eisen MB, Davis RE, et al. Distinct types of diffuse large B-cell lymphoma identified by gene expression profiling. Nature 2000;403:503–11.
15. Rosenwald A and Staudt LM. Clinical translation of gene expression profiling in lymphomas and leukemias. Semin Oncol 2002;29:258–63.
16. Braziel RM, Shipp MA, Feldman AL, et al. Molecular diagnostics. Hematology (Am Soc Hematol Educ Program). 2003;279–93.
17. Sander CA, Medeiros LJ, Abruzzo LV, et al. Lymphoblastic lymphoma presenting in cutaneous sites. A clinicopathologic analysis of six cases. J Am Acad Dermatol 1991;25:1023–31.

18. Borowitz M, Croker B, and Metzgar R. Lymphoblastic lymphoma with the phenotype of common acute lymphoblastic leukemia. Am J Clin Pathol 1983;79:387–91.
19. Lin P, Jones D, Dorfman DM, et al. Precursor B-cell lymphoblastic lymphoma: a predominantly extranodal tumor with low propensity for leukemic involvement. Am J Surg Pathol 2000;24:1480–90.
20. Nathwani B, Diamond L, Winberg C, et al. Lymphoblastic lymphoma: a clinicopathologic study of 95 patients. Cancer 1981;48:2347–57.
21. Lardelli P, Bookman MA, Sundeen J, et al. Lymphocytic lymphoma of intermediate differentiation. Morphologic and immunophenotypic spectrum and clinical correlations. Am J Surg Pathol 1990;14:752–63.
22. Buccheri V, Mihaljevic B, Matutes E, et al. mb-1: a new marker for B-lineage lymphoblastic leukemia. Blood 1993; 82:853–7.
23. Korsmeyer S, Arnold A, Bakhshi A, et al. Immunoglobulin gene rearrangement and cell surface antigen expression in acute lymphocytic leukemias of T-cell and B-cell precursor origins. J Clin Invest 1983;71:301–13.
24. Torlakovic E, Torlakovic G, Nguyen PL, et al. The value of anti-pax–5 immunostaining in routinely fixed and paraffin-embedded sections: a novel pan pre-B and B-cell marker. Am J Surg Pathol 2002;26:1343–50.
25. Nishii K, Kita K, Miwa H, et al. Expression of B cell–associated transcription factors in B-cell precursor acute lymphoblastic leukemia cells: association with PU.1 expression, phenotype, and immunogenotype. Int J Hematol 2000;71:372–8.
26. Saez AI, Artiga MJ, Sanchez-Beato M, et al. Analysis of octamer-binding transcription factors Oct2 and Oct1 and their coactivator BOB.1/OBF.1 in lymphomas. Mod Pathol 2002;15:211–20.
27. Ozdemirli M, Fanburg-Smith JC, Hartmann DP, et al. Precursor B-Lymphoblastic lymphoma presenting as a solitary bone tumor and mimicking Ewing's sarcoma: a report of four cases and review of the literature. Am J Surg Pathol 1998;22:795–804.
28. Ross ME, Zhou X, Song G, et al. Classification of pediatric acute lymphoblastic leukemia by gene expression profiling. Blood 2003;102:2951–9.
29. Pangalis G, Nathwani B, and Rappaport H. Malignant lymphoma, well differentiated lymphocytic: its relationship with chronic lymphocytic leukemia and macroglobulinemia of Waldenstrom. Cancer 1977;39:999–1010.
30. Dick F and Maca R. The lymph node in chronic lymphocytic leukemia. Cancer 1978;41:283–92.
31. Pombo de Oliveira MS, Jaffe ES, and Catovsky D. Leukemic phase of mantle zone (intermediate) lymphoma: its characterization in 11 cases. J Clin Pathol 1989;42:962–72.
32. Perry D, Bast M, Armitage J, et al. Diffuse intermediate lymphocytic lymphoma: a clinicopathologic study and comparison with small lymphocytic lymphoma and diffuse small cleaved cell lymphoma. Cancer 1990;66:1995– 2000.
33. Zukerberg L, Medeiros L, Ferry J, et al. Diffuse low-grade B-cell lymphomas: four clinically distinct subtypes defined by a combination of morphologic and immunophenotypic features. Am J Clin Pathol 1993;100:373–85.
34. Kumar S, Green GA, Teruya-Feldstein J, et al. Use of CD23 (BU38) on paraffin sections in the diagnosis of small lymphocytic lymphoma and mantle cell lymphoma. Mod Pathol 1996;9:925–929.
35. Campo E, Raffeld M, and Jaffe ES. Mantle-cell lymphoma. Semin Hematol 1999;36:115–27.
36. Hamblin TJ, Davis Z, Gardiner A, et al. Unmutated Ig V(H) genes are associated with a more aggressive form of chronic lymphocytic leukemia. Blood 1999;94:1848–54.
37. Bahler DW, Aguilera NS, Chen CC, et al. Histological and immunoglobulin VH gene analysis of interfollicular small lymphocytic lymphoma provides evidence for two types. Am J Pathol 2000;157:1063–70.
38. Oscier DG, Thompsett A, Zhu D, et al. Differential rates of somatic hypermutation in V(H) genes among subsets of chronic lymphocytic leukemia defined by chromosomal abnormalities. Blood 1997;89:4153–60.
39. Wiestner A, Rosenwald A, Barry TS, et al. ZAP-70 expression identifies a chronic lymphocytic leukemia subtype with unmutated immunoglobulin genes, inferior clinical outcome, and distinct gene expression profile. Blood 2003;101:4944–51.
40. Crespo M, Bosch F, Villamor N, et al. ZAP-70 expression as a surrogate for immunoglobulin-variable-region mutations in chronic lymphocytic leukemia. N Engl J Med 2003;348: 1764–75.
41. Orchard JA, Ibbotson RE, Davis Z, et al. ZAP-70 expression and prognosis in chronic lymphocytic leukaemia. Lancet 2004;363:105–11.
42. Krober A, Seiler T, Benner A, et al. V(H) mutation status, CD38 expression level, genomic aberrations, and sur-vival in chronic lymphocytic leukemia. Blood 2002;100:1410–16.
43. Damle RN, Wasil T, Fais F, et al. Ig V gene mutation status and CD38 expression as novel prognostic indicators in chronic lymphocytic leukemia. Blood 1999;94:1840–7.
44. Matutes E, Oscier D, Garcia-Marco J, et al. Trisomy 12 defines a group of CLL with atypical morphology: correlation between cytogenetic, clinical and laboratory features in 544 patients. Br J Haematol 1996;92:382–8.
45. Richter M. Generalized reticular cell sarcoma of lymph nodes associated with lymphocytic leukemia. Am J Pathol 1928;4:285–92.
46. Williams J, Schned A, Cotelingam JD, et al. Chronic lymphocytic leukemia with coexistent Hodgkin's disease: implications for the origin of the Reed–Sternberg cell. Am J Surg Pathol 1991;15:33–42.
47. Brecher M and Banks P. Hodgkin's disease variant of Richter's syndrome: report of eight cases. Am J Clin Pathol 1990;93: 333–9.
48. Momose H, Jaffe ES, Shin SS, et al. Chronic lymphocytic leukemia/small lymphocytic lymphoma with Reed–Sternberg-like cells and possible transformation to Hodgkin's disease. Mediation by Epstein–Barr virus. Am J Surg Pathol 1992;16:859–67.
49. Ben-Ezra J, Burke J, Swartz W, et al. Small lymphocytic lymphoma: a clinicopathologic analysis of 268 cases. Blood 1989;73:579–87.
50. Lennert K, Tamm I, and Wacker H-H. Histopathology and immunocytochemistry of lymph node biopsies in chronic lymphocytic leukemia and immunocytoma. Leuk Lymphoma 1991;7(Suppl):157–60.
51. Hall PA, D'Ardenne AJ, Richards MA, et al. Lymphoplasmacytoid lymphoma: an immunohistological study. J Pathol 1987;153:213–23.
52. Lennert K and Feller A. Histopathology of Non-Hodgkin's Lymphomas, 2nd edition. 1992; New York: Springer-Verlag.
53. Stein H, Lennert K, Feller A, et al. Immunohistological analysis of human lymphoma: correlation of histological and immunological categories. Adv Cancer Res 1984;42:67–147.
54. Harris N and Bhan A. B-cell neoplasms of the lymphocytic, lymphoplasmacytoid, and plasma cell types: immunohistologic analysis and clinical correlation. Hum Pathol 1985;16: 829–37.
55. Andriko JA, Swerdlow SH, Aguilera NI, et al. Is lymphoplasmacytic lymphoma/immunocytoma a distinct entity?: a clinicopathologic study of 20 cases. Am J Surg Pathol 2001;25:742–51.

56. Sundeen J, Longo D, and Jaffe E. CD5 expression in B-cell small lymphocytic malignancies: correlations with clinical presentation and sites of disease. Am J Surg Pathol 1992; 16:130–7.
57. Aoki H, Takishita M, Kosaka M, et al. Frequent somatic mutations in D and/or JH segments of Ig gene in Waldenstrom's macroglobulinemia and chronic lymphocytic leukemia (CLL) with Richter's syndrome but not in common CLL. Blood 1995;85:1913–9.
58. Iida S, Rao PH, Nallasivam P, et al. The t(9;14)(p13;q32) chromosomal translocation associated with lymphoplasmacytoid lymphoma involves the PAX-5 gene. Blood 1996;88: 4110–7.
59. Iida S, Rao PH, Ueda R, et al. Chromosomal rearrangement of the PAX-5 locus in lymphoplasmacytic lymphoma with t(9;14)(p13;q32). Leuk Lymphoma 1999;34:25–33.
60. Thieblemont C, Felman P, Callet-Bauchu E, et al. Splenic marginal-zone lymphoma: a distinct clinical and pathological entity. Lancet Oncol 2003;4:95–103.
61. Melo J, Hegde U, Parreira A, et al. Splenic B cell lymphoma with circulating villous lymphocytes: differential diagnosis of B cell leukaemias with large spleens. J Clin Pathol 1987;40:642–51.
62. Isaacson PG, Matutes E, Burke M, et al. The histopathology of splenic lymphoma with villous lymphocytes. Blood 1994;84:3828–34.
63. Thieblemont C, Felman P, Berger F, et al. Treatment of splenic marginal zone B-cell lymphoma: an analysis of 81 patients. Clin Lymphoma 2002;3:41–7.
64. Hollema H, Visser L, and Poppema S. Small lymphocytic lymphomas with predominant splenomegaly: a comparison of immunophenotypes with cases of predominant lymphadenopathy. Mod Pathol 1991;4:712–7.
65. Mollejo M, Menarguez J, Lloret E, et al. Splenic marginal zone lymphoma: a distinctive type of low-grade B-cell lymphoma. A clinicopathological study of 13 cases. Am J Surg Pathol 1995;19:1146–57.
66. Neiman RS, Sullivan AL, and Jaffe R. Malignant lymphoma simulating leukemic reticuloendotheliosis: a clinicopathologic study of ten cases. Cancer 1979;43:329–42.
67. Pittaluga S, Verhoef G, Criel A, et al. "Small" B-cell non-Hodgkin's lymphomas with splenomegaly at presentation are either mantle cell lymphoma or marginal zone cell lymphoma. A study based on histology, cytology, immunohistochemistry, and cytogenetic analysis. Am J Surg Pathol 1996;20:211–23.
68. Schmid C, Kirkham N, Diss T, et al. Splenic marginal zone cell lymphoma. Am J Surg Pathol 1992;16:455–66.
69. Camacho FI, Mollejo M, Mateo MS, et al. Progression to large B-cell lymphoma in splenic marginal zone lymphoma: a description of a series of 12 cases. Am J Surg Pathol 2001;25:1268–76.
70. Mateo M, Mollejo M, Villuendas R, et al. 7q31-32 allelic loss is a frequent finding in splenic marginal zone lymphoma. Am J Pathol 1999;154:1583–89.
71. Boonstra R, Bosga-Bouwer A, van Imhoff GW, et al. Splenic marginal zone lymphomas presenting with splenomegaly and typical immunophenotype are characterized by allelic loss in 7q31-32. Mod Pathol 2003;16:1210–17.
72. Callihan TT, Holbert JM, and Berard CW. (1983) Neoplasms of terminal B-cell differentiation: the morphologic basis of functional diversity. In: Malignant Lymphomas: A Pathology Annual Monograph. (eds. S. Sommers and P.P. Rosen), pp. 169–268. Appleton-Century Crofts, Norwalk, CT.
73. Falini B, De Solas I, Levine A, et al. Emergence of B-immunoblastic sarcoma in patient with multiple myeloma: a clinicopathologic study of 10 cases. Blood 1982;59: 923–33.
74. Zukerberg L, Ferry J, Conlon M, et al. Plasma cell myeloma with cleaved, multilobated, and monocytoid nuclei. Am J Clin Pathol 1990;93:657–61.
75. Colomo L, Loong F, Rives S, et al. Diffuse large B-cell lymphomas with plasmablastic differentiation represent a heterogeneous group of disease entities. Am J Surg Pathol 2004;28(6):736–47.
76. Kronland R, Grogan T, Spier C, et al. Immunotopographic assessment of lymphoid and plasma cell malignancies in the bone marrow. Hum Pathol 1985;16:1247–54.
77. Ridley RC, Xiao H, Hata H, et al. Expression of syndecan regulates human myeloma plasma cell adhesion to type I collagen. Blood 1993;81:767–74.
78. Mason DY, Cordell JL, Brown MH, et al. CD79a: a novel marker for B-cell neoplasms in routinely processed tissue samples. Blood 1995;86:1453–9.
79. Durie BG and Grogan TM. CALLA-positive myeloma: an aggressive subtype with poor survival. Blood 1985;66:229–32.
80. Van Camp B, Durie B, Spier C, et al. Plasma cells in multiple myeloma express a natural killer cell–associated antigen: CD56 (NHK-1; Leu-19). Blood 1990;76:377–82.
81. Sawyer JR, Waldron JA, Jagannath S, et al. Cytogenetic findings in 200 patients with multiple myeloma. Cancer Genet Cytogenet 1995;82:41–9.
82. Hoyer JD, Hanson CA, Fonseca R, et al. The (11;14) (q13;q32) translocation in multiple myeloma. A morphologic and immunohistochemical study. Am J Clin Pathol 2000;113:831–7.
83. Soverini S, Cavo M, Cellini C, et al. Cyclin D1 overexpression is a favorable prognostic variable for newly diagnosed multiple myeloma patients treated with high-dose chemotherapy and single or double autologous transplantation. Blood 2003;102:1588–94.
84. Claudio JO, Masih-Khan E, and Stewart AK. Insights from the gene expression profiling of multiple myeloma. Curr Hematol Rep 2004;3:67–73.
85. De Vos J, Thykjaer T, Tarte K, et al. Comparison of gene expression profiling between malignant and normal plasma cells with oligonucleotide arrays. Oncogene 2002;21: 6848–57.
86. Isaacson P and Spencer J. Malignant lymphoma of mucosa-associated lymphoid tissue. Histopathology 1987;11:445–62.
87. Isaacson P and Wright D. Malignant lymphoma of mucosa associated lymphoid tissue. A distinctive B cell lymphoma. Cancer 1983;52:1410–16.
88. Isaacson P, Wotherspoon A, Diss T, et al. Follicular colonization in B cell lymphoma of mucosa associated lymphoid tissue. Am J Surg Pathol 1991;15:819–28.
89. Pelstring R, Essell J, Kurtin P, et al. Diversity of organ site involvement among malignant lymphomas of mucosa-associated tissues. Am J Clin Pathol 1991;96:738–45.
90. Parveen T, Navarro-Roman L, Medeiros LJ, et al. Low-grade B-cell lymphoma of mucosa-associated lymphoid tissue arising in the kidney. Arch Pathol Lab Med 1993;117:780–3.
91. Ortiz-Hidalgo C and Wright DH. The morphological spectrum of monocytoid B-cell lymphoma, and its relationship to lymphomas of mucosa-associated lymphoid tissue. Histopathology 1992;21:555–61.
92. Nizze H, Cogliatti S, von Schilling C, et al. Monocytoid B-cell lymphoma: morphological variants and relationship to low-grade B-cell lymphoma of the mucosa-associated lymphoid tissue. Histopathology 1991;18:403–14.
93. Shin S, Sheibani K, Fishleder A, et al. Monocytoid B-cell lymphoma in patients with Sjogren's syndrome: a clinicopathologic study of 13 patients. Hum Pathol 1991;22:422–30.
94. Cogliatti S, Lennert K, Hansmann M, et al. Monocytoid B cell lymphoma: clinical and prognostic features of 21 patients. J Clin Pathol 1990;43:619–25.

95. Campo E, Miquel R, Krenacs L, et al. Primary nodal marginal zone lymphomas of splenic and MALT type. Am J Surg Pathol 1999;23:59–68.
96. Hussell T, Isaacson PG, Crabtree JE, et al. The response of cells from low-grade B-cell gastric lymphomas of mucosa-associated lymphoid tissue to Helicobacter pylori. Lancet 1993;342:571–4.
97. Wotherspoon A, Doglioni C, Diss T, et al. Regression of primary low-grade B-cell gastric lymphoma of mucosa-associated lymphoid tissue type after eradication of Helicobacter pylori. Lancet 1993;342:575–7.
98. Ferry JA, Yang WI, Zukerberg LR, et al. CD5+ extranodal marginal zone B-cell (MALT) lymphoma. A low grade neoplasm with a propensity for bone marrow involvement and relapse. Am J Clin Pathol 1996;105:31–7.
99. Wenzel C, Dieckmann K, Fiebiger W, et al. CD5 expression in a lymphoma of the mucosa-associated lymphoid tissue (MALT)–type as a marker for early dissemination and aggressive clinical behaviour. Leuk Lymphoma 2001;42: 823–9.
100. Ballesteros E, Osborne BM, and Matsushima AY. CD5+ low-grade marginal zone B-cell lymphomas with localized presentation. Am J Surg Pathol 1998;22:201–7.
101. Dierlamm J, Pittaluga S, Wlodarska I, et al. Marginal zone B-cell lymphomas of different sites share similar cytogenetic and morphologic features. Blood 1996;87: 299–307.
102. Horsman D, Gascoyne R, Klasa R, et al. t(11;18)(q21;q21.1): a recurring translocation in lymphomas of mucosa-associated lymphoid tissue (MALT)? Genes Chromosomes Cancer 1992;4:183–7.
103. Auer IA, Gascoyne RD, Connors JM, et al. t(11;18)(q21;q21) is the most common translocation in MALT lymphomas. Ann Oncol 1997;8:979–85.
104. Ott G, Katzenberger T, Greiner A, et al. The t(11;18) (q21;q21) chromosome translocation is a frequent and specific aberration in low-grade but not high-grade malignant non-Hodgkin's lymphomas of the mucosa-associated lymphoid tissue (MALT–) type. Cancer Res 1997;57:3944–8.
105. Dierlamm J, Baens M, Wlodarska I, et al. The apoptosis inhibitor gene API2 and a novel 18q gene, MLT, are recurrently rearranged in the t(11;18)(q21;q21) associated with mucosa-associated lymphoid tissue lymphomas. Blood 1999;93:3601–9.
106. Willis TG, Jadayel DM, Du MQ, et al. Bcl10 is involved in t(1;14)(p22;q32) of MALT B cell lymphoma and mutated in multiple tumor types. Cell 1999;96:35–45.
107. Ohshima K, Muta H, Kawasaki C, et al. Bcl10 expression, rearrangement and mutation in MALT lymphoma: correlation with expression of nuclear factor–kappaB. Int J Oncol 2001;19:283–9.
108. Ye H, Dogan A, Karran L, et al. BCL10 expression in normal and neoplastic lymphoid tissue. Nuclear localization in MALT lymphoma. Am J Pathol 2000;157:1147–54.
109. Lucas PC, Yonezumi M, Inohara N, et al. Bcl10 and MALT1, independent targets of chromosomal translocation in malt lymphoma, cooperate in a novel NF-kappa B signaling pathway. J Biol Chem 2001;276:19012–9.
110. Lucas PC, McAllister-Lucas LM, and Nunez G. NF-kappaB signaling in lymphocytes: a new cast of characters. J Cell Sci 2004;117:31–9.
111. Streubel B, Lamprecht A, Dierlamm J, et al. T(14;18) (q32;q21) involving IGH and MALT1 is a frequent chromosomal aberration in MALT lymphoma. Blood 2003;101: 2335–9.
112. Du M, Diss TC, Xu C, et al. Ongoing mutation in MALT lymphoma immunoglobulin gene suggests that antigen stimulation plays a role in the clonal expansion. Leukemia 1996;10:1190–7.
113. Tierens A, Delabie J, Pittaluga S, et al. Mutation analysis of the rearranged immunoglobulin heavy chain genes of marginal zone cell lymphomas indicates an origin from different marginal zone B lymphocyte subsets. Blood 1998;91:2381–6.
114. de Jong D, Boot H, van Heerde P, et al. Histological grading in gastric lymphoma: pretreatment criteria and clinical relevance. Gastroenterology 1997;112:1466–74.
115. Rosenwald A, Ott G, Stilgenbauer S, et al. Exclusive detection of the t(11;18)(q21;q21) in extranodal marginal zone B cell lymphomas (MZBL) of MALT type in contrast to other MZBL and extranodal large B cell lymphomas. Am J Pathol 1999;155:1817–21.
116. Starostik P, Patzner J, Greiner A, et al. Gastric marginal zone B-cell lymphomas of MALT type develop along 2 distinct pathogenetic pathways. Blood 2002;99:3–9.
117. Ott MM, Rosenwald A, Katzenberger T, et al. Marginal zone B-cell lymphomas (MZBL) arising at different sites represent different biological entities. Genes Chromosomes Cancer 2000;28:380–6.
118. Harris NL, Jaffe ES, Diebold J, et al. The World Health Organization classification of neoplastic diseases of the haematopoietic and lymphoid tissues: report of the Clinical Advisory Committee Meeting, Airlie House, Virginia, November 1997. Histopathology 2000;36:69–86.
119. Sheibani K, Burke J, Swartz W, et al. Monocytoid B cell lymphoma. Clinicopathologic study of 21 cases of a unique type of low-grade lymphoma. Cancer 1988;62:1531–8.
120. Nathwani BN, Drachenberg MR, Hernandez AM, et al. Nodal monocytoid B-cell lymphoma (nodal marginal–zone B-cell lymphoma). Semin Hematol 1999;36:128–38.
121. Camacho FI, Algara P, Mollejo M, et al. Nodal marginal zone lymphoma: a heterogeneous tumor: a comprehensive analysis of a series of 27 cases. Am J Surg Pathol 2003;27:762–71.
122. Berger F, Felman P, Thieblemont C, et al. Non-MALT marginal zone B-cell lymphomas: a description of clinical presentation and outcome in 124 patients. Blood 2000;95: 1950–6.
123. Ngan B-Y, Warnke R, Wilson M, et al. Monocytoid B-cell lymphoma: a study of 36 cases. Hum Pathol 1991;22: 409–41.
124. Nathwani BN, Anderson JR, Armitage JO, et al. Clinical significance of follicular lymphoma with monocytoid B cells. Non-Hodgkin's Lymphoma Classification Project. Hum Pathol 1999;30:263–8.
125. Come ES, Jaffe ES, Andersen JC, et al. Non-Hodgkin's lymphomas in leukemic phase: clinicopathologic correlations. Am J Med 1980;69:667–74.
126. Hu E, Weiss L, Hoppe R, et al. Follicular and diffuse mixed small cleaved and large cell lymphoma—a clinicopathologic study. J Clin Oncol 1985;3:1183–7.
127. Mann R and Berard C. Criteria for the cytologic subclassification of follicular lymphomas: a proposed alternative method. Hematol Oncol 1982;1:187–92.
128. Ott G, Katzenberger T, Lohr A, et al. Cytomorphologic, immunohistochemical, and cytogenetic profiles of follicular lymphoma: 2 types of follicular lymphoma grade 3. Blood 2002;99:3806–12.
129. Bosga-Bouwer AG, van Imhoff GW, Boonstra R, et al. Follicular lymphoma grade 3B includes 3 cytogenetically defined subgroups with primary t(14;18), 3q27, or other translocations: t(14;18) and 3q27 are mutually exclusive. Blood 2003;101:1149–54.
130. Horning SJ, Weiss LM, Nevitt JB, et al. Clinical and pathologic features of follicular large cell (nodular histiocytic) lymphoma. Cancer 1987;59:1470–74.
131. Hans CP, Weisenburger DD, Vose JM, et al. A significant diffuse component predicts for inferior survival in grade 3

follicular lymphoma, but cytologic subtypes do not predict survival. Blood 2003;101:2363–7.
132. Longo DL. What's the deal with follicular lymphomas? J Clin Oncol 1993;11:202–8.
133. Croce C and Nowell P. Molecular basis of human B cell neoplasia. Blood 1985;65:1–7.
134. Hockenbery D, Zutter M, Hickey W, et al. BCL2 protein is topographically restricted in tissues characterized by apoptotic cell death. Proc Natl Acad Sci U S A 1991;88: 6961–5.
135. Gaulard P, d'Agay M, Peuchmaur M, et al. Expression of the bcl-2 gene product in follicular lymphoma. Am J Pathol 1992;140:1089–95.
136. Zha H, Raffeld M, Charboneau L, et al. Similarities of prosurvival signals in Bcl-2-positive and Bcl-2-negative follicular lymphomas identified by reverse phase protein microarray. Lab Invest 2004;84:235–44.
137. Jager U, Bocskor S, Le T, et al. Follicular lymphomas' BCL-2/IgH junctions contain templated nucleotide insertions: novel insights into the mechanism of t(14;18) translocation. Blood 2000;95:3520–9.
138. Cong P, Raffeld M, Teruya-Feldstein J, et al. In situ localization of follicular lymphoma: description and analysis by laser capture microdissection. Blood 2002;99: 3376–82.
139. Stein H, Gerdes J, and Mason D. The normal and malignant germinal centre. Clin Haematol 1982;11:531–59.
140. Dogan A, Du MQ, Aiello A, et al. Follicular lymphomas contain a clonally linked but phenotypically distinct neoplastic B-cell population in the interfollicular zone. Blood 1998;91:4708–14.
141. Cattoretti G, Chang CC, Cechova K, et al. BCL-6 protein is expressed in germinal–center B cells. Blood 1995;86: 45–53.
142. Jaffe ES, Shevach EM, Frank MM, et al. Nodular lymphoma—evidence for origin from follicular B lymphocytes. N Engl J Med 1974;290:813–9.
143. Warnke R and Levy R. Immunopathology of follicular lymphomas. A model of B-lymphocyte homing. N Engl J Med 1978;298:481–86.
144. Jaffe ES, Raffeld M, and Medeiros LJ. Histopathologic subtypes of indolent lymphomas: caricatures of the mature B-cell system. Semin Oncol 1993;20:3–30.
145. Kuppers R, Zhao M, Hansmann ML, et al. Tracing B cell development in human germinal centres by molecular analysis of single cells picked from histological sections. EMBO J 1993;12:4955–67.
146. Garcia CF, Weiss LM, Warnke RA, et al. Cutaneous follicular lymphoma. Am J Surg Pathol 1986;10:454–63.
147. Santucci M, Pimpinelli N, and Arganini L. Primary cutaneous B-cell lymphoma: a unique type of low-grade lymphoma. Clinicopathologic and immunologic study of 83 cases. Cancer 1991;67:2311–26.
148. Sander CA, Flaig MJ, and Jaffe ES. Cutaneous manifestations of lymphoma: a glinical guide based on the WHO classification. Clin Lymphoma 2001;2:86–100.
149. Pinto A, Hutchison RE, Grant LH, et al. Follicular lymphomas in pediatric patients. Mod Pathol 1990;3:308–13.
150. Finn LS, Viswanatha DS, Belasco JB, et al. Primary follicular lymphoma of the testis in childhood. Cancer 1999;85: 1626–35.
151. Banks P, Chan J, Cleary M, et al. Mantle cell lymphoma: a proposal for unification of morphologic, immunologic, and molecular data. Am J Surg Pathol 1992;16:637–40.
152. Raffeld M and Jaffe, ES bcl-1 t(11;14), and mantle cell derived neoplasms. Blood 1991;78:259–63.
153. Jaffe ES, Bookman MA, and Longo DL. Lymphocytic lymphoma of intermediate differentiation—mantle zone lymphoma: a distinct subtype of B-cell lymphoma. Hum Pathol 1987;18:877–80.
154. Weisenburger DD, Kim H, and Rappaport H. Mantle zone lymphoma: a follicular variant of intermediate lymphocytic lymphoma. Cancer 1982;49:1429–38.
155. Velders GA, Kluin-Nelemans JC, De Boer CJ, et al. Mantle-cell lymphoma: a population–based clinical study. J Clin Oncol 1996;14:1269–74.
156. Teodorovic I, Pittaluga S, Kluin-Nelemans JC, et al. Efficacy of four different regimens in 64 mantle–cell lymphoma cases: clinicopathologic comparison with 498 other non-Hodgkin's lymphoma subtypes. European Organization for the Research and Treatment of Cancer Lymphoma Cooperative Group. J Clin Oncol 1995;13:2819–26.
157. Norton AJ, Matthews J, Pappa V, et al. Mantle cell lymphoma: natural history defined in a serially biopsied population over a 20-year period. Ann Oncol 1995;6:249–56.
158. Fisher RI, Dahlberg S, Nathwani BN, et al. A clinical analysis of two indolent lymphoma entities: mantle cell lymphoma and marginal zone lymphoma (including the mucosa-associated lymphoid tissue and monocytoid B-cell subcategories): a Southwest Oncology Group study. Blood 1995;85:1075–82.
159. O'Briain D, Kennedy M, Daly P, et al. Multiple lymphomatous polyposis of the gastrointestinal tract: a clinicopathologically distinctive form of non-Hodgkin's lymphoma of centrocytic type. Am J Surg Pathol 1989;13:691–9.
160. Ott G, Kalla J, Hanke A, et al. The cytomorphological spectrum of mantle cell lymphoma is reflected by distinct biological features. Leuk Lymphoma 1998;32:55–63.
161. Zoldan MC, Inghirami G, Masuda Y, et al. Large-cell variants of mantle cell lymphoma: cytologic characteristics and p53 anomalies may predict poor outcome. Br J Haematol 1996; 93:475–86.
162. Ott G, Kalla J, Ott MM, et al. Blastoid variants of mantle cell lymphoma: frequent bcl-1 rearrangements at the major translocation cluster region and tetraploid chromosome clones. Blood 1997;89:1421–9.
163. Bosch F, Lopez-Guillermo A, Campo E, et al. Mantle cell lymphoma: presenting features, response to therapy, and prognostic factors. Cancer 1998;82:567–75.
164. Argatoff LH, Connors JM, Klasa RJ, et al. Mantle cell lymphoma: a clinicopathologic study of 80 cases. Blood 1997;89:2067–78.
165. Rosenwald A, Wright G, Wiestner A, et al. The proliferation gene expression signature is a quantitative integrator of oncogenic events that predicts survival in mantle cell lymphoma. Cancer Cell 2003;3:185–97.
166. Medeiros LJ, van Krieken JH, Jaffe ES, et al. Association of bcl-1 rearrangements with lymphocytic lymphoma of intermediate differentiation. Blood 1990;76:2086–90.
167. Zukerberg LR, Yang WI, Arnold A, et al. Cyclin D1 expression in non-Hodgkin's lymphomas. Detection by immunohistochemistry. Am J Clin Pathol 1995;103:756–60.
168. Swerdlow SH, Yang WI, Zukerberg LR, et al. Expression of cyclin D1 protein in centrocytic/mantle cell lymphomas with and without rearrangement of the BCL1/cyclin D1 gene. Hum Pathol 1995;26:999–1004.
169. de Boer CJ, Schuuring E, Dreef E, et al. Cyclin D1 protein analysis in the diagnosis of mantle cell lymphoma. Blood 1995;86:2715–23.
170. Jares P, Campo E, Pinyol M, et al. Expression of retinoblastoma gene product (pRb) in mantle cell lymphomas. Correlation with cyclin D1 (PRAD1/CCND1) mRNA levels and proliferative activity. Am J Pathol 1996;148:1591–1600.
171. Greiner TC, Moynihan MJ, Chan WC, et al. p53 mutations in mantle cell lymphoma are associated with variant cytology and predict a poor prognosis. Blood 1996;87: 4302–10.

172. Louie DC, Offit K, Jaslow R, et al. p53 overexpression as a marker of poor prognosis in mantle cell lymphomas with t(11;14)(q13;q32). Blood 1995;86:2892–9.
173. Quintanilla-Martinez L, Thieblemont C, Fend F, et al. Mantle cell lymphomas lack expression of p27Kip1, a cyclin-dependent kinase inhibitor. Am J Pathol 1998;153:175–82.
174. Hernandez L, Fest T, Cazorla M, et al. p53 gene mutations and protein overexpression are associated with aggressive variants of mantle cell lymphomas. Blood 1996;87:3351–9.
175. Pinyol M, Cobo F, Bea S, et al. p16(INK4a) gene inactivation by deletions, mutations, and hypermethylation is associated with transformed and aggressive variants of non-Hodgkin's lymphomas. Blood 1998;91:2977–84.
176. Longo DL, Duffey PL, DeVita VJ, et al. Treatment of advanced-stage Hodgkin's disease: alternating noncrossresistant MOPP/CABS is not superior to MOPP. J Clin Oncol 1991;9:1409–20.
177. Warnke RA, Strauchen JA, Burke JS, et al. Morphologic types of diffuse large cell lymphoma. Cancer 1982;50:690–5.
178. Engelhard M, Brittinger G, Huhn D, et al. Subclassification of diffuse large B-cell lymphomas according to the Kiel classification: distinction of centroblastic and immunoblastic lymphomas is a significant prognostic risk factor. Blood 1997;89:2291–7.
179. O'Hara C, Said J, and Pinkus G. Non-Hodgkin's lymphoma, multilobated B cell type. Hum Pathol 1986;17:593–9.
180. Rudiger T, Gascoyne RD, Jaffe ES, et al. Workshop on the relationship between nodular lymphocyte predominant Hodgkin's lymphoma and T cell/histiocyte-rich B cell lymphoma. Ann Oncol 2002;13:44–51.
181. Delabie J, Vandenberghe E, Kennes C, et al. Histiocyte-rich B-cell lymphoma. A distinct clinicopathologic entity possibly related to lymphocyte predominant Hodgkin's disease, paragranuloma subtype. Am J Surg Pathol 1992;16: 37–48.
182. Skinnider BF, Connors JM, and Gascoyne RD. Bone marrow involvement in T-cell-rich B-cell lymphoma. Am J Clin Pathol 1997;108:570–8.
183. Chittal S, Brousset P, Voigt J, et al. Large B-cell lymphoma rich in T-cells and simulating Hodgkin's disease. Histopathology 1991;19:211–20.
184. Lim MS, Beaty M, Sorbara L, et al. T-cell/histiocyte-rich large B-cell lymphoma: a heterogeneous entity with derivation from germinal center B cells. Am J Surg Pathol 2002;26: 1458–66.
185. Ramsay A, Smith W, and Isaacson P. T-cell-rich B-cell lymphoma. Am J Surg Pathol 1988;12:433–43.
186. Jaffe E. Post-thymic lymphoid neoplasia. In: E. Jaffe (ed.), Surgical Pathology of the Lymph Nodes and Related Organs, Vol. 16, pp. 218–48. Philadelphia: W. B. Saunders, 1985.
187. Miller TP, Grogan TM, Dahlberg S, et al. Prognostic significance of the Ki-67 associated proliferative antigen in aggressive non-Hodgkin's lymphomas: a prospective Southwest Onocology Group trial. Blood 1994;83:1460–66.
188. Wilson WH, Teruya-Feldstein J, Fest T, et al. Relationship of p53, bcl-2, and tumor proliferation to clinical drug resistance in non-Hodgkin's lymphomas. Blood 1997;89:601–9.
189. Gascoyne RD, Adomat SA, Krajewski S, et al. Prognostic significance of Bcl-2 protein expression and Bcl-2 gene rearrangement in diffuse aggressive non-Hodgkin's lymphoma. Blood 1997;90:244–51.
190. Hermine O, Haioun C, Lepage E, et al. Prognostic significance of bcl-2 protein expression in aggressive non-Hodgkin's lymphoma. Groupe d'Etude des Lymphomes de l'Adulte (GELA). Blood 1996;87:265–72.
191. Mounier N, Briere J, Gisselbrecht C, et al. Rituximab plus CHOP (R-CHOP) overcomes bcl-2–associated resistance to chemotherapy in elderly patients with diffuse large B-cell lymphoma (DLBCL). Blood 2003;101:4279–84.
192. Offit K, Lo CF, Louie DC, et al. Rearrangement of the bcl-6 gene as a prognostic marker in diffuse large-cell lymphoma. N Engl J Med 1994;331:74–80.
193. Rosenwald A, Wright G, Chan WC, et al. The use of molecular profiling to predict survival after chemotherapy for diffuse large-B-cell lymphoma. N Engl J Med 2002;346: 1937–47.
194. Hans CP, Weisenburger DD, Greiner TC, et al. Confirmation of the molecular classification of diffuse large B-cell lymphoma by immunohistochemistry using a tissue microarray. Blood 2004;103:275–82.
195. Addis B and Isaacson P. Large cell lymphoma of the mediastinum: a B-cell tumor of probable thymic origin. Histopathology 1986;10:379–90.
196. Moller P, Moldenhauer G, Momburg F, et al. Mediastinal lymphoma of clear cell type is a tumor corresponding to terminal steps of B cell differentiation. Blood 1987;69:1087–95.
197. Lamarre L, Jacobson J, Aisenberg A, et al. Primary large cell lymphoma of the mediastinum. Am J Surg Pathol 1989; 13:730–9.
198. Hofmann WJ, Momburg F, and Moller P. Thymic medullary cells expressing B-lymphocyte antigens. Hum Pathol 1988; 19:1280–7.
199. Kanavaros P, Gaulard P, Charlotte F, et al. Discordant expression of immunoglobulin and its associated molecule mb-1/CD79a is frequently found in mediastinal large B-cell lymphomas. Am J Pathol 1995;146:735–41.
200. Higgins JP and Warnke RA. CD30 expression is common in mediastinal large B-cell lymphoma. Am J Clin Pathol 1999;112:241–7.
201. Pileri SA, Gaidano G, Zinzani PL, et al. Primary mediastinal B-cell lymphoma: high frequency of BCL-6 mutations and consistent expression of the transcription factors OCT-2, BOB.1, and PU.1 in the absence of immunoglobulins. Am J Pathol 2003;162:243–53.
202. Rudiger T, Jaffe ES, Delsol G, et al. Workshop report on Hodgkin's disease and related diseases ('grey zone' lymphoma). Ann Oncol 1998;9(suppl 5):S31–8.
203. Jundt F, Kley K, Anagnostopoulos I, et al. Loss of PU.1 expression is associated with defective immunoglobulin transcription in Hodgkin and Reed–Sternberg cells of classical Hodgkin disease. Blood 2002;99:3060–2.
204. Kuppers R. Molecular biology of Hodgkin's lymphoma. Adv Cancer Res 2002;84:277–312.
205. Jaffe ES and Muller-Hermelink HK. Relationship between Hodgkin's disease and non-Hodgkin's lymphomas. In: P. Mauch, J. Armitage, V. Diehl, R. Hoppe, and L. Weiss (eds.), Hodgkin's Disease, pp. 181–94. Philadelphia, PA: Lippincott Raven, 1999.
206. Zarate OA, Medeiros LJ, Longo DL, et al. Non-Hodgkin's lymphomas arising in patients successfully treated for Hodgkin's disease. A clinical, histologic, and immunophenotypic study of 14 cases. Am J Surg Pathol 1992;16: 885–95.
207. Rosenwald A, Wright G, Leroy K, et al. Molecular diagnosis of primary mediastinal B cell lymphoma identifies a clinically favorable subgroup of diffuse large B cell lymphoma related to Hodgkin lymphoma. J Exp Med 2003;198:851–62.
208. Savage KJ, Monti S, Kutok JL, et al. The molecular signature of mediastinal large B-cell lymphoma differs from that of other diffuse large B-cell lymphomas and shares features with classical Hodgkin lymphoma. Blood 2003;102:3871–9.
209. Jacobson J, Aisenberg A, Lamarre L, et al. Mediastinal large cell lymphoma: an uncommon subset of adult lymphoma curable with combined modality therapy. Cancer 1988;62: 1893–8.
210. Zinzani PL, Martelli M, Magagnoli M, et al. Treatment and clinical management of primary mediastinal large B-cell lym-

phoma with sclerosis: MACOP-B regimen and mediastinal radiotherapy monitored by (67)Gallium scan in 50 patients. Blood 1999;94:3289–93.
211. DiGiuseppe JA, Nelson WG, Seifter EJ, et al. Intravascular lymphomatosis: a clinicopathologic study of 10 cases and assessment of response to chemotherapy. J Clin Oncol 1994;12:2573–9.
212. Rubin MA, Cossman J, Freter CE, et al. Intravascular large cell lymphoma coexisting within hemangiomas of the skin. Am J Surg Pathol 1997;21:860–4.
213. Cesarman E, Chang Y, Moore PS, et al. Kaposi's sarcoma-associated herpesvirus-like DNA sequences in AIDS-related body–cavity based lymphomas. N Engl J Med 1995;332: 1186–91.
214. Nador RG, Cesarman E, Chadburn A, et al. Primary effusion lymphoma: a distinct clinicopathologic entity associated with the Kaposi's sarcoma-associated herpes virus. Blood 1996;88:645–56.
215. Cobo F, Hernandez S, Hernandez L, et al. Expression of potentially oncogenic HHV-8 genes in an EBV-negative primary effusion lymphoma occurring in an HIV-seronegative patient. J Pathol 1999;189:288–93.
216. Teruya-Feldstein J, Zauber P, Setsuda JE, et al. Expression of human herpesvirus-8 oncogene and cytokine homologues in an HIV-seronegative patient with multicentric Castleman's disease and primary effusion lymphoma. Lab Invest 1998; 78:1637–42.
217. DePond W, Said JW, Tasaka T, et al. Kaposi's sarcoma-associated herpesvirus and human herpesvirus 8 (KSHV/HHV8)–associated lymphoma of the bowel. Report of two cases in HIV-positive men with secondary effusion lymphomas. Am J Surg Pathol 1997;21:719–24.
218. Carbone A, Gaidano G, Gloghini A, et al. Differential expression of BCL-6, CD138/syndecan-1, and Epstein–Barr virus–encoded latent membrane protein-1 identifies distinct histogenetic subsets of acquired immunodeficiency syndrome–related non-Hodgkin's lymphomas. Blood 1998;91: 747–55.
219. Beaty MW, Kumar S, Sorbara L, et al. A biophenotypic human herpesvirus 8–associated primary bowel lymphoma [letter; comment]. Am J Surg Pathol 1999;23:992–4.
220. Matolcsy A, Nador RG, Cesarman E, et al. Immunoglobulin VH gene mutational analysis suggests that primary effusion lymphomas derive from different stages of B cell maturation. Am J Pathol 1998;153:1609–14.
221. Hollingsworth HC, Stetler SM, Gagneten D, et al. Immunodeficiency-associated malignant lymphoma. Three cases showing genotypic evidence of both T- and B-cell lineages. Am J Surg Pathol 1994;18:1092–1101.
222. Dupin N, Fisher C, Kellam P, et al. Distribution of human herpesvirus-8 latently infected cells in Kaposi's sarcoma, multicentric Castleman's disease, and primary effusion lymphoma. Proc Natl Acad Sci U S A 1999;96:4546–51.
223. Delecluse HJ, Anagnostopoulos I, Dallenbach F, et al. Plasmablastic lymphomas of the oral cavity: a new entity associated with the human immunodeficiency virus infection. Blood 1997;89:1413–20.
224. Dupin N, Diss TL, Kellam P, et al. HHV-8 is associated with a plasmablastic variant of Castleman disease that is linked to HHV-8–positive plasmablastic lymphoma. Blood 2000;95: 1406–12.
225. Engels EA, Pittaluga S, Whitby D, et al. Immunoblastic lymphoma in persons with AIDS-associated Kaposi's sarcoma: a role for Kaposi's sarcoma–associated herpesvirus. Mod Pathol 2003;16:424–9.
226. Delsol G, Lamant L, Mariame B, et al. A new subtype of large B-cell lymphoma expressing the ALK kinase and lacking the 2; 5 translocation. Blood 1997;89:1483–90.
227. Onciu M, Behm FG, Downing JR, et al. ALK-positive plasmablastic B-cell lymphoma with expression of the NPM-ALK fusion transcript: report of 2 cases. Blood 2003;102: 2642–44.
228. De Paepe P, Baens M, van Krieken H, et al. ALK activation by the CLTC-ALK fusion is a recurrent event in large B-cell lymphoma. Blood 2003;102:2638–41.
229. Magrath I and Shiramizu B. Biology and treatment of small non-cleaved cell lymphoma. Oncology 1989;3:41–53.
230. Ballerini P, Gaidano G, Gong JZ, et al. Multiple genetic lesions in acquired immunodeficiency syndrome–related non-Hodgkin's lymphoma. Blood 1993;81:166–76.
231. Yano T, van Krieken JH, Magrath IT, et al. Histogenetic correlations between subcategories of small noncleaved cell lymphomas. Blood 1992;79:1282–90.
232. Pelicci PG, Knowles DM 2nd, Arlin ZA, et al. Multiple monoclonal B cell expansions and c-myc oncogene rearrangements in acquired immune deficiency syndrome–related lymphoproliferative disorders. Implications for lymphomagenesis. J Exp Med 1986;164:2049–60.
233. Cavdar AO, Gozdasoglu S, Yavuz G, et al. Burkitt's lymphoma between African and American types in Turkish children: clinical, viral (EBV), and molecular studies. Med Pediatr Oncol 1993;21:36–42.
234. Goldschmidts WL, Bhatia K, Johnson JF, et al. Epstein–Barr virus genotypes in AIDS-associated lymphomas are similar to those in endemic Burkitt's lymphomas. Leukemia 1992;6: 875–8.
235. Garcia CF, Weiss LM, and Warnke RA. Small noncleaved cell lymphoma: an immunophenotypic study of 18 cases and comparison with large cell lymphoma. Hum Pathol 1986;17: 454–61.
236. Raphael M, Gentilhomme O, Tulliez M, et al. Histopathologic features of high-grade non-Hodgkin's lymphomas in acquired immunodeficiency syndrome. The French Study Group of Pathology for Human Immunodeficiency Virus–Associated Tumors. Arch Pathol Lab Med 1991;115: 15–20.
237. Karsan A, Gascoyne RD, Coupland RW, et al. Combination of t(14;18) and a Burkitt's type translocation in B-cell malignancies. Leuk Lymphoma 1993;10:433–41.
238. Yano T, Jaffe ES, Longo DL, et al. MYC rearrangements in histologically progressed follicular lymphomas. Blood 1992;80:758–67.
239. Gauwerky CE, Hoxie J, Nowell PC, et al. Pre–B-cell leukemia with a t(8; 14) and a t(14; 18) translocation is preceded by follicular lymphoma. Oncogene 1988;2:431–5.
240. Hao S, Sanger W, Onciu M, et al. Mantle cell lymphoma with 8q24 chromosomal abnormalities: a report of 5 cases with blastoid features. Mod Pathol 2002;15:1266–72.
241. Jaffe ES, Chan JK, Su IJ, et al. Report of the Workshop on Nasal and Related Extranodal Angiocentric T/Natural Killer Cell Lymphomas. Definitions, differential diagnosis, and epidemiology. Am J Surg Pathol 1996;20:103–11.
242. Lipford EH, Margolick JB, Longo DL, et al. Angiocentric immunoproliferative lesions: a clinicopathologic spectrum of post-thymic T cell proliferations. Blood 1988;5: 1674–81.
243. Guinee DJ, Jaffe E, Kingma D, et al. Pulmonary lymphomatoid granulomatosis. Evidence for a proliferation of Epstein–Barr virus infected B-lymphocytes with a prominent T-cell component and vasculitis. Am J Surg Pathol 1994;18: 753–64.
244. Katzenstein A-L and Peiper S. Detection of Epstein–Barr genomes in lymphomatoid granulomatosis: analysis of 29 cases by the polymerase chain reaction. Mod Pathol 1990;3: 435–41.
245. Teruya-Feldstein J, Jaffe ES, Burd PR, et al. The role of Mig, the monokine induced by interferon-gamma, and

IP-10, the interferon-gamma-inducible protein-10, in tissue necrosis and vascular damage associated with Epstein–Barr virus–positive lymphoproliferative disease. Blood 1997;90: 4099–5105.
246. Koss MN, Hochholzer L, Langloss JM, et al. Lymphomatoid granulomatosis: a clinicopathologic study of 42 patients. Pathology 1986;18:283–8.
247. Wilson WH, Kingma DW, Raffeld M, et al. Association of lymphomatoid granulomatosis with Epstein–Barr viral infection of B lymphocytes and response to interferon-alpha 2b. Blood 1996;87:4531–7.
248. Jaffe ES, Krenacs L, Kumar S, et al. Extranodal peripheral T-cell and NK-cell neoplasms. Am J Clin Pathol 1999; 111(suppl 1):S46–55.
249. Chan JKC, Sin VC, Wong KF, et al. Nonnasal lymphoma expressing the natural killer cell marker CD56: a clinicopathologic study of 49 cases of an uncommon aggressive neoplasm. Blood 1997;89:4501–13.
250. Kumar S, Krenacs L, Elenitoba-Johnson K, et al. Subcutaneous panniculitic T-cell lymphoma is a tumor of cytotoxic T-lymphocytes. Hum Pathol 1998;29:397–403.
251. Stein H, Foss HD, Durkop H, et al. CD30(+) anaplastic large cell lymphoma: a review of its histopathologic, genetic, and clinical features. Blood 2000;96:3681–95.
252. Nathwani B, Kim H, and Rappaport H. Malignant lymphoma, lymphoblastic. Cancer 1976;38:964–83.
253. Gouttefangeas C, Bensussan A, and Boumsell L. Study of the CD3-associated T-cell receptors reveals further differences between T-cell acute lymphoblastic lymphoma and leukemia. Blood 1990;74:931–4.
254. Baer R. TAL1, TAL2 and LYL1: a family of basic helix-loop-helix proteins implicated in T cell acute leukaemia. Semin Cancer Biol 1993;4:341–7.
255. Berger R, Dastugue N, Busson M, et al. t(5;14)/HOX11L2-positive T-cell acute lymphoblastic leukemia. A collaborative study of the Groupe Francais de Cytogenetique Hematologique (GFCH). Leukemia 2003;17:1851–7.
256. Ferrando AA, Neuberg DS, Staunton J, et al. Gene expression signatures define novel oncogenic pathways in T cell acute lymphoblastic leukemia. Cancer Cell 2002;1:75–87.
257. Matutes E, Brito-Babapulle V, Swansbury J, et al. Clinical and laboratory features of 78 cases of T-prolymphocytic leukemia. Blood 1991;78:3269–74.
258. Brouet J, Sasportes M, Flandrin G, et al. Chronic lymphocytic leukemia of T cell origin. Lancet 1975;ii:890–3.
259. Loughran T. Clonal diseases of large granular lymphocytes. Blood 1993;82:1–14.
260. Oshimi K, Yamada O, Kenako T, et al. Laboratory findings and clinical courses of 33 patients with granular lymphocyte–proliferative disorders. Leukemia 1993;7:782–8.
261. Uchiyama T, Yodoi J, Sagawa K, et al. Adult T-cell leukemia: clinical and hematologic features of 16 cases. Blood 1977; 50:481–92.
262. Poiesz B, Ruscetti F, and Gazdar A. Detection and isolation of type C retrovirus particles from fresh and cultured lymphocytes of a patient with cutaneous T-cell lymphoma. Proc Natl Acad Sci U S A 1980;77:7415–9.
263. Swerdlow S, Habeshaw J, Rohatiner A, et al. Caribbean T-cell lymphoma/leukemia. Cancer 1984;54:687–96.
264. Manns A, Cleghorn FR, Falk RT, et al. Role of HTLV-I in development of non-Hodgkin lymphoma in Jamaica and Trinidad and Tobago. The HTLV Lymphoma Study Group. Lancet 1993;342:1447–50.
265. Jaffe ES, Blattner WA, Blayney DW, et al. The pathologic spectrum of adult T-cell leukemia/lymphoma in the United States. Am J Surg Pathol 1984;8:263–75.
266. Levine PH, Manns A, Jaffe ES, et al. The effect of ethnic differences on the pattern of HTLV-I–associated T-cell leukemia/lymphoma (HATL) in the United States. Int J Cancer 1994;56:177–81.
267. Levine PH, Cleghorn F, Manns A, et al. Adult T-cell leukemia/lymphoma: a working point-score classification for epidemiological studies. Int J Cancer 1994;59:491–93.
268. Abrams M, Sidawy M, and Novich M. Smoldering HTLV-associated T-cell leukemia. Arch Intern Med 1985;145: 2257–8.
269. Kikuchi M, Mitsui T, Takeshita M, et al. Virus associated adult T-cell leukemia (ATL) in Japan: clinical, histological and immunological studies. Hematol Oncol 1987;4:67.
270. Duggan D, Ehrlich G, Davey F, et al. HTLV-I induced lymphoma mimicking Hodgkin's disease. Diagnosis by polymerase chain reaction amplification of specific HTLV-I sequences in tumor DNA. Blood 1988;71:1027–32.
271. Ohshima K, Kikuchi M, Yoshida T, et al. Lymph nodes in incipient adult T-cell leukemia-lymphoma with Hodgkin's disease–like histologic features. Cancer 1991;67:1622–8.
272. Chan J, Ng C, Lau W, et al. Most nasal/nasopharyngeal lymphomas are peripheral T cell neoplasms. Am J Surg Pathol 1987;11:418–29.
273. Ho F, Choy D, Loke S, et al. Polymorphic reticulosis and conventional lymphomas of the nose and upper aerodigestive tract—a clinicopathologic study of 70 cases, and immunophenotypic studies of 16 cases. Hum Pathol 1990;21: 1041–50.
274. Ferry JA, Sklar J, Zukerberg LR, et al. Nasal lymphoma: a clinicopathologic study with immunophenotypic and genotypic analysis. Am J Surg Pathol 1991;15:268–79.
275. Imamura N, Kusunoki Y, Kawa-Ha K, et al. Aggressive natural killer cell leukaemia/lymphoma: report of four cases and review of the literature. Possible existence of a new clinical entity originating from the third lineage of lymphoid cells. Br J Haematol 1990;75:49–59.
276. Jaffe ES, Costa J, Fauci AS, et al. Malignant lymphoma and erythrophagocytosis simulating malignant histiocytosis. Am J Med 1983;75:741–9.
277. Arber DA, Weiss LM, Albujar PF, et al. Nasal lymphomas in Peru. High incidence of T-cell immunophenotype and Epstein–Barr virus infection. Am J Surg Pathol 1993;17: 392–9.
278. Jaffe ES, Chan JKC, Su IJ, et al. Report of the workshop on nasal and related extranodal angiocentric T/NK cell lymphomas: definitions, differential diagnosis, and epidemiology. Am J Surg Pathol 1996;20:103–11.
279. Medeiros LJ, Peiper SC, Elwood L, et al. Angiocentric immunoproliferative lesions: a molecular analysis of eight cases. Hum Pathol 1991;22:1150–7.
280. Ho F, Srivastava G, Loke S, et al. Presence of Epstein–Barr virus DNA in nasal lymphomas of B and T cell type. Hematol Oncol 1990;8:271–81.
281. Tsang WY, Chan JK, Yip TT, et al. In situ localization of Epstein–Barr virus encoded RNA in non-nasal/nasopharyngeal CD56-positive and CD56-negative T-cell lymphomas. Hum Pathol 1994;25:758–65.
282. Isaacson PG, O'Connor NT, Spencer J, et al. Malignant histiocytosis of the intestine: a T-cell lymphoma. Lancet 1985;2:688–91.
283. Murray A, Cuevas EC, Jones DB, et al. Study of the immunohistochemistry and T cell clonality of enteropathy-associated T cell lymphoma. Am J Pathol 1995;146:509–19.
284. Daum S, Weiss D, Hummel M, et al. Frequency of clonal intraepithelial T lymphocyte proliferations in enteropathy-type intestinal T cell lymphoma, coeliac disease, and refractory sprue. Gut 2001;49:804–12.
285. Spencer J, Cerf-Bensussan N, Jarry A, et al. Enteropathy—associated T-cell lymphoma is recognized by a monoclonal antibody (HML-1) that defines a membrane molecule

on human mucosal lymphocytes. Am J Pathol 1988;132: 1–5.

286. Krenacs L, Smyth MJ, Bagdi E, et al. The serine protease granzyme M is preferentially expressed in NK-cell, gamma delta T-cell, and intestinal T-cell lymphomas: evidence of origin from lymphocytes involved in innate immunity. Blood 2003;101:3590–3.
287. Quintanilla-Martinez L, Lome-Maldonado C, Ott G, et al. Primary non-Hodgkin's lymphoma of the intestine: high prevalence of Epstein–Barr virus in Mexican lymphomas as compared with European cases. Blood 1997;89:644–51.
288. de Bruin PC, Jiwa M, Oudejans JJ, et al. Presence of Epstein–Barr virus in extranodal T-cell lymphomas: differences in relation to site. Blood 1994;83:1612–8.
289. Liang R. Diagnosis and management of primary nasal lymphoma of T-cell or NK-cell origin. Clin Lymphoma 2000; 1:33–7.
290. Gale J, Simmonds PD, Mead GM, et al. Enteropathy-type intestinal T-cell lymphoma: clinical features and treatment of 31 patients in a single center. J Clin Oncol 2000;18:795–803.
291. Daum S, Hummel M, Weiss D, et al. Refractory sprue syndrome with clonal intraepithelial lymphocytes evolving into overt enteropathy-type intestinal T-cell lymphoma. Digestion 2000;62:60–5.
292. Howell WM, Leung ST, Jones DB, et al. HLA-DRB, -DQA, and -DQB polymorphism in celiac disease and enteropathy-associated T-cell lymphoma. Common features and additional risk factors for malignancy. Hum Immunol 1995;43: 29–37.
293. Chott A, Dragosics B, and Radaszkiewicz T. Peripheral T-cell lymphomas of the intestine. Am J Pathol 1992;141:1361–71.
294. Spencer J, Isaacson PG, MacDonald TT, et al. Gamma/delta T cells and the diagnosis of coeliac disease. Clin Exp Immunol 1991;85:109–13.
295. Bagdi E, Diss TC, Munson P, et al. Mucosal intra-epithelial lymphocytes in enteropathy-associated T-cell lymphoma, ulcerative jejunitis, and refractory celiac disease constitute a neoplastic population. Blood 1999;94:260–4.
296. Baumgartner AK, Zettl A, Chott A, et al. High frequency of genetic aberrations in enteropathy-type T-cell lymphoma. Lab Invest 2003;83:1509–16.
297. Gaulard P, Zafrani ES, Mavier P, et al. Peripheral T-cell lymphoma presenting as predominant liver disease: a report of three cases. Hepatology 1986;6:864–8.
298. Farcet J, Gaulard P, Marolleau J, et al. Hepatosplenic T-cell lymphoma: sinusal/sinusoidal localization of malignant cells expressing the T-cell receptor $\gamma\delta$. Blood 1990;75: 2213–9.
299. Gaulard P, Bourquelot P, Kanavaros P, et al. Expression of the alpha/beta and gamma/delta T-cell receptors in 57 cases of peripheral T-cell lymphomas. Identification of a subset of gamma/delta T-cell lymphomas. Am J Pathol 1990;137: 617–28.
300. Cooke CB, Krenacs M, Stetler-Stevenson M, et al. Hepatosplenic gamma/delta T-cell lymphoma: a distinct clinicopathologic entity of cytotoxic gamma/delta T-cell origin. Blood 1996;88:4265–74.
301. Macon WR, Levy NB, Kurtin PJ, et al. Hepatosplenic alphabeta T-cell lymphomas: a report of 14 cases and comparison with hepatosplenic gammadelta T-cell lymphomas. Am J Surg Pathol 2001;25:285–96.
302. Kumar S, Lawlor C, and Jaffe ES. Hepatosplenic T-cell lymphoma of alpha-beta lineage. Am J Surg Pathol 2001;25: 970–1.
303. Suarez F, Wlodarska I, Rigal-Huguet F, et al. Hepatosplenic alphabeta T-cell lymphoma: an unusual case with clinical, histologic, and cytogenetic features of gammadelta hepatosplenic T-cell lymphoma. Am J Surg Pathol 2000;24: 1027–32.
304. Kanavaros P, Boulland ML, Petit B, et al. Expression of cytotoxic proteins in peripheral T-cell and natural killer-cell (NK) lymphomas: association with extranodal site, NK or Tgammadelta phenotype, anaplastic morphology and CD30 expression. Leuk Lymphoma 2000;38:317–26.
305. Wang CC, Tien HF, Lin MT, et al. Consistent presence of isochromosome 7q in hepatosplenic T gamma/delta lymphoma: a new cytogenetic-clinicopathologic entity. Genes Chromosomes Cancer 1995;12:161–4.
306. Alonsozana EL, Stamberg J, Kumar D, et al. Isochromosome 7q: the primary cytogenetic abnormality in hepatosplenic gamma delta T cell lymphoma. Leukemia 1997;11:1367–72.
307. Wlodarska I, Martin-Garcia N, Achten R, et al. Fluorescence in situ hybridization study of chromosome 7 aberrations in hepatosplenic T-cell lymphoma: isochromosome 7q as a common abnormality accumulating in forms with features of cytologic progression. Genes Chromosomes Cancer 2002;33: 243–51.
308. Gouttefangeas C, Bensussan A, and Boumsell L. Utilization of two different T-cell receptors by T-cell acute lymphoblastic lymphoma and leukemia. Nouv Rev Fr Hematol 1990; 32:337–40.
309. Gonzalez CL, Medeiros LJ, Braziel RM, et al. T-cell lymphoma involving subcutaneous tissue: a clinicopathologic entity commonly associated with hemophagocytic syndrome. Am J Surg Pathol 1991;15:17–27.
310. Burg G, Dummer R, Wilhelm M, et al. A subcutaneous delta-positive T-cell lymphoma that produces interferon gamma. N Engl J Med 1991;325:1078–81.
311. Salhany KE, Macon WR, Choi JK, et al. Subcutaneous panniculitis-like T-cell lymphoma: clinicopathologic, immunophenotypic, and genotypic analysis of alpha/beta and gamma/delta subtypes. Am J Surg Pathol 1998;22: 881–93.
312. Toro JR, Liewehr DJ, Pabby N, et al. Gamma-delta T-cell phenotype is associated with significantly decreased survival in cutaneous T-cell lymphoma. Blood 2003;101: 3407–12.
313. Teruya-Feldstein J, Setsuda J, Yao X, et al. MIP-1alpha expression in tissues from patients with hemophagocytic syndrome. Lab Invest 1999; 79:1583–90.
314. Arnulf B, Copie-Bergman C, Delfau-Larue MH, et al. Non-hepatosplenic gamma-delta T-cell lymphoma: a subset of cytotoxic lymphomas with mucosal or skin localization. Blood 1998;91:1723–31.
315. Janeway CA, Jr Jones B, and Hayday A. Specificity and function of T cells bearing gamma delta receptors. Immunol Today 1988;9:73–6.
316. Colby T, Burke J, and Hoppe R. Lymph node biopsy in mycosis fungoides. Cancer 1981;47:351–9.
317. Burke J, Khalil S, and Rappaport H. Dermatopathic lymphadenopathy. An immunophenotypic comparison of cases asssociated and unassociated with mycosis fungoides. Am J Pathol 1986;123:256–63.
318. Ralfkiaer E. Immunohistological markers for the diagnosis of cutaneous lymphomas. Semin Diagn Pathol 1991;8: 62–72.
319. Ashton-Key M, Diss TC, Du MQ, et al. The value of the polymerase chain reaction in the diagnosis of cutaneous T-cell infiltrates. Am J Surg Pathol 1997;21:743–7.
320. Scarisbrick JJ, Woolford AJ, Russell-Jones R, et al. Loss of heterozygosity on 10q and microsatellite instability in advanced stages of primary cutaneous T-cell lymphoma and possible association with homozygous deletion of PTEN. Blood 2000;95:2937–42.
321. Scarisbrick JJ, Woolford AJ, Calonje E, et al. Frequent abnormalities of the p15 and p16 genes in mycosis fungoides and sezary syndrome. J Invest Dermatol 2002;118:493–9.

322. Navas IC, Algara P, Mateo M, et al. p16(INK4a) is selectively silenced in the tumoral progression of mycosis fungoides. Lab Invest 2002;82:123–32.
323. Mao X, Lillington D, Scarisbrick JJ, et al. Molecular cytogenetic analysis of cutaneous T-cell lymphomas: identification of common genetic alterations in Sezary syndrome and mycosis fungoides. Br J Dermatol 2002;147:464–75.
324. Whittaker SJ and Luzzatto L. HTLV-1 provirus and mycosis fungoides. Science 1993;259:1470; author reply 1471.
325. DeCoteau JF, Butmarc JR, Kinney MC, et al. The t(2;5) chromosomal translocation is not a common feature of primary cutaneous CD30+ lymphoproliferative disorders: comparison with anaplastic large-cell lymphoma of nodal origin. Blood 1996;87:3437–41.
326. de Bruin PC, Beljaards RC, van Heerde P, et al. Differences in clinical behaviour and immunophenotype between primary cutaneous and primary nodal anaplastic large cell lymphoma of T-cell or null cell phenotype. Histopathology 1993;23:127–35.
327. Wellmann A, Otsuki T, Vogelbruch M, et al. Analysis of the t(2;5) (p23;q35) translocation by reverse trasnscription-polymerase chain reaction in CD 30+ anaplastic large-cell lymphomas, in other non-Hodgkin's lymphomas of T-cell phenotype, and in Hodgkin's disease. Blood 1995;86:2321–8.
328. Willemze R and Beljaards RC. Spectrum of primary cutaneous CD30 (Ki-1)-positive lymphoproliferative disorders. A proposal for classification and guidelines for management and treatment. J Am Acad Dermatol 1993;28:973–80.
329. Bekkenk MW, Geelen FA, van Voorst Vader PC, et al. Primary and secondary cutaneous CD30(+) lymphoproliferative disorders: a report from the Dutch Cutaneous Lymphoma Group on the long-term follow-up data of 219 patients and guidelines for diagnosis and treatment. Blood 2000;95:3653–61.
330. Paulli M, Berti E, Rosso R, et al. CD30/Ki-1-positive lymphoproliferative disorders of the skin—clinicopathologic correlation and statistical analysis of 86 cases: a multicentric study from the European Organization for Research and Treatment of Cancer Cutaneous Lymphoma Project Group. J Clin Oncol 1995;13:1343–54.
331. Frizzera G, Moran E, and Rappaport H. Angio-immunoblastic lymphadenopathy with dysproteinemia. Lancet 1974;i:1070–3.
332. Weiss L, Strickler J, Dorfman R, et al. Clonal T-cell populations in angioimmunoblastic lymphadenopathy and angioimmunoblastic lymphadenopathy-like lymphoma. Am J Pathol 1986;122:392–7.
333. Feller A, Griesser H, Schilling C, et al. Clonal gene rearrangement patterns correlate with immunophenotype and clinical parameters in patients with angioimmunoblastic lymphadenopathy. Am J Pathol 1988;133:549–56.
334. Attygalle A, Al-Jehani R, Diss TC, et al. Neoplastic T cells in angioimmunoblastic T-cell lymphoma express CD10. Blood 2002;99:627–33.
335. Patsouris D, Noel H, and Lennert K. AILD type of T-cell lymphoma with a high content of epithelioid cells. Histopathology and comparison with lymphoepithelioid cell lymphoma. Am J Surg Pathol 1989;13:161–75.
336. Weiss LM, Jaffe ES, Liu XF, et al. Detection and localization of Epstein–Barr viral genomes in angioimmunoblastic lymphadenopathy and angioimmunoblastic lymphadenopathy-like lymphoma. Blood 1992;79:1789–95.
337. Zettl A, Lee SS, Rudiger T, et al. Epstein–Barr virus-associated B-cell lymphoproliferative disorders in angioimmunoblastic T-cell lymphoma and peripheral T-cell lymphoma, unspecified. Am J Clin Pathol 2002;117:368–79.
338. Quintanilla-Martinez L, Fend F, Moguel LR, et al. Peripheral T-cell lymphoma with Reed–Sternberg–like cells of B-cell phenotype and genotype associated with Epstein–Barr virus infection. Am J Surg Pathol 1999;23:1233–40.
339. Patsouris E, Noel H, and Lennert K. Histological and immunohistological findings in lymphoepithelioid cell lymphoma (Lennert's lymphoma). Am J Surg Pathol 1988;12: 341–50.
340. Kim H, Jacobs C, Warnke R, et al. Malignant lymphoma with a high content of epithelioid histiocytes: a distinct clinicopathologic entity and a form of so–called "Lennert's lymphoma." Cancer 1978;41:620–35.
341. Suchi T, Lennert K, and Tu L-Y. Histopathology and immunohistochemistry of peripheral T-cell lymphomas: a proposal for their classification. J Clin Pathol 1987;40: 995–1015.
342. Rudiger T, Ichinohasama R, Ott MM, et al. Peripheral T-cell lymphoma with distinct perifollicular growth pattern: a distinct subtype of T-cell lymphoma? Am J Surg Pathol 2000;24: 117–22.
343. Coiffier B, Brousse N, Peuchmaur M, et al. Peripheral T-cell lymphomas have a worse prognosis than B-cell lymphomas: a prospective study of 361 immunophenotyped patients treated with the LNH-84 regimen. Ann Oncol 1990;1: 45–50.
344. Lippman S, Miller T, Spier C, et al. The prognostic significance of the immunotype in diffuse large-cell lymphoma: a comparative study of the T-cell and B-cell phenotype. Blood 1988;72:436–41.
345. Armitage J, Greer J, Levine A, et al. Peripheral T-cell lymphoma. Cancer 1989;63:158–63.
346. Picker L, Weiss L, Medeiros L, et al. Immunophenotypic criteria for the diagnosis of non-Hodgkin's lymphma. Am J Pathol 1987;128:181–201.
347. Stein H, Mason D, Gerdes J, et al. The expression of the Hodgkin's disease associated antigen Ki-1 in reactive and neoplastic lymphoid tissue: evidence that Reed–Sternberg cells and histiocytic malignancies are derived from activated lymphoid cells. Blood 1985;66:848–58.
348. Jaffe ES. Anaplastic large cell lymphoma: the shifting sands of diagnostic hematopathology. Mod Pathol 2001;14: 219–28.
349. Benharroch D, Meguerian-Bedoyan Z, Lamant L, et al. ALK-positive lymphoma: a single disease with a broad spectrum of morphology. Blood 1998;91:2076–84.
350. Pileri S, Falini B, Delsol G, et al. Lymphohistiocytic T-cell lymphoma (anaplastic large cell lymphoma CD30+/Ki1+) with a high content of reactive histiocytes. Histopathology 1990;16:383–91.
351. Kinney M, Collins R, Greer J, et al. A small-cell–predominant variant of primary Ki-1 (CD30)+ T-cell lymphoma. Am J Surg Pathol 1993;17:859–68.
352. Kadin ME, Sako D, Berliner N, et al. Childhood Ki-1 lymphoma presenting with skin lesions and peripheral lymphadenopathy. Blood 1986;68:1042–9.
353. Agnarsson B and Kadin M. Ki-1 positive large cell lymphoma: a morphologic and immunologic study of 19 cases. Am J Surg Pathol 1988;12:264–74.
354. Piris M, Brown D, Gatter K, et al. CD30 Expression in non-Hodgkin's lymphoma. Histopathology 1990;17: 211–8.
355. Krenacs L, Wellmann A, Sorbara L, et al. Cytotoxic cell antigen expression in anaplastic large cell lymphomas of T- and null-cell type and Hodgkin's disease: evidence for distinct cellular origin. Blood 1997;89:980–9.
356. Delsol G, Al Saati T, Gatter K, et al. Coexpression of epithelial membrane antigen (EMA), Ki-1, and interleukin-2 receptor by anaplastic large cell lymphomas: diagnostic value in so-called malignant histiocytosis. Am J Pathol 1988;130: 59–70.

357. Morris SW, Kirstein MN, Valentine MB, et al. Fusion of a kinase gene, ALK, to a nucleolar protein gene, NPM, in non-Hodgkin's lymphoma. Science 1994;263:1281–4, [erratum in Science 1995;265:316–7].
358. Pulford K, Lamant L, Morris SW, et al. Detection of anaplastic lymphoma kinase (ALK) and nucleolar protein nucleophosmin (NPM)–ALK proteins in normal and neoplastic cells with the monoclonal antibody ALK1. Blood 1997;89: 1394–1404.
359. Falini B, Pulford K, Pucciarini A, et al. Lymphomas expressing ALK fusion protein(s) other than NPM-ALK. Blood 1999;94:3509–15.
360. Shiota M, Nakamura S, Ichinohasama R, et al. Anaplastic large cell lymphomas expressing the novel chimeric protein p80NPM/ALK: a distinct clinicopathologic entity. Blood 1995;86:1954–60.
361. Falini B, Pileri S, Zinzani PL, et al. ALK+ lymphoma: clinico-pathological findings and outcome. Blood 1999;93:2697–706.
362. Gascoyne RD, Aoun P, Wu D, et al. Prognostic significance of anaplastic lymphoma kinase (ALK) protein expression in adults with anaplastic large cell lymphoma. Blood 1999;93:3913–21.
363. Lukes R, Butler J, and Hicks E. Natural history of Hodgkin's disease as related to its pathological picture. Cancer 1966;19: 317–44.
364. Kaplan HS. Hodgkin's Disease, 2nd ed. Cambridge, MA: Harvard University Press, 1980.
365. Stein H, Marafioti T, Foss HD, et al. Down-regulation of BOB.1/OBF.1 and Oct2 in classical Hodgkin disease but not in lymphocyte predominant Hodgkin disease correlates with immunoglobulin transcription. Blood 2001;97:496–501.
366. Torlakovic E, Tierens A, Dang HD, et al. The transcription factor PU.1, necessary for B-cell development is expressed in lymphocyte predominance, but not classical Hodgkin's disease. Am J Pathol 2001;159:1807–14.
367. Anagnostopoulos I, Hansmann ML, Franssila K, et al. European Task Force on Lymphoma project on lymphocyte predominance Hodgkin disease: histologic and immunohistologic analysis of submitted cases reveals 2 types of Hodgkin disease with a nodular growth pattern and abundant lymphocytes. Blood 2000;96:1889–99.
368. Hansmann M, Stein H, Fellbaum C, et al. Nodular paragranuloma can transform into high-grade malignant lymphoma of B type. Hum Pathol 1989;20:1169–75.
369. Boudova L, Torlakovic E, Delabie J, et al. Nodular lymphocyte–predominant Hodgkin lymphoma with nodules resembling T-cell/histiocyte-rich B-cell lymphoma: differential diagnosis between nodular lymphocyte–predominant Hodgkin lymphoma and T-cell/histiocyte-rich B-cell lymphoma. Blood 2003;102:3753–8.
370. Shimodaira S, Hidaka E, and Katsuyama T. Clonal identity of nodular lymphocyte–predominant Hodgkin's disease and T-cell-rich B-cell lymphoma. N Engl J Med 2000;343: 1124–5.
371. Laumen H, Nielsen PJ, and Wirth T. The BOB.1/OBF.1 co-activator is essential for octamer–dependent transcription in B cells. Eur J Immunol 2000;30:458–69.
372. Marafioti T, Hummel M, Foss HD, et al. Hodgkin and Reed–Sternberg cells represent an expansion of a single clone originating from a germinal center B-cell with functional immunoglobulin gene rearrangements but defective immunoglobulin transcription. Blood 2000;95:1443–50.
373. Brauninger A, Hansmann ML, Strickler JG, et al. Identification of common germinal-center B-cell precursors in two patients with both Hodgkin's disease and non-Hodgkin's lymphoma. N Engl J Med 1999;340:1239–47.
374. Kant JA, Hubbard SM, Longo DL, et al. The pathologic and clinical heterogeneity of lymphocyte-depleted Hodgkin's disease. J Clin Oncol 1986;4:284–94.
375. MacLennan K, Bennett M, Tu A, et al. Relationship of histopathologic features to survival and relapse in nodular sclerosing Hodgkin's disease. Cancer 1989;64:1686–93.
376. Axtell L, Myers M, Thomas L, et al. Prognostic indicators in Hodgkin's disease. Cancer 1972;29:1481–8.
377. Colby T, Hoppe R, and Warnke R. Hodgkin's disease: a clinicopathologic study of 659 cases. Cancer 1981;49:1848–58.
378. Brousset P, Chittal S, Schlaifer D, et al. Detection of Epstein–Barr virus messenger RNA in Reed–Sternberg cells of Hodgkin's disease by in situ hybridization with biotinylated probes on specially processed modified acetone methyl benzoate xylene (ModAMeX) sections. Blood 1991;77: 1781–6.
379. Weiss L, Chen Y, Liu X, et al. Epstein–Barr virus and Hodgkin's disease: a correlative in situ hybridization and polymerase chain reaction study. Am J Pathol 1991;139: 1259–65.
380. Ashton-Key M, Thorpe PA, Allen JP, et al. Follicular Hodgkin's disease. Am J Surg Pathol 1995;19:1294–9.
381. Diehl V, Sextro M, Franklin J, et al. Clinical presentation, course, and prognostic factors in lymphocyte-predominant Hodgkin's disease and lymphocyte-rich classical Hodgkin's disease: report from the European Task Force on Lymphoma Project on Lymphocyte-Predominant Hodgkin's Disease. J Clin Oncol 1999;17:776–83.
382. Uccini S, Monardo F, Stoppacciaro A, et al. High frequency of Epstein–Barr virus genome detection in Hodgkin's disease of HIV-positive patients. Int J Cancer 1990;46:581–85.
383. Kaufman D and Longo D. Hodgkin's disease. Crit Rev Oncol/Hematol 1992;13:135–87.
384. Bennett M, MacLennan K, Hudson G, et al. Non-Hodgkin's lymphoma arising in patients treated for Hodgkin's disease in the BNLI: a 20-year experience. Ann Oncol 1991;2(suppl 2):83–92.
385. Kingma DW, Medeiros LJ, Barletta J, et al. Epstein–Barr virus is infrequently identified in non-Hodgkin's lymphomas associated with Hodgkin's disease. Am J Surg Pathol 1994;18:48–61.
386. Sundeen JT, Cossman J, and Jaffe ES. Lymphocyte predominant Hodgkin's disease, nodular subtype with coexistent "large cell lymphoma." Histological progression or composite malignancy? Am J Surg Pathol 1988;12: 599–606.
387. Wickert RS, Weisenburger DD, Tierens A, et al. Clonal relationship between lymphocytic predominance Hodgkin's disease and concurrent or subsequent large-cell lymphoma of B lineage. Blood 1995;86:2312–20.
388. Greiner TC, Gascoyne RD, Anderson ME, et al. Nodular lymphocyte–predominant Hodgkin's disease associated with large-cell lymphoma: analysis of Ig gene rearrangements by V-J polymerase chain reaction. Blood 1996;88: 657–66.

2

Cytogenetic Analysis of Malignant Lymphoma

Doug Horsman, M.D.

Cytogenetic analysis has made important contributions to our understanding of the acquired genetic alterations that are associated with malignant lymphoma. The identification of chromosomal translocations that are closely associated with specific subtypes of lymphoma have been pivotal discoveries leading to the identification of gene deregulations directly involved in the pathogenesis of lymphomas and other types of cancer. Although often discredited in the molecular era for its dependency of viable tissue, low resolution and difficulty in obtaining high-quality metaphases, cytogenetic analysis has provided remarkably consistent data across institutions and countries for many types of cancer. This is reflected in the abundant published karyotype data that have been assembled in the Mitelman Database of Chromosomal Aberrations in Cancer, where lymphoma ranks second only to leukemia in the number of entries.[1]

The methodology of cancer cytogenetic analysis and the nomenclature used to describe chromosomal alterations is beyond the scope of this chapter, and the interested reader is referred to appropriate monographs for detailed information on these topics.[2,3] The terminology used in this discussion will adhere to International System for Cytogenetic Nomenclature guidelines, but will be as concise and descriptive as possible for the benefit of the nonexpert. A brief presentation of some of the technical aspects of chromosome analysis is required, however, to set the stage for the discussion to follow.

The majority of lymphoma specimens are obtained by sampling of blood, marrow, lymph node, and spleen, and will yield representative metaphases at the hands of an experienced cancer cytogenetic technologist. Biopsy specimens of nonhematopoietic tissue that are infiltrated by lymphomatous proliferations are more challenging specimens from which to obtain representative metaphases. Most lymphomas are characterized by a dominant clone, or stem line, in which all metaphases have the same or closely related chromosomal changes. Clonally related sidelines may be evident with additional changes that appear to arise through a process of sequential acquisition and clonal selection, referred to as clonal evolution. Cell-to-cell variation may be evident and extreme in some cases, rendering the definition of a distinct clone and/or sidelines difficult if not impossible. The degree of genetic instability as visualized at the cytogenetic level is quite variable within and between subtypes of lymphoma, and generally increases in parallel with the clinical progression of the disease. Despite this morphologic variability and the associated interpretive challenges, the majority of lymphomas can be shown to have clonal karyotypes when sufficient metaphases are examined, usually a minimum of 20 or more. The chromosome complement of such clones is usually in the diploid to high hyperdiploid (46 to 69) range. Stem lines and sidelines may also have polyploid chromosome complements (+/−92). In other situations, individual metaphases are abnormal, but distinct from each other, which are referred to as nonclonal changes. Occasionally, two or more apparently unrelated clones may be present. These later two situations are quite uncommon in lymphomas. The proportion of normal to abnormal metaphases identified in the analysis may reflect the degree of infiltration or the relative proliferative capacity of the malignant clone in the sampled tissue. However, this may be influenced by poorly understood in vivo and in vitro factors and may not represent a reliable prognostic factor.

A chromosomal alteration that is recurrent in multiple cases of the same subtype of lymphoma, and often seen as the sole change, is referred to as the primary chromosomal alteration, and usually are balanced translocations that are closely associated with specific types of lymphoma. The primary changes in lymphomas are most often accompanied by an assortment of secondary numerical and structural chromosome changes that vary from case to case, but when multiple cases are examined a recurrent pattern becomes apparent that is characteristic for a subtype of lymphoma. These secondary changes may be whole chromosome gains and losses, balanced translocation and inversions or unbalanced derivatives of these changes, and simple or complex deletions and duplications. Complex rearrangements may generate novel chromosomes whose makeup cannot be determined by the banding pattern, and are called marker chromosomes or unresolved chromosomal additions. While much attention has been focused on the molecular dissection of primary balanced translocations, less attention has been addressed to the numerical or unbalanced structural alterations that are associated with clonal expansion and disease progression. The ability to decipher the complexity of this information has been hampered by the lack of appropriate analytical tools to deal with multiple karyotypes and low-frequency correlation. Such analytical software is now being developed and applied, and will greatly facilitate the analysis and interpretation of this information.[4] The recent development of whole genome scanning techniques will provide much higher-resolution capability, but will generate data on an even higher order of magnitude.[5] The ability to interpret this data and integrate it with gene expression and proteomic analysis will represent an enormous challenge.

Supplemental molecular cytogenetic techniques have been developed recently that permit further refinement and resolution of cytogenetic changes. Of greatest importance is the development of fluorescent in situ hybridization (FISH) techniques that allow interrogation of specific chromosome changes with fluorescence-labeled DNA probes. Such probes are available to identify individual chromosomes, as well as locus-specific sites throughout the length of each chromosome, and are useful for enumerating chromosomal dosage changes or rearrangements within interphase nuclei from fresh or archived tumor samples, or on metaphase spreads to help determine the precise location and possible rearrangement of specific genes. Whole chromosome painting probes have been developed that render a fluorescent color to the whole length of an individual chromosome. Multicolor karyotyping allows color-coded identification of all individual chromosomes within a metaphase spread. The two available techniques, referred to as spectral karyotyping (SKY) and multicolor FISH (MFISH), vary somewhat in methodology but provide essentially the same information.[6,7] A shortcoming of these techniques is their inability to identify the origin of small segments of relocated chromosome material due to lack of a banding correlate. This is being addressed by the development of multicolor chromosome banding reagents for each individual chromosome.[8] The ultimate FISH reagent will allow simultaneous multicolor visualization of chromosome and band specific landmarks in a metaphase spread.[9,10] The combined application of fluorescent probe analysis with immunohistochemistry allows chromosome locus interrogation in parallel with identification of cellular morphologic and phenotypic features.[11]

The development and application of chromosomal genomic hybridization (CGH) represents an important technique for the assessment of dosage alterations in lymphoma and other cancers.[12] Importantly, it can be applied to fresh as well as archival specimens, overcoming the need for viable tissue samples and allowing the retrospective analysis of formalin-fixed, paraffin-embedded tissue. CGH, however, will not detect balanced rearrangements and is limited in its ability to detect deletions or duplications smaller than 10 to 15 MB in size, and requires 50% of the cell population to share the same alteration in order for it to be detected. Further development of CGH will involve the creation of arrays or matrices of small DNA targets bound to a glass slide, containing dispersed or contiguous representation of the DNA from a chromosome region or the entire genome. Whole genome arrays will provide the ultimate in level of resolution for the investigation of unbalanced chromosome alterations in constitutional or cancer cell populations.[5]

The consideration of the cytogenetic analysis of malignant lymphoma presented in this chapter will be based on the recent World Health Organization (WHO) classification of hematologic malignancies.[13] Reference to historical classifications will be made where appropriate to aid in interpretation of cytogenetic data that predate the WHO classification. Abundant use will be made of the Web-based resources of karyotype data contained in the Mitelman Database of Chromosome Aberrations in Cancer (http://cgap.nci.nih.gov/Chromosomes/Mitelman) and the Atlas of Genetics and Cytogenetics in Oncology and Haematology (http://babbage.infobiogen.fr/services/chromcancer/index.html). Historical as well as recent information based on traditional chromosome banding methods will be reviewed, with an emphasis placed on supplemental data obtained through the application of molecular cytogenetic techniques of FISH, multicolor karyotyping, and CGH. The sequence of presentation will begin with the B-cell lymphomas, followed by T-cell lymphomas and conclude with Hodgkin's disease. Within each subgroup, individual entities will be addressed in an order designed to introduce important cytogenetic alterations that are associated with specific subtypes of lymphoma but also present in a less common or secondary event in other subtypes of lymphoma. For a number of rare lymphomas included in the WHO classification where limited cytogenetic data are available, or where a relationship between specific changes and clinical features has not been established, the discussion will be minimal or omitted. Those diseases for which a lymphomatous presentation represents a minor clinical manifestation of the disease, as compared to the more common leukemic presentations, will also be omitted.

B-CELL LYMPHOMAS

Burkitt's Lymphoma

Cytogenetic data on Burkitt's leukemia/lymphoma (BL) has been accumulating since the early 1970s, reflecting the ease of obtaining high-quality metaphases from this highly proliferative B-cell lymphoma. An association with a derivative 14q+ chromosome was initially recognized in 1972,[14] which was shortly thereafter recognized to be the result of a balanced t(8;14)(q24;q32).[15] High-resolution chromosome banding refined the breakpoint locations to 8q24.13 and 14q32.33, respectively.[16] The loci disrupted at these breakpoints were determined to involve the MYC gene at 8q24 and the immunoglobulin heavy-chain gene (IGH) at 14q32.[17,18] Variant translocations were subsequently identified, implicating an IG lambda–MYC rearrangement in the t(8;22)(q24;q11)[19] and an IG kappa-MYC rearrangement in the t(2;8)(p12;q24)[20,21] (Fig. 2–1). The relative frequencies of these three translocations is 75% to 85% for the t(8;14), t(8;22) in 10% to 15%, and t(2;8) in 5% to 10%.[22] The deregulation of MYC by one or other of these translocations is generally considered synonymous for the "typical" form of BL, regardless of lymphomatous or leukemia presentation.

The t(8;14) or variant is the primary alteration associated with BL and is found in endemic, sporadic, and AIDS-associated cases. Unusual among lymphomas, up to 30% of cases show an IG-MYC translocation as the only karyotypic alteration evident at diagnosis. The use of FISH methods based on development of DNA probes specific for the participating genes has enhanced the ability to detect these translocations in a variety of clinical specimens.[23] Additional genetic mutations involving deletions and mutations of MYC regulatory elements, as well as alterations affecting other genes such as p53 and BCL6 may be necessary for the full expression of the malignant phenotype.[24] Evidence of these secondary mutations may be found in the karyotype, or may be cryptic or below the resolution level of chromosome banding. Similar to other lymphomas, an enormous amount of research has been focused on the primary rearrangement, with much less attention addressed to the role of secondary chromosomal changes in the clinical manifestations of the disease. It had been suggested in early studies, however, that these secondary changes may influence disease behavior.[25]

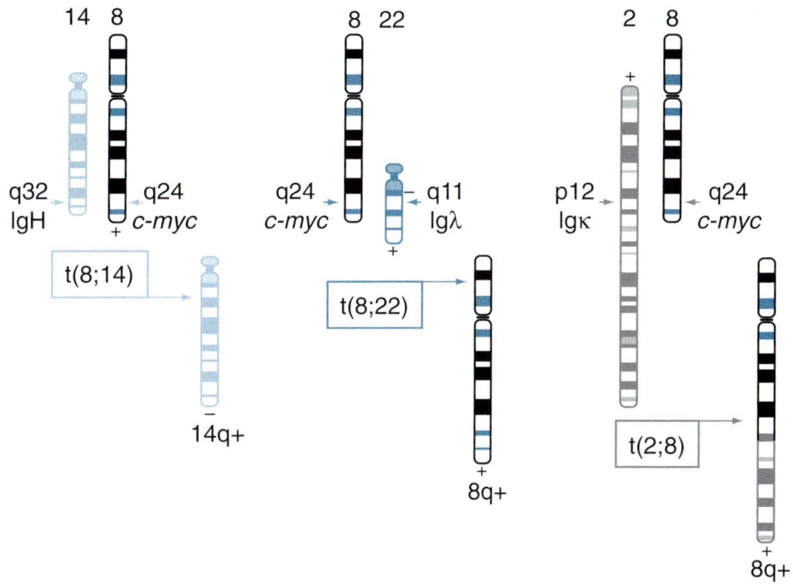

Figure 2–1. Ideogram drawing of the appearance of MYC translocations in Burkitt's lymphoma. In the classic t(8;14), the MYC gene is placed in apposition to the immunoglobulin heavy-chain locus on the derivative chromosome 14. In the variant translocations t(2;8) and t(8;22), the light-chain loci are placed in proximity to the MYC gene on the derivative chromosome 8. The orientation of the translocated segment of each derivative chromosome is denoted by an asterisk. (Adapted from Hecht JL, Aster JC. Molecular biology of Burkitt's lymphoma. J Clin Oncol 2000;18:3707–21, with permission.)

The largest review of the karyotypic changes associated with BL included a single series of 22 cases and a review of 148 published cases.[26] In this large group, the t(8;14) was present in 62% of the total cases, with t(8;22) present in 12% and t(2;8) in 9%. Five cases had normal metaphases only, and 25 did not have a "classic" translocation. The chromosomal complements of the clonal karyotypes were predominantly near-diploid, with all but two cases having 45 to 53 chromosomes. The presence of sidelines and cell-to-cell heterogeneity was uncommon, seen in seven cases only, reflecting low level of genetic instability. The most common trisomies included +7, +8, +12, and +18, and the most common monosomies included −8, −17, and −22. Recurrent structural alterations involved chromosome bands or regions 1q2, 6q11-14, and 17p1, with alterations resulting in duplication of 1q evident in 27 cases, frequently involving a breakpoint at 1q11. This review confirmed 1q alterations as the most frequent secondary change in BL, and also determined that duplication 1q and trisomy 7 were associated with a less favorable clinical outcome, and that patients with BL with variant translocations had poor survival compared to those with the more common t(8;14). In a separate study, deletion of 6q has also been identified to be a negative prognostic change.[27]

A comprehensive review of the secondary chromosomal changes found in lymphomas published prior to 1995 identified 245 published karyotypes with t(8;14) or variant.[28] This analysis determined that 71% had secondary changes (175 of 245), with an average of 3.8 additional alterations per case. Recurrent chromosomal gains and losses that were observed at the 5% or greater level included: duplication 1q (17%), +7 (13%), +12 (7%), deletion 6q (7%), and +3 (6%). Recurrent breakpoints associated with structural alterations involved 1q32 (11%), 1q21 (10%), 14q32 (9%), 1q12 (6%), and 18q21 (5%). The involvement of 14q32 exclusive of its role in t(8;14) most often represented the presence of a t(3;14)(q27;q32), or a t(14;18)(q32;q21) in combination with t(8;14) in an unusual variant of aggressive BL or transformed follicular lymphoma (see Follicular Lymphoma section, aggressive transformation). From this analysis there did not appear to be any difference in the pattern of secondary changes associated with t(8;14) versus the variant translocations. This analysis does not take into consideration the chromosomal regions participating in marker chromosomes or chromosome additions, which would not be possible without enhanced multicolor karyotyping or CGH. Currently, there is no substantial MFISH or SKY data available for BL, other than a few single case reports.

A single large series of BL cases has been studied by CGH, including 46 cases investigated with a combination of G-banding and chromosomal CGH.[29] This revealed the most frequent gains to be duplication of 12q (26%), Xq (22%), 22q (17%), and 9q (15%), and the most frequent sites of deletion to be 13q (17%) and 4q (9%). High-level amplifications were identified at 1q23-1q31 (three cases), and 6p12-p25 and 8p22-p23 in one case each. The study also determined that leukemic BL had more chromosomal changes per case than nodal BL (4.3 vs. 2.7). Structural alterations and duplications of 1q and 7q were associated with a shorter survival, thus confirming previous findings based purely on banding data.[26] The increased frequency and different pattern of secondary alteration seen by CGH possibly indicates the presence of major undisclosed sidelines as well as incorporation of the content of markers and additions into the gain–loss profiles, thus providing more comprehensive dosage data than is possible with standard chromosome banding techniques. The identification of high-level amplifications also indicates an additional mechanism of dosage alteration and genome instability in this disease.

The t(8;14) in AIDS-associated BL has been shown at the molecular level to be similar to endemic BL.[30,31] Variant translocations are seen at a higher frequency than in sporadic BL, especially t(8;22). Duplication of 1q is again seen as the most common secondary alteration, and trisomy 12 may be more frequent in AIDS-associated BL than in sporadic BL.[26,32]

Follicular Lymphoma

Abundant cytogenetic information is available on the chromosomal alterations associated with follicular lymphoma (FL), being one of the most frequent lymphomas represented in the Mitelman database.[1] FL is characterized by the t(14;18) in a majority of cases, and although this translocation is seen in other subtypes of malignant lymphoma its close association with FL has rendered it synonymous with this disease. The t(14;18) was first recognized in 1979.[33] The breakpoints on the derivative chromosomes were shown by high-resolution chromosome banding to involve 14q32.3 and 18q21.1 involving the immunoglobulin heavy-chain gene (IGH) and BCL2 gene, respectively.[34] The resulting IGH–BCL2 fusion on the derivative 14 chromosome represents the primary deregulation associated with this disease, resulting in BCL2 deregulation through proximity to the IGH enhancer element.[35] Variant translocations t(2;18) and t(8;22) in which kappa and lambda, respectively, are rearranged with BCL2 may account for 5% to 10% of cases.[22] The development of FISH probes that specifically target IGH and BCL2 have assisted in the assembly of accurate frequency data and confirmation of the true incidence of t(14;18)-negative FL.

The frequency with which the t(14;18) is found in FL varies considerably from study to study, and may be influenced by geography as well as variation in case selection and the methodology used to detect the translocation. In North America, a frequency of 80% to 90% is observed,[36,37] which is consistently higher than in European centers where it is reported in 70% to 80% of cases,[38] while the lowest frequency is reported in Asia at 40% to 60%.[39,40] In Europe and North America, when defined by uniform diagnostic criteria such as the WHO classification, and where karyotype and FISH analyses are used to provide objective evidence of the t(14;18) or variant, the incidence is probably close to 90%.[36,37,41–43]

The t(14;18) is considered to be the primary genetic alteration associated with FL. Deregulation of BCL2 alone, however, is insufficient to produce clinical disease. Experiments in model systems have shown that additional mutations are required to achieve the fully malignant phenotype.[44] This multistep pathogenesis is reflected clinically by the presence of secondary chromosomal alterations in the great majority of cases studied at diagnosis and during disease progression.[42] In fact, all cases of FL are associated with karyotypic alterations[45] with 5% to 10% having the t(14;18) as the sole alteration.[22,46] Cases of FL without secondary changes are confined mainly to morphologic Grades 1 and 2; however, the disease course in such cases may be similar to those with overt secondary changes, implying that cryptic mutations must be present in these simple karyotypes.

The pattern of secondary chromosomal changes associated with FL at diagnosis has been thoroughly defined. A comprehensive review of the secondary chromosomal changes associated with FL based on published karyotypes available up to 1995 has been reported.[42] In addition, a compilation of the secondary alterations associated with low- and intermediate-grade lymphomas bearing a t(14;18) has been extracted from all published karyotypes in the Mitelman Database.[28] These data have shown that the number of secondary changes average 5.6 per karyotype. With all grades combined, the most common secondary alterations were: +7 (24%), +X (15%), +12 (17%), deletion 6q13-q26 (16%), +18 or +der(18) (10 and 8%), and i(17q) (7%). A representative G-banded karyotype of FL is shown in Fig. 2–2. These recurrent chromosomal participants in the clonal evolution of FL have been confirmed in a number of recent large single-institution studies, with some variation in the frequency of individual chromosome involvement, largely due to the inclusion or exclusion of cases without the t(14;18).[45,46] The significance of this factor varies with the frequency of t(14;18)-negative cases in different studies, and has recently been the focus of a number of studies addressing the low frequency of t(14;18) seen in Grade 3 disease, with the observation that different clinical and cytogenetic features are associated with t(14;18)-negative FL.[47–50] At the cytogenetic level, two subtypes of t(14;18)-negative FL may exist, one group without the translocation that shows evidence of bcl2 over-expression and another group that is both translocation and bcl2 negative. The latter group is characterized by a different pattern of secondary chromosomal alterations, including frequent BCL6 rearrangements and more complex karyotypes, but may be associated with a superior prognosis. In contrast, in the t(14;18)-negative but bcl2-positive cases, bcl2 is apparently deregulated through alternative mechanisms such as increased dosage.

Further resolution of the cytogenetic changes associated with FL has been obtained by CGH and multicolor karyotyping. Three large CGH studies have assessed the chromosomal dosage alterations in FL at presentation.[51–53] In aggregate, these studies have identified dosage alterations in up to 80% of cases, with gains being twice as common as losses, in a pattern very reminiscent of karyotype data. In addition, the CGH studies have helped to better define the minimal regions affected by segmental duplication and deletions, and have identified high-level amplifications that appear to involve diverse loci and to be patient specific. The application of MFISH to a large group of FL selected for

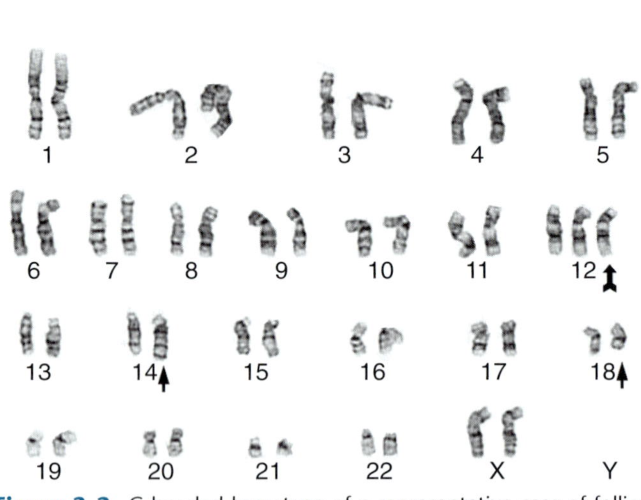

Figure 2–2. G-banded karyotype of a representative case of follicular lymphoma with a single secondary chromosomal alteration involving +12. The *arrowheads* indicate the derivative 14 and derivative 18 chromosomes. The *arrow* indicates the secondary trisomy for chromosome 12.

study based on the presence of unresolved markers and additions confirmed that the chromosomal content of these structural alterations could be further identified, although precise regional identification of involved chromosomal segments may require additional FISH analysis with locus-specific probes or multicolor fluorescent banding probes.[54,55] This study showed a higher frequency of alterations compared to that seen by regular karyotyping, mostly affecting 1p36, 3q27-q29, 12q, 17q, +18/18q+, and +21. The use of the SKY technique on a group of FL cases has also highlighted the recurrent alterations involving loss or rearrangement of 1p36, deletion 6q, +7, +12, duplication or triplication of 12q13-q22, +der(18), and +21.[56]

The sequence of development of secondary chromosomal alterations in FL is poorly understood. Alterations seen as the sole event in addition to the t(14;18) include +der(18), +7, deletion of 6q and 1p, and rearrangement of 3q27.[46] The number of abnormalities, the frequency of alterations such as deletion of 1p36 and 6q, +7, and +der(18), and overall karyotypic complexity increase with disease grade. A computation analysis of 350 published karyotypes at diagnosis has defined a number of distinct pathways of preclinical clonal evolution characterized by +7/+8, +18/18q+/+der(18), +1q, or 6q−. These pathways merge into a common set of deletions that appear to accumulate at a later stage of clonal expansion.[57] A correlation between these distinct pathways and different clinical behaviors was not shown. Whether the post-diagnosis karyotype acquisitions follow these same pathways requires confirmation by multiple time-point studies during the clinical evolution of the disease.

The majority of FL, between 25% and 60%, will eventually transform to more aggressive lymphoma, which is associated with more rapid progression, increase in clinical symptoms, and eventual fatal outcome.[58] Most FL transformations result in the development of diffuse large B-cell lymphoma (DLBCL). An uncommon form of transformation that is more dramatic and with dire clinical consequences involves the acquisition of a secondary t(8;14) or variant Burkitt-type translocation.[59,60] This event is characterized by the development of an aggressive-morphology "blastic" lymphoma that is unresponsive to standard chemotherapy and marrow transplantation. The genetic mechanisms that underlie the more common DLBCL form of transformation event appear to be heterogeneous. Numerous studies have examined the role of secondary chromosomal alterations in the transformation to DLBCL, but only a few of these have been based on documentation of serial karyotypes obtained during disease evolution from indolent to transformed stage.[61,62] The number and type of chromosomal alterations present at diagnosis may be associated with an increased risk for or the occurrence of transformation. These include +7, deletion of 6q23-q26 and 17p, and duplication of 12q.[45,63–67] CGH has also been used to address the issue of FL transformation, assessing paired samples prior to and after transformation to DLBCL.[68,69] These studies have found the standard assortment of secondary changes plus a recurring theme of high-level amplification, often involving 2p13-p16 containing REL/BCL11A. A combined array CGH and gene expression study using a commercial array with 2400 dispersed DNA targets was used to assess pre- and post-transformation specimens.[70] This revealed a variable spectrum of genomic imbalances with over- and under-expression of a large variety of genes, suggesting that a combination of different genetic alterations may be involved. Clearly, the process of FL transformation to DLBCL is a complex phenomenon that will require a combination of gene dosage and expression analyses to enhance our understanding of the process.

The demonstration of a correlation between the occurrence of specific secondary chromosomal alterations in FL and disease prognosis has been elusive. Much of the information overlaps with the propensity to transform, as discussed above. An early analysis indicated that a poor prognosis was associated with duplication of 2p, deletion of 13q32, and the presence of gene amplification.[36] Subsequent studies have not confirmed these findings but have identified other possible associations. The absence of residual normal metaphases, a higher complexity of karyotypes, and deletion of 1p32-36, 6q23-q26, and 17p, have all been linked with shorter survival in one or more studies.[45,71–75] Deletion 1p36 and duplication of 18q have also been shown to correlate with outcome in a group of cases selected for complex karyotypes with markers chromosomes and additions resolved by MFISH.[54] A relationship between extra copies of 12q and outcome has also been identified.[57,76] Further data on the relationship between specific chromosomal alterations and clinical features and outcome of FL will be required to resolve the discrepancies between these numerous studies.

Diffuse Large B-Cell Lymphoma

Diffuse large B-cell lymphoma (DLBC) is a subtype of malignant lymphoma that is heterogeneous at the clinical, morphologic, and genetic level. It includes a number of morphologic variants including centroblastic, immunoblastic, plasmablastic, T-cell/histiocyte-rich, and anaplastic types. In addition, the initial presentation may be de novo or represent transformation from a preexisting indolent lymphoproliferative disorder.[77] A disease-specific primary chromosomal alteration has not been associated with DLBCL. A number of genetic subtypes having translocations such as t(3;14), t(8;14), and t(14;18) are frequently encountered; however, their principal association is with other subtypes of lymphoma, and their occurrence in DLBCL may represent either de novo or transformed disease. Although abundant karyotypic data are available on this disease and a great variety of chromosomal alterations have been identified,[1] detailed analysis of this data is challenged by the diversity of subtypes and presentations of DLBCL.

Until recently, most reports of DLBCL karyotypes have come from large, single-institution series that have combined data from a variety of low, intermediate-, and high-grade lymphomas, based on a variety of different classification systems, and included data from diagnostic, progressed, and post-treatment specimens, including both B-cell and T-cell subtypes. A review of the published data available as of 1998 determined that the most common alterations in DLBCL, present in more than 10% of patients, involve structural changes affecting chromosome or chromosome arm 1, 2p, 3, 5, 6q, 9, 14q, 17, and 18q, with numerical abnormalities such as +X, +3, +5, +6, +7, +12, −17, +18, and +21, and a number of recurrent translocations, primarily t(3;14), t(8;14), and t(14;18).[78] Recurrent alterations that have been shown to be of negative prognostic significance include breaks at 1p32-p36 and 1q21-q23, and deletion of 6q21-q25 and 17p, as well as high karyotypic complexity. Although these data provide an overall picture of the pattern of chromosome changes in DLBCL, they do not give a clear picture of what karyotype changes are associated with the currently recognized morphologic subtypes of DLBCL.

A recent large cytogenetic study that addressed DLBCL as a single entity based on the REAL classification, considered 215 abnormal karyotypes, of which 140 were obtained at diagnosis and 75 post-therapy.[273] The treated group showed a significantly higher frequency of alterations affecting chromosomes 7, 3q27, 1q25, 6p23, and 19q13 compared to the untreated group; however, the data from the two groups were combined as a significant difference in the overall pattern or frequency of changes between the two groups could not be detected. A specific primary change was not found in this group of cases. Only 15% of the karyo-types showed a single abnormality, of which only dup(1)(q21q32), t(8;14), and t(14;18) occurred in more than one instance. Hyperdiploidy was found in 72% of cases. The most common whole chromosome gains or losses were +7 and +12 (17%), +X (13%), −X, −6 and +11 (11%), −Y, and +3 and +18 (10%). Deletions most commonly affected chromosomes 1, 3, 6, and 7, with 36 instances of regional 6q deletion affecting 6q23-q24 (31%), 6q21 (29%), and 6q15 (22%). A total of 1021 breakpoints were identified involving 174 distinct chromosome bands; however, only 10 of these comprised 35% of all breakpoints. The most frequent breakpoint was at 14q32, accounting for 10% of breakpoints and present in 50% of karyotypes. A diversity of other breakpoint sites were found, but only those affecting 1p36, 1p22, 1q21, 3p21, 3q27, 6q21, 8q24, 18q21, and 22q11 were seen in more than 2% of cases. The frequent14q32 rearrangements mostly represented translocations t(3;14), t(8;14), or t(14;18). A number of novel recurrent translocations such as t(1;19)(q21;q13), t(1;6)(q21;q21), and t(10;12)(q24;q22) were found. Interestingly, the presence of any rearrangement of 14q32 was significantly associated with the presence of additional balanced translocations, whereas the absence of a 14q32 rearrangement was associated with unbalanced deletions and or duplications. A hypermutation mechanism has been identified that may underlie the propensity for the development and association of chromosomal translocations in certain subtypes of B-cell lymphoma.[79] This important study has thus confirmed a number of previously established as well as novel nonrandom cytogenetic associations in DLBCL and represents an important contribution to the standard chromosome banding information available for this disease.

CGH analysis has contributed further insight into the chromosomal changes associated with DLBCL. A number of small series, ranging from 9 to 54 cases, including diagnostic as well as recurrent post-therapy lymphomas, have been published.[80–84] Abnormal dosage changes were found generally in 80% to 90% of cases, with a higher frequency and greater randomness of changes seen in the post-therapy specimens. These studies have shown a strong correlation with the pattern of gains and losses detected by standard karyotype analysis but with a higher frequency of events, due to the incorporation of the dosage alterations within marker chromosomes and additions into the CGH profiles. The findings were generally similar between studies, with minor differences most likely due to variability in case selection and the small size of the studies.

The most significant finding in the CGH studies of DLBCL was the identification of recurrent high-level amplifications in 10% to 20% of cases. Chromosomal evidence of gene amplification in the form of double minute (dmin) chromosomes and homogeneously stained regions (hsr) are uncommon in lymphoma. A CGH investigation of a DLBCL with dmin chromosomes revealed high-level amplification of the REL gene located at 2p23-p25.[85] Further investigations of REL in a large series of cases confirmed its amplification 23% of cases, of which 19 were primary extranodal cases of DLBCL.[83] The cases with REL amplification also showed other chromosome changes that are associated with disease progression. These high-level amplifications have been identified at a wide variety of other chromosomal sites by different investigators.[82–84] The common amplified regions in these studies include REL, MYC, MDM2, and BCL2. A recent array CGH study using 496 dispersed gene targets identified 15 different high-level amplifications in 10 of 16 samples, including BCL2, REL, CCND1, CCND2, JAK2, FGF4, and MDM2.[86] Four of these 15 amplicons were not detected by concurrent chromosomal CGH, indicating that high-level amplification may be more frequent and involve more regions than previously demonstrated, and that higher-resolution platforms are required to thoroughly assess the role of this phenomenon in DLBCL.

A number of enhanced cytogenetic studies of DLBCL using multicolor karyotyping techniques have been reported.[56,87,88] These investigations have shown a much higher level of karyotype complexity than revealed by standard banding analysis. One study of 46 cases found 295 chromosomal breaks detected by G banding, as compared to 551 breaks revealed by SKY analysis.[87] Many of the derivative and marker chromosomes contained material derived from multiple sources. A representative MFISH karyotype of a case of DLBCL is shown in Fig. 2–3. Novel recurrent breakpoints and regions of gain and loss, as well as new translocations were identified, including der(14)t(3;14)(q21;q32), t(1;13)(p32;q14), t(1;7)(q21;q22), and der(6)t(6;8)(q11;q11). This higher-resolution analysis was able to confirm a correlation of recurring breakpoint sites with clinical features, including an association of 7q11 with female sex 3p21 with male sex, and 2q31, 3q27, and 7q22 with advanced disease and poor outcome, of which 2q31 and 7q22 had not previously been described. A higher frequency of translocations involving B-cell lymphoma-associated genes other than BCL2 and BCL6 has also been demonstrated.[88] Combined with the CGH studies, these findings confirm a "picture of impressive genetic instability of DLBCL at the cytogenetic level,"[87] and highlight the insufficiency of standard chromosome banding methods to reveal the karyotypic complexity associated with this disease. This observation in DLBCL may in part account for the inconsistency in the literature as to the pattern of chromosomal changes. It is clear that the cytogenetic analysis of malignant lymphomas will have

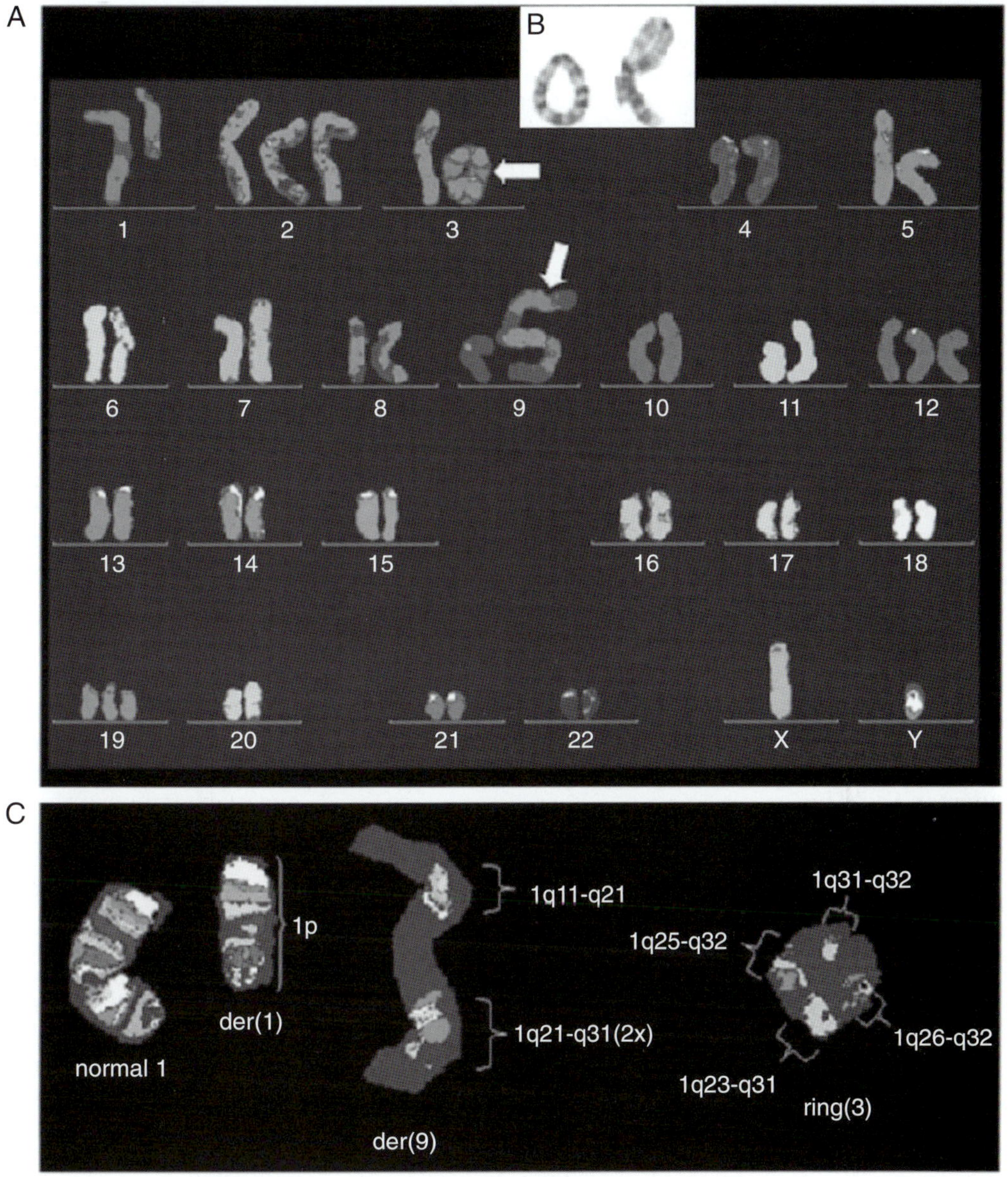

Figure 2–3. Multicolor karyotype (MFISH) of a representative case of diffuse, large B-cell lymphoma. **A:** The karyotype reveals a deletion of the q arm of chromosome 1, trisomy for chromosomes 2, 12, and 19, and two complex rearrangements (*white arrows*) representing a large-ring chromosome 3 composed of alternating segments of material from chromosome 1 and chromosome 3, and a large derivative chromosome 9 composed of alternating segments of material from chromosomes 1, 3, and 9. **B:** G-banded image of ring (3) and der (9). **C:** Multicolor banding pattern of the chromosome 1 segments of der (1), der (9), and ring (3). Normal chromosome 1 is shown on the left. (See color insert.)

to be revisited using these modern molecular cytogenetic techniques.

Although a specific primary genetic event has not been associated with DLBCL, there are a number of genetic subtypes characterized by the presence of the t(14;18), t(3;14), or t(8;14), and related variant translocations. The t(14;18) is seen in 20% to 25% of DLBCL.[22,89–91] A portion of these cases represents transformation from a previous FL, whereas another group represents true de novo presentation without evidence of antecedent lymphoma. Although BCL2 deregulation by an IG translocation is well recognized as a genetic mutation associated with bcl2 over-expression, it has become evident that bcl2 over-expression may result from a variety of mechanisms, including chromosomal dosage gains or amplification of BCL2.[92] Bcl2 over-expression in these cases is associated with a poor prognosis, whereas BCL2 deregulation via a t(14;18) may not be.[90,93–97] The occurrence of t(14;18) within reactive tissues, tonsils, and spleens has been identified.[98,99] These clones may persist and undergo clonal expansion.[100] It is possible that the development of FL and DLBCL may originate from this resource of mutated B-cells through accumulation of critical secondary mutations. Alternatively, such cells may become involved in clonal expansion through a bystander phenomenon, due to their relatively high frequency within the lymphocyte compartment. In this regard, a different gene expression profile has been shown for t(14;18)-positive DLBCL that arises from FL transformation, as compared to de novo t(14;18)-positive DLBCL,[93] which may in part explain the disparate clinical outcomes associated with various mechanisms of BCL2 deregulation.

The t(3;14) or variant translocations involving IGK and IGL may be found in 30% to 35% of DBLCL.[22,101,102] Multiple other partner chromosomes are also involved in translocations with BCL6. In all cases, deregulation is the result of promoter substitution leading to deregulated expression of the bcl6 protein product. BCL6 translocation may be the sole event in rare cases, indicating that it may represent a primary event giving rise to lymphoma, but it is most commonly found in association with other secondary chromosomal changes. These secondary changes are typical of those that accompany other germinal center–derived B-cell lymphomas. The involvement of BCL6 in translocations or rearrangements involving non-IG sites is a frequent occurrence. Complex rearrangements as well as deletions, additions, insertions, and inversions have been described. The use of FISH probes has enhanced the ability to detect and confirm such heterogeneous 3q27 rearrangements, expanding the number of partner chromosomes and involved genes.[103–105] A list of identified rearrangements of 3q27 and BCL6 is provided in Table 2–1.

The prognostic significance of a BCL6 rearrangement in DLBCL remains under investigation. It has been suggested that BCL6 rearrangements in general may be associated with more favorable outcomes, although this has not been confirmed in other studies.[106] The influence of BCL6 rearrangements may be complicated by mechanistic factors, such as whether non-IG BCL6 translocations have a worse prognostic implication than IG-BCL6 translocations.[107] Further studies are required to resolve this issue; however, the importance of 3q27 and BCL6 in DLBCL is underscored by the sheer frequency of its association with this disease, being the most common recurrent genetic alteration, found in up to 50% of cases. The heterogeneous mechanisms of BCL6 deregulation make this the most common mutation target in DLBCL.

The t(8;14) is rarely found in typical DLBCL. Given its close connection with the morphologic and clinical features of Burkitt's lymphoma, an apparent association with the DLBCL may be questioned. Although the involvement of 8q24 may be identified at the cytogenetic level as a translocation or other rearrangement, at the molecular level it may not actually involve the MYC gene, and may be implicated in the deregulation of other genes in the 8q24 neighborhood.[108]

Despite the large volume of cytogenetic data available on DLBCL, interpretation of the clinical implications of this information represents an unresolved challenge. Some resolution may be possible through new opportunities to subcategorize DLBCL by gene expression analysis, which has already identified two major subtypes with germinal center B-cell or activated B-cell gene expression signatures.[109] Correlation of chromosomal alterations with these gene expression profiles may provide new insights into the relationship between specific chromosome alterations and specific subtypes of this disease.[93]

Intravascular Lymphoma

Intravascular lymphoma (IVL) is a rare form of diffuse lymphoma characterized by the presence of focal aggregates of malignant lymphoid cells within vascular lumen.[110] Up to 90% of cases are of B-cell origin, with rare cases of T-cell derivation. An "Asian" variant of IVL has been described characterized by hemophagocytosis and hepatosplenomegaly, but absence of skin and neurologic signs and frequent bone marrow involvement.[111] Karyotypic data on intravascular lymphoma are rare, largely because the diagnosis may not be suspected at the time of tissue sampling. However, a number of cases have been successfully karyotyped from blood and marrow samples, and often show complex chromosomal alterations.[110,112,113] Most of these karyotypes represent the "Asian" variety of IVL. A review of the published cases did not reveal any recurrent primary alterations or breakpoint sites involving immunoglobulin genes or known lymphoma-specific genes.[113] Recurrent secondary alterations were predominantly dosage alterations, most frequently involving monosomy 6 or deletion 6q (59% of cases) and trisomy 18 or duplication of 18q (41% of cases). The commonly deleted region of 6q was 6q21-q23, similar to DLBCL. Duplication of 18q may include amplification of a region including 18q21, possibly implicating BCL2 or other genes located in this region.[82,113] Bcl2 overexpression has been demonstrated in up to half of studied cases. A distinctive pattern of karyotypic alterations associated with the Asian variant has been suggested but additional data will be necessary to confirm this observation.[114] In general, the karyotypic alterations found in this rare form of lymphoma are highly reminiscent of those associated with DLBCL.

Table 2–1. BCL6 Translocations with Confirmed Partner Genes*

Translocation	Gene Fusion	Reference
t(2;3)(p12;q27)	*BCL6/IGK*	Ohshima et al, Leuk Lymphoma 1997;27:329–334
t(3;4)(q27;p13)	*BCL6/RHOH*	Chen et al, Blood 1998;91:603–607
t(3;6)(q27;p21)	*BCL6/PIM1*	Kaneita et al, Br J Haematol 2001;113:803–806
t(3;6)(q27;p21)	*BCL6/SFRS3*	Chen et al, Genes Chromosomes Cancer 2001;32:281–284
t(3;6)(q27;p21)	*BCL6/HIST1H4I*	Akasaka et al, Cancer Res 1997;57:7–12
t(3;7)(q27;p11-13)	*BCL6/ZNFN1A1*	Hosokawa et al, Blood 2000;95:2719–2721
t(3;11)(q27;q23)	*BCL6/POU2AF1*	Galiegue-Zouitina et al, Leukemia 1996;10:579–587
t(3;12)(q27;p13)	*BCL6/GAPD*	Montesinos-Rongen et al, Brain Pathol 2003;13:534–538,
t(3;13)(q27;q14)	*BCL6/LCP1*	Galiegue-Zouitina et al, Genes Chromosomes Cancer 1999;26:97–105
t(3;14)(q27;q32)	*BCL6/IGH*	Baron et al, Proc Natl Acad Sci USA 1993;90:5262–5266
t(3;14)(q27;q32)	*BCL6/HSPCA*	Montesinos-Rongen et al, Brain Pathol 2003;13:534–538
t(3;16)(q27;p11)	*BCL6/IL21R*	Ueda et al, Oncogene 2002;21:368–376
t(3;16)(q27;p13)	*BCL6/MHC2TA*	Kaneita et al, Br J Haematol 2001;113:803–806
t(3;22)(q27;q11)	*BCL6/IGL*	Baron et al, Proc Natl Acad Sci USA 1993;90:5262–5266

*Compiled from Mitelman Database of Chromosome Aberrations in Cancer http://cgap.nci.nih.gov/Chromosomes/Mitelman.

Primary CNS Lymphomas

Primary central nervous system lymphomas (PCSNLs) represent a clinical variant of DLBCL. Very few cytogenetic studies of this type of lymphoma have been reported.[115] The largest amount of information has come from CGH studies.[116–118] Eight cases studied by this technique revealed copy number changes in all cases. The most frequent changes were +12 (63%), +18 (50%), +20q (38%), and deletion of 6q (75%). Deletion 6q is seen at a higher frequency than in systemic DLBCL, suggesting that loss of 6q may be implicated in development of DLBCL in immunologically sequestrated sites.[118,119]

Primary Mediastinal B-Cell Lymphoma

Primary mediastinal B-cell lymphoma (PMBCL) is a rare form of lymphoma that is considered separate from DLBCL based on distinctive clinical features. It presents preferentially in young adults as a bulky mediastinal mass with frequent extrathoracic extension.[120] The malignant cells have a characteristic immunophenotypic profile and are considered to arise from thymic B-cells. Karyotypic information is extremely limited, largely due to the difficulty in obtaining tissue samples. Most of the information on chromosomal alterations in PMBCL has come from CGH and molecular methods targeting specific genes. CGH analysis of 26 cases has revealed chromosomal gains to be much more frequent than losses (110 vs. 10), involving chromosome arm 9p, Xq, and all of chromosome 12.[121] A number of high-level amplifications were also seen, involving REL at 2p13 in two cases. A second CGH study investigated 43 cases, and also showed gains of 9p and Xq in 56% and 40% of cases, respectively.[122] Supplemental locus-specific FISH showed a higher involvement of these two chromosomes, which were both involved in more than 70% of cases. A molecular approach using arbitrary primed PCR has shown a similar pattern of chromosomal changes but involving a larger number of chromosome regions, including X, 2, 5, 7, 9p, and 12 in more than 50% of cases, with a higher frequency of imbalances per case than detected by CGH.[123] Array-based allelotyping has also shown genomic imbalances involving 6p and 9p.[124] Thus, despite a lack of standard karyotype data, a highly characteristic pattern of chromosomal imbalances has been detected in this disease by molecular cytogenetic studies. Duplication or amplification of 9p appears to be the most frequent alteration associated with this disease and may represent a disease-specific alteration. The characteristic combination of Xq and 9p amplification is distinct from other B-cell lymphomas, suggesting a unique pathway of genetic changes associated with PMBCL.

Mantle Cell Lymphoma

Mantle cell lymphoma (MCL) is a subtype of lymphoma characterized by distinctive primary as well as secondary cytogenetic alterations. Virtually all cases in which a clonal karyotype is obtained will show the t(11;14)(p13;q32), which is the primary genetic alteration associated with this neoplasm, first described in 1979.[21] The close association of this translocation with MCL has become more firmly established as the disease profile has been more precisely defined by consensus morphologic and immunophenotypic criteria. The supplemental use of FISH analysis with locus-specific probes for the IGH and BCL1 genes has verified the high frequency of t(11;14) in MCL.[125,126] Unlike FL and BL, variant translocations involving the immunoglobulin light-chain genes are particularly rare, with only two cases of t(11;22)(q13;q11) involving IG lambda having been described.[127,128] A small number of cases do not show the characteristic t(11;14), due to "masking" of the typical features of the der(14) or der(11) by secondary changes, or because of cryptic insertion of BCL1 gene into the IGH locus.[129–131] However, the existence of a true t(11;14)-negative MCL variant has been confirmed to occur in up to 10% of cases by gene expression studies. These atypical cases do not have cyclin D1 over-expression or IGH-BCL1 translocations, but do show other gene expression patterns typical of this lymphoma.[132,133] It may be that other cyclin genes are deregulated in these cases, producing a phenocopy neoplasm that has the usual secondary genetic alterations associated with standard MCL.

In vitro culture of MCL tissue has not yielded good-quality karyotype data. Generally, the cell samples grow poorly with use of standard culture procedures, and though a majority may yield a clonal karyotype, the metaphases are often few and of inferior morphology. Consequently, the cytogenetic data are compromised by the poor quality of the karyotypes. A small minority reveal an isolated t(11;14); however, these cases most likely harbor subcytogenetic alterations at critical loci required for clonal expansion and clinical manifestation of the disease, as it has been demonstrated that the t(11;14) alone is insufficient to generate a fully malignant clonal proliferation.[134]

The great majority of MCLs show secondary chromosomal alterations, the spectrum of which include alterations common to other types of B-cell lymphoma, but a number of specific features render an overall profile of gains and losses that is quite characteristic for MCL. Prior to 1995, only small series of cases of MCL had been reported, either as a component of larger groups of malignant lymphoma karyotypes or in small disease-specific studies. The cytogenetic features of all published cases with the t(11;14) were reviewed in 1995.[28] This analysis revealed that recurrent alterations occurred in more than 10% of cases, and most commonly involved −Y, +3, deletion of 6q and −13, with recurrent breakpoints at 6p31, 6q21, 8q24, and 13q14. An increased number and complexity of secondary alterations have been directly correlated with higher-grade or aggressive disease.[135,136] This is particularly apparent in the blastoid variants, which are frequently associated with complex and polyploid karyotypes.[137]

Since 1995, a number of large studies have focused on the cytogenetic characteristics of MCL, and have been reviewed by Au et al.[138] These studies have confirmed the profile of secondary alterations characteristic of MCL to include deletion of 1p13, 6q, 8p, 9p, 10q, 11q, 13q, and 17p, and duplication of 3q and 12q. The frequent duplications at 3q27 and 12q represent the only recurring dosage gains associated with this disease, both of which are associated with higher-grade disease and poor outcome. The 3q site may implicate a gene other than BCL6, as amplifications and rearrangements of this gene have not been demonstrated in MCL. In contrast, deletions are much more common in MCL and involve a number of sites that are also implicated in other subtypes of B-cell lymphoma, such as 6q, 9p, 11q24, 13q, and 17p.

FISH analysis using probes specific for t(11;14) have important clinical utility for the differential diagnosis of MCL. The highly specific association of the t(11;14) with MCL is of practical value in distinguishing MCL from atypical chronic lymphocytic leukemia, and to distinguish prolymphocytic leukemia from the blastoid variant of MCL.[129–131,139] A representative image of locus-specific FISH probes applied to a case of MCL is shown in Fig. 2–4. A number of studies have used FISH analysis to further interrogate the sites of recurrent gain or loss.[135,136,138,140–142] These FISH investigations have revealed a higher incidence of these secondary alterations compared to what is detected by standard cytogenetic analysis, indicating the presence of small deletions and duplications not identifiable or overlooked by metaphase analysis, or exposing the unresolved duplications present in the frequently additions and marker chromosomes.

An unusual feature of MCL is the rarity of balanced translocations other than t(11;14). In other subtypes of lymphoma, it is common to find secondary balanced translocations involving the immunoglobulin genes or other recombinations. The lack of such translocations may indicate a different form of genetic instability than what is associated with DLBCL, BL, and FL.[79] However, the incidence of such translocations may be underreported due to the poor karyotype quality that is typical of this disease.

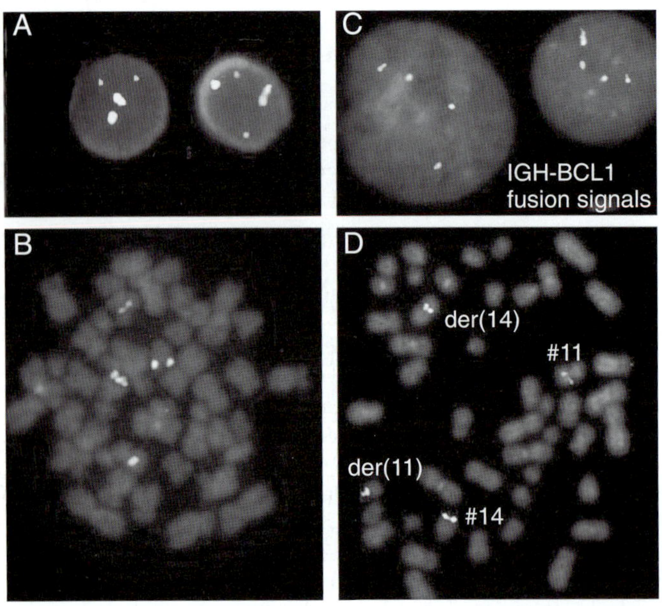

Figure 2–4. Locus-specific FISH images of a representative case of mantle cell lymphoma obtained with a commercial Vysis LSI IGH/BCL1 dual-color, dual-fusion translocation probe. The normal pattern of two BCL1 (red) and two IGH (green) signals are evident in **(A)**, an interphase nucleus, and **(B)**, a metaphase. An abnormal pattern of one BCL1 signal (red), one IGH signal (green), and two IGH-BCL1 fusion signals are evident in **(C)**, an interphase nucleus, and **(D)**, in a metaphase containing the t(11;14) of MCL (normal and derivative chromosomes indicated with *white lettering*). (See color insert.)

Further insight into this finding may be provided in the future by multicolor karyotyping, as cryptic balanced rearrangement may be disguised in the many markers and chromosomal additions. Such enhanced karyotype data have not yet been reported for MCL.

A number of clinical and morphologic variants of MCL are recognized, including a leukemic and a blastoid form of the disease. The few cases of leukemic MCL for which karyotype information is available suggest that there are differences from standard MCL in the pattern of secondary changes, most consistently involving an increased frequency of deletion of 17p, possibly implicating p53 loss or mutation.[143–145] The blastoid variant of MCL may have a de novo presentation (20%) or develop as a transformation event (35%).[146] The blastoid variants have different chromosome changes than standard MCL, characterized by a high proportion of polyploid clones, up to 36% in the classic blastoid variant and 80% in the pleomorphic variant.[147,148] Alterations affecting 8q24 have also been described, including t(8;14), t(2;8), and other translocation partners.[149] Studies assessing the involvement of MYC in these MCL-related 8q24 rearrangements have given inconsistent results, suggesting that MYC deregulation may not be directly involved in these rearrangements.[137,143,149–151] Gene expression studies have indicated that alteration of specific cell-cycle control genes may define blastoid MCL from standard MCL.[152]

The cytogenetic and FISH data have been supplemented by CGH analyses to provide further refinement of the gain and loss profiles associated with MCL. This has been of particular value in this disease because of the high proportion of cases that do not yield high-quality information through chromosome banding efforts.[137,153–158] These CGH studies, similar to targeted FISH analysis, have confirmed a higher frequency of the characteristic deletions and duplications, in which regional losses are consistently more frequent than gains. A higher frequency of duplications was identified as compared to the karyotype data, resulting from resolution of the markers and additions that are typically composed of complex, unbalanced translocations. These studies have significantly refined and narrowed the region of duplication or deletion at a number of sites, such as 3q28-29, 6q25, 9p, 10q, 12q13, 13q14, and 17p. In addition, high-level amplifications were identified at a number of chromosomal sites, a novel feature not previously identified by karyotyping. These amplifications were correlated with specific recurrent regions of duplication (3q28-29, 8q24, Xq26-28), but also showed an association with known fragile sites.[137] An increased number and characteristic pattern of changes was found in the blastoid variant, such as deletion of 9p and 17p, and duplication of 12q, as well as more frequent high-level amplifications.[137]

A recent array-based CGH study that used a dispersed targeted array consisting of 812 selected DNA targets varying in density from 46 clones for chromosome 1 and 18 and two clones for chromosome 21, with a maximum spacing of 15 MB.[159] The analysis of 53 patients identified 50% more dosage alterations than detected by chromosomal CGH performed on the same samples. In addition, novel sites of gain and loss were identified and consensus regions were more precisely defined, allowing a more focused identification of candidate genes in the affected

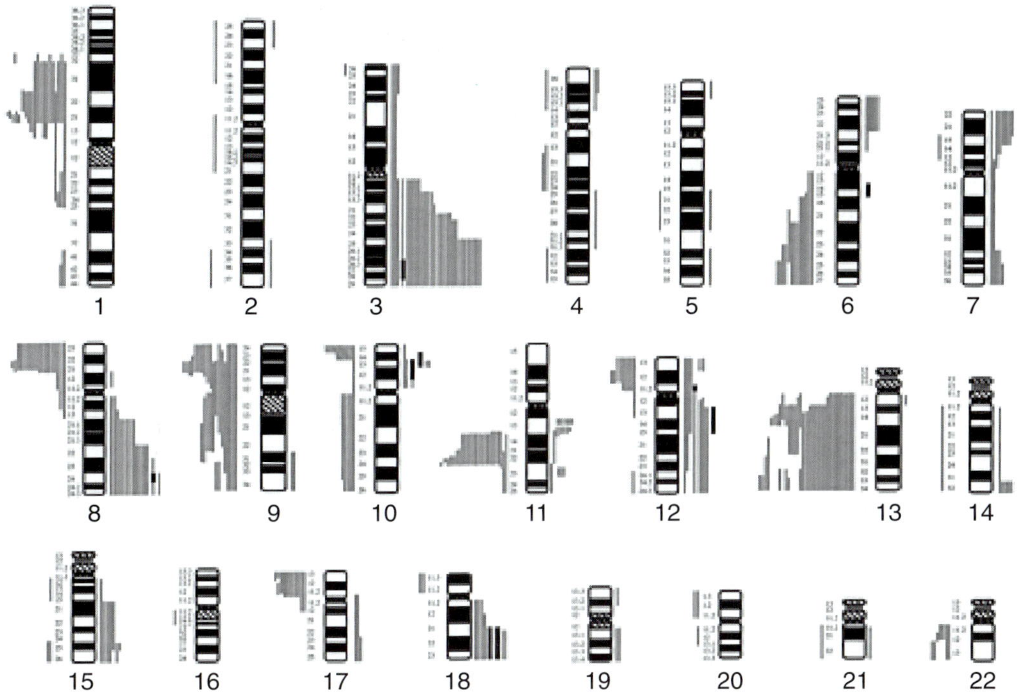

Figure 2–5. Depiction of regions of genomic duplication and deletion detected by array CGH in 53 cases of mantle cell lymphoma. The vertical lines to the *left* of the chromosome ideograms indicate loss of chromosomal material, and the lines to the *right* indicate gains of chromosomal material. Black squares represent high-level DNA amplifications. Since the DNA targets on the array are dispersed, the existence of gain or loss between adjacent targets within a region is inferred but not proven by this method. (Adapted from Kohlhammer H, Schwaenen C, Wessendorf S, et al. Genomic DNA-chip hybridization in t(11;14)-positive mantle cell lymphomas shows a high frequency of aberrations and allows a refined characterization of consensus regions. Blood 2004;104:795–801, with permission.)

regions, due to the much higher level of resolution afforded by this technique. A depiction of the delineated consensus regions of chromosomal gains and losses in MCL is provided in Fig. 2–5. This study clearly demonstrates the potential to obtain a more refined view of the dosage alterations associated with this disease. The stage has been set for the next generation of molecular cytogenetic analysis, using whole-genome tiling path arrays.[5] This will provide a complete and accurate picture of the genomic dosage alterations associated with MCL, and allow direct correlation with gene expression studies.[159]

Marginal Zone Lymphomas

Marginal zone B-cell lymphomas that are listed in the WHO classification include extranodal MALT-type lymphoma, splenic marginal zone lymphoma, and nodal marginal zone lymphoma. These three subtypes of lymphomas arise from mantle zone B-cells and share morphologic, immunophenotypic, and cytogenetic features. The published karyotype data have verified that these entities, although showing morphologic similarities, are clinically and genetically distinct. They will be discussed individually.

Extra Nodal MZL (MALT Lymphomas)

Cytogenetic data on MALT lymphomas have been slow to accumulate, largely due to the sequestered nature of most lesions and the small size of clinical biopsy specimens. The need for cytogenetic analysis may not be a primary consideration at the time of tumor tissue triage. When obtained, such tissue samples may grow poorly in culture with a slow proliferation rate and poor yield of analyzable metaphases. The first cytogenetic study of MALT lymphomas identified structural rearrangements of 1p and trisomies of chromosomes 3 and 7 in nine clonal karyotypes, but found no evidence of a specific recurrent change.[160] A number of subsequent reports confirmed the high incidence of trisomy 3 as well as other chromosomal trisomies.[161–163] The picture has since been clarified significantly, with the current recognition of two cytogenetic subtypes, the more common group characterized by chromosomal aneuploidy, most often involving trisomy 3 and a supporting cast of whole or partial trisomies and deletions, and a second smaller group defined exclusively by a t(11;18)(q21;q21).[164–166] It has become apparent that the aneuploid group tend to be genetically unstable and show a propensity to progress or transform into a more aggressive type of lymphoma, whereas the t(11;18) represents the genetic signature for a subtype of low-grade extra nodal lymphoma that does not progress or transform.[166,167]

The aneuploid subtype of MALT lymphoma is characterized primarily by duplication of chromosomes 3 or 3q, 5, 12, 18, or 18q, and deletion 6q and 17p, with variation in this pattern depending on anatomic site. The recurrent involvement of these specific chromosomes has been verified by studies using FISH probes. Trisomy 3 may be found in 60% to 85% of extranodal MALT lymphomas, although some studies have found a lower frequency.[162,168,169] Regional duplication of 3q may involve two sites at 3q21-23 and 3q25-29.[170] A number of cases have been described that contain a t(3;14)(q27;q32), and the involvement of BCL6 by rearrangement or amplification has been demonstrated through FISH and molecular studies.[171] High-level amplification of 18q may involve BCL2 and MALT1.[172] In general, cases with simple karyotypes are associated with indolent behavior, while more complex hyperdiploid karyotypes and deletions of 17p are associated with aggressive behavior. The pattern of karyotypic alterations in the aneuploid group is shared with nodal and splenic MZL, as well as with DLBCL affecting marginal zone sites, indicating that this subtype of MALT lymphoma may transform into DLBCL. Chromosome changes that arise at transformation to DLBCL may include t(8;14), deletion of 6q, and partial and whole gains of chromosomes 3, 7, 18, and 21.[166] Of additional note, the gastric MALT lymphomas that are responsive to *Helicobacter pylori* eradication are more commonly of the aneuploid subtype.

Extranodal MALT lymphomas with the t(11;18) represent a remarkably uniform subtype of B-cell lymphoma. They have an indolent disease course and do not transform to diffuse lymphoma.[173] Initial cytogenetic studies showed that up to 50% of low-grade MALT lymphoma may have a t(11;18), most commonly found in the gastrointestinal tract and lung, but also reported occasionally at other sites.[166,174–178] A remarkable feature of MALT lymphomas bearing the t(11;18) is the virtual lack of secondary chromosomal alterations. This may reflect a degree of genetic stability that correlates with the lack of propensity to transform or behave in an aggressive manner. Of the 27 MALT karyotypes with t(11;18) that are recorded in the Mitelman Database, only three show additional alterations, one with +3 in a separate stemline,[165] one with inv(16)(p13q22),[179] and one with +3 that was detected by FISH in interphase cells but not in the clonal metaphases.[180] The additional trisomy 3 found in two of these cases may represent either a divergent clone from a common precursor stem line or a second MALT lymphoma in the same tissue. The lack of secondary changes has been corroborated by numerous FISH studies. A single complex variant of t(11;18) has been reported, involving chromosome 12 in an apparently balanced three-way translocation.[181,182]

Cloning of the t(11;18) has identified the involvement of the API2 gene at 11q21, and the MALT1 gene at 18q21, which is located 200 KB centromeric of BCL2.[179,183–185] The pathogenesis of this translocation may be linked to VDJ recombinase activity, and results in the creation of a unique API2-MALT1 fusion transcript.[186,187] This discovery has allowed the development of FISH and RT-PCR assays to improve the detection of this translocation in retrospective and uncultured cases.[187] Application of these detection methods to large series of MZL lymphomas has confirmed the exclusivity of this translocation for extranodal MALT lymphoma, predominantly associated with gastric (50%) and lung (60%) sites and found less commonly elsewhere.[188–191]

Insight into the role of the t(11;18) and the MALT1 gene in the pathogenesis of MZL lymphoma has been provided by the description of two other recurrent translocations in MZL, one involving MALT1 and the other involving BCL10 on chromosome 1, each participating in translocations with the IGH gene. The t(14;18)(q32;q21) results in MALT1 deregulation through an IGH-MALT1 rearrangement.[172,192] A t(1;14)(p22;q32) found in a nodal MZL lymphoma leads to deregulation of BCL10 by the IGH enhancer.[193,194] These disparate chromosomal translocations are part of a common pathway linking over-expression of BCL10 and MALT1 to the development of lymphoma through activation of the NFkB pathway.[195,196] Although t(1;14) and t(14;18) share this mechanistic link to t(11;18), they appear to share a phenotypic link with the aneuploid subtype of MZL, in that they are associated with secondary chromosomal alterations and high-grade transformation. In two of the cases with an IGH-MALT1 fusion, one showed +3 and the other showed +1 and +3 and multiple structural rearrangements, including a t(14;19)(q32;p13).[172] In the cases reported by Streubel et al.,[192] one case showed +X, +3, +4, +13, and +18, and the second showed multiple structural alterations, involving 1q, 6q, 13q, and other sites.

The discovery of the IGH-MALT1 translocation may explain many if not all of the cases of t(14;18) that have been associated with MZL. Up to 18% of low-grade MALT show t(14;18).[192] Also of interest is the distinctive anatomic sites linked to this translocation as compared to the t(11;18). The t(14;18) is found predominantly in non-gastrointestinal or lung sites, and most frequently in the liver. One study has shown t(14;18) in 4 of 4 liver, 3 of 8 ocular, 3 of 11 skin, and 2 of 11 salivary gland MALT lymphomas, but none in stomach, intestine, lung, thyroid, or breast, and none in splenic MZL.[192,197] The t(1;14) is seen in a variety of extranodal MALT lymphoma sites as well as in nodal MZL. All cases of t(1;14) reported by Zhang et al.[194] showed +3 and +18. The biologic mechanisms underlying the mutual exclusivity of the t(11;18) and t(14;18) and the anatomic and clinical phenotypic differences are unknown at this time. It would appear that t(11;18) represents a primary alteration and may preserve a stable genotype, whereas the t(14;18) and t(1;14) appear to arise as secondary alterations in a clonal proliferation that is already characterized by genetic instability and perhaps a high proliferation rate, wherein the apoptosis-generating mechanism provides an additional growth advantage.

Splenic MZL Section

Karyotypic alterations are found in the majority of splenic MZL, although a substantial minority may not yield clonal metaphases, most likely due to a low proliferation rate in a portion of these tumors.[161] The Mitelman Database contains approximately 120 published karyotypes.[1] These data reveal a number of features in common with other subtypes of MZL, as well as showing some specific associations. The most common alterations are unbalanced translocations or deletions of 7q, which are found in up to 40% of cases.[198–201] More than one specific region of 7q may be involved, and biallelic loss has been demonstrated.[202,203] This alteration may define one subset of splenic MZL, as distinct from a second subset characterized by trisomy 3 or duplication of 3q, which is seen in up to 30% to 40% of splenic MZL but rarely if ever in combination deletion of 7q.[199] Recurrent unbalanced alterations such as duplication of a deleted 3p13 chromosome and duplication of 3q via isochromosome formation indicate that the critical dosage alteration involves a locus on the q arm.[163] Other recurrent alterations include structural changes of chromosome 1, +12, deletion 13q, monosomy 17, or deletion of 17q and +18. Focused FISH and molecular analysis seeking 17p deletions have shown a low frequency of p53 losses in splenic MZL, but when present, may identify patients with more aggressive disease.[204,205] Translocations involving 14q32 and BCL1, BCL2, BCL6, and MYC are generally not encountered, although a few cases with undefined addition at 14q32 or translocation with 3q27, 9p13, and 19q13 have been described. An unusual case of aggressive SMZL showed a combination of t(2;8)(p12;q24) and t(14;18)(q32;q21),[206] which may represent the only reported case of a Burkitt-type translocation with involvement of MYC in splenic MZL, whereas the t(14;18) in this case and a few other instances may represent the IGH-MALT1 rearrangement associated with extranodal MALT lymphomas. A number of cases with a t(11;14)(q11;q32) have been described, mostly in reports emanating shortly after the definition of the entity. These cases quite likely represent leukemic MCL, although different breakpoint sites at 11q13 have been suggested.[207,208] A recurrent t(11;14)(p11;q32) has been described in a number of patients, combined with deletion of 7q or 17p in patients with high-grade disease and aggressive disease course.[209] Further descriptions of cases with this translocation will be required to determine if it defines a distinct subset of splenic MZL.

Two studies using chromosomal CGH to refine the karyotype data have been reported.[170,210] These have confirmed the karyotype data, showing that the number of dosage gains exceed losses, with the most frequent gains involving the whole chromosome 3 or 3q arm, 12q, and 18, and the most frequent losses involving 7q and 17p. Similar to CGH analysis of other types of lymphoma, high-level amplifications were described in each study, but involving unique regions in different cases. Narrowing of the recurrent regions of loss and gain was achieved. Refined karyotype data based on multicolor karyotyping have not been reported to date.

Correlation of chromosomal alterations with clinical features and outcome has not shown definitive associations.[207] Deletion of 17p and p53 mutation has been associated with poor prognosis in more than one study. A "blastic" or aggressive variant of splenic MZL has been reported, but no consistent karyotypic alterations have been linked to this form of the disease.[206,211,212] A shorter time to progression has been demonstrated for patients in whom a clonal karyotype was detected as compared to those without an abnormal karyotype, but this did not translate into a survival advantage.[213] A CGH study indicated that cases with genomic losses had an inferior survival outcome.[210]

Nodal MZL

Nodal MZL appears to be genetically distinct from both extranodal and splenic MZL[214]; however, a common set of secondary alterations has been observed in all MZL subtypes.[168] Published cytogenetic data are available on only 38 cases.[1] These reveal simple to complex karyotypes that are mainly hyperdiploid, with one triploid and one tetraploid clone. The recurring numerical alterations include +3 (9 cases), seen as the only alteration in two karyotypes, +18 (7 cases), +7 (5 cases), and +12 (4 cases). Trisomy 3 has been reported in up to 60% of cases from single institutions, either as the sole change or accompanied by other nonrecurrent structural alterations[163]; however, this high incidence is not sustained in other series[169] or in the compiled data. Regional duplications of 3q have been identified, which may point to important loci associated with MZL.[171,215] Trisomy 3 and 18 have been found together in a number of cases. Trisomy 13 has been identified, in one instance as a sole change, and twice in complex clones.[216] A variety of structural alterations have also been observed, most of which were unbalanced rearrangements. These most commonly involve chromosome 1, but affect a number of different breakpoint sites. Recurrent balanced translocations have included t(3;14) (2 cases), t(14;18) (2 cases), and t(11;14) (1 case). The recent identification of t(14;18) with a IGH-MALT1 fusion[172,192] may account for all instances of this look-alike translocation in MZL. The 14q32 locus has also been found in a number of unbalanced translocations between 1q21, 12p11, and 12q13.

The features of clonal evolution seen in nodal and other subtypes of MZL are typical of clonal progression in B-cell lymphomas, and in particular, are reminiscent of those associated with extranodal MALT lymphomas of the aneuploid subtype. Karyotypes associated with transformation of low-grade nodal MZL to high-grade disease have been reported in three cases, which revealed complex karyotypes containing deletions of 6q, 11q, and 17p, and trisomy 12.[217] Additional information on the karyotypic alterations associated with nodal MZL is required, but at the present time, a primary rearrangement in nodal MZL has not been identified.

Cutaneous B-Cell Lymphoma

Cutaneous B-cell lymphoma may represent a primary or secondary lymphoma. Distinguishing primary from secondary lymphoma may be a challenging task, and the definition may not be obvious at first presentation. Secondary involvement of a skin site can be associated with FL, DLBCL, and MZL, and such cases may show any of the characteristic chromosomal alterations associated with the nodal counterpart of those diseases, including the t(14;18), t(3;14), or t(8;14). In this regard, a case of t(14;18) with an IGH-MALT1 rearrangement has been described in a cutaneous manifestation of DLBCL.[218] The karyotypic alterations of so-called primary cutaneous B-cell lymphoma may have a distinctive cytogenetic signature, and this finding has been substantiated by CGH studies. A study of 19 such cases has shown 41% to have detectable dosage alterations with gains exceeding losses.[219] The common gains have included +18 or +18q (50%), +7 or +7q (42%), +3 or +3q and +20 (30% each), +19, and +13 or +13q (25% each).

Lymphoplasmacytic Lymphoma with del(7q)

The association of deletion of 7q with lymphoplasmacytic lymphoma has been reported by a number of investigators. Deletion of 7q may be seen within a more complex karyotype in a number of subtypes of B-cell lymphoma, but when present as a single karyotypic alteration is closely associated with a clinical hematologic syndrome characterized by advanced age and marked splenomegaly with circulating and nodal lymphocytes showing lymphoplasmacytic morphology. The region of 7q that is deleted in these cases appears to be confined to 7q31-32, which may contain a gene whose disruption or loss may be closely linked to the pathogenesis of this subtype of lymphoma.[201,220] An association of a t(9;14)(p13;q32) resulting in a IGH-PAX5 fusion with lymphomas showing lymphoplasmcytic features has been made, but this appears to be a rare finding, and this translocation has also been described in lymphomas that do not show this morphologic feature.[221]

T-CELL LYMPHOMAS

Adult T-Cell Leukemia/Lymphoma

Chromosomal alterations associated with adult T-cell leukemia/lymphoma (ATLL) have demonstrated a high degree of diversity and complexity, characterized by multiple structural rearrangements. The most common breakpoint sites associated with these rearrangements affect 14q32 (28%), 14q11 (14%), and 6q (23%), the latter associated with interstitial deletions. Most karyotypes are consequently near diploid, with the most common numerical changes being trisomy 3 (21%), trisomy 7 (10%), monosomy X (35%), and loss of Y (17%). The lymphomatous version of ATLL is characterized by aneuploid changes with a higher number of numerical and structural changes and marker chromosomes. Cases with changes involving monosomy X, trisomy 3, deletion of 6q21 and 10p, and rearrangements of 11q23 are associated with more aggressive behavior. Oncogenes deregulated by translocation with T-cell receptor genes may not play a major role in the development of ATLL.[222,223]

Anaplastic Large-Cell Lymphoma

The cytogenetic characterization of anaplastic large-cell lymphoma (ALCL) has progressed in parallel with the definition of its clinical and morphologic features. Shortly after the initial description of ALCL,[224] the first karyotype associated with this disease was obtained from tumor cells and a permanent cell line (Karpas 299) derived from a large-cell lymphoma showing predominant sinusoidal distribution.[225] The t(2;5)(p23;q35) present in this karyotype has subsequently become synonymous with this disease. The molecular cloning of the t(2;5) was accomplished in 1994,[226] which identified participation of the ALK gene at 2p23 and the NPM gene at 5q25. Consistent breakpoints in the fusion gene has permitted the development of simple PCR and RT-PCR strategies, as well as FISH probes, to assist in identification of the translocation in clinical specimens.[227,228] The translocation leads to an NPM–ALK fusion that has been determined to be confined to ALCL, and this close association has contributed to the precise definition of the disease.[229–232]

Typical cases of ALCL have been described that do not have the normal t(2;5), due to cryptic and complex variants of this translocation.[233] However, the occurrence of variant translocations involving recombination of ALK at 2p23 with other partner chromosomes account for an important clinical variation of this disease. A review of the variant translocations associated with ALCL has been reported.[234] The common molecular theme of these rearrangements is the creation of fusion genes that encode self-associating and constitutively active chimeric ALK proteins that activate transcription of downstream effector proteins leading to cellular transformation.[235] A compilation of these variant translocations and the associated genes involved, where known, is provided in Table 2–2.

A characteristic pattern of secondary chromosomal alterations is associated with ALK rearrangements. There are approximately 100 published karyotypes with t(2;5) or known variant translocations, which include five cases of cutaneous ALCL.[1] Analysis of the secondary chromosomal alterations within the karyotype data reveals recurrent regions of duplication and deletion that occur in more than 10% of cases, including duplication of X, 1q21-q44, 5q14-q35, 7, and 12, and regional deletions affecting 10q25-26, 17p13, and Yq12. Polyploid clones or sidelines and the presence of other balanced and unbalanced translocations as well as marker chromosomes are frequent. The clinical implications of these secondary chromosomal alterations have not been determined.

Little in the way of refined karyotype data on ALCL is available from CGH or multicolor karyotyping studies. Three cell lines (SUDHL-1, Karpas 299, DEL) have been studied by CGH that showed high-level amplification of 1q21-q44 in DEL and 1q12-q22 in Karpas 299.[236]

Numerous associations have been demonstrated between the chromosomal alterations of ALCL and clinical-pathologic features. Up to 40% of cases are shown to have the t(2;5), including 83% of pediatric cases and 31% of adult cases.[234] The t(2;5) is more common in nodal than extranodal disease, and also shows additional breakpoints at 1p36, 6p25, and 8q24.[237] The t(2;5) is more common in monomorphic and small-cell variants of ALCL, and is rare in primary cutaneous ALCL.[238] In five cases of the cutaneous variant, the karyotypes showed complex changes with only one showing a variant of the t(2;5), consisting of an ins(2;5)(p23;q22q35).[237,239,240] A leukemic form of ALCL[241,242] and an aggressive variant have also been described.[243] Of interest from the biological perspective is

Table 2–2. ALK Translocations with Confirmed Partner Genes in ALCL*

Translocation	Gene Fusion	Reference
t(X;2)(q11-12;p23)	*MSN/ALK*	Tort et al, Lab Invest 2001;81:419–426
t(1;2)(q21;p23)	*TPM3/ALK*	Lamant et al, Blood 1999;93:3088–3095
t(2;5)(p23;q35)	*NPM1/ALK*	Morris et al, Science 1994;263:1281–1284
inv(2)(p23q35)	*ATIC/ALK*	Colleoni et al, Am J Pathol 2000;156:781–789
t(2;3)(p23;q11-12)	*TFG/ALK*	Hernandez et al, Blood 1999;94:3265–3268
t(2;11;2)(p23;p15;q31)	*CARS/ALK*	Cools et al, Genes Chromosomes Cancer 2002;34:354–362
t(2;17)(p23;q25)	*KIAA168/ALK*	Cools et al, Genes Chromosomes Cancer 2002;34:354–362
t(2;19)(p23;p13)	*TPM4/ALK*	Meech et al, Blood 2001;98:1209–1216
t(2;22)(p23;q11)	*CLTCL1/ALK*	Touriol et al, Blood 2000;95:3204–3207
t(2;22)(p23;q13)	*MY119/ALK*	Lamant et al, Genes Chromosomes Cancer 200337:427–432

*Compiled from Mitelman Database of Chromosome Aberrations in Cancer http://cgap.nci.nih.gov/Chromosomes/Mitelman.

the observation of the t(2;5) and other ALK rearrangements in inflammatory myofibroblastic tumors.[244,245]

Angioimmunoblastic Lymphadenopathy

Angioimmunoblastic lymphadenopathy (AILD) is a lymphoproliferative disorder that appears to evolve from a benign lymphoproliferation into a peripheral T-cell, or rarely B-cell, lymphoma. It is unusual at the cytogenetic level due to the characteristic finding of unrelated abnormal metaphases with single trisomies. The disease may have an underlying defect in genetic stability or a failure of a critical apoptotic pathway that tolerates the persistence of cells with chromosomal imbalances. The disease has been shown to progress from an indolent phase with multiple, clonally unrelated aberrant cells to a more progressed stage with established oligoclonal lymphocyte populations, in which clones with trisomy of X, 3, or 15 predominate. FISH analyses have confirmed that these trisomies exist as distinct clones with no common precursor stem line. Cases that progress to a fully malignant stage show gradual establishment of a major clone, those with indolent behavior often having trisomy X or 15, while more aggressive disease is associated with clones bearing trisomy 3.[246]

Enteropathy-Associated T-Cell Lymphoma

Most of the cytogenetic information on enteropathy-associated T-cell lymphoma has come from CGH studies. The largest of these revealed imbalances in 87% of 38 cases with a high frequency of 9q gains (58%), primarily focused on bands 9q33-q34. This finding was confirmed with FISH probes for 9q and showed multiple copies in some cases. In this study, loss of 9p was seen in 18% of cases. Those specimens with more than three imbalances did poorly.[247] Further evidence for the association of loss of 9p21 with this disease has been shown by loss of heterozygosity (LOH) studies, with increased frequency of 9p loss found in cases with a large-cell component (56%), and associated with loss of p16 expression in all cases that demonstrated LOH.[248] Duplication of 5q33.3-34 and 7q31 was seen in more than 30% of cases, with losses evident at 6p24, 7p21, 17q23-25, and 17p13. Two subgroups were defined by these studies, one with duplication of 9q34 and a smaller group with allelic imbalances at 3q27.[249]

Hepatosplenic Gamma/Delta T-Cell Lymphoma

Hepatosplenic gamma/delta T-cell lymphoma (HSTCL) is a rare T-cell lymphoma characterized by infiltration of liver and spleen by malignant post-thymic T-cells. Most cases present in young males, although occasionally affecting older males and females. Cytogenetic studies have confirmed a consistent association of this type of lymphoma with extra copies of 7q, most often in the form of one or more isochromosomes 7q.[250–253] Trisomy 8 is also frequently present. Disease progression is characterized by acquisition of additional copies of 7q, either through duplication of the i(7q) and unbalanced rearrangements affecting the other 7q homologue. The presence of multiple copies of 7q has been verified in 10 of 12 cases investigated by FISH probes targeting 7p and 7q.[254]

NK/T-Cell Lymphoma

This rare form of T-cell lymphoma has a variety of presentations, principally involving the aerodigestive tract, but also presenting in a variety of other sites, including skin. Few cytogenetic studies have been reported, but the available information confirms a nonrandom pattern of chromosomal alterations.[255–257] The most frequent alterations involve deletion of 6q21-q23 and trisomy 7. Isochromosome formation resulting in whole arm duplication of 1q, 6p, 6q, 7q, and 17q is frequently seen, as well as 11q23 rearrangement. Deletion of 6q has been shown by FISH to be confined to the clonal CD56+ CD3− clonal T-cells.[255–257] CGH has shown variable changes in various studies from different countries.[258,259] The frequency of gains is equal to losses, and the pattern of changes is similar in the nasal and cutaneous type of disease. Deletions have been shown to affect numerous sites including 1p, 9p, 13q, and 17p, although there has been inconsistency among studies in this regard. Additional studies are required to further define the consistency and frequency of these proposed recurrent changes in NK/T-cell lymphoma.

Primary Cutaneous T-Cell Lymphoma

Cutaneous T-cell lymphoma (CTCL) may represent involvement of skin by other, primarily nodal-based T-cell lymphoma, such as ALCL, or a primary malignancy associated with mycosis fungoides or parapsoriasis en plaque or other T-cell lymphoproliferations. Little information is available due to the difficulty in obtaining metaphases from skin biopsy specimens. A number of studies have demonstrated complex chromosome changes in early-stage disease, which are often nonclonal and primarily numerical, but may also involve structural alterations. As the disease progresses, the emergence of a pure clonal proliferation can be demonstrated. The aggressiveness of the disease is paralleled by an increasing complexity of the chromosome changes. FISH studies have verified this sequence of emergence of clonal populations. Cytogenetic studies may be of diagnostic and prognostic value in CTCL, but a disease-specific karyotypic alteration has not yet been identified.[260,261]

HODGKIN'S LYMPHOMA

The accumulation of cytogenetic data for Hodgkin's lymphoma has been a challenging task. This has been complicated by a number of factors, including paucity of the malignant Hodgkin's cells in tumor specimens, prominent polyclonal proliferation of B- and T-cells that develops in response to the malignancy, propensity for "secondary" B- or T-cell lymphomas to develop within the involved lymph nodes, and morphologic overlap with other lymphoma entities. Application of routine methods has generally resulted in failure to obtain metaphases or only normal metaphases derived from the reactive lymphocyte population. This difficulty is exemplified in two relatively large studies in which only 20% to 40% of cases yielded clonal karyotypes; this low yield contrasts quite markedly with other subtypes of lymphoma.[262,263] In the successful cases, both clonal and nonclonal karyotypes were obtained that showed heterogeneous changes, often with complex, high-ploidy chromosome complements. Recurrent alterations were shown to involve chromosomal regions that are typically altered in B-cell lymphomas, such as 1p, 1q, 6q, 8q, 9p, and 14q, leading to the speculation that the origin of the malignant Hodgkin's cells was from a B lymphocyte. The frequent occurrence of polyploidy in the Hodgkin's cells has been confirmed by in situ FISH studies, confirming that polyploid complements are confined to these cells and represents the principal malignant proliferation in these tumors.[264] If large numbers of metaphases are screened using standard culturing methods, the frequency of detection of abnormal clones can be increased. This has confirmed a characteristic pattern of genetic instability and a high level of karyotype complexity associated with Hodgkin's disease, with a preponderance of hyperdiploid clones, and a recurrent pattern of associated breakpoints in the structural alterations. A higher frequency of structural alterations is seen in advanced-stage disease.[265] Despite this accumulation of karyotype data, a disease-characteristic primary chromosomal change has not been identified.

Of primary importance in the interpretation of data obtained from standard cytogenetic cultures techniques is the low number of Hodgkin's and Reed–Sternberg cells in the tumors, their low proliferation potential, and the inability to determine by karyotype analysis if the obtained metaphases actually represent the malignant clone. The presence of clonal abnormalities in the "reactive" lymphocyte population has been confirmed by FISH studies to assess aneuploidy in the non-Hodgkin's cells using multiple probes for chromosomes frequently affected by trisomy or monosomy in other lymphomas. The presence of clonal alterations was identified in 1% to 12% of nuclei that were morphologically normal. The significance of these cells in relation to karyotype studies, their role in the primary malignancy, and the possibility that secondary lymphomas develop from such clones have not been determined.

Perhaps more information is currently available on what cytogenetic alterations do not occur in Hodgkin's disease! Application of molecular genetic methods and immunohistochemistry in the 1990s attracted much attention to the possible presence of the t(14;18) of follicular lymphoma and the t(2;5) of anaplastic large-cell lymphoma in Hodgkin's disease. The demonstration of bcl2 overexpression in a proportion of cases spawned a number of reports that used sensitive PCR methods to demonstrate the presence of GH-BCL2 rearrangement in Hodgkin's tumors and support assertions for a causative role in the disease. The contemporary demonstration of t(14;18) positive cells in reactive lymphoid tissue raised the possibility that bystander, nonmalignant B cells may underlie this apparent association.[99] Subsequently, carefully performed studies including single-cell dissections have been able to discredit an etiologic relationship between the t(14;18)-bearing lymphocytes and the Hodgkin's malignant cells.[266,267] On a similar theme, controversy reigned for a number of years regarding the possible relationship between CD30+ Hodgkin's disease and anaplastic large-cell lymphoma with the associated t(2;5) and NPM-ALK fusion protein. The subsequent verification of the specific association of this translocation with ALCL represents an important contribution to the distinction between these two disease entities that share common features at the morphologic and immunophenotypic level, but which are genetically distinct.[230,232]

Abundant information has accumulated recently on the use of CGH on primary tumor specimens and by targeted approaches to collect individual Hodgkin's and Reed–Sternberg cells by laser microdissection. This has confirmed the frequent amplification of a region of 2p, containing REL and BCL11A, as well as 9q, 12q, 17p, and 17q, and consistent regions of loss affecting 6q, 11q, and 13q. An association between the presence of specific changes and different morphologic subtypes of Hodgkin's disease, as well as specific prognostic correlations has been suggested.[268–270] CGH and multicolor karyotyping methods applied to a number of existing Hodgkin's disease cell lines have substantiated the high complexity of the karyotype changes associated with this disease.[271,272] These recent advances demonstrate that significant progress has been made in defining the genetic alterations associated with this complex disease, and setting the stage for correlative studies with gene expression analysis.

References

1. Mitelman F, Johansson B, Mertens R, eds. Mitelman Database of Chromosome Aberrations in Cancer (2001). National Cancer Institute and John Wiley & Sons. Available at: http://cgap.nci.nih.gov/Chromosomes/Mitelman. Accessed.
2. Barch MJ, ed. The ACT Cytogenetic Laboratory Manual, 2nd ed. New York: Raven Press, 1991.
3. International System for Cytogenetic Nomenclature. Basil: Karger, 1995.
4. Hoglund M, Gisselsson D, Sall T, et al. Coping with complexity: multivariate analysis of tumour karyotypes. Cancer Genet Cytogenet 2002;135:103–9.
5. Ishkanian AS, Malloff CA, Watson SK, et al. A tiling resolution DNA microarray with complete coverage of the human genome. Nat Genet 2004;36:299–303.
6. Schrock E, du Manoir S, Veldman T, et al. Multicolor spectral karyotyping of human chromosomes. Science 1996;273:494–7.
7. Speicher MR, Gwyn Ballard S, Ward DC. Karyotyping human chromosomes by combinatorial multi-fluor FISH. Nat Genet 1996;12:368–75.
8. Chudoba I, Plesch A, Lorch T, et al. High resolution multi-color-banding: a new technique for refined FISH analysis of human chromosomes. Cytogenet Cell Genet 1999;84: 156–60.
9. Weise A, Heller A, Starke H, et al. Multitude multicolor chromosome banding (mMCB)—a comprehensive one-step multicolor FISH banding method. Cytogenet Genome Res 2003;1033:34–9.
10. Kakazu N, Bar-Am I, Hada S, et al. A new chromosome banding technique, spectral color banding (SCAN), for full characterization of chromosomal abnormalities. Genes Chromosomes Cancer 2003;37:412–6.
11. Martin-Subero JI, Chudoba I, Harder L, et al. Multicolor-FICTION: expanding the possibilities of combined morphologic, immunophenotypic, and genetic single cell analyses. Am J Pathol 2002;161:413–20.
12. Lichter P, Fischer K, Joos S, et al. Efficacy of current molecular cytogenetic protocols for the diagnosis of chromosome

aberrations in tumor specimens. Cytokines Mol Ther 1996;2:163–9.
13. World Health Organization. World Health Organization Classification of Tumours: Pathology and Genetics of Haematopoietic and Lymphoid Tissues. Lyon: IARC Press, 2001.
14. Manolov G, Manolova Y. Marker band in one chromosome 14 from Burkitt's lymphomas. Nature 1972;237:33–4.
15. Zech L, Haglund U, Nilsson K, et al. Characteristic chromosomal abnormalities in biopsies and lymphoid-cell lines from patients with Burkitt's and non-Burkitt's lymphomas. Int J Cancer 1976;17:47–56.
16. Zhang S, Zech L, Klein G. High-resolution analysis of chromosome markers in Burkitt's lymphoma cell lines. Int J Cancer 1982;29:153–7.
17. Dalla-Favera R, Bregni M, Erikson J, et al. Human c-myc onc gene is located on the region of chromosome 8 that is translocated in Burkitt's lymphoma cells. Proc Natl Acad Sci U S A 1982;79:7824–7.
18. Taub R, Kirsch I, Morton C, et al. Translocation of the c-myc gene into the immunoglobulin heavy chain locus in human Burkitt's lymphoma and murine plasmacytoma cells. Proc Natl Acad Sci U S A 1982;79:7837–41.
19. Berger R, Bernheim A, Weh HJ, et al. A new translocation in Burkitt's tumor cells. Hum Genet 1979;53:111–2.
20. Hiraki MS, Miyamoto KD, Sato J:2/8 Translocation in a Japanese Burkitt's lymphoma. Expermentia 1979;35:742–3.
21. Van Den Berghe H, Parloir C, David G, et al. A new characteristic karyotypic anomaly in lymphoproliferative disorders. Cancer 1979;44:188–95.
22. Heim S, Mitelman F. Cancer Cytogenetics: Chromosomal and Molecular Genetic Aberrations of Tumor Cells, vol. 2. New York: Wiley-Liss, 1995.
23. Siebert R, Matthiesen P, Harder S, et al. Application of interphase fluorescence in situ Hybridization for the detection of the Burkitt's translocation t(8;14)(q24;q32) in B-cell lymphomas. Blood 1998;91:984–90.
24. Hecht JL, Aster JC. Molecular biology of Burkitt's lymphoma. J Clin Oncol 2000;18:3707–21.
25. Sigaux F, Berger R, Bernheim A, et al. Malignant lymphomas with band 8q24 chromosome abnormality: a morphologic continuum extending from Burkitt's to immunoblastic lymphoma. Br J Haematol 1984;57:393–405.
26. Kornblau SM, Goodacre A, Cabanillas F. Chromosomal abnormalities in adult non-endemic Burkitt's lymphoma and leukemia:22 new reports and a review of 148 cases from the literature. Hematol Oncol 1991;9:63–78.
27. Parsa NZ, Gaidano G, Mukherjee AB, et al. Cytogenetic and molecular analysis of 6q deletions in Burkitt's lymphoma cell lines. Genes Chromosomes Cancer 1994;9:13–8.
28. Johansson B, Mertens F, Mitelman F. Cytogenetic evolution patterns in non-Hodgkin's lymphoma. Blood 1995; 86: 3905–14.
29. Garcia JL, Hernandez JM, Gutierrez NC, et al. Abnormalities on 1q and 7q are associated with poor outcome in sporadic Burkitt's lymphoma. A cytogenetic and comparative genomic hybridization study. Leukemia 2003;17:2016–24.
30. Bernheim A, Berger R. Cytogenetic studies of Burkitt's lymphoma-leukemia in patients with acquired immunodeficiency syndrome. Cancer Genet Cytogenet 1988;32:67–74.
31. Haluska FG, Russo G, Andreeff M, et al. Molecular analysis of an AIDS-associated Burkitt's lymphoma: near-identity with endemic cases. Curr Top Microbiol Immunol 1988; 141:75–9.
32. Polito P, Cilia AM, Gloghini A, et al. High frequency of EBV association with non-random abnormalities of the chromosome region 1q21–25 in AIDS-related Burkitt's lymphoma-derived cell lines. Int J Cancer 1995;61:370–4.
33. Fukuhara S, Rowley JD, Variakojis D, et al. Chromosome abnormalities in poorly differentiated lymphocytic lymphoma. Cancer Res 1979;39:3119–28.
34. Yunis JJ, Oken MM, Theologides A, et al. Recurrent chromosomal defects are found in most patients with non-Hodgkin's-lymphoma. Cancer Genet Cytogenet 1984; 13:17–28.
35. Bakhshi A, Wright JJ, Graninger W, et al. Mechanism of the t(14;18) chromosomal translocation: structural analysis of both derivative 14 and 18 reciprocal partners. Proc Natl Acad Sci U S A 1987;84:2396–400.
36. Yunis JJ, Frizzera G, Oken MM, et al. Multiple recurrent genomic defects in follicular lymphoma. A possible model for cancer. N Engl J Med 1987;316:79–84.
37. Offit K. Chromosome analysis in the management of patients with non-Hodgkin's lymphoma. Leuk Lymphoma 1992; 7:275–82.
38. Pezzella F, Ralfkiaer E, Gatter KC, et al. The 14;18 translocation in European cases of follicular lymphoma: comparison of Southern blotting and the polymerase chain reaction. Br J Haematol 1990;76:58–64.
39. Chen PM, Lin SH, Seto M, et al. Rearrangement of bcl-2 genes in malignant lymphomas in Chinese patients. Cancer 1993;72:3701–6.
40. Amakawa R, Fukuhara S, Ohno H, et al. Involvement of bcl-2 gene in Japanese follicular lymphoma. Blood 1989;73: 787–91.
41. Poetsch M, Weber-Matthiesen K, Plendl HJ, et al. Detection of the t(14;18) chromosomal translocation by interphase cytogenetics with yeast-artificial-chromosome probes in follicular lymphoma and nonneoplastic lymphoproliferation. J Clin Oncol 1996;14:963–9.
42. Knutsen T. Cytogenetic mechanisms in the pathogenesis and progression of follicular lymphoma. Cancer Surv 1997; 30:163–92.
43. Horsman DE, Gascoyne RD, Coupland RW, et al. Comparison of cytogenetic analysis, southern analysis, and polymerase chain reaction for the detection of t(14;18) in follicular lymphoma. Am J Clin Pathol 1995;103:472–8.
44. McDonnell TJ, Korsmeyer SJ. Progression from lymphoid hyperplasia to high-grade malignant lymphoma in mice transgenic for the t(14;18). Nature 1991;349:254–6.
45. Tilly H, Rossi A, Stamatoullas A, et al. Prognostic value of chromosomal abnormalities in follicular lymphoma. Blood 1994;84:1043–9.
46. Horsman DE, Connors JM, Pantzar T, et al. Analysis of secondary chromosomal alterations in 165 cases of follicular lymphoma with t(14;18). Genes Chromosomes Cancer 2001;30:375–82.
47. Bosga-Bouwer AG, van Imhoff GW, Boonstra R, et al. Follicular lymphoma grade 3B includes 3 cytogenetically defined subgroups with primary t(14;18), 3q27, or other translocations: t(14;18) and 3q27 are mutually exclusive. Blood 2003;101:1149–54.
48. Horsman DE, Okamoto I, Ludkovski O, et al. Follicular lymphoma lacking the t(14;18)(q32;q21): identification of two disease subtypes. Br J Haematol 2003;120:424–33.
49. Jardin F, Gaulard P, Buchonnet G, et al. Follicular lymphoma without t(14;18) and with BCL-6 rearrangement: a lymphoma subtype with distinct pathological, molecular and clinical characteristics. Leukemia 2002;16:2309–17.
50. Ott G, Katzenberger T, Lohr A, et al. Cytomorphologic, immunohistochemical, and cytogenetic profiles of follicular lymphoma:2 types of follicular lymphoma grade 3. Blood 2002;99:3806–12.
51. Viardot A, Martin-Subero JI, Siebert R, et al. Detection of secondary genetic aberrations in follicle center cell derived lymphomas: assessment of the reliability of comparative

genomic hybridization and standard chromosome analysis. Leukemia 2001;15:177–83.
52. Avet-Loiseau H, Vigier M, Moreau A, et al. Comparative genomic hybridization detects genomic abnormalities in 80% of follicular lymphomas. Br J Haematol 1997; 97:119–22.
53. Bentz M, Dohner H, Werner CA, et al. Identification of genetic imbalances in malignant lymphoma using comparative genomic hybridization. Stem Cells 1995;13:83–7.
54. Lestou VS, Gascoyne RD, Sehn L, et al. Multicolour fluorescence in situ hybridization analysis of t(14;18)-positive follicular lymphoma and correlation with gene expression data and clinical outcome. Br J Haematol 2003;122:745–59.
55. Lestou VS, Gascoyne RD, Salski C, et al. Uncovering novel inter- and intrachromosomal chromosome 1 aberrations in follicular lymphomas by using an innovative multicolor banding technique. Genes Chromosomes Cancer 2002; 34:201–10.
56. Fan YS, Rizkalla K. Comprehensive cytogenetic analysis including multicolor spectral karyotyping and interphase fluorescence in situ hybridization in lymphoma diagnosis. a summary of 154 cases. Cancer Genet Cytogenet 2003;143:73–9.
57. Hoglund M, Sehn L, Connors JM, et al. Identification of cytogenetic subgroups and karyotypic pathways of clonal evolution in follicular lymphomas. Genes Chromosomes Cancer 2004;39:195–204.
58. Horning SJ. Follicular lymphoma: have we made any progress? Ann Oncol 2000;11(Suppl 1):23–7.
59. Voorhees PM, Carder KA, Smith SV, et al. Follicular lymphoma with a Burkitt's translocation—predictor of an aggressive clinical course: a case report and review of the literature. Arch Pathol Lab Med 2004;128:210–3.
60. Karsan A, Gascoyne RD, Coupland RW, et al. Combination of t(14;18) and a Burkitt's type translocation in B-cell malignancies. Leuk Lymphoma 1993;10:433–41.
61. Sanger WG, Armitage JO, Bridge J, et al. Initial and subsequent cytogenetic studies in malignant lymphoma. Cancer 1987;60:3014–9.
62. Whang-Peng J, Knutsen T, Jaffe ES, et al. Sequential analysis of 43 patients with non-Hodgkin's lymphoma: clinical correlations with cytogenetic, histologic, immunophenotyping, and molecular studies. Blood 1995;85:203–16.
63. Richardson ME, Chen QG, Filippa DA, et al. Intermediate-to high-grade histology of lymphomas carrying t(14;18) is associated with additional nonrandom chromosome changes. Blood 1987;70:444–7.
64. Saad Z, Bramwell VH, Wilson SM, et al. Expression of genes that contribute to proliferative and metastatic ability in breast cancer resected during various menstrual phases. Lancet 1998;351:1170–3.
65. Sander CA, Yano T, Clark HM, et al. p53 mutation is associated with progression in follicular lymphomas. Blood 1993;82:1994–2004.
66. Lo Coco F, Gaidano G, Louie DC, et al. p53 mutations are associated with histologic transformation of follicular lymphoma. Blood 1993;82:2289–95.
67. Hough RE, Goepel JR, Alcock HE, et al. Copy number gain at 12q12-14 may be important in the transformation from follicular lymphoma to diffuse large B cell lymphoma. Br J Cancer 2001;84:499–503.
68. Goff LK, Neat MJ, Crawley CR, et al. The use of real-time quantitative polymerase chain reaction and comparative genomic hybridization to identify amplification of the REL gene in follicular lymphoma. Br J Haematol 2000; 111:618–25.
69. Boonstra R, Bosga-Bouwer A, Mastik M, et al. Identification of chromosomal copy number changes associated with transformation of follicular lymphoma to diffuse large B-cell lymphoma. Hum Pathol 2003;34:915–23.
70. Martinez-Climent JA, Alizadeh AA, Segraves R, et al. Transformation of follicular lymphoma to diffuse large cell lymphoma is associated with a heterogeneous set of DNA copy number and gene expression alterations. Blood 2003; 101:3109–17.
71. Offit K, Wong G, Filippa DA, et al. Cytogenetic analysis of 434 consecutively ascertained specimens of non-Hodgkin's lymphoma: clinical correlations. Blood 1991;77:1508–15.
72. Levine EG, Arthur DC, Frizzera G, et al. Cytogenetic abnormalities predict clinical outcome in non-Hodgkin lymphoma. Ann Intern Med 1988;108:14–20.
73. Schouten HC, Sanger WG, Weisenburger DD, et al. Chromosomal abnormalities in untreated patients with non-Hodgkin's lymphoma: associations with histology, clinical characteristics, and treatment outcome. The Nebraska Lymphoma Study Group. Blood 1990;75:1841–7.
74. Levine EG, Juneja S, Arthur D, et al. Sequential karyotypes in non-Hodgkin lymphoma: their nature and significance. Genes Chromosomes Cancer 1990;1:270–80.
75. Kristoffersson U, Heim S, Mandahl N, et al. Prognostic implication of cytogenetic findings in 106 patients with non-Hodgkin lymphoma. Cancer Genet Cytogenet 1987;25: 55–64.
76. Wlodarska I, Mecucci C, Vandenberghe E, et al. dup(12) (q13–qter) in two t(14;18)-negative follicular B–non-Hodgkin's lymphomas. Genes Chromosomes Cancer 1992; 4:302–8.
77. Jaffe ES, Harris NL, Stein H, et al., eds. WHO Classification of Tumours: Pathology and Genetics of Tumours of Haematopoietic and Lymphoid Tissues. Lyon: IARC Press, 2001.
78. Knutsen T. Cytogenetic changes in the progression of lymphoma. Leuk Lymphoma 1998;31:1–19.
79. Pasqualucci L, Neumeister P, Goossens T, et al. Hypermutation of multiple proto-oncogenes in B-cell diffuse large-cell lymphomas. Nature 2001;412:341–6.
80. Berard CW, Greene MH, Jaffe ES, et al. NIH conference. A multidisciplinary approach to non-Hodgkin's lymphomas. Ann Intern Med 1981;94:218–35.
81. Berglund M, Enblad G, Flordal E, et al. Chromosomal imbalances in diffuse large B-cell lymphoma detected by comparative genomic hybridization. Mod Pathol 2002;15:807–16.
82. Monni O, Joensuu H, Franssila K, et al. DNA copy number changes in diffuse large B-cell lymphoma—comparative genomic hybridization study. Blood 1996;87:5269–78.
83. Rao PH, Houldsworth J, Dyomina K, et al. Chromosomal and gene amplification in diffuse large B-cell lymphoma. Blood 1998;92:234–40.
84. Palanisamy N, Abou-Elella AA, Chaganti SR, et al. Similar patterns of genomic alterations characterize primary mediastinal large-B-cell lymphoma and diffuse large–B-cell lymphoma. Genes Chromosomes Cancer 2002;33:114–22.
85. Houldsworth J, Mathew S, Rao P, et al. REL proto-oncogene is frequently amplified in extranodal diffuse large cell lymphoma. Blood 1996;87:25–9.
86. Wessendorf S, Schwaenen C, Kohlhammer H, et al. Hidden gene amplifications in aggressive B-cell non-Hodgkin lymphomas detected by microarray-based comparative genomic hybridization. Oncogene 2003;22:1425–9.
87. Nanjangud G, Rao PH, Hegde A, et al. Spectral karyotyping identifies new rearrangements, translocations, and clinical associations in diffuse large B-cell lymphoma. Blood 2002;99:2554–61.
88. Dave BJ, Nelson M, Pickering DL, et al. Cytogenetic characterization of diffuse large cell lymphoma using multi-color

fluorescence in situ hybridization. Cancer Genet Cytogenet 2002;132:125–32.

89. Yunis JJ, Mayer MG, Arnesen MA, et al. bcl-2 and other genomic alterations in the prognosis of large-cell lymphoma. N Engl J Med 1989;320:1047–54.
90. Offit K, Koduru PR, Hollis R, et al. 18q21 rearrangement in diffuse large cell lymphoma: incidence and clinical significance. Br J Haematol 1989;72:178–83.
91. Offit K, Chaganti RS. Chromosomal aberrations in non-Hodgkin's lymphoma. Biologic and clinical correlations. Hematol Oncol Clin North Am 1991;5:853–69.
92. Monni O, Joensuu H, Franssila K, et al. BCL2 overexpression associated with chromosomal amplification in diffuse large B-cell lymphoma. Blood 1997;90:1168–74.
93. Huang JZ, Sanger WG, Greiner TC, et al. The t(14;18) defines a unique subset of diffuse large B-cell lymphoma with a germinal center B-cell gene expression profile. Blood 2002;99:2285–90.
94. Gascoyne RD, Adomat SA, Krajewski S, et al. Prognostic significance of Bcl-2 protein expression and Bcl-2 gene rearrangement in diffuse aggressive non-Hodgkin's lymphoma. Blood 1997;90:244–51.
95. Jacobson JO, Wilkes BM, Kwaiatkowski DJ, et al. bcl-2 rearrangements in de novo diffuse large cell lymphoma. Association with distinctive clinical features. Cancer 1993;72:231–6.
96. Weisenburger DD, Gascoyne RD, Bierman PJ, et al. Clinical significance of the t(14;18) and BCL2 overexpression in follicular large cell lymphoma. Leuk Lymphoma 2000; 36:513–23.
97. Rantanen S, Monni O, Joensuu H, et al. Causes and consequences of BCL2 overexpression in diffuse large B-cell lymphoma. Leuk Lymphoma 2001;42:1089–98.
98. Limpens J, Stad R, Vos C, et al. Lymphoma-associated translocation t(14;18) in blood B cells of normal individuals. Blood 1995;85:2528–36.
99. Limpens J, de Jong D, van Krieken JH, et al. Bcl-2/JH rearrangements in benign lymphoid tissues with follicular hyperplasia. Oncogene 1991;6:2271–6.
100. Liu Y, Hernandez AM, Shibata D, et al. BCL2 translocation frequency rises with age in humans. Proc Natl Acad Sci USA 1994;91:8910–4.
101. Lo Coco F, Ye BH, Lista F, et al. Rearrangements of the BCL6 gene in diffuse large cell non-Hodgkin's lymphoma. Blood 1994;83:1757–9.
102. Bastard C, Tilly H, Lenormand B, et al. Translocations involving band 3q27 and Ig gene regions in non-Hodgkin's lymphoma [see comments]. Blood 1992;79:2527–31.
103. Sanchez-Izquierdo D, Siebert R, Harder L, et al. Detection of translocations affecting the BCL6 locus in B cell non-Hodgkin's lymphoma by interphase fluorescence in situ hybridization. Leukemia 2001;15:1475–84.
104. Roumier C, Galiegue-Zouitina S, Bastard C, et al. FISH analysis with a YAC probe improves detection of LAZ3/BCL6 rearrangement in non-Hodgkin's lymphoma. Hematol J 2000;1:117–25.
105. Martin-Subero JI, Harder L, Gesk S, et al. Interphase FISH assays for the detection of translocations with breakpoints in immunoglobulin light chain loci. Int J Cancer 2002; 98:470–4.
106. Offit K, Louie DC, Parsa NZ, et al. BCL6 gene rearrangement and other cytogenetic abnormalities in diffuse large cell lymphoma. Leuk Lymphoma 1995;20:85–9.
107. Akasaka T, Ueda C, Kurata M, et al. Nonimmunoglobulin (non-Ig)/BCL6 gene fusion in diffuse large B-cell lymphoma results in worse prognosis than Ig/BCL6. Blood 2000; 96:2907–9.
108. Ladanyi M, Offit K, Jhanwar SC, et al. MYC rearrangement and translocations involving band 8q24 in diffuse large cell lymphomas. Blood 1991;77:1057–63.
109. Alizadeh AA, Eisen MB, Davis RE, et al. Distinct types of diffuse large B-cell lymphoma identified by gene expression profiling. Nature 2000;403:503–11.
110. Molina A, Lombard C, Donlon T, et al. Immunohistochemical and cytogenetic studies indicate that malignant angioendotheliomatosis is a primary intravascular (angiotropic) lymphoma. Cancer 1990;66:474–9 [erratum in Cancer 1990;66:683].
111. Murase T, Nakamura S, Kawauchi K, et al. An Asian variant of intravascular large B-cell lymphoma: clinical, pathological and cytogenetic approaches to diffuse large B-cell lymphoma associated with haemophagocytic syndrome. Br J Haematol 2000;111:826–34.
112. Davey DD, Munn R, Smith LW, et al. Angiotrophic lymphoma. Presentation in uterine vessels with cytogenetic studies. Arch Pathol Lab Med 1990;114:879–82.
113. Khoury H, Lestou VS, Gascoyne RD, et al. Multicolor karyotyping and clinicopathological analysis of three intravascular lymphoma cases. Mod Pathol 2003;16:716–24.
114. Murase T, Nakamura S, Tashiro K, et al. Malignant histiocytosis-like B-cell lymphoma, a distinct pathologic variant of intravascular lymphomatosis: a report of five cases and review of the literature. Br J Haematol 1997;99:656–64.
115. Zattara-Cannoni H, Horshowski N, Figarella-Branger D, et al. Unusual chromosome abnormalities in primary central nervous system lymphoma. Leuk Lymphoma 1996;21: 515–7.
116. Weber T, Weber RG, Kaulich K, et al. Characteristic chromosomal imbalances in primary central nervous system lymphomas of the diffuse large B-cell type. Brain Pathol 2000;10:73–84.
117. Rickert CH, Dockhorn Dworniczak B, Simon R, et al. Chromosomal imbalances in primary lymphomas of the central nervous system. Am J Pathol 1999;155:1445–51.
118. Boonstra R, Koning A, Mastik M, et al. Analysis of chromosomal copy number changes and oncoprotein expression in primary central nervous system lymphomas: frequent loss of chromosome arm 6q. Virchows Arch 2003;443:164–9.
119. Itoyama T, Sadamori N, Tsutsumi K, et al. Primary central nervous system lymphomas. Immunophenotypic, virologic, and cytogenetic findings of three patients without immune defects. Cancer 1994;73:455–63.
120. Barth TF, Leithauser F, Joos S, et al. Mediastinal (thymic) large B-cell lymphoma: where do we stand? Lancet Oncol 2002;3:229–34.
121. Joos S, Otano-Joos MI, Ziegler S, et al. Primary mediastinal (thymic) B-cell lymphoma is characterized by gains of chromosomal material including 9p and amplification of the REL gene. Blood 1996;87:1571–8.
122. Bentz M, Barth TF, Bruderlein S, et al. Gain of chromosome arm 9p is characteristic of primary mediastinal B-cell lymphoma (MBL): comprehensive molecular cytogenetic analysis and presentation of a novel MBL cell line. Genes Chromosomes Cancer 2001;30:393–401.
123. Scarpa A, Taruscio D, Scardoni M, et al. Nonrandom chromosomal imbalances in primary mediastinal B-cell lymphoma detected by arbitrarily primed PCR fingerprinting. Genes Chromosomes Cancer 1999;26:203–9.
124. Rigaud G, Moore PS, Taruscio D, et al. Alteration of chromosome arm 6p is characteristic of primary mediastinal B-cell lymphoma, as identified by genome-wide allelotyping. Genes Chromosomes Cancer 2001;31:191–5.
125. Coignet LJ, Schuuring E, Kibbelaar RE, et al. Detection of 11q13 rearrangements in hematologic neoplasias by double-

color fluorescence in situ hybridization. Blood 1996;87: 1512–9.
126. Vaandrager JW, Schuuring E, Zwikstra E, et al. Direct visualization of dispersed 11q13 chromosomal translocations in mantle cell lymphoma by multicolor DNA fiber fluorescence in situ hybridization. Blood 1996;88:1177–82.
127. Brito-Babapulle V, Pittman S, Melo JV, et al. Cytogenetic studies on prolymphocytic leukemia. 1. B-cell prolymphocytic leukemia. Hematol Pathol 1987;1:27–33.
128. Komatsu H, Yoshida K, Seto M, et al. Overexpression of PRAD1 in a mantle zone lymphoma patient with a t(11;22)(q13;q11) translocation. Br J Haematol 1993; 85:427–9.
129. Siebert R, Matthiesen P, Harder S, et al. Application of interphase cytogenetics for the detection of t(11;14)(q13;q32) in mantle cell lymphomas. Ann Oncol 1998;9:519–26.
130. Mohamed AN, Ali W, Kopptich F, et al. Banded chromosomes versus fluorescence in situ hybridization in the diagnosis of mantle cell lymphoma: a lesson from three cases. Cancer Genet Cytogenet 2002;136:108–12.
131. Aventin A, Nomdedeu J, Briones J, et al. Insertion of the CCND1 gene into the IgH locus in a case of leukaemic small cell mantle lymphoma with normal chromosomes 11 and 14. J Clin Pathol 2003;56:798–800.
132. Rosenwald A, Wright G, Wiestner A, et al. The proliferation gene expression signature is a quantitative integrator of oncogenic events that predicts survival in mantle cell lymphoma. Cancer Cell 2003;3:185–97.
133. Hui P, Howe JG, Crouch J, et al. Real-time quantitative RT-PCR of cyclin D1 mRNA in mantle cell lymphoma: comparison with FISH and immunohistochemistry. Leuk Lymphoma 2003;44:1385–94.
134. Bodrug SE, Warner BJ, Bath ML, et al. Cyclin D1 transgene impedes lymphocyte maturation and collaborates in lymphomagenesis with the myc gene. EMBO J 1994;13: 2124–30.
135. Cuneo A, Bigoni R, Rigolin GM, et al. Cytogenetic profile of lymphoma of follicle mantle lineage: correlation with clinicobiologic features. Blood 1999;93:1372–80.
136. Woroniecka R, Pienkowska-Grela B, Grygalewicz B, et al. Significance of chromosomal markers in the diagnosis of mantle cell lymphoma (MCL). J Appl Genet 2002; 43:545–53.
137. Bea S, Ribas M, Hernandez JM, et al. Increased number of chromosomal imbalances and high-level DNA amplifications in mantle cell lymphoma are associated with blastoid variants. Blood 1999;93:4365–74.
138. Au WY, Gascoyne RD, Viswanatha DS, et al. Cytogenetic analysis in mantle cell lymphoma: a review of 214 cases. Leuk Lymphoma 2002;43:783–91.
139. Dubus P, Young P, Beylot-Barry M, et al. Value of interphase FISH for the diagnosis of t(11:14)(q13;q32) on skin lesions of mantle cell lymphoma. Am J Clin Pathol 2002; 118:832–41.
140. Bigoni R, Cuneo A, Milani R, et al. Secondary chromosome changes in mantle cell lymphoma: cytogenetic and fluorescence in situ hybridization studies. Leuk Lymphoma 2001;40:581–90.
141. Espinet B, Sole F, Woessner S, et al. Translocation (11;14)(q13;q32) and preferential involvement of chromosomes 1, 2, 9, 13, and 17 in mantle cell lymphoma. Cancer Genet Cytogenet 1999;111:92–8.
142. Wlodarska I, Pittaluga S, Hagemeijer A, et al. Secondary chromosome changes in mantle cell lymphoma. Haematologica 1999;84:594–9.
143. Au WY, Horsman DE, Viswanatha DS, et al. 8q24 translocations in blastic transformation of mantle cell lymphoma. Haematologica 2000;85:1225–7.
144. Onciu M, Schlette E, Medeiros LJ, et al. Cytogenetic findings in mantle cell lymphoma cases with a high level of peripheral blood involvement have a distinct pattern of abnormalities. Am J Clin Pathol 2001;116:886–92.
145. Schlette E, Lai R, Onciu M, et al. Leukemic mantle cell lymphoma: clinical and pathologic spectrum of twenty-three cases. Mod Pathol 2001;14:1133–40.
146. Raty R, Franssila K, Jansson SE, et al. Predictive factors for blastoid transformation in the common variant of mantle cell lymphoma. Eur J Cancer 2003;39:321–9.
147. Ott G, Kalla J, Ott MM, et al. Blastoid variants of mantle cell lymphoma: frequent bcl-1 rearrangements at the major translocation cluster region and tetraploid chromosome clones. Blood 1997;89:1421–9.
148. Khoury JD, Sen F, Abruzzo LV, et al. Cytogenetic findings in blastoid mantle cell lymphoma. Hum Pathol 2003;34: 1022–9.
149. Hao S, Sanger W, Onciu M, et al. Mantle cell lymphoma with 8q24 chromosomal abnormalities: a report of 5 cases with blastoid features. Mod Pathol 2002;15:1266–72.
150. Tirier C, Zhang Y, Plendl H, et al. Simultaneous presence of t(11;14) and a variant Burkitt's translocation in the terminal phase of a mantle cell lymphoma. Leukemia 1996; 10:346–50.
151. Vaishampayan UN, Mohamed AN, Dugan MC, et al. Blastic mantle cell lymphoma associated with Burkitt-type translocation and hypodiploidy. Br J Haematol 2001;115: 66–8.
152. de Vos S, Krug U, Hofmann WK, et al. Cell cycle alterations in the blastoid variant of mantle cell lymphoma (MCL-BV) as detected by gene expression profiling of mantle cell lymphoma (MCL) and MCL-BV. Diagn Mol Pathol 2003;12:35–43.
153. Allen JE, Hough RE, Goepel JR, et al. Identification of novel regions of amplification and deletion within mantle cell lymphoma DNA by comparative genomic hybridization. Br J Haematol 2002;116:291–8.
154. Bentz M, Plesch A, Bullinger L, et al. t(11;14)-positive mantle cell lymphomas exhibit complex karyotypes and share similarities with B-cell chronic lymphocytic leukemia. Genes Chromosomes Cancer 2000;27:285–94.
155. Monni O, Oinonen R, Elonen E, et al. Gain of 3q and deletion of 11q22 are frequent aberrations in mantle cell lymphoma. Genes Chromosomes Cancer 1998;21:298–307.
156. Stokke T, DeAngelis P, Smedshammer L, et al. Loss of chromosome 11q21–23.1 and 17p and gain of chromosome 6p are independent prognostic indicators in B-cell non-Hodgkin's lymphoma. Br J Cancer 2001;85:1900–13.
157. Werner CA, Dohner H, Joos S, et al. High-level DNA amplifications are common genetic aberrations in B-cell neoplasms. Am J Pathol 1997;151:335–42.
158. Rosenwald A, Ott G, Krumdiek AK, et al. A biological role for deletions in chromosomal band 13q14 in mantle cell and peripheral T-cell lymphomas? Genes Chromosomes Cancer 1999;26:210–4.
159. Kohlhammer H, Schwaenen C, Wessendorf S, et al. Genomic DNA-chip hybridization in t(11;14)-positive mantle cell lymphomas shows a high frequency of aberrations and allows a refined characterization of consensus regions. Blood 2004;104:795–801.
160. Wotherspoon AC, Pan LX, Diss TC, et al. Cytogenetic study of B-cell lymphoma of mucosa-associated lymphoid tissue. Cancer Genet Cytogenet 1992;58:35–8.
161. Wotherspoon AC, Finn TM, Isaacson PG. Trisomy 3 in low-grade B-cell lymphomas of mucosa-associated lymphoid tissue. Blood 1995;85:2000–4.
162. Brynes RK, Almaguer PD, Leathery KE, et al. Numerical cytogenetic abnormalities of chromosomes 3, 7, and 12 in

marginal zone B-cell lymphomas. Mod Pathol 1996; 9:995–1000.
163. Dierlamm J, Michaux L, Wlodarska I, et al. Trisomy 3 in marginal zone B-cell lymphoma: a study based on cytogenetic analysis and fluorescence in situ hybridization. Br J Haematol 1996;93:242–9.
164. Griffin CA, Zehnbauer BA, Beschorner WE, et al. t(11;18) (q21;q21) is a recurrent chromosome abnormality in small lymphocytic lymphoma. Genes Chromosomes Cancer 1992;4:153–7.
165. Horsman D, Gascoyne R, Klasa R, et al. t(11;18)(q21;q21.1): a recurring translocation in lymphomas of mucosa-associated lymphoid tissue (MALT)? Genes Chromosomes Cancer 1992;4:183–7.
166. Ott MM, Müller-Hermelink HK. The t(11;18)(q21;q21) chromosome translocation is a frequent and specific aberration in low-grade but not high-grade malignant non-Hodgkin's lymphomas of the mucosa-associated lymphoid tissue (MALT-) type. Cancer Res 1997;57:3944–8.
167. Schreuder MI, Hoeve MA, Hebeda KM, et al. Mutual exclusion of t(11;18)(q21;q21) and numerical chromosomal aberrations in the development of different types of primary gastric lymphomas. Br J Haematol 2003;123:590–9.
168. Dierlamm J, Pittaluga S, Wlodarska I, et al. Marginal zone B-cell lymphomas of different sites share similar cytogenetic and morphologic features. Blood 1996;87:299–307.
169. Ott G, Kalla J, Steinhoff A, et al. Trisomy 3 is not a common feature in malignant lymphomas of mucosa-associated lymphoid tissue type. Am J Pathol 1998;153:689–94.
170. Dierlamm J, Rosenberg C, Stul M, et al. Characteristic pattern of chromosomal gains and losses in marginal zone B cell lymphoma detected by comparative genomic hybridization. Leukemia 1997;11:747–58.
171. Dierlamm J, Pittaluga S, Stul M, et al. BCL6 gene rearrangements also occur in marginal zone B-cell lymphoma. Br J Haematol 1997;98:719–25.
172. Sanchez-Izquierdo D, Buchonnet G, Siebert R, et al. MALT1 is deregulated by both chromosomal translocation and amplification in B-cell non-Hodgkin lymphoma. Blood 2003;101:4539–46.
173. Rosenwald A, Stilgenbauer S, Kalla J, et al. Exclusive detection of the t(11;18)(q21;q21) in extranodal marginal zone B cell lymphomas (MZBL) of MALT type in contrast to other MZBL and extranodal large B cell lymphomas. Am J Pathol 1999;155:1817–21.
174. Auer IA, Gascoyne RD, Connors JM, et al. t(11;18)(q21;q21) is the most common translocation in MALT lymphomas. Ann Oncol 1997;8:979–85.
175. Kobayashi Y, Nakata M, Maekawa M, et al. Detection of t(I 1;18) in MALT-type lymphoma with dual-color fluorescence in situ hybridization and reverse transcriptase-polymerase chain reaction analysis. Diagn Mol Pathol 2001;10:207–13.
176. Matteucci C, Galieni P, Leoncini L, et al. Typical genomic imbalances in primary MALT lymphoma of the orbit. J Pathol 2003;200:656–60.
177. Okabe M, Inagaki H, Ohshima K, et al. API2-MALT1 fusion defines a distinctive clinicopathologic subtype in pulmonary extranodal marginal zone B-cell lymphoma of mucosa-associated lymphoid tissue. Am J Pathol 2003;162:1113–22.
178. Yonezumi M, Suzuki R, Suzuki H, et al. Detection of AP12-MALT1 chimaeric gene in extranodal and nodal marginal zone B-cell lymphoma by reverse transcription polymerase chain reaction (PCR) and genomic long and accurate PCR analyses. Br J Haematol 2001;115:588–94.
179. Akagi T, Motegi M, Tamura A, et al. A novel gene, MALT1 at 18q21, is involved in t(11;18) (q21;q21) found in low-grade B-cell lymphoma of mucosa-associated lymphoid tissue. Oncogene 1999;18:5785–94.
180. Hosaka S, Akamatsu T, Nakamura S, et al. Mucosa-associated lymphoid tissue (MALT) lymphoma of the rectum with chromosomal translocation of the t(11;18)(q21;q21) and an additional aberration of trisomy 3. Am J Gastroenterol 1999;94:1951–4.
181. Kubonishi I, Sugito S, Kobayashi M, et al. A unique chromosome translocation, t(11;12;18)(q21;q13;q21) [correction of t(11;12;18)(q13;q13;q12)], in primary lung lymphoma. Cancer Genet Cytogenet 1995;82:54–6.
182. Dierlamm J, Murga Penas EM, Daibata M, et al. The novel t(11;12;18)(q21;q13;q21) represents a variant translocation of the t(11;18)(q21;q21) associated with MALT-type lymphoma. Leukemia 2002;16:1863–4.
183. Mobarak MA, Brody JI. Natural evolution and pathological alterations of lymphoid cell proteins. Immunochemical characteristics of soluble antigens. Clin Chim Acta 1970;30: 609–19.
184. Morgan JA, Yin Y, Borowsky AD, et al. Breakpoints of the t(11;18)(q21;q21) in mucosa-associated lymphoid tissue (MALT) lymphoma lie within or near the previously undescribed gene MALT1 in chromosome 18. Cancer Res 1999;59:6205–13.
185. Dierlamm J, Baens M, Wlodarska I, et al. The apoptosis inhibitor gene API2 and a novel 18q gene, MLT, are recurrently rearranged in the t(11;18)(q21;q21)p6ssociated with mucosa-associated lymphoid tissue lymphomas. Blood 1999;93:3601–9.
186. Sato Y, Akiyama Y, Tanizawa T, et al. Molecular characterization of the genomic breakpoint junction in the t(11;18) (q21;q21) translocation of a gastric MALT lymphoma. Biochem Biophys Res Commun 2001;280: 301–6.
187. Baens M, Steyls A, Dierlamm J, et al. Structure of the MLT gene and molecular characterization of the genomic breakpoint junctions in the t(11;18)(q21;q21) of marginal zone B-cell lymphomas of MALT type. Genes Chromosomes Cancer 2000;29:281–91.
188. Baens M, Maes B, Steyls A, et al. The product of the t(11;18), an API2-MLT fusion, marks nearly half of gastric MALT type lymphomas without large cell proliferation. Am J Pathol 2000;156:1433–9.
189. Inagaki H, Okabe M, Seto M, et al. API2-MALT1 fusion transcripts involved in mucosa-associated lymphoid tissue lymphoma: multiplex RT-PCR detection using formalin-fixed paraffin-embedded specimens. Am J Pathol 2001;158: 699–706.
190. Maes M, Depardieu C, Dargent JL, et al. Primary low-grade B-cell lymphoma of MALT-type occurring in the liver: a study of two cases. J Hepatol 1997;27:922–7.
191. Remstein ED, James CD, Kurtin PJ. Incidence and subtype specificity of API2-MALT1 fusion translocations in extranodal, nodal, and splenic marginal zone lymphomas. Am J Pathol 2000;156:1183–8.
192. Streubel B, Lamprecht A, Dierlamm J, et al. T(14;18) (q32;q21) involving IGH and MALT1 is a frequent chromosomal aberration in MALT lymphoma. Blood 2003;101: 2335–9.
193. Willis TG, Jadayel DM, Du MQ, et al. Bcl10 is involved in t(1;14)(p22;q32) of MALT B cell lymphoma and mutated in multiple tumor types. Cell 1999;96:35–45.
194. Zhang Q, Siebert R, Yan M, et al. Inactivating mutations and overexpression of BCL10, a caspase recruitment domain-containing gene, in MALT lymphoma with t(1;14)(p22;q32). Nat Genet 1999;22:63–8.
195. Lucas PC, Yonezumi M, Inohara N, et al. Bcl10 and MALT1, independent targets of chromosomal translocation in malt lymphoma, cooperate in a novel NF-kappa B signaling pathway. J Biol Chem 2001;276:19012–9.

196. Uren AG, O'Rourke K, Aravind LA, et al. Identification of paracaspases and metacaspases: two ancient families of caspase-like proteins, one of which plays a key role in MALT lymphoma. Mol Cell 2000;6:961–7.
197. Murga Penas EM, Hinz K, Roser K, et al. Translocations t(11;18)(q21;q21) and t(14;18)(q32;q21) are the main chromosomal abnormalities involving MLT/MALT1 in MALT lymphomas. Leukemia 2003;17:2225–9.
198. Offit K, Louie DC, Parsa NZ, et al. Del (7)(q32) is associated with a subset of small lymphocytic lymphoma with plasmacytoid features. Blood 1995;86:2365–70.
199. Sole F, Salido M, Espinet B, et al. Splenic marginal zone B-cell lymphomas: two cytogenetic subtypes, one with gain of 3q and the other with loss of 7q. Haematologica 2001; 86:71–7.
200. Sole F, Woessner S, Florensa L, et al. Frequent involvement of chromosomes 1, 3, 7 and 8 in splenic marginal zone B-cell lymphoma. Br J Haematol 1997;98:446–9.
201. Hernandez JM, Mecucci C, Michaux L, et al. del(7q) in chronic B-cell lymphoid malignancies. Cancer Genet Cytogenet 1997;93:147–51.
202. Mateo M, Mollejo M, Villuendas R, et al.7q31–32 allelic loss is a frequent finding in splenic marginal zone lymphoma. Am J Pathol 1999;154:1583–9.
203. Gruszka-Westwood AM, Hamoudi R, Osborne L, et al. Deletion mapping on the long arm of chromosome 7 in splenic lymphoma with villous lymphocytes. Genes Chromosomes Cancer 2003;36:57–69.
204. Gruszka-Westwood AM, Hamoudi RA, Matutes E, et al. p53 abnormalities in splenic lymphoma with villous lymphocytes. Blood 2001;97:3552–8.
205. Baldini L, Fracchiolla NS, Cro LM, et al. Frequent p53 gene involvement in splenic B-cell leukemia/lymphomas of possible marginal zone origin. Blood 1994;84:270–8.
206. Batanian JR, Dunphy CH, Richart JM, et al. Simultaneous presence of t(2;8)(p12;q24) and t(14;18)(q32;q21) in a B-cell lymphoproliferative disorder with features suggestive of an aggressive variant of splenic marginal-zone lymphoma. Cancer Genet Cytogenet 2000;120:136–40.
207. Thieblemont C, Felman P, Callet-Bauchu E, et al. Splenic marginal-zone lymphoma: a distinct clinical and pathological entity. Lancet Oncol 2003;4:95–103.
208. Troussard X, Mauvieux L, Radford Weiss I, et al. Genetic analysis of splenic lymphoma with villous lymphocytes: a Groupe Francais d'Hematologie Cellulaire (GFHC) study. Br J Haematol 1998;101:712–21.
209. Cuneo A, Bardi A, Wlodarska I, et al. A novel recurrent translocation t(11;14)(p11;q32) in splenic marginal zone B cell lymphoma. Leukemia 2001;15:1262–7.
210. Hernandez JM, Garcia JL, Gutierrez NC, et al. Novel genomic imbalances in B-cell splenic marginal zone lymphomas revealed by comparative genomic hybridization and cytogenetics. Am J Pathol 2001;158:1843–50.
211. Lloret E, Mollejo M, Mateo MS, et al. Splenic marginal zone lymphoma with increased number of blasts: an aggressive variant? Hum Pathol 1999;30:1153–60.
212. Martinez-Climent JA, Sanchez-Izquierdo D, Sarsotti E, et al. Genomic abnormalities acquired in the blastic transformation of splenic marginal zone B-cell lymphoma. Leuk Lymphoma 2003;44:459–64.
213. Thieblemont C, Felman P, Berger F, et al. Treatment of splenic marginal zone B-cell lymphoma: an analysis of 81 patients. Clin Lymphoma 2002;3:41–7.
214. Ott MM, Rosenwald A, Katzenberger T, et al. Marginal zone B-cell lymphomas (MZBL) arising at different sites represent different biological entities. Genes Chromosomes Cancer 2000;28:380–6.
215. Gazzo S, Baseggio L, Coignet L, et al. Cytogenetic and molecular delineation of a region of chromosome 3q commonly gained in marginal zone B-cell lymphoma. Haematologica 2003;88:31–8.
216. Elenitoba-Johnson KS, Kumar S, Lim MS, et al. Marginal zone B-cell lymphoma with monocytoid B-cell lymphocytes in pediatric patients without immunodeficiency. A report of two cases. Am J Clin Pathol 1997;107:92–8.
217. Cuneo A, Bigoni R, Roberti MG, et al. Molecular cytogenetic characterization of marginal zone B-cell lymphoma: correlation with clinicopathologic findings in 14 cases. Haematologica 2001;86:64–70.
218. Cook JR, Sherer M, Craig FE, et al. T(14;18)(q32;q21) involving MALT1 and IGH genes in an extranodal diffuse large B-cell lymphoma. Hum Pathol 2003;34:1212–5.
219. Mao X, Lillington D, Child F, et al. Comparative genomic hybridization analysis of primary cutaneous B-cell lymphomas: identification of common genomic alterations in disease pathogenesis. Genes Chromosomes Cancer 2002; 35:144–55.
220. Dascalescu CM, Peoc'h M, Callanan M, et al. Deletion 7q in B-cell low-grade lymphoid malignancies: a cytogenetic/fluorescence in situ hybridization and immunopathologic study. Cancer Genet Cytogenet 1999;109:21–8.
221. Cook JR, Aguilera NI, Reshmi-Skarja S, et al. Lack of PAX5 rearrangements in lymphoplasmacytic lymphomas: reassessing the reported association with t(9;14). Hum Pathol 2004;35:447–54.
222. Itoyama T, Chaganti RS, Yamada Y, et al. Cytogenetic analysis and clinical significance in adult T-cell leukemia/lymphoma: a study of 50 cases from the human T-cell leukemia virus type-1 endemic area, Nagasaki. Blood 2001;97: 3612–20.
223. Kamada N, Sakurai M, Miyamoto K, et al. Chromosome abnormalities in adult T-cell leukemia/lymphoma: a karyotype review committee report. Cancer Res 1992;52: 1481–93.
224. Stein H, Mason DY, Gerdes J, et al. The expression of the Hodgkin's disease associated antigen Ki-1 in reactive and neoplastic lymphoid tissue: evidence that Reed–Sternberg cells and histiocytic malignancies are derived from activated lymphoid cells. Blood 1985;66:848–58.
225. Fischer P, Nacheva E, Mason DY, et al. A Ki-1 (CD30)-positive human cell line (Karpas 299) established from a high-grade non-Hodgkin's lymphoma, showing a 2;5 translocation and rearrangement of the T-cell receptor beta-chain gene. Blood 1988;72:234–40.
226. Morris SW, Kirstein MN, Valentine MB, et al. Fusion of a kinase gene, ALK, to a nucleolar protein gene, NPM, in non-Hodgkin's lymphoma. Science 1995;267:316–7.
227. Johnson PW, Leek J, Swinbank K, et al. The use of fluorescent in situ hybridization for detection of the t(2;5)(p23;q35) translocation in anaplastic large-cell lymphoma. Ann Oncol 1997;8:65–9.
228. Mathew P, Sanger WG, Weisenburger DD, et al. Detection of the t(2;5)(p23;q35) and NPM-ALK fusion in non-Hodgkin's lymphoma by two-color fluorescence in situ hybridization. Blood 1997;89:1678–85.
229. Elmberger PG, Lozano MD, Weisenburger DD, et al. Transcripts of the npm-alk fusion gene in anaplastic large cell lymphoma, Hodgkin's disease, and reactive lymphoid lesions. Blood 1995;86:3517–21.
230. Herbst H, Anagnostopoulos J, Heinze B, et al. ALK gene products in anaplastic large cell lymphomas and Hodgkin's disease. Blood 1995;86:1694–700.
231. Lamant L, Meggetto F, al Saati T, et al. High incidence of the t(2;5)(p23;q35) translocation in anaplastic large cell

lymphoma and its lack of detection in Hodgkin's disease. Comparison of cytogenetic analysis, reverse transcriptase-polymerase chain reaction, and P-80 immunostaining. Blood 1996;87:284–91.
232. Weiss LM, Lopategui JR, Sun LH, et al. Absence of the t(2;5) in Hodgkin's disease. Blood 1995;85:2845–7.
233. Pittaluga S, Wlodarska I, Pulford K, et al. The monoclonal antibody ALK1 identifies a distinct morphological subtype of anaplastic large cell lymphoma associated with 2p23/ALK rearrangements. Am J Pathol 1997;151:343–51.
234. Drexler HG, Gignac SM, von Wasielewski R, et al. Pathobiology of NPM-ALK and variant fusion genes in anaplastic large cell lymphoma and other lymphomas. Leukemia 2000;14:1533–59.
235. Kutok JL, Aster JC. Molecular biology of anaplastic lymphoma kinase-positive anaplastic large-cell lymphoma. J Clin Oncol 2002;20:3691–702.
236. Gogusev J, Telvi L, Nezelof C. Molecular cytogenetic aberrations in CD30+ anaplastic large cell lymphoma cell lines. Cancer Genet Cytogenet 2002;138:95–101.
237. Ott G, Katzenberger T, Siebert R, et al. Chromosomal abnormalities in nodal and extranodal CD30+ anaplastic large cell lymphomas: infrequent detection of the t(2;5) in extranodal lymphomas. Genes Chromosomes Cancer 1998;22:114–21.
238. Kinney MC, Kadin ME. The pathologic and clinical spectrum of anaplastic large cell lymphoma and correlation with ALK gene dysregulation. Am J Clin Pathol 1999;111: S56–67.
239. Chou WC, Su IJ, Tien HF, et al. Clinicopathologic, cytogenetic, and molecular studies of 13 Chinese Patients with Ki-1 anaplastic large cell lymphoma. Special emphasis on the tumor response to 13-cis retinoic acid. Cancer 1996;78: 1805–12.
240. Weisenburger DD, Gordon BG, Vose JM, et al. Occurrence of the t(2;5)(p23;q35) in non-Hodgkin's lymphoma. Blood 1996;87:3860–8.
241. Chhanabhai M, Britten C, Klasa R, et al. t(2;5) positive lymphoma with peripheral blood involvement. Leuk Lymphoma 1998;28:415–22.
242. Onciu M, Behm FG, Raimondi SC, et al. ALK-positive anaplastic large cell lymphoma with leukemic peripheral blood involvement is a clinicopathologic entity with an unfavorable prognosis. Report of three cases and review of the literature. Am J Clin Pathol 2003;120:617–25.
243. Hodges KB, Collins RD, Greer JP, et al. Transformation of the small cell variant Ki-1+ lymphoma to anaplastic large cell lymphoma: pathologic and clinical features. Am J Surg Pathol 1999;23:49–58.
244. Lemes A, De La Iglesia S, Santana C, et al. t(2;5) associated with a histiocytic-monocytic neoplasm. Leuk Lymphoma 2001;41:429–33.
245. Cools J, Wlodarska I, Somers R, et al. Identification of novel fusion partners of ALK, the anaplastic lymphoma kinase, in anaplastic large-cell lymphoma and inflammatory myofibroblastic tumor. Genes Chromosomes Cancer 2002;34: 354–62.
246. Godde-Salz E, Feller AC, Lennert K. Chromosomal abnormalities in lymphogranulomatosis X (LgrX)/angioimmunoblastic lymphadenopathy (AILD). Leuk Res 1987; 11:181–90.
247. Zettl A, Ott G, Makulik A, et al. Chromosomal gains at 9q characterize enteropathy-type T-cell lymphoma. Am J Pathol 2002;161:1635–45.
248. Obermann EC, Diss TC, Hamoudi RA, et al. Loss of heterozygosity at chromosome 9p21 is a frequent finding in enteropathy-type T-cell lymphoma. J Pathol 2004;202: 252–62.
249. Baumgartner AK, Zettl A, Chott A, et al. High frequency of genetic aberrations in enteropathy-type T-cell lymphoma. Lab Invest 2003;83:1509–16.
250. Alonsozana EL, Stamberg J, Kumar D, et al. Isochromosome 7q: the primary cytogenetic abnormality in hepatosplenic gammadelta T cell lymphoma. Leukemia 1997;11:1367–72.
251. Jonveaux P, Daniel MT, Martel V, et al. Isochromosome 7q and trisomy 8 are consistent primary, non-random chromosomal abnormalities associated with hepatosplenic T gamma/delta lymphoma. Leukemia 1996;10:1453–5.
252. Rossbach HC, Chamizo W, Dumont DP, et al. Hepatosplenic gamma/delta T-cell lymphoma with isochromosome 7q, translocation t(7;21), and tetrasomy 8 in a 9-year-old girl. J Pediatr Hematol Oncol 2002;24:154–7.
253. Wang CC, Tien HF, Lin MT, et al. Consistent presence of isochromosome 7q in hepatosplenic T gamma/delta lymphoma: a new cytogenetic-clinicopathologic entity. Genes Chromosomes Cancer 1995;12:161–4.
254. Wlodarska I, Martin-Garcia N, Achten R, et al. Fluorescence in situ hybridization study of chromosome 7 aberrations in hepatosplenic T-cell lymphoma: isochromosome 7q as a common abnormality accumulating in forms with features of cytologic progression. Genes Chromosomes Cancer 2002; 33:243–51.
255. Zhang Y, Wong KF, Siebert R, et al. Chromosome aberrations are restricted to the CD56+, CD3- tumour cell population in natural killer cell lymphomas: a combined immunophenotyping and FISH study. Br J Haematol 1999;105:737–42.
256. Tien HF, Su IJ, Tang JL, et al. Clonal chromosomal abnormalities as direct evidence for clonality in nasal T/natural killer cell lymphomas. Br J Haematol 1997;97: 621–5.
257. Mao X, Onadim Z, Price EA, et al. Genomic alterations in blastic natural killer/extranodal natural killer-like T cell lymphoma with cutaneous involvement. J Invest Dermatol 2003;121:618–27.
258. Siu LL, Wong KF, Chan JK, et al. Comparative genomic hybridization analysis of natural killer cell lymphoma/ leukemia. Recognition of consistent patterns of genetic alterations. Am J Pathol 1999;155:1419–25.
259. Ko YH, Choi KE, Han JH, et al. Comparative genomic hybridization study of nasal-type NK/T-cell lymphoma. Cytometry 2001;46:85–91.
260. Whang-Peng J, Bunn PA Jr, Knutsen T, et al. Clinical implications of cytogenetic studies in cutaneous T-cell lymphoma (CTCL). Cancer 1982;50:1539–53.
261. Karenko L, Hyytinen E, Sarna S, et al. Chromosomal abnormalities in cutaneous T-cell lymphoma and in its premalignant conditions as detected by G-banding and interphase cytogenetic methods. J Invest Dermatol 1997;108:22–9.
262. Cabanillas F, Pathak S, Trujillo J, et al. Cytogenetic features of Hodgkin's disease suggest possible origin from a lymphocyte. Blood 1988;71:1615–7.
263. Ladanyi M, Parsa NZ, Offit K, et al. Clonal cytogenetic abnormalities in Hodgkin's disease. Genes Chromosomes Cancer 1991;3:294–9.
264. Pringle JH, Shaw JA, Gillies A, et al. Numerical chromosomal aberrations in Hodgkin's disease detected by in situ hybridisation on routine paraffin sections. J Clin Pathol 1997;50:553–8.
265. Falzetti D, Crescenzi B, Matteuci C, et al. Genomic instability and recurrent breakpoints are main cytogenetic findings in Hodgkin's disease. Haematologica 1999;84:298–305.
266. Poppema S, Kaleta J, Hepperle B. Chromosomal abnormalities in patients with Hodgkin's disease: evidence for frequent involvement of the 14q chromosomal region but infrequent

bcl-2 gene rearrangement in Reed–Sternberg cells. J Natl Cancer Inst 1992;84:1789–93.
267. Gravel S, Delsol G, Al Saati T. Single-cell analysis of the t(14;18)(q32;q21) chromosomal translocation in Hodgkin's disease demonstrates the absence of this translocation in neoplastic Hodgkin and Reed–Sternberg cells. Blood 1998;91:2866–74.
268. Joos S, Menz CK, Wrobel G, et al. Classical Hodgkin lymphoma is characterized by recurrent copy number gains of the short arm of chromosome 2. Blood 2002;99:1381–7.
269. Chui DT, Hammond D, Baird M, et al. Classical Hodgkin lymphoma is associated with frequent gains of 17q. Genes Chromosomes Cancer 2003;38:126–36.
270. Martin-Subero JI, Gesk S, Harder L, et al. Recurrent involvement of the REL and BCL11A loci in classical Hodgkin lymphoma. Blood 2002;99:1474–7.
271. Berglund M, Flordal E, Gullander J, et al. Molecular cytogenetic characterization of four commonly used cell lines derived from Hodgkin lymphoma. Cancer Genet Cytogenet 2003;141:43–8.
272. Joos S, Granzow M, Holtgreve-Grez H, et al. Hodgkin's lymphoma cell lines are characterized by frequent aberrations on chromosomes 2p and 9p including REL and JAK2. Int J Cancer 2003;103:489–95.
273. Cigudosa JC, Parsa NZ, Louie DC, et al. Cytogenetic analysis of 363 consecutively ascertained diffuse large B-cell lymphomas. Genes Chromosomes Cancer 1999;25(2):123–33.

3

Molecular Biology of Lymphoma

Vassaliki I. Pappa, M.D.
Bryan D. Young, Ph.D.

Recent advances in molecular genetics have led to the identification of a series of genes affected by chromosomal translocations in lymphoma. It is now clear that the proteins encoded by these genes play important roles in the control of apoptosis and cell cycle progression. The timing and frequency of tumors in animals made transgenic for a single event, such as a translocation, has highlighted the requirement for subsequent genetic changes that act in a cooperative manner to create the fully transformed cell. It is now clear that the control mechanisms of both apoptosis and cell cycle progression involve a complex series of dynamic protein–protein interactions. Disruptions to these interactions, whether by translocation, mutation, or gene deletion can be expected to have profound effects on the behavior of cells. The complex nature of these interactions suggests that it may be possible to reach full tumorigenicity by several different routes. Thus, although there are clear associations between certain chromosomal translocations and lymphoma sub-groups (see Chapter 2), there may well exist underlying cooperative genetic changes that provide full tumorigenicity.

Molecular analysis of translocations in lymphoma, leukemia, and certain solid tumors[1] has shown that they fall into two general classes. The first type involves the activation of a proto-oncogene by juxtaposition into the immunoglobulin (Ig) or T-cell receptor (TCR) genes, usually resulting in aberrant expression from the coding exons that are normally intact. The second type involves breakage and rejoining of intronic sequence in such a way that an in-frame fused mRNA is expressed, resulting in a fused chimeric protein. Both types of event are found in lymphomas. The identification of the molecular basis of these events has provided a wide range of investigative techniques, including the polymerase chain reaction for the junctional sequences and immunohistochemical staining for the proteins encoded by genes involved in translocations. The addition of these approaches to conventional chromosome analysis has helped to clarify the contribution of these events to the various pathologic subtypes of lymphomas.

BURKITT'S LYMPHOMA

C-myc Activation

Burkitt's lymphoma has characteristic chromosomal translocations that involve a recombination between the Ig heavy-chain locus and the *c-myc* oncogene.[2–8] The human immunoglobulin heavy-chain locus is oriented on chromosome 14 with the variable regions telomeric to the constant regions. The breakpoint on chromosome 14 is often in the switch region located 5' to the Cμ constant region gene. The breakpoints on chromosome 8 are usually in or around the first noncoding exon of the *c-myc* gene. The usual result of this translocation is to create a fusion sequence with *c-myc* joined with the Sμ region in opposite transcriptional directions. The two variant chromosome translocations, t(2;8) and t(8;22), observed in about 10% of Burkitt's lymphoma are due to a recombination between the *c-myc* locus and the kappa light-chain gene (Igk)[9] on chromosome 2 or the lambda light-chain gene (Igl)[10] on chromosome 22. In contrast to the heavy-chain locus, both light-chain loci are oriented with their variable regions centromeric to their constant regions, and the breakpoints usually lie 5' to the joining region segments, thus leaving the J region enhancer sequences intact. The corresponding breakpoints on chromosome 8 occur 3' to the *c-myc* gene at a distance that can range from 400 bp to over 100 kb from the *c-myc* polyadenylation site.[11–13] Occasionally the distance can be sufficient to result in a cytogenetically different breakpoint on chromosome 8,[14] and it remains possible that a different gene may be involved. Indeed, the analogous variant translocation in murine plasmacytomas involves a locus other than *c-myc*, named *pvt-1* (plasmacytoma variant translocation).[15]

A further consequence of translocation of the *c-myc* locus can be the introduction of point mutations into its promoter region, the first noncoding exon,[16,17] or either of the two coding exons.[18] Additional evidence of somatic mutation, particularly in the endemic form of Burkitt's lymphoma has been demonstrated by restriction enzyme mapping. PvuII restriction enzyme digestion of DNA from 13 endemic lymphomas revealed 10 abnormally sized *c-myc* alleles indicating a high level of point mutation around the site of transcription termination.[17] Somatic mutation is a common means of generating antibody diversity during normal VDJ rearrangement, and similar mechanisms may be directed at the translocated *c-myc* allele. Since the other *c-myc* allele on chromosome 8 is usually in a germ-line configuration, it can be used an internal control to evaluate the deregulation of the translocated allele. Most studies indicate that the translocated allele continues to be expressed, whereas the normal allele is switched off.[19–21] The extinction of the normal allele and expression of the translocated allele appear to happen independently of whether the breakpoint is within or 5' to the *c-myc* gene.[22,23] A similar analysis of a variant t(2;8) translocation indicated that the rearranged allele continued to be expressed.[9] Although this deregulation leads to more *c-myc* mRNA[24,25] and more c-Myc protein[26,27] in Burkitt's lymphoma cells than other lymphoblastoid cell lines, such quantitative changes may be less important than the inability of the rearranged gene to respond normally to regulatory factors. The point mutations are scattered over a large part of the coding sequence of the translocated allele, but with a concentration in the Myc box 1 in the N-terminal domain. The most frequently mutated residue is Thr-58, the phosphorylation of which targets c-Myc for degradation by the ubiquitin-proteasome pathway.[28] Mutation of Thr-58 causes decreased proteasome-mediated turnover of c-Myc and increased half-life.[29] The resulting disturbance of c-Myc levels could be an important part of tumor progression.

There is epidemiologic and clinical evidence that there are two distinct forms of Burkitt's lymphoma: endemic and sporadic.[30] Although both forms have the typical chromosome translocations, there appear to be subtle differences in the mode of activation, with the sporadic form often involving deletion of *c-myc* regulatory sequences, whereas the endemic form frequently involves point mutations or insertions.[17] It has been suggested that cells from the endemic cases may be derived from the germinal center of lymph nodes, and that cells from the sporadic cases may be derived from the bone marrow.[30] It can be speculated that the endemic form is derived from cells at an earlier stage in the B-cell lineage than the sporadic form. Thus, the endemic translocations, which have a proportion of light-chain Ig gene involvement and a high rate of mutation, could represent errors in VDJ recombination, an event that takes place early in B-cell development.[31] The t(8;14) translocation found in AIDS-associated Burkitt's lymphoma appears to resemble more closely that found in the endemic form.[32,33]

Direct evidence that deregulated *c-myc* genes may have a causative role in Burkitt's lymphoma has come from the study of transgenic mice. Animals transgenic for *c-myc* linked to a steroid inducible promoter often have breast carcinomas,[34] whereas mice transgenic for *c-myc* linked to an Ig enhancer frequently get lymphomas.[35] It is interesting that there is a definite latency period for tumor development, during which further genetic changes take place, implying that c-myc activation alone is insufficient for full tumorigenicity.

The *c-myc* gene encodes a 47-Kd protein that is concentrated in the nucleus, and which is known to have DNA binding properties, albeit at a high concentration.[36] It is highly conserved between mouse and human, and is part of a gene family that includes *N-myc* and *L-myc*. Many studies have shown that c-Myc promotes cell cycle progression and inhibits differentiation (see review by Packham and Cleveland[37]). Withdrawal of growth factors from normal cells results in the down-regulation of c-Myc and the accumulation of cells at the G1/S boundary.[38,39] Enforced c-Myc expression can overcome such cell cycle arrest and drive cells into S phase.[40] Ablation of c-Myc by antisense oligonucleotides or expression constructs blocks entry into S phase.[41,42] c-Myc protein may therefore be regarded as a positive regulator of cell cycle progression with its function being essential for progression through G1 into S phase.

The presence of two sequence motifs in c-Myc that mediate protein–protein interactions implies that c-Myc functions as a transcription factor. In particular, the heptad repeat of leucine residues (leucine zipper or LZ) and the helix-loop-helix (HLH) domain are both features known to mediate protein–protein interactions between transcription factors. c-Myc also contains an adjacent basic region (b region), which makes direct sequence-specific interactions with DNA. Thus, c-Myc contains an extended bHLH-LZ region of a type also found in a group of closely related transcription factors, including USF,[43] TFE3,[44] TFEB,[45] AP-4,[46] and the c-Myc dimerization partner Max.[47,48]

c-Myc protein is known to form heterodimers with Max,[49] an interaction that greatly enhances the sequence specific binding of c-Myc to DNA.[50] Max can homodimerize[50] and heterodimerize with two additional bHLH-LZ proteins, Mxil[51] and Mad,[52] forming complexes that can bind to DNA. Although the c-Myc/Max interaction is central to c-Myc function, other interactions with c-Myc have been demonstrated. For example, c-Myc has been shown to interact with the retinoblastoma-related protein P107 (a suppressor of cell growth).[53,54] Interactions between c-Myc and P107 require the N terminus of c-myc, and, in some Burkitt's lymphomas, mutations in the N terminus of c-Myc have been shown to render c-Myc resistant to P107-mediated suppression.[53] Thus, events that free c-Myc from the negative regulation of P107 may contribute to tumorigenesis in some lymphomas. The N-terminal domain of c-Myc has been shown to interact with a protein called TRRAP,[55] and this interaction appears to be essential for c-myc's oncogenic activity.[56] The TRRAP protein is known to recruit GCN5, a histone acetyltransferase, giving rise to the hypothesis that c-Myc-Max heterodimers activate transcription through recruitment of histone acetyltransferases, histone acetylation, and chromatin remodeling.

A number of experimental systems have been used to demonstrate that the enforced expression of c-Myc not only results in cell cycle progression, but can also induce apoptosis. For example, enforced c-Myc expression in 32D.3 myeloid progenitor cells induces apoptosis in the absence of IL3.[38] Upon withdrawal of IL3, these cells normally down-regulate c-Myc and accumulate at the G0/G1 boundary. These and other experiments have led to the idea that c-Myc expression, in circumstances when the cell would normally be quiescent, leads to apoptosis.[37,57] It may seem paradoxical that activation of c-Myc, which can lead to apoptosis, is so strongly linked to tumors such as Burkitt's lymphoma. However, it is clear from c-Myc transgenic mice that additional events are required before tumors develop. Additionally, a series of genes (*bcl-2*, *pim-1*, *bmi1*, *raf-1*, *ras*, and *abl*) has been identified as cooperating with c-Myc to accelerate tumorigenesis (37). Some of these genes (*bcl-2*, *pim-1*, *raf-1*) can suppress apoptosis, and it would seem likely therefore that c-Myc–mediated tumorigenesis is due to c-Myc–induced cell cycle progression with concomitant suppression of apoptosis provided by other genetic events.

p53, pRb Tumor Suppressor Pathways and the INK4a/ARF Locus

p53 is mutated in at least half of all human tumors, in at least 30% of Burkitt's lymphoma biopsies,[58] and in most Burkitt cell lines.[59] The distribution of mutations is similar to that of other tumors, and includes those known to affect p53 function. In the absence of a p53 mutation, other ways to disrupt the p53 pathway may be in operation. Overexpression of MDM2 has been found in some Burkitt's lymphoma,[60] and shown to compromise p53 function by increasing export of p53 into the cytoplasm for proteasome-mediated degradation.[61] c-Myc–induced apoptosis is mediated in part via the p53 pathway.[62] The activation of c-Myc by a chromosomal translocation could thus create conditions for the selection of p53 inactivation by mutation, leading to enhanced cell survival and further tumor progression.

The INK4a/ARF locus encodes two tumor suppressor genes, p14ARF and p16(INK4), which are the target for homozygous deletions and point mutations in many tumors.[63] P14ARF inhibits MDM2, thus stabilizing p53. p16INK4a binds and inhibits cyclin D-Cdk4/6, thus preventing phosphorylation of pRb. Although p14ARF is infrequently deleted homozygously in Burkitt's lymphoma (3/47 cell lines),[64] this event seems to be associated with wild-type p53. Similarly elevated levels of MDM2 protein also seem to be associated with wild-type p53. Thus, most Burkitt's lymphomas with wild-type p53 appear to have acquired alternative lesions leading to loss of p14ARF or MDM2 overexpression. p16INK4a is most commonly inactivated in Burkitt's lymphoma by promoter methylation, although some examples of homozygous deletion and point mutation have been observed.[65] Thus, the pRb pathway is a target for inactivation in Burkitt's lymphoma. pRb itself appears to be normally functional,[66] although mutations in the nuclear localization signal of a related protein pRB2 have been reported.[67]

MANTLE CELL LYMPHOMA

bcl-1/PRAD-1 Gene Rearrangement

The t(11;14)(q13;q32) was identified as a recurring cytogenetic abnormality in the lymphoproliferative diseases,[68] and subsequently shown to be associated with a subset of diffuse small B-cell, non-Hodgkin's lymphomas variously described as centrocytic lymphoma, mantle zone lymphoma, intermediate differentiated lymphocytic lymphoma, and presently under the term mantle cell lymphoma.[69–72] The t(11;14) translocation has been found also in 2% to 6% of B-CLL, in approximately 18% of B-PLL, multiple myeloma,[73] and in approximately 15% of splenic lymphoma with villous lymphocytes.[74]

The breakpoints were cloned in 1984 from cases reported to be CLL and diffuse large-cell lymphoma.[75,76] The breakpoints on chromosome 11q13 showed tight clustering in a region called *bcl-1* (B-cell lymphoma/leukemia 1).[77] Most of them involve a 2-kb locus called MTC (major translocation cluster).[78–80] The breakpoints on chromosome 14 involve the immunoglobulin heavy-chain joining regions (J_H), and it was hypothesized that the juxtaposition to enhancer elements associated with the IgH locus would affect the transcription of a gene near the *bcl-1* locus. However, despite intensive searches surrounding the breakpoint and substantial chromosomal walks, no deregulated transcriptional unit could be readily identified.

A number of parathyroid adenomas are characterized by clonal rearrangements of the parathyroid hormone gene at 11p15. This proved to be an interchromosomal translocation with 11q13 that over-expressed a newly identified gene located in this region, designated PRAD-1 (parathyroid adenomatosis) gene.[81] PRAD-1 encodes a protein of 295 amino acids with sequence similarities to cyclins, and which can complex with p34cdc2 and induce its kinase activity.[82] The PRAD-1 gene was considered a good candidate for the bcl-1 linked oncogene, especially as the same gene had been identified in two other systems. A p36cyl has been observed in mouse macrophages, and is induced by CSF-1 in the G1 phase of the cell cycle.[83] p36cyl is the murine equivalent of PRAD-1 and also associates with a cdc2-related polypeptide. Additionally, genes from a human glioblastoma introduced into a budding yeast strain, mutant in all three of the known yeast G1 cyclins, complemented the defect, and revealed a new subclass, cyclin D1.[84] Cyclin D1 is abundant in human glioblastoma and is identical to PRAD-1.

The PRAD-1/cyclinD1 (CCND1) gene on 11q13 is located 120kb telomeric from the bcl-1/MTC locus,[82,85–87] although there are two minor translocation clusters (mTCs) that are less frequently involved. mTC1 is localized 22kb telomeric of MTC,[88] and mTC2 maps to the 5' flanking region of cyclin D1 gene.[89] Southern blots using probes spanning the 110-kb distance between the *bcl-1* MTC and the PRAD-1 gene can detect *bcl-1* rearrangements in up to 73% of cases of mantle cell lymphomas.[90,91] The relatively tight clustering of *bcl-1* MTC breakpoints suggests that the polymerase chain reaction may be a suitable technique for the detection of the t(11;14) in clinical samples, providing a diagnostic tool for the differential diagnosis of mantle cell lymphomas.[92]

Cyclin D1 mRNA is over-expressed in B-cell malignancies[93,94] with 11q13 abnormalities and in the majority of mantle cell lymphomas analyzed so far.[85,95] Recent evidence suggests that the t(11;14)(q13;q32) identifies a cytologically atypical subset of B-CLL, characterized by a frequent cytological and cytogenetic evolution, and by a distinct immunophenotype with a bright-staining pattern for surface immunoglobulins (SIg), CD5 positivity, and rare CD23 expression, sharing some biological features with mantle cell lymphoma.[96] Moreover, the cyclin D1 protein has been recently shown by monoclonal and polyclonal cyclin D1 antibodies to be over-expressed in all cases of mantle cell lymphomas examined with no expression in control tissue.[97] The cyclin D1 gene is normally silent in T and B lymphocytes.[98] The tight linkage of the cyclin D1 gene with *bcl-1*, without intervening CpG islands, and its over-expression in B-cell lymphomas with *bcl-1* rearrangement and cell lines with the t(11;14)(q13;q32) provide strong evidence that the cyclin D1 gene is the *bcl-1* oncogene.

The fact that cyclin D1 over-expression has been shown in almost all cases of mantle cell lymphomas,[85,94,95,99] even in the absence of the t(11;14)(q13;q32), raises questions about the mechanisms of cyclin D1 over-expression in these cases. In some examples, the cyclin D1 transcript is truncated at its 3' untranslated region, resulting in loss of AUUUA sequences involved in mRNA stability. The consequence is the production of more stable transcripts, implying a mechanism of post transcriptional derangement in the activation of cyclin D1.[94,100,101] This mechanism may account in part for the over-expression of the cyclin D1 mRNA in the absence of chromosomal translocations, which is observed in some B-cell tumors and breast cancers.

Furthermore, over-expressed cyclin D1 transcripts seem to contain no mutations.[102]

Overexpression of cyclin D1 has also been reported in numerous solid tumors, including breast cancer,[103–105] esophageal carcinoma,[106] colon cancer,[107] and hepatocarcinoma.[108] It is therefore likely that over-expression of cyclin D1 is associated with the pathogenesis of these diseases. Overexpression of cyclin D1 in rat embryo fibroblasts by retroviral transduction resulted in a decrease in the duration of the G1 phase and decreased cell size. These cells produced tumors when injected into nude mice, but with a long latency period, and perturbed the expression of several cellular growth-related genes including *c-myc*, *c-jun*, and cyclin A, but not cyclin D3.[109] Furthermore, transfection of a G1 cyclin into fibroblasts or myeloid cell lines results in a shortening of G1 phase, but the total length of the cell cycle remains unchanged because of a compensatory prolongation of the S phase.[110,111] Moreover, microinjection of cyclin D1 antibodies into fibroblasts arrests the cell at the G1 phase.[112] The transforming activity of cyclin D1 has been shown in primary rat embryonic fibroblasts by co-transfection with *c-myc* or Ha-ras genes. Cyclin D1, together with Ha-ras, has been shown to transform primary cells and enable them to grow fibrosarcomas in nude mice.[113] Cyclin D1 can also transform BRK cells in the presence of activated Ha-ras and an altered E1A protein.[114]

Strong evidence was provided, using osteosarcoma cells deficient for the retinoblastoma-suppressing protein pRB, that all three D-type cyclins may exert their function as parts of a multiprotein complex involving interaction with pRB.[115–118] It has been suggested that cyclin D1 functions by inactivating the inhibitory effect of Rb on cell cycle progression. There is conflicting evidence though, on the ability of cyclin D1 to phosphorylate Rb in vivo, in mammalian cells.[115,116] The observation that D-type cyclins contain the C-X-L-X-E motif, also found in the DNA viral oncoproteins SV40 T antigen, adenovirus E1A, and human papilloma virus E7, may provide a clue to the mechanism of interaction of cyclin D1 with Rb.[119] This motif is required for the binding of cyclin D1 to Rb.[115] The same regions of the Rb protein interact with the E2F transcription factor that regulates the expression of several cellular genes involved in progression through the cell cycle.[120] Cyclin D1 might affect the equilibration between the Rb-E2F complex and free E2F, acting as a dominant transcription repressor.[121] Over-expression of cyclin D1 would increase the amount of free E2F or decrease the amount of Rb-E2f complex, which might enhance the expression of several genes like *c-myc*, *c-jun*, and cyclin A. This hypothesis is supported by the observation that transient over-expression of cyclin D1 decreases the amount of Rb-E2F complex in mammalian and insect cell systems.[116,118]

The oncogenic potential of the cyclin D1 gene has been demonstrated in Eμ-cyclin D1 transgenic mice that over-express cyclin D1, in B and T lymphocytes.[122,123] The cell cycle activity of these lymphocytes, and their size and mitogen responsiveness are normal, but young transgenic animals contain fewer mature B and T cells. Although spontaneous tumors are infrequent, lymphomagenesis was more rapid in mice over-expressing cyclin D1 with c-Myc compared to mice expressing either transgene alone. Moreover, the spontaneous lymphomas of *c-myc* transgenic animals often expressed the endogenous cyclin D1.[122] Similarly, in another study, the cyclin D1/N-myc or L-myc double transgenic mice developed clonal pre-B and B-cell lymphomas. Furthermore, the crossing of cyclin D1 transgenic mice, with Eμ/L-myc transgenics that over-express L-myc in B and T-cell populations, but predominantly develop T-cell tumors, leads in double transgenics to B-cell neoplasia. These findings establish cyclin D1 as a proto-oncogene whose activity depends on a specific cell type, as well as on a specific cooperating partner.[123]

FOLLICULAR LYMPHOMA

t(14;18) and bcl-2

The t(14;18)(q32;q21) translocation, the most common translocation within human lymphoid malignancies,[124,125] characterizes approximately 85% of follicular and 20% of diffuse B-cell lymphomas.[125,126] Molecular cloning of the t(14;18) breakpoint revealed a putative proto-oncogene, *bcl-2* on chromosome 18q21,[127–129] juxtaposed to one of the six immunoglobulin heavy-chain joining regions at 14q32. The *bcl-2* gene consists of three exons. The first intron is 220 bp, and a second intron of 370 kb separates the two coding exons II and III. Two proteins are potentially encoded from the 5.5-kb and the 3.5-kb mRNA transcripts: one encoding a 29-kD 239–amino acid Bcl-2a protein, and the other a 205–amino acid Bcl-2b protein that lacks a hydrophobic carboxyl tail, although this protein has never been seen in vivo in any appreciable amounts.[130] The region of 19 hydrophobic amino acids near the carboxyl terminus is followed by two charged residues that may serve to anchor the protein in membranes.[131] The Bcl-2 protein resides in the nuclear envelope, parts of the endoplasmic reticulum (ER), and outer mitochondrial membrane, but not in a variety of other intracellular membrane compartments including the plasma membrane.[131,132]

In 60% of cases, the breakpoint on chromosome 18 falls in a 500-bp area in the 3' untranslated portion of the third exon of *bcl-2* known as mbr (major breakpoint region),[133,134] and in 25% of cases, it occurs 20 kb downstream in an untranscribed region known as mcr (minor cluster region).[135,136] The breakpoints on chromosome 14 occur adjacent to the joining region of the immunoglobulin heavy-chain gene. Although the open reading frame of *bcl-2* remains intact during the translocation, somatic mutations within it have been described.[137] The t(14;18) is not confined to follicular lymphomas, as it has also been reported in a small percentage of B-CLL with breakpoints mapping between mbr and mcr,[138] in de novo ALL of L2 or L3 FAB subtype,[139–141] and in a number of cases of Hodgkin's disease.[142–144] There are also conflicting reports about the detection of the t(14;18) in cases of benign follicular hyperplasia.[145,146]

Variant t(2;18)(p11;q21) and t(18;22)(q21;q11) translocations have also been described in B-cell chronic lymphocytic leukemias[147] and in follicular lymphomas.[148,149] Molecular studies of these variant translocations have shown that the chromosomal breakpoints consistently map to the 5' region of the *bcl-2* gene (known as the VCR region for variant cluster region) on chromosome 18 and within the κ or λ light-chain loci on chromosomes 2 and 22, respectively.[147,150,151] A variant t(2;18)(p11;q21) translocation was described in a follicular lymphoma resulting in the juxtaposition of a JK segment to a chromosome 18 transcriptional unit located 10 kb upstream of *bcl-2*, termed the FVT-1 (for follicular variant translocation) gene.[152] Moreover, evidence has been found for multiple rearrangements affecting the mbr, mcr, and VCR regions.[153,154]

The reciprocal partner on chromosome 14, the immunoglobulin heavy-chain locus (IgH) on the derivative 14 chromosome, has been demonstrated to bear deletions in 76% of follicular lymphomas, probably as a consequence of nonphysiologic activation of the recombinases involved in class switching.[155] The lack of Ig detection, despite the mature origin of follicular lymphomas, may be explained in some of the cases by the inactivation of both IgH chain genes due to translocation of one allele in combination with deletions or defective rearrangements of the other allele.[156]

The tight clustering of breakpoints on chromosomes 14 and 18 during the translocation has allowed the use of the PCR technique for the detection of t(14;18)-bearing cells using genomic tumor DNA. The level of sensitivity obtained (up to 10^6) make this approach valuable for the detection of minimal residual disease.[157–162] The presence of the translocation can be demonstrated also by Southern blotting using probes to various *bcl-2* breakpoints, the main limitation being the requirement of frozen tissue for high-molecular-weight DNA extraction and the reduced sensitivity compared to PCR.[166,163] Since PCR examines shorter lengths of DNA than Southern analysis, PCR-based tests may be more susceptible to microheterogeneity in breakpoint location.[163] Most studies indicate the use of a combination of cytogenetics, Southern analysis, and PCR for the most reliable detection of the t(14;18).[163–165] Additionally, pulsed field gel electrophoresis has proved to be the most informative process compared with standard methodology.[166]

The PCR technique has allowed the detection of t(14;18) translocation bearing cells in the peripheral blood or bone marrow in patients with localized (stage I and II) disease at diagnosis and in long-term remission after radiation therapy.[167,168] Moreover, the presence of the t(14;18) translocation has been demonstrated at the completion of treatment as well as in long-term remission of advanced-stage disease.[166–172] The prognostic significance of the t(14;18) translocation has been the subject of controversy due probably to differences in the levels of sensitivity obtained by PCR. In some studies, the presence of the t(14;18) translocation has been associated with a poor response to treatment and short survival,[125] although for others the t(14;18) translocation and high Bcl-2 protein expression did not correlate with clinical outcome.[171–175] Other cytogenetic abnormalities, such as chromosomal breaks higher than 6, abnormalities of chromosome regions 1p21-22, 6q23-26, or 17p, have been recently associated with short survival.[175] The detection of the t(14;18) translocation in the reinfused bone marrow autograft in patients with follicular lymphoma treated with high-dose treatment is associated with shorter remission duration,[176–178] and its presence at follow-up, but probably not early after transplantation, is associated with a higher risk of relapse.[178]

It has been postulated that the t(14;18)(q32;q21) translocation event takes place in early B cells at the time of the D to J rearrangement. At the junction on both der14 and der18 chromosomes, short segments of random insertions, up to 24 nucleotides in length, have been observed and considered to represent N insertions, normally found at the VD and DJ junctions after IgH rearrangement.[134] This supports the hypothesis that VDJ recombinase is involved in the generation of the breakpoints on chromosome 14.[127] However the *bcl-2* regions on chromosome 18 possess no combining heptamer-spacer-nonamer motifs surrounding these breakpoints. The mbr region contains several sequence elements that could potentially infer genetic instability or facilitate homologous recombination. A polypurine–polypyrimidine stretch, with a potential to form alternative DNA structures (H-DNA or triplicates), is present in both the mbr and mcr regions. These polypurine tracts can act as targets for mammalian endonucleases and are found around other genetic hot spots.[179–181] Similar repeats of G-rich tetranucleotides have been implicated in immunoglobulin class switching.[182,183] The mbr region contains a Chi-like octamer similar to the recombination signal in *Escherichia coli*, and the human minisatellite core sequence that could activate a Rec BCD-like mechanism.[184–186] More recently, an S1 nuclease–sensitive site was found, which can be the target of an endogenous nuclease present in early B cells. A 45-Kd protein has been identified that binds to the Chi-like polypurine–polypyrimidine tract within mbr and mcr as well as to corresponding Ig sequences, and may play a role in homologous site-specific recombination.[187]

The juxtaposition of the *bcl-2* oncogene with powerful enhancer elements within the IgH locus markedly deregulates the gene by altering both its transcription and the efficiency of RNA processing, resulting in elevated amounts of *bcl-2*/Ig chimeric RNA, giving rise to over-expression of the Bcl-2 protein.[188–190] In normal lymph nodes, the Bcl-2 protein is most abundant in the long-lived recirculating B cells of the follicular mantle.[190–192] Bcl-2 is absent from the centroblasts and centrocytes destined to die within the dark zone and basal light zone. In parallel, surviving T cells within the medulla of the thymus demonstrate substantial Bcl-2 staining, while those in the cortex are negative.[191,192] Over-expression of the Bcl-2 protein has also been shown in follicular and diffuse B-cell lymphomas without concurrent *bcl-2* rearrangement in small lymphocytic, mantle zone lymphomas, chronic lymphocytic leukemia, plasma cell dyscrasias, chronic and acute myelogenous leukemia, and breast cancer suggesting other mechanisms of deregulation of bcl-2.[193–196] As recently shown, the distribution of *bcl-2* mRNA is roughly reciprocal to that of the protein with intense hybridization signal in germinal centers and almost absent in mantle zones. Discordant *bcl-2* RNA and protein levels were also observed in tonsilar epithelial cells and cortical thymocytes. Importantly, follicular lymphomas and cell lines with the t(14;18) have concordant and abundant *bcl-2* mRNA and protein expression, suggesting disruption of translational control mechanisms in follicular lymphomas.[193]

Over-expression of Bcl-2 protein results in prevention of apoptosis or programmed cell death in selected hematopoietic cell lines following deprivation of IL-3, IL-4, or GM-CSF.[197–201] Moreover, studies of Bcl-2 function in cultured postmitotic neurons have established a role for this gene in the suppression of apoptosis in complete absence of cell proliferation. Microinjection of Bcl-2 expression plasmids into nerve growth factor (NGF)–dependent neurons has been shown to markedly delay the rate of cell death that occurs upon removal of the neurotrophic factors from cultures.[202] Over-expression of Bcl-2 can block apoptosis induced by γ-irradiation, glucocorticoids, and a variety of chemotherapeutic agents.[203–206] Bcl-2 also blocks apoptosis that accompanies terminal differentiation of myeloid leukemic cell lines without affecting the differentiation process.[207] Bcl-2 has also been implicated in positive selection of thymocytes and in maintenance of B-cell memory through its effect on survival at specific stages of lymphoid development and differentiation.[208–210] A distinct biological effect of the Bcl-2 protein in different cell types has been demonstrated by a paradoxical inhibition of cell growth in solid tumor cell lines.[211] Bcl-2 has also been implicated in the development of viral persistence and the pathogenesis of virus-associated malignancies, as shown through induction of Bcl-2 expression by the Epstein–Barr virus (EBV) latent membrane protein 1, resulting in protection from apoptosis of B cells.[212]

Genetic analysis of apoptosis in the nematode worm *Caenorhabditis elegans* has identified three genes that regulate cell death: *ced-3*, *ced-4*, and *ced-9*. *ced-9* suppresses apoptosis and has sequence similarity to *bcl-2*, and human *bcl-2* can rescue *ced-9*–deficient worms.[213,214] Thus, some functions of Bcl-2 are extremely well conserved throughout phylogeny. In contrast to *ced-9* and *bcl-2*, *ced-3* and *-4* are involved in the initiation or execution of cell death, as loss of function mutations in these genes results in adult worms with additional cells.[215]

The oncogenic potential of the t(14;18) translocation and resulting Bcl-2 over-expression have been demonstrated by transfection of *bcl-2* constructs into NIH3T3 fibroblasts that develop tumors when injected into mice with a latency period of approximately 4 weeks.[216] Moreover, *bcl-2*/IgH transgenic mice develop a polyclonal follicular lymphoproliferation of small resting IgM/IgD cells that progress to immunoblastic lymphoma, by additional genetic alterations involving *c-myc* rearrangement.[217,218] Most of the lymphomas developing in the Eμ/*bcl-2* transgene involve predominantly the B-cell lineage, and their immunophenotype (Sca-1, CD4, Thy-1, CD34, CD45) is consistent with an origin very early in B-lymphoid development.[219] These observations suggest that the t(14;18) forms a basis for lymphomagenesis, but is not sufficient itself to trigger the neoplastic process. In support of this hypothesis is the observation that the t(14;18) translocation can also be found in blood B cells of normal individuals, and that the frequency increases in the spleen and the blood with age, suggesting a multistep process of lymphomagenesis involving the t(14;18).[220,221] In a *bcl-2* transgenic line expressing high levels of Bcl-2 protein in both cortical and medullary thymocytes, the immature thymocytes are resistant to apoptotic stimuli and have prolonged survival. It was also found that a proportion of thymocytes and peripheral T cells escape the process of negative antigenic selection, eliminating normally autoreactive T cells during thymocyte maturation.[222] T cells in the peripheral lymphoid tissues are moderately elevated despite enhanced survival in vitro, and there is a relatively high proportion of thymocytes with a mature phenotype.[223] Moreover, a *bcl-2* transgene driven by the *lck* promoter results in mice that over-express Bcl-2 within the thymus and in the peripheral T cells, and which develop peripheral T-cell lymphomas predominantly of the diffuse large-cell type at a mean age of 18 months.[224] These data emphasize the tumorigenic potential of repression of cell death in multiple lineages.

The role of Bcl-2 in the normal control of tissue homeostasis was assessed in *bcl-2* knockout mice, which complete embryonic development but display growth retardation and early postnatal mortality. As expected, differentiation of the lymphoid lineage is initially normal, but thymus and spleen undergo massive apoptotic involution, resulting in lymphopenia. The animals die as a consequence of renal failure, the result of severe polycystic kidney disease, and display hypopigmented hair, indicating a defect in redox-regulated melanin synthesis.[225]

The mechanism through which Bcl-2 exerts its antiapoptotic function is not known, but several possibilities have been explored. The localization of Bcl-2 protein in the membranes of nuclear envelope and ER compartments in patches is highly reminiscent of nuclear pore complexes (NPCs),[226] raising the possibility of a role for Bcl-2 in some aspect of nuclear transport, NPC formation, or nuclear envelope assembly and maintenance. The relevance of oxidative phosphorylation to the antiapoptotic function of Bcl-2 has been assessed in human fibroblast cell lines that lack mitochondrial DNA. These experiments showed no requirement for oxidative phosphorylation for the induction of apoptosis or for the death repressor activity of Bcl-2.[227] Bcl-2 overproduction in a rat pheochromocytoma cell line, PC12, did not correlate with the levels of ATP or oxygen consumption, despite their resistance to apoptosis.[228] However Bcl-2 over-expression and increased mitochondrial activity are closely related properties of cell lines resistant to apoptosis induced by glucocorticoids.[229] Another important aspect is the role of Ca2+ in apoptosis, since Ca2+-dependent endonucleases may be involved in the internucleosomal DNA digestion typical of apoptotic cells. Bcl-2 blocks Ca2+ ionophore–induced apoptosis in thymocytes, T-cell leukemia lines, and PC12 cells. Overproduction of Bcl-2, however, does not prevent rises in intracellular Ca2+, suggesting that Bcl-2 blocks apoptosis downstream of this event. Moreover, lymphokine withdrawal in IL-3–dependent cell lines results in gradual loss of Ca2+ from the ER and increase in the Ca2+ in the mitochondria. Over-expression of Bcl-2 reverses these effects, suggesting that Bcl-2 can influence Ca2+ partitioning.[230] In favor of this hypothesis are the observations that glucocorticoid treatment of T cells results in massive loss of Ca2+ from the ER prior to apoptosis,[231] and over-expression of an ER Ca2+-binding protein, calbindin-D, in glucocorticoid-sensitive T-cells delays apoptosis presumably by allowing ER to retain its Ca2+.[232] Another attractive hypothesis is the role of oxidative injury in the induction of cell death, and the finding that Bcl-2 blocks the accumulation of lipid peroxides and possibly other reactive oxygen species in at least some settings.[233]

The concept of Bcl-2 regulating apoptosis through a dynamic process of positive and negative interactions with other proteins led to a search for other proteins with a structural similarity to Bcl-2. Viral Bcl-2 homologues like the BHRF1 in the EBV[234] and the LMW5-HL in the African swine fever virus[235] can both prevent apoptosis, perhaps explaining the latency and persistence of some viral infections. However, cDNAs have been recently cloned for several novel human genes, revealing a family of *bcl-2*–related members. One of these, called *bax*, has a six-exon structure, and demonstrates a complex pattern of alternative RNA splicing that would encode several membrane and cytosolic proteins. Bax protein has been shown to homodimerize and heterodimerize with Bcl-2 in vivo. Bax over-expression accelerates apoptosis induced by cytokine deprivation in IL-3–dependent cell lines and counters the antiapoptotic function of Bcl-2. The ratio of Bcl-2 to Bax determines survival or death upon apoptotic stimuli.[236] Another member of the family termed *bcl-x* produces, by alternative splicing, two distinct *bcl-x* mRNAs and encodes a 241–amino acid protein with 74% homology to Bcl-2. The protein product of the large mRNA, Bcl-xL, stably transfected into IL-3–dependent cell lines, inhibits cell death as effectively as Bcl-2. The second mRNA species, *bcl-xS*, encodes a protein that inhibits the ability of Bcl-2 to enhance the survival of growth factor–deprived cells.[237] Other members of the family include the *mcl-1* gene and the A1 gene isolated from cDNA libraries derived from myeloid leukemic and normal cells, respectively.[238–240] Additionally, the *bad* gene encodes a 204–amino acid protein that forms heterodimers with Bcl-2 and Bcl-xL. Its over-expression in IL-3–dependent cells abolishes the protective effect of Bcl-xL on IL-3 deprivation, and promotes apoptosis probably by competing with Bax for Bcl-xL, resulting in reduction of the Bcl-xL/Bax heterodimers and an increase in the amount of the death-accelerating protein Bax.[241] Another new member of the *bcl-2* family is the *bak* gene, encoding a protein of 211 amino acids, 25% identical to Bcl-2. Three closely related *bak* genes exist: *bak* mapping to chromosome 6, *bak-2* to chromosome 20, and *bak-3* to chromosome 11. Like Bax, the Bak gene product enhances apoptosis following apoptotic stimuli, and unlike Bax, it inhibits cell death in an EBV-transformed cell line. The Bak protein can also bind to an apoptosis-inhibiting adenovirus protein, E1B19K.[242–244]

In the emerging family of Bcl-2–related proteins, two domains, termed Bcl-2 homology 1 and 2 (BH1 and BH2), have been identified.[245] Site-specific mutagenesis of *bcl-2* established these two domains as novel dimerization motifs. Substitution of Gly 145 in the BH1 domain or Trp 188 in BH2 completely abrogates the death repressor activity of Bcl-2 upon apoptotic stimuli, such as IL-3 deprivation, γ-irradiation, and glucocorticoids. Mutations that affected the function of Bcl-2 also disrupted its heterodimerization with Bax while preserving its ability to form homodimers, suggesting that these domains are functionally important and that Bcl-2 exerts its function through heterodimerization with Bax.[245]

Bcl-6 Gene Rearrangements

The reciprocal translocation t(3;22)(q27;q11) was first identified[246] in nine examples from a large lymphoma series (187 specimens). Most of these tumors had in common a diffuse morphology and predominantly a large cell type. Subsequent cytogenetic analysis confirmed[247] and extended[248] these results to include t(3;14)(q27;q32) and t(2;3)(p12;q32) translocations. Molecular analysis with DNA probes from the IGH locus[249] resulted in the identification of a gene at the breakpoint on chromosome 3 by four independent groups. This gene, which has been named *bcl-6*,[250,251] *laz-3*,[252] and *bcl-5*,[253] contains a Kruppel-type COOH-terminal Cys2-His2 zinc finger region. This region has been shown to bind DNA, and a consensus DNA-binding sequence has been identified[254] as (T/A)NCTTTC-NAGG(A/G)AT, a sequence that can be found in the 5′ region of certain genes. Bcl-6 also contains a NH_2-terminal region with significant homology[250] to other zinc finger transcription factors such as the ZFPJS protein, which regulates the major histocompatibility complex II promoter, the Tramtrack (ttk) and Broad-complex (Br-c) proteins in *Drosophila* that regulate developmental transcription,[255] the human KUP protein,[256] and the human PLZF protein that is involved in the t(11;17) variant translocation in acute promyelocytic leukemia.[257] This evolutionarily conserved feature has been named the BTB domain, and may be present in up to 40 different *Drosophila* genes.[258] *bcl-6* mRNA has been detected in cell lines derived from mature B cells, but not from pro-B cells or plasma cells, T cells, or other hemopoietic lineages or other tissues. This restricted range of normal expression has been taken[250] to suggest that Bcl-6 is a transcription factor involved in the control of normal B-cell differentiation and lymphoid organ development.

The genomic structure of *bcl-6* encompasses about 26 kb,[259] and consists of nine exons. *bcl-6* rearrangements with IGH,[249,260] IGκ,[261] and IGλ[253] have now been molecularly analyzed, and it is clear that all these events consistently break *bcl-6* in the same cluster region of about 10 kb at the 5′ end of the gene. Breakpoints are clustered around the first exon, and the putative regulatory region of the *bcl-6* gene is removed during translocation, leading to over-expression of the presumably intact coding region of the gene. Evidence has been found that biallelic rearrangements of *bcl-6* can occur.[262] The fact that the IGH and IGλ rearrangements occur in the same region of *bcl-6* contrasts with the rearrangements affecting *bcl-2* and *c-myc*. IGH rearrangements occur 5′ to *c-myc* and 3′ to *bcl-2*, whereas IGL rearrangements occur 3′ to *c-myc* and 5′ to *bcl-2*. Thus, the configuration of both *bcl-2* and *c-myc* in relation to the Ig loci seems to be important, whereas the removal of the 5′ untranslated region appears to be the important feature of *bcl-6* activation. It is now clear, however, that the *bcl-6* gene can be rearranged with not only the immunoglobulin loci, but with a range of other chromosomal sites (see Chapter 2).

Molecular analysis of the t(3;11)(q27;q23) in a cell line has shown[263] that this translocation results in a fusion between Bcl-6 and BOB1/OBF1, the B-cell specific co-activator of octamer binding transcription factors. The regulatory regions upstream of the noncoding exon two of *bcl-6* are replaced by those of BOB1/OBF1, leaving the coding sequence of bcl-6 intact. Similar analysis of the t(3;4)(q27;p11) translocation in a cell line identified the gene product TTF[264] fused to Bcl-6. TTF, which is only expressed in hemopoietic cells, has homology to the RAS superfamily, and may define a new subgroup of RHO-like proteins. Sequence analysis of the *bcl-6* gene coding sequence in both rearranged and nonrearranged cases found no evidence that mutation plays a role in *bcl-6* activation.[265]

A series of large-scale investigations of the incidence and clinical significance of *bcl-6* rearrangements in lymphoma has been reported.[266–268] Approximately 15% to 20% of all lymphomas were found to have *bcl-6* rearrangements, assessed by Southern analysis. As expected from previous cytogenetic studies, the greatest incidence (30%,[268] 45%[266]) was found in tumors classified as diffuse large-cell lymphomas (DLCL). However, rearrangements have also been found in follicular lymphomas[266,268] and in a case of CLL.[267] In a study[269] of 102 patients with DLLC, 23 cases with *bcl-6* rearrangements and 21 cases with *bcl-2* rearrangements were found. From the clinical follow-up, it was concluded that rearrangement of *bcl-6* may be a favorable prognostic marker when compared to rearrangement of *bcl-2* in this series. The incidence of *bcl-6* rearrangements in AIDS-related lymphomas has also been investigated,[270] and these data showed that about 20% of AIDS-DLCL carried rearrangements to *bcl-6*.

BCL-6 protein expression is normally tightly regulated during B-cell development, being expressed in germinal center B cells, but not in pre–B cells or in differentiated cells such as plasma cells. Thus, its down-regulation, disrupted in lymphoma, may be necessary for normal B-cell differentiation. It is now clear that BCL-6 has a major role in the repression of gene expression, its targets including the B lymphocyte-induced maturation protein (blimp-1),[271] the cell cycle control genes p27kip1 and cyclin D2,[272] and the programmed cell death-2 protein (PDCD2).[273] The N terminal BTB domain (also known as the POZ domain) of BCL-6, which is required for its repression activity, is known to interact with the SMRT and N-CoR co-repressor proteins within histone deacetylase complexes. Specific conserved 17 residues of the BTB domain are responsible for the interactions with these co-repressors. Crytalographic analysis has shown that this region directly binds to a "lateral groove" motif specific to the BCL-6 BTB domain.[274] On the basis of this evidence, a peptide was designed to bind to BCL-6 and thus block recruitment of co-repressors.[275] This inhibitor has been shown to disrupt BCL-6–mediated gene repression, reactivating BCL-6 target genes, and to induce apoptosis and cell cycle arrest in BCL-6-positive lymphoma cells. Thus, such peptide inhibitors are potentially novel therapeutic agents for lymphomas.

EXTRANODAL LYMPHOMAS

Mucosa-Associated Lymphoid Tissue (MALT) Lymphomas

MALT lymphomas (see review by Isaacson and Du[276]) account for about 50% of primary gastric lymphomas, although they can arise in other extranodal sites. These lymphomas are associated with chronic infectious conditions such as *Helicobacter pylori* gastritis, leading to the suggestion that the infection provides the antigenic stimulus for sustaining growth of the lymphoma. However, it is apparent that the immunoglobulin produced by the tumor does not directly recognize *H. pylori*, and shows a pattern of somatic hypermutation typical of antigen selection in the germinal center. Intraclonal variation of the immunoglobulin sequences has been observed, suggesting that there may be adaptation to the long-term antigen stimulation of the chronic infection.

The t(11;18)(q21;21) translocation was first described in 1989,[277] and was subsequently found to be associated with MALT lymphomas.[278] The t(11;18) is present in about one-third of cases and can be found in MALT lymphomas from a variety of anatomic sites. The molecular cloning of this translocation revealed that it resulted in the fusion of the API2 gene on chromosome 11 with the MALT1 gene on chromosome 18.[279] There is evidence that the API2–MALT1 fusion is more frequent in tumors that have disseminated beyond the stomach, and also seems to be associated with failure to eradicate *H. pylori*. It is also clear that this translocation occurs specifically in MALT lymphomas, and not in closely related nodal or splenic marginal zone lymphomas. At the molecular level, the consistently expressed transcript is the API2–MALT1 mRNA, suggesting that this is the transforming protein. Indeed, some fusions at the genomic level could give rise to out-of-frame transcripts, but these are consistently spliced out of the final fusion transcript. This suggests that the API2–MALT1 protein is critical for transformation. Other translocations have been observed in MALT lymphomas. The t(1;14)(p22;q32) is seen in approximately 5% of MALT lymphomas, and has been shown to place the BCL10 gene under the control of the Ig heavy-chain enhancer.[280] This typically results in up-regulated BCL10 protein expression in the nucleus. Another event associated with MALT lymphomas is the t(14;18)(q32;q21) translocation. This places the MALT1 gene under control of the heavy-chain enhancer, resulting in its over-expression.[281] This event seems to be more common in nongastrointestinal lymphomas.

Although these three translocations associated with MALT lymphomas seem on the surface rather different, subsequent studies suggest that there may be common links. API2, which contains three baculovirus IAP repeats (BIRs), a caspase recruitment domain (CARD), and a zinc-binding RING domain, is thought to have an antiapoptotic role, inhibiting caspases 3, 7, and 9. MALT1 has an N-terminal death domain, two IG-like domains, and a caspase-like domain, and is involved in receptor-mediated activation NF-kB. The translocations consistently fuse the BIR domains of API2 with the caspase-like domain of MALT1. The API2–MALT1 fusion protein has been shown to activate the NF-kB pathway, and it has been suggested that this could be a consequence of oligomerization via the BIR domains of API2. Significantly, it has also been shown that MALT1 can form a complex with BCL10, which can result in activation of NF-kB.[282] BCL10 knockout mice have been used to show that BCL10 specifically transduces antigen-receptor signaling to activate the NF-kB pathway.[283] Studies of MALT1 knockout mice indicated that MALT1 operates downstream of BCL10 in the activation of NF-kB.[284]

Given the involvement of both MALT1 and BCL10 in NF-kB signaling, it is possible to speculate on how the different chromosomal translocations may induce transformation.[276] The t(1;14) translocation causes over-expression of BCL10 that could oligomerize via its CARD domain, and thus trigger aberrant NF-kB signaling. In lymphomas with the t(14;18), MALT1 is over-expressed. However, it is unlikely that MALT1 can oligomerize alone, and probably can only do so in association with BCL10. It is significant that t(14;18)-bearing lymphomas have high levels of BCL10 expression,[285] and this may facilitate the dimerization and activation of NF-kB. Lymphomas with the t(11;18) translocation express the API2–MALT1 fusion protein that can dimerize and activate NF-kB. An interesting and unexplained feature of BCL10 is that it is normally expressed in the cytoplasm of B cells. However, in lymphomas with the t(1;14) it is predominantly seen in the nucleus, and this aberrant localization may have an additional role in transformation.

Anaplastic Lymphoma Kinase (ALK) Gene Fusions

Early cytogenetic investigations identified the t(2;5) translocation as a recurring event[286] in tumors referred to as malignant histiocytosis.[287] Subsequent analysis[288–290] has shown that these tumors should be reinterpreted as large-cell anaplastic lymphomas. A particular characteristic of this group is the presence of the Ki-1 (CD-30) surface antigen, and it is now clear that a proportion of this group carry the t(2;5) translocation,[291] particularly where there is evidence of T-cell origin.[292]

It was shown[293] that the translocation results in the in-frame fusion of a gene encoding a protein known as nucleophosmin (NPM) on chromosome 5 to a receptor tyrosine kinase gene (ALK) on chromosome 2. The normal ALK protein is a membrane-spanning tyrosine kinase receptor, the fusion resulting in a chimeric NPM–ALK protein from which the membrane and putative extracellular domains have been lost. RT-PCR analysis of cells known to contain the t(2;5) translocation indicates that breakpoints occur in the same introns of the *npm* and *alk* genes, resulting in identical fusion junctions in the mRNA. The normal NPM protein is a nucleolar phosphoprotein that is involved in the assembly of the small and large ribosomal subunits. NPM expression is cell cycle regulated with a peak before entry into S phase. Since the *alk* gene is normally silent in lymphoid cells, a critical consequence of its fusion to *npm* is the up-regulation of an activated ALK tyrosine-kinase domain.[293] The portion of NPM fused to ALK includes an oligomerization motif that enables NPM–ALK to form homodimers and hetrodimers with wild-type NPM.[294] Heterodimerization with NPM allows NPM–ALK to enter the nucleus and the nucleolus. However, entry of NPM–ALK into the nucleolus does not appear to be required for transformation.[295] The NPM–ALK fusion proteins are heavily phosphorylated on tyrosine residues, which is consistent with activation of the ALK tyrosine kinase.[294]

As detailed earlier (see Chapter 2), a series of chromosomal translocations resulting in ALK fusions have now been identified. Tropomysin3 (TPM3) and tropomysin4 (TMP4) have both been found fused to ALK.[296,297] Similarly the gene TFG has been shown to be fused to ALK as the consequence of a t(2;3)(p23;q21) translocation.[298] Further fusion partners for ALK in ALCL include ATIC,[299] CLTC,[300] MSN,[301] ALO17,[302] and MYH9.[303] The NPM–ALK protein localizes partly to the nucleus and nucleolus since the N-terminal portion of NPM still functions as a nucleolar transporter. However, the variant ALK fusion proteins differ in that TPM3-ALK, TFG-ALK, ATIC-ALK, and CLTC-ALK all show a cytoplasmic localization. A possible common feature of the ALK fusion proteins may be the ability to self-associate. Both TPM3 and TFG contain coiled-coil domains that self-associate, and when fused to ALK result in constitutive tyrosine kinase activity in vitro.[296,304] The possible role of self-association has been further investigated by the construction of an artificial ALK fusion protein in which ALK is joined to the N-terminal of the TPR protein.[295] TPR is involved in chromosomal translocations that result in a TPR–MET kinase fusion in thyroid carcinomas but which has never been found in ALCL. The artificial TPR–ALK fusion had transforming activity comparable to that of NPM–ALK. This experiment and the nature of the ALK fusion proteins suggest that any protein with sufficient self association could function as a partner for ALK.

Although the major occurrence of ALK gene fusion is in T cells, the broad transforming activity of NPM–ALK in vitro suggests that other cell types could be targets. The expression of NPM–ALK in murine bone marrow progenitor cells results in B-cell lymphomas.[305] Furthermore, it has been established that inflammatory myofibroblastic tumors (IMT), which are of a mesenchymal spindle-cell origin, have a high frequency of ALK gene fusions.[306] Three of the fusion partners, TPM3, TPM4, and CLTC, are also fused to ALK in ALCL, whereas two others, RANBP and CARS, have so far only been found in IMT.[302,307] Most gene fusions found in hematopoietic malignancies are rarely, if ever, found in tumors of other tissues. ALK fusions are therefore unusual in the spectrum of target tissues that can be affected.

The various ALK fusions all appear to result in constitutively activated tyrosine kinase activity, the NPM–ALK activity having been shown to be essential for transformation.[308] Downstream effectors that can dock with autophosphorylated sites include phospholipase C-gamma (PLC-γ) and SHC, the p85 subunit of phosphoinositol-3'-kinase (PI3K). The expression of NPM–ALK in cell lines has been shown to result in the phosphorylation and translocation of STAT5 to the nucleus.[309] Another potential downstream target for NPM–ALK is the PI3K/akt pathway. NPM–ALK activates PI3K that in turn activates the antiapoptotic PKB/akt pathway.[310] Significantly, the transformation ability of NPM–ALK can be reversed by treatment with the PI3K inhibitor wortmannin.

Although the expression of CD30, a member of the TNFR superfamily, is a key distinguishing feature of ALCL, its role in the malignant transformation has been in doubt. It is also expressed in Hodgkin's lymphoma where it has been shown to result in activation of NF-kB. Although a physical association has been shown between NPM–ALK and CD30,[311] the activation of CD30 does not lead to enhanced NPM–ALK autophosphorylation.[312] It has recently been shown that NPM–ALK impedes CD30 signaling and NF-kB activation.[313] In this study, the variant ALK fusions TPM3-ALK and the TFG-ALK were unable to inhibit CD30 signaling. NPM–ALK, when transduced into Hodgkin's lymphoma cell lines, produces an ALCL like phenotype and inhibits CD30 signaling. Hence, it appears that the phenotype of CD30 expressing cells can be critically influenced by the presence or absence of the NPM–ALK protein.

GENE MUTATIONS IN LYMPHOMA

Frequent and nonrandom chromosome 17p alterations and p53 mutations have been observed in patients with lymphoproliferative diseases, suggesting an important role in lymphomagenesis and disease progression. Thirty-seven percent of patients with large-cell lymphoma have been reported to have either loss of whole chromosome 17 or of part of 17 (17p–) or all of the short arm (i17q).[314] Other investigators have reported chromosome 17 abnormalities in 31% to 44% of patients with large-cell lymphoma,[315,316] and such abnormalities were correlated with a grave prognosis and a short survival.[317,318]

Over-expression of p53 has been shown by immunostaining in 20% to 50% of diffuse high-grade lymphomas.[319–323] The incidence of mutations of the p53 gene varies from 20% to 30% among different studies,[324–326] but as recently shown, the percentage of p53 mutations in the group of high-grade non-Hodgkin's lymphomas is higher (45%) if the analysis includes exons 2 to 11, and not only the "hot spot" region (exons 5 to 8) where most mutations are known to occur.[327] Moreover, staining for p53 is not predictive of mutations since cases over-expressing p53 in the absence of mutations have been described.[327,328] Within the group of high-grade B-cell lymphomas, the reported frequency of p53 mutations in Burkitt's lymphomas varies between 35% and 45%.[58,328] Almost all cases of Burkitt's lymphoma have a translocation involving the *c-myc* gene, and therefore activation of both p53 and c-Myc may be critical in the development of these tumors. The coexistence of c-Myc and p53 alterations has also been shown in 3/8 and 1/11 diffuse large-cell lymphoma cell lines and tumors, respectively.[329] In Burkitt's lymphoma cell lines, a high frequency of p53 alterations (up to 60%) has also been described.[59,324,330,331] The majority of these cell lines contained only mutant versions of the p53 gene, and most of the mutations were missense, and occasionally nonsense and frame shift. There was no correlation with the type of translocation, ethnic origin of the patients, or EBV status. The expression of p53 in a group of 119 patients with high-grade B-cell NHL has been shown to be an independent poor prognostic factor for survival. Simultaneous expression of bcl-2 and p53 was associated with a poorer prognosis than p53 alone, particularly in the subgroup of nodal lymphomas.[332]

A high frequency of p53 mutations has also been observed in patients with acquired immunodeficiency syndrome (AIDS)–related lymphomas. Although these patients have an increased incidence of B-cell immunoblastic lymphoma, the incidence or type of p53 mutations does not differ when compared with B-cell immunoblastic lymphomas in individuals without HIV infection.[333] Interestingly, in other studies over-expression of p53 was observed in 10/45 of cases analyzed, mainly clustering in the small non-cleaved cell and Ki-1 anaplastic large-cell subtypes. A diffuse or clustered pattern of p53-positive neoplastic cells was seen in the small non-cleaved lymphomas, consequent upon p53 mutations. In contrast, in Ki-1 anaplastic large cell lymphomas p53 immunohistochemical reactivity was limited to scattered tumor cells, but no p53 gene alterations could be detected.[334,335]

Low-grade non-Hodgkin's lymphomas rarely have p53 alterations. Higher frequencies of p53 mutations have recently been shown in the splenic B-cell leukemia/lymphoma of possible marginal origin, where p53 gene alterations involving exons 5, 6, and 8 were found in 40% of cases examined. These mutations were missense or frame shift, and the wild-type sequence at the mutation sites was barely visible, implying the loss of the normal p53 allele in leukemic cells.[336] Most of the p53 alterations in the group of low-grade non-Hodgkin's lymphomas have been associated with progression to high-grade lymphoma. Serial biopsies of patients with follicular lymphoma who underwent histologic transformation showed that a p53 mutation was observed in one-third of the transformed samples, and this was not detected at the follicular stage of the disease.[337] Another study revealed that four of five cases of follicular lymphoma transformed to diffuse large-cell lymphoma were associated with p53 mutations.[338] Interestingly, in one of these positive cases, the same mutation was also present in the pre-transformation biopsy, correlating with the presence of diffuse-type areas within a predominantly follicular pattern.[339] p53 immunoreactivity was observed in 50% of low-grade non-Hodgkin's lymphomas, and was higher in tumors of T-cell origin.[339] There was a positive association between p53 staining and the proliferation state as expressed by PCNA. Another study, however, revealed variable p53 immunostaining in follicular lymphomas between biopsies and between individual follicles within the same tumor, with no correlation with the state of cell proliferation.[340]

Peripheral T-cell lymphomas seem to have a low incidence of p53 mutations, ranging from 3% to 9% of cases examined.[324,341] p53 over-expression was observed in 50% of the cases and did not correlate with cell proliferation as assessed by Ki67 expression.[341] However, within the group of peripheral T-cell lymphomas, the adult T-cell leukemia/lymphoma associated with human T-cell leukemia virus type I (HTLV-1) infection, seems to have a much higher incidence of p53 gene alterations, ranging from 30% to 50% in various studies.[342–345] On the basis of the evaluation of at least 51 patients, it was postulated that p53 alteration represents one of the genetic changes responsible for the progression of the disease.[342–345] The mutations found were mainly missense, nonsense, silent, and frame shift, and the majority of those found in patients with the acute type of disease occurred in highly conserved regions of p53. Moreover, cells carrying p53 mutations showed loss of the other p53 allele.[342–345] p53 mutations correlated with an altered pattern of p53 expression as assessed by immunohistochemical staining.[344,345] The frequency of p53 gene alterations in the acute phase of adult T-cell leukemia/lymphoma was significantly higher than that in the chronic type, suggesting a possible involvement of p53 gene alterations in the disease progression.[346]

Over-expression of p53 protein as assessed by immunohistochemical staining has been detected in about 60% to 80% of cases with mixed cellularity and nodular sclerosing type of Hodgkin's disease.[319,321,323,347] Immunoreactivity is localized to the nuclei of the Reed–Sternberg (RS) cells or its mononuclear variants, and the number of positive cells vary between 10% to 60% of RS cells. Mutations of p53 have been detected in enriched RS cell preparations.[348,349] No correlation has been found between EBV infection and p53 reactivity in RS cells. The background of small lymphocytes, plasma cells, eosinophils, and histiocytes in Hodgkin's samples are unstained for p53. This finding supports the idea that the RS cell is the neoplastic component of Hodgkin's disease. Moreover, no p53 staining was observed in lymphocyte-predominant Hodgkin's disease, suggesting that this disease may be a form of B-cell lymphoma rather than a subtype of Hodgkin's disease.

Although the occurrence of p53 mutations in lymphoma has been the focus of many investigations, it remains possible that alterations to other genes may be equally important in lymphomagenesis. The murine double minute-2 (MDM2) gene encodes a protein that binds to and inactivates p53. MDM2 over-expression has been observed in about 50% of low-grade lymphomas and in about 10% of intermediate/high-grade lymphomas.[350] It has been suggested that accumulation of wt p53 could promote the over-expression of the MDM2 gene product, and that the ratio of MDM2/P53 could play a critical role in lymphoma progression.[351] p53 is known to mediate expression of the P21(p21waf1/cip1) gene whose protein product is involved in growth arrest. The coding sequence of P21 has been investigated for mutations in Burkitt's lymphoma samples. No mutations were found in the clinical samples, but a mutation in Burkitt's cell line was found and shown to result in a loss of function of p21.[352] The CDKN2 gene located on chromosome 9p21 encodes the cyclin dependent kinase 4 inhibitor p16. This gene is a putative tumor suppressor because of its frequent alteration in many kinds of tumor cells. Several studies have investigated the prevalence of CDKN2 alterations and between 6% and 14% of NHL samples have been shown to have acquired alterations.[353–355] It is not yet possible to determine whether CDKN2 alterations are associated with a particular subgroup or grade of lymphoma, although a high frequency of alteration (35%) to CDKN2 and the neighboring gene MTS2 has been noted in T-ALL/lymphoblastic lymphoma.[356]

References

1. Rabbitts TH. Chromosomal translocations in human cancer. Nature 1994;372:143–9.
2. Taub R, Kirsch I, Morton C, et al. Translocation of the c-myc gene into the immunoglobulin heavy chain locus in human Burkitt lymphoma and murine plasmacytoma cells. Proc Natl Acad Sci U S A 1982;79:7837–41.
3. Adams JM, Gerondakis S, Webb E, et al. Cellular myc oncogene is altered by chromosome translocation to an immunoglobulin locus in murine plasmacytomas and is rearranged similarly in human Burkitt lymphomas. Proc Natl Acad Sci U S A 1983;80:2146–50.
4. Erikson J, Ar-Rushdi A, Drwinga HL, et al. Transcriptional activation of the translocated c-myc oncogene in Burkitt lymphoma. Proc Natl Acad Sci U S A 1983;80: 1707–11.
5. Hamlyn PH and Rabbitts TH. Translocation joins c-myc and immunoglobulin gamma 1 genes in a Burkitt lymphoma revealing a third exon in the c-myc oncogene. Nature 1983;304:172–4.
6. Dalla-Favera R, Westin E, Gelmann EP, et al. The human onc gene c-myc: structure, expression, and amplification in the human promyelocytic leukemia cell line HL-60. Nature 1983;304:135–9.
7. Battey J, Moulding C, Taub R, et al. The human c-myc oncogene: structural consequences of translocation into the IgH locus in Burkitt lymphoma. Cell 1983;34:779–87.
8. Croce CM, Tsujimoto Y, Erikson J, et al. Chromosome translocations and B cell neoplasia. Nature 1984;310: 655–60.
9. Emanuel BS, Selden JR, Chaganti RS, et al. The 2p breakpoint of a 2;8 translocation in Burkitt lymphoma interrupts the V kappa locus. Proc Natl Acad Sci U S A 1984;81: 2718–22.
10. Hollis GF, Mitchell KF, Battey J, et al. A variant translocation places the lambda immunoglobulin genes 3' to the c-myc oncogene in Burkitt's lymphoma. Nature 1984; 307:752–5.
11. Rappold GA, Hameister H, Cremer T, et al. The myc proteins are not associated with chromatin in mitotic cells. EMBO J 1984;3:2951–5.
12. Davis M, Malcolm S, and Rabbitts TH. A variant translocation places the lambda immunoglobulin genes 3' to the c-myc oncogene in Burkitt's lymphoma. Nature 1984; 308:286–8.
13. Malcolm S, Davis M, and Rabbitts TH. Breakage on chromosome 2 brings the CK gene to a region 3' of c-myc in a Burkitt's lymphoma line carrying a (2;8) translocation. Cytogenet Cell Genet 1985;39:168–72.
14. Manolov G, Manolova Y, Klein G, et al. Alternative involvement of two cytogenetically distinguishable breakpoints on chromosome 8 in Burkitt's lymphoma associated translocations. Cancer Genet Cytogenet 1986;20:95–9.
15. Cory S, Graham M, Webb E, et al. Variant (6;15) translocation in murine plasmacytomas involves a chromosome 15 locus at least 72 kb from the c-myc oncogene. EMBO J 1985;4:675–81.
16. Rabbitts TH, Forster A, Hamlyn P, et al. Effect of somatic mutation within translocated c-myc genes in Burkitt lymphoma cells. Nature 1984;309:592–7.
17. Pelicci PG, Knowles D, Magrath I, et al. Chromosomal breakpoints and structural alterations of the c-myc locus differ in endemic and sporadic forms of Burkitt lymphoma. Proc Natl Acad Sci U S A 1986;83:2984–8.
18. Murphy W, Sarid J, Taub R, et al. A translocated human c-myc oncogene is altered in a conserved coding sequence. Proc Natl Acad Sci U S A 1986;83:2939–43.
19. Ar-Rushdi A, Nishikura K, Erikson J, et al. Differential expression of the translocated and the untranslocated c-myc oncogene in Burkitt lymphoma. Science 1983;222: 390–3.
20. Taub R, Moulding C, Battey J, et al. Activation and somatic mutation of the translocated c-myc gene in Burkitt lymphoma cells. J Exp Med 1984;159:276–91.
21. Wiman KG, Clarkson B, Hayday AC, et al. Activation of a translocated c-myc gene: role of structural alterations in the upstream region. Proc Natl Acad Sci U S A 1984;81: 6798–802.
22. Nishikura K, Ar-Rushdi A, Erikson J, et al. Differential expression of the normal and of the translocated human c-myc oncogenes in B cells. Proc Natl Acad Sci U S A 1983;80:5107–11.
23. Croce CM, Erikson J, Ar-Rushdi A, et al. Translocated c-myc oncogene of Burkitt lymphoma is transcribed in plasma cells and repressed in lymphoblastoid cells. Proc Natl Acad Sci U S A 1984;81:3547–51.
24. Maguire RT, Robins TS, Thorgeirsson SS, et al. Expression of cellular myc and mos genes in undifferentiated B cell lym-

phomas of Burkitt and non-Burkitt types. Proc Natl Acad Sci U S A 1983;80:1982–6.

25. Reed JC, Nowell PC, and Hoover RG. Regulation of c-myc mRNA levels in normal human lymphocytes by modulators of cell proliferation. Proc Natl Acad U S A 1985;82: 4221–4.
26. Hahn SR and Eisenman RN. Proteins encoded by the human c-myc oncogene: Differential expression in neoplastic cells. Mol Cell Biol 1984;4:2486–97.
27. Ramsay G, Evan GI, and Bishop JM. The protein encoded by the human proto-oncogene c-myc. Proc Natl Acad U S A 1984;81:7742–6.
28. Gregory MA and Hann SR. c-Myc proteolysis by the ubiquitin-proteasome pathway: stabilization of c-Myc in Burkitt's lymphoma cells. Mol Cell Biol 2000;20:2423–35.
29. Bahram F, von der Lehr N, Cetinkaya C, et al. c-Myc hot spot mutations in lymphomas result in inefficient ubiquitination and decreased proteasome-mediated turnover. Blood 2000; 95:2104–10.
30. Favrot MC, Philip I, Philip T, et al. Possible duality in Burkitt's lymphoma origin. Lancet 1984;1:745–7.
31. Morse B, South VJ, Rothberg PG, et al. Somatic mutation and transcriptional deregulation of myc in endemic Burkitt's lymphoma disease: heptamer-nonamer recognition mistakes? Mol Cell Biol 1989;9:74–82.
32. Haluska FG, Russo G, Andreeff M, et al. Molecular analysis of an AIDS-associated Burkitt's lymphoma: near-identity with endemic cases. Curr Top Microbiol Immunol 1988; 141:75–9.
33. Haluska FG, Russo G, Kant J, et al. Molecular resemblance of an AIDS-associated lymphoma and endemic Burkitt lymphomas: implications for their pathogenesis. Proc Natl Acad Sci U S A 1989;86:8907–11.
34. Leder A, Pattengale PK, Kuo A, et al. Consequences of widespread deregulation of the c-myc gene in transgenic mice: Multiple neoplasms and normal development. Cell 1986; 45:485–95.
35. Adams JM, Harris AW, Pinkert CA, et al. The c-myc oncogene driven by immunoglobulin enhancers induces lymphoid malignancy in transgenic mice. Nature 1985; 318:533–8.
36. Persson H and Leder P. Nuclear localisation and DNA binding of a protein expressed by human c-myc oncogene. Science 1984;225:718–21.
37. Packham G and Cleveland JL. c-Myc and apoptosis. Biochim Biophys Acta 1995;1242:11–28.
38. Spencer CA and Groudine M. Control of c-myc regulation in normal and neoplastic cells. Adv Cancer Res 1991;56: 1–48.
39. Marcu KB, Bossone SA, and Patel AJ. myc function and regulation. Annu Rev Biochem 1992;61:809–60.
40. Askew DS, Ashmun RA, Simmons BC, et al. Constitutive c-myc expression in an IL-3-dependent myeloid cell line suppresses cell cycle arrest and accelerates apoptosis. Oncogene 1991;6:1915–22.
41. Heikkila R, Schwab G, Wickstrom E, et al. A c-myc antisense oligodeoxynucleotide inhibits entry into S phase but not progress from G0 to G1. Nature 1987;328:445–9.
42. Prochownik EV, Kukowska J, and Rodgers C. c-myc antisense transcripts accelerate differentiation and inhibit G1 progression in murine erythroleukemia cells. Mol Cell Biol 1988;8:3683–95.
43. Gregor PD, Sawadogo M, and Roeder RG. The adenovirus major late transcription factor USF is a member of the helix-loop-helix group of regulatory proteins and binds to DNA as a dimer. Genes Dev 1990;4:1730–40.
44. Beckmann H, Su LK, and Kadesch T. TFE3: a helix-loop-helix protein that activates transcription through the immunoglobulin enhancer muE3 motif. Genes Dev 1990; 4:167–79.
45. Carr CS and Sharp PA. A helix-loop-helix protein related to the immunoglobulin E box-binding proteins. Mol Cell Biol 1990;10:4384–8.
46. Hu YF, Luscher B, Admon A, et al. Transcription factor AP–4 contains multiple dimerization domains that regulate dimer specificity. Genes Dev 1990;4:1741–52.
47. Blackwood EM and Eisenman RN. Max: a helix-loop-helix zipper protein that forms a sequence-specific DNA-binding complex with Myc. Science 1991;251:1211–7.
48. Prendergast GC, Lawe D, and Ziff EB. Association of Myn, the murine homolog of max, with c-Myc stimulates methylation-sensitive DNA binding and ras cotransformation. Cell 1991;65:395–407.
49. Littlewood TD, Amati B, Land H, et al. Max and c-Myc/Max DNA-binding activities in cell extracts. Oncogene 1992; 7:1783–92.
50. Berberich SJ and Cole MD. Casein kinase II inhibits the DNA-binding activity of Max homodimers but not Myc/Max heterodimers. Genes Dev 1992;6:166–76.
51. Zervos AS, Gyuris J, and Brent R. Mxi1, a protein that specifically interacts with Max to bind Myc-Max recognition sites. Cell 1993;72:223–32 [erratum in Cell 1994;79:following 388].
52. Ayer DE, Kretzner L, and Eisenman RN. Mad: a heterodimeric partner for Max that antagonizes Myc transcriptional activity. Cell 1993;72:211–22.
53. Schneider JW, Gu W, Zhu L, et al. Reversal of terminal differentiation mediated by p107 in Rb–/– muscle cells. Science 1994;264:1467–71.
54. Beijersbergen RL, Hijmans EM, Zhu L, et al. Interaction of c-Myc with the pRb-related protein p107 results in inhibition of c-Myc-mediated transactivation. EMBO J 1994;13:4080–6.
55. McMahon SB, Wood MA, and Cole MD. The essential cofactor TRRAP recruits the histone acetyltransferase hGCN5 to c-Myc. Mol Cell Biol 2000;20:556–62.
56. Park J, Kunjibettu S, McMahon SB, et al. The ATM-related domain of TRRAP is required for histone acetyltransferase recruitment and Myc-dependent oncogenesis. Genes Dev 2001;15:1619–24.
57. Harrington EA, Fanidi A, and Evan GI. Oncogenes and cell death. Curr Opin Genet Dev 1994;4:120–9.
58. Bhatia KG, Gutierrez MI, Huppi K, et al. The pattern of p53 mutations in Burkitt's lymphoma differs from that of solid tumors. Cancer Res 1992;52:4273–6.
59. Farrell PJ, Allan GJ, Shanahan F, et al. p53 is frequently mutated in Burkitt's lymphoma cell lines. EMBO J 1991; 10:2879–87.
60. Capoulade C, Bressac-de Paillerets B, Lefrere I, et al. Overexpression of MDM2, due to enhanced translation, results in inactivation of wild-type p53 in Burkitt's lymphoma cells. Oncogene 1998;16:1603–10.
61. Tao W and Levine AJ. Nucleocytoplasmic shuttling of oncoprotein Hdm2 is required for Hdm2-mediated degradation of p53. Proc Natl Acad Sci U S A 1999; 96:3077–80.
62. Hermeking H and Eick D. Mediation of c-Myc-induced apoptosis by p53. Science 1994;265:2091–3.
63. Sherr CJ. The INK4a/ARF network in tumour suppression. Nat Rev Mol Cell Biol 2001;2:731–7.
64. Lindstrom MS, Klangby U, and Wiman KG. p14ARF homozygous deletion or MDM2 overexpression in Burkitt lymphoma lines carrying wild type p53. Oncogene 2001; 20:2171–7.
65. Klangby U, Okan I, Magnusson KP, et al. p16/INK4a and p15/INK4b gene methylation and absence of p16/INK4a

mRNA and protein expression in Burkitt's lymphoma. Blood 1998;91:1680–7.
66. Sinclair AJ and Frost V. Loss of functional pRB is not a ubiquitous feature of B-cell malignancies. Br J Cancer 1999;80:670–5.
67. Cinti C, Leoncini L, Nyongo A, et al. Genetic alterations of the retinoblastoma-related gene RB2/p130 identify different pathogenetic mechanisms in and among Burkitt's lymphoma subtypes. Am J Pathol 2000;156:751–60.
68. Van den Berghe H, Parloir C, David G, et al. A new characteristic karyotypic anomaly in lymphoproliferative disorders. Cancer 1979;44:188–95.
69. Leroux D, Le-Marc'Hadour F, Gressin R, et al. Non-Hodgkin's lymphomas with t(11;14)(q13;q32): a subset of mantle zone/intermediate lymphocytic lymphoma? Br J Haematol 1991;77:346–53.
70. Vandenberghe E, De-Wolf-Peeters C, Wlodarska I, et al. Chromosome 11q rearrangements in B non Hodgkin's lymphoma. Br J Haematol 1992;81:212–17.
71. Weisenburger DD and Chan WC. Lymphomas of follicles. Mantle cell and follicle center cell lymphomas. Am J Clin Pathol 1993;99:409–20.
72. Shivdasani RA, Hess JL, Skarin AT, et al. Intermediate lymphocytic lymphoma: clinical and pathologic features of a recently characterized subtype of non-Hodgkin's lymphoma. J Clin Oncol 1993;11:802–111.
73. Brito-Babapulle V, Ellis J, Matutes E, et al. Translocation t(11;14)(q13;q32) in chronic lymphoid disorders. Genes Chromosomes Cancer 1992;5:158–65.
74. Oscier DG, Matutes E, Gardiner A, et al. Cytogenetic studies in splenic lymphoma with villous lymphocytes. Br J Haematol 1993;85:487–91.
75. Tsujimoto Y, Yunis J, Onorato-Showe L, et al. Molecular cloning of the chromosomal breakpoint of B-cell lymphomas and leukemias with the t(11;14) chromosome translocation. Science 1984;224:1403–6.
76. Tsujimoto Y, Jaffe E, Cossman J, et al. Clustering of breakpoints on chromosome 11 in human B-cell neoplasms with the t(11;14) chromosome translocation. Nature 1985; 315:340–3.
77. Erikson J, Finan J, Tsujimoto Y, et al. The chromosome 14 breakpoint in neoplastic B cells with the t(11;14) translocation involves the immunoglobulin heavy chain locus. Proc Natl Acad Sci U S A 1984;81:4144–8.
78. Ince C, Blick M, Lee M, et al. Bcl-1 gene rearrangements in B cell lymphoma. Leukemia 1988;2:343–6.
79. Medeiros LJ, Van-Krieken JH, Jaffe ES, et al. Association of bcl-1 rearrangements with lymphocytic lymphoma of intermediate differentiation. Blood 1990;76:2086–90.
80. Williams ME, Westermann CD, and Swerdlow SH. Genotypic characterization of centrocytic lymphoma: frequent rearrangement of the chromosome 11 bcl-1 locus. Blood 1990;76:1387–91.
81. Arnold A, Kim HG, Gaz RD, et al. Molecular cloning and chromosomal mapping of DNA rearranged with the parathyroid hormone gene in a parathyroid adenoma. J Clin Invest 1989;83:2034–40.
82. Motokura T, Bloom T, Kim HG, et al. A novel cyclin encoded by a bcl1-linked candidate oncogene. Nature 1991;350: 512–15.
83. Matsushime H, Roussel MF, Ashmun RA, et al. Colony-stimulating factor 1 regulates novel cyclins during the G1 phase of the cell cycle. Cell 1991;65:701–13.
84. Xiong Y, Connolly T, Futcher B, et al. Human D-type cyclin. Cell 1991;65:691–9.
85. Rosenberg CL, Wong E, Petty EM, et al. PRAD1, a candidate BCL1 oncogene: mapping and expression in centrocytic lymphoma. Proc Natl Acad Sci U S A 1991;88:9638–42.
86. Withers DA, Harvey RC, Faust JB, et al. Characterization of a candidate bcl-1 gene. Mol Cell Biol 1991;11:4846–53.
87. Williams ME, Swerdlow SH, Rosenberg CL, et al. Chromosome 11 translocation breakpoints at the PRAD1/cyclin D1 gene locus in centrocytic lymphoma. Leukemia 1993;7: 241–5.
88. Meeker TC, Sellers W, Harvey R, et al. Cloning of the t(11;14)(q13;q32) translocation breakpoints from two human leukemia cell lines. Leukemia 1991;5:733–7.
89. Rimokh R, Berger F, Delsol G, et al. Rearrangement and overexpression of the BCL-1/PRAD-1 gene in intermediate lymphocytic lymphomas and in t(11q13)-bearing leukemias. Blood 1993;81:3063–7.
90. Williams ME, Swerdlow SH, Rosenberg CL, et al. Characterization of chromosome 11 translocation breakpoints at the bcl-1 and PRAD1 loci in centrocytic lymphoma. Cancer Res 1992;52:5541s–4s.
91. Williams ME, Meeker TC, and Swerdlow SH. Rearrangement of the chromosome 11 bcl-1 locus in centrocytic lymphoma: analysis with multiple breakpoint probes. Blood 1991; 78:493–8.
92. Molot RJ, Meeker TC, Wittwer CT, et al. Antigen expression and polymerase chain reaction amplification of mantle cell lymphomas. Blood 1994;83:1626–31.
93. Delmer A, Ajchenbaum-Cymbalista F, Tang R, et al. Overexpression of cyclin D1 in chronic B-cell malignancies with abnormality of chromosome 11q13. Br J Haematol 1995;89: 798–804.
94. Seto M, Yamamoto K, Iida S, et al. Gene rearrangement and overexpression of PRAD1 in lymphoid malignancy with t(11;14)(q13;q32) translocation. Oncogene 1992;7: 1401–6.
95. Raynaud SD, Bekri S, Leroux D, et al. Expanded range of 11q13 breakpoints with differing patterns of cyclin D1 expression in B cell malignancies. Genes Chromosomes Cancer 1993;8:80–7.
96. Cuneo A, Balboni M, Piva N, et al. Atypical chronic lymphocytic leukaemia with t(11;14)(q13;q32): karyotype evolution and prolymphocytic transformation. Br J Haematol 1995;90:409–16.
97. Yang WI, Zukerberg LR, Motokura T, et al. Cyclin D1 (Bcl-1, PRAD1) protein expression in low-grade B-cell lymphomas and reactive hyperplasia. Am J Pathol 1994;145:86–96.
98. Palmero I, Holder A, Sinclair AJ, et al. Cyclins D1 and D2 are differentially expressed in human B-lymphoid cell lines. Oncogene 1993;8:1049–54.
99. Bosch F, Jares P, Campo E, et al. PRAD-1/cyclin D1 gene overexpression in chronic lymphoproliferative disorders: a highly specific marker of mantle cell lymphoma. Blood 1994; 84:2726–32.
100. Lebwohl DE, Muise-Helmericks R, Sepp-Lorenzino L, et al. A truncated cyclin D1 gene encodes a stable mRNA in a human breast cancer cell line. Oncogene 1994;9:1925–9.
101. Rimokh R, Berger F, Bastard C, et al. Rearrangement of CCND1 (BCL1/PRAD1) 3' untranslated region in mantle-cell lymphomas and t(11q13)-associated leukemias. Blood 1994;83:3689–96.
102. Rosenberg CL, Motokura T, Kronenberg HM, et al. Coding sequence of the overexpressed transcript of the putative oncogene PRAD1/cyclin D1 in two primary human tumors. Oncogene 1993;8:519–21.
103. Buckley MF, Sweeney KJ, Hamilton JA, et al. Expression and amplification of cyclin genes in human breast cancer. Oncogene 1993;8:2127–33.
104. Keyomarsi K and Pardee AB. Redundant cyclin overexpression and gene amplification in breast cancer cells. Proc Natl Acad Sci U S A 1993;90:1112–16.

105. Gillett C, Fantl V, Smith R, et al. Amplification and overexpression of cyclin D1 in breast cancer detected by immunohistochemical staining. Cancer Res 1994;54:1812–17.
106. Tsuruta H, Sakamoto H, Onda M, et al. Amplification and overexpression of EXP1 and EXP2/Cyclin D1 genes in human esophageal carcinomas. Biochem Biophys Res Commun 1993;196:1529–36.
107. Leach FS, Elledge SJ, Sherr CJ, et al. Amplification of cyclin genes in colorectal carcinomas. Cancer Res 1993;53:1986–9.
108. Zhang YJ, Jiang W, Chen CJ, et al. Amplification and overexpression of cyclin D1 in human hepatocellular carcinoma. Biochem Biophys Res Commun 1993;196:1010–16.
109. Jiang W, Kahn SM, Zhou P, et al. Overexpression of cyclin D1 in rat fibroblasts causes abnormalities in growth control, cell cycle progression and gene expression. Oncogene 1993;8:3447–57.
110. Quelle DE, Ashmun RA, Shurtleff SA, et al. Overexpression of mouse D-type cyclins accelerates G1 phase in rodent fibroblasts. Genes Dev 1993;7:1559–71.
111. Resnitzky D, Gossen M, Bujard H, et al. Acceleration of the G1/S phase transition by expression of cyclins D1 and E with an inducible system. Mol Cell Biol 1994;14:1669–79.
112. Baldin V, Lukas J, Marcote MJ, et al. Cyclin D1 is a nuclear protein required for cell cycle progression in G1. Genes Dev 1993;7:1010–16.
113. Lovec H, Sewing A, Lucibello FC, et al. Oncogenic activity of cyclin D1 revealed through cooperation with Ha-ras: link between cell cycle control and malignant transformation. Oncogene 1994;9:323–6.
114. Hinds PW, Dowdy SF, Eaton EN, et al. Function of a human cyclin gene as an oncogene. Proc Natl Acad Sci U S A 1994;91:709–13.
115. Dowdy SF, Hinds PW, Louie K, et al. Physical interaction of the retinoblastoma protein with human D cyclins. Cell 1993;73:499–511.
116. Ewen ME, Sluss HK, Sherr CJ, et al. Functional interactions of the retinoblastoma protein with mammalian D-type cyclins. Cell 1993;73:487–97.
117. Hall FL, Williams RT, Wu L, et al. Two potentially oncogenic cyclins, cyclin A and cyclin D1, share common properties of subunit configuration, tyrosine phosphorylation and physical association with the Rb protein. Oncogene 1993; 8:1377–84.
118. Kato J, Matsushime H, Hiebert SW, et al. Direct binding of cyclin D to the retinoblastoma gene product (pRb) and pRb phosphorylation by the cyclin D-dependent kinase CDK4. Genes Dev 1993;7:331–42.
119. Weinberg RA. Tumor suppressor genes. Science 1991; 254:1138–46.
120. Nevins JR. E2F: a link between the Rb tumor suppressor protein and viral oncoproteins. Science 1992;258:424–9.
121. Weintraub SJ, Prater CA, and Dean DC. Retinoblastoma protein switches the E2F site from positive to negative element. Nature 1992;358:259–61.
122. Bodrug SE, Warner BJ, Bath ML, et al. Cyclin D1 transgene impedes lymphocyte maturation and collaborates in lymphomagenesis with the myc gene. EMBO J 1994;13: 2124–30.
123. Lovec H, Grzeschiczek A, Kowalski MB, et al. Cyclin D1/bcl-1 cooperates with myc genes in the generation of B-cell lymphoma in transgenic mice. EMBO J 1994;13:3487–95.
124. Offit K, Wong G, Filippa DA, et al. Cytogenetic analysis of 434 consecutively ascertained specimens of non-Hodgkin's lymphoma: clinical correlations. Blood 1991;77: 1508–15.
125. Yunis JJ, Frizzera G, Oken MM, et al. Multiple recurrent genomic defects in follicular lymphoma. A possible model for cancer. N Engl J Med 1987;316:79–84.
126. Fukuhara S, Rowley JD, Variakojis D, et al. Chromosome abnormalities in poorly differentiated lymphocytic lymphoma. Cancer Res 1979;39:3119–28.
127. Tsujimoto Y, Gorham J, Cossman J, et al. The t(14;18) chromosome translocations involved in B-cell neoplasms result from mistakes in VDJ joining. Science 1985;229:1390–3.
128. Bakhshi A, Jensen JP, Goldman P, et al. Cloning the chromosomal breakpoint of t(14;18) human lymphomas: clustering around JH on chromosome 14 and near a transcriptional unit on 18. Cell 1985;41:899–906.
129. Cleary ML and Sklar J. Nucleotide sequence of a t(14;18) chromosomal breakpoint in follicular lymphoma and demonstration of a breakpoint-cluster region near a transcriptionally active locus on chromosome 18. Proc Natl Acad Sci U S A 1985;82:7439–43.
130. Tsujimoto Y and Croce CM. Analysis of the structure, transcripts, and protein products of bcl-2, the gene involved in human follicular lymphoma. Proc Natl Acad Sci U S A 1986;83:5214–18.
131. Cazals-Hatem DL, Louie DC, Tanaka S, et al. Molecular cloning and DNA sequence analysis of cDNA encoding chicken homologue of the Bcl-2 oncoprotein. Biochim Biophys Acta 1992;1132:109–13.
132. Monaghan P, Robertson D, Amos TA, et al. Ultrastructural localization of bcl-2 protein. J Histochem Cytochem 1992;40:1819–25.
133. Cleary ML, Smith SD, and Sklar J. Cloning and structural analysis of cDNAs for bcl-2 and a hybrid bcl-2/immunoglobulin transcript resulting from the t(14;18) translocation. Cell 1986;47:19–28.
134. Bakhshi A, Wright JJ, Graninger W, et al. Mechanism of the t(14;18) chromosomal translocation: structural analysis of both derivative 14 and 18 reciprocal partners. Proc Natl Acad Sci U S A 1987;84:2396–400.
135. Cleary ML, Galili N, and Sklar J. Detection of a second t(14;18) breakpoint cluster region in human follicular lymphomas. J Exp Med 1986;164:315–20.
136. Ngan BY, Nourse J, and Cleary ML. Detection of chromosomal translocation t(14;18) within the minor cluster region of bcl-2 by polymerase chain reaction and direct genomic sequencing of the enzymatically amplified DNA in follicular lymphomas. Blood 1989;73:1759–62.
137. Tanaka S, Louie DC, Kant JA, et al. Frequent incidence of somatic mutations in translocated BCL2 oncogenes of non-Hodgkin's lymphomas. Blood 1992;79:229–37.
138. Dyer MJ, Zani VJ, Lu WZ, et al. BCL2 translocations in leukemias of mature B cells. Blood 1994;83:3682–8.
139. Mufti GJ, Hamblin TJ, Oscier DG, and et al. Common ALL with pre-B-cell features showing (8;14) and (14;18) chromosome translocations. Blood 1983;62:1142–6.
140. Lillington DM, Monard S, Johnson PW, et al. The t(14;18) in a patient with de novo acute lymphoblastic leukemia is associated with t(8;9). Leukemia 1994;8:560–3.
141. Kramer MH, Raghoebier S, Beverstock GC, et al. De novo acute B-cell leukemia with translocation t(14;18): an entity with a poor prognosis. Leukemia 1991;5:473–8.
142. LeBrun DP, Ngan BY, Weiss LM, et al. The bcl-2 oncogene in Hodgkin's disease arising in the setting of follicular non-Hodgkin's lymphoma. Blood 1994;83:223–30.
143. Gupta RK, Lister TA, and Bodmer JG. The t(14;18) chromosomal translocation and Bcl-2 protein expression in Hodgkin's disease. Leukemia 1994;8:1337–41.
144. Stetler-Stevenson M, Crush-Stanton S, and Cossman J. Involvement of the bcl-2 gene in Hodgkin's disease. J Natl Cancer Inst 1990;82:855–8.
145. Limpens J, de Jong D, van Krieken JH, et al. Bcl-2/JH rearrangements in benign lymphoid tissues with follicular hyperplasia. Oncogene 1991;6:2271–6.

146. Segal GH, Scott M, Jorgensen T, et al. Standard polymerase chain reaction analysis does not detect t(14;18) in reactive lymphoid hyperplasia. Arch Pathol Lab Med 1994; 118:791–4.
147. Adachi M, Tefferi A, Greipp PR, et al. Preferential linkage of bcl-2 to immunoglobulin light chain gene in chronic lymphocytic leukemia. J Exp Med 1990;171:559–64.
148. Aventin A, Mecucci C, Guanyabens C, et al. Variant t(2;18) translocation in a Burkitt conversion of follicular lymphoma. Br J Haematol 1990;74:367–9.
149. Leroux D, Monteil M, Sotto JJ, et al. Variant t(2;18) translocation in a follicular lymphoma. Br J Haematol 1990; 75:290–2.
150. Adachi M and Tsujimoto Y. Juxtaposition of human bcl-2 and immunoglobulin lambda light chain gene in chronic lymphocytic leukemia is the result of a reciprocal chromosome translocation between chromosome 18 and 22. Oncogene 1989;4:1073–5.
151. Hillion J, Mecucci C, Aventin A, et al. A variant translocation t(2;18) in follicular lymphoma involves the 5' end of bcl-2 and Ig kappa light chain gene. Oncogene 1991; 6:169–72.
152. Rimokh R, Gadoux M, Bertheas MF, et al. FVT–1, a novel human transcription unit affected by variant translocation t(2;18)(p11;q21) of follicular lymphoma. Blood 1993; 81:136–42.
153. Mikraki V, Ladanyi M, and Chaganti RS. Structural alterations in the 5' region of the BCL2 gene in follicular lymphomas with BCL2-MBR or BCL2-MCR rearrangements. Genes Chromosomes Cancer 1991;3:117–21.
154. Seite P, Hillion J, d'Agay MF, et al. BCL2 complex rearrangement in follicular lymphoma: translocation mbr/JH and deletion in the vcr region of the same BCL2 allele. Oncogene 1993;8:3073–80.
155. Zelenetz AD, Cleary ML, and Levy R. A submicroscopic interstitial deletion of chromosome 14 frequently occurs adjacent to the t(14;18) translocation breakpoint in human follicular lymphoma. Genes Chromosomes Cancer 1993; 6:140–50.
156. de Jong D, Voetdijk BM, van Ommen GJB, et al. Translocation t(14;18) in B cell lymphomas as a cause for defective immunoglobulin production. J Exp Med 1989;169:613–24.
157. Lee MS, Chang KS, Cabanillas F, et al. Detection of minimal residual cells carrying the t(14;18) by DNA sequence amplification. Science 1987;237:175–8.
158. Stetler-Stevenson M, Raffeld M, Cohen P, et al. Detection of occult follicular lymphoma by specific DNA amplification. Blood 1988;72:1822–5.
159. Crescenzi M, Seto M, Herzig GP, et al. Thermostable DNA polymerase chain amplification of t(14;18) chromosome breakpoints and detection of minimal residual disease. Proc Natl Acad Sci U S A 1988;85:4869–73.
160. Cotter F, Price C, Zucca E, et al. Direct sequence analysis of the 14q+ and 18q- chromosome junctions in follicular lymphoma. Blood 1990;76:131–5.
161. Corbally N, Grogan L, Dervan PA, et al. The detection of specific gene rearrangements in non-Hodgkin's lymphoma using the polymerase chain reaction. Br J Cancer 1992;66:805–9.
162. Cotter FE, Price C, Meerabux J, et al. Direct sequence analysis of 14q+ and 18q- chromosome junctions at the MBR and MCR revealing clustering within the MBR in follicular lymphoma. Ann Oncol 1991;2:93–7.
163. Pezzella F, Ralfkiaer E, Gatter KC, et al. The 14;18 translocation in European cases of follicular lymphoma: comparison of Southern blotting and the polymerase chain reaction. Br J Haematol 1990;76:58–64.
164. Ladanyi M and Wang S. Detection of rearrangements of the BCL2 major breakpoint region in follicular lymphomas. Correlation of polymerase chain reaction results with Southern blot analysis. Diagn Mol Pathol 1992;1:31–5.
165. Benitez J, Robledo M, Santon A, et al. Correlation between cytogenetic and molecular analysis of t(14;18) in follicular lymphomas. Cancer Genet Cytogenet 1992;59:68–72.
166. Zelenetz AD, Chu G, Galili N, et al. Enhanced detection of the t(14;18) translocation in malignant lymphoma using pulsed-field gel electrophoresis. Blood 1991;78:1552–60.
167. Lambrechts AC, Hupkes PE, Dorssers LC, et al. Translocation (14;18)-positive cells are present in the circulation of the majority of patients with localized (stage I and II) follicular non-Hodgkin's lymphoma. Blood 1993;82: 2510–6.
168. Finke J, Slanina J, Lange W, et al. Persistence of circulating t(14;18)-positive cells in long-term remission after radiation therapy for localized-stage follicular lymphoma. J Clin Oncol 1993;11:1668–73.
169. Price CG, Meerabux J, Murtagh S, et al. The significance of circulating cells carrying t(14;18) in long remission from follicular lymphoma. J Clin Oncol 1991;9:1527–32.
170. Gribben JG, Freedman A, Woo SD, et al. All advanced stage non-Hodgkin's lymphomas with a polymerase chain reaction amplifiable breakpoint of bcl-2 have residual cells containing the bcl-2 rearrangement at evaluation and after treatment. Blood 1991;78:3275–80.
171. Lambrechts AC, Hupkes PE, Dorssers LC, et al. Clinical significance of t(14; 18)-positive cells in the circulation of patients with stage III or IV follicular non-Hodgkin's lymphoma during first remission. J Clin Oncol 1994;12:1541–6.
172. Berinstein NL, Jamal HH, Kuzniar B, et al. Sensitive and reproducible detection of occult disease in patients with follicular lymphoma by PCR amplification of t(14;18) both pre- and post-treatment. Leukemia 1993;7:113–9.
173. Levine EG, Arthur DC, Frizzera G, et al. Cytogenetic abnormalities predict clinical outcome in non-Hodgkin lymphoma. Ann Intern Med 1988;108:14–20.
174. Pezzella F, Jones M, Ralfkiaer E, et al. Evaluation of bcl-2 protein expression and 14;18 translocation as prognostic markers in follicular lymphoma. Br J Cancer 1992;65:87–9.
175. Tilly H, Rossi A, Stamatoullas A, et al. Prognostic value of chromosomal abnormalities in follicular lymphoma. Blood 1994;84:1043–9.
176. Gribben JG, Freedman AS, Neuberg D, et al. Immunologic purging of marrow assessed by PCR before autologous bone marrow transplantation for B-cell lymphoma. N Engl J Med 1991;325:1525–33.
177. Johnson PW, Price CG, Smith T, et al. Detection of cells bearing the t(14;18) translocation following myeloablative treatment and autologous bone marrow transplantation for follicular lymphoma. J Clin Oncol 1994;12:798–805.
178. Gribben JG, Neuberg D, Freedman AS, et al. Detection by polymerase chain reaction of residual cells with the bcl-2 translocation is associated with increased risk of relapse after autologous bone marrow transplantation for B-cell lymphoma. Blood 1993;81:3449–57.
179. Conrad MN, Wright JH, Wolf AJ, et al. RAP1 protein interacts with yeast telomeres in vivo: overproduction alters telomere structure and decreases chromosome stability. Cell 1990;63:739–50.
180. Wahls WP, Wallace LJ, and Moore PD. Hypervariable minisatellite DNA is a hotspot for homologous recombination in human cells. Cell 1990;60:95–103.
181. Boehm T, Mengle-Gaw L, Kees UR, et al. Alternating purine-pyrimidine tracts may promote chromosomal translocations seen in a variety of human lymphoid tumours. EMBO J 1989;8:2621–31.
182. Nikaido T, Yamawaki-Kataoka Y, and Honjo T. Nucleotide sequences of switch regions of immunoglobulin C epsilon

and C gamma genes and their comparison. J Biol Chem 1982;257:7322–9.
183. Gerstein RM, Frankel WN, Hsieh CL, et al. Isotype switching of an immunoglobulin heavy chain transgene occurs by DNA recombination between different chromosomes. Cell 1990;63:537–48.
184. Jeffreys AJ, Wilson V, and Thein SL. Hypervariable 'minisatellite' regions in human DNA. Nature 1985;314:67–73.
185. Krowczynska AM, Rudders RA, and Krontiris TG. The human minisatellite consensus at breakpoints of oncogene translocations. Nucleic Acids Res 1990;18:1121–7.
186. Wyatt RT, Rudders RA, Zelenetz A, et al. BCL2 oncogene translocation is mediated by a chi-like consensus. J Exp Med 1992;175:1575–88.
187. Jaeger U, Purtscher B, Karth GD, et al. Mechanism of the chromosomal translocation t(14;18) in lymphoma: detection of a 45-Kd breakpoint binding protein. Blood 1993;81: 1833–40.
188. Ngan BY, Chen LZ, Weiss LM, et al. Expression in non-Hodgkin's lymphoma of the bcl-2 protein associated with the t(14;18) chromosomal translocation. N Engl J Med 1988;318:1638–44.
189. Gaulard P, d'Agay MF, Peuchmaur M, et al. Expression of the bcl-2 gene product in follicular lymphoma. Am J Pathol 1992;140:1089–95.
190. Seite P, Hillion J, d'Agay MF, et al. BCL2 gene activation and protein expression in follicular lymphoma: a report on 64 cases. Leukemia 1993;7:410–17.
191. Pezzella F, Tse AG, Cordell JL, et al. Expression of the bcl-2 oncogene protein is not specific for the 14;18 chromosomal translocation. Am J Pathol 1990;137:225–32.
192. Hockenbery DM, Zutter M, Hickey W, et al. BCL2 protein is topographically restricted in tissues characterized by apoptotic cell death. Proc Natl Acad Sci U S A 1991;88:6961–5.
193. Chleq-Deschamps CM, LeBrun DP, Huie P, et al. Topographical dissociation of BCL-2 messenger RNA and protein expression in human lymphoid tissues. Blood 1993; 81:293–8.
194. Zutter M, Hockenbery D, Silverman GA, et al. Immunolocalization of the Bcl-2 protein within hematopoietic neoplasms. Blood 1991;78:1062–8.
195. Pettersson M, Jernberg-Wiklund H, Larsson LG, et al. Expression of the bcl-2 gene in human multiple myeloma cell lines and normal plasma cells. Blood 1992;79:495–502.
196. Silvestrini R, Veneroni S, Daidone MG, et al. The Bcl-2 protein: a prognostic indicator strongly related to p53 protein in lymph node-negative breast cancer patients. J Natl Cancer Inst 1994;86:499–504.
197. Vaux DL, Cory S, and Adams JM. Bcl-2 gene promotes haemopoietic cell survival and cooperates with c-myc to immortalize pre-B cells. Nature 1988;335:440–2.
198. Nunez G, London L, Hockenbery D, et al. Deregulated Bcl-2 gene expression selectively prolongs survival of growth factor-deprived hemopoietic cell lines. J Immunol 1990; 144:3602–10.
199. Lotem J and Sachs L. Induction of dependence on hematopoietic proteins for viability and receptor upregulation in differentiating myeloid leukemic cells. Blood 1989;74:579–85.
200. Hockenbery D, Nunez G, Milliman C, et al. Bcl-2 is an inner mitochondrial membrane protein that blocks programmed cell death. Nature 1990;348:334–6.
201. Campana D, Coustan-Smith E, Manabe A, et al. Prolonged survival of B-lineage acute lymphoblastic leukemia cells is accompanied by overexpression of bcl-2 protein. Blood 1993;81:1025–31.
202. Allsopp TE, Wyatt S, Paterson HF, et al. The proto-oncogene bcl-2 can selectively rescue neurotrophic factor-dependent neurons from apoptosis. Cell 1993;73:295–307.
203. Miyashita T and Reed JC. bcl-2 gene transfer increases relative resistance of S49.1 and WEHI7.2 lymphoid cells to cell death and DNA fragmentation induced by glucocorticoids and multiple chemotherapeutic drugs. Cancer Res 1992; 52:5407–11.
204. Lotem J and Sachs L. Regulation by bcl-2, c-myc, and p53 of susceptibility to induction of apoptosis by heat shock and cancer chemotherapy compounds in differentiation-competent and -defective myeloid leukemic cells. Cell Growth Differ 1993;4:41–7.
205. Reed JC, Kitada S, Takayama S, et al. Regulation of chemoresistance by the bcl-2 oncoprotein in non-Hodgkin's lymphoma and lymphocytic leukemia cell lines. Ann Oncol 1994;1:61–5.
206. Miyashita T and Reed JC. Bcl-2 oncoprotein blocks chemotherapy-induced apoptosis in a human leukemia cell line. Blood 1993;81:151–7.
207. Naumovski L and Cleary ML. Bcl2 inhibits apoptosis associated with terminal differentiation of HL-60 myeloid leukemia cells. Blood 1994;83:2261–7.
208. Strasser A, Whittingham S, Vaux DL, et al. Enforced BCL2 expression in B-lymphoid cells prolongs antibody responses and elicits autoimmune disease. Proc Natl Acad Sci U S A 1991;88:8661–5.
209. Sentman CL, Shutter JR, Hockenbery D, et al. bcl-2 inhibits multiple forms of apoptosis but not negative selection in thymocytes. Cell 1991;67:879–88.
210. Nunez G, Hockenbery D, McDonnell TJ, et al. Bcl-2 maintains B cell memory. Nature 1991;353:71–3.
211. Pietenpol JA, Papadopoulos N, Markowitz S, et al. Paradoxical inhibition of solid tumor cell growth by bcl2. Cancer Res 1994;54:3714–17.
212. Henderson S, Rowe M, Gregory C, et al. Induction of bcl-2 expression by Epstein–Barr virus latent membrane protein 1 protects infected B cells from programmed cell death. Cell 1991;65:1107–15.
213. Vaux DL, Weissman IL, and Kim SK. Prevention of programmed cell death in Caenorhabditis elegans by human bcl-2. Science 1992;258:1955–7.
214. Yuan J and Horvitz HR. The Caenorhabditis elegans cell death gene ced-4 encodes a novel protein and is expressed during the period of extensive programmed cell death. Development 1992;116:309–20.
215. Ellis HM and Horvitz HR. Genetic control of programmed cell death in the nematode C. elegans. Cell 1986;44:817–29.
216. Reed JC, Cuddy M, Slabiak T, et al. Oncogenic potential of bcl-2 demonstrated by gene transfer. Nature 1988; 336:259–61.
217. McDonnell TJ, Deane N, Platt FM, et al. bcl-2-immunoglobulin transgenic mice demonstrate extended B cell survival and follicular lymphoproliferation. Cell 1989;57:79–88.
218. McDonnell TJ and Korsmeyer SJ. Progression from lymphoid hyperplasia to high-grade malignant lymphoma in mice transgenic for the t(14; 18). Nature 1991;349:254–6.
219. Strasser A, Harris AW, and Cory S. E mu-bcl-2 transgene facilitates spontaneous transformation of early pre-B and immunoglobulin-secreting cells but not T cells. Oncogene 1993;8:1–9.
220. Limpens J, Stad R, Vos C, et al. Lymphoma-associated translocation t(14;18) in blood B cells of normal individuals. Blood 1995;85:2528–36.
221. Liu Y, Hernandez AM, Shibata D, et al. BCL2 translocation frequency rises with age in humans. Proc Natl Acad Sci U S A 1994;91:8910–14.
222. Siegel RM, Katsumata M, Miyashita T, et al. Inhibition of thymocyte apoptosis and negative antigenic selection in bcl- 2 transgenic mice. Proc Natl Acad Sci U S A 1992;89: 7003–7.

223. Katsumata M, Siegel RM, Louie DC, et al. Differential effects of Bcl-2 on T and B cells in transgenic mice. Proc Natl Acad Sci U S A 1992;89:11376–80.
224. Linette GP, Hess JL, Sentman CL, et al. Peripheral T-cell lymphoma in lck(pr)-bcl-2 transgenic mice. Blood 1995; 86:1255–60.
225. Veis DJ, Sorenson CM, Shutter JR, et al. Bcl-2-deficient mice demonstrate fulminant lymphoid apoptosis, polycystic kidneys, and hypopigmented hair. Cell 1993;75:229–40.
226. Krajewski S, Tanaka S, Takayama S, et al. Investigation of the subcellular distribution of the bcl-2 oncoprotein: residence in the nuclear envelope, endoplasmic reticulum, and outer mitochondrial membranes. Cancer Res 1993;53:4701–14.
227. Jacobson MD, Burne JF, King MP, et al. Bcl-2 blocks apoptosis in cells lacking mitochondrial DNA. Nature 1993; 361:365–9.
228. Mah SP, Zhong LT, Liu Y, et al. The protooncogene bcl-2 inhibits apoptosis in PC12 cells. J Neurochem 1993; 60:1183–6.
229. Smets LA, Van-den-Berg J, Acton D, et al. BCL-2 expression and mitochondrial activity in leukemic cells with different sensitivity to glucocorticoid-induced apoptosis. Blood 1994;84:1613–19.
230. Baffy G, Miyashita T, Williamson JR, et al. Apoptosis induced by withdrawal of interleukin-3 (IL-3) from an IL-3–dependent hematopoietic cell line is associated with repartitioning of intracellular calcium and is blocked by enforced Bcl-2 oncoprotein production. J Biol Chem 1993;268:6511–19.
231. Lam M, Dubyak G, and Distelhorst CW. Effect of glucocorticosteroid treatment on intracellular calcium homeostasis in mouse lymphoma cells. Mol Endocrinol 1993;7:686–93.
232. Dowd DR, MacDonald PN, Komm BS, et al. Stable expression of the calbindin-D28K complementary DNA interferes with the apoptotic pathway in lymphocytes. Mol Endocrinol 1992;6:1843–8.
233. Kane DJ, Sarafian TA, Anton R, et al. Bcl-2 inhibition of neural death: Decreased generation of reactive oxygen species. Science 1993;262:1274–7.
234. Henderson S, Huen D, Rowe M, et al. Epstein–Barr virus-coded BHRF1 protein, a viral homologue of Bcl-2, protects human B cells from programmed cell death. Proc Natl Acad Sci U S A 1993;90:8479–83.
235. Neilan JG, Lu Z, Afonso CL, et al. An African swine fever virus gene with similarity to the proto-oncogene bcl-2 and the Esptein-Barr virus gene BHRF1. J Virol 1993;67:4391–4.
236. Oltvai ZN, Milliman CL, and Korsmeyer SJ. Bcl-2 heterodimerizes in vivo with a conserved homolog, Bax, that accelerates programmed cell death. Cell 1993;74:609–19.
237. Boise LH, Gonzalez-Garcia M, Postema CE, et al. bcl-x, a bcl-2-related gene that functions as a dominant regulator of apoptotic cell death. Cell 1993;74:597–608.
238. Kozopas KM, Yang T, Buchan HL, et al. MCL1, a gene expressed in programmed myeloid cell differentiation, has sequence similarity to BCL2. Proc Natl Acad Sci U S A 1993;90:3516–20.
239. Craig RW, Jabs EW, Zhou P, et al. Human and mouse chromosomal mapping of the myeloid cell leukemia-1 gene: MCL1 maps to human chromosome 1q21, a region that is frequently altered in preneoplastic and neoplastic disease. Genomics 1994;23:457–63.
240. Lin EY, Orlofsky A, Berger MS, and Prystowsky MB. Characterization of A1, a novel hemopoietic-specific early-response gene with sequence similarity to bcl-2. J Immunol 1993;151:1979–88.
241. Yang E, Zha J, Jockel J, Boise LH, Thompson CB, and Korsmeyer SJ. Bad, a heterodimeric partner for Bcl-XL and Bcl-2, displaces Bax and promotes cell death. Cell 1995;80:285–91.
242. Farrow SN, White JH, Martinou I, et al. Cloning of a bcl-2 homologue by interaction with adenovirus E1B 19K. Nature 1995;374:731–3.
243. Chittenden T, Harrington EA, O'Connor R, et al. Induction of apoptosis by the bcl-2 homologue Bak. Nature 1995; 374:733–6.
244. Kiefer MC, Brauer MJ, Powers VC, et al. Modulation of apoptosis by the widely distributed bcl-2 homologue Bak. Nature 1995;374:736–9.
245. Yin XM, Oltvai ZN, and Korsmeyer SJ. BH1 and BH2 domains of Bcl-2 are required for inhibition of apoptosis and heterodimerization with Bax. Nature 1994;369:321–3.
246. Offit K, Jhanwar S, Ebrahim SA, et al. t(3;22)(q27;q11): a novel translocation associated with diffuse non-Hodgkin's lymphoma. Blood 1989;74:1876–9.
247. Leroux D, Stul M, Sotto JJ, et al. Translocation t(3;22)(q23;q11) in three patients with diffuse large B cell lymphoma. Leukemia 1990;4:373–6.
248. Bastard C, Tilly H, Lenormand B, et al. Translocations involving band 3q27 and Ig gene regions in non-Hodgkin's lymphoma. Blood 1992;79:2527–31.
249. Ye BH, Rao PH, Chaganti RS, et al. Cloning of bcl-6, the locus involved in chromosome translocations affecting band 3q27 in B-cell lymphoma. Cancer Res 1993;53:2732–5.
250. Ye BH, Lista F, Lo Coco F, et al. Alterations of a zinc finger-encoding gene, BCL-6, in diffuse large-cell lymphoma. Science 1993;262:747–50.
251. Baron BW, Nucifora G, McCabe N, et al. Identification of the gene associated with the recurring chromosomal translocations t(3;14)(q27;q32) and t(3;22)(q27;q11) in B-cell lymphomas. Proc Natl Acad Sci U S A 1993;90:5262–6.
252. Kerckaert JP, Deweindt C, Tilly H, et al. LAZ3, a novel zinc-finger encoding gene, is disrupted by recurring chromosome 3q27 translocations in human lymphomas. Nat Genet 1993;5:66–70.
253. Miki T, Kawamata N, Arai A, et al. Molecular cloning of the breakpoint for 3q27 translocation in B-cell lymphomas and leukemias. Blood 1994;83:217–22.
254. Kawamata N, Miki T, Ohashi K, et al. Recognition DNA sequence of a novel putative transcription factor, BCL6. Biochem Biophys Res Commun 1994;204:366–74.
255. Harrison SD and Travers AA. The tramtrack gene encodes a Drosophila finger protein that interacts with the ftz transcriptional regulatory region and shows a novel embryonic expression pattern. EMBO J 1990;9:207–16.
256. Chardin P, Courtois G, Mattei MG, et al. The KUP gene, located on human chromosome 14, encodes a protein with two distant zinc fingers. Nucleic Acids Res 1991;19: 1431–6.
257. Chen Z, Brand NJ, Chen A, et al. Fusion between a novel Kruppel-like zinc finger gene and the retinoic acid receptor-alpha locus due to a variant t(11;17) translocation associated with acute promyelocytic leukaemia. EMBO J 1993; 12:1161–7.
258. Zollman S, Godt D, Prive GG, et al. The BTB domain, found primarily in zinc finger proteins, defines an evolutionarily conserved family that includes several developmentally regulated genes in Drosophila. Proc Natl Acad Sci U S A 1994;91:10717–21.
259. Kawamata N, Miki T, Fukuda T, et al. The organization of the BCL6 gene. Leukemia 1994;8:1327–30.
260. Deweindt C, Kerckaert JP, Tilly H, et al. Cloning of a breakpoint cluster region at band 3q27 involved in human non-Hodgkin's lymphoma. Genes Chromosomes Cancer 1993; 8:149–54.
261. Suzuki K, Miki T, Kawamata N, et al. Variant translocation of the BCL6 gene to immunoglobulin kappa light chain gene in B-cell lymphoma. Jpn J Cancer Res 1994;85:911–17.

262. Nakamura Y, Miki T, Kawamata N, et al. Biallelic DNA rearrangements and deletions within the BCL-6 gene in B-cell non-Hodgkin's lymphoma. Br J Haematol 1995; 90:404–8.
263. Galiegue-Zouitina S, Quief S, Hildebrand MP, et al. The B-cell transcriptional coactivator BOB1/OBF1 gene fuses to the LAZ3/BCL6 gene by t(3;11)(q27;q23.1) chromosomal translocation in a B-cell leukaemia line (Karpas231). Blood 1995;86:38a.
264. Dallery E, Galiegue-Zouitina S, Collyn-d'Hooghe M, et al. TTF, a gene encoding a novel small G protein, fuses to the lymphoma-associated LAZ3 gene by t(3;4) chromosomal translocation. Oncogene 1995;10:2171–8.
265. Otsuki T, Yano T, Clark HM, et al. Analysis of LAZ3 (BCL-6) status in B-cell non-Hodgkin's lymphomas: results of rearrangement and gene expression studies and a mutational analysis of coding region sequences. Blood 1995;85: 2877–84.
266. Lo Coco F, Ye BH, Lista F, et al. Rearrangements of the BCL6 gene in diffuse large cell non-Hodgkin's lymphoma. Blood 1994;83:1757–9.
267. Ohno H, Kerckaert JP, Bastard C, et al. Heterogeneity in B-cell neoplasms associated with rearrangement of the LAZ3 gene on chromosome band 3q27. Jpn J Cancer Res 1994;85:592–600.
268. Bastard C, Deweindt C, Kerckaert JP, et al. LAZ3 rearrangements in non-Hodgkin's lymphoma: correlation with histology, immunophenotype, karyotype, and clinical outcome in 217 patients. Blood 1994;83:2423–7.
269. Offit K, Lo Coco F, Louie DC, et al. Rearrangement of the bcl-6 gene as a prognostic marker in diffuse large-cell lymphoma. N Engl J Med 1994;331:74–80.
270. Gaidano G, Lo Coco F, Ye BH, et al. Rearrangements of the BCL-6 gene in acquired immunodeficiency syndrome-associated non-Hodgkin's lymphoma: association with diffuse large-cell subtype. Blood 1994;84:397–402.
271. Shaffer AL, Lin KI, Kuo TC, et al. Blimp–1 orchestrates plasma cell differentiation by extinguishing the mature B cell gene expression program. Immunity 2002;17:51–62.
272. Shaffer AL, Yu X, He Y, et al. BCL-6 represses genes that function in lymphocyte differentiation, inflammation, and cell cycle control. Immunity 2000;13:199–212.
273. Baron BW, Anastasi J, Thirman MJ, et al. The human programmed cell death-2 (PDCD2) gene is a target of BCL6 repression: implications for a role of BCL6 in the down-regulation of apoptosis. Proc Natl Acad Sci U S A 2002; 99:2860–5.
274. Ahmad KF, Melnick A, Lax S, et al. Mechanism of SMRT corepressor recruitment by the BCL6 BTB domain. Mol Cell 2003;12:1551–64.
275. Polo JM, Dell'oso T, Ranuncolo SM, et al. Specific peptide interference reveals BCL6 transcriptional and oncogenic mechanisms in B-cell lymphoma cells. Nat Med 2004; 10:1329–35.
276. Isaacson PG and Du MQ. MALT lymphoma: from morphology to molecules. Nat Rev Cancer 2004;4:644–53.
277. Levine EG, Arthur DC, Machnicki J, et al. Four new recurring translocations in non-Hodgkin lymphoma. Blood 1989;74:1796–800.
278. Horsman D, Gascoyne R, Klasa R, et al. t(11;18)(q21;q21.1): a recurring translocation in lymphomas of mucosa-associated lymphoid tissue (MALT)? Genes Chromosomes Cancer 1992;4:183–7.
279. Dierlamm J, Baens M, Wlodarska I, et al. The apoptosis inhibitor gene API2 and a novel 18q gene, MLT, are recurrently rearranged in the t(11;18)(q21;q21)p6ssociated with mucosa-associated lymphoid tissue lymphomas. Blood 1999;93:3601–9.
280. Willis TG, Jadayel DM, Du MQ, et al. Bcl10 is involved in t(1;14)(p22;q32) of MALT B cell lymphoma and mutated in multiple tumor types. Cell 1999;96:35–45.
281. Streubel B, Lamprecht A, Dierlamm J, et al. T(14;18) (q32;q21) involving IGH and MALT1 is a frequent chromosomal aberration in MALT lymphoma. Blood 2003;101: 2335–9.
282. Lucas PC, Yonezumi M, Inohara N, et al. Bcl10 and MALT1, independent targets of chromosomal translocation in malt lymphoma, cooperate in a novel NF-kappa B signaling pathway. J Biol Chem 2001;276:19012–19.
283. Ruland J, Duncan GS, Elia A, et al. Bcl10 is a positive regulator of antigen receptor-induced activation of NF-kappaB and neural tube closure. Cell 2001;104:33–42.
284. Ruland J, Duncan GS, Wakeham A, et al. Differential requirement for Malt1 in T and B cell antigen receptor signaling. Immunity 2003;19:749–58.
285. Sanchez-Izquierdo D, Buchonnet G, Siebert R, et al. MALT1 is deregulated by both chromosomal translocation and amplification in B-cell non-Hodgkin lymphoma. Blood 2003;101:4539–46.
286. Morgan R, Hecht BK, Sandberg AA, et al. Chromosome 5q35 breakpoint in malignant histiocytosis. N Engl J Med 1986;314:1322.
287. Benz-Lemoine E, Brizard A, Huret JL, et al. Malignant histiocytosis: a specific t(2;5)(p23;q35) translocation? Review of the literature. Blood 1988;72:1045–7.
288. Rimokh R, Magaud JP, Berger F, et al. A translocation involving a specific breakpoint (q35) on chromosome 5 is characteristic of anaplastic large cell lymphoma ('Ki-1 lymphoma'). Br J Haematol 1989;71:31–6.
289. Mason DY, Bastard C, Rimokh R, et al. CD30-positive large cell lymphomas ('Ki-1 lymphoma') are associated with a chromosomal translocation involving 5q35. Br J Haematol 1990;74:161–8.
290. Kaneko Y, Frizzera G, Edamura S, et al. A novel translocation, t(2;5)(p23;q35), in childhood phagocytic large T-cell lymphoma mimicking malignant histiocytosis. Blood 1989;73:806–13.
291. Le Beau MM, Bitter MA, Larson RA, et al. The t(2;5)(p23;q35): a recurring chromosomal abnormality in Ki-1-positive anaplastic large cell lymphoma. Leukemia 1989;3:866–70.
292. Fischer P, Nacheva E, Mason DY, et al. A Ki-1 (CD30)-positive human cell line (Karpas 299) established from a high-grade non-Hodgkin's lymphoma, showing a 2;5 translocation and rearrangement of the T-cell receptor beta-chain gene. Blood 1988;72:234–40.
293. Morris SW, Kirstein MN, Valentine MB, et al. Fusion of a kinase gene, ALK, to a nucleolar protein gene, NPM, in non-Hodgkin's lymphoma. Science 1994;263:1281–4.
294. Bischof D, Pulford K, Mason DY, et al. Role of the nucleophosmin (NPM) portion of the non-Hodgkin's lymphoma-associated NPM-anaplastic lymphoma kinase fusion protein in oncogenesis. Mol Cell Biol 1997;17:2312–25.
295. Mason DY, Pulford KA, Bischof D, et al. Nucleolar localization of the nucleophosmin-anaplastic lymphoma kinase is not required for malignant transformation. Cancer Res 1998;58:1057–62.
296. Lamant L, Dastugue N, Pulford K, et al. A new fusion gene TPM3-ALK in anaplastic large cell lymphoma created by a (1;2)(q25;p23) translocation. Blood 1999;93:3088–95.
297. Meech SJ, McGavran L, Odom LF, et al. Unusual childhood extramedullary hematologic malignancy with natural killer cell properties that contains tropomyosin 4—anaplastic lymphoma kinase gene fusion. Blood 2001;98:1209–16.
298. Hernandez L, Bea S, Bellosillo B, et al. Diversity of genomic breakpoints in TFG-ALK translocations in anaplastic large

cell lymphomas: identification of a new TFG-ALK(XL) chimeric gene with transforming activity. Am J Pathol 2002;160:1487–94.
299. Colleoni GW, Bridge JA, Garicochea B, et al. ATIC-ALK: a novel variant ALK gene fusion in anaplastic large cell lymphoma resulting from the recurrent cryptic chromosomal inversion, inv(2)(p23q35). Am J Pathol 2000;156:781–9.
300. Touriol C, Greenland C, Lamant L, et al. Further demonstration of the diversity of chromosomal changes involving 2p23 in ALK-positive lymphoma: 2 cases expressing ALK kinase fused to CLTCL (clathrin chain polypeptide-like). Blood 2000;95:3204–7.
301. Tort F, Pinyol M, Pulford K, et al. Molecular characterization of a new ALK translocation involving moesin (MSN-ALK) in anaplastic large cell lymphoma. Lab Invest 2001;81:419–26.
302. Cools J, Wlodarska I, Somers R, et al. Identification of novel fusion partners of ALK, the anaplastic lymphoma kinase, in anaplastic large-cell lymphoma and inflammatory myofibroblastic tumor. Genes Chromosomes Cancer 2002;34: 354–62.
303. Lamant L, Gascoyne RD, Duplantier MM, et al. Non-muscle myosin heavy chain (MYH9): a new partner fused to ALK in anaplastic large cell lymphoma. Genes Chromosomes Cancer 2003;37:427–32.
304. Hernandez L, Pinyol M, Hernandez S, et al. TRK-fused gene (TFG) is a new partner of ALK in anaplastic large cell lymphoma producing two structurally different TFG-ALK translocations. Blood 1999;94:3265–8.
305. Kuefer MU, Look AT, Pulford K, et al. Retrovirus-mediated gene transfer of NPM–ALK causes lymphoid malignancy in mice. Blood 1997;90:2901–10.
306. Griffin CA, Hawkins AL, Dvorak C, et al. Recurrent involvement of 2p23 in inflammatory myofibroblastic tumors. Cancer Res 1999;59:2776–80.
307. Ma Z, Hill DA, Collins MH, et al. Fusion of ALK to the Ran-binding protein 2 (RANBP2) gene in inflammatory myofibroblastic tumor. Genes Chromosomes Cancer 2003;37: 98–105.
308. Bai RY, Dieter P, Peschel C, et al. Nucleophosmin-anaplastic lymphoma kinase of large-cell anaplastic lymphoma is a constitutively active tyrosine kinase that utilizes phospholipase C-gamma to mediate its mitogenicity. Mol Cell Biol 1998;18:6951–61.
309. Nieborowska-Skorska M, Slupianek A, Xue L, et al. Role of signal transducer and activator of transcription 5 in nucleophosmin/ anaplastic lymphoma kinase-mediated malignant transformation of lymphoid cells. Cancer Res 2001; 61:6517–23.
310. Bai RY, Ouyang T, Miething C, et al. Nucleophosmin-anaplastic lymphoma kinase associated with anaplastic large-cell lymphoma activates the phosphatidylinositol 3-kinase/Akt antiapoptotic signaling pathway. Blood 2000;96:4319–27.
311. Shiota M, Fujimoto J, Semba T, et al. Hyperphosphorylation of a novel 80 kDa protein-tyrosine kinase similar to Ltk in a human Ki-1 lymphoma cell line, AMS3. Oncogene 1994;9:1567–74.
312. Hubinger G, Scheffrahn I, Muller E, et al. The tyrosine kinase NPM–ALK, associated with anaplastic large cell lymphoma, binds the intracellular domain of the surface receptor CD30 but is not activated by CD30 stimulation. Exp Hematol 1999;27:1796–805.
313. Horie R, Watanabe M, Ishida T, et al. The NPM–ALK oncoprotein abrogates CD30 signaling and constitutive NF-kappaB activation in anaplastic large cell lymphoma. Cancer Cell 2004;5:353–64.
314. Cabanillas F, Pathak S, Trujillo J, et al. Frequent nonrandom chromosome abnormalities in 27 patients with untreated large cell lymphoma and immunoblastic lymphoma. Cancer Res 1988;48:5557–64.
315. Bloomfield CD, Arthur CD, Frizzera G, et al. Nonrandom chromosome abnormalities in lymphoma. Cancer Res 1983;43:2975–84.
316. Yunis JJ, Oken MM, Kaplan ME, et al. Distinctive chromosomal abnormalities in histologic subtypes of non-Hodgkin's lymphoma p53 and bcl-2 expression in high-grade B-cell lymphomas: correlation with survival time. N Engl J Med 1982;307:337–41.
317. Schouten HC, Sanger WG, Weisenburger DD, et al. Chromosomal abnormalities in untreated patients with non-Hodgkin's lymphoma: associations with histology, clinical characteristics, and treatment outcome. The Nebraska Lymphoma Study Group. Blood 1990;75:1841–7.
318. Cabanillas F, Pathak S, Grant G, et al. Refractoriness to chemotherapy and poor survival related to abnormalities of chromosomes 17 and 7 in lymphoma. Am J Med 1989; 87:167–72.
319. Doglioni C, Pelosio P, Mombello A, et al. Immunohistochemical evidence of abnormal expression of the antioncogene-encoded p53 phosphoprotein in Hodgkin's disease and CD30+ anaplastic lymphomas. Hematol Pathol 1991; 5:67–73.
320. Pezzella F, Morrison H, Jones M, et al. Immunohistochemical detection of p53 and bcl-2 proteins in non-Hodgkin's lymphoma. Histopathology 1993;22:39–44.
321. Said JW, Barrera R, Shintaku IP, et al. Immunohistochemical analysis of p53 expression in malignant lymphomas. Am J Pathol 1992;141:1343–8.
322. Soini Y, Paakko P, Alavaikko M, et al. p53 expression in lymphatic malignancies. J Clin Pathol 1992;45:1011–4.
323. Villuendas R, Piris MA, Orradre JL, et al. P53 protein expression in lymphomas and reactive lymphoid tissue. J Pathol 1992;166:235–41.
324. Gaidano G, Ballerini P, Gong JZ, et al. p53 mutations in human lymphoid malignancies: association with Burkitt lymphoma and chronic lymphocytic leukemia. Proc Natl Acad Sci U S A 1991;88:5413–7.
325. Ichikawa A, Hotta T, Takagi N, et al. Mutations of p53 gene and their relation to disease progression in B-cell lymphoma. Blood 1992;79:2701–7.
326. Shiraishi Y. p53 mutation in fresh lymphocytes, B-lymphoblastoid cell lines and their transformed cell lines originating from Bloom syndrome patients. Cancer Genet Cytogenet 1993;68:70–3.
327. Kocialkowski S, Pezzella F, Morrison H, et al. Mutations in the p53 gene are not limited to classic 'hot spots' and are not predictive of p53 protein expression in high-grade non-Hodgkin's lymphoma. Br J Haematol 1995;89:55–60.
328. Villuendas R, Piris MA, Algara P, et al. The expression of p53 protein in non-Hodgkin's lymphomas is not always dependent on p53 gene mutations. Blood 1993;82: 3151–6.
329. Farrugia MM, Duan LJ, Reis MD, et al. Alterations of the p53 tumor suppressor gene in diffuse large cell lymphomas with translocations of the c-MYC and BCL-2 proto-oncogenes. Blood 1994;83:191–8.
330. Wiman KG, Magnusson KP, Ramqvist T, et al. Mutant p53 detected in a majority of Burkitt lymphoma cell lines by monoclonal antibody PAb240. Oncogene 1991;6: 1633–9.
331. Duthu A, Debuire B, Romano J, et al. p53 mutations in Raji cells: characterization and localization relative to other Burkitt's lymphomas. Oncogene 1992;7:2161–7.
332. Piris MA, Pezella F, Martinez-Montero JC, et al. p53 and bcl-2 expression in high-grade B-cell lymphomas: correlation with survival time. Br J Cancer 1994;69:337–41.

333. Nakamura H, Said JW, Miller CW, et al. Mutation and protein expression of p53 in acquired immunodeficiency syndrome-related lymphomas. Blood 1993;82:920–6.
334. De-Re V, Carbone A, De-Vita S, et al. p53 protein overexpression and p53 gene abnormalities in HIV-1-related non-Hodgkin's lymphomas. Int J Cancer 1994;56:662–7.
335. Ballerini P, Gaidano G, Gong JZ, et al. Multiple genetic lesions in acquired immunodeficiency syndrome-related non-Hodgkin's lymphoma. Blood 1993;81:166–76.
336. Baldini L, Fracchiolla NS, Cro LM, et al. Frequent p53 gene involvement in splenic B-cell leukemia/lymphomas of possible marginal zone origin. Blood 1994;84:270–8.
337. Sander CA, Yano T, Clark HM, et al. p53 mutation is associated with progression in follicular lymphomas. Blood 1993;82:1994–2004.
338. Lo Coco F, Gaidano G, Louie DC, et al. p53 mutations are associated with histologic transformation of follicular lymphoma. Blood 1993;82:2289–95.
339. Korkolopoulou P, Oates J, Kittas C, et al. p53, c-myc p62 and proliferating cell nuclear antigen (PCNA) expression in non-Hodgkin's lymphomas. J Clin Pathol 1994;47:9–14.
340. Barrans S, Randerson J, Evans P, et al. Heterogeneity in cell proliferation and expression of p53 and bcl-2 during the indolent phase of germinal centre cell lymphoma: an explanation for clinical variability. Br J Haematol 1995;90:830–6.
341. Matsushima AY, Cesarman E, Chadburn A, et al. Post-thymic T cell lymphomas frequently overexpress p53 protein but infrequently exhibit p53 gene mutations. Am J Pathol 1994;144:573–84.
342. Sakashita A, Hattori T, Miller CW, et al. Mutations of the p53 gene in adult T-cell leukemia. Blood 1992;79:477–80.
343. Sugito S, Yamato K, Sameshima Y, et al. Adult T-cell leukemia: structures and expression of the p53 gene. Int J Cancer 1991;49:880–5.
344. Nagai H, Kinoshita T, Imamura J, et al. Genetic alteration of p53 in some patients with adult T-cell leukemia. Jpn J Cancer Res 1991;82:1421–7.
345. Cesarman E, Chadburn A, Inghirami G, et al. Structural and functional analysis of oncogenes and tumor suppressor genes in adult T-cell leukemia/lymphoma shows frequent p53 mutations. Blood 1992;80:3205–16.
346. Nishimura S, Asou N, Suzushima H, et al. p53 gene mutation and loss of heterozygosity are associated with increased risk of disease progression in adult T cell leukemia. Leukemia 1995;9:598–604.
347. Gupta RK, Norton AJ, Lister TA, et al. p53 protein expression in Reed–Sternberg cells of Hodgkin's disease. Leukemia 1993;7:S31–3.
348. Trumper LH, Brady G, Bagg A, et al. Single-cell analysis of Hodgkin and Reed–Sternberg cells: molecular heterogeneity of gene expression and p53 mutations. Blood 1993; 81:3097–115.
349. Gupta RK, Patel K, Bodmer WF, et al. Mutation of p53 in primary biopsy material and cell lines from Hodgkin disease. Proc Natl Acad Sci U S A 1993;90:2817–21.
350. Watanabe T, Hotta T, Ichikawa A, et al. The MDM2 oncogene overexpression in chronic lymphocytic leukemia and low-grade lymphoma of B-cell origin. Blood 1994;84: 3158–65.
351. Maestro R, Gloghini A, Doglioni C, et al. MDM2 overexpression does not account for stabilization of wild-type p53 protein in non-Hodgkin's lymphomas. Blood 1995;85: 3239–46.
352. Bhatia K, Fan S, Spangler G, et al. A mutant p21 cyclin-dependent kinase inhibitor isolated from a Burkitt's lymphoma. Cancer Res 1995;55:1431–5.
353. Ogawa S, Hangaishi A, Miyawaki S, et al. Loss of the cyclin-dependent kinase 4-inhibitor (p16; MTS1) gene is frequent in and highly specific to lymphoid tumors in primary human hematopoietic malignancies. Blood 1995;86: 1548–56.
354. Uchida T, Watanabe T, Kinoshita T, et al. Mutational analysis of the CDKN2 (MTS1/p16ink4A) gene in primary B-cell lymphomas. Blood 1995;86:2724–31.
355. Duro D, Flexor MA, Bernard O, et al. Alterations of the putative tumor suppressor gene p16/MTS1 in human hematological malignancies. Comptes Rendus Acad Sci Iii 1994; 317:913–9.
356. Otsuki T, Clark HM, Wellmann A, et al. Involvement of CDKN2 (p16INK4A/MTS1) and p15INK4B/MTS2 in human leukemias and lymphomas. Cancer Res 1995;55: 1436–40.

4

Molecular Monitoring of Lymphoma

Jacques J.M. van Dongen, M.D., Ph.D.
Anton W. Langerak, Ph.D.
Tomasz Szczepański, M.D., Ph.D.
Vincent H.J. van der Velden, Ph.D.

The appropriate diagnosis and classification of lymphomas form the basis of clinical patient management, particularly for the choice of treatment protocol. The possibilities for accurate classification of lymphomas have substantially increased over the last decade, particularly by the inclusion of specific immunophenotyping and oncogenetic characteristics. It can be anticipated that the novel developments in the field of gene expression profiling will further improve the classification of lymphomas, with better correlation to outcome.

Despite more accurate classification and better establishment of prognosis in subsets of lymphomas, it is difficult to predict at initial presentation what the treatment effectiveness will be in each individual patient. Treatment effectiveness depends on many factors, such as compliance to the treatment protocol (by the doctor and the patient), intestinal resorption of the drug, efficiency of cytotoxic drug metabolism, condition of the patient (including liver and kidney function), occurrence of infection or other complications, drug resistance of the lymphoma cells, and many other factors as scored in the international prognostic index (IPI).[1]

Over the last decade several large-scale clinical studies have evaluated treatment effectiveness in leukemia patients by measuring the kinetics of disappearance of "minimal residual disease" (MRD) in bone marrow (BM) or peripheral blood (PB) samples during and after treatment.[2] Particularly in acute lymphoblastic leukemia (ALL), MRD diagnostics during the first 3 months of treatment has resulted in the recognition of three MRD-based risk groups, which differ significantly in outcome (6-year event-free survival of 98%, 75%, and 20%).[3,4]

Consequently, also in lymphoma patients, the actual disappearance of malignant cells from PB and BM might be a good surrogate marker to evaluate treatment effectiveness and predict outcome in individual patients. Such MRD monitoring might be particularly helpful in lymphoma types with a high tendency of dissemination to PB and BM, such as small lymphocytic lymphoma, lymphoplasmacytic lymphoma, follicular lymphoma (FL), and mantle cell lymphoma (MCL). In less disseminating lymphomas, such as diffuse large B-cell lymphoma (DLBCL) and anaplastic large-cell lymphoma (ALCL), MRD monitoring in BM or PB might be less informative.

Over the past 15 years, multiple techniques have been evaluated for their potential of detecting MRD with sufficiently high specificity and sensitivity. In practice only flow cytometry and polymerase chain reaction (PCR) techniques appeared to be useful. Flow cytometry uses lymphoma-associated immunophenotypes, oncogene (over)expression (e.g., BCL2 or ALK), and potentially single immunoglobulin (Ig) light-chain (Igκ or Igλ) expression in case of a B-cell lymphoma. PCR techniques exploit rearranged Ig and T-cell receptor (TCR) genes or chromosome aberrations as targets.

Flow cytometry is fast and relatively cheap, but has the disadvantage of a limited sensitivity of one malignant cell in 1000 to 10,000 normal cells (10^{-3} to 10^{-4}) in many types of lymphomas. In some lymphomas the sensitivity is only 10^{-2} to 10^{-3}. This implies that the "dynamic range" of MRD detection in PB and BM is not more than three logs, which limits the possibility to accurately assess the kinetics of tumor load decrease.

PCR–based MRD techniques are more sensitive (10^{-4} to 10^{-6}), but are slower and generally more expensive than flow-cytometric MRD detection, particularly when PCR targets are used, which need to be precisely identified per patient, such as Ig and TCR gene rearrangements or breakpoint fusion regions at the DNA level. Despite these disadvantages most clinical MRD studies in lymphoma patients use PCR techniques for MRD monitoring, because they are applicable in the majority of patients with a high sensitivity.

MRD monitoring potentially has high clinical relevance in curable types of lymphoma, even if only a small subgroup of the patients has a long-term event-free survival. Recognition of this subgroup versus the group of relapsing patients should be the aim of clinical MRD studies, because this would allow treatment stratification in future therapy protocols.

The strategy of MRD monitoring might be different per type of lymphoma: what type of sample is needed for monitoring (PB, BM, or other?); how frequently should the sampling be performed (each week, each month, or other?); and for how long should the MRD monitoring continue (initial treatment phase vs. long-term monitoring, even after withdrawal of treatment?). Logically, early treatment intervention needs detailed MRD information at multiple time points during the first 3 to 6 months of treatment, while long-term MRD monitoring might be relevant for indolent lymphomas with treatment modification in later phases.

This chapter provides the background information of the PCR targets for molecular MRD monitoring (i.e., Ig/TCR gene rearrangements and chromosome aberrations), explains how these targets can be identified, and which real-time quantitative (RQ)-PCR techniques are currently available for MRD monitoring in lymphoma patients. Finally, we summarize the clinical relevance of molecular MRD monitoring in non–Hodgkin's lymphomas, based on the results of published clinical studies.

BACKGROUND INFORMATION ON TARGETS FOR MOLECULAR MONITORING OF LYMPHOMA

Ig/TCR Molecules and Their Encoding Genes

The ability of human lymphocytes to specifically recognize millions of different antigens and antigenic epitopes is based on the enormous diversity (at least 10^{10}) of their antigen-specific receptors, better known as Ig and TCR molecules.[5–7] Being distinct per lymphocyte, each single B or T lymphocyte expresses approximately 10^5 Ig/TCR molecules with identical antigen specificity.

Ig molecules consist of two disulfide-bonded Ig heavy (IgH) chains and two Ig light chains. Ig class or subclass is determined by the isotype of the involved IgH chain, irrespective of the type of light chain. Each B lymphocyte or B-lymphocyte clone expresses only one type of light chain (Igκ or Igλ), whereas multiple IgH isotypes can be expressed.[8] TCR molecules consist of two generally disulfide-linked chains. Two different types of TCR are known: the "classic" TCRαβ receptor, consisting of a TCRα and a TCRβ chain, and the "alternative" TCRγδ receptor, composed of a TCRγ and TCRδ chain.[6,9] Most mature T lymphocytes (85% to 98%) in PB and in most lymphoid tissues are TCRαβ$^+$, while only a minority (2% to 15%) express TCRγδ.[9] Surface membrane–bound Ig (SmIg) molecules and TCR molecules are closely associated with CD79 and CD3 protein chains, required for transmembrane signal transduction of the SmIg-CD79 and TCR-CD3 complexes, respectively (Fig. 4–1).[7]

Each Ig/TCR chain consists of two domains—one variable domain involved in actual recognition of antigens, and one constant domain that mediates the effector function resulting in signaling through the CD79 or CD3 complex. In order to recognize all antigenic epitopes, an extensive repertoire of variable domains of Ig/TCR molecules is needed. If this entire repertoire would be encoded by separate genes, these would occupy a major part of the human genome. However, since the variable domains are encoded by a single exon that is formed through distinct combinations of gene segments, only a limited set of gene segments is sufficient to encode the required diversity of Ig/TCR molecules.[6,10] In the cases of the *IGH*, *TCRB*, and *TCRD* loci, this concerns the combination of variable (V), diversity (D), and joining (J) gene segments, whereas the *IGK*, *IGL*, *TCRA*, and *TCRG* gene complexes only contain V and J gene segments (see Fig. 4–2A,B and Table 4–1 for further details).[6,9,11–19]

Ig/TCR Gene Rearrangement or V(D)J Recombination

During early lymphoid differentiation V, (D), and J gene segments from the germline repertoire of the various Ig/TCR gene complexes are coupled via a tightly regulated process (see later); this process is called Ig/TCR gene rearrangement or V(D)J recombination. The resulting specific combination of V, (D), and J segments in each lymphocyte is also known as V(D)J exon.[5,6,10,20] V(D)J recombination is a complex process involving several proteins, which together form the recombinase enzyme system. Next to regulatory DNA binding proteins, the products of the lymphoid-specific recombinase–activating genes 1 and 2 (RAG1 and RAG2 proteins) are the main constituents of the recombinase complex.[21–23] RAG 1 and RAG 2 specifically bind to the recombination signal sequences (RSS), which flank the 3' side of V gene segments, both sides of D gene segments and the 5' side of J gene segments.[24–26] These RSS elements consist of conserved palindromic heptamer (CACAGTG) and nonamer (ACAAAAACC) sequences, separated by either 12- or 23-bp spacer regions.[24–26] Following the introduction of double-strand breaks (dsb)

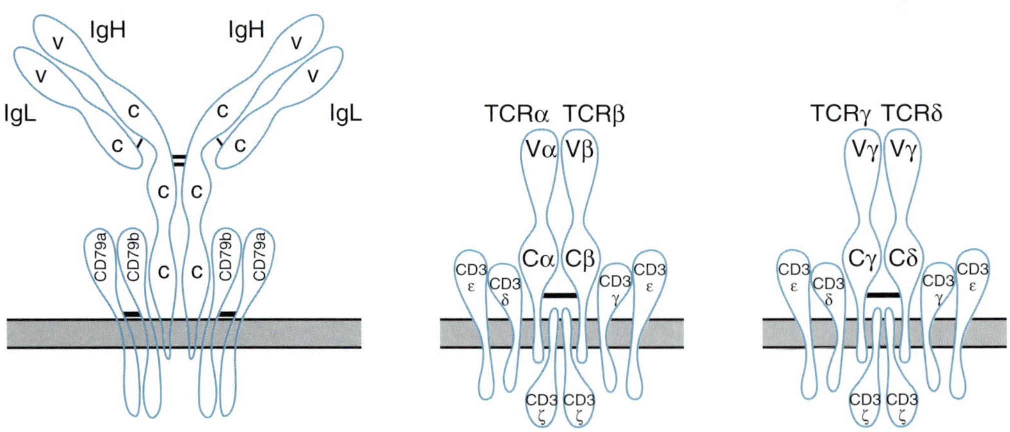

Figure 4–1. Schematic diagram of human Ig/TCR molecules. SmIg molecules are closely associated with disulfide-linked CD79 protein chains, whereas TCRαβ and TCRγδ molecules are associated with CD3 protein chains. CD79 and CD3 are involved in transducing signals upon antigen-induced activation of the SmIg and TCR molecules. The two IgH chains in SmIg molecules as well as the TCRα and TCRβ chains in TCRαβ molecules are connected via disulfide bonds; proteins of the TCRγδ receptor are disulfide linked when derived from Cγ1 sequences, but this interchain disulfide bond is lacking when the TCRγ chain is derived from Cγ2 sequences. V and C, variable and constant domains of Ig or TCR chains.

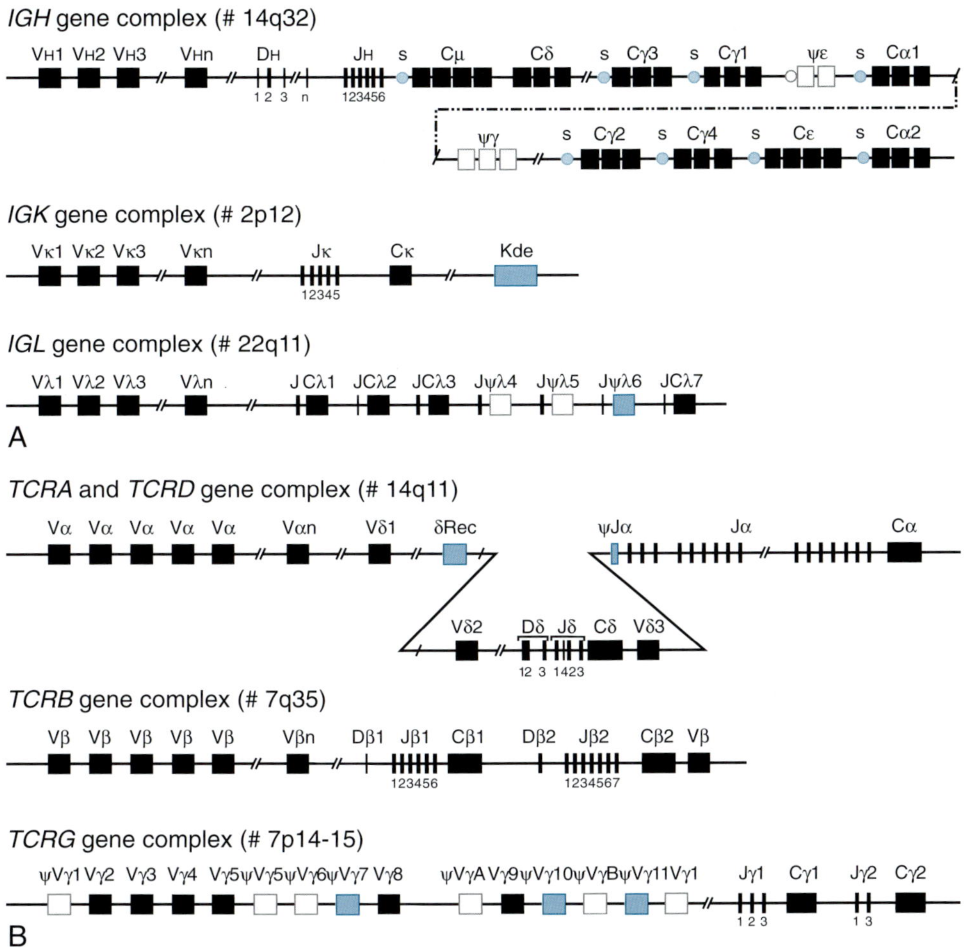

Figure 4–2. Schematic diagram of the human Ig/TCR gene complexes. **A**: Human Ig loci. The *IGH* gene complex comprises ~45 functional V gene segments, 27 functional D gene segments, 6 functional J gene segments, and several C gene segments encoding the various IgH class and subclass constant domains. The switch region that precedes most C gene segments plays a role in IgH (sub)class switching. The *IGK* gene complex consists of ~35 functional V gene segments, 5 J gene segments, and a single C gene segment. The Kde (κ-deleting element) plays a role in the deletion of the Jκ-Cκ or Cκ gene regions in B cells, which rearrange their *IGL* genes. The *IGL* gene complex contains ~30 functional V gene segments and 4 functional C genes, all of which are preceded by a J gene segment. Pseudogenes (ψ) are indicated as open symbols. **B**: Human TCR loci. The *TCRA* gene complex consists of ~45 functional V gene segments, a stretch of 61 J gene segments (50 of which are functional), and a single C gene segment. The *TCRB* gene complex contains ~45 functional V gene segments and 2 C gene segments, both of which are preceded by a D gene segment, and 6 or 7 J gene segments. The *TCRG* gene complex consists of a restricted number of V gene segments (6 functional V gene segments and 9 pseudogenes) and 2 C gene segments, each preceded by 2 or 3 J gene segments. The *TCRD* gene complex comprises 6 V, 3 D, and 4 J gene segments, and a single C gene segment. The major part of the *TCRD* gene complex is located between the Vα and Jα gene segments, and is flanked by the δREC and ψJα gene segments, which are involved in *TCRD* gene deletions that occur prior to *TCRA* gene rearrangements. Pseudogenes (ψ) are indicated as open symbols.

Table 4–1. Estimation of Potential Primary Repertoire of Human Ig/TCR Molecules

	Ig Molecules			TCRαβ Molecules		TCRγδ Molecules	
	IGH	*IGK*	*IGL*	*TCRA*	*TCRB*	*TCRG*	*TCRD*
Number of functional gene segments[a]							
— *V* gene segments	40–46	34–37	27–30	45	44–47	6	6
— *D* gene segments	27[b]	—	—	—	2[b]	—	3[b]
— *J* gene segments	6	5	4	50	13	5	4
Combinatorial diversity		$>1.5 \times 10^6$		$>2 \times 10^6$		>5000	
Junctional diversity[c]	++	±	±	+	++	+	+++
Estimation of total repertoire		$>10^{12}$		$>10^{12}$		$>10^{12}$	

[a] Numbers of functional gene segments are based on the international IMGT (ImMunoGeneTics) database (Lefranc et al[38]).
[b] In *TCRD* gene rearrangements, multiple D segments might be used; this implies that the number of junctions can vary from one to four. In *IGH* and *TCRB* gene rearrangements, generally only one *D* gene segment is used.
[c] ±, one junction with few N-nucleotides; +, one junction with several N-nucleotides; ++, two junctions with several N-nucleotides; +++, two, three or even four junctions with several N-nucleotides.

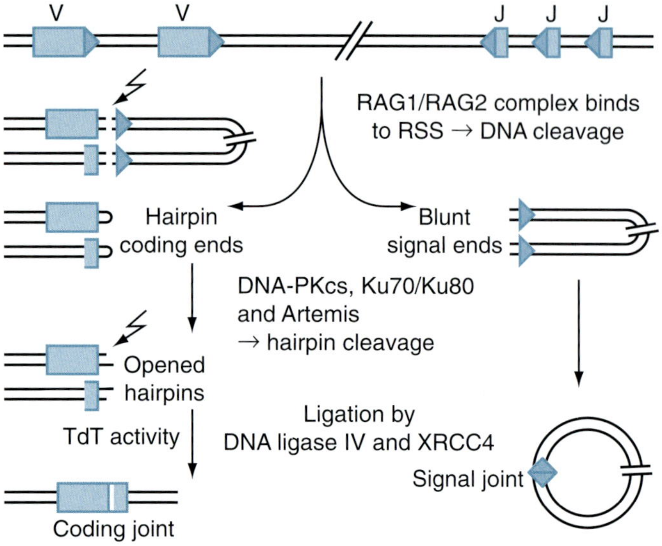

Figure 4–3. Scheme of the V(D)J recombination mechanism. RAG1 and RAG2 proteins bind to RSS resulting in double strand breaks (dsb). After cleavage hairpin structures are formed at the coding ends, whereas the RSS blunt ends fuse to form a signal joint, generally without deletions or insertions of nucleotides. These signal joints together with all intervening sequences will generally be removed from the genome in the form of a so-called excision circle. Processing of the coding ends results in opening of the hairpins via several enzymes known to be involved in dsb repair (DNA-PKCS, Ku70/Ku80, and Artemis). Finally, opened hairpins are relegated (involving DNA ligase IV and XRCC4) to a coding joint, and further diversified by the action of TdT, which introduces nucleotides in a template-independent way.

between the RSS and the rearranging gene segment, a hairpin structure is formed at the coding end of the break (Fig. 4–3). This hairpin has to be opened before relegation to another gene segment can occur via several enzymes known to be involved in dsb repair, which results in the so-called coding joint (Fig. 4–3). During the coding joint formation, deletion and random insertion of nucleotides can occur, leading to imprecise coupling of gene segments. The RSS ends of the breaks fuse head to head (generally without deletion or insertion of nucleotides), and form the so-called signal joint, which is generally removed from the genomic DNA in the form of an excision circle (Fig. 4–3).[6,24,25] Such B- and T-cell receptor excision circles (BRECs and TRECs) are relatively stable molecules, which do not replicate upon cell division; consequently, they are diluted out upon proliferation of the developing lymphoid cells. This characteristic has prompted the development of quantitative assays for analysis of TREC levels as measure for thymic output of recent thymic emigrants.[27,28] TREC analysis has been used to study thymic output in different age groups and different pathophysiologic conditions (e.g., during HIV-1 infection).[27,29]

In Figure 4–4 an example of an *IGH* gene rearrangement is illustrated. Initially a coding joint is formed between a JH gene segment and one of the DH gene segments, whereas the 3' DH RSS and the JH RSS form a signal joint in the excision circle or BREC. In a second rearrangement step, coupling of one of many VH gene segments results in a complete V(D)J exon as well as another BREC with the signal joint of the VH RSS and the 5' DH RSS. The rearranged gene is subsequently transcribed into a precursor mRNA, which is further processed into mature mRNA by splicing out all intronic, noncoding sequences, and coupling of the V(D)J exon and the C exons (Fig. 4–4).[6] Similar rearrangement and transcription processes occur in all other Ig/TCR loci as well. Although the signal joints that are formed during Ig/TCR gene recombination are generally present on excision circles, this is not the case for one exceptional type of rearrangement. Upon inversional rearrangement, which occurs in case of V gene segments in inverted orientation (e.g., the Vβ20, Vδ3, and half of the Vκ gene segments),[18] the signal joint and other intervening sequences between the two coding elements are not removed as TREC or BREC but are preserved in the genome.

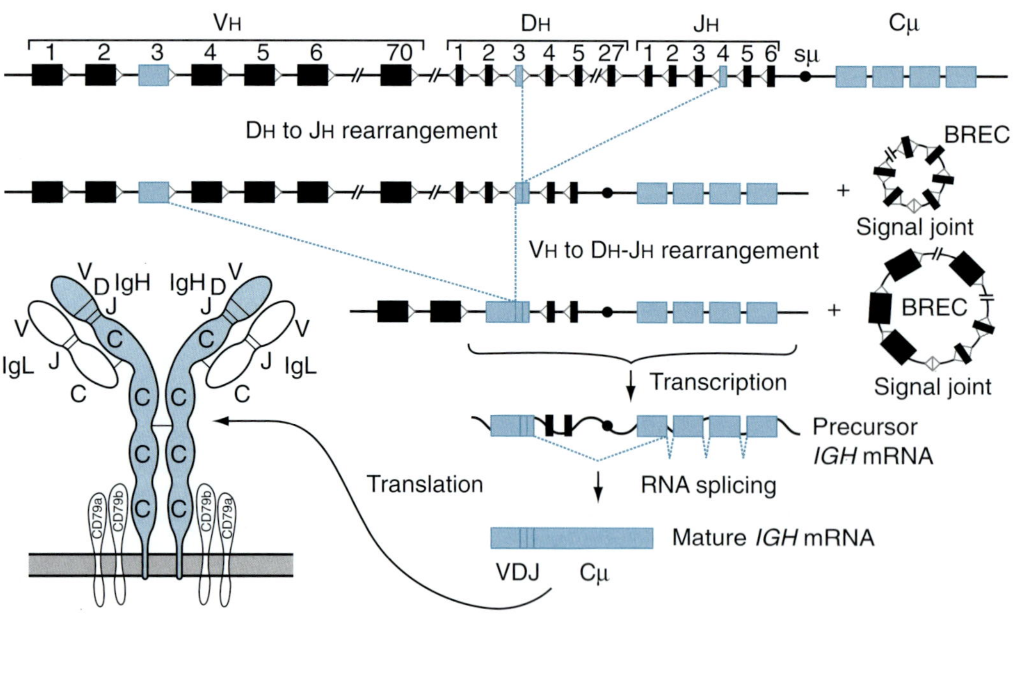

Figure 4–4. Schematic diagram of sequential rearrangement steps, transcription, and translation of the *IGH* gene. In this example, first a DH to JH rearrangement occurs, followed by VH to DH-JH rearrangement, resulting in the formation of a VH-DH-JH coding joint. The rearranged *IGH* gene is transcribed into precursor mRNA, spliced into mature mRNA, and finally translated into a IgH protein. The two extrachromosomal B-cell receptor excision circles (BRECs) that are formed during this recombination process are indicated as well; they contain the D-J signal joint and V-D signal joint, respectively.

As Ig/TCR recombinations are complex processes with imprecise joining of gene segments, approximately two out of three joinings will be out-of-frame.[5] This high frequency of out-of-frame rearrangements may explain why most B cells have biallelic *IGH* rearrangements, and why most T cells have biallelic *TCRB* and *TCRG* gene rearrangements.[10,30] In addition, secondary gene rearrangements appear to occur that are assumed to rescue precursor cells with nonproductive Ig/TCR genes. In *IGH*, *TCRB*, and *TCRD* loci, this concerns secondary D-J rearrangements, whereas secondary V-J rearrangements replace pre-existing V-J joinings in *TCRA*, *TCRG*, *IGK*, and *IGL* genes.[31–33] Both types of rearrangements can occur repeatedly in the same Ig/TCR gene complex as long as appropriate germline V, (D), and J gene segments are available. Another type of secondary rearrangement concerns V segment replacement in a complete V(D)J exon by an upstream V gene segment. This process is mediated via an internal heptamer RSS in the 3′ part of the V gene segments.[34–36] So far, V replacements have especially been observed in *IGH* and *TCRB* genes. Secondary rearrangements have also been found to replace pre-existing productive rearrangements,[37] suggesting that they are also involved in selection processes of immature B cells in BM, and immature T cells in the thymus.[31,37]

Ig/TCR Repertoire

The complete repertoire of Ig/TCR molecules is shaped by V(D)J recombination mechanisms in the Ig/TCR loci. The extent of this potential primary Ig/TCR repertoire is determined by two levels of diversity: combinatorial diversity (different V(D)J combinations) and junctional diversity (due to imprecise joining of V, D, and J gene segments).[5]

Combinatorial diversity results from all possible combinations of available functional V, D, and J gene segments per locus, and the pairing of two different functional protein chains per Ig/TCR molecule (IgH with Igκ or Igλ, TCRα with TCRβ, and TCRγ with TCRδ).[5] As the *IGH* gene complex probably contains at least 40 functional VH gene segments, 27 rearranging DH gene segments, and 6 functional JH gene segments, coupling will result in approximately 6000 possible VH-DH-JH combinations (Table 4–2). Together with the estimated 175 and 115 V-J combinations of the *IGK* and *IGL* genes, respectively, a potential combinatorial diversity of more than 1.5×10^6 can be obtained.[38] A similar diversity can be obtained for TCRαβ molecules (Table 4–2).[38] The combinatorial diversity of TCRγδ molecules is less extensive due to the limited number of functional V, (D), and J gene segments in the encoding gene complexes.[38] Still, because of multiple Dδ gene segment usage, a potential combinatorial repertoire of more than 5000 TCRγδ molecules can be produced.

The aforementioned numbers are based on the assumption of random usage of the available functional V, (D), and J gene segments. However, there are several indications for preferential gene segment usage. For example, fetal B cells use a restricted set of VH gene segments, related to JH proximity,[39,40] TCRαβ$^+$ cells tend to use Jβ2 gene segments more frequently than Jβ1 gene segments,[41] and peripheral TCRγδ$^+$ T lymphocytes exhibit preferential usage of Vγ9-Jγ1.2 and Vδ2-Jδ1 gene segments.[42,43] Alternatively, gene segment usage might be random, but over-representation of certain receptor types might be explained by clonal selection and expansion of particular receptor specificities in peripheral tissues.[44]

The other type of diversity, *junctional diversity*, is based on deletion of nucleotides at the ends of the rearranging gene segments as well as random insertion of nucleotides (N region nucleotides) between the coupled gene segments (junctional region). Insertion of N region nucleotides at the 3' ends of DNA breakpoints is mediated by terminal deoxynucleotidyl transferase (TdT) and occurs in a template-independent way.[45] Absence or decrease in TdT activity during Ig/TCR gene rearrangements leads to the virtual absence of N region insertion, as is found in early fetal thymocytes.[46,47] Rearranged *IGK* and *IGL* genes in mature B cells also have lower levels of N region insertion,[5,20,48] suggesting that the *IGK* and *IGL* genes rearrange in the presence of minimal TdT activity. This is in contrast to the junctional regions of rearranged TCR genes in late fetal and postnatal thymocytes, which all contain N regions.[47] The junctional regions of Ig/TCR genes encode the so-called complementarity-determining regions 3 (CDR3), which are involved in antigen recognition and which function as unique lymphocyte-specific ("fingerprint-like") sequences. N region insertion thus drastically increases diversity of antigen recognition by Ig/TCR chains and molecules. This especially holds true for *IGH*, *TCRB*, and *TCRD* gene rearrangements where multiple couplings (V-D, D-J, and even D-D) can be present within a junctional region. The enormous junctional diversity of TCRδ chains thereby compensates for the relatively low number of different V, D, and J combinations in TCRγδ molecules (Table 4–2).

The repertoire of Ig molecules can be further increased and adapted via antigen-induced somatic hypermutations in the V(D)J exons of rearranged Ig genes.[49,50] These point mutations occur in B lymphocytes that are present in secondary follicles (germinal center reaction), and hence are

Table 4–2. Estimated Number of Human V, (D), and J Gene Segments That Can Potentially Be Involved in Ig/TCR Gene Rearrangements[a]

Gene Segment	*IGH*	*IGK*	*IGL*	*TCRA*	*TCRB*	*TCRG*	*TCRD*
V (family)	~70 (7)	~60 (7)	~40 (11)	~60 (32)	~65 (30)	9 (4)	7[c]
D (family)	~27 (7)	—	—	—	2	—	3
J (family)	6	5	5[b]	61[c]	13	5 (3)	4

[a] Numbers are based on the international IMGT (ImMunoGeneTics) database (Lefranc[38]).
[b] Two of the seven Jλ gene segments have never been observed to be involved in *IGL* gene rearrangements, probably because of their inefficient recombination signal sequences.
[c] These numbers include the nonfunctional δREC gene segment (*TCRD* locus) and the ψJα gene segment (*TCRA* locus).

not found in naive B lymphocytes.[49,50] They are assumed to serve affinity maturation and clonal selection, and to precede or coincide with IgH isotype/class switching.

Rearrangement of Ig/TCR Genes during Lymphoid Differentiation

Rearrangements of Ig/TCR genes start early during lymphoid differentiation, and occur in an hierarchical order that is tightly regulated by transcription factors, such as E2A and HEB, that have been shown to mediate differential accessibility of Ig/TCR loci during differentiation.[51,52]

During B-cell differentiation, *IGH* genes rearrange first, followed by *IGK* genes. If the latter rearrangements are nonfunctional, the *IGL* genes will start to rearrange.[8,10,20] This is, for example, reflected by more frequent Igκ expression on mature B cells; Igλ-positive B-lymphocytes occur less frequently (Igκ/Igλ ratio 1.4). Generally, *IGL* gene rearrangements occur after or coincide with *IGK* gene deletions.[53,54] Virtually all *IGK* gene deletions are mediated via rearrangement of the so-called kappa-deleting element (Kde), which is located downstream of the Cκ gene segment (Fig. 4–2).[55–57] This Kde sequence rearranges either to an isolated heptamer RSS in the Jκ-Cκ intron, thereby deleting the Cκ gene segment, or to a Vκ gene segment, thereby removing both the Jκ and Cκ gene segments (Fig. 4–5).[56,58] Following antigen-induced activation of B lymphocytes, somatic mutations and *IGH* isotype rearrangements can occur.[8,10]

In T-cell differentiation, the *TCRD* genes rearrange first, followed by the *TCRG* genes. This might result in TCRγδ^{+} T lymphocytes, provided that the rearrangements are functional. TCRαβ^{+} T lymphocytes most probably develop via a separate differentiation lineage with *TCRB* gene rearrangements taking place prior to *TCRA* gene rearrangements.[10,59] *TCRA* gene rearrangements are preceded by deletion of the *TCRD* gene, which for the largest part is located between Vα and Jα gene segments (Fig. 4–2).[12,17,18] This *TCRD* gene deletion process is primarily mediated via rearrangement of the flanking δREC and ψJα gene segments.[47,60,61] Virtually all TCRαβ^{+} T lymphocytes have rearranged *TCRG* genes, whereas a large part of the TCRγδ^{+} T lymphocytes have rearranged *TCRB* genes.[10]

Ig/TCR Rearrangements as Clonal Markers of Lymphoid Malignancies

Lymphoid malignancies (i.e., the various types of lymphoid leukemias and non–Hodgkin's lymphomas) are considered to be the malignant counterparts of normal lymphoid (precursor) cells.[62–65] Hence, the majority of lymphoid malignancies also contain rearranged Ig and/or TCR genes. Since they are derived from a single malignantly transformed lymphoid cell, all cells of a lymphoid malignancy have identically rearranged Ig/TCR genes. Analogously to (post)follicular B lymphocytes, follicular and postfollicular B-cell malignancies (e.g., FL, DLBCL, multiple myeloma) harbor somatic hypermutations in their rearranged *IGH* genes and to a lesser extent in their *IGK* and/or *IGL* genes.[66,67] The fact that lymphoid malignancies contain clonal Ig/TCR gene rearrangements can be employed in clonality assessment as well as for target identification for molecular monitoring of patients during and after therapy.[30]

Aberrant and Oncogenic Ig/TCR Gene Rearrangements and Chromosome Aberrations

It has become increasingly clear in recent years that Ig/TCR loci are not only subjected to physiological rearrangements, but can be also involved in so-called illegitimate or aberrant rearrangements. One type of aberrant rearrangement is found in ataxia telangiectasia (AT) and Nijmegen breakage syndrome (NBS) patients, as well as in T-cell neoplasms that develop in AT and NBS patients. This concerns the so-called trans-rearrangements between *TCRB* and *TCRG* loci through t(7;7), or inversion 7 and t(14;14) and/or t(7;14) aberrations.[68–71] However, these trans-rearrangements are not believed to play a direct role in oncogenesis; they are rather considered to be a general indicator of genomic instability with increased risk of lymphoma development.

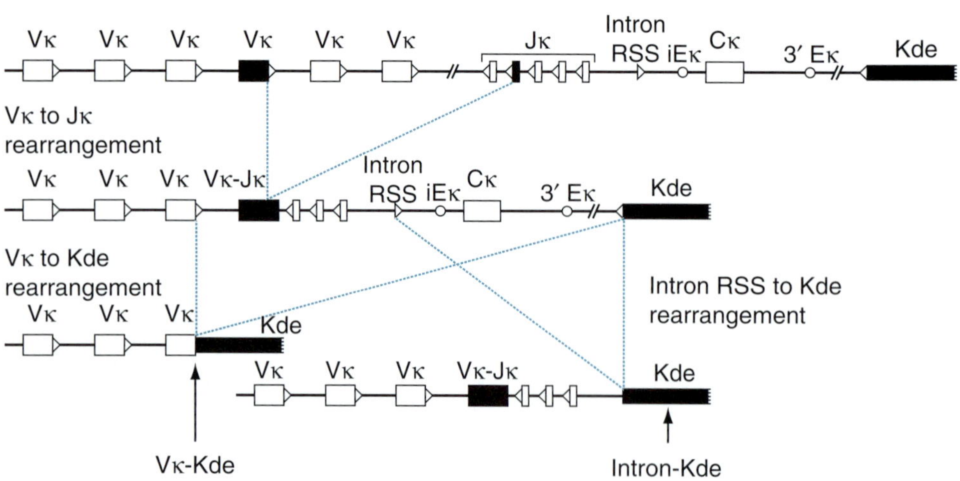

Figure 4–5. Consecutive rearrangements in the *IGK* locus, resulting in the two main types of Kde rearrangements. Generally, recombination starts with Vκ-Jκ rearrangement. Expression of the Vκ-Jκ rearranged allele can be disrupted by rearrangement of Kde (kappa-deleting element) to an intronic RSS, resulting in deletion of the Cκ gene segment, or to any of the Vκ gene segments, resulting in deletion of the entire Vκ-Jκ-Cκ region. Both types of Kde rearrangements result in deletion of the two *IGK* gene enhancers (iEκ and 3′Eκ), most likely precluding further rearrangements in the *IGK* locus.

Another type concerns the oncogenic rearrangements between Ig/TCR loci and (proto)oncogenes that are often located on distinct chromosomes (Table 4–3). Classic examples involving the Ig genes include t(8;14)(q24;q32) and the t(2;8)(q11;q24) and t(8;22)(q24;q11) variants in Burkitt's lymphoma, in which *IGH* (or *IGK* or *IGL*) during the normal V(D)J recombination or class switch recombination processes are erroneously coupled to the *MYC* gene. Other well-known Ig aberrations are t(11;14)(q13;q32) (with coupling of *IGH* J gene segments to *BCL1/CCDN1*) in MCL and t(14;18)(q32;q21) (with coupling of *IGH* J gene segments to *BCL2*) in FL (reviewed in Willis et al.[72]).

IGH chromosome aberrations are also frequent in multiple myeloma. However, these aberrations involve switch regions of the *IGH* genes rather than the V(D)J region. Similar to the V(D)J recombination related aberrations, the final result of these aberrant switch recombination processes often also is over-expression of the involved oncogenes.[73–75]

In precursor T-cell lymphoblastic lymphomas (T-LBL), similar TCR-associated chromosome aberrations can be detected as in T-ALL (e.g., 1p32 aberrations involving the *TAL1* locus, and t(11;14)(p15;q11)/t(11;14)(p13;q11) involving the *LMO1* and *LMO2* loci, respectively), although it should be noted that T-ALL has been studied much more extensively. Virtually all TCR-gene–related aberrations result in over-expression of the involved genes, which often encode transcription factors that are normally not expressed in the T-cell lineage. Remarkably, in the more mature types of T-cell lymphoma, TCR-associated aberrations are virtually not found. The frequency of well-described oncogenic aberrations in these T-cell lymphomas is scarce. Nevertheless, an important recurrent chromosome aberration in ALCL concerns t(2;5)(p13;q35) in which an *NPM-ALK* fusion gene is formed, as well as variant translocations involving the *ALK* gene and different partners (Table 4–3).

It can be predicted that in the coming years yet other Ig/TCR gene translocations may be found through new experimental approaches including FISH, spectral karyotyping analysis, and ligation-mediated PCR (LM-PCR) or long-distance inverse PCR (LDI-PCR) methods. Although their exact prognostic value remains to be established, it can be anticipated that these illegitimate Ig/TCR gene recombinations may be important not only for further classification of lymphoid malignancies but also for molecular monitoring.

IDENTIFICATION OF PCR TARGETS FOR MOLECULAR MONITORING OF LYMPHOMA

PCR Amplification of Ig/TCR Gene Rearrangements

In order to identify clonal Ig/TCR gene rearrangements as molecular targets in the various types of lymphomas, two main approaches have been followed: classic Southern blot analysis and PCR–based techniques.[10,76] This chapter focuses on PCR analysis of Ig/TCR gene rearrangements, which is based on amplification of rearranged Ig/TCR genes including their junctional regions. Such amplification is only possible when the Ig/TCR gene segments are juxtaposed through rearrangement, as the distance between these gene segments in the germline configuration is far too large for efficient amplification.

Table 4–3. Most Important Recurrent Chromosome Aberrations in Human B- and T-Cell Lymphomas

Chromosome Aberration	Involved Genes	Protein Expression	Mechanism	Associated Lymphoma
t(11;14)(q13;q32)	*IGH, BCL1/CCND1*	Cyclin D1	V(D)J	MCL (>95%)
t(14;18)(q32;q21)[a]	*IGH, BCL2*	BCL2	V(D)J	FL (~80%) DLBCL (~20%)
t(8;14)(q24;q32)[a]	*IGH, MYC*	c-MYC	V(D)J/CSR	BL (>98%)
t(3;14)(q27;q32)	*IGH, BCL6*	BCL6/LAZ3	V(D)J	DLBCL (5%–10%)
t(9;14)(p13;q32)	*IGH, PAX5*	PAX-5	V(D)J	LL (~50%)
t(11;18)(q21;q21)	*MALT, API2*	MALT-API2 fusion	?	MZL-MALT (25%–50%)
t(11;14)(q13;q32)	*IGH, BCL1/CCND1*	Cyclin D1	CSR	MM (20%–25%)
t(4;14)(p16;q32)	*IGH, FGFR3/MMSET*	FGFR3	CSR	MM (20%–25%)
t(14;16)(q32;q23)	*IGH, MAF*	c-MAF	CSR	MM (20%–25%)
t(6;14)(p25;q32)	*IGH, IRF4*	IRF4	CSR	MM (~20%)
t(1;14)(q21;q32)	*IGH, MUM2/3*	MUM2/3	CSR	MM (<5%)
t(6;14)(p21;q32)	*IGH, CCND3*	CCND3	CSR	MM (<5%)
t(14;14)(q11;q32) inv14(q11q32)	*TCRD/A, TCL1*	TCL1	V(D)J	T-PLL (70%–75%)
t(X;14)(q28;q11)	*TCRD/A, MCTP1*	MCTP1	V(D)J	T-PLL (~5%)
t(2;5)(p13;q35)[b]	*NPM, ALK*	NPM-ALK fusion	?	ALCL (~75%)

[a] Variants involving the *IGK* (2p12) and *IGL* (22q11) light-chain genes have been described.
[b] Variants involving the *ALK* gene and the *TPM3* (1q21), *TPM4* (19p13), *TFG* (3q12), *CLTC* (17q23), and *ATIC* (2q35) genes, all resulting in ALK fusion proteins, have been described to occur at lower frequencies.
ALCL, anaplastic large-cell lymphoma; BL, Burkitt's lymphoma; CLL, chronic lymphocytic leukemia; CSR, class-switch recombination related; DLBCL, diffuse large B-cell lymphoma; FL, follicular lymphoma; LL, lymphoplasmacytic lymphoma; MALT, mucosa-associated lymphoid tissue; MCL, mantle cell lymphoma; MM, multiple myeloma; MZL, marginal zone lymphoma; T-PLL, T-cell prolymphocytic leukemia; V(D)J, V(D)J recombination related.

Since most Ig/TCR PCR studies in leukemias and lymphomas are performed at the DNA level, PCR primers are normally complementary to exon and/or intron sequences of V, (D), and J gene segments.[77–83] Obviously, the choice of primers depends on the exact Ig/TCR locus and the involved rearranged gene segments. In some protocols general or consensus primers have been used, which recognize, for example, all V or J gene segments of a particular Ig/TCR gene complex. Alternatively family-specific primers, which recognize families of V or J gene segments, can be employed. A third option is to make use of segment-specific primers, which recognize individual gene segments.[77–85]

It should be noted that the Ig/TCR genes not only contain functional V, (D), and J gene segments (Table 4–1), but also nonfunctional (pseudo) gene segments. These can also be involved in gene rearrangements, if they are flanked by proper RSS elements. In order to detect all possible (functional and nonfunctional) Ig/TCR gene rearrangements (see Table 4–2), the primer sets should thus be able to recognize virtually all V, (D), and J gene segments. This would imply that many different primer sets have to be designed, which would be very inefficient for routine PCR–based analysis of Ig/TCR gene rearrangements. In the case of *IGH*, *IGK*, and *IGL* gene rearrangements, the use of primers for the relatively limited number of VH, Vκ, and Vλ families (Table 4–2) would already lead to a reduction in the number of required primers. A further reduction has been achieved by the elegant multiplex strategies developed in the European BIOMED-2 Concerted Action BMH4-CT98-3936, entitled "PCR-Based Clonality Studies for Early Diagnosis of Lymphoproliferative Disorders."[76] The BIOMED-2 multiplex tubes contain multiple primers in one PCR reaction mixture, which couple broad recognition of virtually all segments to an efficient and reliable assay.[76] PCR analysis of *TCRA* and *TCRB* gene rearrangements would also require many primers, given the many different V and J gene segments of these loci (Table 4–2 and Fig. 4–2).[12,13,86–91] RT-PCR strategies in which VαJα-Cα and VβDβJβ-Cβ transcripts are analyzed only partly solve this problem, as many different Vα or Vβ primers still need be used in combination with a single Cα or Cβ primer.[88–90] A similar robust BIOMED-2 multiplex approach as for the Ig loci has now also proven to be highly reliable for analyzing both incomplete Dβ-Jβ and complete Vβ-Jβ gene rearrangements.[76,92] Finally, although *TCRG* and *TCRD* gene rearrangements can relatively easily be analyzed with only a restricted number of PCR primers due to the limited number of individual V and J gene segments (see also Table 4–2 and Fig. 4–2),[15,18,93,94] efficient BIOMED-2 multiplex approaches are now also available for the *TCRG* and *TCRD* loci.[76] Standardized and quality-controlled BIOMED-2 multiplex PCR tubes for *IGH*, *IGK*, *IGL*, *TCRB*, *TCRG*, and *TCRD* genes are available from IVS Technologies, San Diego, CA.

Despite obvious advantages (speed, low amount of DNA required, applicability on DNA from any type of material), PCR–based Ig/TCR gene analysis might also harbor several drawbacks as compared to Southern blot analysis. One is the risk of false-negative results due to inappropriate recognition of all Ig/TCR gene segments that can potentially be involved in rearrangements, by the applied primer sets. This has now largely been overcome by the aforementioned standardized multiplex assays for analysis of all types of Ig/TCR gene rearrangements.[76] Another important pitfall of PCR analysis is the risk of false-positive results due to the fact that clonally rearranged Ig/TCR genes cannot be amplified in a specific way, but are rather amplified in the same way as normal, polyclonal Ig/TCR gene rearrangements. Hence, discrimination between monoclonal (leukemia-derived) and polyclonal (reactive) PCR products is essential to avoid false-positive interpretations, which emphasizes the need to further analyze the PCR-amplified rearranged gene products.

Analysis of PCR Amplified Ig/TCR Products

PCR–based detection of clonal Ig/TCR gene rearrangements is relatively easy if the tumor cell percentage is high (e.g., >90%). In such cell samples, the background of Ig/TCR gene rearrangements derived from normal polyclonal cells generally does not hamper interpretation. However, if a sample contains substantial numbers of polyclonal B or T cells, such as in most lymph node samples, many additional polyclonal Ig/TCR PCR products will be present. In such samples, discrimination between monoclonal and polyclonal PCR products via standard gel electrophoresis can be difficult, as it implies the need to identify clonal PCR products as dominant bands within a background of multiple weaker products/bands.[81,82] One can facilitate the cumbersome analysis by exploiting the junctional region heterogeneity of Ig/TCR rearrangements. As junctional regions are "fingerprint-like" sequences that differ between lymphocytes or lymphocyte clones, they thus represent specific markers for each individual leukemia.[77–80,84,85] Several strategies have been developed that employ the Ig/TCR junctional region heterogeneity to discriminate between polyclonal and clonal cell populations: direct sequencing of the PCR products,[95] single-strand conformation polymorphism (SSCP) analysis,[96,97] denaturing gradient gel electrophoresis (DGGE),[98,99] temperature-gradient gel electrophoresis (TGGE),[100] heteroduplex analysis,[101,102] and GeneScan analysis.[103,104]

Especially the latter two methods have proven their utility. Originally designed for mutation detection of genetic diseases, heteroduplex analysis, after modification, can also be applied to analysis of Ig/TCR PCR products. In heteroduplex analysis, PCR products are denatured (94°C) and subsequently cooled (4°C) to induce formation of homoduplexes (with identical, clonal junctions) or heteroduplexes (with different junctional regions), which can then be separated from each other by polyacrylamide gel electrophoresis based on differences in conformation (Fig. 4–6).[102] Application of heteroduplex analysis makes it possible to discern between PCR products derived from monoclonal (homoduplex bands) and polyclonal (smear of heteroduplexes) cell populations. In GeneScan analysis, in which fluorochrome-labeled Ig/TCR PCR products are analyzed on high-resolution polyacrylamide gels, monoclonal Ig/TCR PCR products give rise to fragments of identical size, whereas polyclonal products result in PCR products showing a Gaussian distribution of junctional region sizes (Fig. 4–6). Although slightly better detection limits have

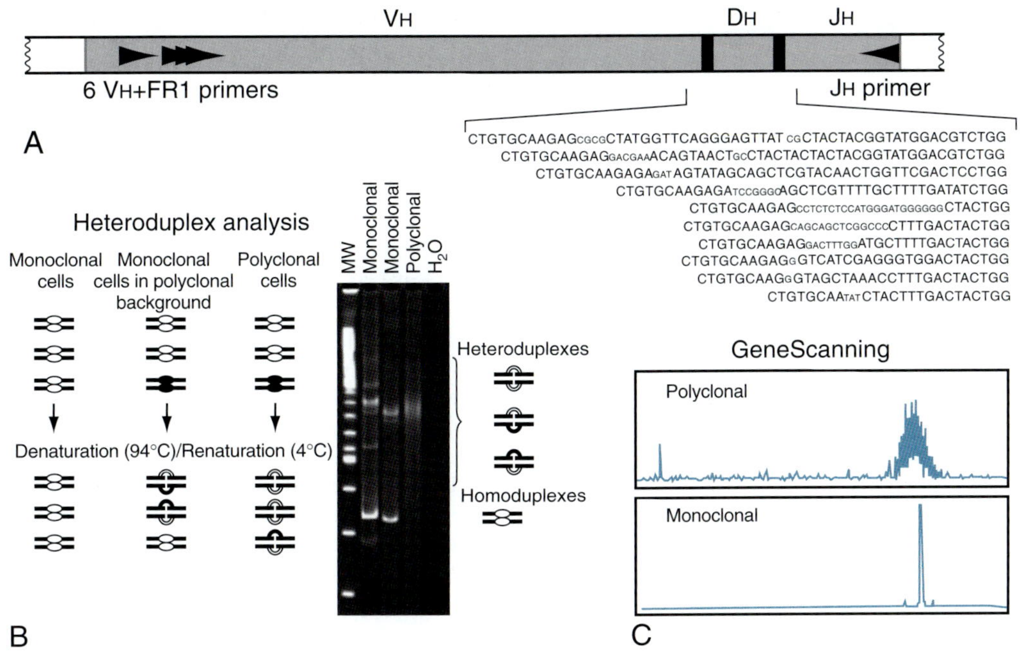

Figure 4–6. Schematic diagram of heteroduplex analysis and GeneScan analysis techniques. Rearranged *IGH* genes show heterogeneity (in size and nucleotide composition) in their junctional regions. This heterogeneity of rearranged *IGH* PCR products is employed in heteroduplex analysis (size and composition) and GeneScan analysis (size) to discern between products derived from monoclonal and polyclonal lymphoid cell populations. In heteroduplex analysis, PCR products are heat denatured (5 min, 94°C) and subsequently rapidly cooled (1 hour, 4°C) to induce duplex (homo- or hetero-duplex) formation. In cell samples consisting of clonal lymphoid cells, the PCR products of rearranged *IGH* genes give rise to homoduplexes after denaturation and renaturation, whereas in samples that contain polyclonal lymphoid cell populations the single-strand PCR fragments will mainly form heteroduplexes, which result in a background smear of slowly migrating fragments upon electrophoresis. In GeneScan analysis, fluorochrome-labeled rearranged *IGH* products are first denatured prior to high-resolution fragment analysis of the resulting single-strands fragments. Monoclonal cell samples will give rise to PCR products of identical size, whereas in polyclonal samples many different *IGH* PCR products will be formed, which show a characteristic Gaussian size distribution.

been found for GeneScan analysis than for heteroduplex analysis, the latter technique is easy, cheap, and probably more reliable in case of Ig/TCR targets showing relatively small junctional regions (e.g., Vκ-Jκ or Vλ-Jλ rearrangements). This has to do with the fact that in GeneScan analysis only size is evaluated, whereas in heteroduplex analysis the heterogeneity of PCR products reflects size and composition of the junctional regions.

Multicenter studies to evaluate informativity of the multiplex Ig/TCR PCR heteroduplex and/or GeneScan strategies in lymphomas have recently been performed within the frame of the European BIOMED-2 program. Initial results in the most important (WHO-defined[105]) B-cell lymphoma entities illustrate that both *IGH* and *IGK* analyses are highly informative with respect to identification of clonal Ig rearrangements that can be used as targets for molecular monitoring (Table 4–4) (Evans PAS, Salles G, Groenen PJTA, manuscript in preparation). Apart from MCL that contained clonal *IGH* and *IGK* PCR products in 100% of cases, also FL, DLBCL, and marginal zone lymphoma scored high (around 80% of cases for both loci). Incomplete DH-JH and *IGL* rearrangements appeared to occur much less frequently in all B-cell lymphoma entities (Table 4–4). In order to reduce the risk of false-negativity caused by improper annealing to gene segments and by somatic hypermutations, multiple loci (e.g., *IGH* and *IGK*) should be analyzed to increase the chances of finding targets for monitoring. Clear findings also emerged from a study on T-cell lymphoma entities (WHO classification), in which both *TCRB* (73% to 98%, depending on the T-cell lymphoma entity) and *TCRG* (68% to 93%) analysis appeared highly informative, whereas *TCRD* was less frequently rearranged (Table 4–5) (Brüggemann M, White H, Gaulard P, manu-

Table 4–4. Analysis of Ig Gene Rearrangements as PCR Targets for Molecular Monitoring in Human B-Cell Lymphomas

	Informativity			
NHL Type	***IGH* (V-J)**	***IGH* (D-J)**	***IGK***	***IGL***
DLBCL	++	+	++	+
FL	++	±	++	±
MCL	+++	±	+++	+
MZL	++	+	++	+

±, <25% of cases; +, 26%–50% of cases; ++, 51%–90% of cases; +++, >90% of cases.

DLBCL, diffuse large B-cell lymphoma; FL, follicular lymphoma; MCL, mantle cell lymphoma; MZL, marginal zone lymphoma.

Table 4–5. Analysis of TCR Gene Rearrangements as PCR Targets for Molecular Monitoring in Human T-Cell Lymphomas

	Informativity		
NHL Type	*TCRB*	*TCRG*	*TCRD*
ALCL	++	++	±
AIL-T	++	+++	+[a]
PTCL-NOS	+++	+++	±[a]

[a] Frequency higher in TCRγδ$^+$ cases.
±, <25% of cases; +, 26%–50% of cases; ++, 51%–90% of cases; +++, >90% of cases.
ALCL, anaplastic large-cell lymphoma; AIL-T, angioimmunoblastic T-cell lymphoma; PTCL-NOS, peripheral T-cell lymphoma not otherwise specified.

script in preparation). The data further reveal the strength of analyzing both *TCRB* and *TCRG* rearrangements to find enough reliable targets for molecular monitoring of T-cell lymphomas.

PCR-Based Analysis of Oncogenic (Ig/TCR) Aberrations

PCR–based analysis of Ig/TCR-related chromosome aberrations is easier than identifying clonal Ig/TCR rearrangements, as the oncogenic rearrangements specifically occur in the lymphoma cells and in principle not in normal lymphocytes at substantial levels. Hence, there is no background from nonlymphoma cells to be taken into account. These chromosome aberrations generally do not result in fusion gene transcripts, but rather lead to over-expression of the involved (onco)gene irrespective of the exact, mostly unique, breakpoint. This has prompted the development of PCR strategies at the genomic level, employing Ig or TCR specific primers in combination with one or multiple primers in the partner gene region, depending on the number of involved breakpoint cluster regions. In the case of t(14;18)/*BCL2-IGH*, this has resulted in highly informative multiplex strategies in which a consensus JH primer is used with multiple primers around *BCL2* breakpoint cluster areas.[76] However, for some aberrations such as t(11;14)/*BCL1-IGH* or t(8;14)//*MYC-IGH* not all breakpoints are nicely clustered, implying that many additional primers are needed to identify all aberrations for monitoring purposes. In others, too few data about individual breakpoints are available yet to develop reliable assays. An attractive alternative for t(8;14) identification might be initial amplification of the *MYC*-CH fusion using multiplex LD-PCR with subsequent sequencing of the precise breakpoint region.[106,107]

Finally, some aberrations do result in fusion gene transcripts (*MALT-API2*; *NPM-ALK*), which makes their identification breakpoint-independent and therefore more simple, although for actual monitoring it is often preferred to employ the unique patient- and lymphoma-specific breakpoint area at the genomic level to prevent false-positivity through cross-contamination.

MOLECULAR MONITORING OF LYMPHOMA: DETECTION OF MINIMAL RESIDUAL DISEASE

Techniques for MRD monitoring should meet several criteria in order to obtain reliable results[2]:

- Sensitivity of at least 10^{-3} (one malignant cell within thousand normal cells), but sensitivities of 10^{-4} to 10^{-6} are preferred.
- Tumor specificity (discrimination between malignant and normal cells, without false-positive results).
- Stability of tumor-specific markers (no false-negative results owing to loss of the MRD targets during the course of the disease).
- Intralaboratory and interlaboratory reproducibility (essential for multicenter treatment protocols).
- Feasibility (easy standardization and rapid collection of results for clinical application).
- Precise quantification of MRD levels should be possible.

PCR analysis of Ig genes, TCR genes, and chromosome aberrations fulfill these criteria. Furthermore, one or more of these PCR targets can be detected in virtually all non–Hodgkin's lymphomas.

Until 5 years ago, MRD quantification by PCR analysis of Ig/TCR gene rearrangements and chromosome aberrations was mainly performed using semiquantitative PCR analyses, such as limiting dilution PCR and competitive PCR. For MRD detection using chromosome aberrations, even qualitative approaches were applied, based on positivity/negativity of nested PCR. The complex and time-consuming PCR analyses for quantification of the involved target have recently been replaced by RQ-PCR.[108] In contrast to PCR endpoint quantification techniques, RQ-PCR permits accurate quantification during the exponential PCR amplification phase. Because of the real-time detection, the RQ-PCR method has a very large dynamic detection range over five orders of magnitude. Quantitative data can be obtained in a short period of time, since post-PCR processing is not necessary.

Principles of the Real-Time Quantitative PCR Analysis (RQ-PCR)

Three RQ-PCR technologies are most commonly used (see Fig. 4–7). The first technology is based on hydrolysis (TaqMan) probes and exploits the 5′ → 3′ nuclease activity of the Taq polymerase to detect and quantify specific PCR products as the reaction proceeds. Upon amplification, an internal target-specific hydrolysis probe conjugated with a reporter and a quencher dye is degraded, resulting in emission of a fluorescent signal by the reporter dye that accumulates during the consecutive PCR cycles (Fig. 4–7B). The second technology uses hybridization probes and exploits the fluorescence resonance energy transfer (FRET) technology. This method requires two hybridization probes complementary to neighboring sequences, one labeled with a fluorochrome at the 3′ end, and the other carrying a fluorochrome at the 5′ end (Fig. 4–7C). One fluorochrome is a donor fluorochrome, whereas the other fluorochrome (acceptor) emits fluorescent light, if it is positioned close to the donor dye. Maximal fluorescence is measured during

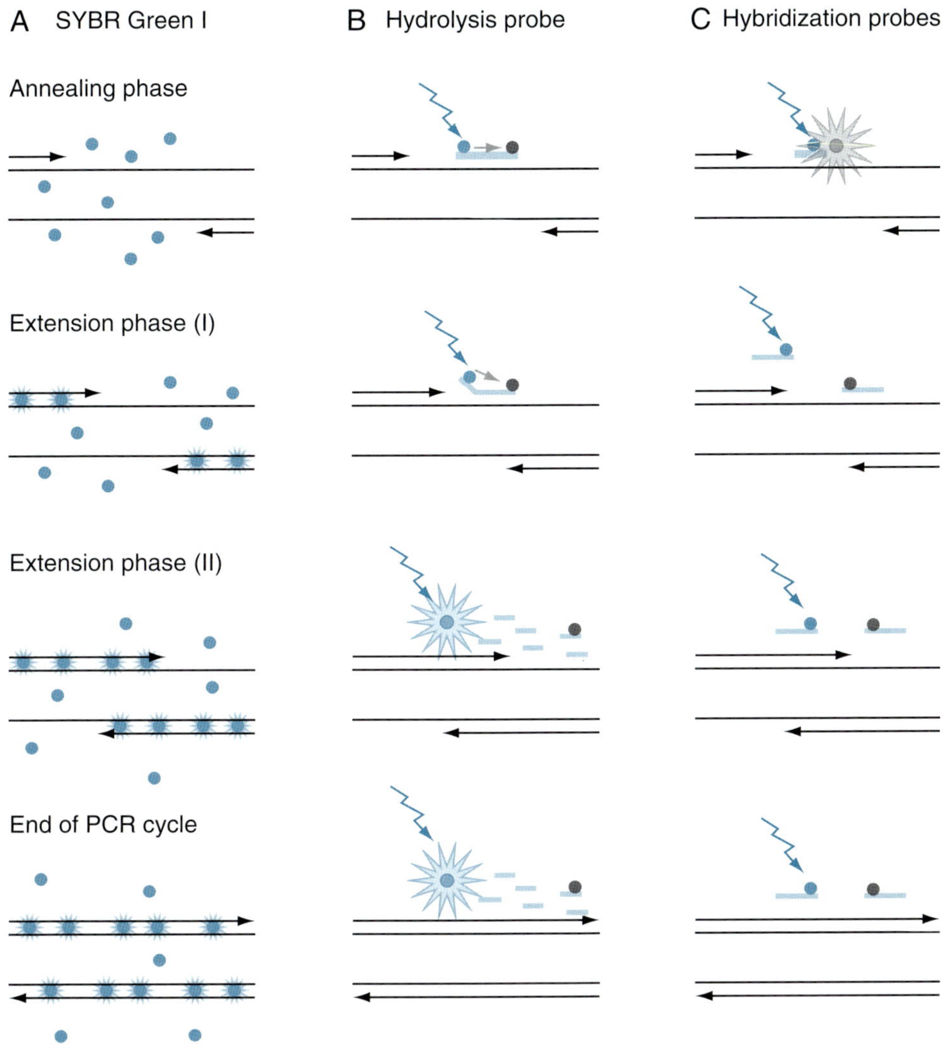

Figure 4–7. Principles of real-time quantitative PCR (RQ-PCR) techniques. **A**: SYBR Green I technique. SYBR Green I fluorescence is enormously increased upon binding to double-stranded DNA. During the extension phase, more and more SYBR Green I will bind to the PCR product, resulting in an increased fluorescence. Consequently, during each subsequent PCR cycle, more fluorescence signal will be detected. **B**: Hydrolysis probe technique. The hydrolysis probe is conjugated with a quencher fluorochrome, which absorbs the fluorescence of the reporter fluorochrome as long as the probe is intact. However, upon amplification of the target sequence, the hydrolysis probe is displaced and subsequently hydrolyzed by the Taq polymerase. This results in the separation of the reporter and quencher fluorochrome and consequently the fluorescence of the reporter fluorochrome becomes detectable. During each consecutive PCR cycle, this fluorescence will further increase because of the progressive and exponential accumulation of free reporter fluorochromes. **C**: Hybridization probes technique. In this technique, one probe is labeled with a donor fluorochrome at the 3′ end and a second probe is labeled with an acceptor fluorochrome. When the two fluorochromes are in close vicinity (i.e., within one to five nucleotides), the emitted light of the donor fluorochrome will excite the acceptor fluorochrome. This results in the emission of fluorescence, which subsequently can be detected during the annealing phase and first part of the extension phase of the PCR reaction. After each subsequent PCR cycle, more hybridization probes can anneal, resulting in higher fluorescence signals.

the annealing step of each PCR cycle, when both probes hybridize to adjacent target sequences on the same strand. A third technology for RQ-PCR is based on the detection of SYBR green I (DNA intercalating dye) during PCR employing patient-specific primers (Fig. 4–7A). The SYBR Green I dye binds to the minor groove of double-stranded DNA, which greatly enhances its fluorescence. During the consecutive PCR cycles, the amount of double-stranded PCR product will increase, and therefore more SYBR Green I dye can bind to DNA and emit its fluorescence. Maximal SYBR Green I dye binding will occur at the end of the elongation phase of each PCR cycle. RQ-PCR analysis using nonspecific detection should always include a melting curve analysis in order to discriminate between specific PCR products and nonspecific PCR products.

RQ-PCR Approaches

For RQ-PCR–based detection of MRD in lymphoma patients several strategies can be chosen for positioning of

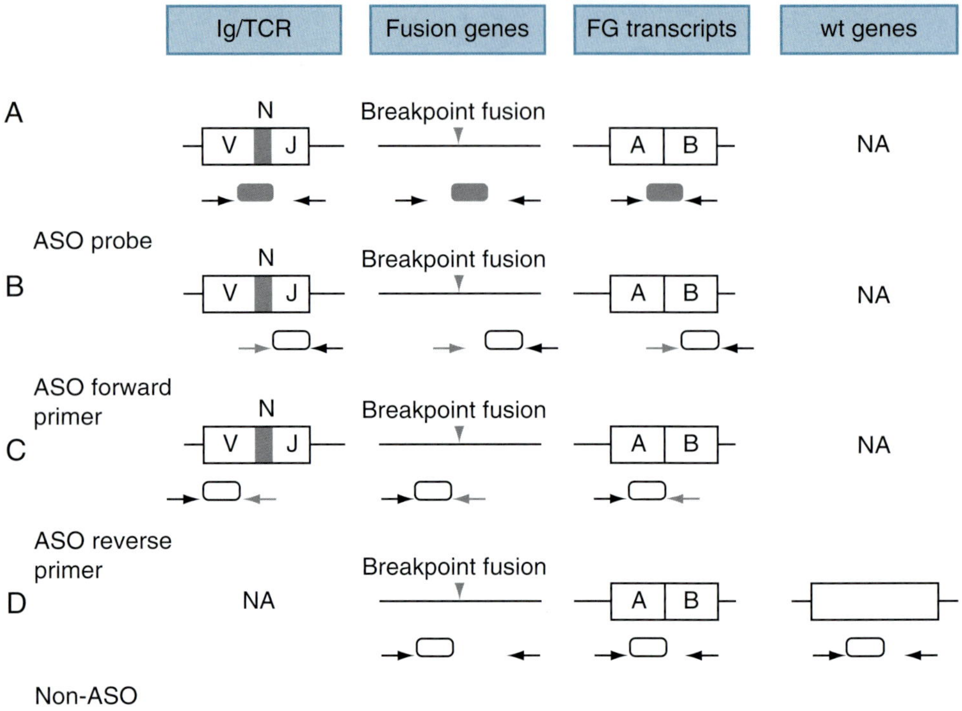

Figure 4–8. RQ-PCR approaches. **A**: ASO probe approach. **B**: ASO forward primer approach. **C**: ASO reverse primer approach. **D**: Non-ASO approach. The four approaches are shown for the different types of MRD-PCR targets. Primers are indicated as arrows, whereas the probe (either one hydrolysis probe or two hybridization probes) is indicated by the oval symbol; the ASO probe or primer is indicated in gray. NA: not applicable; FG, fusion gene; wt, wild type.

the oligonucleotides in order to achieve patient-specific/lymphoma-specific amplification (See Fig. 4–8).[108]

ASO Probe Approach

In the allele-specific oligonucleotide (ASO) probe approach (see Fig. 4–8A), the probe is positioned at the tumor-specific sequence, such as the junctional region of Ig/TCR gene rearrangements or the breakpoint area of fusion genes.[109] The probe is used in combination with a forward and reverse primer, which are positioned in germline sequences opposite of the tumor-specific sequence. Although good sensitivities can be obtained by this approach, a major drawback is that for each individual tumor-specific MRD-PCR target a fluorogenic probe has to be designed and ordered.

ASO Forward or ASO Reverse Primer Approach

The ASO forward primer approach (see Fig. 4–8B) employs a forward primer positioned in the tumor-specific sequence in combination with a germline reverse primer and a germline probe (e.g., in the J gene segment) (Fig. 4–9). The ASO reverse primer approach (Fig. 4–8C) is comparable to the ASO forward primer approach, but with opposite location of the germline primer and probe relative to the tumor-specific sequence. Instead of a germline probe, the SYBR Green I dye can be used to detect the PCR product. However, a nested PCR approach may be needed for reaching sufficiently high sensitivity.[110]

Allele-Nonspecific (Germline) Primer and Probe Approach

For tumor-specific MRD-PCR targets that are not found in normal cells, such as fusion gene transcripts, it is not necessary to apply ASO primers or ASO probes (Fig. 4–8D). If aberrant expression of a gene (e.g., *CCND1*) is analyzed, primers and probe are designed on the wild-type (germline) nucleotide sequence of the involved gene.[111–116] Germline primers and probes can also be applied for fusion gene transcripts; in these cases the forward primer is located in an exon from one fusion gene partner, whereas the reverse primer is located in an exon of the other fusion gene partner. Also for fusion genes, which in principle are patient specific, germline primer and probes can be used, because such fusion genes are not, or only at very low levels, present in normal cells.[117–124]

Ig/TCR Genes as MRD-PCR Targets in Lymphoma Patients

For MRD analysis using (RQ-)PCR techniques, two types of patient-specific sequences are most frequently used in lymphoma patients: junctional regions of rearranged Ig and TCR genes and breakpoint fusion regions of chromosome aberrations. Other MRD-PCR targets include fusion gene transcripts associated with chromosomal abnormalities and aberrantly expressed genes; these will only be discussed briefly.

MRD Monitoring by PCR Analysis of Rearranged Ig/TCR Genes

MRD monitoring is possible in virtually all mature lymphoid malignancies via PCR analysis of Ig/TCR gene rearrangements. The junctional regions of rearranged Ig and TCR genes are unique "fingerprint-like" sequences, which are assumed to be different in each lymphoid cell, and thus also in each lymphoid malignancy.[2] Therefore, junctional regions can be used as tumor-specific targets for MRD-PCR analysis. The presence of clonal Ig/TCR gene rearrange-

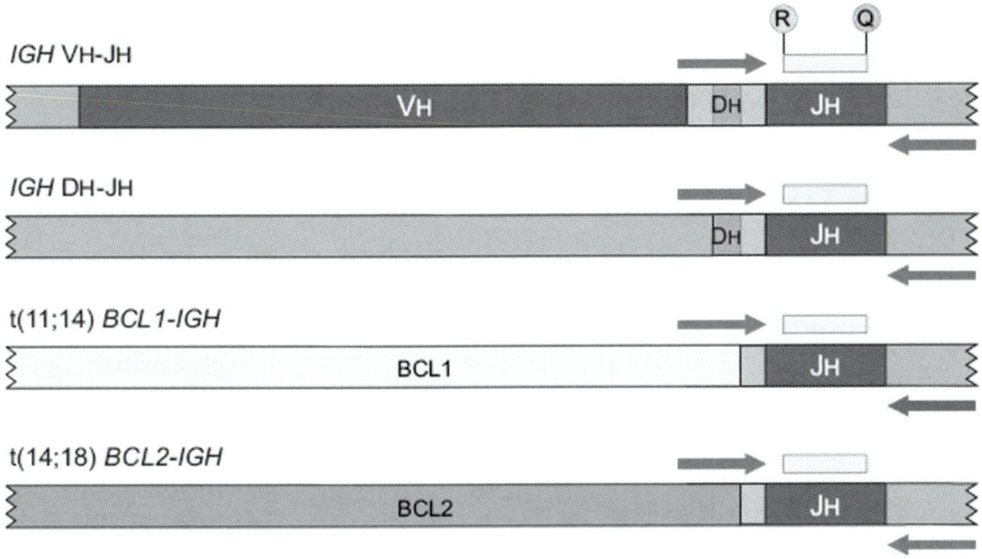

Figure 4–9. Common germ-line JH primer/probe set for RQ-PCR analysis of various types of normal and aberrant *IGH* genes. Schematic representation of a complete IGH gene rearrangement (**A**), incomplete IGH gene rearrangement (**B**), *BCL2-IGH* rearrangement (**C**), and *BCL1-IGH* rearrangement (**D**). It is possible to use a single set of a germline JH hydrolysis probes and JH reverse primers in RQ-PCR MRD assay for all these different rearrangements. Allele-specific forward primers are designed for each patient, being located on the junctional regions and downstream parts of VH, DH, *BCL2*, and *BCL1*, respectively.

ments can be analyzed by heteroduplex analysis or GeneScan analysis. Subsequently, the precise nucleotide sequence of the junctional regions can be determined. This sequence information allows the design of junctional region-specific oligonucleotides (either ASO probes or ASO primers), which can be used to detect malignant cells among normal lymphoid cells during follow-up of patients.

Ig Gene Rearrangements as MRD-PCR Targets in B-Lineage Lymphomas

For MRD studies in lymphoma patients, *IGH* gene rearrangements are frequently used, because they are present in virtually all lymphoma patients.[76] Also *IGK* and *IGL* gene rearrangements can be applied as MRD-PCR target in lymphoma patients.[125,126]

A limitation of Ig gene rearrangements as the MRD-PCR target is the occurrence of somatic hypermutations in many B-NHL, especially FL and post-follicular B-NHL.[50] Of importance, in FL the somatic mutation process can still be active, resulting in the formation of subclones with different specificities of the Ig molecules.[127] Such subclones may no longer be recognized by the applied primer/probe set, resulting in false-negative MRD results. In post-follicular B-NHL, such false-negative MRD results are less likely, because their V-(D-)J exons are assumed to remain stable throughout the disease course. It should be noted that approximately 60% of B-cell lymphomas contain at least one deleted *IGK* allele, and approximately 30% contain an incomplete *IGH* gene rearrangement. These *IGK*-Kde and DH-JH rearrangements are not prone to somatic hypermutations, and therefore theoretically are preferred targets for MRD analysis.

Most secondary rearrangements (e.g., D-J replacements in the *IGH* gene, V-J replacements in *IGK*, *IGL*, *TCRA*, and *TCRG* genes, and replacement of the V gene segment in the *IGH*, *TCRB*, and *TCRG* genes) occur only in immature B- and T-cells. Consequently, this phenomenon does not hamper MRD monitoring in lymphomas.[31,39,128]

If *IGH* gene rearrangements are chosen as MRD-PCR target, the ASO forward primer approach (generally using a probe located in the J gene segments) has several advantages over the ASO reverse primer approach (generally using a probe located in the V gene segments). First, the number of J gene segments is lower than the number of V gene segments, and consequently a lower number of probes need to be made. Second, the germline JH primer and probe can be applied for both complete (V-D-J) and incomplete (D-J) gene rearrangements. Third, somatic hypermutations particularly occur in the V gene segment and this may result in less optimal primer and probe annealing.[129] By sequencing the entire V(D)J exon using downstream-located JH primers, it can be checked whether the available JH germline primer and probe can indeed be applied in a particular patient. On the other hand, the ASO reverse primer approach might theoretically be more sensitive in some cases, due to the higher number of V gene segments as compared to J gene segments, but this is not supported by our data or data in the literature.[130–134]

Several primer/probe sets for RQ-PCR–based detection of leukemia-specific *IGH* gene rearrangements have been described, particularly for application in ALL patients.[109,130–132,135–139] In principle, these sets can also be applied for MRD studies in lymphoma patients, although the presence of somatic hypermutations might particularly hamper efficient annealing of germline VH primers and probes. As indicated above, sequencing of the *IGH* gene rearrangement may be necessary to confirm that the relevant VH germline primer and probe can still bind to the mutated gene. To increase the applicability of germline probes, one can consider using 3'-minor groove binding (MGB) probes. These MGB probes are shorter than conventional probes, thereby allowing their design in small areas of the VH gene segments that are less susceptible to somatic hypermutations.[140]

IGK gene rearrangements are less frequently applied as MRD-PCR target in lymphoma patients.[125,126] However, particularly *IGK*-Kde rearrangements may be ideal MRD-PCR targets because they are not prone to somatic hypermutations and are stable throughout the course of the disease, and only one germline primer/probe set is required for MRD detection in all patients.[138]

IGL gene rearrangements have hardly been used as MRD-PCR target.[126] Nevertheless, they can be used in all Igλ-positive patients, although somatic hypermutations may limit their detection and their use as MRD-PCR target.

TCR Gene Rearrangements as MRD-PCR Targets in T-Lineage Lymphomas

Like Ig gene rearrangements in B cells, TCR gene rearrangements in T-cells can be considered as unique "*fingerprint-like*" sequences that can be applied as PCR target for detection of MRD in T-cell malignancies. The mature T-cell malignancies should be discerned from T-ALL and T-LBL, which are regarded to be thymus-derived malignancies based on their positivity for TdT. Mature (post-thymic) T-cell malignancies do not have TdT expression and frequently express TCR molecules. Most T-NHL belong to the TCRαβ lineage, although small categories of TCRγδ$^+$ T-NHL have been identified (e.g., hepatosplenic T-cell lymphoma).

TCRG gene rearrangements are found in virtually all mature T-lineage malignancies. Southern blot analysis showed that all malignancies belonging to the TCRαβ lineage have *TCRB* gene rearrangements and most of them have biallelic *TCRD* gene deletions.[141] Thus, MRD studies in mature T-cell malignancies can generally use junctional regions of rearranged *TCRG* and *TCRB* genes as PCR targets, whereas *TCRD* gene rearrangements are less often available. Using the newly developed BIOMED-2 multiplex PCR strategy for *TCRB* detection, it is possible to identify Vβ-Jβ and Dβ-Jβ joinings in virtually all patients with Southern blot detectable *TCRB* gene rearrangements.[76,92] Alternatively, it is possible to determine the precise *TCRB* gene rearrangement via RT-PCR analysis of *TCRB* gene transcripts using multiple Vβ family primers in combination with a single Cβ primer.[142]

As soon as the involved V, (D), and J gene segments as well as the junctional region are identified via sequencing, a patient-specific primer can be designed and used for MRD-PCR studies. For *TCRG*,[130] *TCRD*,[139] and *TCRB*,[143] several germline primer/probe sets have been designed; in combination with patient-specific primers sensitivities of 10^{-4} can generally be reached (see below).

In mature T-cell malignancies, TCR genes are not affected by somatic mutations and are not susceptible to ongoing or secondary rearrangements. Consequently, one MRD-PCR target should be sufficient for reliable monitoring of mature T-cell malignancies during and after treatment.

Sensitivity of PCR Analysis of Junctional Regions

The sensitivity of MRD-PCR analysis of junctional regions is dependent on the type of rearrangement, on the size of the junctional region, and on the "background" of normal lymphoid cells with comparable Ig/TCR gene rearrangements.[108,130–132,138,143,144] Junctional regions of complete V-D-J rearrangements (*IGH*, *TCRB*, *TCRD*) are extensive, whereas junctional regions of V-J rearrangements (*IGK*, *IGL*, *TCRG*) are three to four times smaller. Normal cells can contain the same rearranged gene segments as the leukemic cells. For instance, if rearrangements involving JH4, JH5, or JH6 are used as MRD-PCR target, background amplification is frequently observed, whereas this is hardly seen in case of rearrangements involving JH1, JH2, or JH3.[131] This probably can be explained by the fact that JH1, JH2, and JH3 are rarely used in pediatric or adult peripheral B cells.[145–148] VγI-Jγ1.3 and VγI-Jγ2.3 rearrangements occur in many T-cell malignancies, but they are also found in a large fraction (70% to 90%) of normal PB T-cells. This might significantly influence sensitivity levels, particularly taking into account the abundance of polyclonal Vγ-Jγ joinings in normal T-cells in post-induction follow-up samples.[149] Similarly, substantial expansions of normal precursor-B cells with polyclonal *IGH* gene rearrangements in regenerating BM after cessation of therapy might affect the sensitivity of MRD detection using Ig gene rearrangements as PCR targets.[150,151]

Breakpoint Fusion Regions of Chromosome Aberrations as MRD-PCR Targets

In approximately 30% of B-NHL patients, chromosome aberrations can be employed as tumor-specific MRD-PCR targets in which the PCR primers are chosen at opposite sides of the breakpoint fusion region.[152,153] In B-NHL, chromosomal aberrations frequently involve Ig genes, such as t(14;18) in FL, t(11;14) in MCL, and t(8;14), t(2;8), and t(8;22) in Burkitt's lymphoma (Table 4–3).[154–156] In all these B-NHL types, the breakpoints generally occur outside coding regions, implying that these translocations are not amenable to RT-PCR analysis for MRD detection, but should be studied at the DNA level. An advantage of using fusion genes as tumor-specific PCR targets for MRD detection is their stability during the disease course.

In T-NHL, only a few well-defined translocations are known so far. This concerns the *NPM-ALK* fusion gene that is observed in ALCL with t(2;5) and that can be used for RT-PCR analysis, and potentially in some cases for PCR analysis at the DNA level as well (Table 4–3).[157] Furthermore, T-LBL in childhood might have the same chromosome aberrations as found in T-ALL, such as *TAL1* deletions.

It should be noted that MRD detection of chromosome aberrations by PCR is not always applicable, because in many lymphoid malignancies no specific chromosome aberrations have been identified yet.

MRD Detection via PCR Analysis of BCL2-IGH Fusion Gene Derived from t(14;18)

One of the most widely studied chromosomal translocations is t(14;18), involving the *BCL2* and *IGH* genes, which occurs in 80% of patients with FL, 20% of patients with DLBCL and which is detectable by standard PCR procedures in 60% to 70% of cases with t(14;18).[76,158] The resulting *BCL2-IGH* fusion gene is widely used as marker for detection of MRD in patients with FL. Because most breakpoints cluster within the MBR of the *BCL2* gene, patients can be monitored using one primer located upstream of the MBR in the *BCL2* gene and one primer located within the JH region of the *IGH* gene. For RQ-PCR–based detection of *BCL2-IGH* fusion genes, several approaches have been reported. Most studies apply a forward *BCL2* primer, located upstream of the MBR or MCR, and a common JH reverse primer in combination with a fluorogenic probe located in the *BCL2* gene.[117,119–122,159] Alternatively, these primers can be used in combination with one or more JH probes (Fig. 4–9),[160] or in combination with SYBR Green I.[161] The use of JH probes has the advantage that these probes can be used in all t(14;18)-positive patients, irrespective of the exact location of the breakpoint in the *BCL2* gene. This may particularly be useful for patients in whom the *BCL2* breakpoints are not located within the MBR or MCR, which comprise approximately 25% of all FL patients.[162,163] In such cases, the exact location of the breakpoint can be determined using LD-PCR.[164]

It should be noted that positive results in sensitive *BCL2-IGH* PCR studies should be interpreted with caution, because the presence of non-neoplastic *BCL2-IGH* rearrangements has also been reported in PB, BM, and other tissues of healthy individuals, although at low levels ($<10^{-4}$) in most subjects.[165–167] Surprisingly, circulating t(14;18)-positive cells were detected in patients in long-term clinical remission after radiation therapy for localized FL.[168] The extensive RQ-PCR–based analyses estimated the overall incidence of *BCL2-IGH* positivity in healthy individuals and cancer patients at diagnosis at 10% to 25%.[166,167] In contrast, *BCL2-IGH* rearrangements were extremely rare after chemotherapy, indicating that non-neoplastic *BCL2-IGH*-positive cells cannot act as major confounding factors for PCR in chemotherapy-treated patients.[166] Interestingly, in the study of Ladetto et al., two out of eight patients converting to MRD-positivity after high-dose sequential chemotherapy followed by autologous PB stem cell transplantation (SCT) had different *BCL2-IGH* junctions. In both cases, the molecular recurrence was relatively late and both patients remained in clinical remission.[169] Another very illustrative case report showed persistence of donor-derived t(14;18)-positive nonmalignant B cells in FL patients treated with allogeneic BMT.[170] Moreover, an international multicenter study revealed a high variability of *BCL2-IGH* PCR results between different laboratories, with an unexpectedly high frequency of false-positive results.[171] Such false-positive results due to normal $t(14;18)^+$ cells or intralaboratory contamination can be prevented by routine design of patient-specific oligonucleotides directed against the fusion-region sequence of the *BCL2-IGH* junction (Fig. 4–9).[160,172] Alternatively, RQ-PCR followed by high-resolution capillary electrophoresis may be used to determine the size of the PCR product in order to check for contamination.[173]

MRD Detection via PCR Analysis of BCL1-IGH Fusion Gene Derived from t(11;14)

The t(11;14) is characteristic for most MCL and involves the *BCL1* and *IGH* genes. In 30% to 40% of MCL patients, the breakpoints are clustered within a restricted area (the MTC region), allowing easy identification at the DNA level by standard PCR analysis with one primer located upstream of the MTC in the *BCL1* gene and one primer located within the JH region of the *IGH* gene.[76,174] In these cases, the *BCL1-IGH* fusion gene is an attractive MRD-PCR target. For RQ-PCR–based detection of *BCL1-IGH* fusion genes, several approaches, comparable to those for *BCL2-IGH*, have been reported. A forward *BCL1* primer and fluorogenic probe, both located upstream of the MTC region, in combination with a common JH reverse primer are most often used.[122,123] The same primers can also be used in combination with one or more JH probes,[124] or in combination with SYBR Green I.[175] Instead of applying germline primers only, one could also design one patient-specific oligonucleotide directed against the fusion-region sequence of the *BCL1-IGH* (Fig. 4–9). The use of JH probes has the advantage that these probes can be used in all t(11;14)-positive patients, irrespective of the exact location of the breakpoint in the *BCL1* gene. This may particularly be useful for patients in which the *BCL1* breakpoints are not located within the MTC.[176]

MRD Detection via PCR Analysis of MYC-Ig Fusion Genes Derived from t(8;14), t(2;8), or t(8;22)

Due to the great variability of the breakpoint region in t(8;14) involving the *IGH* and *MYC* genes, a standard PCR assay is generally not sufficient for detection of this translocation, but long-distance (LD)-PCR is frequently successful.[177] The LD-PCR approach was also applied for MRD detection in Burkitt's lymphoma patients, reaching a sensitivity of 10^{-4}.[106]

MRD Detection via PCR Analysis of the SIL-TAL1 Fusion Gene Derived from del(1)(p32p32)

The microdeletion on 1p32 is the most frequent chromosome aberration found in T-LBL, present in 10% to 20% of patients. This microdeletion involves the *TAL1* gene and the *SIL* gene (*SCL* interrupting locus), which is located approximately 90 kb upstream. As a result, the *TAL1* reading frame is placed under the control of the *SIL* promoter, which is expressed in T cells. The *SIL-TAL1* fusion gene can easily be detected by PCR, and therefore is an attractive target for MRD analysis.[178] By using a reverse primer and probe in the *TAL1* gene in combination with a (patient-specific) forward primer located within the *SIL* gene, sensitivities of at least 10^{-4} are generally obtained.

MRD Detection via PCR Analysis of Other Fusion Genes

In many chromosome aberrations, the breakpoints of different patients are scattered over large areas up to 200 kb or more.[179,180] This concerns both chromosome aberrations with aberrantly expressed genes and chromosome aberrations leading to fusion genes with fusion gene transcripts (e.g., *NPM-ALK*).[181] New techniques for rapid and efficient screening of relatively large breakpoint regions, such as long-distance PCR and long-distance inverse PCR,[164,182,183] should render such genomic breakpoint fusion sites into more feasible MRD-PCR targets.

Fusion Gene Transcripts and Aberrantly Expressed Genes

In some lymphomas, fusion gene transcripts or aberrantly expressed genes can theoretically be used for MRD detection. Examples include the *NPM-ALK* fusion gene transcript in ALCL with t(2;5), expression of *CCND1* transcripts in MCL with t(11;14), and over-expression of *MYC* in Burkitt's lymphomas with t(2;8), t(8;14), or t(8;22). Although RQ-PCR assays for such transcripts have been reported,[111–116,184] they have not yet been used for MRD detection. However, theoretically this might be possible, although transcripts in normal cells may limit the sensitivity of the MRD analysis.[185]

Because of the high sensitivity of PCR techniques, cross-contamination of RT-PCR products between patient samples is a major pitfall in RT-PCR–mediated MRD studies, resulting in up to 20% of false-positive results.[186] Such cross-contamination is difficult to recognize, since leukemia-specific fusion gene transcript–derived PCR products and wild-type transcript–derived PCR products are not patient-specific. This is in contrast to PCR products obtained from genomic breakpoint fusion regions, such as in t(14;18) and *TAL1* deletions, which can be identified by use of patient-specific oligonucleotide probes.

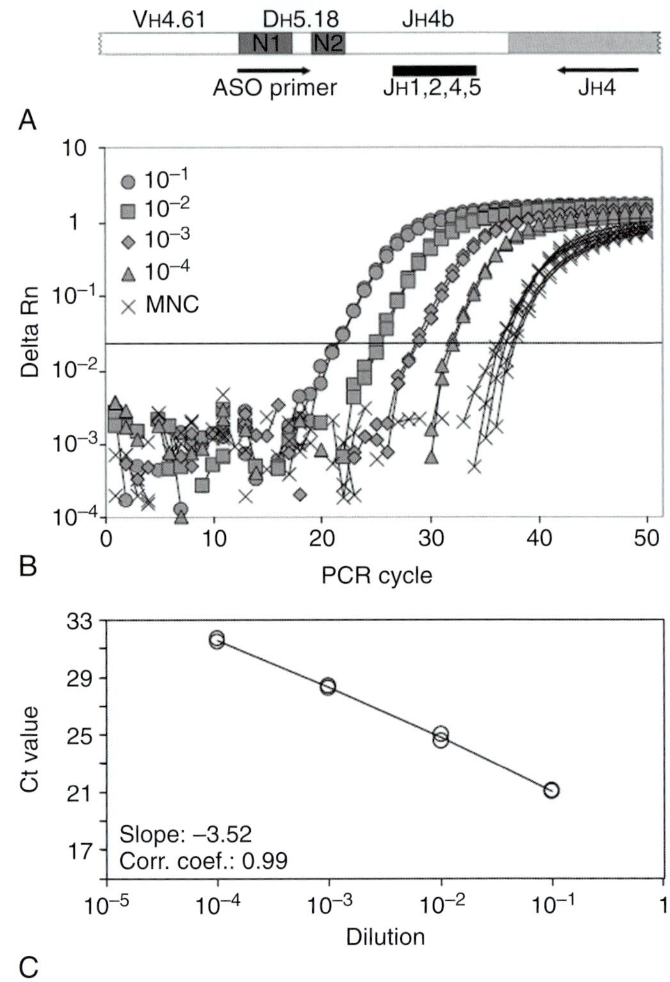

Figure 4–10. RQ-PCR assay for detection of MRD using VH-JH gene rearrangement as a patient-specific target. **A:** Schematic representation of a complete *IGH* gene rearrangement. A patient-specific forward primer was designed for this patient, and used in combination with a germline JH1,2,4,5 hydrolysis probe and germline JH4 reverse primer. **B:** Amplification plot of the RQ-PCR analysis of the rearrangement shown in (**A**). Due to hydrolysis of the TaqMan probe during each PCR cycle the amount of fluorescence increases exponentially, until a plateau phase is reached. Based on the background fluorescence observed within the first 3-15 PCR cycles, a threshold can be set. The cycle at which the fluorescence exceeds this threshold is referred to as the cycle threshold (CT). If a standard curve is prepared using 10-fold dilutions of a diagnostic sample, the CT values of two subsequent dilutions should differ by 3.3 (i.e., 2log(10)). **C:** By plotting the dilution against the CT value, a standard curve is obtained. Based on the CT value of an unknown sample, this standard curve can be used to calculate the relative amount of template present in the unknown sample.

Quantification of MRD Levels

Determining Sensitivity

For MRD analysis, it is not only important to obtain quantitative data, but the assay should also be sufficiently sensitive. The required sensitivity is dependent on the clinical application, but generally a sensitivity of at least 10^{-3}, but preferably 10^{-4} to 10^{-5} should be reached. To determine the sensitivity of the RQ-PCR assay, dilution experiments should be performed, generally using diagnostic material of the patient. By plotting the logarithmic value of the dilution against the CT, a standard curve with a slope of −3.3 should be obtained (see Fig. 4–10). For the analysis of the sensitivity, several criteria (including reproducibility of the measurement, the difference between specific and nonspecific amplification, slope and correlation coefficient of the standard curve) should be taken into account.[108]

Interpretation of MRD Data

Although RQ-PCR is a quantitative technique, it does not mean that the obtained data can be quantified in each case. Particularly low MRD levels, below the reproducible range of the assay, are not reproducible and therefore cannot be quantified appropriately. In addition, discrimination between MRD positivity and MRD negativity can be difficult, particularly for MRD-PCR targets with background amplification. In order to compare data between different studies and/or different laboratories, it is essential to have uniform guidelines for experimental set-up and data interpretation. For Ig/TCR–based MRD data in ALL, such guidelines are currently being developed within the European Study Group on MRD detection in ALL (ESG-MRD-ALL, a consortium of 26 international laboratories, coordinated by J.J.M. van Dongen and V.H.J. van der Velden).[108] These guidelines should be evaluated for use in monitoring of lymphoma as well.

Control Genes

To obtain quantitative MRD-PCR data, it is crucial that control genes are included in the analysis to correct for the quantity and quality of the DNA. One should select a control gene that is located on a chromosome that is not frequently gained or lost in the studied type of lymphoma. The albumin gene, located on chromosome 4, is often used, but other genes (e.g., β-actin, β-globin, and *GAPDH*) can be used as well (reviewed in Van der Velden et al.[108]). Selection of an appropriate control gene for RNA/cDNA targets requires additional criteria, including a similar expression level in different cell types, no relationship with cell cycle or cell activation, a stability comparable to the MRD-PCR target, an expression level comparable to the MRD-PCR target, and the absence of processed pseudogenes. Since genomic DNA frequently contaminates RNA preparations, it is essential to ensure that the primers employed are specific to cDNA.

After having analyzed the control gene, the MRD level as determined by the MRD-PCR target can be corrected for the amount and "amplifiability" of DNA present in the sample. Such correction is usually performed using the standard curve method or the comparative CT method.[108] If the control gene RQ-PCR shows a lower template amount than expected, special caution should be taken for several reasons. First, this lower value can be the result of inhibition. One should note that the degree of inhibition of the control gene RQ-PCR is not always identical to the degree of inhibition in the MRD target RQ-PCR, and consequently an overestimation or underestimation of the MRD level can be made.[187] Addition of bovine serum albumin (BSA) prevents inhibition, and we therefore recommend the routine addition of 0.04% BSA to all RQ-PCR reactions.[187] Second, a lower input of template DNA will result in loss of sensitivity. This especially will be relevant in follow-up samples that seem to be MRD negative. For such samples, it is important to estimate the maximal MRD level that can be detected. Alternatively, one could establish acceptable ranges for control gene values and use these ranges for exclusion of poor samples.

Expression of MRD Data

At present, at least three possibilities exist for the expression of MRD data. First, MRD levels can be determined relative to the diagnostic sample. This method is often used for tumor-specific MRD-PCR targets at the DNA level, such as Ig/TCR gene rearrangements and fusion genes, because calibrators (either cell lines or plasmids) are routinely not available. Second, MRD levels can be expressed relative to a calibrator, such as a cell line known to express the MRD-PCR target of interest. This method is frequently used for MRD-PCR targets that are not patient-specific, such as fusion gene transcripts or *CCND1* expression. By making a standard curve of the calibrator, the MRD level of an unknown sample can be determined relative to the calibrator. Third, data can be expressed as copy numbers by using plasmid standard curves, which is most frequently used for fusion gene transcripts. Plasmids have the advantage of being stable and robust, and thus can be used for the analysis of intra- and inter-laboratory RQ-PCR variations. On the other hand, using plasmids greatly increases the risk of contamination and thereby of false-positive results.[108]

CLINICAL RELEVANCE OF MOLECULAR MONITORING OF NON–HODGKIN'S LYMPHOMAS

The principles of MRD monitoring have been developed in acute leukemias, which are malignant proliferations originating or heavily disseminating into BM compartment and frequently present in PB (reviewed in Szczepanski and Van Dongen[188]). In lymphoma patients, it is generally not possible to monitor minimal residual disease at the original site of disease. However, cytomorphologic evaluation of BM aspirations and trephine biopsies, preferably done bilaterally,[189,190] shows that in proportion of lymphomas malignant cells can be clearly detected in BM at diagnosis (Table 4–6). In a smaller proportion of NHL patients, lymphoma cells are also detectable in PB. In particular, circulating lymphoma cells are frequently found in BM and PB in the subgroup of high- and intermediate-grade lymphomas. Molecular studies can, on the one hand, contribute to better recognition of minimal BM infiltration at diagnosis, undetectable with cytomorphologic analyses. On the other hand, the presence of MRD in BM and to lesser extent in PB might constitute a surrogate marker for treatment effectiveness.

Detection of BM Involvement During Initial Staging of NHL

Molecular detection of BM and/or PB involvement has not yet been routinely implemented into clinical staging of NHL. Nevertheless, several studies demonstrated the presence of aberrant $CD5^+/TdT^+$ cells in BM of most children with T-LBL.[191,192] Also using patient-specific TCR gene rearrangements, it is possible to detect circulating lymphoma cells in BM/PB in virtually all patients with T-LBL.[193] Similarly, it is possible to identify BM monoclonal B-cell subsets characterized by monotypic Ig light-chain expression in an additional 10% to 15% of B-NHL patients without morphological BM involvement.[194] In addition, preliminary results of a PCR–based MRD study of *IGH* genes in B-NHL confirmed a higher incidence of BM involvement than suggested by cytomorphologic findings.[194,195] BM involvement detected by *BCL2-IGH* PCR analysis is a constant feature, not only of advanced stage FL with t(14;18), but also in patients with localized stages I and II.[196,197] Using long-distance PCR for t(8;14), BM involvement was found in more than one-third of samples from children with Burkitt's lymphoma. This mainly concerned patients without morphologic BM involvement, but with advanced-stage disease.[106,107]

Molecular staging might have prognostic significance. This was demonstrated for DLBCL, where it was possible to identify a subset of patients with negative BM histology and positive Ig PCR results characterized by significantly lower complete remission rate and significantly poorer overall survival as compared with patients, in whom both BM histology and PCR results were negative.[198] Further prospective studies should reveal whether detection of submicroscopic BM involvement with sensitivities of 10^{-3} to 10^{-5} would improve prediction of clinical outcome in lymphoma patients. If so, patients with detectable high MRD levels in BM at diagnosis might require more intensive treatment.

Clinical Relevance of MRD Monitoring in FL Patients

Limited Value of MRD Monitoring in PB in FL Patients Treated with Conventional Chemotherapy

The majority of clinical studies concentrated on FL with t(14;18) using the *BCL2-IGH* fusion gene as DNA target for PCR–based MRD analysis (reviewed in Szczepanski and Van Dongen,[188] Corradini et al.,[199] and Darby and Johnson[200]).

Table 4–6. Possibilities for Molecular Monitoring in Most Frequently Occurring Non–Hodgkin's Lymphomas

Type of Lymphoma	Relative Frequency[a]	Dissemination to		Occurrence of Somatic Hypermutation	Availability of MRD-PCR Targets		
		Peripheral Blood[b]	Bone Marrow[a]		Ig/TCR[c]	Chromosome Breakpoint Fusions[d]	Fusion Gene Transcripts
B-cell lymphomas							
Small lymphocytic lymphoma/B-CLL	6.7%	++	~70%	>50%	>98%	–	–
Lymphoplasmacytic lymphoma	1.2%	++	~70%	100%	>95%	–	–
MALT lymphoma	7.6%	±	~10%	100%	85%–90%	30%	30%
Nodal marginal zone lymphoma	1.8%	+	~40%	75%[e]	>95%	–	–
Follicular lymphoma	22.1%	+	~40%	100%	>95%	70%–80%	–
Mantle cell lymphoma	6.0%	+	~60%	<5%	>98%	30%–40%	–
Diffuse large B-cell lymphoma	30.6%	±	~20%	100%	90%–95%	–	–
Mediastinal large B-cell lymphoma	2.4%	–	<5%	100%	>65%	–	–
Burkitt's lymphoma	2.1%	+	~30%	100%	>80%	70%	–
T-cell lymphomas							
Precursor T-cell lymphoblastic lymphoma	1.7%	+	~40%	NA	>95%	15%	–
Anaplastic large-cell lymphoma	2.4%	±	~10%	NA	75%–80%	20%	75%
Mature T-cell lymphomas (except ALCL)	7.6%	+	~40%	NA	>98%	–	–

[a] Based on Jaffe ES, Harris NL, Stein H, et al., eds. World Health Organization Classification of Tumours: Pathology and Genetics of Tumours of Haematopoietic and Lymphoid Tissues. Lyon: IARC Press, 2001[105]; and The Non–Hodgkin's Lymphoma Classification Project. A clinical evaluation of the International Lymphoma Study Group classification of non–Hodgkin's lymphoma. Blood 1997;89:3909–3918.[234]

[b] ++, detectable in >60% of cases; +, detectable in 30%–60% of cases; ±, detectable in 10%–30% of cases; –, detectable in <10% of cases.

[c] Deduced from preliminary results of BIOMED-2 Concerted Action (Evans PAS, Salles G, Groenen PJTA, manuscript in preparation; Brüggemann M, White H, Gaulard P, manuscript in preparation); Sahota SS, Forconi F, Ottensmeier CH, et al. Typical Waldenstrom macroglobulinemia is derived from a B-cell arrested after cessation of somatic mutation but prior to isotype switch events. Blood 2002;100:1505–1507[235]; Fodinger M, Winkler K, Mannhalter C, et al. Combined polymerase chain reaction approach for clonality detection in lymphoid neoplasms. Diagn Mol Pathol 1999;8:80–91[236]; and Leithauser F, Bauerle M, Huynh MQ, et al. Isotype-switched immunoglobulin genes with a high load of somatic hypermutation and lack of ongoing mutational activity are prevalent in mediastinal B-cell lymphoma. Blood 2001;98:2762–2770.[237]

[d] Chromosome breakpoint fusions as detectable by PCR at the DNA level.

[e] Based on Conconi A, Bertoni F, Pedrinis E, et al. Nodal marginal zone B-cell lymphomas may arise from different subsets of marginal zone B lymphocytes. Blood 2001;98:781–786.[238]

NA, not available.

Most FL patients harbor lymphoma cells in BM or PB at initial presentation (Table 4–6), with BM being more informative for MRD monitoring than PB.[196,197,201] More than half of the patients convert to MRD negativity during the first year of cytotoxic treatment, which is associated with longer relapse-free survival.[202] In patients with advanced t(14;18) positive NHL (stage III/IV) treated with conventional induction therapy, no obvious correlation was found between the presence or absence of t(14;18)-positive cells in circulation and relapse-free survival.[203] Using RQ-PCR, Mandigers et al. prospectively assessed response to induction chemotherapy in PB of FL patients.[121] Half of the patients converted to PCR negativity and another one-third had very low levels of MRD as measured in a *BCL2-IGH* RQ-PCR assay. However, this molecular response in PB seemed not to be associated with better progression-free survival.[121]

Apparently, MRD monitoring in PB has limited value in FL patients, but MRD monitoring in BM might be more valuable.

MRD Kinetics in FL Patients Treated with Chimeric CD20 Antibody

Recently, the combination of chemotherapy and treatment with the chimeric (mouse–human) CD20 antibody (Rituximab) was shown to produce durable clinical remission in a subgroup of FL patients accompanied by PCR-negativity in BM and/or PB.[204,205] Patients who achieved sustained molecular remission had significantly better clinical outcome at 3-year follow-up, as compared to persistently MRD-positive patients or those who converted from negativity to MRD-PCR-positivity.[205]

t(14;18)-positive B cells can even be effectively cleared from PB and/or BM in a subset of patients treated with Rituximab as single front-line treatment.[206] PCR-negativity in PB 1 month after treatment completion can identify patients with a significantly lower rate of disease progression during the first year of follow-up.[206] Although a significant subset of patients remained MRD-negative 1 year after completion of Rituximab treatment, the prognostic significance of such molecular remission should be established after longer follow-up.

MRD Detection in Autologous BM Grafts of FL Patients

PB stem cell (SC) harvests in FL with t(14;18) collected after standard mobilization chemotherapy are frequently contaminated by lymphoma cells, with MRD levels comparable to MRD in BM.[207,208] Even CD34$^+$/CD19$^+$ progenitors with t(14;18) could be identified in BM and PB.[209,210] With the currently available techniques it is possible to effectively *ex vivo/in vitro* purge autologous grafts of FL cells, as assessed by the disappearance of clonal *BCL2-IGH* PCR products.[211–213] In addition, PCR analysis of *IGH* gene junctional regions showed that the purging process in autologous BM harvests can be successful in 50% of the FL cases, while it is generally ineffective in patients with DLBCL.[214] Preliminary RQ-PCR data indicated that successful *in vitro* purging of t(14;18)-positive cells is only possible in patients with a low tumor burden in SC harvests.[120] It is virtually impossible to achieve MRD-negativity after purging when PB-SC aphereses contain more than 1% of CD19$^+$ B cells.[215] With recently developed high-dose sequential chemotherapy, it is possible to harvest MRD-PCR–negative autologous BM grafts in most FL patients and MRD-PCR–negative autologous PB grafts in more than half of the patients.[216,217] Such *in vivo* purging is particularly effective after addition of Rituximab. Preliminary data suggest that combination of high-dose chemotherapy and Rituximab can yield MRD-PCR–negative autografts in virtually all patients.[218]

Initial data suggested that patients transplanted with MRD-PCR–negative autologous grafts showed significantly longer disease-free survival in comparison to those whose BM contained residual clonal lymphoma cells after purging.[219] Recent studies also showed that only a small fraction of patients who received an MRD-PCR–negative autologous grafts collected after high-dose sequential chemotherapy relapsed, while more than half of patients who were treated with MRD-positive grafts relapsed.[216,217] In contrast, several other studies could not demonstrate a significant correlation between FL outcome and PCR status of the reinfused BM.[118,220]

Negativity or Persistence of Low MRD Levels in FL Patients in Complete Remission after SCT

Initial studies in a heterogeneous group of B-NHL showed that persistent MRD-PCR positivity in BM after autologous SCT was associated with impending clinical relapse, whereas all patients with eradication of PCR-detectable lymphoma cells remained in continuous clinical remission.[214] Nevertheless, persistence of patient-specific *IGH* gene rearrangements during long-term complete remission has also been reported.[221]

MRD studies for the presence of *BCL2-IGH* transcripts in patients treated with purged autologous SCT showed that the patients in continuous molecular remission after SCT had significantly higher relapse-free survival as compared to patients with persistent PCR positivity.[220,222] In another group of patients treated with autologous PB-SCT, reappearance of PCR positivity at any time post-transplantation was associated with increased relapse risk.[210] Diametrically different conclusions were drawn from another study, in which the majority of patients after purged autologous SCT remained MRD-PCR–positive, and no correlation was found between the MRD-PCR status and relapse-free survival.[223] Such differences in the clinical significance of MRD in FL patients might be at least partly due to differences in intensity of chemotherapy preceding autologous SCT. A recent study demonstrated that intensified high-dose sequential chemotherapy followed by autologous PB-SCT using unpurged grafts leads to MRD-negativity after SCT in two-thirds of patients.[217]

RQ-PCR data indicate that patients in continuous clinical remission after high-dose chemotherapy supported by autologous BMT might become transiently MRD-negative[118]; in most patients *BCL2-IGH* fusion genes were persistently found with stable levels within one order of magnitude.[118] Sequential MRD monitoring using patient-specific PCR techniques in a group of patients with advanced-stage FL treated with high-dose sequential chemotherapy and autografting showed that virtually all patients with all follow-up samples PCR-negative remained in complete remission.[224] In contrast, most patients, who were persistently MRD-positive, relapsed.

Another treatment option for patients with FL might be allogeneic SCT. Monitoring of the number of *BCL2-IGH*-positive cells in BM/PB after allogeneic SCT significantly reflects the clinical remission status. This information might be used to assess the graft-versus-lymphoma effect of allogeneic SCT and subsequent donor lymphocyte infusions in relapsing patients.[225] Recently, allogeneic SCT with a reduced-intensity conditioning regimen including Rituximab was shown to be effective in a subset of FL patients. Preliminary data suggest that such treatment might result in long-term clinical remission and sustained *BCL2-IGH* negativity.[226]

These combined MRD studies indicate that intensified high-dose sequential chemotherapy followed by transplantation with MRD-negative autologous BM or PB-SC grafts is a promising treatment modality in FL patients. Multicenter clinical studies using well-standardized MRD-PCR techniques are required to establish the quantitative criteria for molecular remission in FL and the potential applicability of MRD information for clinical decision making.

Clinical Relevance of MRD Monitoring in MCL Patients

With the use of *IGH* gene rearrangements and *BCL1-IGH* fusion genes as DNA targets, MCL patients were found to be continuously MRD-positive in BM and/or PB during chemotherapy.[227,228] In the majority of MCL patients MRD levels in BM and PB vary between 10^{-2} and 10^{-3}, indicating extensive dissemination of MCL cells and significant resistance to conventional chemotherapy schemes.[228] With more intensive treatment including a combination of the chimeric CD20 antibody and conventional chemotherapy, approximately one-third of MCL patients can reach an MRD-PCR–negative status.[229] However, in the majority of cases this conversion to PCR-negativity is transient, and this molecular remission is not associated with better progression-free survival.

Until recently, it was virtually impossible to harvest autologous MRD-negative BM or PB-SC grafts in MCL.[216,224,227,228] Some mobilization regimens before PB-SC even resulted in increased PB contamination with tumor cells.[228] In addition, the purging procedure in MCL was generally unsuccessful.[213,227,228] Reinfusion of MRD-positive grafts was uniformly associated with the relapse of MCL.[227] Recently, significant progress has been achieved by "*in vivo* purging" of PB CD34$^+$ autografts using a combination of high-dose chemotherapy followed by immunotherapy with Rituximab.[230] With such a regimen, it was possible to obtain optimal amounts of PCR-MRD–negative PB-SC in virtually all MCL patients.[230,231]

Preliminary data suggested that high-dose chemo-radiotherapy followed by autologous PB-SCT might result in molecular remission in a subset of MCL patients.[224,232] MRD-PCR–negativity after PB-SCT was strongly predictive of progression-free survival.[232] These promising data by Pott and colleagues[232] have been recently confirmed by Gianni and colleagues.[231] After standard debulking chemotherapy followed by high-dose chemotherapy, Rituximab, and autografting with MRD-negative PB-SC, the majority of MCL patients achieved durable clinical and molecular remission.[231]

Allogeneic SCT represents another effective treatment regimen for patients with advanced MCL, and preliminary data show conversion to MRD negativity after SCT, which is related to long-term hematologic remission.[227,233]

Clinical Relevance of MRD Monitoring in Children with Burkitt's Lymphoma

A single study evaluated MRD detection in Burkitt's lymphoma patients, who were molecularly positive in BM at initial diagnosis. Most patients had MRD-negativity as assessed with long-distance PCR for t(8;14) after one cycle of intensive chemotherapy. The only two patients who did not reach molecular remission in BM during the treatment succumbed to disease progression.[106] None of the patients with MRD negativity in BM at diagnosis experienced relapse. Thus, it was suggested that MRD monitoring in Burkitt's lymphoma might be restricted to patients with initial molecular BM involvement.[106] However, another group identified a subset of patients without BM/PB involvement at diagnosis who suffered from disease recurrence.[107]

CONCLUSION AND FUTURE ASPECTS OF MOLECULAR MONITORING OF LYMPHOMA

Lymphoma patients cannot be routinely monitored at the original site of disease for evaluation of treatment effectiveness. Furthermore, in contrast to leukemia patients, the dissemination of malignant cells to BM and PB is much less prominent in lymphoma patients. Still, in many lymphoma patients at diagnosis, lymphoma cells are also found in BM and PB at levels of more than 10^{-2} or even 10^{-1}. Consequently, multiple clinical studies have used molecular monitoring of BM and PB samples to evaluate the effectiveness of various treatment modalities, such as high-dose chemotherapy, CD20 antibody treatment, and transplantation. These studies have shown the clinical value of MRD information. Nevertheless, large-scale multicenter clinical studies are needed to fully assess the value of MRD diagnostics before multicenter, MRD-based treatment protocols can be designed.

It is remarkable to see that the majority of clinical MRD studies in lymphoma patients used DNA breakpoint fusions of chromosome aberrations as MRD-PCR targets. This mainly concerned t(14;18), t(11;14), and rarely t(8;14). Consequently, these studies focused on FL, MCL, and Burkitt's lymphoma. Generally the chromosome breakpoint fusions were not sequenced, implying that the applied PCR technique was not patient-specific, but disease-specific. Such nonspecific application of chromosome aberrations as sensitive MRD-PCR targets might lead to false-positive results due to cross-contaminations of PCR products. This cross-contamination still is an underestimated problem in many laboratories.[171]

The preferential usage of chromosome aberrations as PCR targets was probably caused by initial difficulties to identify a suitable Ig or TCR gene rearrangement in each lymphoma patient. The BIOMED-2 Concerted Action BMH4-CT98-3936 has now solved all pitfalls concerning the detection and identification of Ig/TCR gene rearrangements in mature lymphoid malignancies.[76] Furthermore, RQ-PCR techniques are now available for virtually all types of Ig/TCR gene rearrangements.[108,130,131,138,143,144] Therefore, the forthcoming clinical MRD studies can now exploit the BIOMED-2 multiplex tubes and the available RQ-PCR methods, in order to use Ig/TCR gene rearrangements as MRD-PCR targets in virtually all lymphoma patients.

When designing multicenter (international) MRD-based treatment protocols, it is essential that not only the clinical centers closely collaborate, but also the involved MRD-PCR laboratories. In order to obtain fully comparable MRD results, the MRD-PCR laboratories need to use standardized MRD techniques as well as strict guidelines for interpretation of the RQ-PCR results.

MRD-PCR analysis of Ig genes, TCR genes, and chromosome aberrations is now the gold standard for MRD detection in lymphoid malignancies. However, RQ-PCR analysis of patient-specific targets is time-consuming, expensive, and needs high technical skills. Therefore, it will be attractive to use a faster, easier, and cheaper technique, such as flow cytometry. Thus far, flow cytometry is not yet sufficiently sensitive and cannot yet be applied in the majority of lymphoma patients. It will be a challenge to further improve flow-cytometric MRD detection, but this should be possible with the new generation of multicolor flow cytometers (6 to 10 colors) and the development of new antibodies such as those against new oncogenic markers and novel markers as identified by gene expression profiling.

References

1. The International Non–Hodgkin's Lymphoma Prognostic Factors Project. A predictive model for aggressive non–Hodgkin's lymphoma. N Engl J Med 1993;329: 987–94.

2. Szczepanski T, Orfao A, van der Velden VHJ, et al. Minimal residual disease in leukaemia patients. Lancet Oncol 2001;2:409–17.
3. Van Dongen JJM, Seriu T, Panzer-Grumayer ER, et al. Prognostic value of minimal residual disease in acute lymphoblastic leukaemia in childhood. Lancet 1998;352: 1731–8.
4. Willemse MJ, Seriu T, Hettinger K, et al. Detection of minimal residual disease identifies differences in treatment response between T-ALL and precursor B-ALL. Blood 2002;99:4386–93.
5. Davis MM and Björkman PJ. T-cell antigen receptor genes and T-cell recognition. Nature 1988;334:395–402.
6. Owen MJ and Lamb JR, eds. Immune Recognition. Oxford: IRL Press, 1988.
7. Borst J, Brouns GS, de Vries E, et al. Antigen receptors on T and B lymphocytes: parallels in organization and function. Immunol Rev 1993;132:49–84.
8. Klaus GGB. B Lymphocytes. Oxford: Oxford University Press, 1990.
9. Van Dongen JJM, Comans-Bitter WM, Wolvers-Tettero ILM, et al. Development of human T lymphocytes and their thymus-dependency. Thymus 1990;16:207–34.
10. Van Dongen JJM and Wolvers-Tettero ILM. Analysis of immunoglobulin and T cell receptor genes. Part I. Basic and technical aspects. Clin Chim Acta 1991;198: 1–91.
11. Yoshikai Y, Clark SP, Taylor S, et al. Organization and sequences of the variable, joining and constant region genes of the human T-cell receptor alpha-chain. Nature 1985;316:837–40.
12. Griesser H, Champagne E, Tkachuk D, et al. The human T cell receptor alpha-delta locus: a physical map of the variable, joining and constant region genes. Eur J Immunol 1988;18:641–4.
13. Toyonaga B, Yoshikai Y, Vadasz V, et al. Organization and sequences of the diversity, joining, and constant region genes of the human T-cell receptor beta chain. Proc Natl Acad Sci U S A 1985;82:8624–8.
14. Quertermous T, Strauss WM, Van Dongen JJM, et al. Human T cell gamma chain joining regions and T cell development. J Immunol 1987;138:2687–90.
15. Lefranc MP and Rabbitts TH. The human T-cell receptor gamma (TRG) genes. Trends Biochem Sci 1989;14: 214–8.
16. Zhang XM, Tonnelle C, Lefranc MP, et al. T cell receptor gamma cDNA in human fetal liver and thymus: variable regions of gamma chains are restricted to V gamma I or V9, due to the absence of splicing of the V10 and V11 leader intron. Eur J Immunol 1994;24:571–8.
17. Takihara Y, Tkachuk D, Michalopoulos E, et al. Sequence and organization of the diversity, joining, and constant region genes of the human T-cell delta-chain locus. Proc Natl Acad Sci U S A 1988;85:6097–101.
18. Breit TM, Wolvers-Tettero ILM, Beishuizen A, et al. Southern blot patterns, frequencies and junctional diversity of T-cell receptor d gene rearrangements in acute lymphoblastic leukemia. Blood 1993;82:3063–74.
19. Davodeau F, Peyrat MA, Hallet MM, et al. Characterization of a new functional TCR J delta segment in humans. Evidence for a marked conservation of J delta sequences between humans, mice, and sheep. J Immunol 1994;153:137–42.
20. Tonegawa S. Somatic generation of antibody diversity. Nature 1983;302:575–81.
21. Schatz DG, Oettinger MA, and Baltimore D. The V(D)J recombination activating gene, RAG-1. Cell 1989;59: 1035–48.
22. Oettinger MA, Schatz DG, Gorka C, et al. RAG-1 and RAG-2, adjacent genes that synergistically activate V(D)J recombination. Science 1990;248:1517–23.
23. McBlane JF, van Gent DC, Ramsden DA, et al. Cleavage at a V(D)J recombination signal requires only RAG1 and RAG2 proteins and occurs in two steps. Cell 1995;83:387–95.
24. Lieber MR. The mechanism of V(D)J recombination: a balance of diversity, specificity, and stability. Cell 1992;70:873–6.
25. Lieber MR. The role of site-directed recombinases in physiologic and pathologic chromosomal rearrangements. In Kirsch IR, ed. The Causes and Consequences of Chromosomal Aberrations. Boca Raton, FL: CRC Press, 1993:238–45.
26. van Gent DC, Ramsden DA, and Gellert M. The RAG1 and RAG2 proteins establish the 12/23 rule in V(D)J recombination. Cell 1996;85:107–13.
27. Hazenberg MD, Verschuren MC, Hamann D, et al. T cell receptor excision circles as markers for recent thymic emigrants: basic aspects, technical approach, and guidelines for interpretation. J Mol Med 2001;79:631–40.
28. Ye P and Kirschner DE. Reevaluation of T cell receptor excision circles as a measure of human recent thymic emigrants. J Immunol 2002;168:4968–79.
29. Hazenberg MD, Otto SA, Cohen Stuart JW, et al. Increased cell division but not thymic dysfunction rapidly affects the T-cell receptor excision circle content of the naive T cell population in HIV-1 infection. Nat Med 2000;6: 1036–42.
30. Van Dongen JJM and Wolvers-Tettero ILM. Analysis of immunoglobulin and T cell receptor genes. Part II. Possibilities and limitations in the diagnosis and management of lymphoproliferative diseases and related disorders. Clin Chim Acta 1991;198:93–174.
31. Marolleau JP, Fondell JD, Malissen M, et al. The joining of germ-line V alpha to J alpha genes replaces the preexisting V alpha-J alpha complexes in a T cell receptor alpha, beta positive T cell line. Cell 1988;55:291–300.
32. McCormack WT, Liu M, Postema C, et al. Excision products of TCR V alpha recombination contain in-frame rearrangements: evidence for continued V(D)J recombination in TCR+ thymocytes. Int Immunol 1993;5:801–4.
33. Huang C and Kanagawa O. Ordered and coordinated rearrangement of the TCR alpha locus: role of secondary rearrangement in thymic selection. J Immunol 2001;166: 2597–601.
34. Covey LR, Ferrier P, and Alt FW. VH to VHDJH rearrangement is mediated by the internal VH heptamer. Int Immunol 1990;2:579–83.
35. Kleinfield R, Hardy RR, Tarlinton D, et al. Recombination between an expressed immunoglobulin heavy-chain gene and a germline variable gene segment in a Ly 1+ B-cell lymphoma. Nature 1986;322:843–6.
36. Golub R, Huang CY, Kanagawa O, et al. Valpha gene replacement in a TCRalpha knock-in mouse. Eur J Immunol 2001;31:2919–25.
37. Fondell JD, Marolleau JP, Primi D, et al. On the mechanism of non-allelically excluded V alpha-J alpha T cell receptor secondary rearrangements in a murine T cell lymphoma. J Immunol 1990;144:1094–103.
38. Lefranc MP. IMGT databases, web resources and tools for immunoglobulin and T cell receptor sequence analysis, http://imgt.cines.fr. Leukemia 2003;17:260–6.
39. Alt FW, Blackwell TK, and Yancopoulos GD. Development of the primary antibody repertoire. Science 1987; 238:1079–87.
40. Schroeder HW Jr, Hillson JL, and Perlmutter RM. Early restriction of the human antibody repertoire. Science 1987; 238:791–3.

41. Leiden JM, Dialynas DP, Duby AD, et al. Rearrangement and expression of T-cell antigen receptor genes in human T-lymphocyte tumor lines and normal human T-cell clones: evidence for allelic exclusion of Ti beta gene expression and preferential use of a J beta 2 gene segment. Mol Cell Biol 1986;6:3207–14.
42. Triebel F and Hercend T. Subpopulations of human peripheral T gamma delta lymphocytes. Immunol Today 1989; 10:186–8.
43. Borst J, Wicherink A, Van Dongen JJM, et al. Non-random expression of T cell receptor gamma and delta variable gene segments in functional T lymphocyte clones from human peripheral blood. Eur J Immunol 1989;19:1559–68.
44. Breit TM, Wolvers-Tettero IL, and van Dongen JJ. Unique selection determinant in polyclonal V delta 2-J delta 1 junctional regions of human peripheral gamma delta T lymphocytes. J Immunol 1994;152:2860–4.
45. Desiderio SV, Yancopoulos GD, Paskind M, et al. Insertion of N regions into heavy-chain genes is correlated with expression of terminal deoxytransferase in B cells. Nature 1984;311:752–5.
46. Elliott JF, Rock EP, Patten PA, et al. The adult T-cell receptor delta-chain is diverse and distinct from that of fetal thymocytes. Nature 1988;331:627–31.
47. Breit TM, Wolvers-Tettero ILM, Bogers AJ, et al. Rearrangements of the human TCRD-deleting elements. Immunogenetics 1994;40:70–5.
48. Victor KD and Capra JD. An apparently common mechanism of generating antibody diversity: length variation of the VL-JL junction. Mol Immunol 1994;31:39–46.
49. Berek C and Milstein C. Mutation drift and repertoire shift in the maturation of the immune response. Immunol Rev 1987;96:23–41.
50. Rajewsky K, Forster I, and Cumano A. Evolutionary and somatic selection of the antibody repertoire in the mouse. Science 1987;238:1088–94.
51. Romanow WJ, Langerak AW, Goebel P, et al. E2A and EBF act in synergy with the V(D)J recombinase to generate a diverse immunoglobulin repertoire in nonlymphoid cells. Mol Cell 2000;5:343–53.
52. Langerak AW, Wolvers-Tettero ILM, van Gastel-Mol EJ, et al. Basic helix-loop-helix proteins E2A and HEB induce immature T-cell receptor rearrangements in nonlymphoid cells. Blood 2001;98:2456–65.
53. Hieter PA, Korsmeyer SJ, Waldmann TA, et al. Human immunoglobulin kappa light-chain genes are deleted or rearranged in lambda-producing B cells. Nature 1981; 290:368–72.
54. Korsmeyer SJ, Hieter PA, Sharrow SO, et al. Normal human B cells display ordered light chain gene rearrangements and deletions. J Exp Med 1982;156:975–85.
55. Klobeck HG and Zachau HG. The human CK gene segment and the kappa deleting element are closely linked. Nucleic Acids Res 1986;14:4591–4603.
56. Siminovitch KA, Bakhshi A, Goldman P, et al. A uniform deleting element mediates the loss of kappa genes in human B cells. Nature 1985;316:260–2.
57. Langerak AW, Nadel B, De Torbal A, et al. Unraveling the consecutive recombination events in the human IGK locus. J Immunol 2004;173:3878–88.
58. Graninger WB, Goldman PL, Morton CC, et al. The kappa-deleting element. Germline and rearranged, duplicated and dispersed forms. J Exp Med 1988;167:488–501.
59. Ritter MA and Crispe IN. The Thymus. Oxford: Oxford University Press, 1992.
60. De Villartay JP, Hockett RD, Coran D, et al. Deletion of the human T-cell receptor delta-gene by a site-specific recombination. Nature 1988;335:170–4.
61. Hockett RD, de Villartay JP, Pollock K, et al. Human T-cell antigen receptor (TCR) delta-chain locus and elements responsible for its deletion are within the TCR alpha-chain locus. Proc Natl Acad Sci U S A 1988;85:9694–8.
62. Janossy G, Bollum FJ, Bradstock KF, et al. Cellular phenotypes of normal and leukemic hemopoietic cells determined by analysis with selected antibody combinations. Blood 1980;56:430–41.
63. Foon KA and Todd RF. Immunologic classification of leukemia and lymphoma. Blood 1986;68:1–31.
64. Greaves MF. Differentiation-linked leukemogenesis in lymphocytes. Science 1986;234:697–704.
65. Van Dongen JJM, Adriaansen HJ, and Hooijkaas H. Immunophenotyping of leukaemias and non–Hodgkin's lymphomas. Immunological markers and their CD codes. Neth J Med 1988;33:298–314.
66. Raffeld M, Wright JJ, Lipford E, et al. Clonal evolution of t(14;18) follicular lymphomas demonstrated by immunoglobulin genes and the 18q21 major breakpoint region. Cancer Res 1987;47:2537–42.
67. Cleary ML, Galili N, Trela M, et al. Single cell origin of bigenotypic and biphenotypic B cell proliferations in human follicular lymphomas. J Exp Med 1988;167:582–97.
68. Hinz T, Allam A, Wesch D, et al. Cell-surface expression of transrearranged Vgamma-cbeta T-cell receptor chains in healthy donors and in ataxia telangiectasia patients. Br J Haematol 2000;109:201–10.
69. Kobayashi Y, Tycko B, Soreng AL, et al. Transrearrangements between antigen receptor genes in normal human lymphoid tissues and in ataxia telangiectasia. J Immunol 1991; 147:3201–9.
70. Retiere C, Halary F, Peyrat MA, et al. The mechanism of chromosome 7 inversion in human lymphocytes expressing chimeric gamma beta TCR. J Immunol 1999;162:903–10.
71. Stern MH, Lipkowitz S, Aurias A, et al. Inversion of chromosome 7 in ataxia telangiectasia is generated by a rearrangement between T-cell receptor beta and T-cell receptor gamma genes. Blood 1989;74:2076–280.
72. Willis TG and Dyer MJ. The role of immunoglobulin translocations in the pathogenesis of B-cell malignancies. Blood 2000;96:808–22.
73. Bergsagel PL, Chesi M, Nardini E, et al. Promiscuous translocations into immunoglobulin heavy chain switch regions in multiple myeloma. Proc Natl Acad Sci U S A 1996;93: 13931–6.
74. Nishida K, Tamura A, Nakazawa N, et al. The Ig heavy chain gene is frequently involved in chromosomal translocations in multiple myeloma and plasma cell leukemia as detected by in situ hybridization. Blood 1997;90:526–34.
75. Richelda R, Ronchetti D, Baldini L, et al. A novel chromosomal translocation t(4;14)(p16.3;q32) in multiple myeloma involves the fibroblast growth-factor receptor 3 gene. Blood 1997;90:4062–70.
76. Van Dongen JJM, Langerak AW, Bruggemann M, et al. Design and standardization of PCR primers and protocols for detection of clonal immunoglobulin and T-cell receptor gene recombinations in suspect lymphoproliferations. Report of the BIOMED-2 Concerted Action BMH4-CT98-3936. Leukemia 2003;17:2257–317.
77. Yamada M, Hudson S, Tournay O, et al. Detection of minimal disease in hematopoietic malignancies of the B-cell lineage by using third-complementarity–determining region (CDR-III)-specific probes. Proc Natl Acad Sci USA 1989; 86:5123–7.
78. d'Auriol L, Macintyre E, Galibert F, et al. In vitro amplification of T cell gamma gene rearrangements: a new tool for the assessment of minimal residual disease in acute lymphoblastic leukemias. Leukemia 1989;3:155–8.

79. Macintyre EA, d'Auriol L, Duparc N, et al. Use of oligonucleotide probes directed against T cell antigen receptor gamma delta variable-(diversity)-joining junctional sequences as a general method for detecting minimal residual disease in acute lymphoblastic leukemias. J Clin Invest 1990;86:2125–35.
80. Breit TM, Wolvers-Tettero ILM, Hählen K, et al. Extensive junctional diversity of gd T-cell receptors expressed by T-cell acute lymphoblastic leukemias: implications for the detection of minimal residual disease. Leukemia 1991;5:1076–86.
81. Deane M and Norton JD. Immunoglobulin heavy chain variable region family usage is independent of tumor cell phenotype in human B lineage leukemias. Eur J Immunol 1990;20:2209–17.
82. Deane M, Pappas H, and Norton JD. Immunoglobulin heavy chain gene fingerprinting reveals widespread oligoclonality in B-lineage acute lymphoblastic leukaemia. Leukemia 1991;5:832–8.
83. Veelken H, Tycko B, and Sklar J. Sensitive detection of clonal antigen receptor gene rearrangements for the diagnosis and monitoring of lymphoid neoplasms by a polymerase chain reaction–mediated ribonuclease protection assay. Blood 1991;78:1318–26.
84. Hansen-Hagge TE, Yokota S, and Bartram CR. Detection of minimal residual disease in acute lymphoblastic leukemia by in vitro amplification of rearranged T-cell receptor delta chain sequences. Blood 1989;74:1762–7.
85. Jonsson OG, Kitchens RL, Scott FC, et al. Detection of minimal residual disease in acute lymphoblastic leukemia using immunoglobulin hypervariable region specific oligonucleotide probes. Blood 1990;76:2072–9.
86. Schäble KF and Zachau HG. The variable genes of the human immunoglobulin kappa locus. Biol Chem Hoppe Seyler 1993;374:1001–22.
87. Williams SC and Winter G. Cloning and sequencing of human immunoglobulin V lambda gene segments. Eur J Immunol 1993;23:1456–61.
88. Oksenberg JR, Stuart S, Begovich AB, et al. Limited heterogeneity of rearranged T-cell receptor V alpha transcripts in brains of multiple sclerosis patients. Nature 1991;353:94.
89. Broeren CP, Verjans GM, Van Eden W, et al. Conserved nucleotide sequences at the 5' end of T cell receptor variable genes facilitate polymerase chain reaction amplification. Eur J Immunol 1991;21:569–75.
90. Doherty PJ, Roifman CM, Pan SH, et al. Expression of the human T cell receptor V beta repertoire. Mol Immunol 1991;28:607–12.
91. Wei S, Charmley P, Robinson MA, et al. The extent of the human germline T-cell receptor V beta gene segment repertoire. Immunogenetics 1994;40:27–36.
92. Droese J, Langerak AW, Groenen PJ, et al. Validation of BIOMED-2 multiplex PCR tubes for detection of TCRB gene rearrangements in T-cell malignancies. Leukemia 2004; 18:1531–8.
93. Ravetch JV, Siebenlist U, Korsmeyer S, et al. Structure of the human immunoglobulin mu locus: characterization of embryonic and rearranged J and D genes. Cell 1981; 27:583–91.
94. Matsuda F, Shin EK, Nagaoka H, et al. Structure and physical map of 64 variable segments in the 3'0.8-megabase region of the human immunoglobulin heavy-chain locus. Nat Genet 1993;3:88–94.
95. Van Oostveen JW, Breit TM, de Wolf JT, et al. Polyclonal expansion of T-cell receptor-gd+ T lymphocytes associated with neutropenia and thrombocytopenia. Leukemia 1992; 6:410–8.
96. Davis TH, Yockey CE, and Balk SP. Detection of clonal immunoglobulin gene rearrangements by polymerase chain reaction amplification and single-strand conformational polymorphism analysis. Am J Pathol 1993;142:1841–7.
97. Koch OM, Volkenandt M, Goker E, et al. Molecular detection and characterization of clonal cell populations in acute lymphocytic leukemia by analysis of conformational polymorphisms of cRNA molecules of rearranged T-cell-receptor-gamma and immunoglobulin heavy-chain genes. Leukemia 1994;8:946–52.
98. Bourguin A, Tung R, Galili N, et al. Rapid, nonradioactive detection of clonal T-cell receptor gene rearrangements in lymphoid neoplasms. Proc Natl Acad Sci USA 1990;87: 8536–40.
99. Wood GS, Tung RM, Haeffner AC, et al. Detection of clonal T-cell receptor gamma gene rearrangements in early mycosis fungoides/Sezary syndrome by polymerase chain reaction and denaturing gradient gel electrophoresis (PCR/DGGE). J Invest Dermatol 1994;103:34–41.
100. Linke B, Pyttlich J, Tiemann M, et al. Identification and structural analysis of rearranged immunoglobulin heavy chain genes in lymphomas and leukemias. Leukemia 1995;9:840–7.
101. Bottaro M, Berti E, Biondi A, et al. Heteroduplex analysis of T-cell receptor gamma gene rearrangements for diagnosis and monitoring of cutaneous T-cell lymphomas. Blood 1994;83:3271–8.
102. Langerak AW, Szczepanski T, van der Burg M, et al. Heteroduplex PCR analysis of rearranged T cell receptor genes for clonality assessment in suspect T cell proliferations. Leukemia 1997;11:2192–9.
103. Kneba M, Bolz I, Linke B, et al. Analysis of rearranged T-cell receptor beta-chain genes by polymerase chain reaction (PCR) DNA sequencing and automated high resolution PCR fragment analysis. Blood 1995;86:3930–7.
104. Linke B, Bolz I, Fayyazi A, et al. Automated high resolution PCR fragment analysis for identification of clonally rearranged immunoglobulin heavy chain genes. Leukemia 1997;11:1055–62.
105. Jaffe ES, Harris NL, Stein H, et al, eds. World Health Organization Classification of Tumours: Pathology and Genetics of Tumours of Haematopoietic and Lymphoid Tissues. Lyon: IARC Press, 2001.
106. Mussolin L, Basso K, Pillon M, et al. Prospective analysis of minimal bone marrow infiltration in pediatric Burkitt's lymphomas by long-distance polymerase chain reaction for t(8;14)(q24;q32). Leukemia 2003;17:585–9.
107. Busch K, Borkhardt A, Wossmann W, et al. Combined polymerase chain reaction methods to detect c-myc/IgH rearrangement in childhood Burkitt's lymphoma for minimal residual disease analysis. Haematologica 2004;89: 818–25.
108. Van der Velden VHJ, Hochhaus A, Cazzaniga G, et al. Detection of minimal residual disease in hematologic malignancies by real-time quantitative PCR: principles, approaches, and laboratory aspects. Leukemia 2003;17:1013–34.
109. Pongers-Willemse MJ, Verhagen OJHM, Tibbe GJM, et al. Real-time quantitative PCR for the detection of minimal residual disease in acute lymphoblastic leukemia using junctional regions specific TaqMan probes. Leukemia 1998; 12:2006–14.
110. Nakao M, Janssen JW, Flohr T, et al. Rapid and reliable quantification of minimal residual disease in acute lymphoblastic leukemia using rearranged immunoglobulin and T-cell receptor loci by LightCycler technology. Cancer Res 2000; 60:3281–9.
111. Koiso H, Tsukamoto N, Miyawaki S, et al. Quantitative analysis of cyclin D1 and CD23 expression in mantle cell lymphoma and B-chronic lymphocytic leukemia. Leuk Res 2002;26:809–15.

112. Medeiros LJ, Hai S, Thomazy VA, et al. Real-time RT-PCR assay for quantifying cyclin D1 mRNA in B-cell non–Hodgkin's lymphomas. Mod Pathol 2002;15:556–64.
113. Bijwaard KE, Aguilera NS, Monczak Y, et al. Quantitative real-time reverse transcription-PCR assay for cyclin D1 expression: utility in the diagnosis of mantle cell lymphoma. Clin Chem 2001;47:195–201.
114. Peghini PE and Fehr J. Analysis of cyclin D1 expression by quantitative real-time reverse transcription-polymerase chain reaction in the diagnosis of mantle cell lymphoma. Am J Clin Pathol 2002;117:237–45.
115. Suzuki R, Takemura K, Tsutsumi M, et al. Detection of cyclin D1 overexpression by real-time reverse-transcriptase–mediated quantitative polymerase chain reaction for the diagnosis of mantle cell lymphoma. Am J Pathol 2001; 159:425–9.
116. Elenitoba-Johnson KS, Bohling SD, Jenson SD, et al. Fluorescence PCR quantification of cyclin D1 expression. J Mol Diagn 2002;4:90–6.
117. Estalilla OC, Medeiros LJ, Manning JT Jr, et al. 5′→3′ exonuclease-based real-time PCR assays for detecting the t(14;18)(q32;21): a survey of 162 malignant lymphomas and reactive specimens. Mod Pathol 2000;13:661–6.
118. Hirt C and Dolken G. Quantitative detection of t(14;18)-positive cells in patients with follicular lymphoma before and after autologous bone marrow transplantation. Bone Marrow Transplant 2000;25:419–26.
119. Dolken L, Schuler F, and Dolken G. Quantitative detection of t(14;18)-positive cells by real-time quantitative PCR using fluorogenic probes. Biotechniques 1998;25:1058–64.
120. Ladetto M, Sametti S, Donovan JW, et al. A validated real-time quantitative PCR approach shows a correlation between tumor burden and successful ex vivo purging in follicular lymphoma patients. Exp Hematol 2001;29:183–93.
121. Mandigers CM, Meijerink JP, Mensink EJ, et al. Lack of correlation between numbers of circulating t(14;18)-positive cells and response to first-line treatment in follicular lymphoma. Blood 2001;98:940–4.
122. Olsson K, Gerard CJ, Zehnder J, et al. Real-time t(11;14) and t(14;18) PCR assays provide sensitive and quantitative assessments of minimal residual disease (MRD). Leukemia 1999;13:1833–42.
123. Luthra R, Sarris AH, Hai S, et al. Real-time 5′→3′ exonuclease-based PCR assay for detection of the t(11;14)(q13;q32). Am J Clin Pathol 1999;112:524–30.
124. Andersen NS, Donovan JW, Zuckerman A, et al. Real-time polymerase chain reaction estimation of bone marrow tumor burden using clonal immunoglobulin heavy chain gene and bcl-1/JH rearrangements in mantle cell lymphoma. Exp Hematol 2002;30:703–10.
125. Bertoni F, Zucca E, Genini D, et al. Immunoglobulin light chain kappa deletion rearrangement as a marker of clonality in mantle cell lymphoma. Leuk Lymphoma 1999;36:147–50.
126. Hoogeveen-Westerveld M, Hupkes PE, Doekharan D, et al. Rearranged immunoglobulin light chain genes as minimal residual disease markers in intermediate- and high-grade malignant B cell non–Hodgkin's lymphoma. Leukemia 1998;12:1810–16.
127. Cleary ML, Meeker TC, Levy S, et al. Clustering of extensive somatic mutations in the variable region of an immunoglobulin heavy chain gene from a human B cell lymphoma. Cell 1986;44:97–106.
128. Reth M, Gehrmann P, Petrac E, et al. A novel VH to VHDJH joining mechanism in heavy-chain-negative (null) pre-B cells results in heavy-chain production. Nature 1986; 322:840–2.
129. Ladetto M, Donovan JW, Harig S, et al. Real-time polymerase chain reaction of immunoglobulin rearrangements for quantitative evaluation of minimal residual disease in multiple myeloma. Biol Blood Marrow Transplant 2000;6: 241–53.
130. Van der Velden VHJ, Wijkhuijs JM, Jacobs DCH, et al. T cell receptor gamma gene rearrangements as targets for detection of minimal residual disease in acute lymphoblastic leukemia by real-time quantitative PCR analysis. Leukemia 2002; 16:1372–80.
131. Verhagen OJHM, Willemse MJ, Breunis WB, et al. Application of germline *IGH* probes in real-time quantitative PCR for the detection of minimal residual disease in acute lymphoblastic leukemia. Leukemia 2000;14:1426–35.
132. Bruggemann M, Droese J, Bolz I, et al. Improved assessment of minimal residual disease in B cell malignancies using fluorogenic consensus probes for real-time quantitative PCR. Leukemia 2000;14:1419–25.
133. Donovan JW, Ladetto M, Zou G, et al. Immunoglobulin heavy-chain consensus probes for real-time PCR quantification of residual disease in acute lymphoblastic leukemia. Blood 2000;95:2651–8.
134. Pfitzner T, Engert A, Wittor H, et al. A real-time PCR assay for the quantification of residual malignant cells in B cell chronic lymphatic leukemia. Leukemia 2000;14: 754–66.
135. Rasmussen T, Poulsen TS, Honore L, et al. Quantitation of minimal residual disease in multiple myeloma using an allele-specific real-time PCR assay. Exp Hematol 2000;28: 1039–45.
136. Eckert C, Landt O, Taube T, et al. Potential of LightCycler technology for quantification of minimal residual disease in childhood acute lymphoblastic leukemia. Leukemia 2000; 14:316–23.
137. Gerard CJ, Olsson K, Ramanathan R, et al. Improved quantitation of minimal residual disease in multiple myeloma using real-time polymerase chain reaction and plasmid-DNA complementarity determining region III standards. Cancer Res 1998;58:3957–64.
138. Van der Velden VHJ, Willemse MJ, van der Schoot CE, et al. Immunoglobulin kappa deleting element rearrangements in precursor-B acute lymphoblastic leukemia are stable targets for detection of minimal residual disease by real-time quantitative PCR. Leukemia 2002;16:928–36.
139. Szczepanski T, van der Velden VHJ, and van Dongen JJM. Real-time quantitative (RQ)-PCR for the detection of minimal residual disease in childhood acute lymphoblastic leukemia. Haematologica 2002;87 Suppl. 1:183–91.
140. Uchiyama M, Maesawa C, Yashima-Abo A, et al. Short consensus probes with 3'-minor groove binder of the immunoglobulin heavy-chain gene for real-time quantitative PCR in B-cell non-Hodgkin lymphomas. Lab Invest 2004;84:932–6.
141. Langerak AW, Wolvers-Tettero ILM, and van Dongen JJM. Detection of T cell receptor beta (TCRB) gene rearrangement patterns in T cell malignancies by Southern blot analysis. Leukemia 1999;13:965–74.
142. Langerak AW, van Den Beemd R, Wolvers-Tettero ILM, et al. Molecular and flow cytometric analysis of the Vbeta repertoire for clonality assessment in mature TCRalphabeta T-cell proliferations. Blood 2001;98:165–73.
143. Bruggemann M, Van der Velden VHJ, Raff T, et al. Rearranged T-cell receptor beta genes represent powerful targets for quantification of minimal residual disease in childhood and adult T-cell acute lymphoblastic leukemia. Leukemia 2004;18:709–19.
144. Szczepanski T, Van der Velden VHJ, Hoogeveen PG, et al. Vdelta2-Jalpha rearrangements are frequent in precursor–B-acute lymphoblastic leukemia but rare in normal lymphoid cells. Blood 2004;103:3798–804.

145. Sanz I. Multiple mechanisms participate in the generation of diversity of human H chain CDR3 regions. J Immunol 1991;147:1720–9.
146. Wasserman R, Galili N, Ito Y, et al. Predominance of fetal type DJH joining in young children with B precursor lymphoblastic leukemia as evidence for an in utero transforming event. J Exp Med 1992;176:1577–81.
147. Yamada M, Wasserman R, Reichard BA, et al. Preferential utilization of specific immunoglobulin heavy chain diversity and joining segments in adult human peripheral blood B lymphocytes. J Exp Med 1991;173:395–407.
148. Steenbergen EJ, Verhagen OJ, van Leeuwen EF, et al. B precursor acute lymphoblastic leukemia third complementarity-determining regions predominantly represent an unbiased recombination repertoire: leukemic transformation frequently occurs in fetal life. Eur J Immunol 1994;24:900–8.
149. Van Wering ER, van der Linden-Schrever BEM, van der Velden VHJ, et al. T lymphocytes in bone marrow samples of children with acute lymphoblastic leukemia during and after chemotherapy might hamper PCR–based minimal residual disease studies. Leukemia 2001;15:1031–3.
150. Van Wering ER, van der Linden-Schrever BE, Szczepanski T, et al. Regenerating normal B-cell precursors during and after treatment of acute lymphoblastic leukaemia: implications for monitoring of minimal residual disease. Br J Haematol 2000;110:139–46.
151. Van Lochem EG, Wiegers YM, van den Beemd R, et al. Regeneration pattern of precursor-B-cells in bone marrow of acute lymphoblastic leukemia patients depends on the type of preceding chemotherapy. Leukemia 2000;14:688–95.
152. Breit TM, Beishuizen A, Ludwig WD, et al. tal-1 deletions in T-cell acute lymphoblastic leukemia as PCR target for detection of minimal residual disease. Leukemia 1993;7:2004–11.
153. Gribben JG. Monitoring disease in lymphoma and CLL patients using molecular techniques. Best Pract Res Clin Haematol 2002;15:179–95.
154. Cleary ML and Sklar J. Nucleotide sequence of a t(14;18) chromosomal breakpoint in follicular lymphoma and demonstration of a breakpoint-cluster region near a transcriptionally active locus on chromosome 18. Proc Natl Acad Sci U S A 1985;82:7439–43.
155. Williams ME, Meeker TC, and Swerdlow SH. Rearrangement of the chromosome 11 bcl-1 locus in centrocytic lymphoma: analysis with multiple breakpoint probes. Blood 1991; 78:493–498.
156. Leder P, Battey J, Lenoir G, et al. Translocations among antibody genes in human cancer. Science 1983;222:765–71.
157. Morris SW, Kirstein MN, Valentine MB, et al. Fusion of a kinase gene, ALK, to a nucleolar protein gene, NPM, in non–Hodgkin's lymphoma. Science 1994;263:1281–4.
158. Yunis JJ, Oken MM, Kaplan ME, et al. Distinctive chromosomal abnormalities in histologic subtypes of non–Hodgkin's lymphoma. N Engl J Med 1982;307:1231–6.
159. Luthra R, McBride JA, Cabanillas F, et al. Novel 5' exonuclease-based real-time PCR assay for the detection of t(14;18)(q32;q21) in patients with follicular lymphoma. Am J Pathol 1998;153:63–8.
160. Jenner MJ, Summers KE, Norton AJ, et al. JH probe real-time quantitative polymerase chain reaction assay for Bcl-2/IgH rearrangements. Br J Haematol 2002;118:550–8.
161. Bohling SD, King TC, Wittwer CT, et al. Rapid simultaneous amplification and detection of the MBR/JH chromosomal translocation by fluorescence melting curve analysis. Am J Pathol 1999;154:97–103.
162. Buchonnet G, Jardin F, Jean N, et al. Distribution of BCL2 breakpoints in follicular lymphoma and correlation with clinical features: specific subtypes or same disease? Leukemia 2002;16:1852–6.
163. Albinger-Hegyi A, Hochreutener B, Abdou MT, et al. High frequency of t(14;18)-translocation breakpoints outside of major breakpoint and minor cluster regions in follicular lymphomas: improved polymerase chain reaction protocols for their detection. Am J Pathol 2002;160:823–32.
164. Akasaka T, Muramatsu M, Ohno H, et al. Application of long-distance polymerase chain reaction to detection of junctional sequences created by chromosomal translocation in mature B-cell neoplasms. Blood 1996;88:985–94.
165. Limpens J, Stad R, Vos C, et al. Lymphoma-associated translocation t(14;18) in blood B cells of normal individuals. Blood 1995;85:2528–36.
166. Ladetto M, Drandi D, Compagno M, et al. PCR-detectable nonneoplastic Bcl-2/IgH rearrangements are common in normal subjects and cancer patients at diagnosis but rare in subjects treated with chemotherapy. J Clin Oncol 2003;21: 1398–1403.
167. Summers KE, Goff LK, Wilson AG, et al. Frequency of the Bcl-2/IgH rearrangement in normal individuals: implications for the monitoring of disease in patients with follicular lymphoma. J Clin Oncol 2001;19:420–24.
168. Finke J, Slanina J, Lange W, et al Persistence of circulating t(14;18)-positive cells in long-term remission after radiation therapy for localized-stage follicular lymphoma. J Clin Oncol 1993;11:1668–73.
169. Ladetto M, Mantoan B, Ricca I, et al. Recurrence of Bcl-2/IgH polymerase chain reaction positivity following a prolonged molecular remission can be unrelated to the original follicular lymphoma clone. Exp Hematol 2003;31:784–8.
170. Rosenblum MD, Drobyski WR, Keever-Taylor C, et al. Concurrent presence of both patient and donor t(14;18) in a follicular lymphoma patient after undergoing allogeneic BMT: implications for minimal residual disease detection post-transplant. Bone Marrow Transplant 2003;31:947–9.
171. Johnson PW, Swinbank K, MacLennan S, et al. Variability of polymerase chain reaction detection of the bcl-2-IgH translocation in an international multicentre study. Ann Oncol 1999;10:1349–54.
172. Galoin S, al Saati T, Schlaifer D, et al. Oligonucleotide clonospecific probes directed against the junctional sequence of t(14;18): a new tool for the assessment of minimal residual disease in follicular lymphomas. Br J Haematol 1996; 94:676–84.
173. Sanchez-Vega B, Vega F, Hai S, et al. Real-time t(14;18) (q32;q21) PCR assay combined with high-resolution capillary electrophoresis: a novel and rapid approach that allows accurate quantitation and size determination of bcl-2/JH fusion sequences. Mod Pathol 2002;15:448–53.
174. Tsujimoto Y, Yunis J, Onorato-Showe L, et al. Molecular cloning of the chromosomal breakpoint of B-cell lymphomas and leukemias with the t(11;14) chromosome translocation. Science 1984;224:1403–6.
175. Bohling SD, Wittwer CT, King TC, et al. Fluorescence melting curve analysis for the detection of the bcl-1/JH translocation in mantle cell lymphoma. Lab Invest 1999; 79:337–45.
176. Degan M, Doliana R, Gloghini A, et al. A novel bcl-1/JH breakpoint from a patient affected by mantle cell lymphoma extends the major translocation cluster. J Pathol 2002;197: 256–63.
177. Basso K, Frascella E, Zanesco L, et al. Improved long-distance polymerase chain reaction for the detection of t(8;14)(q24;q32) in Burkitt's lymphomas. Am J Pathol 1999; 155:1479–85.
178. Pongers-Willemse MJ, Seriu T, et al. Primers and protocols for standardized MRD detection in ALL using immunoglobulin and T cell receptor gene rearrangements and TAL1 deletions as PCR targets. Report of the BIOMED-1 Concerted

Action: investigation of minimal residual disease in acute leukemia. Leukemia 1999;13:110–18.
179. Joos S, Haluska FG, Falk MH, et al. Mapping chromosomal breakpoints of Burkitt's t(8;14) translocations far upstream of c-myc. Cancer Res 1992;52:6547–52.
180. Joos S, Falk MH, Lichter P, et al. Variable breakpoints in Burkitt lymphoma cells with chromosomal t(8;14) translocation separate c-myc and the IgH locus up to several hundred kb. Hum Mol Genet 1992;1:625–32.
181. Sarris AH, Luthra R, Papadimitracopoulou V, et al. Amplification of genomic DNA demonstrates the presence of the t(2;5) (p23;q35) in anaplastic large cell lymphoma, but not in other non–Hodgkin's lymphomas, Hodgkin's disease, or lymphomatoid papulosis. Blood 1996;88:1771–9.
182. Reichel M, Gillert E, Breitenlohner I, et al. Rapid isolation of chromosomal breakpoints from patients with t(4;11) acute lymphoblastic leukemia: implications for basic and clinical research. Leukemia 2001;15:286–8.
183. Wiemels JL, Cazzaniga G, Daniotti M, et al. Prenatal origin of acute lymphoblastic leukaemia in children. Lancet 1999;354:1499–1503.
184. Saez AI, Artiga MJ, Romero C, et al. Development of a real-time reverse transcription polymerase chain reaction assay for c-myc expression that allows the identification of a subset of c-myc+ diffuse large B-cell lymphoma. Lab Invest 2003;83:143–52.
185. Maes B, Vanhentenrijk V, Wlodarska I, et al. The NPM-ALK and the ATIC-ALK fusion genes can be detected in non-neoplastic cells. Am J Pathol 2001;158:2185–93.
186. Gabert J, Beillard E, Van der Velden VHJ, et al. Standardization and quality control studies of 'real-time' quantitative reverse transcriptase polymerase chain reaction of fusion gene transcripts for residual disease detection in leukemia—a Europe Against Cancer program. Leukemia 2003;17: 2318–57.
187. Moppett J, van der Velden VHJ, Wijkhuijs AJ, et al. Inhibition affecting RQ-PCR–based assessment of minimal residual disease in acute lymphoblastic leukemia: reversal by addition of bovine serum albumin. Leukemia 2003;17: 268–70.
188. Szczepanski T and Van Dongen JJM. Detection of minimal residual disease. In Henderson ES, Lister TA, Greaves MF, eds. Leukemia. Philadelphia: WB Saunders, 2002: 249–83.
189. Sandlund JT, Downing JR, and Crist WM. Non–Hodgkin's lymphoma in childhood. N Engl J Med 1996;334:1238–48.
190. Evans L and Hancock B. Non–Hodgkin lymphoma. Lancet 2003;362:139–46.
191. Van Dongen JJM, Hooijkaas H, Adriaansen HJ, et al. Detection of minimal residual acute lymphoblastic leukemia by immunological marker analysis: possibilities and limitations. In Hagenbeek A and Löwenberg B, eds. Minimal Residual Disease in Acute Leukemia. Dordrecht: M Nijhoff Publishers, 1986:113–33.
192. Bradstock KF and Kerr A. Immunological detection of covert leukaemic spread in mediastinal T- cell lymphoblastic lymphoma. Leuk Res 1985;9:905–11.
193. Sabesan V, Cairo MS, Lones MA, et al. Assessment of minimal residual disease in childhood non-hodgkin lymphoma by polymerase chain reaction using patient-specific primers. J Pediatr Hematol Oncol 2003;25:109–13.
194. Gomyo H, Shimoyama M, Minagawa K, et al. Morphologic, flow cytometric and cytogenetic evaluation of bone marrow involvement in B-cell lymphoma. Haematologica 2003; 88:1358–65.
195. Kurokawa T, Kinoshita T, Ito T, et al. Detection of minimal residual disease B cell lymphoma by a PCR-mediated RNase protection assay. Leukemia 1996;10:1222–31.
196. Gribben JG, Freedman A, Woo SD, et al. All advanced stage non–Hodgkin's lymphomas with a polymerase chain reaction amplifiable breakpoint of bcl-2 have residual cells containing the bcl-2 rearrangement at evaluation and after treatment. Blood 1991;78:3275–80.
197. Lambrechts AC, Hupkes PE, Dorssers LC, et al. Translocation (14;18)-positive cells are present in the circulation of the majority of patients with localized (stage I and II) follicular non–Hodgkin's lymphoma. Blood 1993;82:2510–16.
198. Mitterbauer-Hohendanner G, Mannhalter C, Winkler K, et al. Prognostic significance of molecular staging by PCR-amplification of immunoglobulin gene rearrangements in diffuse large B-cell lymphoma (DLBCL). Leukemia 2004;18:1102–07.
199. Corradini P, Ladetto M, Pileri A, et al. Clinical relevance of minimal residual disease monitoring in non–Hodgkin's lymphomas: a critical reappraisal of molecular strategies. Leukemia 1999;13:1691–95.
200. Darby AJ and Johnson PW. Molecular remission and non–Hodgkin's lymphoma. Best Pract Res Clin Haematol 2002;15:549–62.
201. Gribben JG, Neuberg D, Barber M, et al. Detection of residual lymphoma cells by polymerase chain reaction in peripheral blood is significantly less predictive for relapse than detection in bone marrow. Blood 1994;83:3800–07.
202. Lopez-Guillermo A, Cabanillas F, McLaughlin P, et al. The clinical significance of molecular response in indolent follicular lymphomas. Blood 1998;91:2955–60.
203. Lambrechts AC, Hupkes PE, Dorssers LC, et al. Clinical significance of t(14;18)-positive cells in the circulation of patients with stage III or IV follicular non–Hodgkin's lymphoma during first remission. J Clin Oncol 1994;12:1541–6.
204. Czuczman MS, Grillo-Lopez AJ, White CA, et al. Treatment of patients with low-grade B-cell lymphoma with the combination of chimeric anti-CD20 monoclonal antibody and CHOP chemotherapy. J Clin Oncol 1999;17:268–76.
205. Rambaldi A, Lazzari M, Manzoni C, et al. Monitoring of minimal residual disease after CHOP and rituximab in previously untreated patients with follicular lymphoma. Blood 2002;99:856–62.
206. Colombat P, Salles G, Brousse N, et al. Rituximab (anti-CD20 monoclonal antibody) as single first-line therapy for patients with follicular lymphoma with a low tumor burden: clinical and molecular evaluation. Blood 2001;97:101–6.
207. Hardingham JE, Kotasek D, Sage RE, et al. Molecular detection of residual lymphoma cells in peripheral blood stem cell harvests and following autologous transplantation. Bone Marrow Transplant 1993;11:15–20.
208. Leonard BM, Hetu F, Busque L, et al. Lymphoma cell burden in progenitor cell grafts measured by competitive polymerase chain reaction: less than one log difference between bone marrow and peripheral blood sources. Blood 1998;91:331–9.
209. Macintyre EA, Belanger C, Debert C, et al. Detection of clonal CD34+19+ progenitors in bone marrow of BCL2-IgH-positive follicular lymphoma patients. Blood 1995; 86:4691–8.
210. Moos M, Schulz R, Martin S, et al. The remission status before and the PCR status after high-dose therapy with peripheral blood stem cell support are prognostic factors for relapse-free survival in patients with follicular non–Hodgkin's lymphoma. Leukemia 1998;12:1971–6.
211. Gribben JG, Saporito L, Barber M, et al. Bone marrows of non–Hodgkin's lymphoma patients with a bcl-2 translocation can be purged of polymerase chain reaction-detectable lymphoma cells using monoclonal antibodies and immunomagnetic bead depletion. Blood 1992;80:1083–9.
212. Di Nicola M, Siena S, Corradini P, et al. Elimination of bcl-2-IgH-positive follicular lymphoma cells from blood trans-

plants with high recovery of hematopoietic progenitors by the miltenyi CD34+ cell sorting system. Bone Marrow Transplant 1996;18:1117–21.

213. Tarella C, Corradini P, Astolfi M, et al. Negative immunomagnetic ex vivo purging combined with high-dose chemotherapy with peripheral blood progenitor cell autograft in follicular lymphoma patients: evidence for long-term clinical and molecular remissions. Leukemia 1999; 13:1456–62.
214. Zwicky CS, Maddocks AB, Andersen N, et al. Eradication of polymerase chain reaction detectable immunoglobulin gene rearrangement in non–Hodgkin's lymphoma is associated with decreased relapse after autologous bone marrow transplantation. Blood 1996;88:3314–22.
215. Straka C, Oduncu F, Drexler E, et al. The CD19+ B-cell counts at peripheral blood stem cell mobilization determine different levels of tumour contamination and autograft purgability in low-grade lymphoma. Br J Haematol 2002;116: 695–701.
216. Corradini P, Astolfi M, Cherasco C, et al. Molecular monitoring of minimal residual disease in follicular and mantle cell non–Hodgkin's lymphomas treated with high-dose chemotherapy and peripheral blood progenitor cell autografting. Blood 1997;89:724–31.
217. Ladetto M, Corradini P, Vallet S, et al High rate of clinical and molecular remissions in follicular lymphoma patients receiving high-dose sequential chemotherapy and autografting at diagnosis: a multicenter, prospective study by the Gruppo Italiano Trapianto Midollo Osseo (GITMO). Blood 2002;100:1559–65.
218. Galimberti S, Guerrini F, Morabito F, et al. Quantitative molecular evaluation in autotransplant programs for follicular lymphoma: efficacy of in vivo purging by Rituximab. Bone Marrow Transplant 2003;32:57–63.
219. Gribben JG, Freedman AS, Neuberg D, et al. Immunologic purging of marrow assessed by PCR before autologous bone marrow transplantation for B-cell lymphoma. N Engl J Med 1991;325:1525–33.
220. Apostolidis J, Gupta RK, Grenzelias D, et al. High-dose therapy with autologous bone marrow support as consolidation of remission in follicular lymphoma: long-term clinical and molecular follow-up. J Clin Oncol 2000; 18:527–536.
221. Scholten C, Hilgarth B, Hilgarth M, et al. Predictive value of clone-specific CDR3 PCR in high-grade non–Hodgkin's lymphoma: long-term persistence of a clone-specific rearrangement in a patient with secondary high-grade NHL in remission after high-dose therapy. Br J Haematol 1997; 97:246–47.
222. Gribben JG, Neuberg D, Freedman AS, et al. Detection by polymerase chain reaction of residual cells with the bcl-2 translocation is associated with increased risk of relapse after autologous bone marrow transplantation for B-cell lymphoma. Blood 1993;81:3449–57.
223. Johnson PW, Price CG, Smith T, et al. Detection of cells bearing the t(14;18) translocation following myeloablative treatment and autologous bone marrow transplantation for follicular lymphoma. J Clin Oncol 1994;12:798–805.
224. Corradini P, Ladetto M, Zallio F, et al. Long-term follow-up of indolent lymphoma patients treated with high-dose sequential chemotherapy and autografting: evidence that durable molecular and clinical remission frequently can be attained only in follicular subtypes. J Clin Oncol 2004;22:1460–68.
225. Mandigers CM, Meijerink JP, Raemaekers JM, et al. Graft-versus-lymphoma effect of donor leucocyte infusion shown by real-time quantitative PCR analysis of t(14;18). Lancet 1998;352:1522–3.
226. Ho AY, Devereux S, Mufti GJ, et alA. Reduced-intensity rituximab-BEAM-CAMPATH allogeneic haematopoietic stem cell transplantation for follicular lymphoma is feasible and induces durable molecular remissions. Bone Marrow Transplant 2003;31:551–7.
227. Andersen NS, Donovan JW, Borus JS, et al. Failure of immunologic purging in mantle cell lymphoma assessed by polymerase chain reaction detection of minimal residual disease. Blood 1997;90:4212–21.
228. Jacquy C, Lambert F, Soree A, et al. Peripheral blood stem cell contamination in mantle cell non-Hodgkin lymphoma: the case for purging? Bone Marrow Transplant 1999;23:681–6.
229. Howard OM, Gribben JG, Neuberg DS, et al. Rituximab and CHOP induction therapy for newly diagnosed mantle-cell lymphoma: molecular complete responses are not predictive of progression-free survival. J Clin Oncol 2002;20:1288–94.
230. Magni M, Di Nicola M, Devizzi L, et al. Successful in vivo purging of CD34-containing peripheral blood harvests in mantle cell and indolent lymphoma: evidence for a role of both chemotherapy and rituximab infusion. Blood 2000;96:864–9.
231. Gianni AM, Magni M, Martelli M, et al. Long-term remission in mantle cell lymphoma following high-dose sequential chemotherapy and in vivo rituximab-purged stem cell autografting (R-HDS regimen). Blood 2003;102:749–55.
232. Pott C, Schrader C, Derner N, et al. Molecular remission predicts progression-free survival in mantle cell lymphoma after peripheral blood stem cell transplantation. Ann Oncol 2002;13:69a.
233. Corradini P, Ladetto M, Astolfi M, et al. Clinical and molecular remission after allogeneic blood cell transplantation in a patient with mantle-cell lymphoma. Br J Haematol 1996;94:376–8.
234. The Non–Hodgkin's Lymphoma Classification Project. A clinical evaluation of the International Lymphoma Study Group classification of non–Hodgkin's lymphoma. Blood 1997;89:3909–18.
235. Sahota SS, Forconi F, Ottensmeier CH, et alFK. Typical Waldenstrom macroglobulinemia is derived from a B-cell arrested after cessation of somatic mutation but prior to isotype switch events. Blood 2002;100:1505–07.
236. Fodinger M, Winkler K, Mannhalter C, et al. Combined polymerase chain reaction approach for clonality detection in lymphoid neoplasms. Diagn Mol Pathol 1999;8:80–91.
237. Leithauser F, Bauerle M, Huynh MQ, et al. Isotype-switched immunoglobulin genes with a high load of somatic hypermutation and lack of ongoing mutational activity are prevalent in mediastinal B-cell lymphoma. Blood 2001;98: 2762–70.
238. Conconi A, Bertoni F, Pedrinis E, et al. Nodal marginal zone B-cell lymphomas may arise from different subsets of marginal zone B lymphocytes. Blood 2001;98:781–6.

5

Molecular Diagnosis of the Lymphomas by Gene Expression Profiling

Louis M. Staudt, M.D., Ph.D.

Throughout the history of cancer diagnosis, new technologies have catalyzed the classification of cancer into biologically and clinically meaningful subgroups. Notable past examples include the development of cytological stains that highlight morphologic differences between cancer types, the development of monoclonal antibodies and their use in flow cytometry and immunohistochemistry, and the application of molecular biological techniques to reveal the activation of oncogenes and the inactivation of tumor suppressor genes. The Human Genome Project has provided a powerful new approach to the molecular diagnosis of cancer known as gene expression profiling.[1] The technological platform for gene expression profiling is the DNA microarray, an ordered array of thousands of genes on a solid support. DNA microarrays are able to simultaneously measure the mRNA expression levels of each gene on the array, resulting in a profile of gene activity in a cell. Differential mRNA expression underlies many fundamental biological processes, including cellular lineage decisions, differentiation, cellular proliferation and survival, and cell–cell interactions. The gene expression profiles of cancer cells can therefore provide information about the cell of origin of the cancer, the mechanisms of malignant transformation, and the interplay between cancer cells and tumor-infiltrating normal cells.

Current diagnostic categories can often be readily associated with characteristic gene expression signatures. Although the majority of cases within a diagnostic category may be accurately diagnosed by current methods, these characteristic gene expression signatures may help solidify the diagnosis or, in a minority of difficult cases, may call the diagnosis into question and suggest an alternative. In addition, gene expression profiling can identify molecularly distinct subgroups of cancer that are indistinguishable by current methodologies. These newly discovered cancer subgroups can have all the hallmarks of distinct diseases: they may have different normal cellular counterparts, different oncogenic lesions, and different clinical outcomes. Such observations provide the basis for suggesting a new taxonomy of cancer that is based on comprehensive molecular analysis, and not solely on morphology.

Indeed, one of the most perplexing problems in cancer diagnosis and treatment is that patients given the same diagnosis can have widely divergent clinical outcomes. The gene expression profiles of cancer biopsies obtained at diagnosis can be used to divide current diagnostic categories into molecular distinct diseases with different responses to therapy and/or different overall survival rates. In addition, gene expression–based predictors of survival can be constructed that further account for the observed clinical heterogeneity. In many cases, the genes that constitute these molecular diagnoses and prognoses reflect underlying biological features of the tumors that influence survival.

Cancer subgroups defined by gene expression profiling can be more molecularly and clinically homogeneous than those defined by current diagnostic methods. In many cases, particular oncogenic events occur selectively in one cancer subgroup, suggesting that therapeutic strategies may ultimately be tailored to the specific molecular features of a patient's tumor. Indeed, gene expression profiling has already uncovered new therapeutic targets in certain lymphoma subgroups. This chapter will provide examples for each of these principles derived from gene expression profiling studies of the lymphomas.

ANALYTIC METHODS FOR GENE EXPRESSION PROFILING

Prior to the advent of DNA microarrays, the molecular analysis of cancer focused on a handful of oncogenes and tumor suppressor genes about which much was known. This "classic" approach has been fruitful, but DNA microarrays now allow a more agnostic view of which genes are important for cancer. Gene expression profiling can provide expression data on virtually all of the roughly 30,000 genes encoded in the human genome, which poses a tremendous interpretive challenge.[2–4]

Two general methods have been applied to gene expression profiling data derived from cancer specimens. In an "unsupervised" approach, the gene expression patterns are used to discover relationships between samples, often resulting in the definition of cancer subgroups that share broad gene expression programs. Various pattern recognition algorithms are used in this effort, each of which begins with a choice of genes whose gene expression levels vary among cancer specimens. The gene set can either be all genes represented on a DNA microarray or a subset of the genes that focuses attention on a particular biological feature of the specimens. The subgroups of cancer that are defined using an unsupervised approach are highly dependent on the gene set used. In general, the value of a cancer subgroup distinction is gauged by whether the subgroups utilize different pathogenetic mechanisms or differ with respect to clinical features such as treatment response and survival.

In the "supervised" approach, external clinical or molecular data are used to identify those genes whose expression patterns vary in a biologically important fashion. Statistical methods are used to correlate the expression of each gene on a DNA microarray with the behavior of an external parameter. Often the external parameter is a clinical variable such as overall survival, response to therapy, tumor stage and anatomic location of disease, or metastatic behavior. Alternatively, the external parameter can be a molecular feature of the tumor such as the presence of a translocation, mutation in a gene, or deletions or amplifications of a chromosomal region. Based on a statistical cutoff, a list of genes is generated that can be used to "predict" the external parameter.

The peril of the supervised approach is that the predictive models that are created may be "over-fit" to the data used to generate them. As a result, the models may perform poorly when tested on independent data sets. One way to minimize this danger is to use a "leave-one-out cross-validation strategy" in which one sample is removed from the data set, a predictive model is created on the remaining samples, and the model is used to predict the nature of the excluded sample. However, the most definitive way to prove that a predictive model has not been over-fit to the data is to divide the cases into a "training" set that is used to create the model, and a "validation" set that is used to test its performance. Gene expression profiling studies that employ this methodology and demonstrate that the derived statistical model performs well in an independent validation set will have the greatest chance of being reproduced using different patient cohorts.

When using either the unsupervised or supervised methods, it is important to derive biological meaning from the lists of genes that are found to discriminate cancer subgroups or predict clinical behavior. A helpful approach to this goal is to make use of gene expression "signatures."[5] Broadly defined, a gene expression signature is a set of genes that are co-regulated in association with a particular biological process. For example, a gene expression signature may be composed of genes that are characteristically expressed in a particular cell lineage or stage of differentiation. Gene expression signatures can also reflect biological processes such as cellular proliferation or the response to nutrient starvation. Discrete gene expression signatures can be also be defined that reflect the action of individual transcription factors or signaling pathways. By measuring the expression of gene expression signature within a cancer sample, it is possible to derive multiple biological insights about the cancer, such as its cell of origin, proliferation rate, and utilization of particular regulatory pathways.[5] Thus, gene expression signature analysis can provide an "executive summary" of the biological features of a cancer sample.

Gene expression signatures are, by definition, composed of co-regulated genes, but the proteins encoded by these genes may have disparate functions. Another way to gain insight into the biology underlying gene expression profiles is to make use of lists of genes whose protein products are functionally linked to a biological process. Large international consortia are engaged in curating lists of genes that function in particular biological processes.[6] However, genes that encode functionally related proteins may or may not be co-regulated. Statistical methods have been developed to detect the enrichment of a set of functionally related genes within a larger group of genes that, for example, discriminate two cancer types.[7] With the variety of analytical tools described above, researchers can use gene expression profiling data to develop new insights into cancer pathogenesis, clinical behavior, and treatment response.

DIFFUSE LARGE B-CELL LYMPHOMA (DLBCL)

Gene Expression Subgroups within DLBCL

DLBCL has long been enigmatic in that roughly 40% of patients can be cured by anthracycline-based combination chemotherapy, whereas the remainder succumb to this disease.[8] This clinical heterogeneity can be traced to molecular heterogeneity in these tumors at diagnosis.[9] In actuality, the diagnostic category of DLBCL is an amalgam of at least three distinct molecular subgroups that are morphologically indistinguishable.[9–13] These three subgroups have been termed germinal center B-cell–like (GCB) DLBCL, activated B-cell–like (ABC) DLBCL, and primary mediastinal B-cell lymphoma (PMBL), and can be readily distinguished from one another by the expression of hundreds of genes (Fig. 5–1A). As detailed below, these DLBCL subgroups can be considered distinct diseases in that they originate from B cells at different stages of differentiation, use distinct oncogenic mechanisms, and differ significantly in their survival rates following chemotherapy.

An early application of DNA microarray technology identified the GCB and ABC DLBCL subgroups, and demonstrated that they differ in the expression of thousands of genes.[9] Several lines of evidence support the view that GCB and ABC DLBCL arise from B cells at different stages of differentiation. First, GCB DLBCLs express hundreds of genes that are characteristically expressed in normal germinal center B cells, whereas ABC DLBCLs have down-regulated these genes.[9,13] These genes encode well-known germinal center B-cell surface markers such as CD10, but also a wide variety of transcription factors and signaling molecules. Thus, GCB DLBCLs have "inherited" the gene expression program of normal germinal center B cells and, by inference, would also share certain biological features with germinal center B cells.

One of the genes that best discriminates GCB and ABC DLBCL is BCL-6, the oncogene that is most frequently deregulated and/or mutated in DLBCL.[14,15] BCL-6 is a transcriptional repressor that blocks expression of a set of B-cell activation genes, the cell cycle inhibitor p27kip1, and the transcriptional repressor Blimp-1.[16,17] Blimp-1 is a powerful regulatory factor that promotes plasmacytic differentiation by, on one hand, blocking the expression of virtually the entire set of mature B-cell differentiation genes and, on the other hand, blocking expression of c-myc and other proliferation associated genes, leading to cell cycle arrest.[18] Thus, the expression of BCL-6 in GCB DLBCLs may serve to promote cell cycle progression by repressing p27kip1 and derepressing c-myc, and may block plasmacytic differentiation by repressing Blimp-1. BCL-6 is also likely to affect other aspects of GC biology, possibly by blocking cellular senescence[19] and interfering with the expression of molecules such as CD80 that influence the interaction of B and T cells.[20]

In contrast, ABC DLBCLs may be derived from a B cell that is in the process of differentiating from a germinal

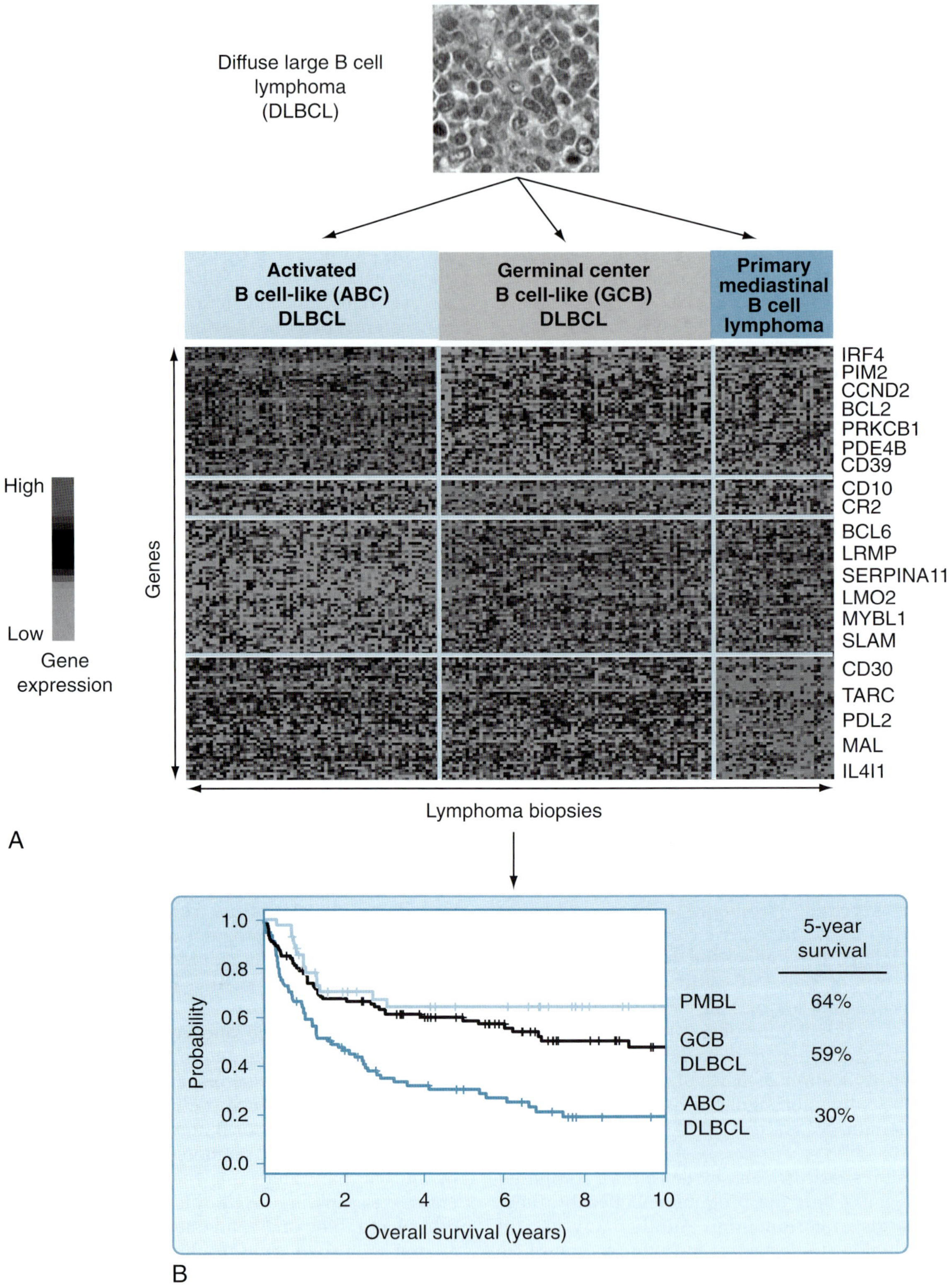

Figure 5–1. Definition of molecularly and clinically distinct subgroups of diffuse large B-cell lymphoma (DLBCL) by gene expression profiling. **A:** Gene expression differences between germinal center B-cell–like (GCB) DLBCL, activated B-cell–like DLBCL, and primary mediastinal B-cell lymphoma (PMBL). Each row represents gene expression data from an individual biopsy sample, and each column represents a single gene on the DNA microarray. Relative gene expression is indicated according to the color bar shown at the left. Representative genes that distinguish the DLBCL subgroups are indicated. Not shown are ~18% of DLBCLs that do not fit any of the three gene expression subgroups well. **B:** DLBCL gene expression subgroups have distinct overall survival rates following chemotherapy. Kaplan–Meier plot showing overall survival of patients in each of the DLBCL subgroups. (Data adapted from Fig. 3A in Rosenwald A, Wright G, Leroy K, et al. Molecular diagnosis of primary mediastinal B cell lymphoma identifies a clinically favorable subgroup of diffuse large B cell lymphoma related to Hodgkin lymphoma. J Exp Med 2003;198:851–62, with permission.) (See color insert.)

center B cell to a plasma cell. A large number of genes that are characteristically expressed in plasma cells are more highly expressed in ABC DLBCLs than in GCB DLBCLs.[13] These include XBP-1, a transcription factor that is responsible for the secretory phenotype of plasma cells.[21] ABC DLBCLs express XBP-1 and various of its target genes that encode endoplasmic reticulum and Golgi apparatus proteins.[13] However, ABC DLBCLs lack expression of other plasma cell genes, and thus are phenotypically different from multiple myeloma.

Analysis of immunoglobulin gene mutations in DLBCLs lends support to the hypothesis that germinal center B cells give rise to GCB DLBCLs, whereas post-germinal center B cells give rise to ABC DLBCLs.[22] GCB DLBCLs were found to have ongoing somatic hypermutation of the rearranged immunoglobulin gene within the malignant clone, which is also a feature of normal germinal center B cells. The immunoglobulin genes of ABC DLBCLs were also highly mutated, suggesting that the cell from which these lymphomas originated had traversed the germinal center. However, ABC DLBCLs were not found to have ongoing somatic hypermutation, in keeping with the notion that they are derived from a post-germinal center B cell that has inactivated the somatic hypermutation mechanism.

The gene expression dichotomy between GCB and ABC DLBCLs has been observed in two subsequent studies that included 58 DLBCL patients[13,23] and 273 DLBCL patients,[10] respectively. An algorithm was devised, based on Bayesian statistics, that determines the probability that a patient's tumor belongs to the GCB or ABC DLBCL subgroup.[13] Although this method was developed using gene expression data from the "Lymphochip" spotted DNA microarray,[24] it was also able to classify DLBCL samples that were profiled using Affymetrix oligonucleotide microarrays. The robustness of this algorithm across different microarray platforms should facilitate the translation of these findings into the clinical setting. Using this algorithm, approximately 40% of DLBCLs belong to the GCB subgroup and 34% belong to the ABC DLBCL subgroup. Among the remaining 26% of DLBCLs, roughly 8% are PMBLs (see below), but the others remain unclassified.

Gene expression profiling was used to develop a molecular diagnosis of PMBL,[11,25] a subgroup of DLBCL that had been previously defined largely by clinical criteria.[26,27] PMBL differs from GCB and ABC DLBCL by the expression of hundreds of genes, which enabled the development of a gene expression–based predictor of this distinction[25] (Fig. 5–1A). Clinically, PMBL patients were younger (median age 33) than patients with GCB or ABC DLBCL (median age over 60), and the tumors involved the mediastinum and other thoracic structures.[25] Although these clinical differences are in accord with the previous studies of PMBL, it is important to emphasize that only 75% of the samples deemed to be PMBL on clinical grounds were found to have the gene expression profile of PMBL.[25] The samples that lacked the PMBL profile were GCB or ABC DLBCLs that happened to involve the mediastinum prominently.

A striking and unanticipated relationship was found between PMBL and Hodgkin's lymphoma by gene expression profiling.[11,25] Over one-third of the genes that were more highly expressed in PMBL than in other DLBCL subgroups were also expressed in Hodgkin's lymphoma cell lines (Fig. 5–2A). These include known markers of PMBL such as Mal[28] and IL4I.[29] Several of these genes encode proteins that have been shown to be highly expressed in primary Hodgkin's Reed–Sternberg cells from nodular sclerosing Hodgkin's lymphoma, including CD30,[30] IL-13 receptor α,[31] TARC,[32] and Mal[25] (Fig. 5–2B).

In the light of this strong molecular resemblance, it is particularly notable that PMBL and Hodgkin's lymphoma share numerous other clinical and pathologic features, including prevalence in young patients, especially women, presentation in the mediastinum, and prominence of sclerosis in the tumors.[33] It has been speculated that the cell of origin of PMBL is the rare B-cell population that resides in the thymus.[28] It is possible that the gene expression similarities between PMBL and Hodgkin's lymphoma indicate that both of these lymphoma types can originate in the thymus from the same type of normal B-cell precursor. Additionally, these lymphomas may use common oncogenic pathways that confer a particular gene expression signature. Indeed, PMBL and Hodgkin's lymphoma express genes that targets of the NF-κB and interferon signaling pathways, suggesting that these pathways are constitutively activated by unknown mechanisms in both lymphoma types[11,25] (Fig. 5–2A). Gain or amplification of chromosome region 9p24 is characteristic of both PMBL and Hodgkin's lymphoma, and is not present in other DLBCLs, providing a further molecular link between these lymphomas[25,34,35] (Fig. 5–3A). Despite these striking molecular similarities, PMBL and Hodgkin's lymphoma can be readily distinguished by gene expression profiling,[25] suggesting that they use some distinct pathogenetic pathways. Nonetheless, given the many important molecular similarities between PMBL and HL, it is conceivable that these lymphomas may respond similarly to certain therapeutic approaches.

Clinical Differences Between DLBCL Subgroups

Importantly, the molecular diagnosis of DLBCL subgroups identifies groups of patients who differ in their survival following treatment with anthracycline-based chemotherapy regimens[9,10,13] (Fig. 5–1B). The 5-year survival rates of PMBL, GCB DLBCL, and ABC DLBCL patients in one patient cohort were found to be 64%, 59%, and 31%, respectively.[13] The GCB DLBCL and ABC DLBCL subgroups identified in a another patient cohort had similarly distinct 5-year survival rates of 62% and 26%, respectively.[13] Several immunohistochemistry studies have approximated the distinction between GCB DLBCL and ABC DLBCL by analyzing the expression of a few proteins, and have confirmed the clinical differences between the subgroups.[36–39] For example, one study used two markers of GCB DLBCL (CD10 and BCL-6), and one marker of ABC DLBCL (IRF4/MUM-1). By immunohistochemistry, this study defined a GCB DLBCL subgroup equivalent (CD10+ or BCL6+/IRF4–), and a non-GCB DLBCL subgroup (CD10–/BCL-6+/IRF4+ or CD10-BCL6–), and these two DLBCL subsets had 5-year survival rates of 76% and 34%, respectively.[39] The fact that no one protein marker was sufficient to differentiate the DLBCL subgroups underscores the virtue of profiling the expression of many genes in parallel on DNA microarrays. The survival differences between the

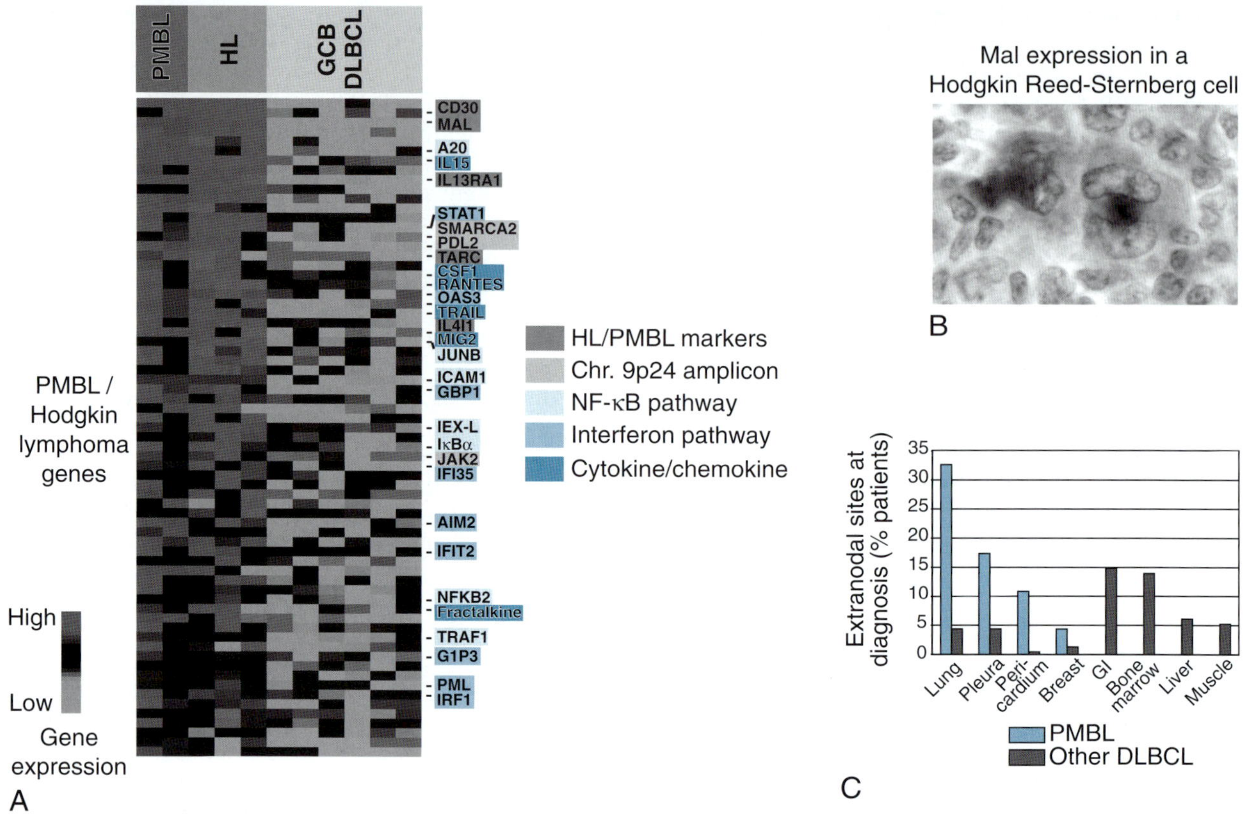

Figure 5–2. Similarities between primary mediastinal B-cell lymphoma (PMBL) and Hodgkin lymphoma. **A:** PMBL and Hodgkin's lymphoma (HL) share a broad gene expression program. The 69 genes depicted are all PMBL "signature" genes that are more highly expressed in PMBL than in other DLBCLs, and are also more highly expressed in HL cell lines than in germinal center B-cell–like (GCB) DLBCL cell lines. Average gene expression levels in primary PMBL tumors (*lane 1*) and in a PMBL cell line, K1106 (*lane 2*), are shown. Also shown are gene expression levels in three HL cell lines and in six GCB DLBCL cell lines. Selected genes are highlighted that have been shown to be characteristically expressed in primary Hodgkin's Reed–Sternberg cells and/or PMBL cells (*black*). Also highlighted are genes that are activated by signaling through the NF-κB (*red*) or interferon (*brown*) pathways. Numerous genes encoding chemokines and cytokines, many of which are activated by the NF-κB pathway, are also indicated (*blue*). PMBL and HL tumors frequently harbor a gain/amplification of chromosome region 9p24, which contains several genes that are characteristically expressed in both lymphoma types (*green*). **B:** Detection of Mal protein expression in a primary Hodgkin's Reed–Sternberg cell by immunohistochemistry. **C:** Frequency of involvement of various extra nodal sites in PMBL and other DLBCLs. PMBL, like HL, frequently extends to various thoracic structures (**left**). Extranodal sites that are frequently involved in other DLBCLs are not involved in cases of PMBL (**right**). (Data are adapted from Figs. 3B, 5A, and 6B in Rosenwald A, Wright G, Leroy K, et al. Molecular diagnosis of primary mediastinal B cell lymphoma identifies a clinically favorable subgroup of diffuse large B cell lymphoma related to Hodgkin lymphoma. J Exp Med 2003;198:851–62, with permission.) (See color insert.)

DLBCL subgroups support the view that they should be viewed as distinct diseases.

The DLBCL subgroup distinction accounts for some, but not all, of the heterogeneity in the response of DLBCL patients to treatment. The remaining clinical heterogeneity can be traced to other molecular differences between the DLBCL tumors (see below) and to clinical factors such as those that are included in the International Prognostic Index (IPI).[40] The DLBCL subgroup distinction is statistically independent of the IPI in predicting survival, demonstrating that these subgroups are not acting simply as surrogates for the clinical variables.[9,10] Nonetheless, there are some statistically significant differences between the DLBCL subgroups with respect to individual components of the IPI. In comparison to patients with GCB DLBCL, patients with ABC DLBCL were more often aged over 60 and had a poorer performance status (ECOG > 2).[10] The majority of patients with PMBL (53%) were aged under 35, whereas the majority of patients with GCB or ABC DLBCL (59%) were over 60.[25] These considerations suggest that clinical trials in DLBCL that selectively enroll patients based on age or performance status may be skewed in their representation of the particular DLBCL subgroups.

The DLBCL subgroups also differ with respect to involvement of extra nodal sites[25] (Fig. 5–2C). The extra nodal sites most often involved in PMBL are the lung, pleura, pericardium, and breast, suggesting that this disease spreads by local extension from the mediastinum to other thoracic structures. These sites are infrequently involved in patients with other forms of DLBCL. By contrast, the frequent sites of extra nodal involvement in GCB and ABC DLBCL are the gastrointestinal tract, bone marrow, liver,

	GCB DLBCL	ABC DLBCL	PMBL
c-rel amplification	16%	0	25%
BCL-2 translocation	45%	0	18%
Gain chromosome 3q	0	24%	5%
Gain/amp chromosome 9p24	0	6%	43%
Constitutive NF- κB activation	–	+	+

A

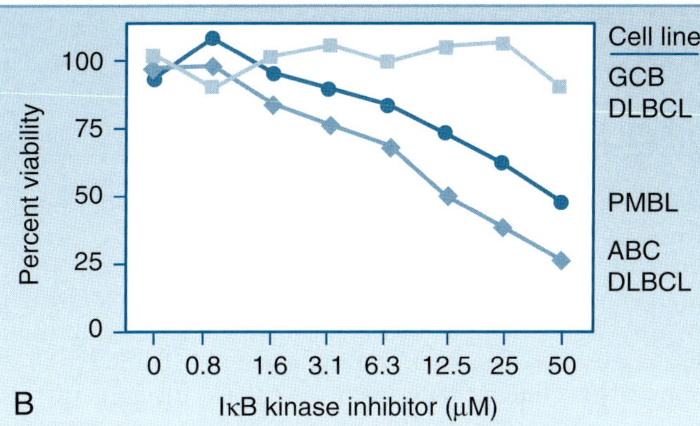

B

Figure 5–3. DLBCL subgroups use distinct pathogenetic mechanisms. **A:** Recurrent oncogenic changes in DLBCL are associated with particular gene expression subgroups. The frequency of the indicated genomic or signaling abnormalities in each DLBCL subgroup is indicated.[10,25,43,45,46] **B:** Constitutive IκB kinase activity is required for survival of ABC DLBCL and PMBL cells, but not GCB DLBCL cells. Cell line models of GCB DLBCL (OCI-Ly7), ABC DLBCL (OCI-Ly3), and PMBL (K1106) were treated with a small molecule inhibitor of IκB kinase, and viability was compared at 48 hours for untreated cells.[46]

and muscle, and these extra nodal sites are not involved in PMBL. Further analysis is needed to uncover the molecular mechanisms accounting for the ability of certain DLBCLs to propagate in specific extra nodal sites.

Distinct Oncogenic Mechanisms in DLBCL Subgroups

Analysis of recurrent translocations, chromosomal abnormalities, and oncogenic signaling pathways has revealed striking differences in the frequency of these oncogenic events in the DLBCL subgroups (Fig. 5–3A). The nonrandom distribution of these abnormalities strongly supports the notion that the DLBCL subgroups represent distinct disease entities that use different pathogenetic mechanisms.

Two recurrent oncogenic abnormalities in DLBCL, the t(14;18) translocation involving *BCL2* and amplification of the *c-rel* locus, were detected in a fraction of GCB DLBCL and PMBL tumors, but never in ABC DLBCL tumors[10,41] (Fig. 5–3A). The t(14;18) increases BCL2 gene and protein expression in those GCB DLBCLs and PMBLs that bear this translocation. By contrast, many ABC DLBCLs have high *BCL2* expression in the absence of the t(14;18) translocation[10] (Fig. 5–1A). The t(14;18) translocation would therefore not provide a selective advantage to ABC DLBCLs, which may explain its absence in this DLBCL subgroup. In fact, the majority of DLBCLs that over-express BCL-2 protein belong to the ABC DLBCL subgroup. Previous studies have associated BCL-2 protein expression, but not the t(14;18), with inferior survival in DLBCL.[42] This finding may be explained by the high expression of *BCL2* in ABC DLBCLs, which have a relatively poor prognosis.

Comparative genomic hybridization analysis revealed that almost one quarter of ABC DLBCL tumors had a gain of the chromosome 3q arm, often in the context of trisomy 3, yet this abnormality was never detected in GCB DLBCL and only rarely in PMBL[43] (Fig. 5–3A). It is currently unclear which molecular pathways are influenced by gains of 3q. However, it is notable that tumors with this abnormality have lower expression of the "lymph node" gene expression signature that reflects tumor-infiltrating host cells (see below), suggesting that 3q gains alter the interaction between the tumor and its microenvironment.[43] The genomic copy number of the chromosome 9p24 region was increased in 43% of PMBLs, but never in GCB DLBCLs and only rarely in ABC DLBCLs.[25] This region contains several genes that are over-expressed as a result of the translocation, including *JAK2* and *PDL2* (Fig. 5–2A). JAK2 tyrosine kinase activity has been detected in PMBL, and may contribute to its unique molecular features.[44] PDL2 is an important modulator of T-cell activation that may play a role in the development of PMBLs within the T-cell–rich milieu of the thymus.[25]

A critical molecular difference between the DLBCL subgroups is the activation of the NF-κB pathway (Fig. 5–3A, B). This key pro-survival pathway was found to be constitutively active in ABC DLBCL, but not GCB DLBCLs.[45] ABC DLBCL cell lines were found to have constitutive activation of the IκB kinase, which leads to the phosphorylation and degradation of IκB, an inhibitor of the NF-κB pathway. Blockade of the NF-κB pathway in ABC DLBCL but not GCB DLBCL cells was lethal, thus validating NF-κB as a molecular target in this subset of DLBCL patients.[45] Recently, PMBL was found to express genes that are activated by the NF-κB transcription factors, and NF-κB was found to be localized to the nucleus in these tumors[11,25] (Fig. 5–3A). Highly selective small-molecule inhibitors of IκB kinase show toxicity for ABC DLBCL and PMBL cell lines, but not GCB DLBCL cell lines[46] (Fig. 5–2B). Thus, both ABC DLBCL and PMBL activate IκB kinase by unknown mechanisms, and depend on this activation for their survival. These results support the further development of IκB kinase inhibitors as potentially new therapies for those lymphomas that rely on NF-κB signaling for their survival. This example highlights how molecular profiling can identify key intracellular pathways that may be attacked therapeutically in particular subgroups of patients.

GENE EXPRESSION–BASED PREDICTION OF SURVIVAL FOLLOWING CHEMOTHERAPY FOR DLBCL

The division of DLBCLs into gene expression subgroups defines distinct diseases within DLBCL that differ with respect to cell of origin, oncogenic abnormalities, and overall survival. These subgroups were discovered using "unsupervised" methods that identified patterns within the gene expression data that distinguished the DLBCL subgroups. No clinical data were used to discern these gene expression subgroups. An alternative "supervised" approach has been applied in DLBCL to identify genes whose expression levels correlate with survival.[10,23] It would be expected that some of the genes discovered by this method would be the same genes that distinguish the DLBCL subgroups, since these subgroups have different overall survival rates. Indeed, two of the genes whose expression levels were most strongly associated with poor outcome in one study,[23] *PRKCB1* (protein kinase Cβ) and *PDE4B* (phosphodiesterase 4B), are genes that are more highly expressed in ABC DLBCL compared with the other DLBCL subgroups.[10,47] Another study used supervised methods to develop a six-gene model of survival in DLBCL.[48] Two genes in this model, BCL6 and LMO2, are characteristically expressed in GCB DLBCL, while two other genes, BCL2 and CCND2, are most highly expressed in ABC DLBCL.[10,47] As described below, a "germinal center B-cell" gene expression signature has been associated with favorable outcome, and this reflects the expression of these genes in GCB DLBCL and, to a lesser degree, PMBL, both of which have a relatively good prognosis.[10]

In addition, the supervised approach identified some genes with expression patterns that are correlated with survival in a manner that is statistically independent of the DLBCL distinction.[10] These genes may reflect biological processes that influence the response to chemotherapy irrespective of the exact type of DLBCL that is being treated.

In one study of 240 DLBCL patients, a supervised approach was used to develop a molecular predictor of survival based on four gene expression signatures[10] (Fig. 5–4). This study identified "survival predictor genes" whose expression patterns were statistically associated with survival, and found that the majority of these genes could be classified into one of four gene expression signatures termed "germinal center B cell," "MHC Class II," "lymph node," and "proliferation." For each patient, the expression levels of the survival predictor genes belonging to the same gene expression signature were averaged, and these gene expression signature averages were used to create a multivariate statistical model of survival, termed the "survival predictor." This model assigned a "survival predictor score" to each patient based on the expression of these four gene expression signatures in the tumor specimen. The patients were ranked according to their survival predictor scores and divided into four equal quartiles that had widely differing 5-year survival rates of 73%, 71%, 36%, and 15%, respectively (Fig. 5–4B).

This gene expression–based model of survival accounts for much, but not all, of the heterogeneity in the survival of DLBCL patients. The remaining heterogeneity can be ascribed, in part, to the clinical prognostic factors of the IPI. This is evident from the observation that the gene expression–based model is statistically independent of the IPI in predicting survival.[10] Thus, the molecular predictor is not acting as a mere surrogate for clinical prognostic factors. Despite the prognostic power of the IPI, it has not proven useful in stratifying patients for different treatment regimens.[49] Since the gene expression–based survival predictor is based on biological differences between the DLBCL tumors, it may be more likely to identify groups of patients who will respond differentially to new treatments.

As mentioned above, the prognostic ability of gene expression–based survival model is related, in part, to the prognostic differences among the DLBCL subgroups. The germinal center B-cell signature is expressed more highly in GCB DLBCL and PMBL than in ABC DLBCL. Thus, the favorable prognostic influence of this signature mirrors the relatively favorable prognosis of GCB DLBCL and PMBL. As detailed below, other gene expression signatures in the survival model reflect biological differences among the DLBCL tumors that are not completely captured by the DLBCL subgroup distinction.

One gene expression signature associated with favorable overall survival is the "lymph node" signature, which reflects the infiltration of the involved lymph nodes in some patients with nonmalignant immune cells. The lymph node signature includes many genes that encode markers of macrophages and NK cells, as well as genes that encode extracellular matrix components.[10] It is important to emphasize that this gene expression signature is not a feature of normal lymph nodes, despite its name. While the lymph node signature is a variable feature among DLBCLs, it is not strongly expressed in other lymphoma types such as mantle cell lymphoma and small lymphocytic lymphoma. GCB DLBCL and PMBL have a higher average expression of the lymph node signature genes than ABC DLBCL.[10,25] Nonetheless, the expression of the lymph node signature varies among ABC DLBCLs and is associated with favorable survival within this subgroup of patients. Thus, the lymph node signature reflects variability in the character and abundance of nonmalignant cells in DLBCL tumors that is at least partially independent of the distinction between the DLBCL subgroups.

One hypothesis to explain the association of the lymph node signature with favorable survival is that it reflects an innate immune response to the lymphoma that contributes to curative responses to chemotherapy. Alternatively, the variable expression of the lymph node signature among DLBCL tumors may reflect differences in the malignant cells that influence their ability to interact with the host microenvironment. Indeed, comparative genomic hybridization analysis of DLBCLs has detected some chromosomal abnormalities that are associated with either high or low expression of the lymph node signature.[43]

The MHC Class II signature is associated with favorable survival and includes all genes that encode this important set of antigen presentation proteins, as well as the gene-encoding invariant chain, which is required for antigen presentation by MHC Class II proteins. Variation in MHC Class II expression is independent of the DLBCL subgroup distinction.[10] Immunohistochemical analysis demonstrated

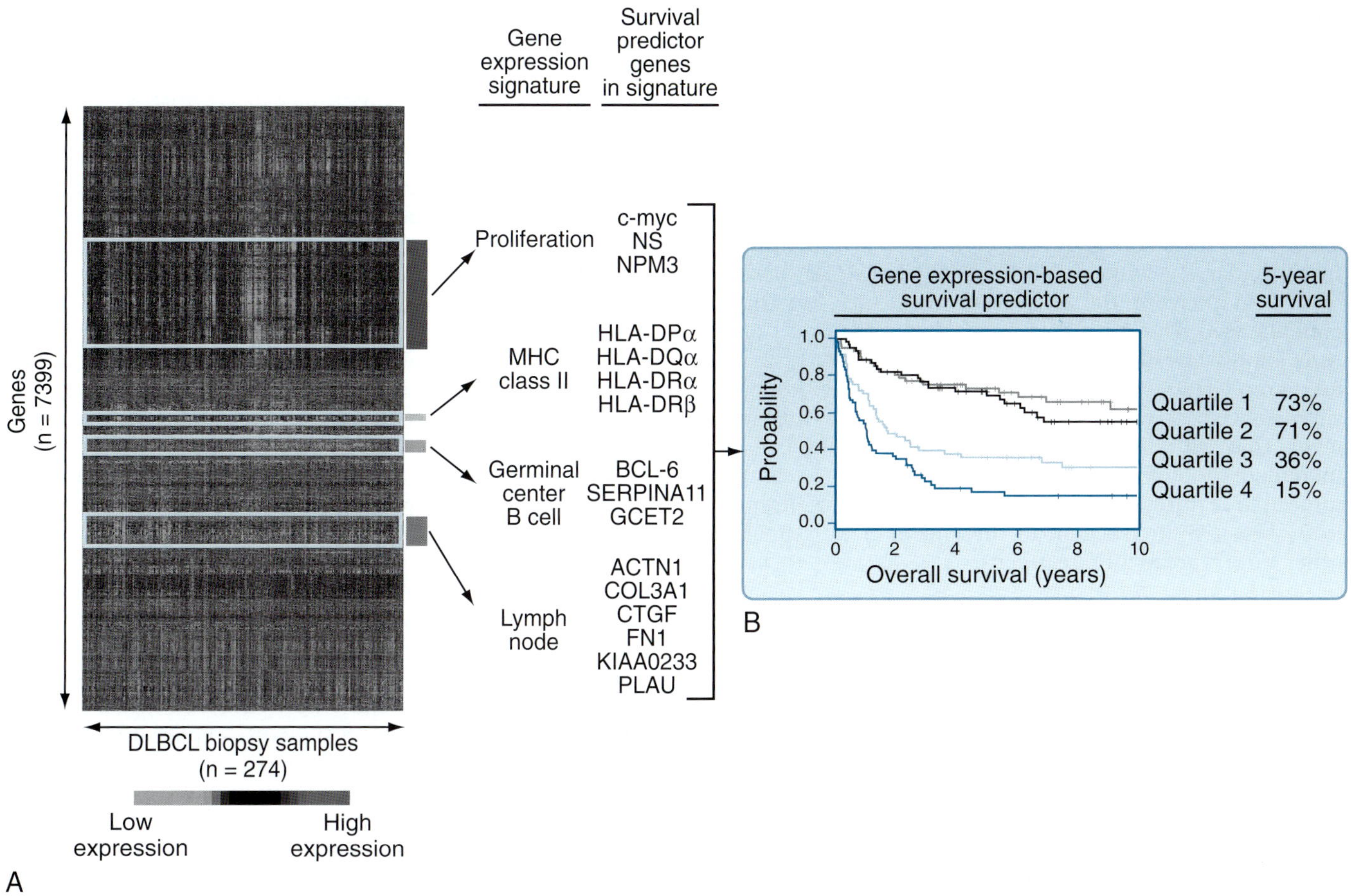

Figure 5–4. A gene expression–based predictor of survival following chemotherapy for DLBCL. **A:** Hierarchical clustering of the gene expression data reveals gene expression signatures containing survival predictor genes. A hierarchical clustering algorithm was used to organize genes based on their expression across 274 DLBCL biopsy samples. Four gene expression signatures are indicated, each of which is composed of coordinately expressed genes that reflect a specific biological aspect of the tumors (see text for details). A supervised method was used to discover genes whose expression patterns were correlated with the length of survival, and the majority of these "survival predictor genes" belonged to one of the four indicated gene expression signatures.[10] Shown are 16 representative survival predictor genes from these four signatures that were used to create a multivariate model of survival. **B:** Kaplan–Meier plot of overall survival of DLBCL patients stratified using the gene expression–based survival predictor. DLBCL patients were assigned to one of four quartiles based on their "survival predictor score," which was calculated using the gene expression–based survival model. (Data are adapted from Fig. 2C in Rosenwald A, Wright G, Chan WC, et al. The use of molecular profiling to predict survival after chemotherapy for diffuse large B-cell lymphoma. N Engl J Med 2002;346:1937–47, with permission.) (See color insert.)

that the variation in expression of this signature is due to differences in MHC Class II expression in the malignant clone, not to differences in the number of MHC Class II–expressing nonmalignant cells.[50,51] Since the MHC Class II genes and the gene-encoding invariant chain reside on different chromosomes, the low expression of the MHC Class II signature in some tumors cannot be explained by a single genomic deletion in the tumor cells. Rather, it is likely that some DLBCLs have a defect in a transcriptional regulatory pathway that reduces the expression of all of the genes in the MHC Class II signature. Tumors with low expression of MHC Class II expression were found to have fewer CD8+ T cells than those with high MHC Class II expression.[50] Although MHC Class II molecules are involved in antigen presentation to CD4+ helper T cells, helper T cells can promote the activation of CD8+ cytotoxic T cells. Thus, it is plausible that variable expression of MHC Class II proteins in DLBCL may affect the host immune response to the tumor, but further work is needed to evaluate whether this mechanism accounts for the association between expression of the MHC Class II signature and survival.

Many of the genes whose expression patterns were associated with poor outcome in DLBCL belong to the proliferation gene expression signature.[10] This signature includes genes that are expressed at high levels in dividing cells and at lower levels in quiescent cells.[5,9] Interestingly, one of the proliferation signature genes that was found to be most strongly associated with poor prognosis in DLBCL is *c-myc*,[10] an oncogene well known to play a role in lymphomagenesis. On average, ABC DLBCLs have higher expression of *c-myc* than GCB DLBCLs or PMBLs. Thus, the poor prognosis associated with expression of the proliferation signature may be partially related to the relatively poor prognosis of ABC DLBCL.

The above-mentioned gene expression–based survival predictors were developed by studying patients treated with anthracycline-based multiagent chemotherapy regimens such as CHOP. Newer therapies for lymphomas are becoming available, and it will be important to test the molecular survival predictors in the context of these new treatments. In particular, the addition of Rituximab to CHOP has been shown to increase the overall survival rate for DLBCL patients aged over 60.[52] It is likely that some or all of the gene expression signatures that are associated with survival following CHOP chemotherapy will retain their prognostic significance for patients treated with CHOP plus Rituximab, given that Rituximab improves the overall survival rate incrementally. It will nevertheless be important to search for molecular features of DLBCL tumors that make them specifically sensitive or resistant to the effects of Rituximab, or other novel therapeutic regimens.

GENE EXPRESSION–BASED PREDICTOR OF SURVIVAL FOLLOWING DIAGNOSIS OF MANTLE CELL LYMPHOMA

In mantle cell lymphoma, survival times range from less than 1 year to more than 10 years following diagnosis. DNA microarrays were used to correlate gene expression in 91 mantle cell lymphoma biopsies with length of survival following diagnosis.[12] The genes whose expression patterns were most significantly associated with short survival belonged to the proliferation gene expression signature, which is a surrogate for tumor proliferation rate (Fig. 5–5A). A molecular predictor of survival based on the average expression of proliferation signature genes was able to stratify patients into four prognostic groups with median survival times of 0.8, 2.3, 3.3, and 6.7 years[12] (Fig. 5–5B). Semiquantitative analysis of proliferation markers such as Ki67 by immunohistochemistry has also demonstrated the association between high tumor proliferation rate and short survival in mantle cell lymphoma.[53–56] However, the prognostic groups identified by immunohistochemistry differed in survival by only 2.1 to 2.7 years.[53–56] The superiority of gene expression profiling in predicting survival is likely due to the more accurate estimation of tumor proliferation rate afforded by the quantitative measurement of proliferation signature gene expression. The ability to accurately predict the length of survival of mantle cell lymphoma patients should prove to be valuable in patient management: Those patients with low expression of the proliferation signature have an indolent form of the disease that can be managed by watchful waiting, whereas patients with high expression of the proliferation signature have an aggressive disease and should be considered for clinical trials involving novel therapies.

The variability in the proliferation rate can be traced to distinct molecular abnormalities in the mantle cell lymphomas that affect cell cycle progression[12] (Fig. 5–5C). Mantle cell lymphoma is typified by a t(11;14) translocation, which deregulates the expression of the *cyclin D1* gene. Cyclin D1, in a complex with either cdk4 or cdk6, promotes transition from G1 phase to S phase in the cell cycle.[57] Unexpectedly, gene expression profiling revealed that mantle cell lymphomas differ in *cyclin D1* mRNA expression levels, despite bearing similar translocations[12] (Fig. 5–4C). Higher expression of *cyclin D1* mRNA expression was associated with higher proliferation rate and shorter survival. One mechanism underlying the differences in *cyclin D1* expression involves the variable expression of *cyclin D1* mRNA isoforms that differ in the 3' untranslated region. The *cyclin D1* 3' untranslated region that contains an mRNA destabilizing element (UTR),[58–60] and some mantle cell lymphomas, have genomic deletions in this region.[58–63] Such deletions result in a short *cyclin D1* mRNA isoform that lacks the 3' UTR and, consequently, is more stable and accumulates to higher levels.

Another molecular abnormality associated with higher expression of the proliferation signature and shorter survival in mantle cell lymphoma was deletion of the INK4a/ARF locus[12] (Fig. 5–5C). This genomic locus encodes p16, which blocks the G1 to S phase transition of the cell cycle by inhibiting the action of cyclin D1/cdk complexes, as well as $p14^{ARF}$, which antagonizes p53.[57] Deletion of the INK4a/ARF locus and increased *cyclin D1* expression were found to be statistically independent in their associations with high proliferation signature expression and short survival.[12] Thus, the proliferation gene expression signature serves as a quantitative integrator of multiple oncogenic events that alter the proliferation rate in mantle cell lymphoma and, consequently, the survival of these patients.

GENE EXPRESSION–BASED PREDICTOR OF SURVIVAL FOLLOWING DIAGNOSIS OF FOLLICULAR LYMPHOMA

The clinical course of follicular lymphoma is highly variable: the median survival is approximately 10 years, but some patients live more than 15 years following diagnosis, whereas others succumb to this disease in less than 5 years.[64,65] In some cases, the malignancy transforms into DLBCL, which is rapidly fatal. Patients with follicular lymphoma are managed by watchful waiting, or are treated with chemotherapy and/or various forms of immunotherapy. However, no definitive evidence has been presented that any of these approaches provide a survival advantage, and therefore there is no consensus as to the best treatment for these patients.[64]

The malignant cells of follicular lymphoma are derived from germinal center B cells. Roughly 90% have these lymphomas bear the t(14;18) translocation that deregulates the expression of BCL2, a potent antiapoptotic protein. A variety of other genomic aberrations have been reported in follicular lymphoma, and some of these have been associated with transformation to DLBCL.[66] However, the heterogeneity in survival of these patients has not been explained by these various molecular abnormalities.

DNA microarray analysis revealed that the length of survival in follicular lymphoma can be predicted by the gene expression profile of the tumor at the time of diagnosis.[67] A supervised analytic method, termed "survival signature

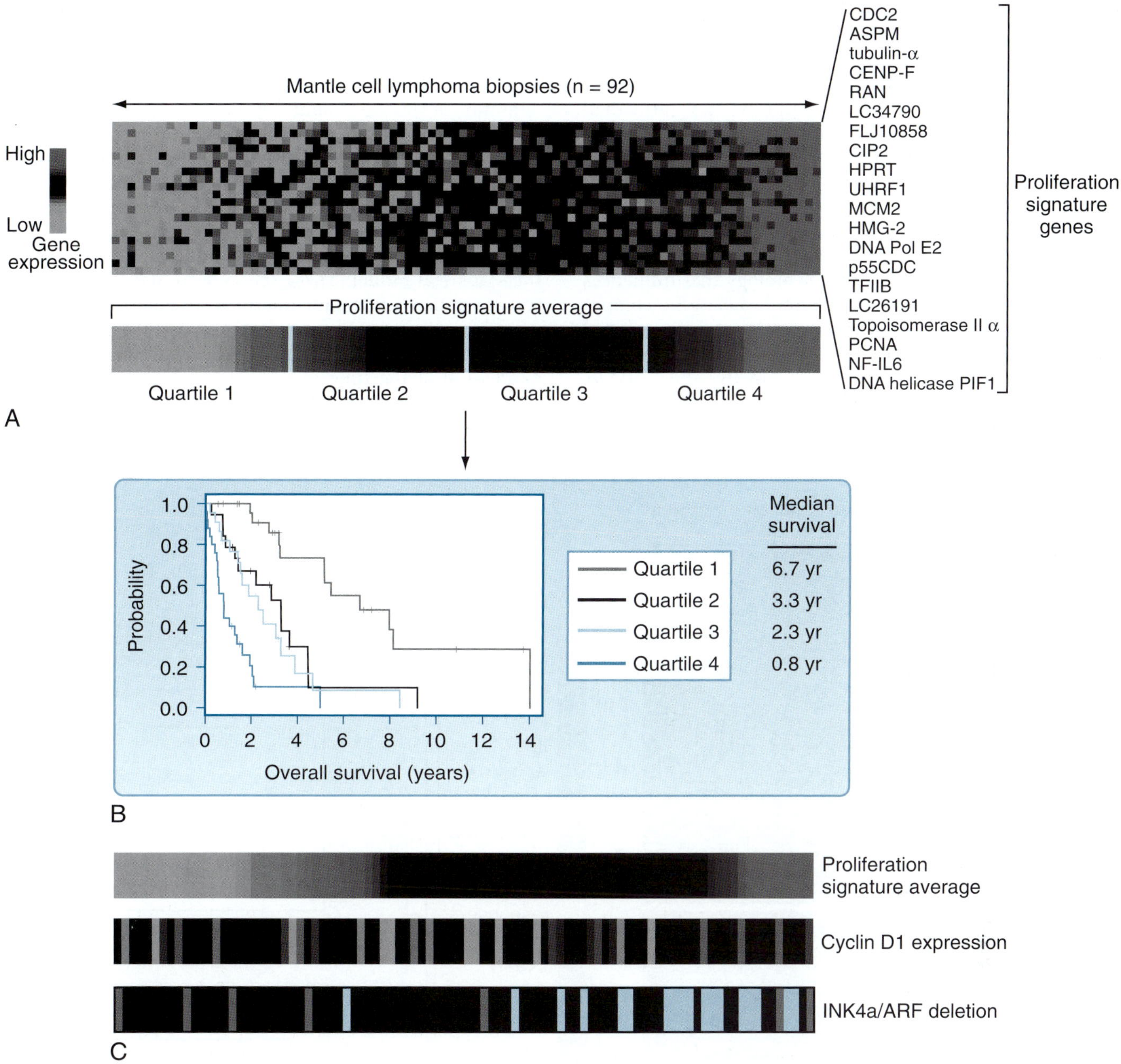

Figure 5–5. The length of survival in mantle cell lymphoma is predicted by gene expression in the tumor at diagnosis. **A:** Development of a gene expression–based survival predictor for mantle cell lymphoma. A supervised method was used to identify genes whose expression patterns were correlated with length of survival following diagnosis of mantle cell lymphoma. The majority of these genes belong to the proliferation gene expression signature, which includes genes that are more highly expressed in proliferating than in quiescent cells. The expression levels of the 20 proliferation signature genes shown were averaged to create a proliferation signature average for each of 92 mantle cell lymphoma patients. Patients were divided into four equal quartiles based on the proliferation signature average. **B:** Kaplan–Meier plot of overall survival of mantle cell lymphoma patients stratified by the proliferation signature average. **C:** The proliferation signature average is a quantitative character of multiple oncogenic events that influence the proliferation rate. A higher expression level of the cyclin D1 mRNA coding region is observed in many tumors with high proliferation signature averages (see text for details). Tumors with deletion of the INK4a/ARF locus encoding p16 and p14ARF are indicated in yellow, and are more commonly observed in tumors with a high proliferation signature average. (Data are adapted from Figs. 2A and B, 4A, and 5A in Rosenwald A, Wright G, Wiestner A, et al. The proliferation gene expression signature is a quantitative integrator of oncogenic events that predicts survival in mantle cell lymphoma. Cancer Cell 2003;3:185–97, with permission.) (See color insert.)

analysis," was used to a discover gene expression signatures that are associated with either short or long survival following diagnosis of follicular lymphoma. Survival signature analysis begins with the division of the samples into a training set and a test set. Within the training set, individual genes are identified whose expression patterns are correlated with the length of survival. Next, a hierarchical clustering algorithm is used to group these genes into "survival signatures" based on their coordinate expression across the samples in the training set. Because of their coordinate expression, the genes within a survival signature are likely to reflect the same aspect of tumor biology that influences the length of survival. The expression levels of the component genes in each survival signature are then averaged, and various multivariate models of survival are created using these survival signature averages. Finally, the survival models are tested for their reproducibility using the independent test set samples.

In the case of follicular lymphoma, this method identified ten survival signatures based on a training set of 93 biopsy samples[67] (Fig. 5–6A). A multivariate model of survival was created from two of these signatures, termed "immune response-1" and "immune response-2." Expression of the immune response-1 signature was associated with long survival, whereas expression of the immune response-2 signature was associated with short survival. Importantly, this survival model predicted the length of survival in an independent test set of 94 cases. Patients in the test set were assigned a survival predictor score based on the statistical model. These scores were used to divide the test set patients into four quartiles that had strikingly disparate median survival rates of 3.9, 10.8, 11.1, and 13.6 years, respectively (Fig. 5–6B). The fact that tumor gene expression at the time of diagnosis predicts the length of survival implies that changes in the tumor cell genome acquired after the time of diagnosis do not have a strong

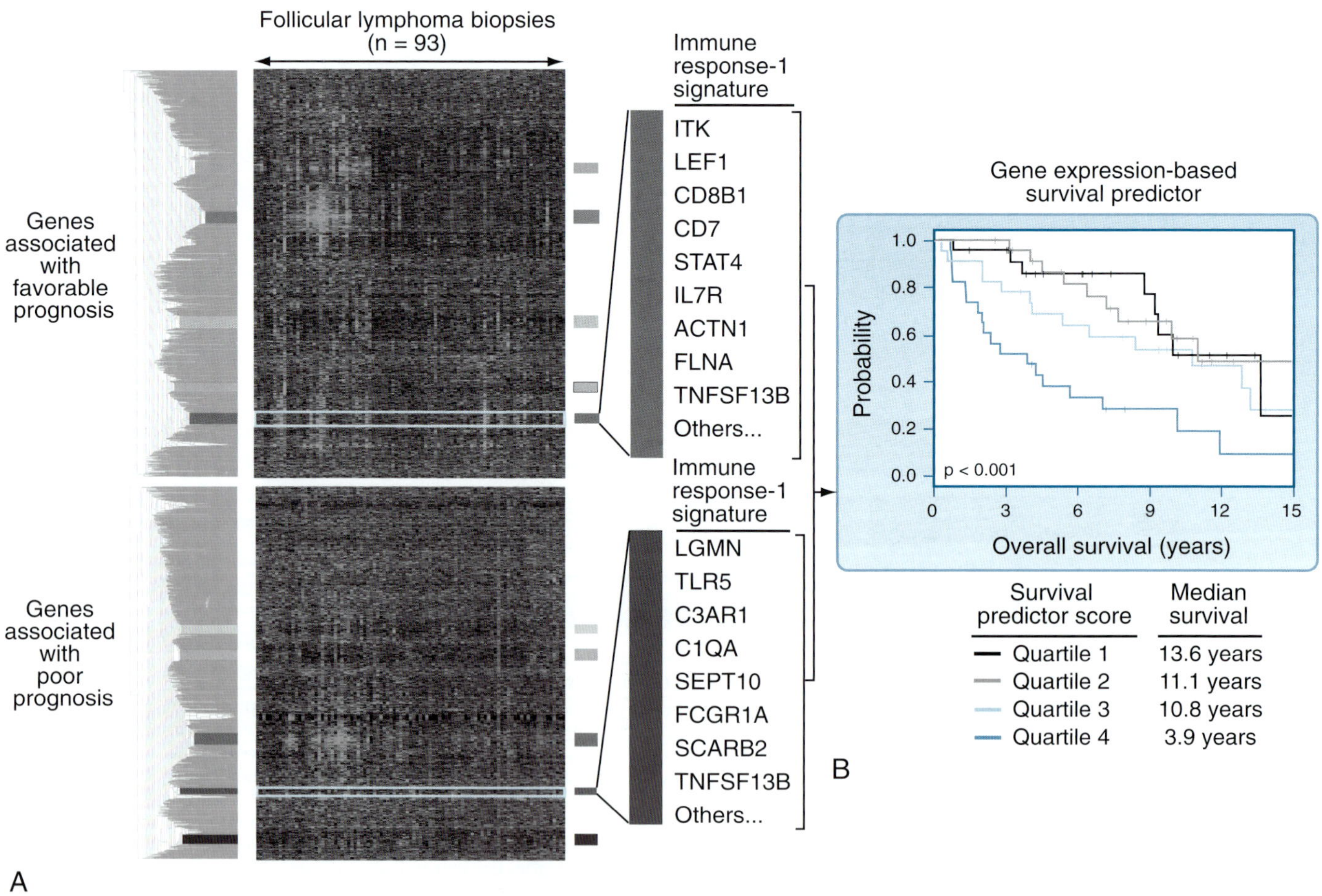

Figure 5–6. A gene expression–based survival model in follicular lymphoma. **A:** Identification of gene expression signatures associated with good or poor prognosis in follicular lymphoma. Genes with expression patterns that correlated with long survival (**top panel**) or short survival (**bottom panel**) following diagnosis were organized by hierarchical clustering across 93 follicular lymphoma biopsy samples. Ten gene expression signatures were identified (*colored bars*), two of which were used to create an optimal model of survival.[67] Representative genes in these two signatures, termed immune response-1 and immune response-2, are shown. **B:** Kaplan–Meier plot of overall survival of follicular lymphoma patients stratified using the gene expression–based survival predictor. Patients were assigned a survival predictor score using the gene expression–based survival predictor, and were divided into four equal quartiles according to the scores. (Data are adapted from Fig. 1C and D in Dave SS, Wright G, Tan B, et al. A molecular predictor of survival following diagnosis of follicular lymphoma based on the profile of non-malignant tumor-infiltrating immune cells. N Engl J Med 2003;351:2159–69, with permission.) (See color insert.)

impact on the length of survival. Rather, the survival signatures appear to reflect aspects of tumor cell biology existing at diagnosis that influence the clinical aggressiveness of follicular lymphoma.

Much, but not all, of the heterogeneity in the survival of follicular lymphoma patients can be predicted based on tumor gene expression. The remaining heterogeneity can be accounted for, in part, by various clinical factors that have been associated with the length of survival in follicular lymphoma, such as the components of the IPI.[67] The gene expression–based survival model was found to be statistically independent of all available clinical prognostic factors, demonstrating that the survival signatures were not acting as mere surrogates of the clinical parameters.[67]

To directly identify which cells in the tumor biopsies were expressing the genes of the immune response-1 and immune response-2 signatures, flow cytometry was used to separate the malignant and nonmalignant cells based on the expression of CD19[67] (Fig. 5–7A). Gene expression profiling of the sorted subpopulations from the tumor biopsies demonstrated that the majority of the genes in the immune response-1 and immune response-2 signatures were expressed preferentially in the CD19-negative nonmalignant infiltrating cells of the tumor. Furthermore, the genes in these two signatures were not preferentially expressed in normal germinal center B cells, the cell of origin of origin of follicular lymphoma, but rather were expressed in either T cells or monocytes (Fig. 5–5B). These findings demonstrate that the character of the tumor-infiltrating immune cells in follicular lymphoma is the predominant feature that predicts the length of survival following diagnosis.

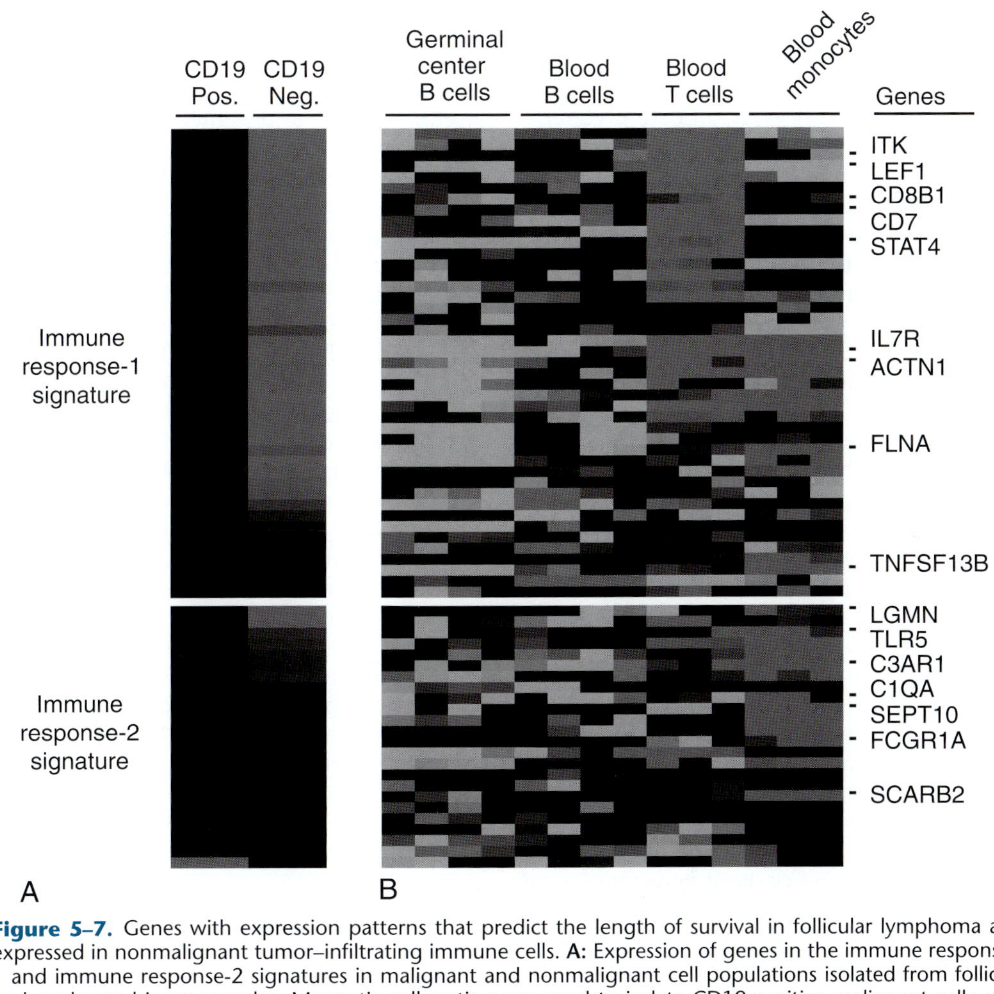

Figure 5–7. Genes with expression patterns that predict the length of survival in follicular lymphoma are expressed in nonmalignant tumor–infiltrating immune cells. **A:** Expression of genes in the immune response-1 and immune response-2 signatures in malignant and nonmalignant cell populations isolated from follicular lymphoma biopsy samples. Magnetic cell sorting was used to isolate CD19-positive malignant cells and CD19-negative nonmalignant cells from follicular lymphoma biopsies. The majority of genes in both the immune response-1 and immune response-2 signatures are more highly expressed (*red*) in the nonmalignant cell fraction. **B:** Expression of the immune response-1 and immune response-2 signature genes in various normal subpopulations of immune cells. Tonsilar germinal center B cells and blood B cells, T cells, and monocytes were analyzed by gene expression profiling. Most genes belonging to the immune response-1 signature are highly expressed in blood T cells or monocytes, whereas the majority of genes in the immune response-2 signature are most highly expressed in monocytes. Neither gene expression signature is highly expressed in germinal center B cells, the cell of origin for follicular lymphoma. (Data are adapted from Figs. 2A and 3B in Dave SS, Wright G, Tan B, et al. A molecular predictor of survival following diagnosis of follicular lymphoma based on the profile of non-malignant tumor-infiltrating immune cells. N Engl J Med 2003;351:2159–69, with permission.) (See color insert.)

The follicular lymphoma survival signatures were named based on the known function of several of their component genes.[67] The immune response-1 signature includes genes encoding well-known T-cell markers such as CD7, CD8B1, and the IL-7 receptor, as well as the T-cell signaling proteins STAT4, LEF, and ITK (Fig. 5–7B). However, this signature does not merely reflect the number of T cells in the biopsy since the expression levels of other pan–T-cell genes (e.g., *CD2*, *LAT*) were not associated with survival. In addition, this signature includes genes characteristically expressed in macrophages, such as *ACTN1*[68] and *TNFSF13B* (*BLYS/BAFF*) (Fig. 5–7B). Thus, the immune response-1 signature reflects a complex mixture of T cells and other immune cells that is associated with long survival in follicular lymphoma.

By contrast, the immune response-2 signature did not include genes expressed preferentially in T cells, but rather included genes expressed in monocytes and/or dendritic cells (Fig. 5–7B). Two genes in this signature, *SEPT10* and *LGMN*, encode, respectively, a septin and a lysosomal protease that are highly expressed in mature dendritic cells.[69,70] Other immune response-2 genes include *TLR5*, *C3AR1*, and *FCGR1A* that encode receptors for flagellin, C3A, and immunoglobulin Fc regions, respectively, and are preferentially expressed in myelomonocytic cells.[71–74] In summary, the immune response-2 signature is associated with short survival in follicular lymphoma, and appears to reflect an immune infiltrate that is relatively low in T-cell content and relatively enriched in cells of the myeloid lineage.

Follicular lymphoma is one of the cancers in which spontaneous regression has been reported, although this occurs rarely.[75] Remissions in the absence of therapy have also been noted in melanoma and renal cell carcinoma, a phenomenon that has been ascribed to an antitumor immune response in some patients. In this regard, the favorable prognosis associated with expression of the immune response-1 signature suggests that this signature may reflect a type of immune response that is capable of limiting the progression of follicular lymphoma. Thus, the immune response-1 signature could represent an adaptive immune response to the lymphoma. By contrast, the genes that constitute the immune response-2 signature do not encode T-cell markers, but rather encode markers of cells in the innate immune system. In follicular lymphomas with high expression of the immune response-2 signature, the infiltrating immune cells may be responding to "danger" signals derived from the malignant cells.

Two hypotheses could account for the variation in immune cell signatures among follicular lymphomas. First, genetic polymorphisms that influence immune responses in general may modulate the nature of the tumor infiltrating immune cells. Alternatively, the malignant cells in the follicular lymphoma may dictate the character of the immune infiltrate. These hypotheses could be evaluated by analyzing gene expression and genomic alterations in purified malignant cells from tumors that are skewed toward either the immune response-1 or immune response-2 phenotypes.

While it is possible that the immune response-1 signature reflects an adaptive immune response to the malignant cells that is associated with longer survival, other models are conceivable. The infiltrating immune cells may provide trophic signals that either increase proliferation or prolong survival of the malignant clone. In this scenario, the malignant clone may be "addicted" to the trophic factors from the immune cells, and this dependence may limit the ability of tumor cells to spread beyond the lymph node to anatomical locations lacking these immune cells. Indeed, certain spontaneously occurring mouse lymphomas have an absolute requirement for their growth on cytokines provided by normal immune cells.[76] An understanding of such interactions in human lymphomas may provide new targets for therapeutic attack.

The prognostic power of the gene expression–based survival predictor should prove helpful in patient management. Watchful waiting is a reasonable clinical approach for those patients in the top three quartiles since they have a rather indolent form of this lymphoma. On the other hand, those patients assigned to the fourth quartile have an aggressive lymphoma, and should be considered for clinical trials involving novel therapies. The gene expression–based survival predictor should be particularly helpful in designing clinical trials in follicular lymphoma. Since the median survival of these patients is roughly 10 years, it has not been possible to conduct clinical trials in follicular lymphoma in which overall survival is the primary endpoint. If a clinical trial is designed to enroll patients in the least favorable quartile of the gene expression–based survival predictor, overall survival could be an achievable endpoint since the median survival of these patients is 3.9 years.

Since the survival-associated gene expression signatures in follicular lymphoma reflect the immune infiltrates in these tumors, it is conceivable that these signatures might also influence the response to various immune-based therapies. Anti-idiotype vaccination holds therapeutic promise in follicular lymphoma,[77–79] and the success of this approach most likely depends on the ability of the vaccine to activate T lymphocytes. Therefore, it is possible that anti-idiotype vaccination will be most effective in those patients with high expression of the immune response-1 signature, since this signature reflects an immune infiltrate in follicular lymphoma that includes T cells. Antibodies to CD20, such as Rituximab, cause tumor regression in some patients with follicular lymphoma,[80–83] and it is possible that expression of the immune response-1 or immune response-2 signatures could influence the response to this therapy. Such speculations need to be tested prospectively in clinical trials in which gene expression profiling of biopsy samples from the patients is performed.

CLINICAL IMPLEMENTATION OF GENE EXPRESSION PROFILING

Current diagnosis of the lymphoid malignancies relies on histological examination of the tumor supplemented with a variety of laboratory tests, including immunohistochemistry, flow cytometry, fluorescence in situ hybridization (FISH), and *in situ* hybridization to detect viral transcripts. Most of these methods are semiquantitative and rely upon the experience of a highly trained hematopathologist. Gene expression profiling using DNA microarrays has the potential to deliver a quantitative and reproducible diagnosis to patients with lymphoid malignancies.[84]

The major types of lymphoma recognized by the WHO can be readily distinguished from one another by their gene expression profiles[84] (Fig. 5–8). An analytical algorithm

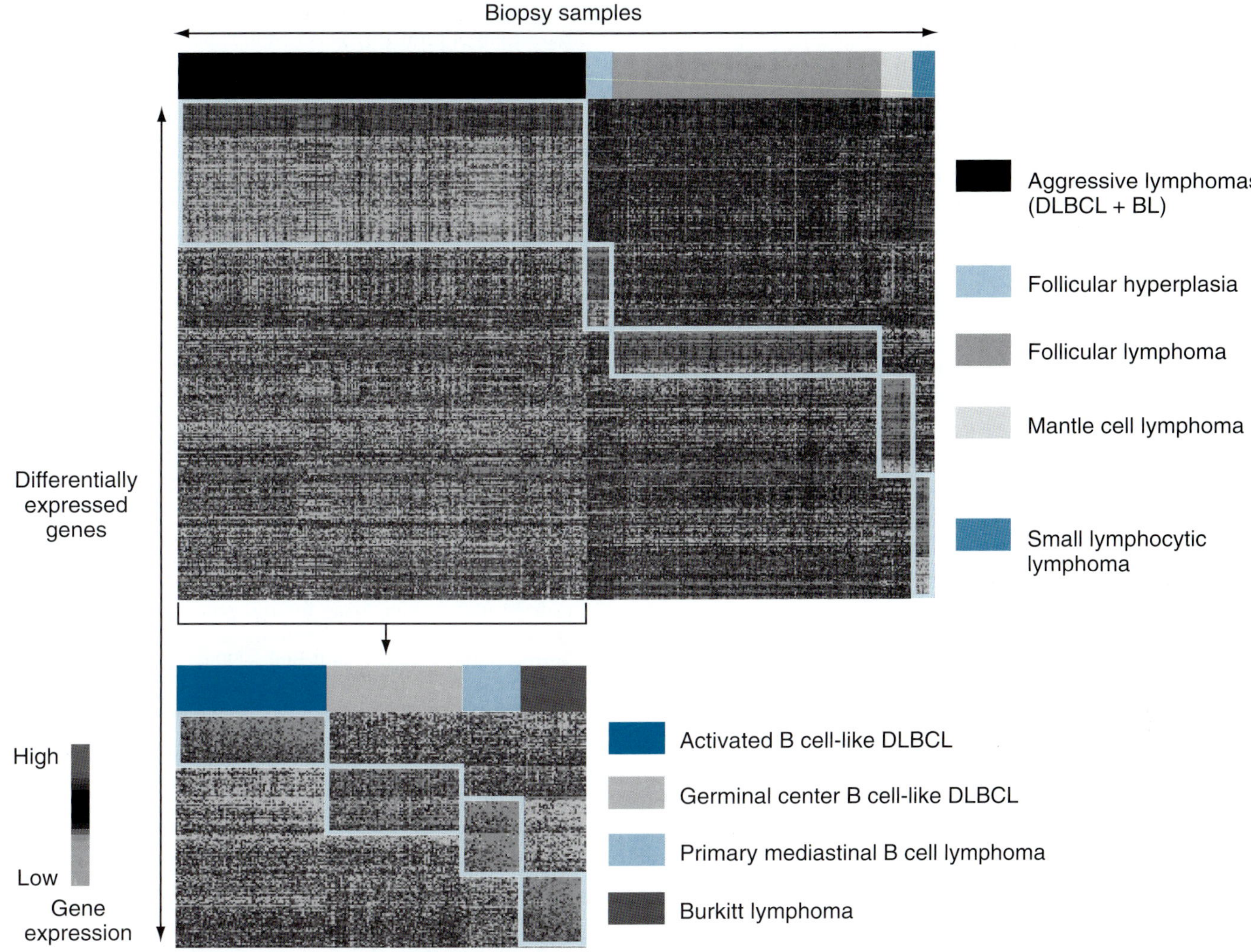

Figure 5–8. Molecular diagnosis of lymphomas by gene expression profiling. Gene expression of several hundred genes can be used to reliably assign a biopsy specimen to a lymphoma type.[84] The first step of the algorithm separates aggressive lymphomas (DLBCL), Burkitt's lymphoma (BL), and other common lymphoma types from one another (**top panel**). The second step distinguishes BL from the three DLBCL subgroups (**bottom panel**). A custom DNA microarray can be used to make these distinctions, and to provide prognostic information for patients with DLBCL, mantle cell lymphoma, and follicular lymphoma. (See color insert.)

based on Bayesian statistics has been constructed that assigns a probability that a biopsy specimen belongs to a particular lymphoma type.[84] The first step of this algorithm distinguishes between aggressive lymphomas (DLBCL/Burkitt's lymphoma), follicular lymphoma, mantle cell lymphoma, small lymphocytic lymphoma, and benign follicular hyperplasia. The second step of the algorithm subdivides aggressive lymphomas into GCB DLBCL, ABC DLBCL, PMBL, and Burkitt's lymphoma. Importantly, this algorithm allows some samples to be declared "unclassified" if they do not have gene expression profiles that correspond well to those of known lymphoma types. The concordance between the diagnosis given by current methodology and the gene expression–based diagnosis ranges from 95% to 100%.[84] In some of the cases in which the two diagnostic methods were found to be discrepant, histological review suggested the coexistence of two lymphoma types, often follicular lymphoma and DLBCL. In such cases, the "true" diagnosis is unclear.

As a first step towards clinical implementation of gene expression profiling, a custom DNA microarray was constructed, termed LymphDx.[84] This oligonucleotide-based microarray is constructed using Affymetrix technology and measures the expression of roughly 2653 genes. The LymphDx microarray includes all of the genes needed to distinguish the various lymphoma types and subgroups. In addition, this microarray includes the genes that are used to create the gene expression–based survival predictors for DLBCL, follicular lymphoma, and mantle cell lymphoma. Potentially, such a diagnostic microarray could supplant most other diagnostic tests currently performed for the diagnosis of lymphoid malignancies. However, it is expected that a pathologist will still perform morphological and histological evaluation of the biopsy specimen, which will help determine whether the specimen contains sufficient tumor cells to yield a reliable gene expression profile. A prospective evaluation of the LymphDx microarray will be needed to carefully assess its performance.

During this evaluation, quality control criteria will be established that can be used to determine the reliability of the gene expression–based diagnoses. In addition, it is anticipated that some cases of lymphoid malignancy will be encountered that have gene expression profiles that do not resemble closely the profiles of any recognized lymphoma type, and these cases will need to be evaluated carefully to see if they may represent novel lymphoma types. The transition to a gene expression–based diagnosis of lymphomas will require certain changes in standard clinical practice, such as the preservation of frozen biopsy material for each patient. Nonetheless, the demonstrated ability of gene expression profiling to provide quantitative and reproducible diagnostic and prognostic information should provide the impetus needed to apply this technology in clinical practice.

References

1. Staudt LM. Molecular diagnosis of the hematologic cancers. N Engl J Med 2003;348:1777–85.
2. Sherlock G. Analysis of large-scale gene expression data. Curr Opin Immunol 2000;12:201–5.
3. Simon R. Diagnostic and prognostic prediction using gene expression profiles in high-dimensional microarray data. Br J Cancer 2003;89:1599–604.
4. Ransohoff DF. Rules of evidence for cancer molecular-marker discovery and validation. Nat Rev Cancer 2004;4:309–14.
5. Shaffer AL, Rosenwald A, Hurt EM, et al. Signatures of the immune response. Immunity 2001;15:375–85.
6. Camon E, Magrane M, Barrell D, et al. The Gene Ontology Annotation (GOA) project: implementation of GO in SWISS-PROT, TrEMBL, and InterPro. Genome Res 2003;13:662–72.
7. Mootha VK, Lindgren CM, Eriksson KF, et al. PGC-1alpha-responsive genes involved in oxidative phosphorylation are coordinately downregulated in human diabetes. Nat Genet 2003;34:267–73.
8. Coiffier B. Diffuse large cell lymphoma. Curr Opin Oncol 2001;13:325–34.
9. Alizadeh AA, Eisen MB, Davis RE, et al. Distinct types of diffuse large B-cell lymphoma identified by gene expression profiling. Nature 2000;403:503–11.
10. Rosenwald A, Wright G, Chan WC, et al. The use of molecular profiling to predict survival after chemotherapy for diffuse large B-cell lymphoma. N Engl J Med 2002;346:1937–47.
11. Savage KJ, Monti S, Kutok JL, et al. The molecular signature of mediastinal large B-cell lymphoma differs from that of other diffuse large B-cell lymphomas and shares features with classical Hodgkin lymphoma. Blood 2003;102:3871–9.
12. Rosenwald A, Wright G, Wiestner A, et al. The proliferation gene expression signature is a quantitative integrator of oncogenic events that predicts survival in mantle cell lymphoma. Cancer Cell 2003;3:185–97.
13. Wright G, Tan B, Rosenwald A, et al. A gene expression–based method to diagnose clinically distinct subgroups of diffuse large B cell lymphoma. Proc Natl Acad Sci U S A 2003;100:9991–6.
14. Staudt LM, Dent AL, Shaffer AL, et al. Regulation of lymphocyte cell fate decisions and lymphomagenesis by BCL-6. Int Rev Immunol 1999;18:381–403.
15. Dalla-Favera R, Migliazza A, Chang CC, et al. Molecular pathogenesis of B cell malignancy: the role of BCL-6. Curr Top Microbiol Immunol 1999;246:257–63.
16. Shaffer AL, Yu X, He Y, et al. BCL-6 represses genes that function in lymphocyte differentiation, inflammation, and cell cycle control. Immunity 2000;13:199–212.
17. Tunyaplin C, Shaffer AL, Angelin-Duclos CD, et al. Direct repression of prdm1 by Bcl-6 inhibits plasmacytic differentiation. J Immunol 2004;173:1158–65.
18. Shaffer AL, Lin KI, Kuo TC, et al. Blimp-1 orchestrates plasma cell differentiation by extinguishing the mature B cell gene expression program. Immunity 2002;17:51–62.
19. Shvarts A, Brummelkamp TR, Scheeren F, et al. A senescence rescue screen identifies BCL6 as an inhibitor of anti-proliferative p19(ARF)-p53 signaling. Genes Dev 2002;16:681–6.
20. Niu H, Cattoretti G, and Dalla-Favera R. BCL6 controls the expression of the B7-1/CD80 costimulatory receptor in germinal center B cells. J Exp Med 2003;198:211–21.
21. Shaffer AL, Shapiro-Shelef M, Iwakoshi NN, et al. XBP1, downstream of Blimp-1, expands the secretory apparatus and other organelles, and increases protein synthesis in plasma cell differentiation. Immunity 2004;21:81–93.
22. Lossos IS, Alizadeh AA, Eisen MB, et al. Ongoing immunoglobulin somatic mutation in germinal center B cell–like but not in activated B cell–like diffuse large cell lymphomas. Proc Natl Acad Sci U S A 2000;97:10209–13.
23. Shipp MA, Ross KN, Tamayo P, et al. Diffuse large B-cell lymphoma outcome prediction by gene-expression profiling and supervised machine learning. Nat Med 2002;8:68–74.
24. Alizadeh A, Eisen M, Davis RE, et al. The Lymphochip: a specialized cDNA microarray for the genomic-scale analysis of gene expression in normal and malignant lymphocytes. Cold Spring Harbor Symp Quant Biol 1999;64:71–8.
25. Rosenwald A, Wright G, Leroy K, et al. Molecular diagnosis of primary mediastinal B cell lymphoma identifies a clinically favorable subgroup of diffuse large B cell lymphoma related to Hodgkin lymphoma. J Exp Med 2003;198:851–62.
26. Barth TF, Leithauser F, Joos S, et al. Mediastinal (thymic) large B-cell lymphoma: where do we stand? Lancet Oncol 2002;3:229–34.
27. Jaffe ES, Harris NL, Stein H, et al. Tumours of Haematopoietic and Lymphoid Tissues. Lyon: IARC Press, 2001.
28. Copie-Bergman C, Plonquet A, Alonso MA, et al. MAL expression in lymphoid cells: further evidence for MAL as a distinct molecular marker of primary mediastinal large B-cell lymphomas. Mod Pathol 2002;15:1172–80.
29. Copie-Bergman C, Boulland ML, Dehoulle C, et al. Interleukin 4-induced gene 1 is activated in primary mediastinal large B-cell lymphoma. Blood 2003;101:2756–61.
30. Schwab U, Stein H, Gerdes J, et al. Production of a monoclonal antibody specific for Hodgkin and Sternberg-Reed cells of Hodgkin's disease and a subset of normal lymphoid cells. Nature 1982;299:65–7.
31. Skinnider BF, Elia AJ, Gascoyne RD, et al. Interleukin 13 and interleukin 13 receptor are frequently expressed by Hodgkin and Reed–Sternberg cells of Hodgkin lymphoma. Blood 2001;97:250–5.
32. van den Berg A, Visser L, Poppema S. High expression of the CC chemokine TARC in Reed–Sternberg cells. A possible explanation for the characteristic T-cell infiltratein Hodgkin's lymphoma. Am J Pathol 1999;154:1685–91.
33. Jaffe ES and Muller-Hermelink K. Relationship between Hodgkin's disease and non-Hodgkin's lymphomas. In: Mauch PM, Armitage JO, Diehl V, et al., eds. Hodgkin's Disease. Philadelphia: Lippincott Williams & Wilkins, 1999:181–91.
34. Joos S, Otano-Joos MI, Ziegler S, et al. Primary mediastinal (thymic) B-cell lymphoma is characterized by gains of chromosomal material including 9p and amplification of the REL gene. Blood 1996;87:1571–8.
35. Joos S, Kupper M, Ohl S, et al. Genomic imbalances including amplification of the tyrosine kinase gene JAK2 in CD30+ Hodgkin cells. Cancer Res 2000;60:549–52.
36. Chang CC, McClintock S, Cleveland RP, et al. Immunohistochemical expression patterns of germinal center and activa-

tion B-cell markers correlate with prognosis in diffuse large B-cell lymphoma. Am J Surg Pathol 2004;28:464–70.
37. de Leval L, Braaten KM, Ancukiewicz M, et al. Diffuse large B-cell lymphoma of bone: an analysis of differentiation-associated antigens with clinical correlation. Am J Surg Pathol 2003;27:1269–77.
38. Tzankov A, Pehrs AC, Zimpfer A, et al. Prognostic significance of CD44 expression in diffuse large B cell lymphoma of activated and germinal centre B cell–like types: a tissue microarray analysis of 90 cases. J Clin Pathol 2003;56:747–52.
39. Hans CP, Weisenburger DD, Greiner TC, et al. Confirmation of the molecular classification of diffuse large B-cell lymphoma by immunohistochemistry using a tissue microarray. Blood 2004;103:275–82.
40. Shipp M. A predictive model for aggressive non-Hodgkin's lymphoma. N Engl J Med 1993;329:987–94.
41. Huang JZ, Sanger WG, Greiner TC, et al. The t(14;18) defines a unique subset of diffuse large B-cell lymphoma with a germinal center B-cell gene expression profile. Blood 2002; 99:2285–90.
42. Gascoyne RD, Adomat SA, Krajewski S, et al. Prognostic significance of Bcl-2 protein expression and Bcl-2 gene rearrangement in diffuse aggressive non-Hodgkin's lymphoma. Blood 1997;90:244–51.
43. Zettl A, Bea S, Wright G, et al. Chromosomal imbalances in germinal center B-cell like and activated B-cell like diffuse large B-cell lymphoma influence gene expression signatures and improve the gene expression–based survival prediction.
44. Guiter C, Dusanter-Fourt I, Copie-Bergman C, et al. Constitutive STAT6 activation in primary mediastinal large B-cell lymphoma. Blood 2004;104:543–9.
45. Davis RE, Brown KD, Siebenlist U, et al. Constitutive nuclear factor kappaB activity is required for survival of activated B cell–like diffuse large B cell lymphoma cells. J Exp Med 2001;194:1861–1874.
46. Lam LT, Davis RE, Pierce J, et al. Small molecule inhibitors of IkB-kinase are selectively toxic for subgroups of diffuse large B cell lymphoma defined by gene expression profiling. Clin Cancer Res 2005;11:1–13.
47. Davis RE and Staudt LM. Molecular diagnosis of lymphoid malignancies by gene expression profiling. Curr Opin Hematol 2002;9:333–8.
48. Lossos IS, Czerwinski DK, Alizadeh AA, et al. Prediction of survival in diffuse large B-cell lymphoma based on the expression of six genes. N Engl J Med 2004;350:1828–37.
49. Shipp MA, Abeloff MD, Antman KH, et al. International Consensus Conference on High-Dose Therapy with Hematopoietic Stem Cell Transplantation in Aggressive Non-Hodgkin's Lymphomas: report of the jury. J Clin Oncol 1999;17:423–9.
50. Rimsza LM, Roberts RA, Miller TP, et al. Loss of MHC class II gene and protein expression in diffuse large B-cell lymphoma is related to decreased tumor immunosurveillance and poor patient survival regardless of other prognostic factors: a follow-up study from the Leukemia and Lymphoma Molecular Profiling Project. Blood 2004;103:4251–8.
51. Miller TP, Lippman SM, Spier CM, et al. HLA-DR (Ia) immune phenotype predicts outcome for patients with diffuse large cell lymphoma. J Clin Invest 1988 82:370–2.
52. Coiffier B, Lepage E, Briere J, et al. CHOP chemotherapy plus rituximab compared with CHOP alone in elderly patients with diffuse large B-cell lymphoma. N Engl J Med 2002; 346:235–42.
53. Argatoff LH, Connors JM, Klasa RJ, et al. Mantle cell lymphoma: a clinicopathologic study of 80 cases. Blood 1997; 89:2067–78.
54. Bosch F, Lopez-Guillermo A, Campo E, et al. Mantle cell lymphoma: presenting features, response to therapy, and prognostic factors. Cancer 1998;82:567–75.
55. Raty R, Franssila K, Joensuu H, et al. Ki-67 expression level, histological subtype, and the International Prognostic Index as outcome predictors in mantle cell lymphoma. Eur J Haematol 2002;69:11–20.
56. Velders GA, Kluin-Nelemans JC, De Boer CJ, et al. Mantle-cell lymphoma: a population-based clinical study. J Clin Oncol 1996;14:1269–74.
57. Sherr CJ and McCormick F. The RB and p53 pathways in cancer. Cancer Cell 2002;2:103–12.
58. Lebwohl DE, Muise-Helmericks R, Sepp-Lorenzino L, et al. A truncated cyclin D1 gene encodes a stable mRNA in a human breast cancer cell line. Oncogene 1994;9:1925–9.
59. Lin S, Wang W, Wilson GM, et al. Down-regulation of cyclin D1 expression by prostaglandin A(2) is mediated by enhanced cyclin D1 mRNA turnover. Mol Cell Biol 2000; 20:7903–13.
60. Rimokh R, Berger F, Bastard C, et al. Rearrangement of CCND1 (BCL1/PRAD1) 3' untranslated region in mantle-cell lymphomas and t(11q13)-associated leukemias. Blood 1994; 83:3689–96.
61. de Boer CJ, van Krieken JH, Kluin-Nelemans HC, et al. Cyclin D1 messenger RNA overexpression as a marker for mantle cell lymphoma. Oncogene 1995;10:1833–40.
62. Seto M, Yamamoto K, Iida S, et al. Gene rearrangement and overexpression of PRAD1 in lymphoid malignancy with t(11;14)(q13;q32) translocation. Oncogene 1992;7:1401–6.
63. Withers DA, Harvey RC, Faust JB, et al. Characterization of a candidate bcl-1 gene. Mol Cell Biol 1991;11:4846–53.
64. Horning SJ. Follicular lymphoma: have we made any progress? Ann Oncol 2000;11(Suppl 1):23–7.
65. Johnson PW, Rohatiner AZ, Whelan JS, et al. Patterns of survival in patients with recurrent follicular lymphoma: a 20-year study from a single center. J Clin Oncol 1995;13:140–7.
66. Lossos IS and Levy R. Higher grade transformation of follicular lymphoma: phenotypic tumor progression associated with diverse genetic lesions. Semin Cancer Biol 2003;13: 191–202.
67. Dave SS, Wright G, Tan B, et al. A molecular predictor of survival following diagnosis of follicular lymphoma based on the profile of non-malignant tumor-infiltrating immune cells. N Engl J Med 2003;351:2159–69.
68. Allen LA and Aderem A. Molecular definition of distinct cytoskeletal structures involved in complement- and Fc receptor-mediated phagocytosis in macrophages. J Exp Med 1996;184:627–37.
69. Li DN, Matthews SP, Antoniou AN, et al. Multistep autoactivation of asparaginyl endopeptidase in vitro and in vivo. J Biol Chem 2003;278:38980–90.
70. Sui L, Zhang W, Liu Q, et al. Cloning and functional characterization of human septin 10, a novel member of septin family cloned from dendritic cells. Biochem Biophys Res Commun 2003;304:393–8.
71. Ames RS, Li Y, Sarau HM, et al. Molecular cloning and characterization of the human anaphylatoxin C3a receptor. J Biol Chem 1996;271:20231–4.
72. Roglic A, Prossnitz ER, Cavanagh SL, et al. cDNA cloning of a novel G protein-coupled receptor with a large extracellular loop structure. Biochim Biophys Acta 1996;1305:39–43.
73. Muzio M, Bosisio D, Polentarutti N, et al. Differential expression and regulation of toll-like receptors (TLR) in human leukocytes: selective expression of TLR3 in dendritic cells. J Immunol 2000;164:5998–6004.
74. Hayashi F, Smith KD, Ozinsky A, et al. The innate immune response to bacterial flagellin is mediated by Toll-like receptor 5. Nature 2001;410:1099–103.
75. Horning SJ and Rosenberg SA. The natural history of initially untreated low-grade non-Hodgkin's lymphomas. N Engl J Med 1984 311:1471–5.

76. Ponzio NM and Thorbecke GJ. Requirement for reverse immune surveillance for the growth of germinal center-derived murine lymphomas. Semin Cancer Biol 2000; 10:331–40.
77. Bendandi M, Gocke CD, Kobrin CB, et al. Complete molecular remissions induced by patient-specific vaccination plus granulocyte-monocyte colony-stimulating factor against lymphoma. Nat Med 1999;5:1171–7.
78. Kwak LW, Campbell MJ, Czerwinski DK, et al. Induction of immune responses in patients with B-cell lymphoma against the surface-immunoglobulin idiotype expressed by their tumors. N Engl J Med 1992;327:1209–15.
79. Timmerman JM, Czerwinski DK, Davis TA, et al. Idiotype-pulsed dendritic cell vaccination for B-cell lymphoma: clinical and immune responses in 35 patients. Blood 2002;99:1517–26.
80. Czuczman MS, Grillo-Lopez AJ, White CA, et al. Treatment of patients with low-grade B-cell lymphoma with the combination of chimeric anti-CD20 monoclonal antibody and CHOP chemotherapy. J Clin Oncol 1999;17:268–76.
81. Maloney DG, Grillo-Lopez AJ, White CA, et al. IDEC-C2B8 (Rituximab) anti-CD20 monoclonal antibody therapy in patients with relapsed low-grade non-Hodgkin's lymphoma. Blood 1997;90:2188–95.
82. Witzig TE, Gordon LI, Cabanillas F, et al. Randomized controlled trial of yttrium-90–labeled ibritumomab tiuxetan radioimmunotherapy versus rituximab immunotherapy for patients with relapsed or refractory low-grade, follicular, or transformed B-cell non-Hodgkin's lymphoma. J Clin Oncol 2002;20:2453–63.
83. Colombat P, Salles G, Brousse N, et al. Rituximab (anti-CD20 monoclonal antibody) as single first-line therapy for patients with follicular lymphoma with a low tumor burden: clinical and molecular evaluation. Blood 2001;97: 101–6.
84. Wright G, Dave SS, Tan B, et al. LymphDx: a custom microarray for molecular diagnosis and prognosis in non-Hodgkin lymphoma. Submitted 2004.

Epidemiology of Hodgkin's and Non-Hodgkin's Lymphomas

Naoko Ishibe, Sc.D.
Margaret Tucker, M.D.

Lymphomas are a heterogeneous group of malignancy of the lymphatic system, broadly classified into two categories: Hodgkin's lymphoma (more commonly known as Hodgkin's disease [HD]) and non-Hodgkin's lymphoma (NHL). HD accounts for approximately 15% of all lymphomas and is common in young adults. Overall incidence rates have held steady and, due to improvements in therapy, is a treatable disease, especially in younger people. NHL, in contrast, has had a largely unexplained rise in incidence and a greater variability in treatment success.[1] In this chapter, we discuss recent findings in the literature on the epidemiology of HD and NHL.

HODGKIN'S LYMPHOMA

Background

HD is an uncommon malignancy of the lymphatic system that was first described by Thomas Hodgkin in 1832. Its characteristic feature is the presence of multinucleated Hodgkin's and Reed–Sternberg cells (World Health Organization), but the etiology and molecular events that result in its malignant transformation remain largely unknown.

Incidence and Mortality Rates

Incidence Rates

HD has a unique bimodal distribution, with the first peak being between the ages of 15 and 34 years and a second peak among individuals over 50 years.[2] In the United States, it is estimated that approximately 7350 new cases of HD will be diagnosed in 2005.[3] The age-adjusted incidence rate with both genders combined was 2.7 per 100,000 person-years from 1997 to 2001.[4] Although the incidence rate has been relatively stable over time, differences in incidence rate have been observed across age groups. An increase of HD incidence among young adults and a decrease among individuals over 40 have been observed.[5,6] The decrease among older HD cases reflects a reduction in the number of misdiagnoses.[7]

In the United States, overall incidence rates are higher in men than in women, with a strong male predominance in pediatric HD cases. Incidence rates are highest in whites, followed by blacks and Hispanics, and lowest in Asians.[4] Internationally, the pattern in HD incidence rates is similar to those observed in the United States. Asians have the lowest rates, with age-adjusted incidence rates of 0.8 per 100,000 in men, and 0.2 per 100,000 in women. In Caucasians, the incidence rates observed are 4.5 per 100,000 in men and 3.0 per 100,000 in women.[8]

Histologically, HD is classified into four subtypes that differ clinically and epidemiologically. The four histologic subtypes delineated by the Rye classification system follow: lymphocyte depleted (LD), lymphocyte predominant (LP), mixed cellularity (MC), and nodular sclerosis (NS). Nodular sclerosis is the most common subtype; based on a study by Glaser, age-adjusted incidence rate of 1.5 per 100,000 was observed.[9] In contrast, the LD subtype is the least common form with an age-adjusted incidence rate of 0.19 per 100,000.[9]

Although all four variants occur across all age groups, race/ethnicities, and genders, the subtypes of HD are distributed differently. NS is most commonly observed in young adults, whereas older adult cases are much more likely to exhibit the less common MC and LD subtypes.[10] Moreover, rates of NS have increased among younger people, especially in women.[7] Although the pattern of histologic subtypes are identical by race/ethnicity (i.e., NS is most common and LD is least common), in African Americans of both genders, the bimodal age-specific pattern is less striking than in whites.[11] The relatively depressed HD rates in blacks at young adult and older adult ages reflect lower rates of NS in young adulthood and of MC and LD subtypes at older ages.[12]

Mortality Rates and Survival

Between the late 1960s and late 1990s, mortality from HD has declined by over 60% in Western Europe, and to an even greater extent in the United States,[12] with resulting mortality rates of 0.5 per 100,000 in men and 0.3 per 100,000 in women. Much of this improvement has been attributed to the development of multiagent chemotherapy and more accurate radiotherapy; patients with early-stage disease having 5-year survival rates of 90% are common.[13]

Even though improvements in treatment have made HD one of the most successfully treated cancers, mortality rates have not declined nearly as appreciably in Eastern European countries, and older adult patients with HD continue to have poorer prognosis than younger adult cases, even when stage and histology are taken into account.[14,15] Five-year relative survival rate for patients diagnosed under age 45 is nearly twice that for persons diagnosed over the age of 65 (89% vs. 45%).[15]

Risk Factors Associated with Hodgkin's Lymphoma

Genetics

Approximately 5% of HD cases have been estimated to occur as familial HD,[16] and the importance of genetic factors in the etiology of HD has been suggested by family and population studies. Studies of familial aggregation of HD have found a threefold increase in risk for developing HD in first-degree relatives.[17–19] This association is stronger among younger cases,[17] males,[17–20] and siblings.[17,21]

Further evidence suggesting a role for shared genetic factors is the elevation in risk of HD among monozygotic twins.[22,23] In a study of 432 sets of monozygotic and dizygotic twins affected by HD, Mack et al. observed 10 pairs of twins concordant for the disease; all 10 pairs who were affected with HD were monozygotic twins.[23]

HD was first associated with the human leukocyte antigen (HLA) type in a study by Amiel.[24] Since then, several studies have weakly, but consistently, associated the HLA Class I region on chromosome 6 to familial HD.[25–28] Although maximum logarithm of the odds (LOD) scores have been modest, ranging from 2.12 to 3.55, depending on the assumptions made (e.g., dominant or recessive models), it appears that a subset of HD families is genetically linked.

More recently, studies have suggested that adult HD is influenced by the HLA Class II antigens,[29–32] although it is not clear which is the main susceptibility locus. In a familial Hodgkin's disease study, evidence for linkage disequilibrium was reported for the *DRB1*1501–DQA1*0102–DQB1*0602* haplotype and the *DRB5-0101* allele, particularly in familial HD cases with nodular sclerosis histologic subtype.[29] In sporadic HD, the *HLA-DPB1* locus has most consistently been found to confer susceptibility to HD, although the associations have been small.[31,32]

Another approach to identify potential susceptibility genes is a whole genome linkage screen. Among 44 high-risk families, 1058 microsatellite markers spaced at approximately 3.5 centimorgans were genotyped.[33] The strongest evidence for linkage was found near marker D4S394 (nominal $p = 0.00002$). The results were consistent with recessive inheritance. Other locations suggestive of linkage were found on chromosomes 2 and 11.

Infectious Agents

Epstein–Barr Virus

For many years, HD has been thought to have an infectious etiology. Epstein–Barr virus (EBV), in particular, has received special attention since the observation by Evans that HD in young adults shares epidemiologic features with infectious mononucleosis (IM).[34] Since then, considerable evidence supporting the role for a chronic EBV infection in HD has emerged. Several cohort studies following up individuals who have had IM have shown a threefold increase in risk of HD.[35–37] Furthermore, elevated anti-EBV antibody titers have been observed to precede the onset of HD,[38] and EBV has been found in the malignant cells of HD (i.e., Hodgkin's/Reed–Sternberg cells),[39,40] suggesting a link between the infectious agent and the disease.

Recent studies investigating the association between EBV and HD have indicated that the association is quite complex. Not only is the prevalence of EBV in HD cases more common in less developed countries than in industrialized nations,[41,42] but it is also more common in the mixed cellularity histologic subtype than in the predominant nodular sclerosis subtype.[43] Furthermore, a number of studies have reported that the association between EBV and HD is more common in childhood and later-onset HD rather than in young adult cases, as first hypothesized.[41,44,45] The majority of HD is of the nodular sclerosis histologic subtype, particularly in young adults, which may partly explain these findings.

However, a few recent studies suggest that the role of EBV in young adults is still unclear. Hjalgrim et al. conducted a large population-based study following patients with IM in Denmark and Sweden and reported the excess risk of HD to be confined to children and young adults.[36] Alexander et al. also reported a statistically significant association between IM and HD that was heightened in EBV-positive HD.[46] Furthermore, the same group found that the association of IM with EBV-positive HD cases was particularly strong in a subgroup with HLA-Class II DPB1*0301 phenotype.[46]

Human Herpesvirus-6

Human herpesvirus-6 (HHV-6) is a T-lymphotropic double-stranded DNA virus that is ubiquitous in human adult population that has been suggested to play a role in the development of HD. Epidemiologic studies have found higher frequency and higher titers of anti–HHV-6 antibodies in patients with HD than in controls,[47] a correlation between antibody titers and the clinical course of HD,[48] and a higher frequency of HHV-6 sequences by PCR and Southern blot analysis in HD.[47,49] However, unlike EBV, HHV-6 DNA has not been detectable in the neoplastic HRS cells,[50] arguing against its pathogenic role in HD.

Human Immunodeficiency Virus-1

Infection with human immunodeficiency virus (HIV) is associated with an increased risk of developing certain cancers, including Kaposi's sarcoma, NHL (see section on NHL), and HD. However, the occurrence of HIV-associated HD has been overshadowed by the strong association observed between HIV infection and NHL. Yet, significant increases in risk of HD, with odds ratios (ORs) ranging between 2.5 and 11.5, have been reported among individuals with or at risk of AIDS.[51–55] In contrast to the histologic type predominant in HIV-negative young adults, the mixed cellularity subtype predominates in individuals with AIDS.[52,56]

Although the information on AIDS-associated lymphomas from less developed countries is limited, the association with HD appears to be specific to individuals living in Western countries. In a case-control study in South Africa, no association was observed between HIV status and HD (OR = 1.4, 95% confidence interval [CI] 0.7–2.8).[57] One explanation for this observation includes the possibility that patients in Africa are dying of other HIV-associated diseases.

Occupational Exposures

WOODWORKING

Studies have addressed whether certain occupational groups are at increased risk of developing HD. Numerous investigations have focused on the woodworking industry since a twofold increase in risk of HD among woodworkers was published in 1967.[58] Although a moderately positive association between HD and woodworking has been reported by five studies,[58–62] an equal number have reported no elevation in risk among those employed in the woodworking industry.[63–67]

CHEMICAL EXPOSURES

Other occupational hazards that have been investigated due to initial reports of an elevated risk of HD include exposure to chemical agents such as benzene, phenoxy herbicides, and chlorophenols. However, subsequent studies have not produced convincing evidence linking these exposures to HD.[68]

NON-HODGKIN'S LYMPHOMA

Background

Non-Hodgkin's lymphomas (NHL) are a heterogeneous group of lymphoproliferative diseases with longstanding confusion as to its classification. In an effort to create a classification system with standardized nomenclature, numerous classification schemes have been proposed. The latest World Health Organization classification of malignant lymphomas emphasizes the importance of using all available features (i.e., morphology, immunophenotype, genetic, and clinical features) in the diagnosis of NHL, and includes follicular lymphoma; diffuse large B-cell lymphoma (DLBCL); Burkitt's lymphoma; mantle cell lymphoma; mucosa-associated lymphoid tissue (MALT) lymphoma; mature T-cell lymphoma; chronic lymphocytic leukemia/small lymphocytic lymphoma (CLL/SLL); mediastinal large B-cell lymphoma; anaplastic large-cell lymphoma; nodal marginal zone lymphoma; and precursor T-lymphoblastic, lymphoplasmacytic lymphoma, and other types.[69]

Incidence and Mortality Rates

Incidence Rates

The most striking feature of NHL is the largely unexplained increase in incidence that has been observed over the last 20 years in the United States and European countries.[6] This increase is partly due to AIDS-associated lymphomas, but these histologic types (central nervous system, Burkitt's, and high-grade immunoblastic) have decreased since the introduction of retroviral therapy[70] in 1995, and risk factors responsible for the observed increase remain largely unknown.

The overall annual incidence rate of NHL estimated from the nine registries that participate in the Surveillance, Epidemiology and End Results (SEER) program of the National Cancer Institute was 19.0 cases per 100,000 persons in 2001,[4] and an estimated 56,390 NHL cases will be diagnosed in the United States in 2005.[3] Age-adjusted incidence

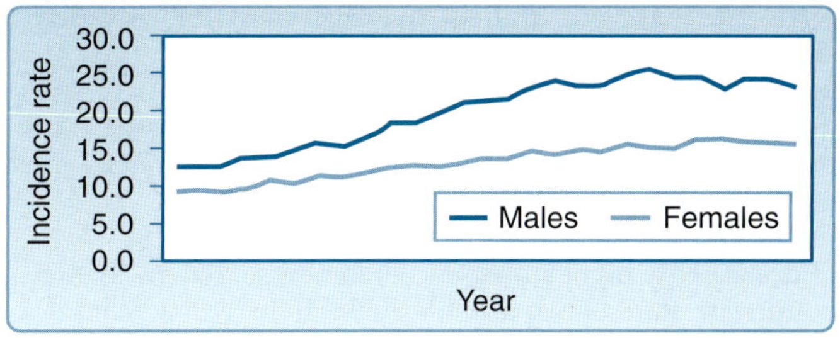

Figure 6–1. Age-adjusted incidence of all non-Hodgkin's lymphoma combined, by gender in Surveillance, Epidemiology and End Results program of National Cancer Institute, 1975–2001.

rates show steady increases in both genders (Fig. 6–1) over this time period, and rates are consistently higher among men than women and in whites compared to nonwhites.

Moreover, time trends in incidence rates show a more complex pattern when histologic type and disease site are taken into account. The data on histology in SEER have varied over time, and the majority of the data are in working formulation classification. The histologic types from other eras can be translated to working formulation for consistency (Fig. 6–2). There is a steady rise in incidence over the entire time period for all of the subtypes, with a small recent decrease in the high grade. The majority of non-Hodgkin's lymphomas arise in lymph nodes, and incidences of follicular and nodular lymphomas have steadily increased. Data obtained from the SEER program suggest that increases in

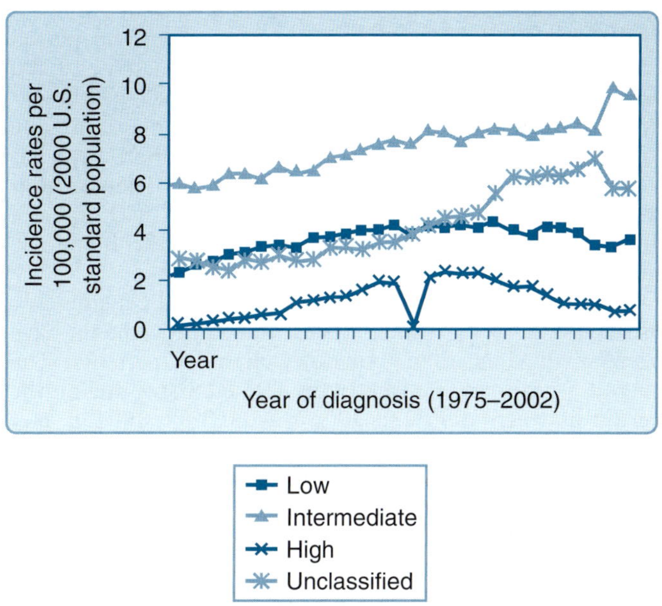

Figure 6–2. Age-adjusted incidence rates for working formulation subtypes in Surveillance, Epidemiology and End Results program of National Cancer Institute, 1975–2001. In this graph, low grade includes ICD-O-2 codes 9670–9671, 9693–9696, 9691–9692; intermediate grade includes 9697–9698, 9672–9676, 9688, 9593, 9680–9683; high grade includes 9684–9687; and unclassified grade includes 9590–9592, 9594–9595, 9677, 9690, 9700–9709, 9710–9717.

NHL incidence are limited to NHL types not considered AIDS-associated and in groups at low risk of AIDS (i.e., men over 55 years of age and women of all ages).[71] When AIDS-associated lymphomas were examined in SEER, these histologic types revealed a peak incidence around 1995 with a subsequent decline in rate.[71]

Internationally, NHL incidence rates vary 8- to 10-fold,[72,73] with higher incidence rates observed in Western countries. Rates are particularly high in North America, Australia, Italy, and Switzerland,[74] and lower in Asian countries. Rates in South America are intermediate between those in Asia and North America.[75] However, incidence rates appear to be increasing across virtually all registries; consistent declines have not been observed in any registry.

In children, particularly high incidence rates have been noted in Egypt, among non-Kuwaitis in Kuwait, in Portugal, in Spain, and in U.S. blacks.[76] Excluding Burkitt's lymphoma, the NHL pattern mirrors those for Hodgkin's lymphoma, where rates are lowest in Asian countries, intermediate in developed countries of North America and Europe, and highest in developing countries in Latin America and the Middle East. Incidence rates are also higher in males than in females.

In the United States, the age-adjusted incidence rates for childhood NHL under the age of 15 years ranged from 0.6 to 1.0 per 100,000 person-years from 1975 to 2001.[4] Similar to pediatric HD, mortality rates in children with NHL have declined substantially between 1975 and 2000 from 0.4 per 100,000 to 0.2 per 100,000.

Mortality and Survival Rates

The mortality rate from NHL in the United States was 8.4 deaths per 100,000 based on estimates from the period between 1997 and 2001,[4] and an estimated 19,200 deaths will result due to this disease in 2005.[3] Although mortality has decreased in children and young adults due to improvements in treatment, overall mortality has increased over time, especially in the elderly.[75] These secular trends may reflect trends in incidence rates, inaccuracy of diagnosis, or improved treatments for specific histologic subtypes.

Population-based 5-year survival improved considerably in the 1970s in the United States, but improvements have been small since then, especially in older patients. The overall 5-year survival rate in the United States during the period between 1995 and 2000 was 60.3%,[4] and Fig. 6–3 illustrates survival trends from 1974 to 2000 by gender and race/ethnicity. Overall, females have slightly better 5-year survival rates than males, and whites have better survival rates than blacks.[4]

However, survival rates differ considerably by histologic subtype. Low-grade lymphomas, such as SLL and follicular lymphoma, have higher survival rates than intermediate-grade lymphomas, such as DLBCL. High-grade lymphomas, such as CNS lymphoma, Burkitt's lymphoma, and immunoblastic lymphoma have the poorest survival rates.[77] Table 6–1 summarizes relative survival rates by NHL subtypes from SEER in working formulation. Survival has improved for each subtype over time.

Table 6–1. Five-Year and 10-Year Relative Survival Rates (%) by Non-Hodgkin Lymphoma Subgroup (Working Formulation) and by Year of Diagnosis from Surveillance Epidemiology and End Results, 1975–1999

	Low	Intermediate	High	Unclassified
5-Year Relative Survival Rates				
1975–1979	63.3	41.9	29.4	50.1
1980–1984	67.1	45.7	38.2	55.6
1985–1989	69.0	48.6	36.2	50.0
1990–1994	71.5	49.7	35.5	49.1
1995–1999	76.6	52.0	44.3	61.0
10-Year Relative Survival Rates				
1975–1979	46.6	34.1	24.1	41.4
1980–1984	49.0	37.8	33.3	46.9
1985–1989	50.1	41.0	31.8	43.1
1990–1994	55.7	43.1	32.6	42.3
1995–1999	NA	NA	NA	NA

NA, not available.

Risk Factors Associated with Non-Hodgkin's Lymphoma

Immunodeficiency

Transplantation

Immunodeficiency, whether congenital or acquired, is associated with an increased risk of NHL. Epidemiologic studies have consistently reported a considerable increase of developing NHL among patients who have been immune suppressed for organ or bone marrow transplantation.[78–80] Relative risks of 10 to 67 have been reported following renal,[80–82] bone marrow,[79] and heart transplantations.[78] In a Swedish study of 5931 patients who underwent transplantation for kidney, liver, heart, and other organs between 1970 and 1997, a marked excess of NHL cases was observed (standardized incidence ratio [SIR] = 5.0; 95% CI 4.4–8.0). This association was particularly strong during the first year following transplantation, transplantation at a young age, and among non–renal-transplant patients.[80] Post-transplant lymphomas commonly have extranodal involvement, particularly of the central nervous system,[81] and histologically, the tumors tend to be diffuse large cells.[82]

Autoimmune Disorders

Patients with autoimmune disorders,[83] such as rheumatoid arthritis,[84,85] Sjögren's syndrome,[86,87] Hashimoto thyroiditis,[88] and systemic lupus,[89,90] also have elevated risk of NHL. The increase in risk has been attributed to the disturbance in immune function found in these patients or to the immunosuppressive therapy used to treat these autoimmune disorders. However, the predominant lymphoma subtype appears to vary by autoimmune disorder (e.g., rheumatoid arthritis and DLBCL; Sjögren's syndrome and MALT lymphoma),[91] suggesting that different mechanisms are involved.

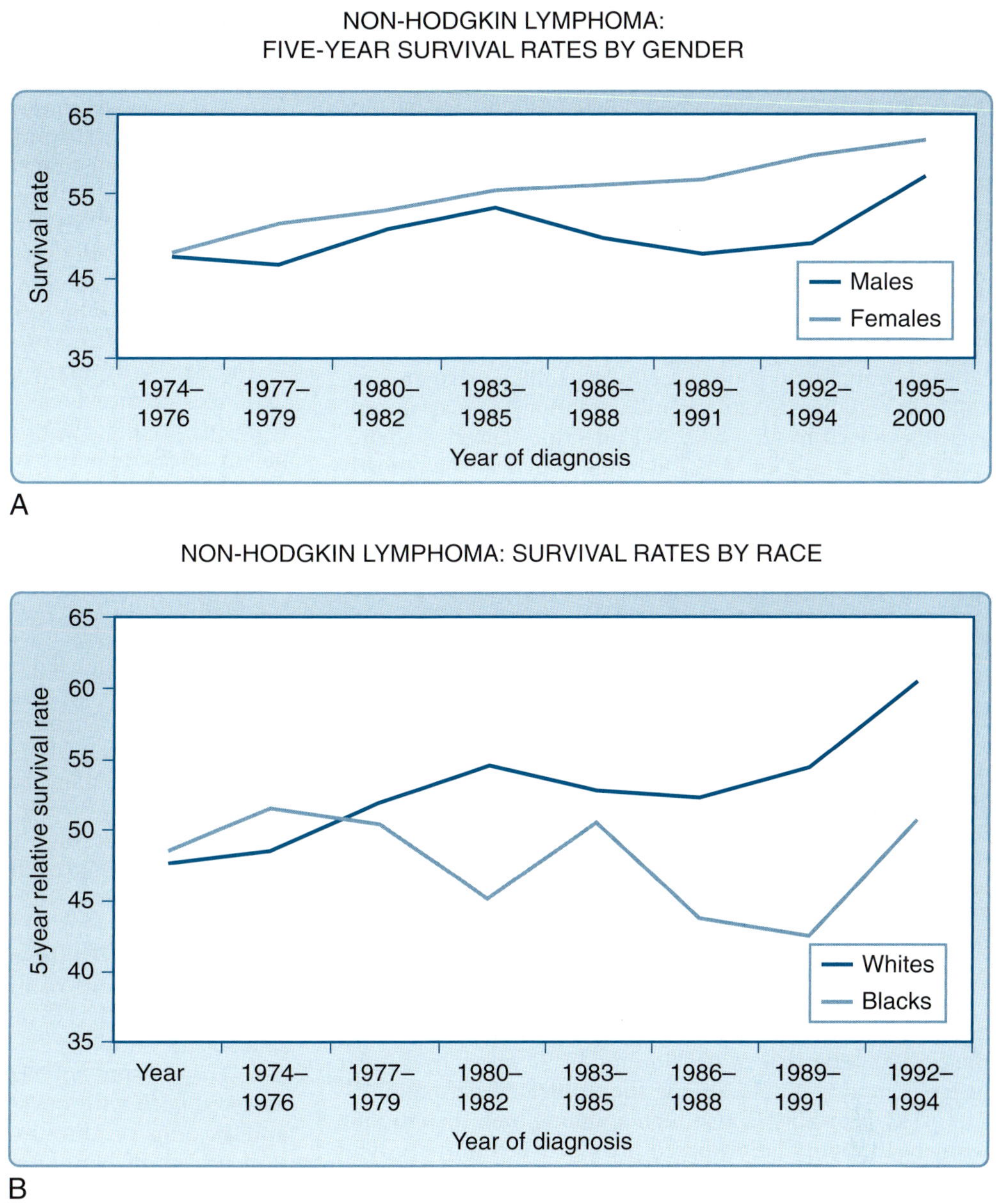

Figure 6–3. **A:** Age-adjusted 5-year relative survival rates of all non-Hodgkin's lymphomas (NHL) combined, by gender, in Surveillance, Epidemiology and End Results program of National Cancer Institute (SEER), 1975–2001. **B:** Age-adjusted 5-year relative survival rates of all NHL combined, by race/ethnicity, in SEER, 1975–2001.

Infectious Agents

Human Immunodeficiency Virus

HIV infection is associated with aggressive, systemic NHL presenting with widespread disease and extranodal involvement with poor prognosis.[92] Compared with high-grade NHL in HIV-negative patients, patients with AIDS-associated NHL have a higher rate of relapse and shorter overall survival.[93]

More specifically, primary brain lymphoma, Burkitt's lymphoma, and immunoblastic NHL have been classified as AIDS-defining illnesses since the beginning of the AIDS epidemic,[94] and approximately 4% to 5% of AIDS patients have NHL as their AIDS-defining illness.[95] With the introduction of highly active antiretroviral therapy (HAART), incidence rates for AIDS-related NHL have declined from 6.2 to 3.6 per 1000 person-years,[70] but NHL as a proportion of AIDS-defining illnesses has also increased.[95] While some studies have reported little improvement in survival in AIDS-related NHL since the introduction of HAART,[96,97] others have demonstrated improved survival.[98–100]

Epstein–Barr Virus

EBV DNA has been observed in 10% to 30% of all NHL tumors,[101] but is most strongly associated with Burkitt's lymphoma. EBV is present 'in essentially all cases of endemic Burkitt's lymphoma (eBL), which occurs in children where malaria is endemic.[102,103] It is the most common pediatric cancer in tropical Africa, accounting for approximately 50% of all childhood cancer,[104] and average annual incidence rates vary from 5 to 10 per 100,000 in children under the age of 15.[105] The age peak of eBL is between 5 and 10 years, and there is a marked decline after age 15 years.[106] It is also more common in boys than girls by a 2:1 ratio, and this preponderance is even stronger in eBL patients with jaw tumors (3:1).[107]

In contrast, only about 15% to 30% of all nonendemic, or sporadic BL (sBL) are EBV related and occur less frequently.[108] In the United States, the incidence rate of sBL is closer to 2 per million,[105] and age at diagnosis is more evenly distributed throughout the first two decades of life. Like eBL, a three-to-one predominance of sBL in males is observed.[107]

Helicobacter pylori

Most gastric mucosa-associated lymphoid tissue (MALT) lymphomas are acquired as a reaction to *H. pylori* infection,[109] and a case–control study reported a six-fold increase in gastric lymphoma risk with previous *H. pylori* infection.[110] MALT lymphomas are thought to originate from cells in the marginal zone of secondary follicles that are generated in response to chronic inflammation, such as chronic gastritis caused by this bacterial infection. Direct evidence confirming its role in MALT lymphomagenesis has mostly been obtained from in vitro experiments and clinical evaluations. Remission of gastric MALT lymphoma can be achieved in 60% to 90% of patients who are treated with antibiotics used to eradicate *H. pylori*.[111,112]

Human T-Cell Lymphotropic Virus-1

Human T-cell lymphotropic virus-1 (HTLV-1) is a major risk factor for adult T-cell lymphoma/leukemia (ATLL) in endemic areas of southern Japan, the Caribbean Basin, West Africa, the Middle East, South America, and Melanesia.[113] Several methods of viral transmission have been well established, including sexual, transfusion related, and through breastfeeding.[114] The latency period from infection to ATLL is quite long. ATLL is thought to be a clonal expansion of HTLV-1 infected CD4+ T lymphocytes. The viral oncoprotein Tax is important in this process. Tax alters signaling pathways, leading to increased cytokine production, lymphocyte proliferation, and accumulation of somatic mutations.[114] The lifetime risk of developing ATLL is small, less than 5%.[115] The risk of developing ATLL varies by gender in Japan, and is higher among those infected perinatally.[116] The ATLL mortality is also higher among men than among women. In a population-based prospective cohort study of the natural history of HTLV-1 infection, significantly higher proviral loads have been found in individuals prior to diagnosis of ATLL than in controls.[117] The natural history of disease in infected individuals varies by population.[113] The rates of ATLL are higher in the Japanese than Jamaicans; in Jamaicans, there is no detectable gender difference. In a comparison of Jamaican and Japanese carriers with similar provirus loads, Jamaican carriers were more likely to have higher antibody titers ($p = 0.002$) and detection of anti-Tax antibody ($p = 0.002$) than Japanese carriers. These findings suggest that the differences in the immune response may explain part of the population differences in rates of ATLL.

Borrelia burgdorferi

Since the early 1990s, an association between the causal agent for Lyme disease and a low-grade cutaneous B-cell lymphoma has been recognized. Histologically, these tumors are similar to mucosa-associated B-cell lymphoma (MALT), frequently related to infection with *H. pylori*.[118] Eradication of *B. burgdorferi* has been associated with resolution of the lymphoma.[119,120] *B. burgdorferi*, however, is rare among the cutaneous B-cell lymphomas.[121]

Occupational and Environmental Exposures

Pesticides

Agricultural workers are exposed to a diverse array of chemical hazards, and a number of epidemiologic studies have reported an association between farming and NHL.[122–125] Although not all studies support these findings,[126,127] the increase in NHL risk may be due, in part, to pesticide use.[128–130] Pesticide exposure is not limited to farmers, and a recent study by Zahm reported an increase in NHL risk among workers who applied pesticide employed at a lawn care company.[130]

Until recently, many of these human studies have relied on surrogate measures, such as occupation or self-reported exposure frequency. In a recent study, direct biologic exposure measurements were made of serum pesticide and polychlorinated biphenyl concentration.[131] Quintana et al. reported a significant increase in NHL with organochlorine pesticide exposure, supporting the previous occupational findings.[131] In a population-based case–control study assessing organochlorines in vacuum cleaner dust, an increase in risk (OR 1.5, 95% CI 1.2–2.0) of NHL was found for polychlorinated biphenyl congeners with a suggestive trend. There was also a small risk in men associated with dichlorodiphenyldichloroethylene.[132]

Within the class of pesticides, the widespread use of herbicides in particular has raised public concern since an initial report of a six-fold risk with NHL was described.[133,134] A number of studies that analyzed cases and controls exposed to phenoxyacetic acids reported a positive association with the most widely used herbicide 2,4-dichlorophenoxyacetic acid (2,4-D),[135,136] but some subsequent studies have not supported these findings.[122,137] A recent study conducted in a cohort of male employees who manufactured the herbicide 2,4-D[138] did not find them to be at increased risk of developing NHL. In a large population-based case–control study of NHL, residential use of herbicides was assessed both with questionnaire data and measured 2,4-D and dicamba residues in vacuum cleaner dust.[139] No elevation in risk of lymphoma was found for residential exposure to these herbicides. Although use of herbicides has been postulated to contribute to the population increase over time, this large study found no evidence to support the hypothesis. However, the Institute of Medicine concluded that there is sufficient evidence to consider herbicides as a risk factor of NHL.[140]

Organic Solvents

Organic solvents, such as benzene and trichloroethylene (TCE), are known carcinogens, and exposure to these chemicals cause lymphatic and hematopoietic tumors in animals.[141,142] Contact with various organic solvents has been reported to be associated with excess NHL risk.[127,143–146] One study found a threefold statistically significant increase in risk among patients with high-grade exposure to organic solvents, as well as a nonsignificant increase in risk among those with low-grade exposure.[143] A study by Blair et al.[144] also observed odds ratio that was slightly larger among those in the higher intensity category, but the association was not statistically significant.

Excesses among occupational groups or industry that are routinely exposed to organic solvents have also been reported. Employment in dry cleaning,[125,147] aircraft maintenance,[148] publishing, petroleum refining, painting,[149] and building cleaning services (e.g., janitors) have all weakly been associated with increased NHL risk.[125]

Ultraviolet Radiation Exposure

Ultraviolet radiation is an established cause of immune suppression and has been hypothesized to increase the risk of NHL. Indirect evidence, most notably ecologic studies, links NHL with exposure to sunlight. Ecologic studies show parallel geographic patterns and temporal trends in NHL,[150,151] and a population-based study in Sweden found a modest association between sunlight and NHL using geographic latitude of residence as a surrogate variable of sun exposure.[126] Others have also reported a relationship between NHL incidence with residing in areas with greater sun exposure,[152,153] but not all studies have confirmed this association.[154–157] A recent large Scandinavian case–control study demonstrated consistent, significant negative associations of sun exposure measures and risk of NHL.[158]

Positive associations with cutaneous malignancies, tumors strongly associated with sun exposure, have also been observed with NHL, providing further support for this hypothesis. A number of studies have demonstrated an increased relative risk for NHL after the diagnosis of skin cancers including melanoma and vice versa.[158–162] Additional studies also suggest that NHL occurs more frequently in individuals with light, nonpigmented skin than those with darker, pigmented skin.[74,163]

Hair Dyes

Since the late 1970s, use of hair dyes has been investigated as a risk factor for NHL. Both occupational and personal use have been assessed with inconsistent findings.[164–169] The inconsistency may be partially explained by a recent finding that risk was only elevated among long-term users who started dying their hair before 1980.[170] In this study, risk of NHL was doubled among those who used darker permanent dyes for more than 25 years. No risk was found in those who started dying their hair after 1980.

Genetics

Genetic Immunodeficiency Syndromes

Patients with genetic immunodeficiency syndromes, such as ataxia-telangiectasia (AT), Wiskott–Aldrich syndrome, and X-linked lymphoproliferative syndrome, have been documented to be predisposed to developing lymphoma.[171–174] Upwards of 25% of patients with these immunodeficiencies will develop cancer, of which NHL accounts for more than 50% of these malignancies.[175]

Familial Aggregation

Apart from these syndromes, familial aggregation of lymphomas has been reported in family and population-based studies. Families with multiple cases of NHL have been described[176,177] in the literature, but no clear mode of inheritance pattern has emerged. The majority of NHL occurring in families has been in sib pairs,[176] although multi-generational pedigrees and parent–child affectation patterns have noted anticipation in these families, suggesting a possible genetic basis. However, being simultaneously exposed to an environmental agent cannot be ruled out. A large population-based study in Scandinavia found apparent evidence of anticipation, but when secular trends of increasing incidence of NHL were accounted for, the evidence for anticipation disappeared.[178]

Population-based studies have also consistently shown NHL cases to be more likely to have a family history of lymphoma than controls.[179–182] In general, the risk of lymphoma among siblings of NHL cases has been stronger and among males.[182,183] However, the associations are modest, and it is unlikely that a major proportion of cases have a strong genetic basis.

CONCLUSIONS

Hodgkin's Lymphoma

Incidence rates have remained stable and improvements in treatment have prolonged survival, and HD apparently is closely linked with infectious agents, such as EBV. Yet, the etiology of HD remains unclear and prevention strategies have not emerged. Epidemiologic studies incorporating molecular techniques are a priority, since they may clarify the role of known risk factors, such as EBV, and identify other causal pathways.

Non-Hodgkin's Lymphoma

The factors leading to the secular increase in NHL rates have yet to be identified, although a number of suspected causes have been identified. One recurring theme that increases the risk of NHL appears to be related to immune dysfunction. Individuals at increased risk include those with primary immunodeficiency diseases, with AIDS, and who are immunosuppressed subsequent to transplantation. Multidisciplinary approaches will need to be utilized to gain a better understanding of this disease.

References

1. Sherr PA, Mueller NE. Non-Hodgkin's lymphomas. In: Schottenfeld D and Fraumeni JF Jr, eds., Cancer Epidemiology and Prevention, 2nd ed. New York: Oxford University Press, 1996:920–45.
2. MacMahon B. Epidemiology of Hodgkin's disease. Cancer Res 1966;26:1189–200.
3. Jemal A, Murray T, Ward E, et al. Cancer Statistics, 2005. CA Cancer J Clin 2005;55:10–30.
4. Ries LAG, Eisner MP, Kosary CL, et al., eds. SEER Cancer Statistics Review, 1975–2001. Bethesda, MD: National Cancer Institute, 2004.
5. Glaser SL. Recent incidence and secular trends in Hodgkin's disease and its histologic subtypes. J Chron Dis 1986;39: 789–98.
6. Hartge P, Devesa SS, Fraumeni JF Jr. Hodgkin's and non-Hodgkin's lymphomas. In: Doll R, Fraumeni JF Jr, Muir CS, eds., Trends in Cancer Incidence and Mortality. Cold Spring Harbor, NY: Cold Spring Harbor Laboratory Press, 1994: 423–53.
7. Glaser SL, Swartz WG. Time trends in Hodgkin's disease incidence: the role of diagnostic accuracy. Cancer 1990;66: 2196–204.

8. Parkin DM, Muir CS, Whelan SL, et al. Cancer Incidence in Five Continents, Vol. VI. IARC Scientific Publications 120. Lyon: International Agency for Research on Cancer, 1992.
9. Glaser SL. Regional variation in Hodgkin's disease incidence by histologic subtype in the U.S. Cancer 1987;60:2841–7.
10. Clarke CC, Glaser SL, Prehn AW. Age-specific survival after Hodgkin's disease in population-based cohort (United States). Cancer Causes Control 2001;12:803–12.
11. Glaser SL. Black-White differences in Hodgkin's disease incidence in the United States by age, sex, histology subtype and time. Int J Epidemiol 1991;20:68–75.
12. Levi F, Lucchini F, Negri E, et al. Trends in mortality from Hodgkin's disease in western and eastern Europe. Br J Cancer 2002;87:291–3.
13. Kennedy BJ, Loeb V, Peterson VM, et al. National survey of patterns of care for Hodgkin's disease. Med Pediatr Oncol 1985;56:2547–56.
14. Walker A, Schoenfeld ER, Lowman JT, et al. Survival of the older patient compared with the younger patients with Hodgkin's disease. Cancer 1990;65:1635–40.
15. Ries LAG, Kosary CL, Hankey BF, et al. SEER Cancer Statistics Review, 1973–1996. Bethesda, MD: National Cancer Institute, 1999.
16. Ferraris AM, Racchi O, Rapezzi D, et al. Familial Hodgkin's disease: a disease of young adulthood? Ann Hematol 1997; 74:131–4.
17. Goldin LR, Pfeiffer RM, Gridley G, et al. Familial aggregation of Hodgkin lymphoma and related tumors. Cancer 2004;100:1902–8.
18. Kerzin-Stoarrar L, Faed MJ, MacGillivray JB, et al. Incidence of familial Hodgkin's disease. Br J Cancer 1983;47:707–12.
19. Bernard SM, Cartwright RA, Darwin CM, et al. Hodgkin's disease: case–control epidemiological study in Yorkshire. Br J Cancer 1987;55:85–90.
20. Hemminki K, Li X. Cancer risks in twins: results from the Swedish Family Cancer Database. Int J Cancer 2002;99: 873–8.
21. Grufferman S, Cole P, Smith PG, et al. Hodgkin's disease in siblings. N Engl J Med 1977;296:248–50.
22. Shibuya H, Tsukada K, Takagi M, et al. Synchronous Hodgkin's disease in monozygotic twins. Acta Radiol Oncol 1984;23:425–8.
23. Mack TM, Cozen W, Shibata DK, et al. Concordance for Hodgkin's disease in identical twins suggesting genetic susceptibility to the young-adult form of the disease. N Engl J Med. 1995;334:413–8.
24. Amiel JL. Study of the leukocyte phenotype in Hodgkin's disease. In: Curtoni ES, Matting PL, Tosi MR, eds., Histocompatibility Testing. Copenhagen: Ejnar Munksgaard, 1967:79–81.
25. Hors J, Dausset J. HLA and susceptibility to Hodgkin's disease. Immunol Rev 1983;70:167–92.
26. Risch N. Assessing the role of HLA-linked and unlinked determinants of disease. Am J Hum Genet 1987;40:1–14.
27. Berberich FR, Berberich MS, King MC, et al. Hodgkin's disease susceptibility: linkage to the HLA locus demonstrated by a new concordance method. Hum Immunol 1983;6:207–17.
28. Shugart YY, Collins A. Combined segregation and linkage analysis of 59 Hodgkin's disease families indicates the role of HLA determinants. Eur J Hum Genet 2000;8: 460–3.
29. Harty LC, Lin AY, Goldstein AM, et al. HLA-DR, HLA-DQ, and TAP genes in familial Hodgkin disease. Blood 2002;99: 690–3.
30. Klitz W, Aldrich CL, Fildes N, et al. Localization of predisposition to Hodgkin's disease in the HLA class II region. Am J Hum Genet 1994;54:497–505.
31. Taylor GM, Gokhale DA, Crowther D, et al. Further investigation of the role of HLA-DPB1 in adult Hodgkin's disease (HD) suggests an influence on susceptibility to different HD subtypes. Br J Cancer 1999;80:1405–11.
32. Alexander FE, Jarrett RF, Cartwright RA, et al. Epstein–Barr virus and HLA-DPB1-*0301 in young adult Hodgkin's disease: evidence of inherited susceptibility to Epstein–Barr virus in cases that are EBV^{+ve}. Cancer Epidemiol Biomarkers Prev 2001;10:705–9.
33. Goldin LR, MccMaster ML, Ter-Minassian M, et al. A genome screen of families at high risk for Hodgkin lymphoma: evidence for a susceptibility gene on chromosome 4. J Med Genet 2005;42:595–601.
34. Evans AS. The spectrum of infections with Epstein–Barr virus: a hypothesis. J Infectious Dis 1971;124:330–7.
35. Gutensohn N, Cole P. Epidemiology of Hodgkin's disease. Semin Oncol 1980;7:92–102.
36. Hjalgrim H, Askling J, Sorensen P, et al. Risk of Hodgkin's disease and other cancers after infectious mononucleosis. J Natl Cancer Inst 2000;92:1522–8.
37. International Agency for Research on Cancer. Epstein–Barr Virus and Kaposi's Sarcoma Herpesvirus/Human Herpesvirus 8. Vol. 70, IARC monographs on the evaluation of carcinogenic risks to humans. Lyon: IARC Press, 1997.
38. Mueller N, Evans A, Harris NL, et al. Hodgkin's disease and Epstein–Barr virus: altered antibody pattern before diagnosis. N Engl J Med 1989;320:689–95.
39. Weiss LM, Movahed LA, Warnke RA, et al. Detection of Epstein–Barr viral genomes in Reed-Sternberg cells of Hodgkin's disease. N Engl J Med 1989;320:502–6,.
40. Pallesen G, Hamilton-Dutoit SJ, Rowe M, et al. Expression of Epstein–Barr virus latent gene products in tumour cells of Hodgkin's disease. Lancet 1991;337:320–2,.
41. Jarrett RF, Armstrong AA, Alexander E. Epidemiology of EBV and Hodgkin's lymphoma. Ann Oncol 1996;7(Suppl):5–10.
42. Chang KL, Albujar PF, Chen YY, et al. High prevalence of Epstein–Barr virus in the Reed-Sternberg cells of Hodgkin's disease occurring in Peru. Blood 1993;81:496–501.
43. Glaser SL, Lin RJ, Stewart SL, et al. Epstein–Barr virus-associated Hodgkin's disease: epidemiologic characteristics in international data. Int J Cancer 1997;70:375–82.
44. Armstrong AA, Alexander FE, Cartwright R, et al. Epstein–Barr virus and Hodgkin's disease: further evidence for the three disease hypothesis. Leukemia 1998;12:1272–6.
45. Glaser SL, Lin RJ, Stewart SL, et al. Epstein–Barr virus-associated Hodgkin's disease: epidemiologic characteristics in international data. Int J Cancer 1997;70:375–82.
46. Alexander FE, Jarrett RF, Lawrence D, et al. Risk factors for Hodgkin's disease by Epstein–Barr virus (EBV) status: prior infection by EBV and other agents. Br J Cancer 2000;82: 1117–21.
47. Torelli G, Marasca R, Luppi M, et al. Human herpesvirus-6 in human lymphomas: identification of specific sequences in Hodgkin's lymphomas by polymerase chain reaction. Blood 1991;77:2251–8.
48. Levine PH, Ebbesen P, Ablashi DV, et al. Antibodies to human herpes virus-6 and clinical course in patients with Hodgkin's disease. Int J Cancer 1992;51:53–7.
49. Di Luca D, Dolcetti R, Mirandola P, et al. Human herpesvirus 6: a survey of presence and variant distribution in normal peripheral lymphocytes and lymphoproliferative disorders. J Infect Dis 1994;170:211–5.
50. Valente G, Secchiero P, Lusso P, et al. Human herpesvirus 6 and Epstein–Barr virus in Hodgkin's disease: a controlled study by polymerase chain reaction and in situ hybridization. Am J Pathol 1996;149:1501–10.
51. Goedert JJ, Cote TR, Virgo P, et al. Spectrum of AIDS-associated malignant disorders. Lancet 1998;351:1833–9.

52. Franceschi S, Dal Maso L, Arniani S, et al. Risk of cancer other than Kaposi's sarcoma and non-Hodgkin's lymphoma in persons with AIDS in Italy. Br J Cancer 1998;78:966–70.
53. Grulich AE, Li Y, McDonald A, et al. Rates of non-AIDS-defining cancers in people with HIV infection before and after AIDS diagnosis. AIDS 2002;16:1155–61.
54. Frisch M, Biggar RJ, Engels EA, et al. Association of cancer with AIDS-related immunosuppression in adults. JAMA 2001;285:1736–45.
55. Gallagher B, Wang Z, Schymura MJ, et al. Cancer incidence in New York State acquired immunodeficiency syndrome patients. Am J Epidemiol 2001;154:544–56.
56. Serraino D, Pezzotti P, Dorrucci M, et al. Cancer incidence in a cohort of human immunodeficiency virus seroconverters. Cancer 1997;79:1004–8.
57. Sitas F, Bezwoda WR, Levin V, et al. Association between human immunodeficiency virus type 1 infection and cancer in the black population of Johannesburg and Soweto, South Africa. Br J Cancer 1997;75:1704–07.
58. Milham S, Hesser JE. Hodgkin's disease in woodworkers. Lancet 1967;2:136–7.
59. Petersen GR, Milham S. Hodgkin's disease: mortality and occupational exposure to wood. J Natl Cancer Inst 1974; 53:957–8.
60. Fonte R, Grigis L, Grigs P, et al. Chemicals and Hodgkin's disease. Lancet 1982;2:50.
61. Greene MH, Brinton LA, Fraumeni JF, et al. Familial and sporadic Hodgkin's disease associated with occupational wood exposure. Lancet 1978;16:626.
62. Acheson ED, Pippard EC, Winter PD. Mortality of English furniture makers. Scand J Work Environ Health 1984;10: 211–7.
63. Milham S. Mortality experience of the AFL-CIO United Brotherhood of Carpenters and Joiners of America, 1969–1970. NIOSH 74–129. Cincinnati, OH. National Institute for Occupational Safety and Health, 1974.
64. Olsen J, Sabroe S. A follow-up study of non-retired and retired workers of the Danish Carpenters/Cabinet Makers Union. Int J Epidemiol 1979;8:379–82.
65. Kirchoff LV, Evans AS, McClelland KE, et al. A case–control study of Hodgkin's disease in Brazil: epidemiological aspects. Am J Epidemiol 1980;112:595–608.
66. Bernard SM, Cartwright RA, Darwin CM, et al. Hodgkin's disease: case–control epidemiological study in Yorkshire. Br J Cancer 1987;55:85–90.
67. LaVecchia C, Negri E, D'Avanzo B, et al. Occupation and lymphoid neoplasms. Br J Cancer 1989;60:385–8.
68. McCunney RJ. Hodgkin's disease, work, and the environment: a review. J Occup Environ Med 1999;41:36–46.
69. Jaffe ES, Harris NL, Stein H, et al., eds. World Health Organization Classification of Tumours. Pathology and Genetics of Tumours of Haematopoietic and Lymphoid Tissues. Lyon: International Agency for Research on Cancer Press, 2001.
70. International Collaboration on HIV and Cancer. Highly active antiretroviral therapy and incidence of cancer in human immunodeficiency virus-infected adults. J Natl Cancer Inst 2000;92:1823–30.
71. Eltom MA, Jemal A, Mbulaiteye SM, et al. Trends in Kaposi's sarcoma and non-Hodgkin's lymphoma incidence in the United States from 1973 through 1998. J Natl Cancer Inst 2002;94:1204–10.
72. Waterhouse J, Muir C, Shanmugaratnam K, et al. Cancer Incidence in Five Continents, Vol. IV. IARC Scientific Publication 42. Lyon: International Agency for Research on Cancer, 1982.
73. Muir C, Waterhouse J, Mack T, et al. Cancer Incidence in Five Continents, Vol. V. IARC Scientific Publication 42. Lyon: International Agency for Research on Cancer, 1987.
74. Parkin DM, Whelan SL, Ferlay J, et al., eds. Cancer Incidence in Five Continents. Lyon: International Agency for Research on Cancer, 1997.
75. Devesa SS, Fears T. Non-Hodgkin's lymphoma time trends: United States and International Data. Cancer Res 1992;52(Suppl):5432s–40s.
76. Parkin DM, Kramárová E, Draper GJ, et al., eds., International Incidence of Childhood Cancer, Vol. II. IARC Scientific Publication 144. Lyon: International Agency for Research on Cancer, 1998.
77. National Cancer Institute. Adult Non-Hodgkin's Lymphoma (PDQ®), June 2005. Available at: www.cancer.gov/cancertopics/pdq/treatment/adult-non-hodgkins/healthprofessional. Accessed June 30, 2005.
78. Opelz G, Henderson R, and Collaborative Transplant Study. Incidence of non-Hodgkin lymphoma in kidney and heart transplant recipients. Lancet 1993;342:1514–6.
79. Curtis RE, Travis LB, Rowlings PA, et al. Risk of lymphoproliferative disorders after bone marrow transplantation: a multi-institutional study. Blood 1999;94:2208–16.
80. Adami J, Gäbel H, Lindolöf B, et al. Cancer risk following organ transplantation: a nationwide cohort study in Sweden. Br J Cancer 2003;89:1221–7.
81. Hoover R, Fraumeni JF Jr. Risk of cancer in renal-transplant recipients. Lancet 1973;2:55–7.
82. Hoover RN. Lymphoma risks in populations with altered immunity: a search for mechanism. Cancer Res 1992; 52(Suppl):5447s–52s.
83. Zhang Y, Holford TR, Leaderer B, et al. Prior medical conditions and medication use and risk of non-Hodgkin lymphoma in Connecticut, United States women. Cancer Causes Control 2004;15:419–28.
84. Gridley G, McLaughlin JK, Ekbom A, et al. Incidence of cancer among patients with rheumatoid arthritis. J Natl Cancer Inst 1993;85:307–11.
85. Thomas E, Brewster DH, Black RJ, et al. Risk of malignancy among patients with rheumatic conditions. Int J Cancer 2000;88:497–502.
86. Kassan SS, Thomas TL, Moutsopoulos HM, et al. Increased risk of lymphoma in Sicca Syndrome. Ann Intern Med 1978;89:888–92.
87. Voulgarelis M, Dafni UG, Isenberg DA, et al. a multicenter, retrospective, clinical study by the European Concerted Action on Sjörgren's Syndrome. Arthritis Rheum 1999;42: 1765–72.
88. Thieblemont C, Mayer A, Dumontet C, et al. Primary thyroid lymphoma is a heterogeneous disease. J Clin Endocrinol Metab 2002;87:105–11.
89. Ragnarsson Ó, Gröndal G, Steinsson K. Risk of malignancy in an unselected cohort of Icelandic patients with systemic lupus erythermatosus. Lupus 2003;12:687–91.
90. Cibere J, Sibley J, Haga M. Systemic lupus erythermatosus and the risk of malignancy. Lupus 2001;10: 394–400.
91. Baecklund E, Sundström C, Ekbom A, et al. Lymphoma subtypes in patients with rheumatoid arthritis. Arthritis Rheum 2003;48:1543–50.
92. Coté TR, Biggar RJ, Rosenberg P, et al. Non-Hodgkin's lymphoma among people with AIDS. Incidence, presentation and public health burden. Int J Cancer 1997;73: 645–50.
93. Vaccher E, Tirelli U, Spina M, et al. Age and serum lactate dehydrogenase level are independent prognostic factors in human immunodeficiency virus-related non-Hodgkin's lymphomas: a single-institute study of 96 patients. J Clin Oncol 1996;14:2217–23.
94. Centers for Disease Control and Prevention. Revision of the case definition of acquired immunodeficiency syndrome for

national reporting—United States. MMWR Morb Mortal Wkly Rep 1985;34:373–5.
95. Dal Maso L, Franceschi S. Epidemiology of non-Hodgkin lymphomas and other haemolymphopoietic neoplasms in people with AIDS. Lancet Oncol 2003;4:110–9.
96. Levine AM, Seneviratne L, Espina BM, et al. Evolving characteristics of AIDS-related lymphoma. Blood 2000;96: 4084–90.
97. Matthews G, Bower M, Mandalia S, et al. Changes in acquired immunodeficiency syndrome-related lymphoma since the introduction of highly active antiretroviral therapy. Blood 2000;96:2730–4.
98. Besson C, Goubar A, Gabarre J, et al. Changes in AIDS-related lymphoma since the era of highly active antiretroviral therapy. Blood 2001;98:2339–44.
99. Robotin MC, Law MG, Milliken S, et al Clinical features and predictors of survival of AIDS-related non-Hodgkin's lymphoma in population-base case series in Sydney, Australia. HIV Med 2004;5:377–84.
100. Spina M, Carbone A, Vaccher E, et al. Outcome in patients with non-Hodgkin lymphoma and with or without human immunodeficiency virus infection. Clin Infect Dis 2004; 38:142–4.
101. Ott G, Ott MM, Feller AC, et al. Prevalence of Epstein–Barr virus DNA in different T-cell entities in a European population. Int J Cancer 1992;51:562–7.
102. de-Thé G, Geser A, Day NE, et al. Epidemiological evidence for causal relationship between Epstein–Barr virus and Burkitt's lymphoma for Ugandan prospective study. Nature 1978;274:756–61.
103. Burkitt DP. The discovery of Burkitt's lymphoma. Cancer 1983;51:1777–86.
104. Carbone A, Canzonieri V, Gloghini A, et al. Burkitt's lymphoma: historical background and recent insights into classification and pathogenesis. Ann Otol Rhinol Laryngol 2000;109:693–702.
105. Rabkin CS, Ward MH, Manns A, et al. Epidemiology of non-Hodgkin's lymphomas. In: Magrath I, ed., The Non-Hodgkin's Lymphoma, 2nd ed. London: Arnold, 1997: 171–86.
106. Magrath IT. Burkitt's lymphoma. In: Mollander D, ed., Diseases of the Lympathic System: Diagnosis and Therapy. New York: Springer Verlag, 1983:103–39.
107. Magrath IT. African Burkitt's lymphoma. Am J Pediatr Hematol Oncol 1991;13:222–46.
108. Evans AS and Mueller N. Epstein-Barr virus and malignant lymphomas. In: Evans AS, Kaslow R, eds., Viral Infections of Humans: Epidemiology and Control, 4th ed. New York: Plenum Medical Book Co., 1995:895–933.
109. Wotherspoon AC, Ortiz Hidalgo C, Falzon MR, et al. Helicobacter pylori-associated gastritis and primary B-cell gastric lymphoma. Lancet 1991;338:1175–6.
110. Parsonnet J, Hansen S, Rodriguez L, et al. Helicobacter pylori infection and gastric lymphoma. N Engl J Med 1994;330: 1267–71.
111. Wotherspoon AC, Doglioni C, Diss TC, et al. Regression of primary low-grade B-cell gastric lymphoma of mucosa-associated lymphoid tissue type after eradication of Helicobacter pylori. Lancet 1993;342:575–7.
112. Sugiyama T, Asaka M, Nakamura T, et al. API2-MALT1 chimeric transcript is a predictive marker for the responsiveness of H. pylori eradication treatment in low-grade gastric MALT lymphoma. Gastroenterology 2001;120: 1884–5.
113. Hisada M, Stuver SO, Okayama A, et al. Persistent paradox of natural history of human T-lymphotropic virus type I. parallel analyses of Japanese and Jamaican carriers. J Infect Dis 2004;190:1605–9.
114. Nicot C. Current views in HTLV-1-associated adult T-cell leukemia/lymphoma. Am J Hematol 2005;78:232–9.
115. Kondo T, Kono H, Miyamoto N, et al. Age- and sex-specific cumulative rate and risk of ATLL for HTLV-1 carriers. Int J Cancer 1989;43:1061–4.
116. Hisada M, Okayama A, Spiegelman D, et al. Sex-specific mortality from adult t-cell leukemia among carriers of human T-lymphotropic virus type I. Int J Cancer 2001;91: 497–9.
117. Okayama A, Stuver S, Matsuoka M, et al. Role of HTLV-1 proviral DNA load and clonality in the development of adult T-cell leukemia/lymphoma in asymptomatic carriers. Int J Cancer 2004;110:621–5.
118. Garbe C, Stein H, Dienemann D, et al. Borrelia burgdorferi–associated B cell lymphoma: clinical and immunohistologic characterization of four cases. J Am Acad Dermatol 1991;24:584–90.
119. Roggero E, Zucca E, Mainetti C, et al. Eradication of Borrelia burgdorferi infection in primary marginal zone B-cell lymphoma of the skin. Hum Pathol 2000;31:263–8.
120. de la Fouchardiere A, Vandenesch F, Berger F. Borrelia-associated primary cutaneous MALT lymphoma in a nonendemic region. Am J Surg Pathol 2003;27:702–3.
121. Kodama K, Massone C, Chott A, et al. Primary cutaneous large B-cell lymphomas: clinicopathologic features, classification, and prognostic factors ina large series of patients. Blood, prepublished online June 9, 2005 [DOI 10.1182/ blood-2005-03-1175, 2005].
122. Woods JS, Polissar L, Severson RK. Soft tissue sarcoma and non-Hodgkin's lymphoma in relation to phenoxy herbicide and chlorophenol exposure in western Washington. J Natl Cancer Inst 1987;78:899–910.
123. Zahm SH, Blair A. Pesticides and non-Hodgkin's lymphoma. Cancer Res 1992;52(Suppl):5485s-8s.
124. Keller-Byrne JE, Khuder SA, Schaub EA, et al. A meta-analysis of non-Hodgkin's lymphoma among farmers in the central United States. Am J Ind Med 1997;31:442–4.
125. Zheng T, Blair A, Zhang Y, et al. Occupation and risk of non-Hodgkin's lymphoma and chronic lymphocytic leukemia. J Occup Environ Med 2002;44:469–74.
126. Adami J, Gridley G, Nyrén O, et al. Sunlight and non-Hodgkin's lymphoma: a population-based cohort study in Sweden. Int J Cancer 1999;80:641–5.
127. Dryver E, Brandt L, Kauppinen T, et al. Occupational exposures and non-Hodgkin's lymphoma in South Sweden. Int J Occup Environ Health 2004;10:13–21.
128. Cantor KP, Blair A, Everett G, et al. Pesticides and other agricultural risk factors for non-Hodgkin's lymphoma among men in Iowa and Minnesota. Cancer Res 1992;52:2447–55.
129. Hardell L, Eriksson M, Nordstrom M. Exposure to pesticides as risk factor for non-Hodgkin's lymphoma and hairy cell leukemia: pooled analysis of two Swedish case–control studies. Leuk Lymphoma 2002;43:1043–9.
130. Zahm SH. Mortality study of pesticide applicators and other employees of a lawn care service company. J Occup Environ Med 1997;39:1055–60.
131. Quintana PJE, Delfino RJ, Korrick S, et al. Adipose tissue levels of organochlorine pesticides and polychlorinated biphenyls and risk of non-Hodgkin's lymphoma. Environ Health Perspect 2004;112:854–61.
132. Colt JS, Severson RK, Lubin J, et al. Organochlorine in carpet dust and non-Hodgkin lymphoma. Epidemiology 2005;16: 516–25.
133. Hardell L. Malignant lymphoma o histiocytic type and exposure to phenoxyacetic acides or chlorophenols. Lancet 1979;1:55.
134. Hardell L, Eriksson M, Lenner P, et al. Malignant lymphoma and exposure to chemicals, especially organic solvents,

chlorophenols and phenoxy acids: a case–control study. Br J Cancer 1981;43:169–76.
135. Hoar SK, Blair A, Holmes FF, et al. Agricultural herbicide use and risk of lymphoma and soft-tissue sarcoma. JAMA 1986;256:1141–7.
136. Hoar Zahm S, Weisenburger DD, Babbitt PA, et al. A case–control study of non-Hodgkin's lymphoma and the herbicide 2,4-dichlorophenoxyacetic acid (2,4-D) in Eastern Nebraska. Epidemiology 1990;1:349–56.
137. Asp S, Riihimaki V, Hernberg S, et al. Mortality and cancer morbidity of Finnish chlorophenoxy herbicide applicators: an 18-year prospective follow-up. Am J Ind Med 1994; 26:243–53.
138. Burns CJ, Beard KK, Cartmill JB. Mortality in chemical workers potentially exposed to 2,4-dichlorophenoxyacetic acid (2,4-D) 1945–1994: an update. Occup Environ Med 2001;58:24–30.
139. Hartge P, Colt JS, Severson RK, et al. Residential herbicide use and risk of non-Hodgkin lymphoma. Cancer Epidemiol Biomarkers Prev 2005;14:934–7.
140. Institute of Medicine. Veterans and Agent Orange: Health Effect of Herbicides Used in Vietnam. Washington, DC: National Academies of Sciences, 1994.
141. International Agency for Research on Cancer. IARC Monographs on the Evaluation of Carcinogenic Risks to Humans. Overall Evaluations of Carcinogenicity: An Updating of IARC Monographs. Vols. 1–42. Lyon: International Agency for Research on Cancer, 1987.
142. Huff JE, Haseman JK, DeMarini DM, et al. Multiple-site carcinogenicity of benzene in Fischer 344 rats and B6C3F1 mice. Environ Health Perspect 1989;82:125–63.
143. Hardell L, Eriksson M, Degerman A. Exposure to phenoxyacetic acids, chlorophenols, or organic solvents in relation to histopathology, stage, and anatomical localization of non-Hodgkin's lymphoma. Cancer Res 1994;54: 2386–9.
144. Blair A, Linos A, Stewart PA, et al. Evaluation of risks for non-Hodgkin's lymphoma by occupation and industry exposures from a case–control study. Am J Ind Med 1993;23: 301–12.
145. Hayes RB, Yin SN, Dosemeci M, et al. Benzene and the dose-related incidence of hematologic neoplasm in China. Chinese Academy of Preventive Medicine—National Cancer Institute Benzene Study Group. J Natl Cancer Inst 1997; 89:1065–71.
146. Rego MA, Sousa CS, Kato M, et al. Non-Hodgkin's lymphomas and organic solvents. J Occup Environ Med 2002; 44:78–881.
147. Blair A, Stewart PA, Tolbert PE, et al. Cancer and other causes of death among a cohort of dry cleaners. Br J Ind Med 1990;47:162–8.
148. Spirtas R, Stewart PA, Lee JS, et al. Retrospective cohort mortality study of workers at an aircraft maintenance facility. Epidemiological results. Br J Ind Med 1991;48: 515–30.
149. Lundberg I, Milatou-Smith R. Mortality and cancer incidence among Swedish paint industry workers with long-term exposure to organic solvents. Scand J Work Environ Health 1998;24:270–5.
150. Cartwright RA, McNally R, Staines A. The increasing incidence of non-Hodgkin's lymphoma (NHL): the possible role of sunlight. Leuk Lymphoma 1994;14:387–94.
151. Bentham G. Association between incidence of non-Hodgkin's lymphoma and solar ultraviolet radiation in England and Wales. BMJ 1996;312:1128–31.
152. McMichael AJ, Giles GG. Have increases in solar ultraviolet exposure contributed to the rise in incidence of non-Hodgkin's lymphoma? Br J Cancer 1996;73:945–50.
153. Bentham G. Association between incidence of non-Hodgkin's lymphoma and solar ultraviolet radiation in England and Wales. BMJ 1996;312:1128–31.
154. Hartge P, Devesa SS, Grauman D, et al. Non-Hodgkin's lymphoma and sunlight. J Natl Cancer Inst 1996;88:298–300.
155. Freedman DM, Zahm SH, Dosemeci M. Residential and occupational exposure to sunlight and mortality from non-Hodgkin's lymphoma: composite (three-fold) case–control study. BMJ 1997;311:750–1.
156. Hu S, Ma F, Collado-Mesa F, et al. Ultraviolet radiation and incidence of non-Hodgkin's lymphoma among Hispanics in the United States. Cancer Epidemiol Biomarkers Prev 2004; 13:59–64.
157. Hughes AM, Armstrong BK, Vajdic CM, et al. Sun exposure may protect against non-Hodgkin lymphoma: a case–control study. Int J Cancer 2004;112:865–71.
158. Smedby KE, Hjalgrim H, Melbye M, et al. Ultraviolet radiation exposure and risk of malignant lymphomas. J Natl Cancer Inst 2005;97:199–209.
159. Hall P, Rosendahl I, Mattsson A, et al. Non-Hodgkin's lymphoma and skin malignancies—shared etiology? Int J Cancer 1995;62:519–22.
160. Adami J, Frisch M, Yuen J, et al. Evidence of an association between non-Hodgkin's lymphoma and skin cancer. BMJ 1995;310:1491–5.
161. Goggins WB, Finkelstein DM, Tsao H. Evidence for an association between cutaneous melanoma and non-Hodgkin's lymphoma. Cancer 2001;91:874–80.
162. McKenna DB, Stockton D, Brewster DH, et al. Evidence for an association between cutaneous malignant melanoma and lymphoid malignancy: a population-based retrospective cohort study in Scotland. Br J Cancer 2003;88:74–8.
163. Hughes AM, Armstrong BK, Vajdic CM, et al. Pigmentary characteristics, sun sensitivity and non-Hodgkin lymphoma. Int J Cancer 2004;110:429–34.
164. HennekensCH, Speizer FE, Rosner B, et al. Use of permanent hair dyes and cancer among registered nurses. Lancet 1979;1:1390–3.
165. Teta MJ, Walrath H, Meigs JW, et al. Cancer incidence among cosmetologists. J Natl Cancer Inst 1984;72:1051–7.
166. Lynge E, Thygesen L. Use of surveillance systems for occupational cancer: data from the Danish national system. Int J Epidemiol 1988;17:493–500.
167. Thun MJ, Altekruse SF, Namboodiri MM, et al. Hair dye use and risk of fatal cancers in U.S. women J Natl Cancer Inst 1994;86:210–5.
168. Benavente Y, Garcia N, Domingo-Domenech E, et al. Regular use of hair dyes and risk of lymphoma in Spain. Int J Epidemiol 2005 (advance access at http://ije.oxfordjournals.org/cgi/reprint/dyi109v1. on May 24, 2005).
169. Tavani A, Negri E, Franceschi S, et al. Hair dye use and risk of lymphoid neoplasms and soft tissue sarcomas. Int J Cancer 2005;113:629–31.
170. Zhang Y, Holford TR, Leaderer B, et al. Hair-coloring product use and risk of non-Hodgkin's lymphoma: a population-based case–control study in Connecticut. Am J Epidemiol 2004;159:148–54.
171. Tibebu M, Polliack A. Familial lymphomas: a review of the literature with report of cases in Jerusalem. Leuk Lymphoma 1990;1:195–201.
172. Horwitz M. The genetics of familial leukemia. Leukemia 1997;11:1347–59.
173. Egler RM, de Kraker J, Slater R, et al. Documentation of Burkitt lymphoma with t(8:14)(q24:q32) in X-linked lymphoproliferative disease. Cancer 1992;70:683–7.
174. Linet MS, Pottern LM. Familial aggregation of hemapoietic malignancies and risk of non-Hodgkin's lymphoma. Cancer Res 1992;52(Suppl):5468s–73s.

175. Filipovich AH, Mathur A, Kamat D, et al. Primary immunodeficiencies: genetic risk factors for lymphoma. Cancer Res 1992;52(Suppl):5465s–7s.
176. Greene MH. Non-Hodgkin's lymphoma and mycosis fugoides. In: Schottenfeld D, Fraumeni JF Jr, eds., Cancer Epidemiology and Prevention. Philadelphia, WB Saunders, 1982:754–78.
177. Wiernik PH, Wang SQ, Hu XP, et al. Age of onset evidence for anticipation in familial non-Hodgkin's lymphoma. Br J Hematol 2000;108:72–9.
178. Daugherty SE, Pfeiffer RM, Mellemkjaer L, et al. No evidence for anticipation in lymphoproliferative tumors in population-based samples. Cancer Epidemiol Biomarkers Prev 2005;14:1245–50.
179. Cartwright RA, McKinney PA, O'Brien C, et al. Non-Hodgkin's lymphoma: case–control epidemiological study in Yorkshire. Leuk Res 1988;12:81–8.
180. Pottern LM, Linet M, Blair A, et al. Familial cancers associated with subtypes of leukemia and non-Hodgkin's lymphoma. Leukemia 1991;15:305–14.
181. Zhu K, Levine RS, Gu Y, Brann EA, et al. Non-Hodgkin's lymphoma and family history of malignant tumors in a case–control study (United States). Cancer Causes Control 1998;9:77–82.
182. Chatterjee N, Hartge P, Cerhan JR, et al. Risk of non-Hodgkin's lymphoma and family history of lymphatic, hematologic, and other cancers. Cancer Epidemiol Biomarkers Prev 2004;13:1416–21.
183. Paltiel O, Schmit T, Adler B, et al. The incidence of lymphoma in first-degree relatives of patients with Hodgkin disease and non-Hodgkin lymphoma. Cancer 2000;88: 2357–66.

7

Paraneoplastic Syndromes

Jennifer R. Brown, M.D., Ph.D.
Arthur T. Skarin, M.D.

Paraneoplastic syndromes are signs and symptoms of a malignancy that are not physically related to the tumor itself. They are quite uncommon, so symptoms resulting directly from the underlying malignancy must always be ruled out first. The "remote effects," or indirect manifestations, of an underlying malignancy have long been a source of fascination, however, and have been extensively reviewed for a variety of cancers.[1,2] The etiology of most paraneoplastic syndromes remains obscure, although the most common underlying mechanisms are thought to be secretion of cytokines by tumor cells, and induction of immune responses against normal tissues.

Paraneoplastic phenomena, which are primarily endocrinologic, neurologic, hematologic, renal, dermatologic, or rheumatologic, are not infrequently a first or early manifestation of malignancy; one series estimated that 7.4% of malignancies present initially with a paraneoplastic syndrome, with an additional 4.6% having a paraneoplastic syndrome as an early finding.[3] In that series, 16.7% of lymphomas presented initially with a paraneoplastic manifestation, most commonly rheumatologic or dermatologic. The syndrome may serve as a sensitive detection mechanism for response to treatment or for relapse, and often will resolve with successful therapy of the underlying neoplasm. Particularly in the case of neurologic phenomena, however, the syndrome may be irreversible, and may therefore dominate the prognosis of the patient. This chapter will focus on paraneoplastic syndromes associated with lymphomas.

ENDOCRINOLOGIC MANIFESTATIONS

The most common paraneoplastic endocrinopathy in patients with lymphoma is hypercalcemia, estimated to occur in approximately 1% of patients with Hodgkin's disease and 4% of patients with non-Hodgkin's lymphoma (NHL).[4,5] The incidence of hypercalcemia in "high-grade" NHLs may approach 30%, while in "low-grade" NHLs, it is only about 1% to 2%.[4] Within NHLs, B-cell lymphomas as well as adult T-cell leukemia/lymphoma are most commonly implicated,[6,7] although hypercalcemia has also been reported in peripheral T-cell lymphoma and angioimmunoblastic lymphadenopathy.[8,9]

Mechanisms for malignancy-induced hypercalcemia commonly include humoral hypercalcemia, mediated by parathyroid hormone-related peptide (PTH-RP), or osteolytic bone destruction. Both of these are less common in lymphomas. The most common mechanism in lymphoma is overproduction of 1,25-dihydroxyvitamin D_3 [$1,25(OH)_2D_3$] (calcitriol).[4,6,7] This mechanism is responsible for almost all described cases of hypercalcemia in Hodgkin's lymphoma, and for at least 30% of cases in NHL.[4] The syndrome is characterized by intestinal hyperabsorption of calcium, normal serum phosphate without urinary phosphate wasting, hypercalciuria, and low or normal levels of PTH.[4,6,7,10] By analogy to sarcoidosis and tuberculosis, elevated calcitriol levels are believed to be due to increased activity of 1α-hydroxylase in normal macrophages. A subclinical dysregulation of calcium metabolism may occur even in normocalcemic patients with non-Hodgkin's lymphoma; one study found hypercalciuria in 71% of such patients, and 18% had abnormally elevated serum calcitriol levels.[11] Calcitriol-mediated hypercalcemia is generally responsive to corticosteroids.[4]

The mechanisms of hypercalcemia in NHL may be multifactorial, and are still being elucidated. One recent study found that 62.5% of hypercalcemic patients with NHL had elevated levels of PTH-RP, as compared to 23% of normocalcemic patients with NHL; elevated PTH-RP levels were seen primarily in patients with advanced stage, high-grade disease.[10] Concomitant suppression of PTH and calcitriol were observed, suggesting that in those cases PTH-RP may be the primary mechanism of hypercalcemia.

The lymphoma most commonly associated with paraneoplastic hypercalcemia is adult T-cell leukemia/lymphoma caused by human T-cell lymphotropic virus (HTLV), Type I. Increased serum calcium levels associated with increased bone turnover are present at diagnosis in 21% to 45% of these patients.[6,12,13] Studies are conflicting as to the exact etiology of hypercalcemia in this lymphoma; elevated calcitriol levels, as well as elevated PTHrP levels with suppressed calcitriol, have both been reported in this disease.[4,6,13] TNF-β and IL-1 made by tumor cells have also been suggested to play a role.[14]

Finally, primary hyperparathyroidism coexisting with lymphoma has been reported in several cases in the literature.[15] Primary hyperparathyroidism is more common in patients with cancer than in the general population, and patients with cancer are more likely to have primary hyperparathyroidism than the general population.[16] The mechanism of this association is unknown.

Scattered case reports have documented other unusual endocrinopathies in lymphoma patients. Autoimmunity to the insulin receptor with resultant hypoglycemia was reported in a patient with Hodgkin's disease (HD).[17] In this case, the hypoglycemia did not respond to azathioprine or plasmapheresis but remitted after the use of prednisolone, and the erythrocyte-receptor binding of insulin became normal. Hypertension has been reported as an unusual paraneoplastic phenomenon in a 14-year-old girl with Stage IIIB Hodgkin's lymphoma. The hypertension was due to an elevated serum renin level that declined with a successful response to combination chemotherapy.[18]

NEUROLOGIC MANIFESTATIONS

The differential diagnosis of neurologic syndromes in patients with lymphoma is quite extensive, including direct effects of disease spread to the central or peripheral nervous systems, toxicity of specific therapies, neurologic manifestations of central nervous system (CNS) infections, metabolic derangements, and paraneoplastic syndromes.[2] The neurologic paraneoplastic syndromes are uncommon, occurring in about 7% of cancer patients; they are most commonly associated with lung cancer,[19] but do have an estimated 2.5% incidence in HD.[20] The most common mechanism is immunologic, with the malignancy inducing formation of antibodies that attack normal neural tissue. These immune responses can result in nervous system damage at any level of the neural axis. Antineuronal antibodies have been reported in 38% of patients with paraneoplastic syndromes with a high specificity of 98.6%.[21] Numerous neurologic syndromes have been described,[2] but the following is a discussion of the more common paraneoplastic syndromes reported in lymphomas.

Central Nervous System

Paraneoplastic cerebellar degeneration (PCD) is one of the most common neurologic syndromes reported in HD, and HD is one of the more common neoplastic causes of PCD, after lung, ovarian and breast cancers.[22] PCD has also been reported in non-Hodgkin's lymphoma.[23] Onset is generally subacute, with ocular dysmetria or nystagmus, and dysarthia or gait ataxia among the earliest findings. Progression may lead to incapacitation and severe disability. In a series of 21 patients, neurologic symptoms followed HD diagnosis by 1 to 54 months in 17 of 21 patients.[22] The activity or stage of HD did not correlate with symptoms, and in fact, six patients developed PCD while in prolonged complete remission of HD. Serum antibodies that react specifically with Purkinje cells were present in six cases but were distinct from those seen in PCD associated with gynecologic cancers (anti-Yo) or small-cell lung cancer (anti-Hu). Subsequent work has identified an anti-Purkinje cell antibody, called anti-TR, in both CSF and serum of patients with PCD and HD, but not in patients with either one alone.[24] At autopsy, extensive Purkinje cell loss is seen.[23] Occasional spontaneous clinical improvement occurs, but corticosteroids, other immunosuppressive therapy, and plasmapheresis have not clearly shown benefit.[22]

Other rare syndromes of the CNS have been reported in HD. Limbic encephalitis, characterized by dementia and memory loss (Ophelia's syndrome), occurs rarely in HD and may reverse with successful therapy of HD.[25] Other paraneoplastic causes of dementia include angioendotheliosis, with magnetic resonance imaging findings consistent with multiple strokes.[26] A paraneoplastic choreiform disorder, associated with an unidentified antineuronal antibody, has been observed in HD,[27] as has a paraneoplastic myelopathy, which responded to intrathecal dexamethasone.[28]

Motor Neuron Disease

A motor neuron disease with characteristic upper and lower motor neuron involvement, as well as involvement of the corticospinal tracts at autopsy, has been associated with both HD and NHL.[29] Clinical features are consistent with amyotrophic lateral sclerosis (ALS). In one series of 34 patients, 66% of the patients had elevated CSF protein without evidence of malignant cells. Forty-three percent had a monoclonal serum paraprotein, and 33% had CSF oligoclonal bands.[29] Nineteen ultimately died of the neurologic disorder, with seven showing improvement and six stable. Treatment was of unclear benefit; several patients improved with chemotherapy for active lymphoma, and several underwent plasmapheresis, without apparent benefit.[29] The overall incidence of lymphoma in patients with ALS is unclear; in a prospective study of patients presenting with motor neuron disease, 4 of 37 (11%) patients had a paraprotein, 1 of whom had lymphoma, and 2 of 37 patients who underwent screening bone marrow biopsy were found to have lymphoma.[30]

Peripheral Nerves

Paraneoplastic disorders involving peripheral nerves include demyelinating neuropathies, isolated sensory neuropathies, and neuropathies due to paraproteins or vasculitis. Guillain-Barré syndrome, ascending acute demyelinating polyneuropathy, has been reported in patients with both HD and NHLs, as has its chronic variant, chronic idiopathic demyelinating polyradiculoneuropathy (CIDP).[31] An unusual brachial plexopathy, characterized by asymmetric weakness and paresthesias of both upper extremities and most likely due to an inflammatory demyelinating plexopathy or neuropathy, responded to corticosteroids in one patient.[32]

Peripheral sensory neuropathy is clearly associated with malignancy. In one study, 363 patients presented with new onset peripheral sensory neuropathy, of whom 53 had no identified cause.[33] Eighteen of 51 developed malignancies between 3 and 72 months following diagnosis of neuropathy, and 3 of these patients had NHL.[33] Scattered autopsy reports of paraneoplastic sensory neuropathies have revealed loss of dorsal root ganglion cells, sometimes with T-cell infiltration.[31]

Peripheral polyneuropathy is associated with serum monoclonal paraproteins, and occurs in about 5% of patients with lymphoplasmacytic lymphoma (Waldenström's macroglobulinemia). Patients with other B-cell lymphomas and paraproteins, most commonly IgM paraproteins, may also develop sensory neuropathies.[31] Antibodies against myelin associated glycoprotein have been identified in some of these patients, and may correlate with the clinical syndrome, but their role in pathogenesis remains controversial.[34] Treatment of the underlying B-cell lymphoma, or corticosteroids or intravenous immunoglobulin may lead to remission of the neuropathy.[31,34]

Paraneoplastic vasculitic neuropathy has also been described and is generally characterized by an asymmetric sensorimotor axonal polyneuropathy.[35] This syndrome has been associated with anti-Hu antibodies in lung cancer patients,[34] but is idiopathic in lymphoma patients.[30] This entity may respond to steroids or cyclophosphamide.[35]

Autonomic Nerves

Clinical paraneoplastic dysfunction of the autonomic nervous system is rarely seen in lymphomas. However, a study of 20 patients with advanced HD or NHL revealed that 80% had subclinical autonomic dysfunction prior to therapy, and 55% had persistent dysfunction following treatment, although most showed some improvement despite neurotoxic chemotherapy.[36] The etiology of these findings is unclear, but is thought to reflect a paraneoplastic process.

Neuromuscular Function

Rare patients with lymphoma may develop Eaton–Lambert syndrome or myasthenia gravis.[37] In one patient with thymic lymphoblastic lymphoma, chemotherapy resulted in a complete remission of lymphoma and myasthenia gravis.[38] Although rare, either of these neuromuscular syndromes may predate the clinical appearance of lymphoma.

HEMATOLOGIC MANIFESTATIONS

In one large series of 317 patients with non-Hodgkin's lymphomas[39], 63% of patients had at least one abnormal blood cell count at diagnosis, regardless of whether the disease involved the bone marrow. Anemia was present in 42%, both thrombocytopenia and thrombocytosis seen in approximately 13%, and leukocytosis in 26% with leukopenia in 6%. Thrombocytopenia and leukopenia were more common in patients with bone marrow disease.[39]

Autoimmune hemolytic anemia (AIHA) due to warm-reacting antibodies occurs mainly in B- or T-cell lymphoproliferative disorders, although it has been reported in HD.[40] The incidence of AIHA in angioimmunoblastic lymphadenopathy with dysproteinemia is as high as 45%, and 20% in chronic lymphocytic leukemia, but more typically 2% to 3% in other lymphomas and HD.[41] Immune-mediated thrombocytopenia[42] may occur, together with AIHA as Evans' syndrome, or in isolation.[43] Mechanisms for the development of these syndromes include tumor production of autoantibodies, or tumor induction of novel antigens that lead to autoantibody production. Effective treatment of the disease will often induce remission.

Other paraneoplastic causes of anemia also occur. AIHA due to cold-reacting autoantibodies (cold agglutinins) is commonly associated with B-cell NHL of many types.[44] One case report of a patient with MALT (mucosal-associated lymphoid tissue) lymphoma of the lung showed that the hemolytic anemia was due to a monoclonal IgM with anti-I cold agglutinin activity,[45] although other specificities have also been reported.[44] The monoclonal gammopathy and AIHA responded to steroid therapy. Severe anemia due to pure red cell aplasia has been reported most commonly in thymomas, but also in T-cell lymphoproliferative disorders. T-cell–mediated suppression of erythropoiesis has been demonstrated, with improvement in the anemia after cyclophosphamide therapy.[46] Microangiopathic hemolytic anemia (MAHA), related to various causes of erythrocyte shearing, is exceedingly rare in lymphomas.[47]

White cell lineages may be affected, but rarely have clinical significance. A paraneoplastic leukemoid reaction has been noted in many patients with malignancy, including HD and NHL. Monocytosis and granulocytosis without infection are asymptomatic; the underlying mechanism is likely tumor production of a relevant growth factor.[48,49] Eosinophilia occurs in about 20% of patients with HD, 21% of patients with acute T-cell leukemia/ lymphoma, 11% of patients with T-cell lymphoma, and 10% of patients with B-cell lymphoma,[2,50] and is of unclear significance. Tumor infiltration by more than 5% eosinophils has been shown to predict decreased survival in HD, but did not correlate with peripheral blood eosinophilia.[51] Peripheral blood eosinophilia with eosinophilic fasciitis has heralded relapse in at least one reported case of peripheral T-cell lymphoma.[52] Eosinophilia is probably related to production of IL-5, a cytokine that promotes eosinophil growth and differentiation. Lymphocytes from three patients with T-cell lymphomas extensively infiltrated by eosinophils were found to express IL-5 mRNA.[53] Enhanced expression of the IL-5 gene has also been reported in HD.[54]

Patients evaluated for thrombocytosis will most commonly have secondary thrombocytosis (88%) rather than primary (12%). Of those with secondary thrombocytosis, approximately 15% will have an underlying malignancy.[55] Estimates of the incidence of thrombocytosis in patients with malignancy range from 13% in NHL[39] to 30% to 40% of all patients.[2] Patients with cancer-related thrombocytosis have been shown to have more frequent anemia with elevated levels of ferritin, lactate dehydrogenase LDH, C-reactive protein, ESR, and IL-1a and IL-6; these factors reflect inflammation, and may be associated with release of a thrombopoietic growth factor.[56] Thrombosis and hemorrhage are rare, and platelet counts decrease to normal with successful therapy of the underlying neoplasm.

Subclinical activation of the clotting cascade, migratory thrombophlebitis (Trousseau's syndrome), and disseminated intravascular coagulation (DIC) occur primarily in patients with solid tumors, although DIC and fibrinolysis are also seen in acute promyelocytic leukemia. Lymphomas are uncommon causes.

RENAL MANIFESTATIONS

Renal abnormalities in lymphomas are most commonly directly related to the disease, but paraneoplastic syndromes are usually manifested as a nephrotic syndrome. In fact, approximately 10% of patients with newly diagnosed idiopathic nephrotic syndrome are found to have a malignancy, usually a carcinoma.[57] Most patients with carcinomas have membranous glomerulonephritis.[57] Fewer than 50 cases of paraneoplastic nephrotic syndrome in HD have been reported.[58] The most common glomerular lesion (80% of cases) is lipoid nephrosis, or minimal change disease. The remaining 20% of cases show typical membranous glomerulonephritis, focal sclerosis, or membranoproliferative glomerulonephritis.[2] Other lymphomas, most commonly chronic lymphocytic leukemia (CLL), have also been associated with nephrotic syndrome; in the case of CLL, 50% of patients have underlying membranoproliferative glomerulonephritis, with the others having membranous glomerulonephritis, minimal-change disease and amyloidosis.[59] These cases are commonly associated with circulating monoclonal immunoglobulins or cryoglobulins and have been reported to improve with treatment of the underlying CLL.[60]

The nephrotic syndrome is less common in NHL, but may be seen in Burkitt's lymphoma or diffuse large-cell lymphoma. In 35 cases, available biopsies showed minimal change lesions in 5, membranous lesions in 7, and membranoproliferative lesions in 7.[58] As in many CLL-related cases, immunoglobulin deposits have been detected, suggesting an immune complex cause of the syndrome.[60,61]

DERMATOLOGIC MANIFESTATIONS

Malignancies have been associated with a great number of paraneoplastic skin lesions.[2] Numerous pigmented lesions and keratoses may occur. Acanthosis nigricans, characterized by symmetric brown areas of hyperpigmentation and hyperkeratosis especially in the axillae, neck flexures, and anogenital area, is usually associated with abdominal adenocarcinomas, but occasional patients with lymphoma have been reported.[62] Tumor secretion of TGF-α may be involved in the pathogenesis. Sweet's syndrome consists of fever, neutrophilia, and multiple cutaneous plaques or nodules that result from intense dermal infiltration by neutrophils. More than 85% of patients with malignancy-associated Sweet's syndrome have a hematologic malignancy, most commonly acute myelogenous leukemia but also HD and T and B cell NHL.[63,64] Steroids induce a rapid clinical response. An unusual dermatosis, in which the epidermal spongiosis is infiltrated by neutrophils, has been reported in a 12-year-old girl with an adjacent diffuse large-cell lymphoma.[65] The lymphoma and dermatosis responded dramatically to chemotherapy. Exfoliative dermatitis has also been reported in HD and NHL, including cutaneous T-cell lymphoma (CTCL).[66]

Bullous lesions have been reported in patients with HD and NHL. Paraneoplastic pemphigus is a distinct and rare autoimmune disease characterized by extensive and painful mucosal ulcerations and skin lesions. The mucocutaneous eruption resembles both erythema multiforme major (Stevens–Johnson syndrome) and pemphigus vulgaris. Autoantibodies against epidermal proteins desmoplakin I and II have been detected by direct immunofluorescent studies on skin biopsy and immunoprecipitation studies on serum, as well as on involved bronchial epithelium of one unfortunate patient.[67,68] The disease is most commonly associated with NHL and CLL, and most patients die in several months regardless of the course of the underlying neoplasm. Rare patients may have prolonged survival.[67,69,70] One patient with follicular lymphoma and paraneoplastic pemphigus resistant to steroids and cyclophosphamide achieved complete remission of the paraneoplastic pemphigus and partial remission of the lymphoma following a course of rituximab therapy.[71]

Lichen planus has been reported in three patients with low-grade lymphomas.[72] A cell-mediated immune response is primarily responsible.

Granuloma annulare (GA) is a chronic dermatosis characterized by annular plaques of skin-colored or violaceous papules typically affecting children or young adults. Recently, a population of patients with associated malignancy has been described, and 56% of these patients had lymphoma, most commonly HD.[73] The median age of this population was significantly older than the typical affected population, and suggests that patients with newly diagnosed GA in middle or later life warrant an evaluation for malignancy.

Miscellaneous paraneoplastic cutaneous lesions include fasciitis panniculitis syndrome (FPS), eosinophilic fasciitis, and progressive atrophying chronic dermohypodermitis (PACGD). FPS is characterized by swelling and patchy induration of the skin of the extremities more often than trunk, and tends to occur in association with hematologic malignancies.[63] Biopsied tissue shows chronic inflammation and fibrous thickening of the subcutaneous septa, fascia, and perimysium. The pathogenesis is unknown.[74] Eosinophilic fasciitis is characterized by painful sclerodermatous lesions without acrosclerosis and has been reported with leukemias, HD, PTCL, and CTCL.[52,75] Histologic features include edema and lymphocytic inflammation in the superficial fascia and dermis with deposition of immune reactants. Peripheral eosinophilia and circulating immune complexes were noted in one patient with CTCL and one with PTCL.[52,75] PACGD has been associated with HD and often predates the clinical onset of HD.[76] This granulomatous skin disease with skin looseness partially responds to corticosteroids as well as azathioprine.[76] The pathogenesis of PACGD is unknown.

GASTROINTESTINAL MANIFESTATIONS

Patients with malignancy often present with anorexia, loss of taste, weight loss, and cachexia. These symptoms predate the tumor and may reverse with proper anticancer therapy. Data from mice have suggested that cachexia may be related to production of TNF-α (cachectin) and IL-1β by tumor cells.[77] TNF-α inhibits lipoprotein lipase activity in peripheral tissues and may facilitate metabolic abnormalities resulting in anorexia-cachexia.[77]

Intestinal obstruction may be the presenting feature of patients with occult lymphoma who have acquired angioedema.[78] In this disorder, which may also be hereditary, there is an acquired deficiency of complement component C1 inhibitor. The resultant angioedema can occur in the face, throat, mouth, larynx, neck, and scrotum and result in peripheral edema and episodes of intestinal pseudo-obstruction. Acquired angioedema occurs most often in low-grade B-cell lymphomas, often with associated circulating paraproteins, and is a consequence of increased consumption or destruction of C1 inhibitor.[79] Danazol may reverse the angioedema by increasing synthesis of the C1 inhibitor.

RHEUMATOLOGIC AND CONNECTIVE TISSUE MANIFESTATIONS

Rheumatoid arthritis, asymmetric polyarthritis, and systemic lupus erythematosus (SLE) have all been associated with lymphomas, but this relationship may be due to the known increased risk of lymphoma in patients previously diagnosed with connective tissue disease.[2,80] One case of SLE diagnosed simultaneously with ovarian adenocarcinoma has been reported, and found to have an unusual pattern of antinuclear antibodies, suggestive of a novel, possibly malignancy-related target.[81] Palmar fasciitis and arthritis are characterized by complete loss of upper extremity function and contracture and have rarely been associated with HD.[82] Immunoglobulin deposits have been seen in the fascial tissue, suggesting an immunologic cause.

Polymyositis (PM) and dermatomyositis (DM) are inflammatory myopathies that can occur in all age groups,[83] and are associated with a five-fold to seven-fold increase in the incidence of malignancies.[84] PM is characterized by the subacute onset of symmetric weakness in proximal muscles, with about one-third of patients also developing dysphagia. DM is similar but includes a characteristic skin rash which is erythematous, pruritic, and scaly in sun-exposed areas. PM has been reported in a child with an occult immunoblastic lymphoma.[85] Both the lymphoma and the PM regressed with systemic chemotherapy. DM is more frequently associated with malignancy but lymphoma is a rare association. In a review of 12 patients with HD and DM, most presented first with DM, and were older and had more advanced HD, than patients without DM.[84] Pathogenesis remains obscure.

The first case of orbital myositis identified as a paraneoplastic syndrome in a patient with large cell lymphoma was recently reported.[86] The patient presented with multiple cranial neuropathies, a sensory polyneuropathy, and serum and spinal fluid paraproteins, but no evidence of malignant involvement. Although the paraneoplastic features responded to immunosuppressive therapy, the lymphoma progressed despite intensive chemotherapy. A T-cell infiltrate was observed in the tissues but no target antigen was identified.

Vasculitic syndromes can occur as rare paraneoplastic syndromes. Primary angiitis of the CNS has been reported in 12 patients with HD.[87] Patients presented with nonspecific symptoms including headache, nausea and vomiting, and were most commonly diagnosed with CNS angiitis simultaneously with or following the diagnosis of HD. Treatment with chemotherapy, steroids and sometimes XRT resulted in 25% having a full recovery, 50% dying, and the remaining 25% suffering permanent severe neurologic deficits. Paraneoplastic Raynaud's phenomenon, sometimes progressing to true acrocyanosis, has also been reported. Approximately 19% of these patients have hematologic malignancies, with half of those diagnosed with lymphoma.[88] The mechanism is unknown, but may be autoimmune or due to cancer-related coagulopathy.[88]

MISCELLANEOUS MANIFESTATIONS

Fever is a relatively common paraneoplastic feature of malignancy, occurring in an estimated 5% of cases.[2] Underlying occult infection and adrenal insufficiency must always be ruled out. Fever occurs primarily in patients with lymphomas but also with myxomas, renal cell carcinoma, and osteosarcoma. The classic Pel–Ebstein fever of HD is uncommon but characterized by days to weeks of persistent fever, alternating with similar periods without fever. The mechanism of fever relates to release of pyrogens, possibly IL-6, which has been shown to be released by tumor cells.[89]

Hypertrophic pulmonary osteoarthropathy (HPO) is a well-recognized syndrome of digital clubbing, periostitis of the long bones, and sometimes polyarthritis, suggestive of rheumatoid arthritis. Although most frequently seen in lung cancer patients, it has been reported in intrathoracic HD. Successful chemotherapy of HD has resulted in complete reversal of HPO.[90]

Amyloidosis is a syndrome of tissue deposition of amyloid, generally composed of monoclonal light chains that form a specific protease-resistant protein conformation, a twisted ß-pleated sheet fibril, and accumulate in tissues, particularly heart, nerves, gastrointestinal tract, skin and tongue.[91] Although most often associated with multiple myeloma (6% to 15% of cases), amyloidosis also occurs in 4% of patients with HD, and 10% of those with B-cell lymphomas.[2]

Unusual paraneoplastic features have been noted in certain patients with T-cell lymphomas. Four patients with isolated bone marrow lymphoma (three T-cell and one large B-cell type) presented with unexplained fever, abnormal liver function tests, polyserositis, and neurologic symptoms.[92] Several patients with extranodal peripheral T-cell lymphomas have been reported who presented with fever, weight loss, liver failure, pancytopenia, and coagulopathy in the absence of lymphadenopathy.[93] The pathogenesis of these paraneoplastic processes may relate in part to circulating cytokines and soluble cytokine receptors that have been described in T-cell lymphomas.[94]

Cancer-associated retinopathy has been well described in patients with solid tumors, but one patient with HD has recently been reported.[95] She developed night blindness and mottling of the retinal pigment epithelium in the fundi of both eyes. A unique antibody specific for photoreceptors was identified in her serum. Despite the apparent cure of her HD, and steroids for her retinopathy, her visual acuity continued to worsen.[95]

References

1. Hall TC, ed. Paraneoplastic syndromes. Ann NY Acad Sci 1974;230:1.
2. Arnold SM, Patchell R, Lowy AM, et al. Paraneoplastic syndromes. In: DeVita VT Jr, Hellmann S, and Rosenberg SA, eds. Cancer: Principles and Practice of Oncology, 6th ed. Philadelphia: Lippincott Williams & Wilkins, 2001: 2511–36.
3. Zuffa M, Kubancok J, Rusnak I, et al. Early paraneoplastic syndrome in medical oncology: clinicopathological analysis of 1694 patients treated over 20 years. Neoplasma 1984;31: 231–6.
4. Seymour JF and Gagel RF. Calcitriol: the major humoral mediator of hypercalcemia in Hodgkin's disease and non-Hodgkin's lymphomas. Blood 1993;82:1383–94.
5. Canellos GP. Hypercalcemia in malignant lymphoma and leukemia. Ann NY Acad Sci 1974;230:240–6.
6. Adams JS, Fernandez M, Gacad MA, et al. Vitamin D metabolite–mediated hypercalcemia and hypercalciuria patients with AIDS and non–AIDS-associated lymphoma. Blood 1989; 73:235–9.
7. Rosenthal N, Insogna KL, Godsall JW, et al. Elevations in circulating 1,25-dihydroxyvitamin D in three patients with lymphoma-associated hypercalcemia. J Clin Endocrinol Metab 1985;60:29–33.
8. Hanson CA, Brunning RD, Gajl-Peczalska KJ, et al. Bone marrow manifestations of peripheral T-cell lymphoma. A study of 30 cases. Am J Clin Pathol 1986;86:449–60.
9. Sworn MJ, Buchanan R, and McGill DA. Angioimmunoblastic lymphadenopathy and hypercalcemia. J Clin Pathol 1979; 32:1072.

10. Kremer R, Shustik C, Tabak T, et al. Parathyroid-hormone-related peptide in hematologic malignancies. Am J Med 1996;100:406–11.
11. Seymour J, Gagel RF, Hagemeister FR, et al. Calcitriol production in hypercalcemic and normocalcemic patients with non-Hodgkin's lymphoma. Ann Intern Med 1994;121:633–40.
12. Shimoyama M, Ota K, Kikuchi M, et al. Major prognostic factors of adult patients with advanced T-cell lymphoma/leukemia. J Clin Oncol 1988;6:1088–97.
13. Bunn PA Jr, Schechter GP, Jaffe E, et al. Clinical course of retrovirus-associated adult T-cell lymphoma in the United States. N Engl J Med 1983;309:257–64.
14. Ishibashi K, Ishitsuka K, Chuman Y, et al. Tumor necrosis factor-β in the serum of adult T-cell leukemia with hypercalcemia. Blood 1991;77:2451–5.
15. Owen CM, Blewitt RW, Harrison PV, et al. Two cases of primary hyperparathyroidism associated with primary cutaneous lymphoma. Br J Dermatol 2000;142:120–3.
16. Skrabanek P, McPartlin J, and Powell D. Tumor hypercalcemia and "ectopic hyperparathyroidism." Medicine 1980;9:262–82.
17. Braund WJ, Williamson DH, Clark A, et al. Autoimmunity to insulin receptor and hypoglycaemia in patient with Hodgkin's disease. Lancet 1987;1:237–40.
18. Singh AP, Charan VD, Desai N, et al. Hypertension as a paraneoplastic phenomenon in childhood Hodgkin's disease. Leuk Lymphoma 1993;11:315–7.
19. Croft P and Wilkinson M. The incidence of carcinomatous neuromyopathy in patients with various types of carcinoma. Brain 1965;88:427–34.
20. Currie S, Henson RA, Morgan HG, et al. The incidence of the nonmetastatic neurological syndromes of obscure origin in the reticuloses. Brain 1970;93:629–40.
21. Moll JWB, Henzen-Logmans SC, Splinter TAW, et al. Diagnostic value of anti-neuronal antibodies for paraneoplastic disorders of the nervous system. J Neurol Neurosurg Psychiatry 1990;53:940–3.
22. Hammack J, Kotanides H, Rosenblum MK, et al. Paraneoplastic cerebellar degeneration. Neurology 1992;42:1938–43.
23. Symonds RP, Hogg RB, and Bone I. Paraneoplastic neurological syndromes associated with lymphomas. Leuk Lymphoma 1994;15:487–90.
24. Graus F, Dalmau J, Valldeoriola F, et al. Immunological characterization of a neuronal antibody (anti-Tr) associated with paraneoplastic cerebellar degeneration and Hodgkin's disease. J Neuroimmunol 1997;74:55–61.
25. Carr I. The Ophelia syndrome: memory loss in Hodgkin's disease. Lancet 1982;1:844–5.
26. Petito CK, Gottlieb GJ, Dougherty JH, et al. Neoplastic angioendotheliosis: ultrastructural study and review of the literature. Ann Neurol 1978;3:393–9.
27. Batchelor TT, Platten M, Palmer-Toy DE, et al. Chorea as a paraneoplastic complication of Hodgkin's disease. J Neuro-Oncol 1998;36:185–9.
28. Hughes M, Ahern V, Kefford R, et al. Paraneoplastic myelopathy at diagnosis in a patient with pathologic stage IA Hodgkin disease. Cancer 1992;70:1598–600.
29. Younger DS, Rowland LP, Latov N, et al. Lymphoma, motor neuron diseases and amyotrophic lateral sclerosis. Ann Neurol 1991;29:78–86.
30. Rowland LP, Sherman WH, Latov N, et al. Amyotrophic lateral sclerosis and lymphoma: bone marrow examination and other diagnostic tests. Neurology 1992;42:1101–2.
31. Hughes RAC, Britton T, and Richards M. Effects of lymphoma on the peripheral nervous system. J R Soc Med 1994;87:526–30.
32. Lachance DH, O'Neill BP, Harper CM Jr, et al. Paraneoplastic brachial plexopathy in a patient with Hodgkin's disease. Mayo Clin Proc 1991;66:97–101.
33. Camerlingo M, Nemni R, Ferraro B, et al. Malignancy and sensory neuropathy of unexplained cause. Arch Neurol 1998;55:981–4.
34. Grisold W and Drlicek M. Paraneoplastic neuropathy. Curr Opin in Neurology 1999;12:617–25.
35. Oh SJ, Slaughter R, and Harrell L. Paraneoplastic vasculitic neuropathy: a treatable neuropathy. Muscle Nerve 1991;14:152–6.
36. Turner ML, Boland OM, Parker AC, et al. Subclinical autonomic dysfunction in patients with Hodgkin's disease and non-Hodgkin's lymphoma. Br J Haematol 1993;84:623–6.
37. Tyler HR. Paraneoplastic syndromes of nerve, muscle, and neuromuscular junction. Ann NY Acad Sci 1974;230:348–57.
38. Liu KL, Herbrecht R, Tranchant C, et al. Malignant thymic lymphoblastic lymphoma and myasthenia gravis: an exceptional association. Nouv Rev Fr Hematol 1992;34:221–3.
39. Conlan MG, Armitage JO, Bast M, et al. Clinical significance of hematologic parameters in non-Hodgkin's lymphoma at diagnosis. Cancer 1991;67:1389–95.
40. Kedar A, Khan AB, Mattern JQA II, et al. Autoimmune disorders complicating adolescent Hodgkin's disease. Cancer 1979;44:112–6.
41. Johnson RA and Roodman GD. Hematologic manifestations of malignancy. Disease-A-Month 1989;35:721–68.
42. Berkman AW, Kickler T, and Braine H. Platelet-associated IgG in patients with lymphoma. Blood 1984;63:944–8.
43. Evans RS, Takahasi K, Duane RT, et al. Primary thrombocytopenic purpura and acquired hemolytic anemia: evidence for a common etiology. Arch Intern Med 1957;87:48–65.
44. Crisp D and Pruzanski W. B-cell neoplasms with homogenous cold-reacting antibodies (cold agglutinins). Am J Med 1982;72:915–22.
45. Liaw Y, Yang P, Su I, et al. Mucosa-associated lymphoid tissue lymphoma of the lung with cold-reacting autoantibody-mediated hemolytic anemia. Chest 1994;105:288–90.
46. Akard LP, Brandt J, Lee L, et al. Chronic T-cell lymphoproliferative disorder and pure red cell aplasia. Am J Med 1987;83:1069–74.
47. Antman KH, Skarin AT, Mayer RJ, et al. Microangiopathic hemolytic anemia and cancer: a review. Medicine (Baltimore) 1979;58:377–84.
48. Hocking W, Goodman J, and Golde D. Granulocytosis associated with tumor production of colony-stimulating factor. Blood 1983;61:600–3.
49. Okabe T, Sato N, Knodo Y, et al. Establishment and characterization of a human cancer cell line that produces human colony-stimulating factor. Cancer Res 1978;38:3910–7.
50. Murata K, Yamada Y, Kamihira S, et al. Frequency of eosinophilia in adult T-cell leukemia/lymphoma. Cancer 1992;69:966–71.
51. von Wasielewski R, Seth S, Franklin J, et al. Tissue eosinophilia correlates strongly with poor prognosis in nodular sclerosing Hodgkin's disease: allowing for known prognostic factors. Blood 2000;95:1207–13.
52. Kim H, Kim MO, Ahn MJ, et al. Eosinophilic fasciitis preceding relapse of peripheral T-cell lymphoma. J Kor Med Sci 2000;15:346–50.
53. Samoszuk M, Ramzi E, and Cooper DL. Interleukin-5 mRNA in three T-cell lymphomas with eosinophilia. Am J Hematol 1993;42:402–4.
54. Samoszuk M and Nansen L. Detection of interleukin-5 messenger RNA in Reed–Sternberg cells of Hodgkin's disease with eosinophilia. Am Soc Hematol 1990;75:13–6.
55. Griesshammer M, Bangerter M, Sauer T, et al. Aetiology and clinical significance of thrombocytosis: analysis of 732 patients with an elevated platelet count. J Intern Med 1999;245:295–300.

56. Alexandrakis MG, Passam FH, Moschandrea IA, et al. Levels of serum cytokines and acute phase proteins in patients with essential and cancer-related thrombocytosis. Am J Clin Oncol 2003;26:135–40.
57. Burstein DM, Korbet SM, and Schwartz MM. Membranous glomerulonephritis and malignancy. Am J Kidney Dis 1993; 22:5–10.
58. Dabbs DJ, Striker L, Mignon F, et al. Glomerular lesions in lymphomas and leukemias. Am J Med 1986;80:63–70.
59. Aslam N, Nseir NI, Viverett JF, et al. Nephrotic syndrome in chronic lymphocytic leukemia: a paraneoplastic syndrome? Clin Nephrol 2000;54:492–7.
60. Moulin B, Ronco PM, Mougenot B, et al. Glomerulonephritis in chronic lymphocytic leukemia and related B-cell lymphomas. Kidney Int 1992;42:127–35.
61. Hyman LR, Burkholder PM, Joo PA, et al. Malignant lymphoma and the nephrotic syndrome: a clinicopathologic analysis with light immunofluorescence and electron microscopy of the renal lesions. J Pediatr 1973;82:207–12.
62. Curth HO. Classification of acanthosis nigricans. Int J Dermatol 1976;15:592–3.
63. Cohen PR and Kurzrock R. Sweet's syndrome and malignancy. Am J Med 1987;82:1220–6.
64. Cohen PR, Talpaz M, and Kurzrock R. Malignancy-associated Sweet's syndrome: review of the world literature. J Clin Oncol 1988;6:1887–97.
65. Tope WT, Fishbein JD, White PF, et al. Large cell lymphoma presenting with a distinctive inflammatory dermatosis. J Am Acad Dermatol 1991;25:912–5.
66. Nicolis GD and Helwig EB. Exfoliative dermatitis: a clinicopathologic study of 135 cases. Arch Dermatol 1973;108: 788–97.
67. Perniciaro C, Kuechle MK, Colon-Otero G, et al. Paraneoplastic pemphigus: a case of prolonged survival. Mayo Clin Proc 1994;69:851–5.
68. Fullerton SH, Woodley DT, Smoller RS, et al. Paraneoplastic pemphigus with autoantibody deposition in bronchial epithelium after autologous bone marrow transplantation. JAMA 1992;267:1500–2.
69. Rybojad M, Leblanc T, Flageul B, et al. Paraneoplastic pemphigus in a child with a T-cell lymphoblastic lymphoma. Br J Dermatol 1993;128:418–2.
70. Tankel M, Tannenbaum S, and Parekh S. Paraneoplastic pemphigus presenting as an unusual bullous eruption. J Am Acad Dermatol 1993;29:825–8.
71. Heizmann M, Itin P, Wernli M, et al. Successful treatment of paraneoplastic pemphigus in follicular NHL with rituximab: report of a case and review of treatment for paraneoplastic pemphigus in NHL and CLL. Am J Hematol 2001;66:142–4.
72. Helm TN, Camisa C, Liu AY, et al. Lichen planus associated with neoplasia: a cell-mediated immune response to tumor antigens? J Am Acad Dermatol 1994;30:219–24.
73. Li A, Hogan DJ, Sanusi ID, et al. Granuloma annulare and malignant neoplasms. Am J Dermatopathol 2003;25:113–6.
74. Naschitz JE, Yeshurun D, Zuckerman E, et al. Cancer-associated fasciitis panniculitis. Cancer 1994;73:231–5.
75. Chan LS, Hanson CA, and Cooper KD. Concurrent eosinophilic fasciitis and cutaneous T-cell lymphoma. Arch Dermatol 1991;127:862–5.
76. Benisovich V, Papadopoulos E, Amorosi EL, et al. The association of progressive, atrophying, chronic granulomatous dermohypodermitis with Hodgkin's disease. Cancer 1988; 62:24252–9.
77. Yoneda T, Alsina MA, Chavez JB, et al. Evidence that tumor necrosis factor plays a role in the paraneoplastic syndromes of cachexia and leukocytosis in a human tumor in nude mice. J Clin Invest 1991;87:977–85.
78. Eck SL, Morse JH, Janssen DA, et al. Angioedema presenting as chronic gastrointestinal symptoms. Am J Gastroenterol 1993;88:436–9.
79. Bain BJ, Catovsky D, and Ewan PW. Acquired angioedema as the presenting feature of lymphoproliferative disorders of mature B lymphocytes. Cancer 1993;72:3318–22.
80. Efremidis A, Eiser AR, Grishman E, et al. Hodgkin's lymphoma in an adolescent with systemic lupus erythematosus. Cancer 1984;53:142–6.
81. Freundlich B, Makover D, and Maul GG. A novel antinuclear antibody associated with a lupuslike paraneoplastic syndrome. Ann Intern Med 1988;109:295–7.
82. Pfinsgraff J, Buckingham RB, Killian PJ, et al. Palmar fasciitis and arthritis with malignant neoplasms: a paraneoplastic syndrome. Semin Arthritis Rheum 1986;16:118–25.
83. Bohan A, Peter JB, Bowman RL, et al. A computer-assisted analysis of 153 patients with polymyositis and dermatomyositis. Medicine 1977;56:255–86.
84. Dowsett RJ, Wong RL, Robert N, et al. Dermatomyositis and Hodgkin's disease. Am J Med 1986;80:719–23.
85. Sherry DD, Haas JE, and Milstein JM. Childhood polymyositis as a paraneoplastic phenomenon. Pediatr Neurol 1993;9: 155–6.
86. Harris GJ, Murphy ML, Schmidt EW, et al. Orbital myositis as a paraneoplastic syndrome. Arch Ophthalmol 1994;112: 380–6.
87. Rosen CL, DePalma L, and Morita A. Primary angiitis of the central nervous system as a first presentation in Hodgkin's disease: a case report and review of the literature. Neurosurgery 2000;46:1508–10.
88. Poszepczynska-Guigne E, Viguier M, Chosidow O, et al. Paraneoplastic acral vascular syndrome: epidemiologic features, clinical manifestations and disease sequelae. J Am Acad Dermatol 2002;47:47–52.
89. Fukumoto S, Matsumoto T, Harada S, et al. Pheochromocytoma with pyrexia and marked inflammatory signs: a paraneoplastic syndrome with possible relation to interleukin-6 production. J Clin Endocrinol Metab 1991;73: 877–81.
90. Atkinson MK, McElwain TJ, Peckham MJ, et al. Hypertrophic pulmonary osteoarthropathy in Hodgkin's disease. Cancer 1976;38:1729–34.
91. Glenner GG. Amyloid deposits and amyloidosis: the β-fibriloses. N Engl J Med 1966;19:539–43.
92. Ponzoni M and Li CY. Isolated bone marrow non-Hodgkin's lymphoma: a clinicopathologic study. Mayo Clin Proc 1994; 69:37–43.
93. Diez-Martin JL, Lust JA, Witzig TE, et al. Unusual presentation of extranodal peripheral T-cell lymphomas with multiple paraneoplastic features. Cancer 1991;68:834–41.
94. Raziuddin S, Sheikha A, Abu-eshy S, et al. Circulating levels of cytokines and soluble cytokine receptors in various T-cell malignancies. Cancer 1994;73:2426–31.
95. To KW, Thirkill CE, Jakobiec FA, et al. Lymphoma-associated retinopathy. Ophthalmology 2002;109:2149–53.

Diagnostic Procedures and Principles of Therapy

2

8

The Approach to the Patient with Malignant Lymphoma

Bruce D. Cheson, M.D.

A number of generalities can be applied to the evaluation and management of patients with lymphomas. However, there are numerous differences that are specific to tumor type, age, performance status, comorbid conditions, and other factors. In the future, strategies may vary on the basis of molecular and genetic features. This chapter will discuss assessment prior to therapy, management during treatment, and long-term follow-up.

PRETREATMENT ASSESSMENT

A patient with lymphoma most commonly presents with an enlarged lymph node, less often with the consequences of involvement of an organ, such as bone marrow, liver, stomach, or brain. If the node is hard and with no identifiable cause, such as a local infection or associated with symptoms, the diagnosis of lymphoma should be suspected. After the suspicious node is biopsied, the most critical first step is to ensure the correct diagnosis. Although concordance among pathologists is very high with some histologies (e.g., follicular non-Hodgkin's lymphoma [NHL]), others may require review by an expert lymphoma pathologist.

Once the diagnosis of the particular subtype of malignant lymphoma has been established, a careful history should be taken, including an assessment of potential epidemiologic risk factors, such as risk for HIV infection. The presence or absence of constitutional symptoms should be noted as they are associated with an unfavorable outcome: fevers greater than 38°C, night sweats, and/or unintentional weight loss of greater than 10% of body weight during the 6 months prior to the time of diagnosis. Other lymphoma-related complaints may include pruritus and, in Hodgkin's lymphoma (HL), alcohol-induced pain, or other symptoms in an involved node bearing area.[1] Other symptoms may signal specific sites of organ involvement. An assessment of Karnovsky, Eastern Cooperative Oncology Group, or World Health Organization performance status is important, especially for patients entering clinical research trials, since eligibility may require a certain level of function, and performance status may influence the results of therapy. A family history may identify other members with a lymphoid malignancy or autoimmune disorder.

Physical examination should include notation of the location and size of all lesions, with accurate measurements in two dimensions, when possible, to reduce the likelihood of intra- and inter-observer variability. At the time of diagnosis, a lymph node that is either larger than 1 cm in its short transverse diameter or hard to palpation should be considered suspicious for involvement by lymphoma. CT scanning and autopsy series have shown that the upper limit of lymph node size in normal individuals was approximately 1.0 cm in the short axis. However, this threshold varies with anatomic location.[2–9] The upper limits of normal mediastinal nodes ranged from 5 mm to 12 mm in the short axis, with greater variation in the long axis. The size of abdominal nodes on CT scans in patients with either blunt trauma, or benign or malignant diseases other than lymphoma, varies by region from 8 mm to 11 mm; however, normal nodes in the pelvis may be as large as 15 mm. Because different radiologists may be reviewing subsequent scans, consistent indicator lesions should be used to minimize interobserver variability.

LIVER AND SPLEEN ASSESSMENT

A spleen or liver that is felt to be enlarged on physical examination should be considered suspicious for involvement by lymphoma. This impression may require confirmation by CT scans to measure the size of the organ and to identify the presence of tumor masses.

Laboratory Studies

A variety of laboratory studies are needed for standard of care, whereas others are investigational and more relevant to the conduct of a clinical research study.

Standard Laboratory Studies

A complete blood count provides a rough assessment of bone marrow reserves. Careful examination of the peripheral blood smear with a white blood cell differential is important to evaluate for the presence of circulating lymphoma cells. A test for the human immunodeficiency virus (HIV) should be performed in patients at high risk for HIV infection and in those patients with an aggressive NHL or HL, because of potential differences in approach to treatment clinical course, and tolerance of therapy.

Other required studies include serum chemistries with a mineral panel, an assessment of hepatic and renal function, and lactate dehydrogenase (LDH) as an indicator of tumor mass. An elevated uric acid level may predict a patient at increased risk for urate nephropathy following initiation of therapy.

A serum protein electrophoresis in patients with small lymphocytic lymphoma, lymphoplasmacytic lymphoma (LPL), or marginal zone NHL may identify the presence of a monoclonal antibody that can be further evaluated with quantitative immunoglobulins. (However, it is unlikely that this information will impact on patient management.)

Gene expression studies using DNA microarray analyses have demonstrated clinically distinct subsets of patients even within histologic type and clinical prognostic group (Figure 8–1).[10–13] While currently investigational, these assays and newer technologies may soon play a major role in treatment decisions.

BONE MARROW ASSESSMENT

A bone marrow aspirate and biopsy are a routine part of the staging of lymphoma patients. Although bilateral bone marrow biopsies have been reported to increase sensitivity of detection of NHL involvement by 10% to 20% compared with a unilateral sampling, even patients with negative bilateral biopsies may have bone marrow involvement. Therefore, a unilateral bone marrow specimen of at least 2 cm in length is generally sufficient.[14,15] A lack of uniformity in interpretation and reporting of the bone marrow sample remains a major problem. The cellularity of the bone marrow should be recorded, especially for patients who are being considered for radioimmunotherapy for whom a threshold of about 15% cellularity may select appropriate candidates. Not only should the marrow be classified as being involved with lymphoma or not, but, if involved, the histologic subtype of lymphoma should be noted, because of the possibility of a discordant histology. Flow cytometry may identify a clonal population of cells not detected morphologically, but this test should not be used as a substitute for careful histologic review. Moreover, the clinical relevance of flow cytometric detection of subclinical NHL has not yet been demonstrated.[16] Immunoperoxidase studies of the bone marrow can be valuable in distinguishing benign from malignant lymphoid nodules.

Magnetic resonance imaging (MRI), immunoscintography, and PET scanning have each been reported to improve the accuracy of detection of bone marrow involvement.[17–20] Moog et al.[19] reported on 78 untreated patients with HL (n = 39) or NHL (n = 39). In 10.3% there was an upgrade in stage based on bone marrow findings. The biopsy detected 5.1% that were PET-negative, whereas PET identified 12.8% that were biopsy negative. However, not all studies support the utility of PET.[21] In general, the role of these studies is unclear, and they should not be used as a substitute for a bone marrow biopsy since they do not provide important information on the status of normal bone marrow precursors nor the histology of the marrow involvement.

Molecular and cytogenetic studies (e.g., bcl-2, bcl-6) of the blood and/or bone marrow, while providing prognostic information, are not currently part of routine patient evaluation since they are expensive and do not yet direct treatment.

Imaging Studies

Standard radiographic assessment includes CT scans of the neck, chest, abdomen, and pelvis, as well as other apparently involved sites (e.g., orbit, central nervous system [CNS]). An MRI may assist in the assessment of bone disease that is equivocal on plain radiographs.[18,22] Because of their limited sensitivity and specificity, chest radiographs are less often performed.

Gallium Scan

Single photon emission computed tomography (SPECT) with gallium scanning compares favorably with CT scans, radiographs, and physical examination.[23–27] SPECT gallium is especially valuable in differentiating lymphoma from benign tissue. The precise role for gallium scans in monitoring disease status in patients with NHL varies with the histology and site of involvement. Whereas gallium scanning may play a role in the evaluation of patients with large

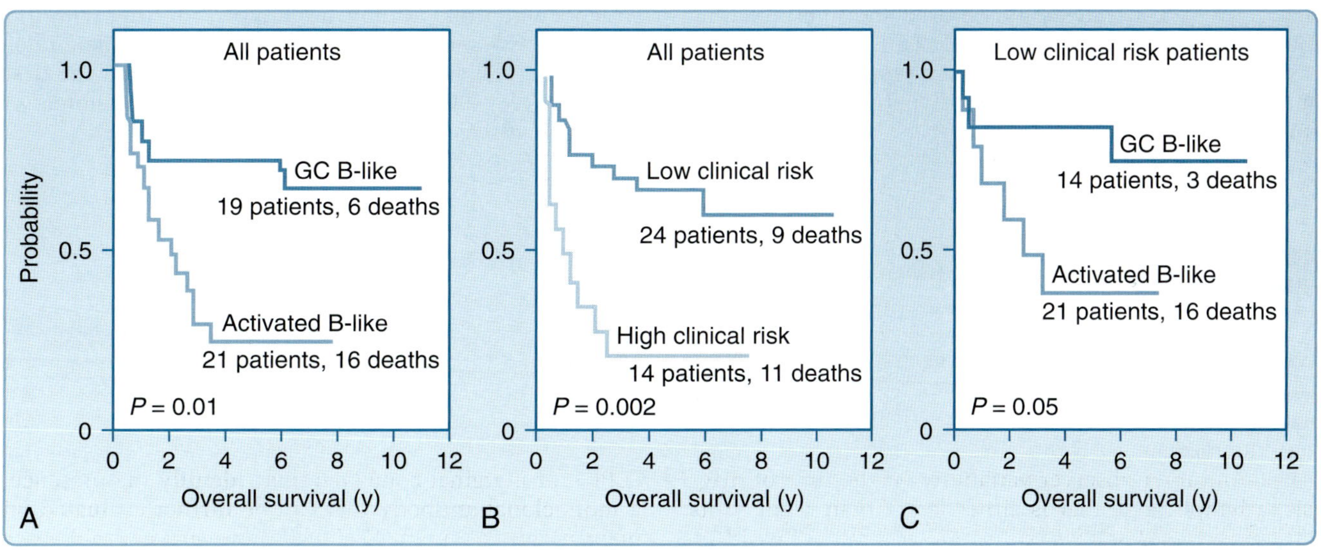

Figure 8–1. Distinct types of DLBC NHL by gene expression profiling.

B-cell NHL, it appears to have limited utility in patients with a low-grade NHL histology.[27]

SPECT gallium scan results following treatment may also predict outcome.[25,27] Vose et al.[27] treated patients with diffuse aggressive NHL using high-dose chemotherapy with autologous transplantation and found that the failure-free survival (FFS) at 1 year for patients with a positive SPECT gallium scan following therapy was 15% compared with a 3-year FFS of 47% for those with a negative scan.

PET Scans

PET scanning is a noninvasive metabolic imaging technique that detects fluorodeoxyglucose (FDG) labeled with fluorine 18 that is taken up by tumor cells, as well as inflammatory tissue (see Chapter 10). PET scanning has replaced gallium scanning because of its better resolution, increased sensitivity, and shorter procedure time.[28] The usefulness of the PET scan varies with histology, and whether it is being used at diagnosis, for restaging after therapy, or for detection of early relapse. Because of its lack of specificity, PET scanning is not useful in making the diagnosis of NHL. Moreover, it is not part of the current staging of patients and PET scans should not currently be included in determining patient stage. The available data thus far suggest that the initial therapy will be altered on the basis of PET scan in fewer than 10% of patients.[21,29] The frequency of a positive PET scan at diagnosis varies with the histologic subtype.[30–32] Some studies suggest that there is a greater likelihood of aggressive lymphomas being PET-positive than low grade.[31] Elstrom et al.[32] found that all of their large-cell and mantle cell lymphomas were positive, 98% of the follicular NHL, but only 67% of marginal zone and 40% of peripheral T-cell NHL. Extranodal marginal zone NHLs are generally negative.[31] A low rate of detection has also been reported for small lymphocytic lymphoma.[21]

Recent studies have suggested a potential role for PET scans in monitoring response to therapy by distinguishing active tumor from fibrotic tissue or an inflammatory process.[33] Although a positive test following therapy is generally considered an accurate predictor of failure, such results lead to changes in therapy in fewer than 10% of patients.[29,34] A PET scan should be used and interpreted in conjunction with history, physical examination, and CT scans. False-positive results have been reported with infection, inflammation, or thymic hyperplasia following therapy.

LUMBAR PUNCTURE

A lumbar puncture is recommended only in patients with signs or symptoms suggestive of central nervous system disease, or for those at high risk for involvement. Van Besien et al.[35] reported a study of 605 patients with aggressive NHL entered into prospective clinical research studies. In univariate analysis, CNS relapse could be predicted by advanced stage, elevated serum LDH, the presence of B symptoms, more than one extranodal site, B-phenotype, bone marrow involvement, involvement of skin, parenchymal organs, subcutaneous tissue, and muscle. However, in multivariate analysis, only LDH and more than one extranodal site predicted CNS relapse.

ENDOSCOPY

In certain histologies of NHL, the bowel is often involved. In mantle cell lymphoma, the characteristic finding by endoscopy is polyposis.[36–38] The diagnosis of mucosa associated lymphoid tissue lymphoma of the stomach, the most common indolent lymphoma involving the stomach, is made by endoscopy, which is also the preferred means of follow-up.[39]

STAGING

Patients are assigned an Ann Arbor stage based on the results of the physical examination, bone marrow, and imaging studies (Table 8–1). Although initially developed for prognosis and treatment planning purposes for patients with HL, the Ann Arbor stage was soon adopted for NHL as well. Patients are further substaged into A and B, reflecting the absence or presence of constitutional symptoms, respectively. Constitutional symptoms occur in only 10% to 20% of patients with Stage I disease but in up to 40% of patients with Stages III or IV disease at diagnosis. The Ann Arbor system has also been modified by subdividing patients with Stage II disease into those without or with bulky disease, defined as a tumor mass exceeding 10 cm in diameter or a mediastinal mass greater than a third of the maximum chest diameter. Those without bulky disease are grouped with the Stage I patients as having limited disease. Patients with bulky tumors are lumped together with those who have advanced-stage disease because of their poorer prognosis. The Cotswold classification included the designation of "X" for patients with Hodgkin's lymphoma who had bulky disease.[40]

Table 8–1. International Index (Patients of All Ages)

Risk Group[a]	Risk Factors	Distribution of Cases (%)	CR Rate (%)	Survival Rate (%) 2-Y	Survival Rate (%) 5-Y
Low	0,1	35	87	84	73
Low-Intermediate	2	27	67	66	51
High-Intermediate	3	22	55	54	43
High	4,5	16	44	34	26

Notes: Factors include age >60, LDH > normal, performance status >1, Stage III/IV, extranodal involvement >1 site.
[a] Score 0 or 1 for each factor: 0 = absent , 1 = present.

However, for a number of reasons the Ann Arbor system is less clinically relevant for NHL than HL. First, NHL spreads in a less predictable manner than HL. Second, the NHL are primarily systemic diseases at presentation as demonstrated by the observation that only 5% to 10% of "indolent" NHL and 20% of "aggressive" NHL patients present with localized disease. Third, the availability of more effective systemic therapies has reduced the use of localized radiation therapy. Finally, more powerful prognostic factors are available for NHL that may have a greater impact on outcome than clinical stage.

The marked heterogeneity even within clinical stage reflects the importance of other prognostic factors. The International Prognostic Index (IPI) was developed on the basis of clinical and laboratory data from 2031 patients with aggressive NHL who had been treated a doxorubicin-containing chemotherapy regimen.[41] Response to therapy and survival were predicted by age, stage, performance status, number of extranodal sites of involvement, and serum LDH (Table 8–1). Although the IPI can also be applied to the indolent histologies,[42,43] few indolent NHL present with poor-risk disease. A better separation into prognostic groups that can be attained with the IPI has been suggested for a follicular lymphoma IPI (FLIPI) using age of greater than 60 years, Stage III–IV, LDH, hemoglobin, and number of extranodal sites.[44] Newer systems using molecular and genetic findings are in development.

Other studies may be dictated by the specific therapeutic agents, including cell surface receptors for targeted therapies (e.g., CD20 for rituximab), cardiac ejection fraction for anthracycline containing regimens, and renal function for platinum-based therapies.

A number of other tests may be of future value but are not currently considered standard practice, including molecular studies (e.g., bcl-2, bcl-6), beta-2-microglobulin, and genetic profiling. Whereas these assays may provide prognostic information, they currently do not impact on patient care.

In the future, a variety of tests may be used to direct therapy. For example, response to rituximab may be predicted by DNA microarray signatures,[12] Fc receptor polymorphisms[45,46] and bcl-2 expression.[47] Full evaluation should be completed within a fortnight of the diagnosis being made, and sooner in the case of the symptomatic ill patient. At this time, a full management plan can be made and discussed with the patient, particular attention being given to whether the anticipated outcome is cure or palliation, and what the treatment options may be. The same applies at the time of progression.

ASSESSMENT DURING TREATMENT

The management of patients undergoing treatment is determined by the histologic subtype of lymphoma and the type of therapy being administered. For example, the frequency of determining blood counts will be more frequent, perhaps weekly, in a patient on an anthracycline-based regimen, but would be less often for a patient receiving single-agent rituximab. Similarly, serum chemistries and liver studies should be performed more often if initially abnormal or if the treatment includes a drug with specific organ toxicities (e.g., pulmonary function studies with bleomycin).

The frequency of imaging studies should also be determined by the context in which treatment is being administered. Patients on a clinical research trial will have predetermined time points for assessment of primary and secondary endpoints (e.g., response, progression-free survival). For patients not in a study, repeating the pretreatment studies is generally not recommended until post-treatment response assessment, unless clinically indicated. As noted above, PET scans performed after one or two cycles may predict subsequent outcome.[48,49] However, there is no information presently available to support the benefit of changing treatment based on that information.

RESPONSE ASSESSMENT

Response in patients with lymphomas is most often defined by regression in the size and number of enlarged lymph nodes or confluent lymph node masses; therefore, it is critical to determine how small an involved node must become following treatment to be considered "normal." The criterion of 1.5 cm in transverse diameter has been established as normal for Hodgkin's disease.[40] Nodes that are ≤1.5 cm but are considered to be abnormal, should decrease to ≤1.0 cm to be considered normal in size. Using the longest transverse diameter appears to provide a more accurate assessment of response than the short axis in patients with NHL.[50] Incrementally reducing the bidimensional requirement from 2.0 cm × 2.0 cm to 1.5 cm × 1.5 cm, and 1.0 cm × 1.0 cm does not appear to reduce the overall response rate, but it does result in a significant decrease in the CR rate.[51]

Lymph nodes may be completely or only partially involved by lymphoma. Following effective treatment, this mass may decrease in size but not necessarily disappear. As tumor-involved nodes shrink in size following treatment, fibrosis, necrosis, or inflammation result in a persistent enlargement of a node that may be histologically uninvolved by tumor.[52] Response assessment of a group of nodes that were initially enlarged and matted together and appeared as a mass, but which broke up into several smaller nodal masses after treatment may be difficult. Thus, persistence of residual masses following chemotherapy does not necessarily indicate residual disease.[53–56] As many as 30% to 50% of patients with a large intra-abdominal mass at presentation may have a residual mass following therapy.[53,55] In a comparison of ProMACE/MOPP with ProMACE/CytaBOM conducted at the NCI, restaging laparotomy was abandoned because 95% of residual abdominal masses did not contain lymphoma.[56]

The presence of residual masses has confounded assignment of patients to response categories. There has been considerable variability among studies; in some series, patients with residual masses were reclassified at a future time, depending on the subsequent behavior of the mass.[57,58] In a trial conducted by the NCI of Canada Clinical Trials Group (NCIC-CTG), a complete remission required a return of all nodes to less than 1 cm, unless larger nodes were negative by histologic examination.[59] Some investigators have used terms such as "probable CR."[60] Coiffier et al.[58] reported that 553 of 737 (75%) patients with aggressive NHL experienced disappearance of clinical and laboratory evidence of disease, although 150 of those (27%) had a persistent mediastinal or abdominal mass on CT scan.

There was no difference in time to relapse or survival between those with or without a residual mass; as a result they retroactively included such cases within the CR category if morphologic evidence of NHL was not available or if the size of the mass did not change after two courses of treatment. Several investigators recommend that a large abdominal or mediastinal mass that undergoes more than 50% reduction in size and remains stable for 2 to 4 months should not prevent classification as a CR given the absence of all other measurable disease,[55–57,60–62] whereas a cut-off of 75% is used by others.[58]

The increasing availability of PET scans has reduced the confusion surrounding the persistent mass.[63] PET appears to be better for monitoring disease than gallium scanning.[64] It is more accurate for supradiaphragmatic disease than CT scans, but may be comparable to CT scans in assessment of subdiaphragmatic disease.[29] Overall, it is more predictive of outcome than CT.[65] Some investigators suggest that the two are complementary and thus both should be performed.[48] The clearest role for PET is in post-treatment assessment.[66] Spaepen et al.[67] studied 93 patients with various lymphomas who underwent PET after treatment and were followed for at least a year. The 56 of 67 with a normal study remained in clinical complete remission (CCR) for a median of 653 days. The 26 who were PET-positive all relapsed at a median of 73 days. Zinzani et al.[34] reported on 44 patients with HL or aggressive NHL presenting with abdominal disease, which was bulky in 41%. Following therapy, none of those with a negative PET and CT relapsed, yet all of those who had a positive CT and PET relapsed. One patient of 24 who was positive by CT but negative by PET relapsed. The 2-year relapse-free survival for those with a positive PET was 0% compared with 95% for those who were PET-negative.

Jerusalem et al.[65] reported on 54 patients with intermediate- or high-grade NHL or HL. Residual masses were noted by CT in 13 of 19 patients with HL and 11 of 35 with NHL. Of the 24 patients with residual masses on CT, 5 had a positive PET compared with only 1 of 30 without a mass. All 6 patients who were PET-positive relapsed compared with 5 of 19 (26%) with a mass on CT but a negative PET, and 3 of 29 with a negative CT and PET. Patients with a positive PET had a 1-year progression-free survival of 0% versus 86% with a negative PET, with an overall survival of 50% versus 92%.

Spaepen et al.[68] evaluated 70 patients with aggressive NHL who underwent a CT scan after three or four cycles of treatment. None of the 33 who were positive sustained a durable remission compared with 31 of the 37 who were negative and remained in remission at 1107 days.

Römer et al.[33] performed PET scans in 11 patients with a variety of histologies of NHL, mostly but not all aggressive, at baseline and at weeks 1 and 6 after chemotherapy was initiated. During the follow-up period of a median of 16 months, six of the patients remained in remission, and these tended to be those with a lower day 7 metabolic rate of FDG, which improved in predictability at day 42.

INTERNATIONAL WORKING GROUP RECOMMENDATIONS

The following criteria were developed by an international group of clinical researchers in NHL.[15]

Complete Remission

Complete remission requires:

1. Complete disappearance of all detectable clinical and radiographic evidence of disease, and disappearance of all disease-related symptoms if present prior to therapy, and normalization of those biochemical abnormalities (e.g., LDH) definitely assignable to NHL.
2. All lymph nodes and nodal masses must have regressed to normal size (<1.5 cm in their greatest transverse diameter for nodes >1.5 cm prior to therapy). Previously involved nodes that were 1.1 to 1.5 cm in their short axis prior to treatment must have decreased to ≤1 cm in their greatest transverse diameter after treatment, or by more than 75% in the sum of the products of the greatest diameters (SPD).
3. The spleen, if considered to be enlarged prior to therapy on the basis of a CT scan, must have regressed in size and must not be palpable on physical examination. However, no normal "size" can be specified because of the difficulties in accurately evaluating splenic and hepatic size. For instance, spleens thought to be of normal size may contain lymphoma, whereas an enlarged spleen may not necessarily reflect the presence of lymphoma, but variations in anatomy, blood volume, the use of hematopoietic growth factors, or other causes. Any macroscopic nodules in any organs detectable on imaging techniques should no longer be present. Similarly, other organs considered to be enlarged prior to therapy due to involvement by lymphoma, such as liver and kidneys, must have decreased in size.
4. If the bone marrow was involved by lymphoma prior to treatment, the infiltrate must be cleared on repeat bone marrow aspirate and biopsy of the same site. The sample on which this determination is made must be adequate (≥20 mm biopsy core). Flow cytometric, molecular or cytogenetic studies are not considered part of routine assessment to document persistent disease at the present time. These studies should only be incorporated in trials examining important research questions.

Complete Remission/Unconfirmed

Complete remission/unconfirmed (CRu) includes those patients who fulfill Criteria 1, 2, and 3 above, but with one or more of the following features:

1. A residual lymph node mass greater than 1.5 cm in greatest transverse diameter, which has regressed by more than 75% in the SPD. Individual nodes that were previously confluent must have regressed by more than 75% in their SPD compared with the size of the original mass.
2. Indeterminate bone marrow (increased number or size of aggregates without cytologic or architectural atypia).

Partial Remission

1. SPD decrease of ≥50% of the six largest dominant nodes or nodal masses. These nodes or masses should be selected according to the following features: (a) they should be clearly measurable in at least two perpendicular dimensions; (b) they should be from as disparate regions of the body as possible; and (c) they should

include mediastinal and retroperitoneal areas of disease whenever these sites are involved.
2. No increase in the size of the other nodes, liver, or spleen.
3. Splenic and hepatic nodules must regress by at least 50% in the SPD.
4. With the exception of splenic and hepatic nodules, involvement of other organs is considered evaluable and not measurable disease.
5. Bone marrow assessment is irrelevant for determination of a partial remission (PR) because it is evaluable and not measurable disease; however, if positive, the cell type should be specified in the report, such as large-cell lymphoma or low-grade lymphoma (i.e., small, lymphocytic, small cleaved or mixed small and large cells).
6. No new sites of disease.

Stable Disease

1. Less than a PR (see above), but not progressive disease (see below).

Relapsed Disease (CR, CRu)

1. Appearance of any new lesion or increase by more than 50% in the size of previously involved sites.
2. A ≥50% increase in greatest diameter of any previously identified node that is greater than 1 cm in its short axis or in the SPD of more than one node.

Progressive Disease (PR, Nonresponders)

1. A ≥50% increase from nadir in the SPD of any previously identified abnormal nodes for PRs or nonresponders.
2. Appearance of any new lesion during or at the end of therapy.

Response Assessment

Response is currently assessed on the basis of clinical, radiologic, and pathologic (i.e., bone marrow) criteria.

1. CT scans remain the standard for evaluation of nodal disease. Thoracic, abdominal, and pelvic CT scans are recommended even if those areas were not initially involved because of the unpredictable pattern of recurrence in NHL. Studies should be performed no later than 2 months after treatment has been completed to assess response. This interval may vary with the type of treatment; for instance, a longer period may be more appropriate for biological agents where the anticipated time to response may be greater.
2. A bone marrow aspirate and biopsy should only be performed to confirm a CR if initially positive, or when it is clinically indicated by new abnormalities in the peripheral blood counts or blood smear.

Table 8–2. Major Endpoints for Clinical Trials

Endpoint	Response Category	Definition
Overall survival	All patients	Death from any cause
Event-free survival	All patients	Failure or death from any cause
Progression-free survival	All patients	Disease progression or death from any cause

Note: All measured from entry into study.

Integration of PET into the International Response Criteria has been evaluated.[63] In a retrospective analysis of 54 patients with aggressive NHL treated with CHOP-based chemotherapy and followed for at least 18 months after therapy. The 18-month progression-free survival was not different if patients were considered a CR by CT or PET and CT. However, the major difference was in patients considered PR for whom the progression-free survival was 70% with the International Workshop recommendation and 22% when PET was included. The use of PET also abolished the subsets of patients who were considered CRu and SD. The use of immunohistochemistry would also reduce the number of indeterminate bone marrows by distinguishing lymphomatous nodules from benign residual lymphoid nodules (Figures 8–2a, b, c).

Endpoints

Whereas response rates are of interest in Phase II studies of new agents, they are generally not the most important endpoint Phase I studies, where toxicity is identified, or Phase III trials, where efficacy endpoints are more important. In Phase III trials, the major endpoints of interest should include progression-free survival, event-free survival (time to treatment failure), freedom from progression, and overall survival (Tables 8–2 and 8–3). Overall survival and failure-free survival are measured from entry onto a trial until death from any cause, or until death or progression of disease, respectively. Progression-free survival for all patients is taken from the time of entry into study until disease progression or death from any cause. This endpoint is more important in aggressive NHL, where it correlates better with survival than in follicular NHL. Secondary endpoints such as disease-free survival or cause-specific survival may also be included, but only when the other endpoints have been reported. Disease-free survival for patients in CR or CRu is measured from the first assessment, which documents that

Table 8–3. Secondary Endpoints

Endpoint	Response	Definition	Measured from
Disease-free survival	CR/CRu	Time to relapse	Documentation of response
Response duration	CR/CRu/PR	Time to relapse or progression	Documentation of response
Cause-specific death	All patients	Death from non-Hodgkin's lymphoma	Death
Time to next treatment	All patients	Time to new treatment	Entry into study

CR, complete remission; CRu, complete remission unconfirmed; PR, progressive disease.

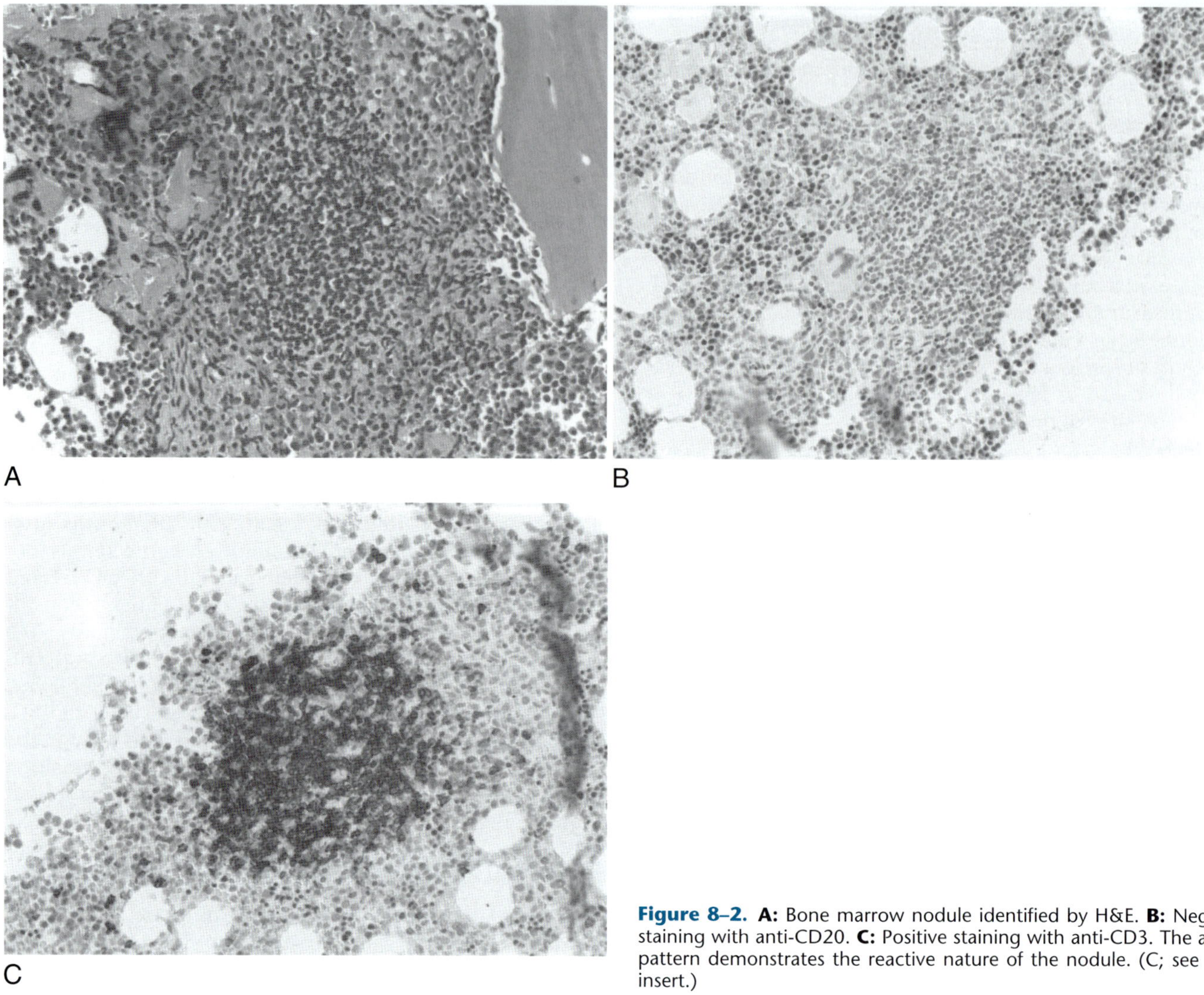

Figure 8–2. A: Bone marrow nodule identified by H&E. **B:** Negative staining with anti-CD20. **C:** Positive staining with anti-CD3. The above pattern demonstrates the reactive nature of the nodule. (C; see color insert.)

response to the date of disease progression. An endpoint that has become increasingly popular is time to next treatment. However, unless the indications for treatment are clearly specified, there can be considerable bias in these determinations.

Follow-up

Patients with a follicular or low-grade NHL who are being managed with a "watch and wait" approach need to be followed for the development of disease-related symptoms or signs of organ involvement. No consensus regarding the frequency of follow-up of such patients exists. However, routine imaging studies are generally not warranted.

The manner in which patients are followed after completing treatment may differ considerably between a clinical trial and clinical practice, and whether treatment is initiated with curative or palliative intent. Good clinical judgment and a careful history and physical examination are the most important components of monitoring patients after treatment. There is little indication for regular surveillance CT or PET scans in the majority of patients. Weeks et al.[69] assessed the role of conventional screening for relapse in patients with NHL. The authors concluded that follow-up strategies based on standard radiographic procedures and blood tests were not effective in detecting preclinical relapse patients with large-cell lymphoma. They recommended that screening studies should not be site-specific and the frequency of study should be determined by the patient's risk for relapse and whether there is a potentially curative salvage therapy. Oh et al.[70] studied 328 patients with previously untreated Stage I follicular NHL, 78 of whom relapsed and were part of the study. They had received a variety of treatments. At a median follow-up of 101 months, only 14% of relapses were picked up by CT scans, and just 4.3% benefitted from the CT. The number of relapses identified by physical examination was similar to CT scans. Minimum testing at follow-up visits should include history, physical examination for lymphadenopathy, abdominal masses, or organomegaly, and blood tests including a complete blood count and serum chemistries, including LDH. Additional blood tests and imaging studies may be added for relevant clinical indications.

In a clinical trial, uniformity of reassessment is necessary to ensure comparability among studies with respect to the major endpoints of event-free survival, disease-free survival, and progression-free survival. It is obvious, for example, that a protocol requiring extensive reevaluation every 2 months will produce different apparent intervals for those endpoints compared to one requiring the same testing annually, even if the true times to events are the same. One recommendation has been to assess patients on clinical trials after completion of treatment at a minimum of every 3 months for 2 years, then every 6 months for 3 years, and then annually for at least 5 years.[15] Few recurrences occur beyond that point for patients with large-cell NHL. However, there is a continuous risk of relapse for patients with a follicular histology. These intervals may vary with specific treatments, protocols, or unique drug characteristics.

CONCLUSIONS

As with diagnosis, classification, and prognosis, staging and response assessment are in a state of transition. Newer technologies such as DNA microarrays have the potential to delineate clinically meaningful patient subsets even within the risk groups of the IPI.[10,11] PET scans already appear to be of value in assessing response. Precise staging has become less important with the availability of more effective systemic agents. Response categories do not necessarily correlate with outcome as attested to the fact that most patients with advanced-stage NHL who attain a complete remission still relapse and die from their disease. More sensitive measures to define the presence of minimal residual disease are needed, with studies to determine if modification of therapy on the basis of that information impacts on patient outcome.

References

1. Cheson BD. Hodgkin's disease, alcohol and vena caval obstruction. JAMA 1978;239:23–4.
2. Dorfman RE, Alpern MB, Gross BH, et al. Upper abdominal lymph nodes: criteria for normal size determined with CT. Radiology 1991;180:319–22.
3. Einstein DM, Singer AA, Chilcote WA, et al. Abdominal lymphadenopathy: spectrum of CT findings. RadioGraphics 1991; 11:457–72.
4. Glazer GM, Gross BH, Quint LE, et al. Normal mediastinal lymph nodes: number and size according to American Thoracic Society mapping. AJR Am J Roentgenol 1985;144: 261–5.
5. Hopper KD, Kasales CJ, Van Slyke MA, et al. Analysis of interobserver and intraobserver variability in CT tumor measurements. AJR Am J Roentgenol 1996;187:851–4.
6. Kiyono K, Sone S, Sakai F, et al. The number and size of normal mediastinal lymph nodes: a postmortem study. AJR Am J Roentgenol 1988;150:771–6.
7. Steinkamp HJ, Hosten N, Richter C, et al. Enlarged cervical lymph nodes at helical CT. Radiology 1994;191:795–8.
8. van den Brekel MWM, Castelijns JA, Snow GB. Detection of lymph node metastases in the neck: radiologic criteria. Radiology 1994;192:617–18.
9. Genereux GP, Howie JL. Normal mediastinal lymph node size and number: CT and anatomic study. AJR Am J Roentgenol 1984;142:1095–100.
10. Alizadeh AA, Eisen MB, Davis RE, et al. Distinct types of diffuse large B-cell lymphoma identified by gene expression profiling. Nature 2000;403:503–11.
11. Rosenwald A, Wright G, Chan WC, et al. The use of molecular profiling to predict survival after chemotherapy for large B-cell lymphoma. N Engl J Med 2002;346:1937–47.
12. Bohen SP, Troyanskaya OG, Alter O, et al. Variation in gene expression patterns in follicular lymphoma and response to rituximab. Proc Natl Acad Sci U S A 2003;100:1926–1930.
13. Savage KJ, Monti S, Kutok JL, et al. The molecular signature of mediastinal large B-cell lymphoma differs from that of other diffuse large B-cell lymphomas and shares features with classical Hodgkin lymphoma. Blood 2003;102:3871–9.
14. Coller BS, Chabner BA, Gralnick HR. Frequencies and patterns of bone marrow involvement in non-Hodgkin's lymphomas: observations on the value of bilateral biopsies. Am J Hematol 1977;3:105–19.
15. Cheson BD, Bennett JM, Kantarjian H, et al. Report of an international working group to standardize response criteria for myelodysplastic syndromes. Blood 2000;96:3671–4.
16. Palacio C, Acebedo G, Navarrete M, et al. Flow cytometry in the bone marrow evaluation of follicular and diffuse large B-cell lymphomas. Haematologica 2001;86:934–40.
17. Hoane BR, Shields AF, Porter BA, et al. Detection of lymphomatous bone marrow involvement with magnetic resonance imaging. Blood 1991;78:728–738.
18. Altehoefer C, Blum U, Bathmann J, et al. Comparative diagnostic accuracy of magnetic resonance imaging and immunoscintography for detection of bone marrow involvement in patients with malignant lymphoma. J Clin Oncol 1997;15:1754–60.
19. Moog F, Bangerter M, Kotzerke J, et al. 18-F-fluorodeoxyglucose-positron emission tomography as a new approach to detect lymphomatous bone marrow. Blood 1998;16:603–9.
20. Carr R, Barrington SF, Madan B, et al. Detection of lymphoma in bone marrow by whole-body positron emission tomography. Blood 1998;91:3340–6.
21. Jerusalem G, Beguin Y, Najjar F, et al. Positron emission tomography (PET) with 18F-fluorodeoxyglucose (18F-FDG) for the staging of low-grade non-Hodgkin's lymphoma (NHL). Ann Oncol 2001;12:825–30.
22. Devizzi L, Maffiolo L, Bonfante V, et al. Comparison of gallium scan, computed tomography, and magnetic resonance in patients with mediastinal Hodgkin's disease. Ann Oncol 1997;8:53–6.
23. Israel O, Front D, Lam M, et al. Gallium 67 imaging in monitoring lymphoma response to treatment. Cancer 1988;61: 2439–43.
24. Kaplan WD, Jochelson MS, Herman TS, et al. Gallium-67 imaging: a predictor of residual tumor viability and clinical outcome in patients with diffuse large-cell lymphoma. J Clin Oncol 1990;8:1966–70.
25. Janicek M, Kaplan W, Neuberg D, et al. Early restaging gallium scans predict outcome in poor-prognosis patients with aggressive non-Hodgkin's lymphoma treated with high-dose CHOP chemotherapy. J Clin Oncol 1997;15:1631–7.
26. Even-Sapir E, Bar-Shalom R, Israel O, et al. Single-photon emission computed tomography quantitation of gallium citrate uptake for the differentiation of lymphoma from benign hilar uptake. J Clin Oncol 1995;13:942–6.
27. Vose JM, Bierman PJ, Anderson JR, et al. Single-photon emission computed tomography gallium imaging versus computed tomography: predictive value in patients undergoing high-dose chemotherapy and autologous stem-cell transplantation for non-Hodgkin's lymphoma. J Clin Oncol 1996;14:2473–9.
28. Wirth A, Seymour JF, Hicks RJ, et al. Fluorine-18 flurordeoxyglucose positron emission tomography, gallium-67 scintigraphy, and conventional staging for Hodgkin's disease and non-Hodgkin's lymphoma. Am J Med 2002;112: 262–8.

29. Buchmann I, Reinhardt M, Elsner K, et al. 2-(fluorine-18)fluoro-2-deoxy-D-glucose positron emission tomography in the detection and staging of malignant lymphoma. A bicenter trial. Cancer 2001;91:889–99.
30. Najjar F, Hustinx R, Jerusalem G, et al. Positron emission tomography (PET) for staging low-grade non-Hodgkin's lymphomas (NHL). Cancer Biother Radiopharm 2001;16: 297–304.
31. Hoffmann M, Kletter K, Diemling M, et al. Positron emission tomography with fluorine-18-2-fluoro-2-deoxy-D-glucose (F18-FDG) does not visualize extranodal B-cell lymphoma of the mucosa-associated lymphoid tissue (MALT)-type. Ann Oncol 1999;10:1185–9.
32. Elstrom R, Guan L, Baker G, et al. Utility of FDG-PET scanning in lymphoma by WHO classification. Blood 2003;101: 3875–6.
33. Römer W, Hahauske A-R, Zieger S, et al. Positron-emission tomography in non-Hodgkin's lymphoma: assessment of chemotherapy with fluorodeoxyglucose. Blood 1998;91: 4464–71.
34. Zinzani PL, Magagnoli M, Chierichetti F, et al. The role of positron emission tomography (PET) in the management of lymphoma patients. Ann Oncol 1999;10:1141–3.
35. van Besien K, Ha CS, Murphy S, et al. Risk factors, treatment, and outcome of central nervous system recurrence in adults with intermediate-grade and immunoblastic lymphoma. Blood 1998;91:1178–4.
36. Zucca E, Roggero E, Pinotti G, et al. Patterns of survival in mantle cell lymphoma. Ann Oncol 1995;6:257–62.
37. Argatoff LH, Connors JM, Klasa RJ, et al. Mantle cell lymphoma: a clinicopathologic study of 80 cases. Blood 1997; 89:2067–78.
38. Hiddemann W, Unterhalt M, Hermann R, et al. Mantle-cell lymphomas have more widespread disease and a slower response to chemotherapy compared with follicle-center lymphomas: results of a prospective comparative analysis of the German Low-Grade Lymphoma Study Group. J Clin Oncol 1998;16:1922–30.
39. Savio A, Franzin G, Wotherspoon AC, et al. Diagnosis and posttreatment follow-up of Helicobacter pylori-positive gastric lymphoma of mucosa-associated lymphoid tissue: Histology, polymerase chain reaction, or both? Blood 1996;87: 1255–60.
40. Lister TA, Crowther D, Sutcliffe SB, et al. Report of a committee convened to discuss the evaluation and staging of patients with Hodgkin's disease: Cotswolds Meeting. J Clin Oncol 1989;7:1630–6.
41. Shipp MA, Harrington DP, Anderson JR, et al. Development of a predictive model for aggressive lymphoma: The International Non-Hodgkin's Lymphoma Prognostic Factors Project. N Engl J Med 1993;329:987–94.
42. Löpez-Guillermo A, Montserrat E, Bosch F, et al. Applicability of the International Prognostic Index for aggressive lymphomas in patients with low-grade lymphoma. J Clin Oncol 1994;12:1343–8.
43. Hermans J, Krol ADG, van Groningen K, et al. International prognostic index for aggressive non-Hodgkin's lymphoma is valid for all malignancy grades. Blood 1995;86: 1460–3.
44. Colombat P, Solal-Celigny P, Roy P. Validity of the Follicular Lymphoma International Prognostic Index (FLIPI) in all age groups. Blood 2002;100:770a(Abstr 3046).
45. Cartron G, Dacheux L, Salles G, et al. Therapeutic activity of humanized anti-CD20 monoclonal antibody and polymorphism in IgG Fc receptor FcgammaRIIIa gene. Blood 2002;99:754–8.
46. Weng WK, Levy R. Two immunoglobulin G fragment C receptor polymorphisms independently predict response to rituximab in patients with follicular lymphoma. J Clin Oncol 2003;21:3940–7.
47. Mounier N, Briere J, Gisselbrecht C, et al. Rituximab plus CHOP (R-CHOP) overcomes bcl-2-associated resistance to chemotherapy in elderly patients with diffuse large B-cell lymphoma (DLBCL). Blood 2003;101:4279–84.
48. Freudenberg LS, Antoch G, Schütt P, et al. FDG-PET/CT in restaging of patients with lymphoma. Eur J Nucl Med Mol Imaging 2004;31:325–9.
49. Kostakoglu L, Coleman M, Somrov S, et al. FDG-PET after one cycle of chemotherapy accurately predicts response to therapy in large cell (aggressive) non-Hodgkin's lymphoma (NHL) and Hodgkin's disease (HD). Proc Soc Nuc Med (Abstr 651533) 2004.
50. Grillo-López AJ, McLaughlin P, Cheson BD, et al. First report on the application of the new response criteria (RC) proposed for NHL: the Rituximab pivotal trial. Proc ASCO 1998.
51. Grillo-López AJ, Cheson B, Horning S, et al. Response criteria (RC) for NHL: importance of "normal" lymph node (LN) size and correlations with response. Ann Oncol 2000;11: 399–408.
52. Lewis E, Bernardino ME, Salvador PG, et al. Post-therapy CT-detected mass in lymphoma patients: is it viable tissue? J Comput Assist Tomogr 1982;6:792–5.
53. Fuks JZ, Aisner J, Wiernik PH. Restaging laparotomy in the management of the non-Hodgkin lymphomas. Med Pediatr Oncol 1982;10:429–38.
54. Stewart FM, Williamson BR, Innes DJ, et al. Residual tumor masses following treatment for advanced histiocytic lymphoma. Cancer 1985;55:620–623.
55. Surbone A, Longo DL, DeVita VT Jr, et al. Residual abdominal masses in aggressive non-Hodgkin's lymphoma after combination chemotherapy: significance and management. J Clin Oncol 1988;6:1832–7.
56. Longo DL, DeVita VT Jr, Duffey PL, et al. Superiority of ProMACE-CytaBOM over ProMACE-MOPP in the treatment of advanced diffuse aggressive lymphoma: Results of a prospective randomized trial. J Clin Oncol 1991;9: 25–38.
57. Waits TM, Greco FA, Greer JP, et al. Effective therapy for poor-prognosis non-Hodgkin's lymphoma with 8 weeks of high-dose–intensity combination chemotherapy. J Clin Oncol 1993;11:943–9.
58. Coiffier B, Gisselbrecht C, Herbrecht R, et al. LNH-84 regimen: a multicenter study of intensive chemotherapy in 737 patients with aggressive malignant lymphoma. J Clin Oncol 1989;7:1018–26.
59. Meyer RM, Quirt IC, Skillings JR, et al. Escalated as compared with standard doses of doxorubicin in BACOP therapy for patients with non-Hodgkin's lymphoma. N Engl J Med 1993; 329:1770–6.
60. Zuckerman KS, Case DC Jr, Gams RA, et al. Chemotherapy of intermediate- and high-grade non-Hodgkin's lymphomas with an intensive epirubicin-containing regimen. Blood 1993; 82:3564–73.
61. Zuckerman KS, LoBuglio AF, Reeves JA. Chemotherapy of intermediate- and high-grade non-Hodgkin's lymphomas with a high-dose doxorubicin-containing regimen. J Clin Oncol 1990;8:248–56.
62. Chopra R, Goldstone AH, Pearce R, et al. Autologous versus allogeneic bone marrow transplantation for non-Hodgkin's lymphoma. A case-controlled analysis of the European Bone Marrow Transplant Group Registry data. J Clin Oncol 1992; 10:1690–5.
63. Juweid ME, Wiseman GA, Menda Y, et al. Integrated PET plus CT-based response assessment of aggressive non-Hodgkin's lymphoma. Blood 2003;102:629a(Abstr 2321).

64. Van Den Bossche B, Lambert B, De Winter F, et al. 18FDG PET versus high-dose 67Ga scintigraphy for restaging and treatment follow-up of lymphoma patients. Nuc Med Comm 2002;23:1079–83.
65. Jerusalem G, Beguin Y, Fassotte MF, et al. Whole-body positron emission tomography using 18F-fluorodeoxyglucose for posttreatment evaluation in Hodgkin's disease and non-Hodgkin's lymphoma has higher diagnostic and prognostic value than classical computed tomography scan imaging. Blood 1999;94:429–33.
66. de Wit M, Bohuslavizki KH, Buchert R, et al. 18FDG-PET following treatment as valid predictor for disease-free survival in Hodgkin's lymphoma. Ann Oncol 2001;12:29–37.
67. Spaepen K, Stroobants S, Dupont P, et al. Prognostic value of positron emission tomography (PET) with fluorine-18 fluorodeoxyglucose ([^{18}F]FDG) after first-line chemotherapy in non-Hodgkin's lymphoma: Is [^{18}F]FDG-PET a valid alternative to conventional diagnostic methods? J Clin Oncol 2001;19:414–9.
68. Spaepen K, Stroobants S, Dupont P, et al. Early restaging positron emission tomography with 18F-fluorodeoxyglucose predicts outcome in patients with aggressive non-Hodgkin's lymphoma. Ann Oncol 2002;13:1356–63.
69. Weeks JC, Yeap BY, Canellos GP, et al. Value of follow-up procedures in patients with large-cell lymphoma who achieve a complete remission. J Clin Oncol 1991;9:1196–203.
70. Oh YK, Ha CS, Samuels BI, et al. Stages I-III follicular lymphoma: Role of CT of the abdomen and pelvis in follow-up studies. Radiology 1999;210:483–6.

9

Differential Diagnosis

Jennifer R. Brown, M.D., Ph.D.
Arthur T. Skarin, M.D.

Although many lymphomas present initially with lymphadenopathy, benign causes of lymphadenopathy are also frequent. Isolated enlarged lymph nodes, particularly in the cervical area, can be found in healthy adults and are often without clinical significance.[1] In one series of 543 patients referred for further evaluation of lymphadenopathy, only 17.5% had an underlying malignant disorder, with 11.4% having a lymphoproliferative disorder and 6.1% a metastatic solid tumor.[2] Of the remainder, 22.1% had no significant lymphadenopathy, 3.9% had benign tumors, 30.9% had benign reactive lymphadenopathy, and 25.6% had miscellaneous non-neoplastic disorders.[2] Malignant lymphoproliferative diseases are more likely to cause generalized lymphadenopathy or associated organomegaly.[3]

The differential diagnosis of lymphadenopathy is broad. Those etiologies warranting further discussion can be divided between benign causes and lymphoproliferative disorders ranging from benign to frankly malignant. Benign causes discussed further below include infections, systemic autoimmune disorders and sarcoidosis, hypersensitivity reactions to drugs or silicone, and unusual reactive primary lymphadenopathies. The atypical lymphoproliferative disorders include Castleman's disease, angioimmunoblastic lymphadenopathy with dysproteinemia, lymphomatoid granulomatosis, and lymphomatoid papulosis.

BENIGN ETIOLOGIES OF SIGNIFICANT LYMPHADENOPATHY

Infections

Significant lymphadenopathy can result from infections of all types. Acute bacterial infections, generally streptococcal or staphylococcal, are seen in the primary care setting and often treated empirically with antibiotics. In one large British referral series, the most common infections identified were toxoplasmosis, tuberculosis, Epstein–Barr virus (EBV), and human immunodeficiency virus (HIV).[2] Previous studies have confirmed the relatively high incidence of toxoplasmosis, tuberculosis, and EBV-induced infectious mononucleosis[4] in patients with persistent multifocal lymphadenopathy.

Lymphotropic viruses such as EBV cause a spectrum of lymphoproliferative disorders (LPDs) that range from benign to malignant. Years ago Dameshek and Gunz stated that infectious mononucleosis (IM) is a regulated neoplasm.[5] In the immunocompetent patient EBV infection of B lymphocytes causes a polyclonal LPD, which is infectious mononucleosis (IM). This disorder, characterized mainly by lymphadenopathy, is controlled by T lymphocytes that recognize the foreign peptides on the surface of the infected B lymphocytes, resulting in their eradication and resolution of the illness within a few weeks. Despite this usual pattern, a large population-based study has recently confirmed that the risk of EBV-associated Hodgkin's lymphoma is increased approximately four-fold following acute infectious mononucleosis.[6] Furthermore, in immunosuppressed patients, fatal IM can occur, as for example, in the X-linked LPD described by Purtilo and Stevenson.[7] EBV is an important co-factor in the development of non-Hodgkin's lymphomas in patients with primary and acquired immunodeficiencies,[8,9] and has been strongly implicated as the etiologic agent in post-transplant LPDs.[10] These LPDs range from benign to malignant, and can be monoclonal or polyclonal.[11] An understanding of the evolution from a benign, polyclonal EBV-infected B-cell population to a malignant monoclonal B-cell lymphoma is critically important, but as yet not worked out.[11]

AUTOIMMUNE LYMPHADENOPATHY

Most autoimmune disorders can be associated with lymphadenopathy and occasionally splenomegaly. Rheumatoid arthritis, systemic lupus erythematosus (SLE), and Sjögren's syndrome are most commonly associated, but lymphadenopathy may also be seen in dermatomyositis, Hashimoto's thyroiditis, Graves' disease, primary biliary cirrhosis, mixed connective tissue disease, and essential mixed cryoglobulinemia.[12] Lymph node biopsy results generally show reactive lymphoid hyperplasia, but should be performed for any suspicious or persistent lymph nodes since these patients do have an elevated risk of lymphoma.

In rheumatoid arthritis, lymphadenopathy may affect up to 75% of patients at some time during the illness. The enlarged nodes may be regional (near inflamed joints) or generalized.[13] Lymph node biopsy shows extensive reactive follicular hyperplasia and interfollicular plasmacytosis. The etiology of this lymphadenopathy remains unclear, with speculation centered on the role of interleukin-6 (IL-6) or chronic immune stimulation.[12] Patients with rheumatoid arthritis are at increased risk of malignant LPDs (usually marginal zone lymphoma or large B-cell lymphoma), particularly with long-standing disease of at least 15 years.[14] Felty's syndrome, a rare complication of severe rheumatoid arthritis that occurs in 1% of patients, consists of splenomegaly, neutropenia, and recurrent infections.[15] In a retrospective review of 906 men with Felty's syndrome from a Veterans Affairs Hospital, the risk for subsequent non-Hodgkin's lymphoma (NHL) was much greater than the twofold risk reported in rheumatoid arthritis and was similar to the risk of lymphoma in Sjögren's syndrome.[16]

Lymphadenopathy in patients with SLE is also common, occurring in 25% to 67% of patients.[17] Patients are generally younger than those with rheumatoid arthritis, and occasionally may present with lymphadenopathy. The most characteristic histologic features are coagulation necrosis, hematoxylin bodies (extracellular amorphous material composed of degenerated cellular contents, mostly DNA), and DNA deposition within vessel walls.[18] The pathogenesis of SLE adenopathy is unknown but apparently is not related to vasculitis. Cancers and lymphomas occur in patients with SLE at variable rates. An early report reviewed lymphomas in 18 cases of SLE, with simultaneous diagnoses in 4, lymphoma predating SLE in 2, and occurring after SLE in 16.[19] More recently, 5 cases of lymphoma were reported in patients with autoimmune disorders, including 2 with SLE.[20] The lymphomas in these reports included Hodgkin's lymphoma, NHL (usually large cell type), and chronic lymphocytic leukemia.[20]

Sjögren's syndrome is an autoimmune disorder characterized by dryness of the eyes and mouth (sicca syndrome), along with serum autoantibodies and abnormal lymphoid infiltration of salivary glands.[21] The disease may be primary or associated with other connective tissue diseases such as rheumatoid arthritis. Lymphadenopathy occasionally occurs in patients with Sjögren's syndrome and may be localized or generalized.[22] The initial biopsy usually shows reactive follicular hyperplasia and interfollicular plasmacytosis, similar to what is seen in rheumatoid arthritis. However, patients are at increased risk of LPD, which has been reported in excised enlarged lymph nodes of 18 of 138 patients.[22] One study has estimated that the incidence of malignant lymphoma in patients with Sjögren's syndrome is increased 44-fold.[23] Types of LPD vary from low-grade small lymphocytic to large-cell B immunoblastic, but marginal zone lymphoma is particularly common.[24–26] Salivary gland enlargement in patients with Sjögren's syndrome may herald development of an LPD, as may hepatosplenomegaly, pulmonary infiltrates, renal insufficiency, or cytopenias. Mikulicz's disease (myoepithelial sialadenitis) describes the classic histopathologic features seen in enlarged salivary glands of patients with Sjögren's syndrome. Although the features appear to be benign, modern immunohistologic and molecular genetic studies have revealed monoclonal B-cell populations that undoubtedly evolve into malignant LPD.[27] The development of Sjögren's syndrome-associated LPD appears to be related to several factors, including chronic immune stimulation, EBV-driven B-cell expansion, genetic alterations, and defective immune surveillance.[12,21]

HYPERSENSITIVITY LYMPHADENOPATHY

Patients may develop lymphadenopathy as a hypersensitivity reaction to medications (Table 9–1). Features such as fever, rash, arthralgias, and eosinophilia are usually present.[12] The classic cause of this hypersensitivity reaction is phenytoin and its related hydantoin derivatives, first described in the classic report of 1959.[28] Most patients with this adenopathy have been on the drug for less than 4 months, although some have had drug exposure for years. Adenopathy is particularly prominent in the cervical lymph nodes. Biopsy most often shows features similar to viral-induced lymphadenopathy, with partial or complete effacement of nodal architecture by a polymorphous infiltrate of immunoblasts, small lymphocytes, eosinophils, and plasma cells.[29] In one review of 25 patients with lymphadenopathy thought to be related to phenytoin exposure, a wide range of histologic features was reported by the Armed Forces Institute of Pathology.[30] The 60% of cases that were benign included follicular and mixed hyperplasias, paracortical immunoblastic proliferations, and LPD resembling AILD. The 40% of cases that were malignant included seven cases of NHL, and three cases of Hodgkin's lymphoma. Serial study of two cases showed progression of atypical hyperplasia to NHL.

Table 9–1. Medications Associated with Lymphadenopathy

Phenytoin	Carbamazepine
Para-amino salicylic acid	Phenylbutazone
Indomethacin	Aspirin
Sulphonamides	Iron dextran
Penicillins	Erythromycin
Gentamicin	Tetracycline
Thiouracil compounds	Sulfasalazine
Griseofulvin	Antithymocyte globulin
OKT-3	Gold
Halothane	Bacillus Calmette-Guerin
Allopurinol	Insulin
Primidone	Methyldopa, levodopa

From Segal G, Clough JD, and Tubbs RR. Autoimmune and iatrogenic causes of lymphadenopathy. Semin Oncol 1993;20:611,[12] with permission.

More than 30 cases of lymphadenopathy related to carbamazepine have also been reported, and generally regress when carbamazepine is discontinued.[12] However, as for phenytoin, long-term follow-up is important, particularly when lymphadenopathy persists or progresses, because of the risk of an evolving malignant LPD.

Multiple factors have been suggested to explain the association of phenytoin and related drugs with subsequent benign and malignant LPDs. Chronic immunosuppression due to the drugs was implied in an epidemiologic study.[31] It was found that 8 (1.6%) of 516 patients with Hodgkin's lymphoma or NHL had a history of phenytoin therapy compared with 3 (0.6%) of 516 patients with other cancers and 2 (0.4%) of 516 tumor-free subjects. Abnormalities of the immune system occur in as many as 70% of patients receiving phenytoin and carbamazepine[12,32,33] and include 1) suppressor T-cell abnormalities, both decreased and increased function; 2) depressed cellular and humoral responses; 3) serum sickness-like (immune complex) disease; 4) abnormal lymphocyte metabolism; 5) autoimmune phenomena; and 6) severe immune dysregulation.[34]

Hypersensitivity to phenytoin has been estimated to occur in about 1 in 10^3 to 10^5 people.[35] An enzyme defect that blocks detoxification of metabolites of aromatic anticonvulsants is inherited in an autosomal recessive manner and may result in genetic predisposition.[35] Of clinical relevance, in vitro tests are available to determine individual susceptibility, which is especially useful in patients with a family history of anticonvulsant-drug hypersensitivity reactions.[35]

SILICONE-ASSOCIATED LYMPHADENOPATHY

Lymphadenopathy related to silicone has become increasingly recognized since silicone-elastomer prostheses became available for joint replacement surgery.[36] Most cases occur in axillary lymph nodes of patients with rheumatoid arthritis who have joint replacement surgery for hand deformities.[37] Inguinal lymphadenopathy has rarely been reported, usually related to insertion of a silicone prosthesis in the lower extremities.[38] Lymph node biopsy shows reactive lymphoid hyperplasia with many multinucleated giant cells, most containing refractile, nonbirefringent material that proves to be silicone.[38] Confluent noncaseating granulomas may also be present.[39] Up to 15% of patients undergoing silicone implant arthroplasty may develop regional lymphadenopathy.[38] Particulate silicone generated by small fractures of the prosthesis is trapped in draining lymph nodes, resulting in slowly progressive asymptomatic enlargement. A lymphoma may be suspected, particularly in patients with underlying rheumatoid arthritis, and biopsy can be justified. Nonsilicone large joint implants using polyester or polyethylene may also result in regional lymphadenopathy by a similar mechanism.[40] Lymph node biopsy shows characteristic sinus histiocytosis with polarizing, birefringent material in the cytoplasm of the histiocytes.

Liquid silicone used in breast augmentation procedures may eventually result in regional lymphadenopathy. Breast prostheses may rupture or particulate silicone may slowly leak from an intact prosthesis, eventually resulting in lymph node enlargement.[41,42] Although axillary nodes are generally asymptomatic, occasional tender nodes have occurred.[38] Histologic findings are less reactive than those related to solid silicone joint prostheses and include only occasional multinucleated giant cells and clear silicone-containing vacuoles.[41]

MISCELLANEOUS BENIGN DISORDERS

A number of other benign disorders may be associated with reactive lymphadenopathy. Histopathologic findings are well described elsewhere, and only certain conditions that may be confused with lymphoma are discussed here.

Sarcoidosis is a multisystem disease of unknown cause, characterized by noncaseating granulomata throughout various tissues and organs. Many clinical presentations occur, but most commonly generalized or bilateral hilar lymphadenopathy or lung involvement. Lymph node biopsy specimens are easily distinguishable from lymphoma, with noncaseating granulomata composed of epithelioid cells, often with Langerhans or foreign body-type giant cells. No excess risk of lymphoma has been observed in patients with sarcoidosis.[43]

Dermatopathic adenopathy (DA) refers to enlarged lymph nodes often found in patients with chronic skin diseases, particularly generalized exfoliative dermatitis and mycosis fungoides. In mycosis fungoides, about 25% of early cases have dermatopathic adenopathy, 70% to 75% of advanced cases, and 90% of patients with generalized erythroderma (Sézary syndrome).[44] Lymph node biopsy shows a normal follicular pattern and an intact capsule. The follicles, however, show slight enlargement of their germinal centers surrounded by a rim of lymphocytes. The paracortical areas stand out as pale patches, due to an increase in large histiocytes or macrophages with abundant pale cytoplasm and large pale nucleoli. Interspersed are small lymphocytes with cerebriform nuclei, which are difficult to distinguish from mycosis fungoides cells. Special studies show that the large, pale cells are composed of dendritic cells, Langerhans cells, and indeterminate cells.[44]

Most patients with *systemic amyloidosis* present with nephrotic syndrome, congestive heart failure, orthostatic hypotension, carpal tunnel syndrome, and peripheral neuropathy. Only occasionally is generalized lymphadenopathy or splenomegaly the presenting feature.[45] Tissue biopsy shows deposition of an amorphous hyaline-like substance that stains pink with hematoxylin and eosin, and under polarized light, Congo red produces an apple-green birefringence. Electron microscopy reveals the diagnostic rigid, linear, nonbranching aggregated fibrils of indefinite length.[45] Systemic amyloidosis refers to a final common pathway for tissue protein deposition and is only associated with underlying lymphomas approximately 4% to 10% of the time.[46,47]

BENIGN LYMPHOPROLIFERATIVE DISORDERS

Inflammatory Pseudo-Tumor of Lymph Nodes

Inflammatory pseudo-tumor of lymph nodes occurs mainly in young adults who present with enlarged lymph nodes in single or multiple sites, with or without systemic complaints.[48,49] The nodes may be quite large (>3 cm) and involve central as well as peripheral sites. Mild anemia and hypergammaglobulinemia are often present. Lymph node biopsy reveals expansion of the hilum and fibrous trabeculae with proliferation of spindle cells and vessels, admixed with lymphocytes and plasma cells. The uninvolved nodal parenchyma shows only nonspecific reactive changes. These features may at times be mistaken for Kaposi's sarcoma (KS), Castleman's disease, Hodgkin's lymphoma, or NHL.[50] The inflammatory pseudo-tumor of lymph nodes probably represents the end result of an inflammatory response to multiple etiologies, including *Pseudomonas* or toxoplasmosis infection.[50] Spontaneous regression occurs in most patients.

HISTIOCYTIC NECROTIZING LYMPHADENITIS (KIKUCHI'S LYMPHADENITIS)

Histiocytic necrotizing lymphadenitis (Kikuchi's lymphadenitis) was first described in Japan in 1972,[51] and is a benign, self-limited disorder that occurs worldwide. Most patients are younger than 40 years of age with a small female predominance. Solitary or multiple lymph nodes are enlarged, most often in the cervical area, usually nontender, and rarely larger than 2 cm in diameter.[50] Constitutional symptoms suggestive of a flu-like illness often occur. Lymph node histopathology consists of a histiocytic proliferation with karyorrhectic foci, often exhibiting a "starry-sky" appearance. The center of the karyorrhectic foci shows coagulative necrosis surrounded by histiocytes, plasmacytoid monocytes, and immunoblasts (T-cell lineage). Characteristic "crescentic histiocytes" are phagocytic cells with eccentrically located crescentic nuclei.[50] The clinical course is self-limited, although corticosteroids may occasionally be indicated.[52] An infectious etiology has been postulated, as well as an autoimmune etiology related to SLE.[53–55] No association has been found with HHV-8, HHV-6, parainfluenza, or EBV, however.[51,53,56,57]

SINUS HISTIOCYTOSIS WITH MASSIVE LYMPHADENOPATHY (ROSAI–DORFMAN DISEASE)

Sinus histiocytosis with massive lymphadenopathy (Rosai–Dorfman disease) is an unusual entity that was initially described in 1969,[58] and is characterized by greatly enlarged, matted lymph nodes in an otherwise healthy person. Rosai–Dorfman disease usually occurs in young adults, with a mean age of about 20 years.[59] About 25% of patients have fever. Up to 40% of cases can occur in extranodal sites, most commonly in the head and neck.[59,60] The systemic features include fever, elevated sedimentation rate, low serum albumin level, polyclonal hypergammaglobulinemia, reversal of CD4-to-CD8 ratio in peripheral blood lymphocytes, and anemia. About 10% of cases have one or more immune disorders preceding or associated with onset of the disease.[59,61] Lymph node biopsy shows a thickened fibrous capsule with distention of the sinuses by large, benign histiocytes characterized by abundant cytoplasm and vesicular nuclei with prominent nucleoli. The etiology of Rosai–Dorfman disease is unknown; speculation has centered on an unusual histiocytic reaction possibly mediated by secretion of cytokines or an as yet unknown infection. Approximately 50% of patients have a self-limited clinical course with spontaneous remission in several weeks.[50,60,62] In most other cases, the disease remains stable without regression or progression, although rare deaths have been reported.[63] Bulky lesions can be resected, and steroids and single agent chemotherapy have been used when necessary.[50,60,62,64]

VASCULAR TRANSFORMATION OF SINUSES

Vascular transformation of sinuses is a rare reactive condition found incidentally in lymph nodes removed at surgery for cancer or lymphoma. The lymph node sinuses become transformed into complex endothelial-lined channels.[65–67] Any cause of lymphatic or vascular obstruction may predispose to this finding, including thrombosis, severe heart failure, and previous regional surgery or radiation therapy. In the rare cases where patients have no obvious predisposing factors, cancer should be sought.[50] Microscopically, vascular transformation of the sinuses shows expansion and sclerosis of nodal sinuses with sparing of the nodal capsule. The normal lymphoid parenchyma shows variable degrees of atrophy. Within the sinuses, vessel proliferation is prominent, with irregular slits or rounded vascular spaces lined by flat endothelium along with solid vascular foci. The differential diagnosis does include Kaposi's sarcoma.[50] Treatment is not indicated.

PROGRESSIVE TRANSFORMATION OF GERMINAL CENTERS

Progressive transformation of germinal centers (PTGC) was initially described in 1975 as a lesion closely associated with nodular lymphocyte–predominant Hodgkin's lymphoma (NLPHD).[68] Subsequent studies suggested that PTGC often predated NLPHD by months to years.[69,70] Retrospective studies ultimately suggested that 1% of cases of NLPHD may be preceded by PTGC, and another 1.5% of cases may be simultaneously or subsequently diagnosed with NLPHD.[71–73] Small prospective studies have shown that the diagnoses of PTGC and HD often coincide, but that only about 2.5% of patients with PTGC go on to develop HD.[71]

Most patients with PTGC present with asymptomatic solitary lymphadenopathy. Histologically, PTGCs are large lymphoid follicles in which mantle zone lymphocytes accumulate and expand the germinal center. In most reported cases, one to several PTGCs are noted in a single cross-section, and most of the lymph node shows reactive changes.[71] Generalized lymph node enlargement is more common in pediatric patients, although florid PTGC, defined as more than nine PTGCs per lymph node cross section, is associated with generalized lymphadenopathy as well as persistent or recurrent lymphadenopathy.[71] Immunohistochemical studies show that PTGCs comprise mainly polyclonal B cells with the immunophenotype of mantle zone lymphocytes. The etiology of PTGC is unknown but may reflect an ineffective immune response to certain antigens. The finding of PTGC in patients with previous or active Hodgkin's lymphoma, as well as hypogammaglobulinemia—both disorders associated with T-cell defects—also supports an immunologic abnormality as causative.[71]

Patients with PTGC require no therapy. Lymphadenopathy either remains stable or regresses spontaneously. Long-term follow-up is indicated due to the small risk for subsequent NLPHD.[71]

ATYPICAL POTENTIALLY MALIGNANT LYMPHOPROLIFERATIVE DISORDERS

These diseases are distinct from the benign lymphoproliferative disorders in that they have significant potential for or have already acquired a malignant phenotype. These include Castleman's disease, lymphomatoid granulomatosis, and lymphomatoid papulosis. Angioimmunoblastic lymphadenopathy with dysproteinemia (AILD) will also be discussed. Although it was previously classified as an atypical lymphoproliferative disorder, AILD likely represents an evolving malignant T-cell clone and is now classified as a true lymphoma because of its malignant clinical course.

Castleman's Disease (Angiofollicular [Giant] Lymph Node Hyperplasia)

In 1956, Castleman and coworkers described a patient with a localized mediastinal mass that on biopsy showed hyperplasia resembling Hassall's corpuscles of the thymus, as well as capillary proliferation and hyalinization.[74] Detailed studies subsequently described two pathologic forms of the same disease, referred to as the hyaline vascular type, similar to that described by Castleman, and representing 90% of cases, and the plasma cell type, characterized by persistent sinuses and sheets of plasma cells in the interfollicular regions and representing 10% of cases.[75] The patients initially described by Castleman had unicentric disease, localized to one lymph node which was often found incidentally on imaging, and most commonly in the mediastinum or hilum, followed by the abdomen. Surgical resection is curative for these patients.[75–77]

First described in 1978, multicentric Castleman's disease (MCD) is a systemic disorder of generalized lymphadenopathy, fevers, sweats, fatigue, and weight loss.[78,79] Pathologically, it is almost always the plasma cell variant. An association has long been noted with Kaposi's sarcoma, which occurs in 13% of patients in historical series from the pre-HIV era,[79] and more recently with HIV. The association with KS led to the discovery that human herpes virus-8, a novel human herpes virus[80,81] first identified as the causative agent of Kaposi's sarcoma (KS), is also highly associated with Castleman's disease. Multiple studies have since confirmed that HHV-8 is universally found in HIV-associated MCD, and also present in approximately 40% to 50% of HIV-negative MCD.[81,82] Unicentric CD is likely a different disease, as only one reported case has been associated with HHV-8.[83–85]

Although HHV-8 is clearly implicated in most cases of MCD, the pathogenesis of those cases that are HHV-8-negative remains unclear and may be related to lymphoproliferation driven by a different, perhaps viral or autoimmune, antigen, and defective immune regulation.[79] Dysregulated IL-6 production by the germinal centers may provide some of the immune stimulus.[86,87] Expression of the IL-6 gene has been detected in Castleman's lymph nodes, and removal of the lymph nodes results in transient relief of symptoms and decreased IL-6 production.[86] Retroviral transduction of IL-6 coding sequences into hematopoietic stem cells has reproduced the clinical and laboratory features of Castleman's disease in mice.[88]

The clinical course of MCD is unfortunately often aggressive. Median survival in the pre-HIV era was 26 months,[50] and HIV-infected patients do even more poorly, with a median survival of 8 to 14 months.[89,90] Patients die of fulminant infection or the development of malignancy, particularly KS or NHL. Fully 70% of HIV+, HHV-8+ patients develop KS.[89–91] Approximately 15% to 20% of MCD patients develop intermediate- to high-grade NHL.[91,92] In one prospective cohort study of HIV+, HHV-8+ patients, the actuarial 2-year incidence of NHL was 24.3%, 15-fold greater than expected for unselected HIV patients.[93]

Limited data are available concerning therapy for MCD. Spontaneous remission occurs occasionally. Steroids, single-agent chemotherapy drugs, and anti-human IL-6 antibody can all reduce symptoms, but responses are generally short-lived.[90,92–94] Standard-dose chemotherapy for intermediate-grade NHL has been reported to induce sustained remissions.[95,96] Single-agent rituximab induced 3- to 12-month remissions in 67% of reported patients, but half of those developed worsened KS.[97]

ANGIOIMMUNOBLASTIC LYMPHADENOPATHY WITH DYSPROTEINEMIA (AILD)

The atypical LPD called AILD was described more than 20 years ago by several investigators.[98–100] Although the histologic features suggest a benign process, the clinical course is aggressive, and clonal T-cell populations can be identified, so AILD is now properly characterized as a T-cell lymphoma. Characteristically, patients present with signs and symptoms of lymphoma, including fevers, sweats, weight loss, and generalized lymphadenopathy; they may also have hepatosplenomegaly, skin rash, Coombs'-positive hemolytic anemia, and polyclonal hypergammaglobulinemia.

Histological features are generally similar to benign viral lymphoproliferations, with a diffuse effacement of architecture by a polymorphous infiltrate of plasma cells, lymphocytes, eosinophils, and epithelioid histiocytes.[99,100] A prominent arborizing vasculature is readily evident, and amorphous pink-staining proteinaceous material is present in the interstitium. Interspersed throughout the lymph node are large immunoblasts, which may form sheets or clusters; however, the extent of clustering does not predict outcome and the disease is now classified as a lymphoma regardless of the presence or absence of this feature.[99,101] Cytogenetic studies have identified trisomy 3, trisomy 5, and +X in patients with AILD, and in approximately half the cases, more than one clone was detected, suggesting that at least initially this disorder can be oligoclonal.[102] Gene rearrangement studies have shown primarily T-cell–receptor gene rearrangements in 70% of cases, with immunoglobulin heavy-chain gene rearrangements occasionally detected, sometimes in the same patient.[101,103–105] Multiple TCR clones can appear and disappear with time in a single lesion.[101,103] If histologic features of true lymphoma emerge, often a dominant clone will appear, usually with the phenotype of a helper CD4+ T cell.[104]

LYMPHOMATOID GRANULOMATOSIS

Lymphomatoid granulomatosis was originally described as a pulmonary angiitis characterized by an angiodestructive polymorphic inflammatory infiltrate with scattered large atypical cells.[106,107] The prevalence of the T cells in the infiltrate initially suggested this to be a T-cell disorder, but no clonality could be demonstrated.[107–109] Subsequently the large atypical lymphoid cells were found to be EBV-infected B cells, at least some of which contained clonal immunoglobulin gene rearrangements. This disorder is therefore now recognized as an EBV-related B-cell lymphoproliferative disorder[108–111] that affects men more than women, generally in the fifth or sixth decade of life.[112–114] Most patients present with respiratory symptoms and bilateral pulmonary nodules, often with cavitation. Extrathoracic manifestations are common and include skin involvement in 37%, and nervous system involvement in 30% of patients.[115]

This disease has an unpredictable clinical course ranging from resolution without treatment to early fatality.[112–114] The largest series of 152 patients reported a 67% mortality and median survival of 14 months,[114] with patients dying of pulmonary complications, infection, central nervous system disease, and lymphoma. Histologic grading of the lesion may help stratify patients by prognosis.[107,110,111] Grade I lesions have very rare EBV-positive cells, Grade II lesions contain scattered EBV positive cells, and Grade III lesions, with sheets of large atypical EBV positive cells, are histologically consistent with frank malignant lymphoma.[107,110,111] This progression of malignant transformation is likely analogous to that seen in post-transplant EBV lymphoproliferative disorders.

The benefit of treatment has been difficult to establish in the early phases of the disease. The two largest older series failed to show a difference in outcome among patients treated with chemotherapy, steroids, or observation.[112,114] The only prospective study did suggest that treatment with cyclophosphamide and steroids could induce prolonged complete remissions.[113] Observation is reasonable for asymptomatic patients with minimal disease burden and low-grade disease, but patients with more aggressive low-grade or Grade III disease should be treated with combination chemotherapy for intermediate-grade lymphoma.[107]

LYMPHOMATOID PAPULOSIS

Lymphomatoid papulosis is a cutaneous T-cell lymphoproliferative disorder that presents as multiple, usually small skin papules or nodules, which may wax and wane for years.[116,117] Despite this clinically indolent course, the histologic appearance is malignant; the lesion is characterized by a population of activated CD4+ CD30+ helper T cells that resemble Reed–Sternberg cells, in a background of small lymphocytes.[118] These CD30+ cells harbor a clonal TCR gene rearrangement,[119,120] making lymphomatoid papulosis (LP) a clonal T-cell lymphoproliferative disorder. Between 20% and 80% of LP patients will eventually develop frank lymphomas with the same underlying TCR gene rearrangement. Hodgkin's lymphoma, cutaneous T-cell lymphomas, and anaplastic large-cell lymphomas are most commonly seen.[118,119,121] Early treatment of the LP is symptomatic because there is no evidence that treatment alters the natural history of the disorder.[117]

Acknowledgment

Dr. Jennifer Brown was supported in part by the Clinical Investigator Training Program: Harvard/MIT Health Sciences and Technology-Beth Israel Deaconess Medical Center, in Collaboration with Pfizer Inc.

References

1. Linet OI and Metzler C. Incidence of palpable cervical nodes in adults. Postgrad Med 1977;62:210.
2. Chau I, Kelleher MT, Cunningham D, Norman AR, et al. Rapid Access Multidisciplinary Lymph Node Diagnostic Clinic: analysis of 550 patients. Br J Cancer 2003;88: 354–61.
3. Abba AA, Bamgboye AE, Afzal M, et al. Lymphadenopathy in adults: a clinicopathological analysis. Saudi Med J 2002;23:282–6.
4. Pangalis GA, Vassilakopoulos TP, Boussiotis VA, et al. Clinical approach to lymphadenopathy. Semin Oncol 1993;20: 570.
5. Dameshek W and Gunz F. Leukemia, 2nd ed. New York: Grune & Stratton, 1964.
6. Hjalgrim H, Askling J, Rostgaard K, et al. Characteristics of Hodgkin's lymphoma after infectious mononucleosis. New Engl J Med 2003;349:1324–32.
7. Purtilo DT and Stevenson M. Lymphotropic viruses as etiologic agents of lymphoma. Hematol Oncol Clin North Am 1991;5:901.
8. Filipovich AH, Mathur A, Kamat D, et al. Primary immunodeficiencies: genetic risk factors for lymphoma. Cancer Res 1992;52(Suppl 19):5465s.
9. Shibata D, Weiss LM, Nathwani BN, et al. Epstein–Barr virus in benign lymph node biopsies from individuals infected with the human immunodeficiency virus is associated with concurrent or subsequent development of non-Hodgkin's lymphoma. Blood 1991;77:1527.
10. Seiden MV and Sklar J. Molecular genetic analysis of post-transplant lymphoproliferative disorders. Hematol Oncol Clin North Am 1993;7:447.
11. Yarbro JW. The Epstein–Barr virus and the distinction between benign and malignant lymphoproliferative processes. Semin Oncol 1993;20:658.
12. Segal G, Clough JD, and Tubbs RR. Autoimmune and iatrogenic causes of lymphadenopathy. Semin Oncol 1993;20:611.
13. Kojima M, Hosomura Y, Itoh H, et al. Reactive proliferative lesions in lymph nodes from rheumatoid arthritis patients: a clinicopathological and immunohistochemical study. Acta Pathol Jpn 1990;40:249.
14. Symmons DPM. Neoplasms of the immune system in rheumatoid arthritis. Am J Med 1985;78(Suppl 1A):22.
15. Rosenstein ED and Kramer N. Felty's and pseudo-Felty's syndrome. Semin Arthritis Rheum 1991;21:129.
16. Gridley G, Klippel JH, Hoover RN, et al. Incidence of cancer among men with the Felty syndrome. Ann Intern Med 1994;120:35.
17. Estes D and Christian CC. The natural history of systemic lupus erythematosus by prospective analysis. Medicine 1971;50:85.
18. Schnitzer B. Reactive lymphoid hyperplasia. In: Jaffe ES, ed. Surgical Pathology of the Lymph Nodes and Related Organs, pp 22–56. Philadelphia: WB Saunders, 1985.
19. Green JA, Dawson AA, and Walker W. Systemic lupus erythematosus and lymphoma. Lancet 1978;2:753.
20. Houssiau FA, Kirkove C, Asherson RA, et al. Malignant lymphoma in systemic rheumatic diseases. A report of five cases. Clin Exp Rheumatol 1991;9:515.
21. Fox RI, Luppi M, Kang HI, et al. Reactivation of Epstein–Barr virus in Sjögren's syndrome. Springer Semin Immunopathol 1991;13:217.
22. McCurley TL, Collins RD, Ball E, et al. Nodal and extranodal lymphoproliferative disorders in Sjögren's syndrome: a clinical and immunopathologic study. Hum Pathol 1990; 21:482.
23. Kassan SS, Thomas T, Moutsopoulos HM, et al. Increased risk of lymphoma in Sicca syndrome. Ann Intern Med 1978;89:888–92.
24. Voulgarelis M, Dafini UG, Isenberg DA, et al. Malignant lymphoma in primary Sjögren's syndrome. Arthritis Rheum 1999;42:1765–72.
25. Tzioufas AG. B-cell lymphoproliferation in primary Sjögren's syndrome. Clin Exp Rheumatol 1996;14 (Suppl 14):65–70.
26. Royer B, Cazals-Hatem D, Sibilia J, et al. Lymphomas in patients with Sjögren's syndrome are marginal zone B-cell neoplasms, arise in diverse extranodal and nodal sites, and are not associated with viruses. Blood 1997;90:766–75.
27. Segal GH, Wittwer CT, Fishleder AJ, et al. Identification of monoclonal B-cell populations by rapid-cycle PCR: a practical screening method for the detection of immunoglobulin gene rearrangements. Am J Pathol 1992;141:1291.

28. Saltzstein SJ and Ackerman LV. Lymphadenopathy induced by anticonvulsant drugs and mimicking clinically and pathologically malignant lymphomas. Cancer 1959;12:164.
29. Harris NL and Widder DJ. Phenytoin and generalized lymphadenopathy. Arch Pathol Lab Med 107:663, 1983.
30. Abbondanzo SL, Irey NS and Frizzera G. Dilantin-associated lymphadenopathy: spectrum of histopathologic patterns [Abstract]. Lab Invest 1992;66:73A.
31. Li FP, Willard DR, Goodman R, et al. Malignant lymphoma after diphenylhydantoin (Dilantin) therapy. Cancer 1975;36: 1359.
32. Sorrell TC and Forbes IJ. Depression of immune competence by phenytoin and carbamazepine: studies in vivo and in vitro. Clin Exp Immunol 1975;20:273.
33. Dosch HM, Jason J, and Gelfand EW. Transient antibody deficiency and abnormal T suppressor cells induced by phenytoin. N Engl J Med 1982;306:406.
34. Sinnige HAM, Boender CA, Kuypers EW, et al. Carbamazepine-induced pseudolymphoma and immune dysregulation. J Intern Med 1990;227:355.
35. Gennis MA, Vemuri R, Burns EA, et al. Familial occurrence of hypersensitivity to phenytoin. Am J Med 1991;91: 631.
36. Swanson AB. Finger joint replacement by silicone rubber implants and the concept of implant fixation by encapsulation. Ann Rheuma Dis 1969;28(Suppl):47.
37. Endo LP, Edwards NL, Longley S, et al. Silicone and rheumatic diseases. Semin Arthritis Rheum 1987;17:112.
38. Paplanus SH and Payne CM. Axillary lymphadenopathy 17 years after silicone implants: study with x-ray microanalysis. J Hand Surg 1988;13a:411.
39. Rogers LA, Longtine J, Garnick MB, et al. Silicone lymphadenopathy in a long distance runner: complication of a Silastic prosthesis. Hum Pathol 1988;19:1237.
40. Gray MH, Talbert ML, Talbert WM, et al. Changes seen in lymph nodes draining the sites of large joint prostheses. Am J Surg Pathol 1989;13:1050.
41. Wintsch W, Smahel J, Clodius L, et al. Local and regional lymph node response to ruptured gel-filled mammary prostheses. Br J Plastic Surg 1978;3l:349.
42. Truong LD, Cartwright J, Goodman MD, et al. Silicone lymphadenopathy associated with augmentation mammoplasty: morphologic features of nine cases. Am J Surg Pathol 1988;12:484.
43. Reich JM, Mullooly JP, and Johnson RE. Linkage analysis of malignancy-associated sarcoidosis. Chest 1995;107:605.
44. Lever WF and Schaumburg-Lever G. Dermatopathic lymphadenopathy. In: Histopathology of the Skin, 7th ed., pp. 113–14. Philadelphia: JB Lippincott, 1990.
45. Kyle RA and Greipp PR. Amyloidosis (AL): clinical and laboratory features in 229 cases. Mayo Clin Proc 1983;58: 665.
46. Stone MJ. Amyloidosis: a final common pathway for protein deposition in tissues. Blood 75:531.
47. Kaplan HS. Hodgkin's Disease, 2nd ed. Cambridge: Harvard University Press, 1980.
48. Davis RE, Warnke RA, and Dorfman RF. Inflammatory pseudotumor of lymph nodes: additional observations and evidence for an inflammatory etiology. Am J Surg Pathol 1991;15:744.
49. Perrone T, de Wolf-Peeters C, and Frizzera G. Inflammatory pseudotumor of lymph nodes: a distinctive pattern of nodal reaction. Am J Surg Pathol 1988;12:351.
50. Chan JKC and Tsang WYW. Uncommon syndromes of reactive lymphadenopathy. Semin Oncol 1993;20:648.
51. Dorfman RF. Histiocytic necrotizing lymphadenitis of Kikuchi and Fujimoto. Arch Pathol Lab Med 1987;111: 1026.
52. Sumiyoshi Y, Kikuchi M, Ohshima K, et al. A case of histiocytic necrotizing lymphadenitis with bone marrow and skin involvement. Virchows Arch A Pathol Anat Histopathol 1992;420:275.
53. Lin H-C, Su C-Y, Huang C-C, et al. Kikuchi's disease: a review and analysis of 61 cases. Otolaryngol Head Neck Surg 2003;128:650–3.
54. Quintas-Cardama A, Fraga M, Cozzi SN, et al. Fatal Kikuchi–Fujimoto disease: the lupus connection. Ann Hematol 2003;82:186–8.
55. Litwin MD, Kirkham B, Henderson DR, et al. Histiocytic necrotizing lymphadenitis in systemic lupus erythematosus. Ann Rheum Dis 1992;51:805–7.
56. Sumiyoshi Y, Kikuchi M, Ohshima K, et al. Human herpesvirus-6 genome in histiocytic necrotizing lymphadenitis (Kikuchi's disease) and other forms of lymphadenitis. Am J Clin Pathol 1993;99:609–14.
57. George TI, Jones CD, Zehnder JL, et al. Lack of human herpesvirus 8 and Epstein–Barr virus in Kikuchi's histiocytic necrotizing lymhadenitis. Hum Pathol 2002;34:130–4.
58. Rosai J and Dorfman RF. Sinus histiocytosis with massive lymphadenopathy: a newly recognized benign clinicopathologic entity. Arch Pathol 1969;87:63.
59. Foucar E, Rosai J, and Dorfman R. Sinus histiocytosis with massive lymphadenopathy (Rosai–Dorfman disease): review of the entity. Semin Diagn Pathol 1990;7:19.
60. Kademani D, Patel SG, Prasad ML, et al. Intraoral presentation of Rosai–Dorfman disease: a case report and review of the literature. Oral Surg Oral Med Oral Pathol Oral Radiol Endod 2002;93:699–701.
61. Foucar E, Rosai J, Dorfman RF, et al. Immunological abnormalities and their significance in sinus histiocytosis with massive lymphadenopathy. Am J Clin Pathol 1984;82:515.
62. Pulsoni A, Anghel G, Falcucci P, et al. Treatment of sinus histiocytosis with massive lymphadenopathy (Rosai–Dorfman disease): report of a case and literature review. Am J Hematol 2002:69:67–71.
63. Foucar E, Rosai J, and Dorfman RF. Sinus histiocytosis with massive lymphadenopathy: an analysis of 14 deaths occurring in a patient registry. Cancer 1984;54:1834–40.
64. Komp DM. The treatment of sinus histiocytosis with massive lymphadenopathy (Rosai–Dorfman disease). Semin Diagn Pathol 1990;7:83.
65. Fayemi AO and Toker C. Nodal angiomatosis. Arch Pathol Lab Med 1975;99:170.
66. Michal M and Koza V. Vascular transformation of lymph node sinuses—a diagnostic pitfall, histopathologic, and immunohistochemical study. Pathol Res Pract 1989;185:441.
67. Haferkamp O, Rosenau W, and Lennert K. Vascular transformation of lymph node sinuses due to venous congestion. Arch Pathol 1971;92:81.
68. Lennert K and Hansmann ML. Progressive transformation of germinal centers: clinical significance and lymphocytic predominance Hodgkin's disease—the Kiel experience. Am J Surg Pathol 1987;11:149.
69. Burns BF, Colby TV, and Dorfman RF. Differential diagnostic features of nodular L&H Hodgkin's disease, including progressive transformation of germinal centers. Am J Surg Pathol 1984;8:253.
70. Osborne BM and Butler JJ. Clinical implications of progressive transformation of germinal centers. Am J Surg Pathol 1984;8:725.
71. Ferry JA, Zukerberg LR and Harris NL. Florid progressive transformation of germinal centers. Am J Surg Pathol 1987;11:149.
72. Verma A, Stock W, Norohna S, et al. Progressive transformation of germinal centers: report of 2 cases and review of the literature. Acta Haematol 2002;108:33–8.

73. Poppema S, Kaiserling, E and Lennert K. Hodgkin's disease with lymphocytic predominance, nodular type (nodular paragranuloma) and progressively transformed germinal centers—a cytohistological study. Histopathology 1979;3/4:295–308.
74. Castleman B, Iverson L, and Menendez VP. Localized mediastinal lymph node hyperplasia resembling thymoma. Cancer 1956;9:822.
75. Keller AR, Hocholzer L, and Castleman B. Hyaline-vascular and plasma-cell types of giant lymph node hyperplasia of the mediastinum and other locations. Cancer 1972;29:670.
76. Chronowski GM, Ha CS, Wilder RB, et al. Treatment of unicentric and multicentric castleman's disease and the role of radiotherapy. Cancer 2001;92:670–6.
77. Bowne WB, Lewis JJ, Filippa DA, et al. The management of unicentric and multicentric Castleman's disease. Cancer 1999;85:706–17.
78. Gaba AR, Stein RS, Sweet DL, et al. Multicentric giant lymph node hyperplasia. Am J Clin Pathol 1978;69:86.
79. Peterson BA and Frizzera G. Multicentric Castleman's disease. Semin Oncol 1993;20:636.
80. Chang Y, Cesarman E, Pessin MS, et al. Identification of herpesvirus-like DNA sequences in AIDS-associated Kaposi's sarcoma. Science 1994;266:1865–9.
81. Gessain A, Briere J, Angelin-Duclos C, et al. Human herpes virus-8 (KSHV) and malignant lymphoproliferations in France: a molecular study of 250 cases including two AIDS-associated body cavity-based lymphomas. Leukemia 1997;11:266–72.
82. Soulier J, Grollet L, Oksenhendler E, et al. Kaposi's sarcoma-associated herpesvirus-like DNA Sequences in multicentric Castleman's disease. Blood 1995;86:1276–80.
83. Chadburn A, Cesarman E, Nador RG, et al. Kaposi's sarcoma-associated herpesvirus sequences in benign lymphoid proliferations not associated with human immunodeficiency virus. Cancer 1997;80:788–97.
84. Luppi M, Barozzi P, Maiorana A, et al. Human herpesvirus-8 DNA sequences in human immunodeficiency virus-negative angioimmunoblastic lymphadenopathy and benign lymphadenopathy with giant germinal center hyperplasia and increased vascularity. Blood 1996;87:3903–9.
85. Kikuta H, Itakura O, Taneichi K, et al. Tropism of human herpesvirus 8 for peripheral blood lymphocytes in patients with Castleman's disease: clinical findings and clinicopathologic correlations in 15 patients. J Clini Oncol 1985;3:1202–16.
86. Yoshizaki K, Matsuda T, Nishimoto H, et al. Pathogenic significance of interleukin-6 (IL-6/BSF-2) in Castleman's disease. Blood 1989;74:1360.
87. Leger-Ravet MB, Peuchmaur M, Devergne O, et al. Interleukin-6 gene expression in Castleman's disease. Blood 1991;78:2923.
88. Brandt SJ, Bodine DM, Dunbar CE, et al. Dysregulated interleukin-6 expression produces a syndrome resembling Castleman's disease in mice. J Clin Invest 1990;86:592.
89. Dupin N, Diss TL, Kellam P, et al. HHV-8 is associated with a plasmablastic variant of Castleman's disease that is linked to HHV-8 positive plasmablastic lymphoma. Blood 2000;95:1406–12.
90. Oksenhendler E, Duarte M, Soulier J, et al. Multicentric Castleman's disease in HIV infection: a clinical and pathological study of 20 patients. AIDS 1996;10:61–7.
91. Weisenburger DD, Nathwani BN, Winberg CD, et al. Multicentric angiofollicular lymph node hyperplasia: a clinicopathologic study of 16 cases. Hum Pathol 1985;16:162–72.
92. Frizzera G, Peterson BA, Bayrd ED, et al. A systemic lymphoproliferative disorder with morphologic features of Castleman's disease: clinical findings and clinicopathologic correlations in 15 patients. J Clin Oncol 1985;3:1202.
93. Oksenhendler E, Boulanger E, Galicier L, et al. High incidence of Kaposi sarcoma–associated herpesvirus-related non–Hodgkin lymphoma in patients with HIV infection and multicentric Castleman diease. Blood 2002;99:2331–6.
94. Beck J, Hsu S, Wijdens J, et al. Alleviation of systemic manifestations of Castleman's disease by monoclonal anti–interleukin-6 antibody. N Engl J Med 1994;330:602.
95. Hall PA, Donaghy M, Cotter FE, et al. An immunohistological and genotypic study of the plasma cell form of Castleman's disease. Histopathology 1989;14:333.
96. Herrada J, Cabanillas F, Rice L, et al. The clinical behavior of localized and multicentric Castleman disease. Ann Intern Med 1998;128:657–62.
97. Marcelin A-G, Aaron L, Mateus C, et al. Rituximab therapy for HIV-associated Castleman's disease. Blood 2003;102:2786–8.
98. Freter CE and Cossman J. Angioimmunoblastic lymphadenopathy with dysproteinemia. Semin Oncol 1993;20:627.
99. Lukes RJ and Tindle BH. Immunoblastic lymphadenopathy. A hyperimmune entity resembling Hodgkin's disease. N Engl J Med 1975;292:1.
100. Frizzera G, Moran EM, and Rappaport H. Angioimmunoblastic lymphadenopathy with dysproteinaemia. Lancet 1974;1:1070.
101. Sallah S and Gagnon GA. Angioimmunoblastic lymphadenopathy with dysproteinemia: emphasis on pathogenesis and treatment. Acta Haematol 1998;99:57–64.
102. Schlegelberger B, Zhang Y, Matthiesen K, et al. Detection of aberrant clones in nearly all cases of angioimmunoblastic lymphadenopathy with dysproteinemia-type T-cell lymphoma by combined interphase and metaphase cytogenetics. Blood 1994;84:2640.
103. Lipford EH, Smith HR, Pittaluga S, et al. Clonality of angioimmunoblastic lymphadenopathy and implications for its evolution to malignant lymphoma. J Clin Invest 1987;79:637.
104. Willenbrock K, Roers A, Seidl C, et al. Analysis of T cell subpopulations in T cell non-Hodgkin's lymphoma of angioimmunoblastic lymphadenopathy with dysproteinemia type by single target gene amplification of T cell receptor beta gene rearrangements. Am J Pathol 2001;158:1851–7.
105. Feller AC, Griesser H, Schilling CV, et al. Clonal gene rearrangement patterns correlate with immunophenotype and clinical parameters in patients with angioimmunoblastic lymphadenopathy. Am J Pathol 1988;133:549–56.
106. Liebow AA, Carrington CRB, and Friedman PJ. Lymphomatoid granulomatosis. Hum Pathol 1972;3:457.
107. Jaffe ES and Wilson WH. Lymphomatoid granulomatosis: pathogenesis, pathology and clinical implications. Cancer Surv 1997;30:233–48.
108. Myers JL, Kurtin PL, Katzenstein A-LA, et al. Lymphomatoid granulomatosis: evidence of immunophenotypic diversity and relationship to Epstein–Barr virus infection. Am J Surg Pathol 1995;19:1300–2.
109. Nicholson AG, Wotherspoon AC, Diss TC, et al. Lymphomatoid granulomatosis: evidence that some cases represent Epstein–Barr virus–associated B-cell lymphoma. Histopathology 1996;29:317–24.
110. Guinee JD, Jaffe ES, Kingma D, et al. Pulmonary lymphomatoid granulomatosis: evidence for a proliferation of Epstein–Barr virus infected B-lymphocytes with a prominent T-cell component and vasculitis. Am J Surg Pathol 1994;18:753–64.

111. Wilson WH, Kingma DW, Raffeld M, et al. Association of lymphomatoid granulomatosis with Epstein–Barr viral infection of B lymphocytes and response to interferon-α2b. Blood 1996;87:4531–7.
112. Koss MN, Hochholzer L, Langloss JM, et al. Lymphomatoid granulomatosis: a clinicopathologic study of 42 patients. Pathology 1986;18:283–8.
113. Fauci AS, Haynes BF, Costa J, et al. Lymphomatoid granulomatosis: prospective clinical and therapeutic experience over 10 years. N Engl J Med 1982;306:68–74.
114. Katzenstein A-LA, Carrington CRB, and Liebow AA. Lymphomatoid granulomatosis: a clinicopathologic study of 152 cases. Cancer 1979;43:360–73.
115. Myers JL. Lymphomatoid granulomatosis: past, present, future? Mayo Clin Proc 1990;65:274.
116. Davis TH, Morton CC, Miller-Cassman R, et al. Hodgkin's disease, lymphomatoid papulosis, and cutaneous T-cell lymphoma derived from a common T-cell clone. N Engl J Med 1992;326:1115–22.
117. Cabanillas F, Armitage J, Pugh WC, et al. Lymphomatoid papulosis: a T-cell dyscrasia with a propensity to transform into malignant lymphoma. Ann Intern Med 1995;122: 210–17.
118. Kadin ME. Common activated helper T-cell origin for lymphomatoid papulosis, mycosis fungoides, and some types of Hodgkin's disease. Lancet 1985;2:864–65.
119. Chott A, Vonderheid EC, Olbricht S, et al. The dominant T cell clone is present in multiple regressing skin lesions and associated T cell lymphomas of patients with lymphomatoid papulosis. J Invest Dermatol 1996;106:696–700.
120. Steinhoff M, Hummel M, Anagnostopoulos I, et al. Single-cell analysis of CD30+ cells in lymphomatoid papulosis demonstrates a common clonal T-cell origin. Blood 2002; 100:578–84.
121. Gniadecki R, Lukowsky A, Rossen K, et al. Bone marrow precursor of extranodal T-cell lymphoma. Blood 2003;102: 3797–9.

10

Diagnostic Radiology

Sarah J. Vinnicombe, B.Sc., M.R.C.P., F.R.C.R.
Rodney H. Reznek, M.B., Ch.B., F.R.C.P., F.R.C.R.

The extraordinary evolution of cross-sectional imaging in the last 20 years has had profound effects on clinical practice in oncology. During this time there have been major changes in the routine imaging of patients with Hodgkin's disease (HD) and non-Hodgkin's lymphoma (NHL). Cross-sectional imaging has become crucial in prognostication and in the appropriate choice of treatment at the time of staging; in the assessment of response to treatment during and at the end of therapy; and in screening for relapse. It is frequently indicated during the course of treatment in order to resolve a clinical problem such as febrile neutropenia or chest consolidation. Finally, it is of critical importance in clinical trials, not only in Phase II studies but also in Phase III studies. In attempting to address these issues, the oncologist is faced with a variety of accurate, reproducible noninvasive cross-sectional technologies including computed tomography (CT), magnetic resonance imaging (MRI), and ultrasound (U/S). Furthermore, in the past decade the increased availability of positron emission tomography (PET) has resulted in a resurgence of interest in the role of functional imaging at every stage in the management of the patient with lymphoma, and a large body of literature focusing on the place of ^{18}fluorodeoxyglucose (FDG)-PET has appeared. This will be discussed elsewhere in Chapter 11.

EVALUATION AND CHOICE OF IMAGING TECHNIQUE

Given the range of techniques available, it can be difficult to choose the most appropriate one and use it in a rational way. In order to do so, the oncologist must be aware that the requirements for an ideal test will vary, depending on the precise clinical question being asked; those for a staging test may be very different from those for evaluation of response to treatment. For a baseline study, consideration should be given as to whether the intention is merely to detect all sites of disease (which may be all that is required for staging), or to define the precise local extent of disease, which may in turn affect therapy through intensification of treatment in the presence of bulk disease, or planning of radiotherapy portals. Whereas most clinicians recognize the importance of a baseline study that evaluates all anatomical areas prior to commencement of treatment, it may only be necessary to obtain a limited interim scan during treatment. Choice of a particular imaging modality will depend not only on the indication for imaging, but also on factors such as the technical performance of the test, its diagnostic accuracy in a given clinical situation, and importantly, on local factors including availability of equipment, local expertise, and funding.

Strategies have been proposed for assessment of the outcome of the use of imaging technologies.[1] The most widely used one, initially developed by Fineberg et al.,[2] was modified by the Institute of Medicine in the United States, resulting in a five-level evaluative hierarchical framework (Fig. 10–1). This hierarchy presupposes that a good performance at any given level is only possible after satisfactory performance has been attained at the preceding levels. Assuming that local factors are not an issue, then the key question is the overall diagnostic accuracy of a test in a particular situation. This comprises the efficacy (technical and diagnostic performance) and effectiveness (diagnostic and therapeutic impact), as well as efficiency, which relates more to economic considerations. The most commonly used measure of the latter is the cost-effectiveness, of which an example might be the cost of a PET scan compared with the effect of incorrectly diagnosing the nature of a residual mass.

The *technical performance* of a test is a measure of its reproducibility and anatomical accuracy, neither of which are in question with modern cross-sectional modalities. The technological advances in CT, U/S, and MRI in the last decade are such that there can be no comparison between the diagnostic accuracy of these machines and first- or second-generation machines. Of more relevance is the *diagnostic performance* of the test, that is, whether the test correctly identifies the presence or absence of disease. The sensitivity and specificity of a test, the so-called intrinsic operating characteristics, are independent of disease prevalence, unlike the positive and negative predictive values, which are dependent on the population to which the test is being applied. This needs to be borne in mind whenever a test is being evaluated. Most of the literature on imaging in lymphoma relates to the diagnostic performance, which will clearly be a major consideration in initial staging of the patient with lymphoma (see next section). Sensitivity and specificity are affected by sampling error and bias, but more importantly, they are altered by changing the threshold for calling a test positive, probably positive, probably negative, or negative: receiver–operator characteristic curve (ROC) analysis. This has been comprehensively reviewed by Goldin et al.[3] and Begg et al.[4] An accurate test is one in which a high sensitivity is combined with a low false-positive rate (high specificity). In deciding the criterion for test positivity, an arbitrary position is adopted that is considered to be the best compromise between sensitivity and specificity. The effects of ROC curve analysis can be

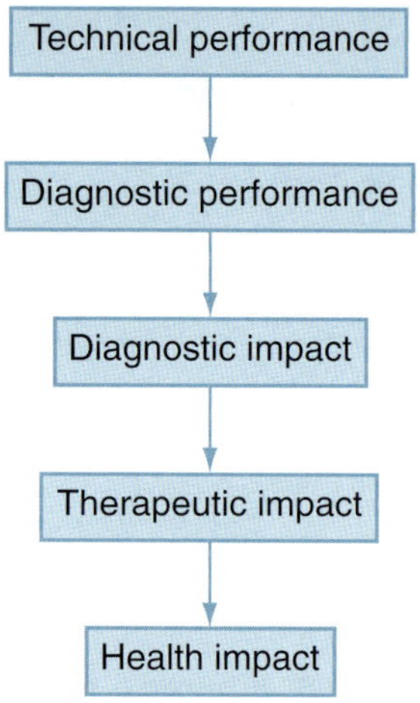

Figure 10–1. An evaluative framework for the use of imaging in lymphoma.

profound—for example, alteration of the size criterion for calling a lymph node normal or enlarged can affect staging and categorization of response to treatment. ROC curve analysis also permits comparison of different imaging tests, but it should of course be borne in mind that with the virtual demise of the staging laparotomy in recent years, true pathologic gold standards against which to judge diagnostic accuracy are generally lacking. It follows from this that all clinicians managing patients with lymphoma should understand the principles of ROC analysis in order to appreciate the implications of a positive or negative imaging result.

The *diagnostic impact* of a test is reflected by the influence of the test on the diagnostic confidence of the clinician, which in turn, will lead to the test displacing older established methods as the gold standard, such as the replacement of lymphangiography (LAG) by CT in staging of lymphoma, the replacement of myelography with craniospinal MRI in the evaluation of the neuraxis, and the increasing use of FDG-PET scanning in the evaluation of the residual mass. However, even when a new test has been shown to have greater diagnostic impact, this is only relevant if it will alter patient management: the *therapeutic impact*. For example, in patients with NHL, the demonstration of splenic or bone marrow infiltration may not be important in terms of therapeutic choices, since most patients will have other evidence of Stage III or IV disease requiring systemic treatment. Rapid acceptance of certain imaging technologies means that the therapeutic impact can be difficult to assess; for example, MRI became widely used before randomized controlled clinical trials had been carried out. In addition, the therapeutic impact can change as an imaging technology develops. This was demonstrated by Fineberg et al.,[5] who showed that CT had a diagnostic impact in 58% of lymphoma patients and a therapeutic impact in 15%, more often in NHL than HD, and that the overall impact increased with time as newer scanners were introduced. The effect of novel imaging modalities on patient outcome, or health impact, is even more difficult to assess because of clustering of tests, parallel diagnostic procedures, and variable response to the test results.

INITIAL STAGING IN MALIGNANT LYMPHOMA

The objective of baseline staging is to define the local extent of overt disease whilst at the same time identifying occult disease elsewhere. The latter is facilitated by knowledge of the variable patterns of spread in the malignant lymphomas and the different patterns of disease seen in HD and NHL, which will affect the likelihood that particular anatomical sites will be affected. Sites often involved should be screened if the diagnostic test chosen is sufficiently accurate. Sites that are rarely involved should be screened only if there is suggestive symptomatology or as dictated by the specific histologic subtype of NHL. If a site is frequently affected but the screening test is insensitive, the vigor of the search will depend on the effect a positive result will have on patient management.

Imaging Modalities and Staging

Prior to the development of modern generation CT scanners, patients with lymphoma were subjected to a battery of imaging tests, virtually none of which, other than chest radiography, are now obtained routinely. The ideal staging test should obviously be a whole-body technique that is sufficiently sensitive and specific, reliable, free of side effects and widely available within a suitable timeframe. CT fulfills most of these criteria, reliably demonstrating nodal enlargement and most extranodal sites of disease. It consistently depicts the full extent of disease and facilitates choice of a suitable lesion for percutaneous biopsy if indicated. Through the demonstration of bulky disease and extranodal involvement, it provides important prognostic information in patients with HD and NHL. It will also highlight potential problems that could influence delivery of treatment, such as central venous occlusion or renal tract obstruction by lymphomatous masses. Finally, it is generally sufficiently accurate to allow radiotherapy planning. For these reasons it has, until very recently, been the single modality of choice for the staging and follow-up of patients with lymphoma. In HD, the choice of treatment will be directly affected by the disease stage, distribution and the presence of bulk disease, as recognized in the Cotswold modification of the Ann Arbor staging classification (Table 10–1). On the other hand, in NHL, treatment choices will depend far more on the specific histologic type of NHL, but nonetheless, the clinical stage (both the extent and distribution of disease) has profound effects on the prognosis; hence the importance of accurate staging in both conditions. In instances of low-grade NHL, CT will identify the 10% to 15% of patients with limited disease who are suitable for treatment with radiotherapy.

In specific situations, other cross-sectional modalities may be the technique of choice, and these will be highlighted.

Nodal Disease

Although HD and NHL are both diseases of the lymph nodes, there are recognizable differences between the imaging findings in the two groups, particularly at presentation. Generally, though both conditions result in nodal enlargement, this is more pronounced in NHL than in HD,

Table 10–1. Staging of Lymphoma (Cotswold Classification)[120]

Stage	Area of Involvement
I	One lymph node region or extralymphatic site
II	Two or more lymph node regions on the same side of the diaphragm
III	Involvement of lymph node region or structures on both sides of diaphragm, subdivided as follows:
III (1[a])	With involvement of spleen and/or splenic hilar, coeliac, and portal nodes
III (2[a])	With para-aortic, iliac, or mesenteric nodes
IV	Extranodal sites beyond those designated E
	Additional Qualifiers
A	No symptoms
B	Fever, sweats, weight loss (to 10% of body weight)
E	Involvement of single extranodal site, contiguous in proximity to a known nodal site
X[a]	Bulky disease Mass >1/3 thoracic diameter at T5 Mass >10 cm maximum dimension
CE[a]	Clinical stage
PS[a]	Pathological stage: PS at a given site denoted by a subscript (i.e., M = marrow, H = liver, L = lung, O = bone, P = pleural, D = skin)

[a]Modifications from Ann Arbor system.

but both can produce large conglomerate nodal masses, or conversely, minimal nodal enlargement, particularly in nodular sclerosing HD. A feature of malignant lymphoma is that tissue planes tend to be preserved, resulting in discrete masses, which displace adjacent structures rather than invade them, but extranodal extension can occur, particularly with aggressive high-grade NHL.

A major limitation of CT scanning in lymphoma is that recognition of nodal disease rests solely on size criteria, the single most helpful measurement being the short axis diameter. With the evolution of CT scanner technology, the recognized upper limits of normal for nodal size have diminished; currently accepted values are shown in Table 10–2. Detection of disease in normal-sized lymph nodes remains impossible, even though clustering of multiple small nodes in sites such as the anterior mediastinum and mesentery is highly suggestive. By the same token, it is generally not possible to distinguish between those lymph nodes that are enlarged as a consequence of reactive hyperplasia and those involved by lymphoma, although preservation of a central fatty hilum, recognizable through its low CT attenuation, is helpful in the former. The use of intravenous contrast medium adds little diagnostic information, most lymph nodes enhancing uniformly and moderately.[6] It does, however, facilitate recognition of nodal enlargement in anatomically complex areas such as the neck and the pelvis, where the presence of multiple vascular structures can be confusing. Though ultrasound will demonstrate nodal enlargement in the neck and upper abdomen, the thorax is not amenable to ultrasound interrogation and often the retroperitoneum cannot be visualized because of overlying bowel gas.[7–10] Lymphomatous involvement typically results in uniformly hypoechoic enlarged lymph nodes with no specific features, though the pattern of vascular perfusion as assessed with power Doppler may suggest the diagnosis.[11] Ultrasound is insufficiently reliable for routine staging but has a problem-solving role in confirming the nodal nature of a palpable mass as well as resolving diagnostic issues affecting the major viscera.[12,13] MRI is as accurate as CT in the depiction of lymph node enlargement, but it has no real advantages and tends to be used as an adjunctive modality in identifying nodal disease and assessing response to treatment.[14–16] As with CT, nodal involvement on MRI can only be predicted on the basis of size, rather than signal characteristics.[17] Currently, MR-specific lymphographic agents in the form of ultra-small superparamagnetic iron oxide particles (USPIO) do not have a role in the identification of small lymphomatous deposits within normal-sized lymph nodes.[18,19]

As indicated above, the major criterion for recognition of nodal involvement by lymphoma with the three main cross-sectional techniques is that of size, which inevitably means that there will be false-positive and -negative examinations. However, this problem does not arise with functional radioisotope studies. With the development of FDG-PET scanning there has been a resurgence of interest in the use of functional imaging as a staging tool, since it obviates some of the problems previously associated with gallium (Ga(67)) scintigraphy. It is clear that FDG-PET is at least as sensitive as CT at nodal staging, with a trend to greater sensitivity on a lesion-by-lesion analysis.[20] It also

Table 10–2. Accepted Upper Limits of Normal for Lymph Node Size (SAD) by Site

Site	Size (SAD) (mm)	Source
Face	Not visible	Tart et al., 1993[140]
Neck	10	Van den Brekel et al., 1990[141]
Mediastinum	10	Glazer et al., 1985[142]
Retrocrural	6	Callen et al., 1977[143]
Porta hepatis	8	Dorfman et al., 1991[144]
Retroperitoneum	10	Dorfman et al., 1991[144]
Pelvis	8	Vinnicombe et al., 1995[145]

SAD, short axis diameter.

appears to have greater sensitivity than Ga^{67} for small masses, masses below the diaphragm, and low-grade NHL.[21,22] This is discussed in greater detail in Chapter 11.

Neck

In the neck, CT often demonstrates far more extensive disease than is evident clinically. It can identify nodes that are impalpable, and it is accurate in the assessment of response to treatment, particularly after radiotherapy, where the resultant induration renders clinical assessment difficult. The neck is one area where the administration of intravenous contrast greatly facilitates interpretation of the study, as it enables differentiation of lymph nodes from adjacent vascular structures. Between 60% and 80% of patients with HD present with a group of enlarged cervical nodes, the internal jugular chain typically being involved first. Nodes greater than 1 cm in short axis diameter are considered enlarged. Spread to adjacent nodal groups is contiguous, and patients with bulky supraclavicular or bilateral cervical adenopathy are at greater risk of infradiaphragmatic disease. In NHL, cervical lymph nodes are less commonly involved, but are often larger. Extranodal involvement of Waldeyer's ring is a common finding. The pattern of nodal involvement is less predictable because of hematogenous spread, and between 40% and 60% of patients with NHL who present with enlarged cervical lymph nodes will have disseminated disease. MRI can be helpful in the assessment of supraclavicular fossa masses, where artifacts from the shoulder can degrade CT images.[15]

Thorax

All nodal groups in the thorax may be involved with HD and NHL, but the frequency and distribution differ in the two conditions. Again, nodes with a short axis diameter greater than 1 cm are considered enlarged. However, the presence of multiple small nodes within the anterior mediastinum should be regarded with suspicion. Thoracic nodal involvement is seen much more commonly at presentation with HD than NHL (60% to 80% vs. 20% to 40%).[23,24] All the mediastinal sites are more frequently involved by HD than NHL except the paracardiac and posterior mediastinal nodes. However, at presentation, patients with HD who have thoracic disease almost always have disease affecting the prevascular and paratracheal stations (84%), and in this situation, other sites (hilar, subcarinal) may be involved as well (Fig. 10–2). Conversely, it is extremely rare for other intrathoracic nodal sites to be involved by HD in the absence of nodal disease in prevascular and paratracheal stations. Nearly all patients with nodular sclerosing HD have anterior mediastinal disease. Though posterior mediastinal disease is rare, occurring in 5% or less, when it is seen, contiguous retrocrural disease should be sought. Nodal enlargement in two or more sites is seen in the majority of patients with HD, whereas in NHL, only one group is involved in nearly 50% of cases. In NHL it is not uncommon to find nodal disease in the absence of disease in the superior mediastinum, the latter being involved in only 34% of cases.[25] This is particularly true when there is bulky intra-abdominal disease, such patients often demonstrating enlargement of low paravertebral and paracardiac nodal groups.

Although even bulky nodal masses tend to displace adjacent structures rather than invade them, vascular and airway compromise can occur, particularly with mediastinal diffuse large B cell lymphoma (DLBCL) and nodular sclerosing HD. Calcification within nodal masses is rare before therapy, being more common in aggressive subtypes of NHL,[26] but is not infrequently seen after therapy. Similarly, cystic degeneration can be seen before therapy in large masses and such cysts can persist after treatment, but in HD at least they do not have any prognostic implications[27] (Fig. 10–3).

Large anterior mediastinal masses usually represent *thymic disease* as well as nodal masses, and occasionally the

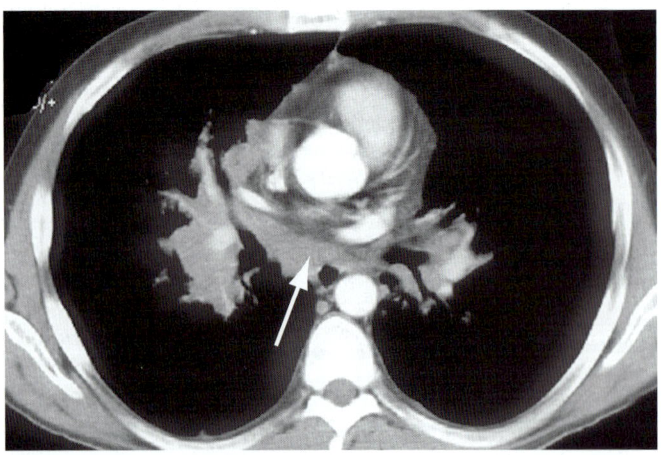

Figure 10–2. Axial contrast-enhanced CT of the thorax, demonstrating subcarinal (*arrowed*) and hilar nodal enlargement in a patient with HD.

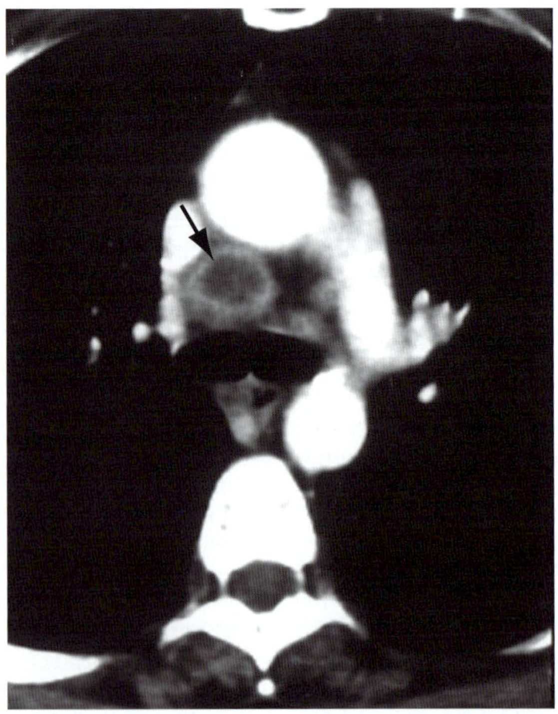

Figure 10–3. Axial contrast-enhanced CT of the thorax in a patient with NS HD. Note cystic change within the precarinal lymph node (*arrowed*).

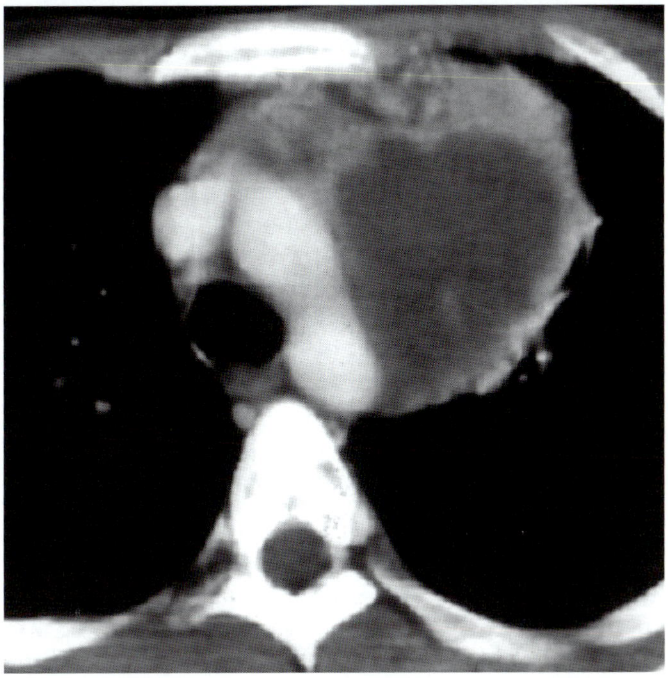

Figure 10–4. Axial contrast-enhanced CT of the thorax demonstrating a large thymic mass with cystic change in a patient with HD.

former can only be diagnosed after treatment, when the thymus resumes its normal configuration.[28,29] Thymic involvement is seen in 30% to 50% of patients with newly diagnosed HD, and is also seen with mediastinal LBCL. As with large nodal masses, cystic change can be recognized with CT and more often with MRI, especially in mediastinal LBCL[30,31] (Fig. 10–4). There is some evidence that high-grade NHL has a more heterogeneous pattern of enhancement after administration of intravenous contrast material than low-grade tumors of comparable size, but the clinical implications of this observation are unclear.[32] Calcification is not uncommon after therapy and is more readily recognized with CT than MRI. A particular problem after chemotherapy is rebound thymic hyperplasia, which is not always distinguishable from relapse even with functional imaging, both Ga-67 and FDG-PET showing increased uptake in thymic hyperplasia.

CT frequently demonstrates impalpable axillary nodal enlargement in HD and NHL. The presence of a fatty hilum within such nodes at CT suggests a diagnosis of reactive hyperplasia rather than malignant involvement. CT will also demonstrate subpectoral nodal enlargement, which is rarely evident clinically. Care should be taken to closely inspect the internal mammary and paracardiac nodal groups at CT, since these often lie outside conventional radiotherapy fields and are common sites for relapse (Fig. 10–5).

It has been repeatedly shown that CT will detect thoracic abnormalities, mostly nodal enlargement, in up to as many as 30% of patients with a normal chest radiograph at presentation.[24,33,34] Patients with HD shown by CT to have even moderate amounts of unsuspected intrathoracic disease have a poorer prognosis.[35] Even in patients who clearly have mediastinal disease on the chest radiograph, CT provides incremental information on the extent of disease and involvement of adjacent structures such as the pericardium and lung parenchyma (see next section). CT has been shown to change the clinical stage in around 15% of patients with HD and NHL, and management may be altered in as many as 25% because of upstaging or demonstration of greater disease extent. This is particularly so where radiotherapy is planned.[24,33,34,36–38] Thus, the therapeutic impact is more pronounced in patients with HD rather than NHL.[24,25] Nonetheless, even in patients with NHL, CT of the chest is routinely carried out for all the reasons indicated in the preceding discussion.

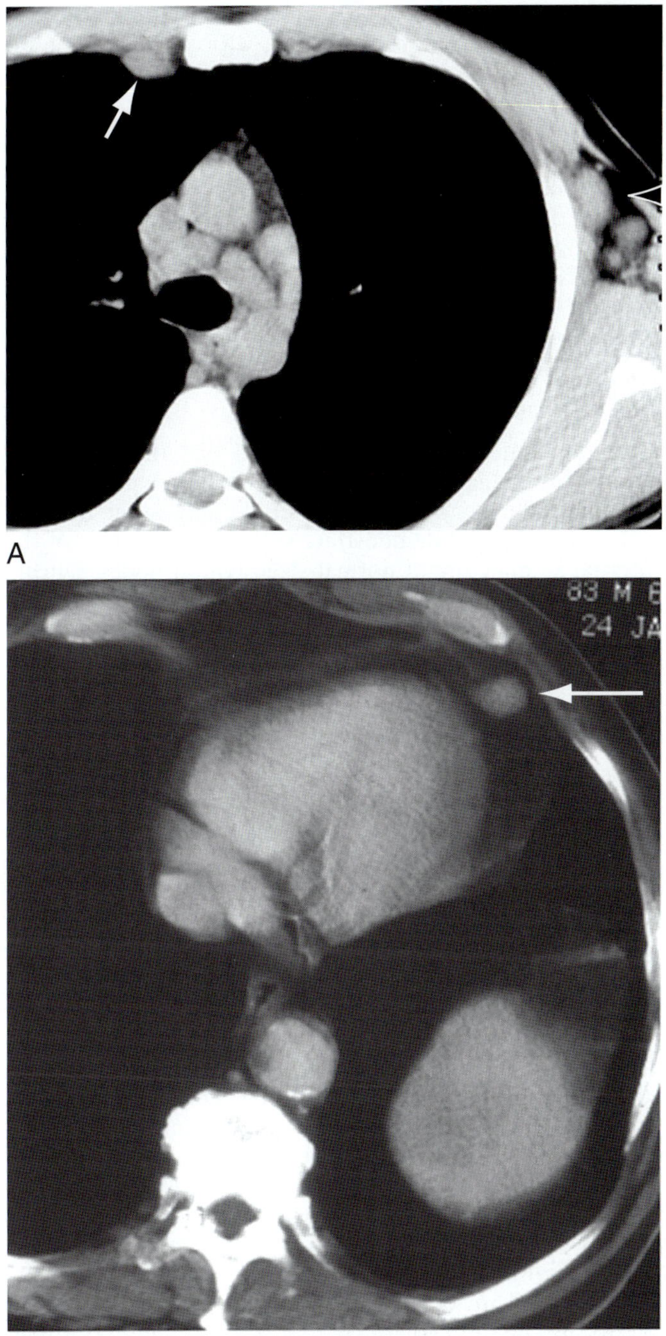

Figure 10–5. Axial CT of the thorax. **A:** At level of aortic arch showing enlarged precarinal, aortopulmonary, internal mammary (*arrow*) and axillary lymph nodes (*arrowhead*). **B:** At left ventricle, showing an enlarged paracardiac lymph node (*arrow*) in a patient with HD.

Although routine MRI of the chest is generally unnecessary, it has been demonstrated that MRI can provide additional information by depicting nodal enlargement in sites that are poorly seen with CT, for example, the low supraclavicular fossa, the subcarinal region, and the aortopulmonary window. In addition, it is superior to CT in the demonstration of disease extension to the chest wall. Finally, there is experimental evidence that MR of large mediastinal masses can provide prognostic information, in as much as heterogeneous high signal on T2-weighted scans tends to be associated with high-grade tumors and a poorer prognosis.[39,40]

Abdomen and Pelvis

Prior to the development of CT, LAG was the method of choice for evaluation of the retroperitoneal lymph nodes, its major advantage being that, unlike any other imaging technique, it could demonstrate subtle disturbances of the internal architecture of normal-sized lymph nodes. During the 1980s, several studies showed that LAG was equal to or slightly superior to CT for detecting nodal lymphoma.[41–49] However, given the very limited spatial, contrast, and temporal resolution of first- and second-generation CT scanners, this is not surprising. In these studies, though CT tended to show the overall extent of disease better, with occasional depiction of "off-axis" lymph nodes, LAG was more likely to change disease stage. However, LAG does have several disadvantages, chiefly its inability to demonstrate lymph nodes above the level of the second lumbar vertebra and outside the retroperitoneum, as well as the true extent of a nodal mass once it has broken through the lymph node capsule. Its advantages have become limited due to the development of newer generation CT scanners, which permit the detection of smaller degrees of lymphadenopathy. Newer generation multidetector scanners are quite capable of detecting lymph nodes of 5 mm or less in diameter, even in locations like the celiac axis and porta hepatis. Since scan times are so fast, movement artifact has become less of a problem; so, for example, small prominent mesenteric lymph nodes are readily seen. Another important factor in the decline of LAG in HD is the increasing efficacy of chemotherapy, which is now able to salvage patients with apparent early stage supradiaphragmatic disease, but who actually harbor microscopic foci of tumor in the infradiaphragmatic lymph nodes. Thus, although LAG remains the only imaging method that visualizes nodal architecture, the complementary yield over CT in HD is negligible. It is estimated that in only 5% of cases of HD will LAG show true positive abnormalities in lymph nodes smaller than 1 cm (i.e., where abdominal CT is unequivocally negative).[49] The large number of false-positive LAG studies as a result of reactive hyperplasia accounts for its low positive predictive value in this situation.[49,50] Stomper et al. demonstrated that, for HD, true positive LAG and gallium scans were seen only when lymph nodes were larger than 10 mm and 20 mm, respectively, that is, when CT would have identified them as abnormal.[49] Inevitably too, there will be some false-negative studies where microscopic tumor deposits are not recognizable.

There are only a small amount of data on the comparative accuracy of LAG and CT as judged against staging laparotomy in patients with NHL.[48] Pond et al. demonstrated that although bone marrow biopsy influenced clinical stage more often than CT or LAG, the latter were much more likely to result in a change of management.[48] Given the frequency with which NHL will affect the mesenteric nodes (which are not opacified by LAG), the greater likelihood of bulky adenopathy, and the higher frequency of extranodal visceral disease, it is not surprising that CT has a very high diagnostic impact. In the past decade, there has been a dramatic decline in the number of LAGs performed for lymphoma in most oncology centers,[51] and this has resulted in a general lack of expertise both in carrying out the procedure and in interpretation of the results. Although some specialized centers continue to undertake LAG in HD, it is generally only recommended when immediate detection of tumor in a normal sized retroperitoneal node is considered essential for patient management and when local expertise is available.[50]

At presentation, the retroperitoneal lymph nodes will be involved in about 35% of patients with HD and up to 55% of patients with NHL.[52,53] Mesenteric lymph nodes will be affected in more than 50% of those with NHL but less than 5% of those with HD. Nodes around the porta hepatis and splenic hilum are also involved in up to 33% of patients with HD, and even more in NHL (Fig. 10–6). In HD, as in the chest, spread is in contiguity from one nodal group to the next via directly connected lymphatic pathways, so that the presence of retrocrural disease should prompt close evaluation of the celiac axis. Involved lymph nodes are often only minimally enlarged, and around the celiac axis, multiple normal-sized nodes may be seen.[49,54] By contrast, in NHL, nodal involvement is frequently noncontiguous, bulky, and commonly associated with extranodal disease. Regional nodal involvement is frequently seen in patients with primary extranodal lymphoma involving an abdominal viscus. Though mesenteric nodal enlargement can be marked, multiple prominent but normal sized nodes should be regarded with suspicion, as should soft tissue nodularity and streakiness within the mesentery. In the pelvis, all nodal groups may be involved in HD and NHL. As in the supradiaphragmatic regions, enhancement after intra-

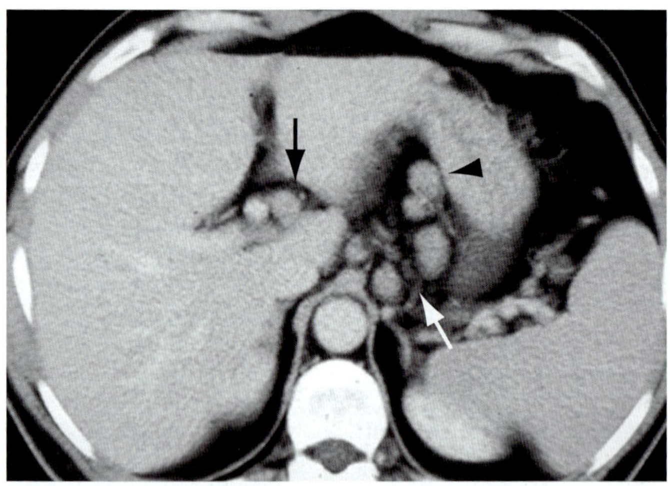

Figure 10–6. Axial contrast-enhanced CT of the abdomen in a patient with HD demonstrating nodal enlargement in the celiac axis (*white arrow*), gastrohepatic ligament (*arrowhead*), and porta hepatis (*black arrow*).

venous contrast is generally mild to moderate, though rim enhancement is occasionally seen. Generally, central necrosis, peripheral, or multilocular enhancement in nodal masses favor infection rather than lymphomatous infiltration.[55] The addition of intravenous contrast medium facilitates recognition of nodal enlargement in patients with a paucity of intra-abdominal fat and helps differentiate lymph nodes from vascular tributaries.

Although MRI can demonstrate nodal enlargement as readily as CT, it does not have a role in routine staging except in a problem-solving capacity, especially in the pelvis, where internal iliac venous tributaries can be difficult to differentiate from lymph nodes. In patients with massive pelvic disease, it can help define the precise extent of tumor.[14,56]

Extranodal Disease

Lymphoma occurs in extranodal sites at the time of presentation in up to 40% of cases, the majority of which are NHL. Extranodal involvement is seen more often in childhood lymphomas and in those associated with immunodeficiency states. Intra-abdominal sites are most commonly affected, though secondary spread of lymph node disease into adjacent structures (the "E" lesion) can occur anywhere and is seen with HD and NHL. For aggressive lymphomas, the presence of extranodal disease is an adverse prognostic factor, as recognized in the International Prognostic Index (IPI)[57] (Table 10–3). The increasing incidence of NHL has been more marked for extranodal sites, especially in the gastrointestinal tract, eye, and central nervous system. It is important therefore to be aware of the protean manifestations of extranodal lymphoma that can be seen at CT, many of which mimic other disease entities. As with nodal disease, CT generally performs well in the depiction of extranodal disease, though there are certain areas where ultrasound and MRI are more accurate. There is increasing evidence for the utility of whole-body FDG-PET scanning compared with CT, chiefly because of its ability to detect bone marrow involvement.[58] However, it has yet to replace CT as a primary staging modality (see Chapter 11).

Thorax

On chest radiography, *parenchymal lung involvement* is thrice as common in HD (12%) as NHL (4%). In HD, secondary involvement of the lung parenchyma is usually by direct invasion from adjacent nodal masses; hence it is usually perihilar or juxta-mediastinal. This "E" lesion, often seen at CT, does not affect stage and rarely alters management (Fig. 10–7). By contrast, in NHL, though this pattern occurs with mediastinal LBCL, pulmonary or pleural lesions can be seen without any mediastinal or hilar nodal enlargement in up to 50% of cases. This is extremely unusual in HD unless there has been prior mediastinal irradiation, in which instance relapse may occur in the lungs alone.[59] Parenchymal involvement is commoner in the presence of widespread extrathoracic disease, especially in AIDS-related lymphoma (ARL).[60]

The radiographic changes are varied and complex. As indicated above, involvement is often paramediastinal. The most common pattern is one or more discrete nodules, usually less well defined than other metastases, which may cavitate (Fig. 10–7). Areas of consolidation with air bronchograms, often subpleural, are also commonly seen.[23,61,62] Spread along the peribronchial lymphatics results in peribronchial nodulation and linear opacity. Occasionally a lymphangitic picture is seen, but this is sufficiently rare in HD to necessitate exclusion of other causes in the first instance. Most primary pulmonary lymphomas are low-grade lymphomas derived from bronchus-associated lymphoid tissue (BALT)[63] (Fig. 10–8). Solitary or multiple lung nodules occur in more than 50%, or there may be single or

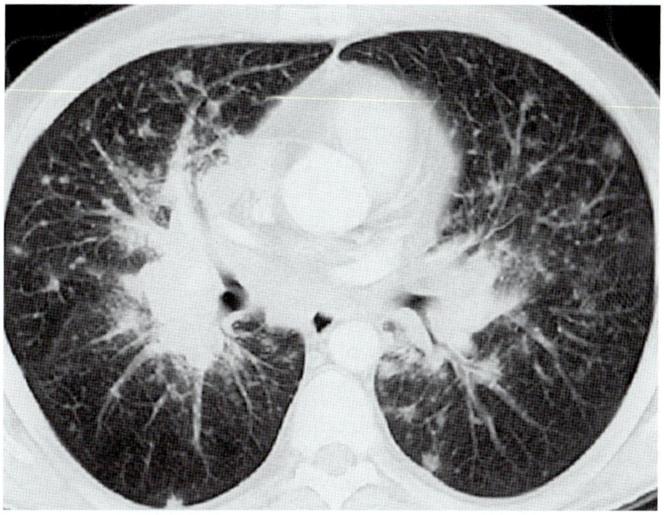

Figure 10–7. Lung windows of the same patient as in Figure 9–2 showing juxtamediastinal involvement of the lung parenchyma (the "E" lesion) with, in addition, widespread noncontiguous nodulation indicating Stage IV disease.

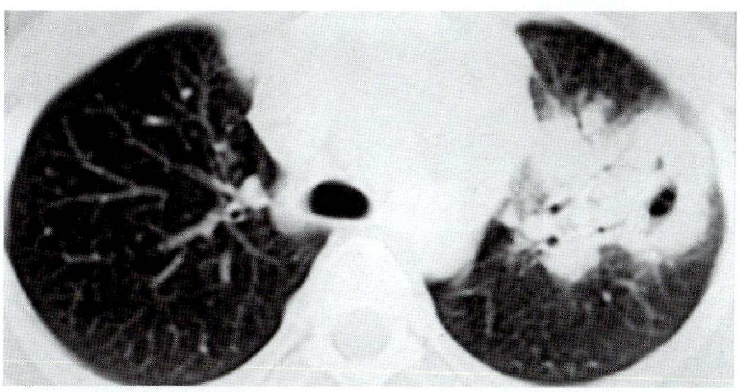

Figure 10–8. Axial CT on lung settings in a patient with primary pulmonary NHL of MALT type. There is a poorly defined mass-like area of consolidation in the left upper lobe with air bronchograms and cavitation.

Table 10–3. Factors Associated with an Adverse Prognosis in Aggressive Lymphoma
Age >60 years
Elevated serum lactate dehydrogenase (LDH)
Eastern Cooperative Oncology Group (ECOG) status >1 (nonambulatory)
Advanced stage (III or IV)
Presence of >1 extranodal site of disease

multiple areas of consolidation with ill-defined alveolar opacities.[64,65] Lesions are often bilateral and indolent, and associated effusions occur in up to 20%. High-grade NHL accounts for the remaining 15% to 20% of primary lung lymphomas and these patients are often symptomatic, with rapidly progressive radiographic abnormalities, which can cause diagnostic confusion. The diverse appearances can pose a diagnostic problem, as can the fact that many patients are at risk for other causes of lung disease such as:

- Opportunistic infection
- Radiation-induced pneumonitis
- Drug-related pulmonary fibrosis

In one study of patients with HIV, the presence of cavitation, nodule size under 1 cm, and a centrilobular distribution favored infection,[66] but though high-resolution CT has a definite role,[67] percutaneous or transbronchial biopsy will often be necessary to establish the diagnosis.

Pleura and Pericardium

Although large pleural effusions are readily recognized on chest radiographs, CT will demonstrate very small pleural and pericardial effusions. The former can be seen on presentation chest radiographs in up to 10% of patients and in as many as 50% of chest CT scans, nearly always with accompanying mediastinal nodal disease. Many such effusions are believed to be secondary to central lymphatic or vascular obstruction, since they resolve after mediastinal irradiation. Solid pleural masses or nodules are more commonly seen in relapsed disease, usually with an associated effusion.[68] Pericardial effusions are seen in up to 6% of patients with HD at presentation and are presumptive evidence of direct involvement from adjacent nodal or thymic masses. The cause of small effusions commonly seen in patients undergoing therapy for HD and NHL is unclear. Direct cardiac involvement is relatively unusual and rarely intracardiac masses occur, usually with high-grade T-cell lymphomas or occasionally DLBCL in the setting of ARL or post-transplant lymphoproliferative disorder (PTLD) (Fig. 10–9). MRI is the method of choice for defining cardiac involvement where necessary.[69]

Chest Wall

Bulky intrathoracic nodal masses commonly abut the chest wall, but direct invasion can also occur, usually from the anterior mediastinum in patients with HD. This is one area where MRI offers distinct advantages over CT, because of the intrinsic differences in signal intensity of the chest wall musculature and lymphomatous tissue on T2-weighted sequences. This can directly affect planning of radiotherapy portals.[70,71]

Primary *breast* lymphoma is rare, accounting for 1% of all breast tumors. Fairly well-defined unilateral masses are seen, though synchronous bilateral masses are well recognized, particularly in secondary disease, where there is usually accompanying axillary nodal involvement.[72] A diffuse inflammatory pattern can also occur, especially during pregnancy and lactation and in Burkitt's lymphoma (BL).

Abdomen and Pelvis

One of the major weaknesses of CT as a staging tool is its relatively poor diagnostic performance in the diagnosis of *splenic* disease, particularly where there is diffuse splenic infiltration. Laparotomy data have shown that the spleen is involved in up to 35% of patients with HD and up to 40% of patients with NHL.[73,74] In 10% of patients with HD clinically confined to supradiaphragmatic sites, it is the sole abdominal focus of disease. The sensitivity of any cross-sectional imaging modality for the detection of splenic HD remains low, largely because deposits usually measure well under 1 cm. Splenomegaly does not necessarily imply infiltration and conversely, disease can be found in normal sized spleens. Nodules over 1 cm in size can be reliably detected with any imaging modality (Fig. 10–10). Earlier studies with pathologic correlation cited sensitivities for CT as low as 11% to 50%, but these were on first and second-generation scanners, either without any intravenous contrast medium or with contrast administered slowly by infusion. Anecdotally, detection of small nodules has improved with the advent of multidetector-CT and the routine use of

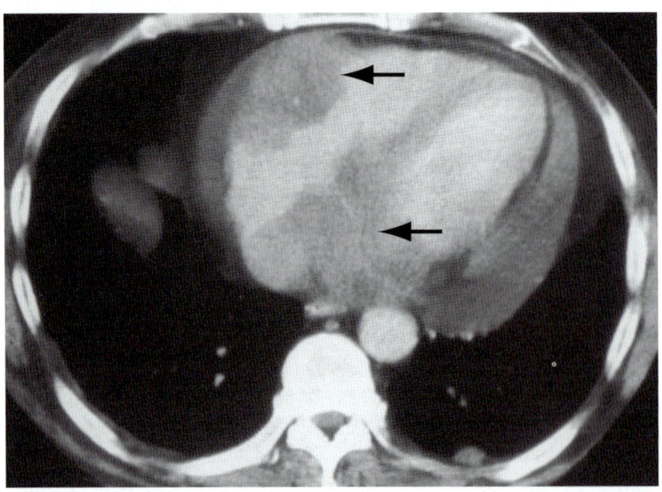

Figure 10–9. Axial contrast-enhanced CT of the thorax in a patient with ARL showing a large pericardial effusion and two intracardiac masses (*arrowed*).

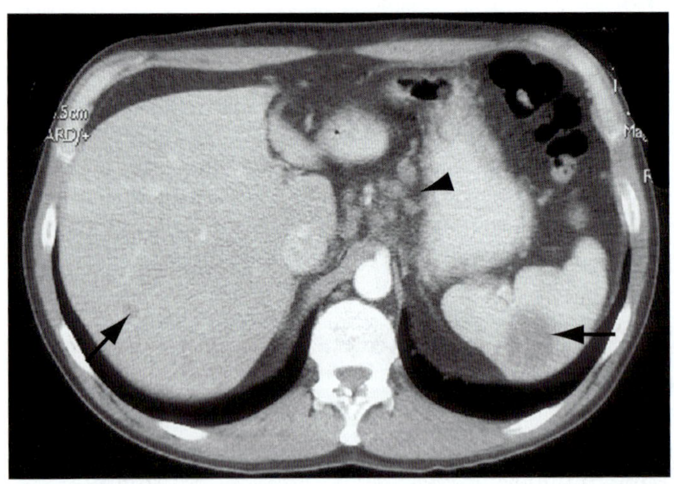

Figure 10–10. Axial contrast-enhanced CT of a patient with HD showing a focal splenic lesion (*right arrow*) and multiple prominent gastrohepatic lymph nodes (*arrowhead*) in addition to a tiny hepatic lesion (*left arrow*).

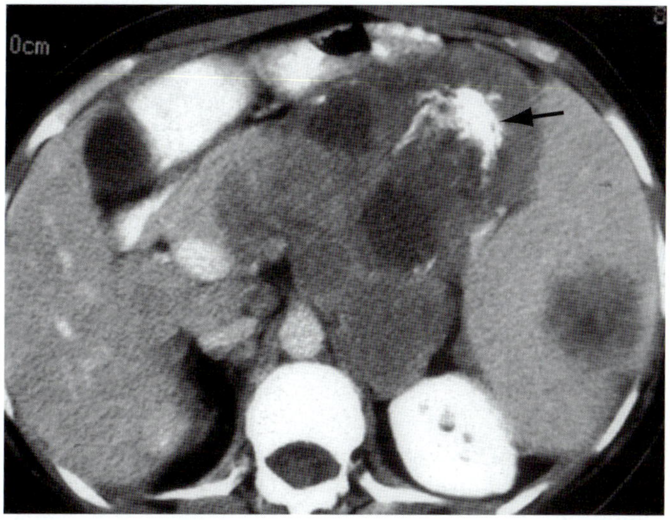

Figure 10–11. A focal splenic deposit in association with massive nodal enlargement involving the splenic hilum and tail of the pancreas in a patient with NHL. Note dystrophic calcification within the nodal mass (*arrowed*).

powered injectors for administration of intravenous contrast medium, since the entire spleen can be imaged when there is optimal parenchymal enhancement. Nodules have a nonspecific appearance, being hypoechoic on ultrasound, hypodense on enhanced CT, and of intermediate T2-signal intensity at MRI. The presence of splenic hilar lymph nodes is highly correlated with splenic involvement. Modern high-resolution ultrasound may be slightly more sensitive than CT for the detection of diffuse infiltration and nodules as small as 3 mm.[78] However, the identification of splenic HD is less critical than before, since patients with early stage disease who relapse because of untreated splenic infiltration can now be salvaged more successfully.

Primary splenic NHL is rare, being seen particularly with mantle cell and splenic marginal zone lymphomas, where there can be massive splenomegaly; infarction is a common complication. Solitary or multiple masses may be recognized (Fig. 10–11), and in NHL diffuse infiltration can be inferred from the presence of splenomegaly. Unfortunately, the intrinsic tissue contrast of MRI is insufficient for detection of infiltration, but intravenous small paramagnetic iron oxide particles may improve detection of focal and diffuse infiltration.[17,75,76] Various splenic volumes and indices have been developed; while some authors have used them to predict involvement with good results, they are generally somewhat cumbersome and have not gained widespread acceptance. Splenic volumes can be normal with obvious focal involvement and can decrease in response to treatment even if previously normal.

Finally there is evidence that whole-body FDG-PET scanning can detect splenic involvement at least as well as CT and probably better than Ga^{67} scans.[58,77] However, it is uncertain how much this would affect management, especially since patients with NHL will usually have other CT evidence of disease below the diaphragm.

Liver

There are similar problems in the reliable detection of hepatic lymphoma with cross-sectional imaging, since in untreated patients, involvement usually takes the form of small macroscopic or microscopic foci of tumor around the portal tracts. Hepatomegaly tends to indicate involvement. In HD, up to 5% of patients have hepatic disease at presentation, nearly always in association with splenic disease. The incidence is three times higher in NHL and even higher in the pediatric population and in recurrent disease. Focal lesions do occur in HD and NHL, and are generally indistinguishable from metastases with any imaging modality (Fig. 10–12). Occasionally, periportal infiltration is seen as low-density soft tissue around the portal tracts, especially in children and in ARL (Fig. 10–13). Primary hepatic NHL

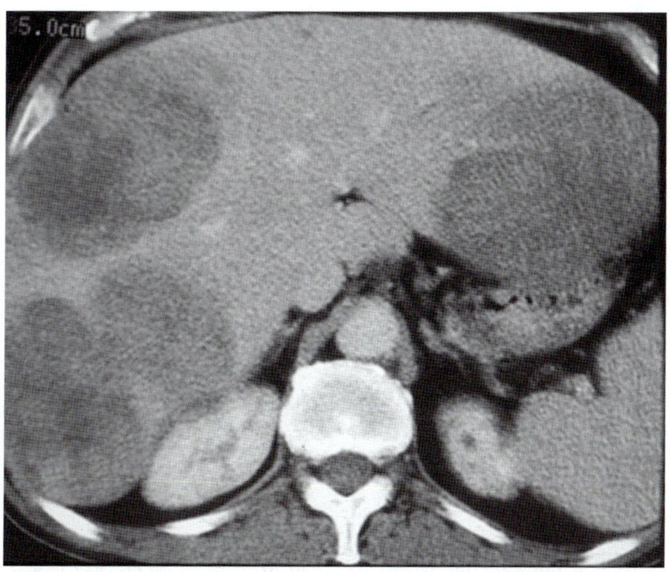

Figure 10–12. Multiple hepatic masses in a patient with NHL. The appearance is indistinguishable from that of metastases.

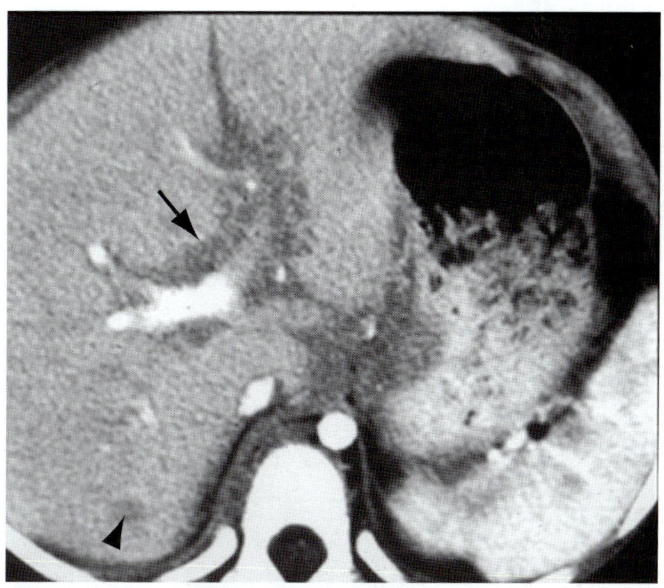

Figure 10–13. Contrast-enhanced CT of a pediatric patient with NHL demonstrating periportal low attenuation (*arrowed*) in addition to a small focal hypodense nodule in the right lobe of the liver (*arrowhead*).

is rare but the incidence is increasing, possibly as a result of its association with chronic hepatitis B and C. It is indistinguishable radiologically from hepatocellular carcinoma.

Gastrointestinal Tract

The gastrointestinal tract is the commonest site of primary extranodal lymphoma (nearly always NHL), being the initial site of disease in 10% to 15% of adult patients with NHL. In HD, involvement is secondary to invasion by adjacent nodal masses, which is well demonstrated by CT. This form of secondary involvement is much commoner in NHL because of its predilection for the mesenteric lymph nodes, and there are often multiple sites of disease. Although barium studies depict mucosal abnormalities better than CT, their role in staging is limited. On the other hand, CT can demonstrate the extent of mural disease, the presence of extramural spread, and regional nodal involvement.[78] Primary gastrointestinal lymphomas develop from lymphoid elements in the lamina propria, and there are two age-related peaks: under 10 years (BL) and between 50 and 60 years (mostly gastrointestinal-associated lymphoid tissue or GALT type, and high-grade, peripheral T-cell type associated with enteropathies). These generally involve only one site, and a modified Ann Arbor staging system recognizes this.[79] In both primary and secondary forms, the stomach is most commonly involved (50%), followed by the small bowel (33%), the colon (16%), and then the esophagus (<1%). In children, the ileum and ileocecal region are nearly always affected, up to 50% being BL, whereas anorectal disease is associated with ARL.

Common imaging features at CT are polypoid nodulation or massive localized or circumferential mural thickening, such as of the stomach or small bowel (Fig. 10–14). The presence of preserved fat planes around hollow viscera suggests a diagnosis of lymphoma rather than carcinoma, as does the presence of bulky retroperitoneal adenopathy. However, gastric mucosa–associated lymphoid tissue (MALT) lymphomas typically result in minimal gastric wall thickening, which may not be identified even with a dedicated gastric CT using an oral water load and intravenous smooth muscle relaxants. In this situation, endoscopic ultrasound is the method of choice for local staging and assessment of response to treatment[80–82] (Fig. 10–15). However, since multiorgan involvement can be present in up to 25% of these patients, extensive staging may be necessary.[83] In the small bowel, a particular advantage of CT is that it can demonstrate the complications of lymphoma

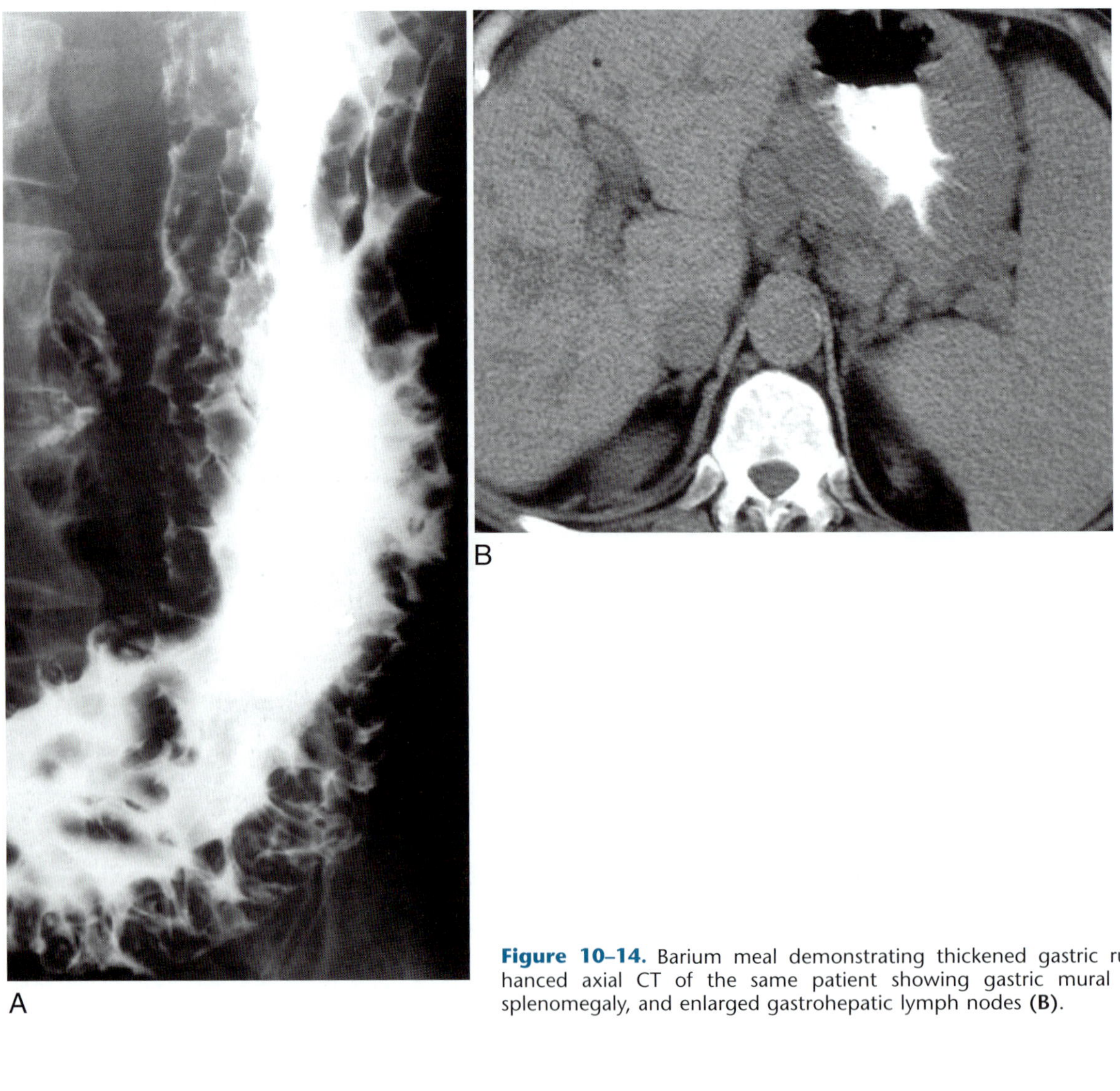

Figure 10–14. Barium meal demonstrating thickened gastric rugal folds **(A)**. Unenhanced axial CT of the same patient showing gastric mural thickening (*arrowed*), splenomegaly, and enlarged gastrohepatic lymph nodes **(B)**.

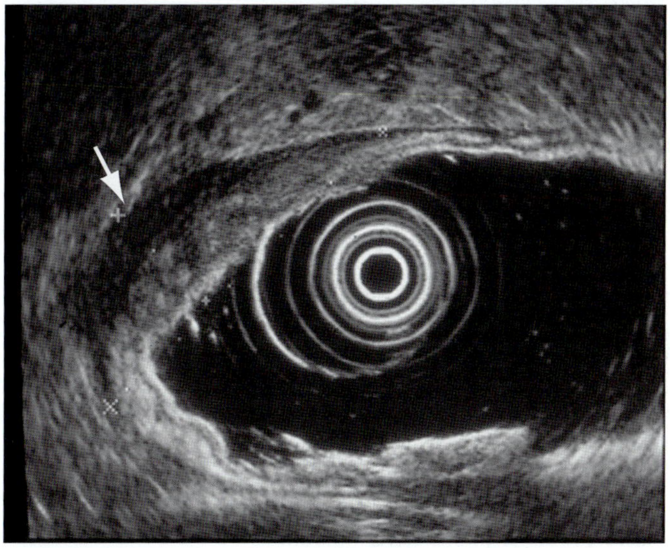

Figure 10–15. Endoscopic ultrasound depicting localized gastric mural thickening in a patient with gastric MALT lymphoma (*arrowed*).

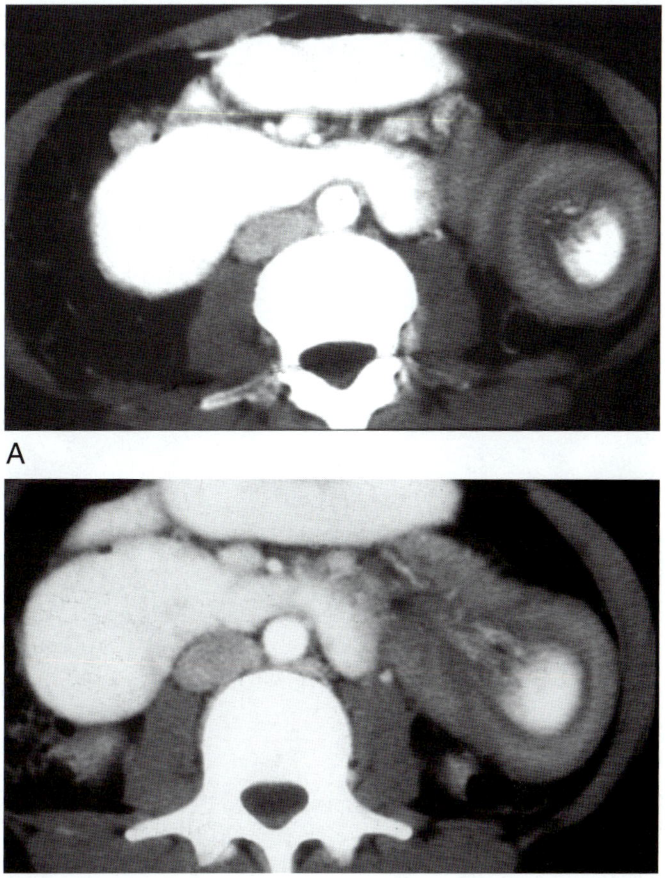

Figure 10–16. "Coiled spring" appearance of jejuno-jejunal intussusception with proximal duodenal obstruction secondary to jejunal lymphoma (*arrowed*) **(A,B)**.

such as obstruction, aneurysmal dilatation, and perforation. The polypoid forms predispose to intussusception, a classic mode of presentation also well demonstrated by CT (Fig. 10–16). Within the colon, CT will detect mural nodules or large masses, which in the cecum can appear identical to cecal carcinoma, a clue to the correct diagnosis being concomitant involvement of the terminal ileum. In advanced disease, CT can demonstrate strictures and fistulae, the latter being a feature of ARL.

Pancreas

Primary *pancreatic* lymphoma is most unusual, although secondary involvement is not infrequently seen as a result of direct invasion from adjacent nodal masses, either localized or diffuse. Intrinsic involvement results in a mass that may be indistinguishable from pancreatic carcinoma with biliary ductal obstruction and vascular encroachment, though again, the presence of nodal disease below the level of the renal veins suggests the correct diagnosis.[84,85] (Fig. 10–17). Occasionally, diffuse enlargement of the entire gland is seen.

Genitourinary Tract

In end-stage lymphoma, 50% or more cases will have some involvement of the genitourinary tract. The testis is most frequently affected, followed by the kidneys and perirenal space. In HD, involvement is nearly always secondary to invasion from adjacent nodal masses, which can be seen at CT. Isolated primary renal lymphoma is extremely rare, but with the routine deployment of contrast-enhanced helical CT, secondary renal tract involvement is increasingly recognized. Most cases are intermediate or high-grade NHL (DLBCL and BL in particular), and only rarely will recognition of renal disease alter disease staging. Renal function is generally preserved, but CT is able to depict diminished perfusion as a result of vascular encasement by nodal masses, and also hydronephrosis. Renal involvement may take many forms:

- Multiple masses (60%) (Fig. 10–17)
- Solitary masses (10% to 20%)
- Direct infiltration from the retroperitoneum (25%) or isolated disease in the perirenal space
- Diffuse renal infiltration (up to 10%)

An important differential diagnosis of the solitary mass is a renal cell carcinoma, particularly since in up to 50% there will be no accompanying retroperitoneal nodal disease.

Rarely isolated involvement of the ureter is seen, but bladder involvement is more frequent, usually secondary to invasion from adjacent nodal masses (seen in up to 15% at autopsy). Both primary and secondary NHL can result in focal or diffuse mural thickening, for which the differential diagnosis is transitional cell carcinoma. MALT-type NHL is seen in older women with a history of chronic cystitis, and can result in solitary or occasionally multiple sessile masses. As with the other pelvic viscera, MRI, with its multiplanar capability, may be of value in assessing the presence of transmural spread and involvement of adjacent organs.

Although primary adrenal NHL is rare, secondary involvement is not infrequently seen and is often bilateral, though adrenal insufficiency as a result is unusual (Fig. 10–18). Bilateral adrenal hyperplasia in association with lymphoma has also been described.[86]

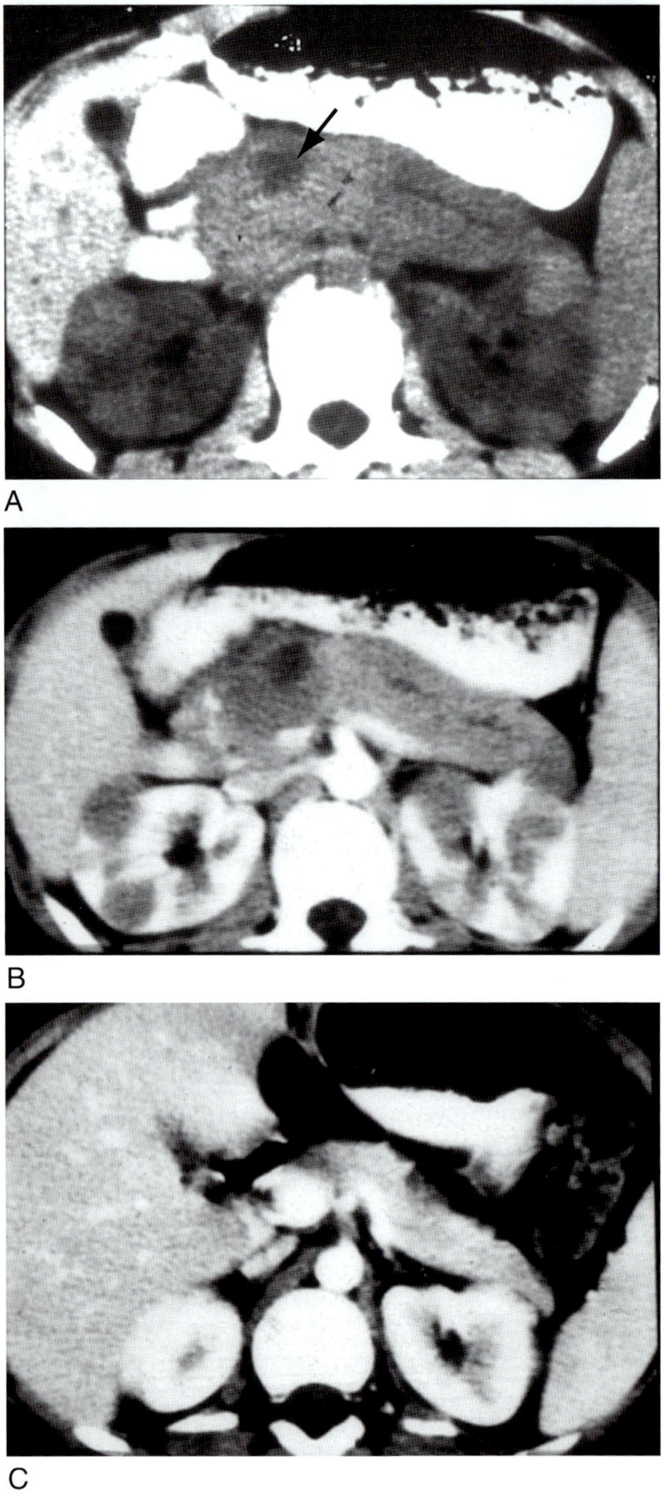

Figure 10–17. Unenhanced axial CT scan demonstrating multiple hyperdense renal masses and a focal mass in the body of the pancreas (*arrowed*) **(A)**. Post-contrast scan demonstrating the "density reversal sign" of the multiple renal lymphomatous masses **(B)**. Post-therapy, the appearances have normalized **(C)**.

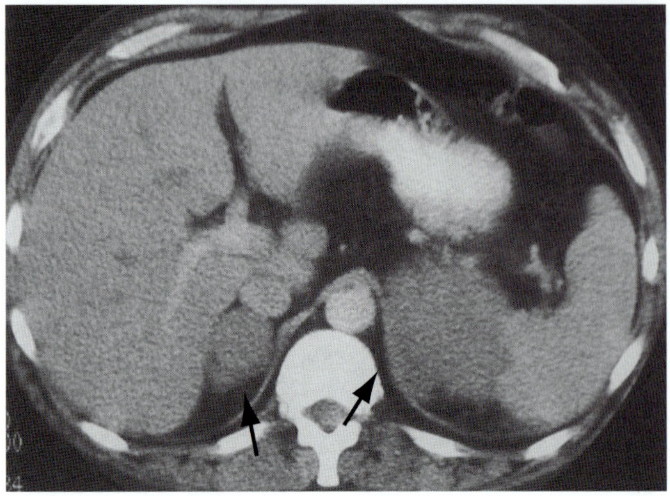

Figure 10–18. Axial CT scan of the same patient as in Figure 9–9 showing bilateral adrenal masses (*arrowed*).

Testicular lymphoma is the commonest testicular neoplasm in men over 60. At presentation the testis is affected in 1% of men with NHL (more in BL and with lymphoma of Waldeyer's ring and the central nervous system). Involvement with HD is extremely rare. Ultrasound will demonstrate focal areas of decreased echogenicity or testicular enlargement with a generalized decrease in reflectivity. MRI appears to offer little advantage over ultrasound.[87]

Primary lymphoma of the *female genital tract* accounts for around 1% of all extranodal NHL, and is primarily DLBCL or BL. Hence there are two age peaks in incidence. The uterine cervix is often affected, with large exophytic masses that are extremely well depicted by MRI, which is also very useful in assessment of response to treatment and follow-up[88] (Fig. 10–19). Ovarian lymphoma can appear identical

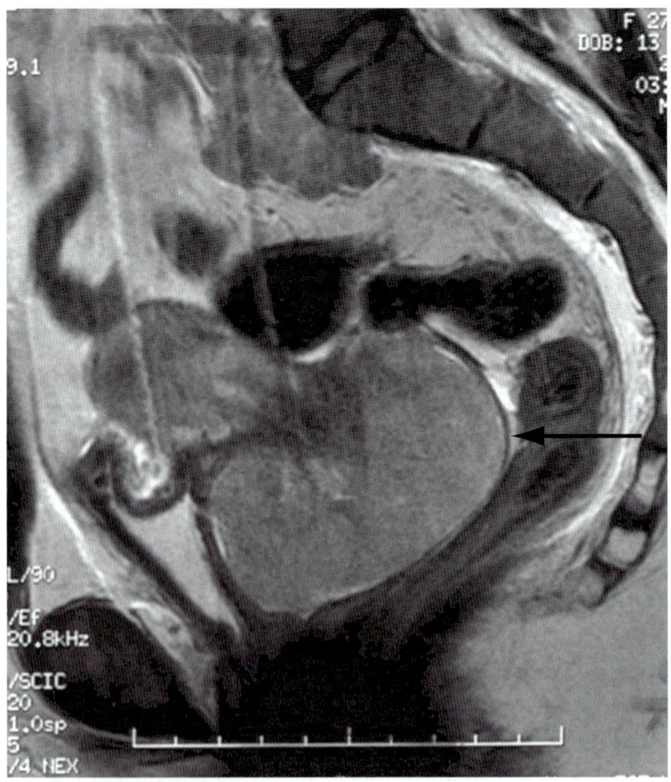

Figure 10–19. Sagittal T2-weighted MRI scan of a patient with cervical NHL showing a large homogeneous exophytic mass (*arrowed*) expanding the vagina and compressing the urinary bladder anteriorly.

to ovarian carcinoma, though the presence of large bilateral masses without hemorrhage or calcification may suggest the diagnosis.[89]

Central Nervous System

Much of the increased incidence of NHL has occurred in the orbit and central nervous system, a phenomenon only partly explained by the association of primary central nervous system lymphoma (PCNSL) with AIDS. Secondary involvement can be seen in up to 15% of patients with NHL at some point during their illness, especially with testicular or ovarian presentations, high-grade T-cell, Burkitt's, and immunoblastic lymphomas. Whereas PCNSL tends to affect the deep white matter and basal ganglia of the cerebral hemispheres, secondary disease tends to affect the extra-axial spaces of the brain and spinal cord.[90] Although MRI and CT have equivalent sensitivities in the detection of PCNSL, MRI has clear advantages over CT in the posterior fossa and spinal canal and contents (Fig. 10–20). In high-risk groups or where symptomatology dictates, screening with craniospinal MRI should be considered. Contrast-enhanced MRI has been shown to be more sensitive than CT in the demonstration of leptomeningeal lymphoma, though there is a significant false-negative rate when compared to leptomeningeal carcinomatosis.[91,92] Although CT will depict extension of retroperitoneal disease through the intervertebral foramina into the spinal canal, MR will detect more subtle disease and more clearly demonstrates the extent and degree of spinal cord or cauda equina compression.

Orbit

Similarly, in the orbit, MR best demonstrates the presence and extent of any intracranial extension, and the intrinsic tissue contrast allows delineation of the relationship of tumor to the intra- and extraconal structures (Fig. 10–21). Extensive staging with CT is still necessary, as around 50% of patients will have disease outside the CNS.

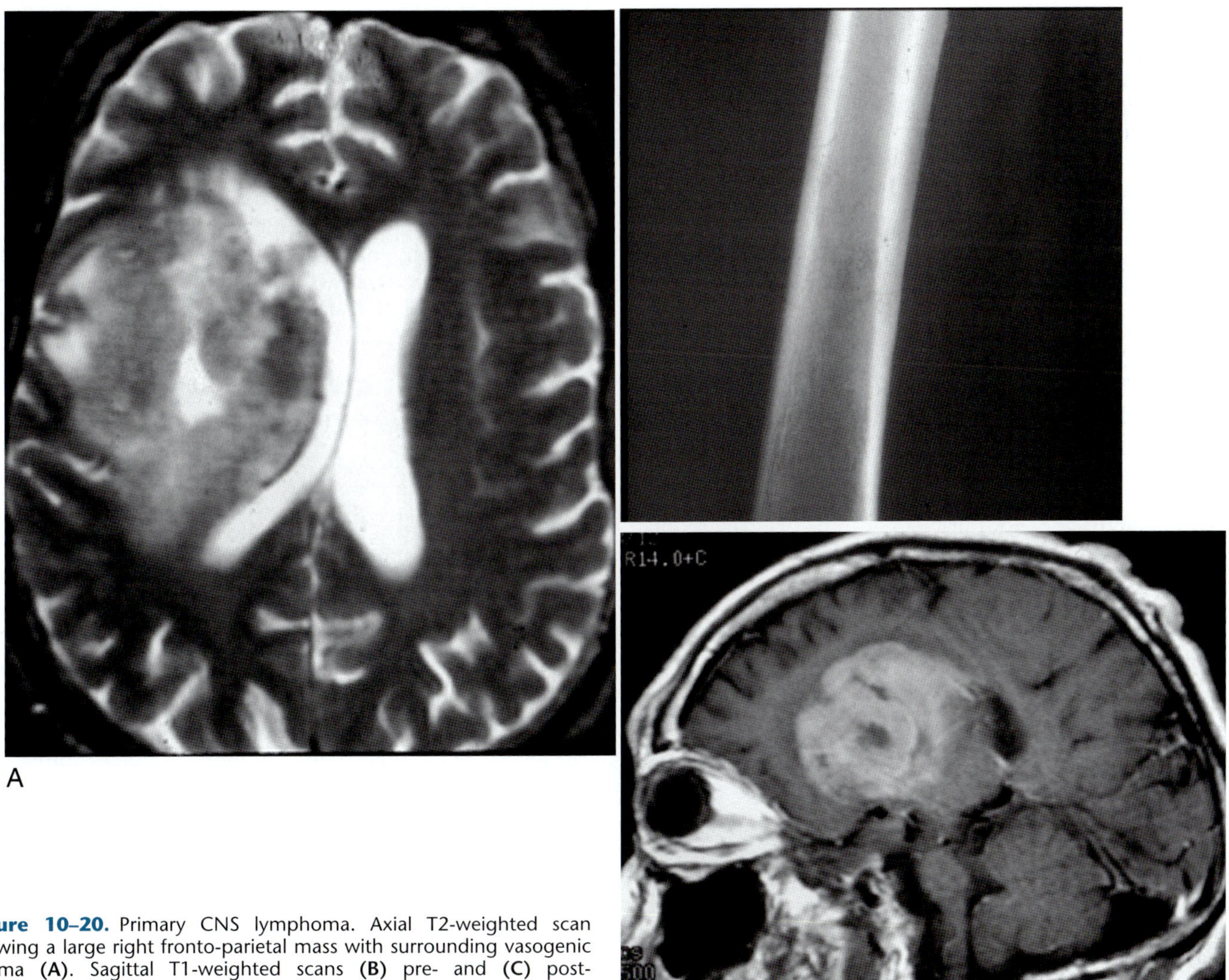

A

C

Figure 10–20. Primary CNS lymphoma. Axial T2-weighted scan showing a large right fronto-parietal mass with surrounding vasogenic edema **(A)**. Sagittal T1-weighted scans **(B)** pre- and **(C)** post-intravenous gadolinium demonstrating marked slightly heterogeneous enhancement of the mass.

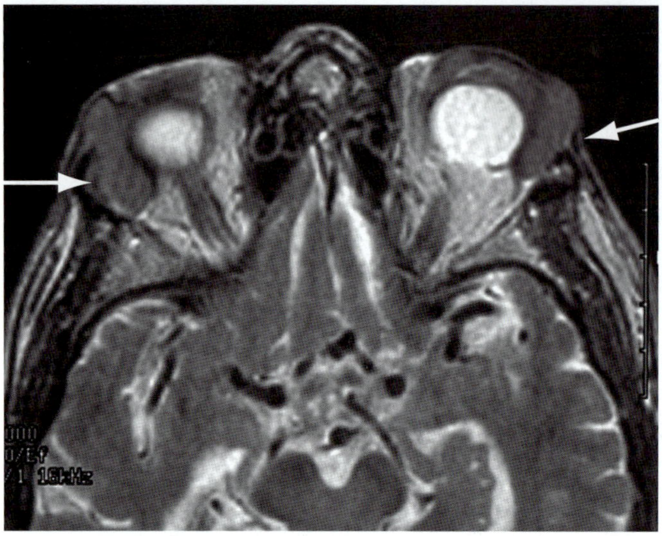

Figure 10–21. Axial T2-weighted MR scan of the orbit in a patient with bilateral lymphomatous masses involving the lacrimal glands (*arrowed*).

Head and Neck

Around 10% of patients with NHL present with extranodal disease in the head and neck, chiefly involving Waldeyer's ring. Many such patients will have synchronous or metachronous involvement of the gastrointestinal tract (possibly a reflection of the fact that many tumors are MALT type), hence many centers include abdominal CT and/or endoscopy as part of staging. MRI is the preferred technique for evaluation of head and neck lymphoma because of excellent tumor-to-background contrast and delineation of spread through the facial region and into the cranial cavity.

Musculoskeletal System

Skeletal involvement can occur in HD and NHL, usually as a result of invasion from adjacent lymph node masses, in which circumstance there is no effect on staging (the "E" lesion). This needs to be distinguished from involvement of osseous bone at the time of presentation or relapse, which can occur in both conditions, and which would qualify as extranodal disease. Both instances can be detected by plain radiography and CT scanning viewed on "bone windows." Osseous involvement is seen in up to 6% of adult patients with NHL (more in children) and 20% of patients with HD. Although isotope scintigraphy is more sensitive in the detection of skeletal involvement, it is not routinely indicated unless the patient is suspected of having primary lymphoma of bone, where it helps exclude clinically occult disease elsewhere. There is some evidence that FDG-PET is more accurate than bone scintigraphy, with a high positive predictive value for osseous involvement.[95]

Primary lymphoma of bone accounts for only 1% of all NHL, and is diagnosed less frequently than before, probably because more sensitive staging techniques are capable of detecting synchronous disease elsewhere. MRI is again the technique of choice for local staging, since it can demonstrate the extent of cortical bone disease, muscle infiltration, and underlying marrow involvement with ease[96] (Fig. 10–22).

Although it is often possible to detect intramuscular masses with CT because of expansion of the muscle and loss of fat planes, MRI excels because of the high contrast between the low T2 signal of muscle and intermediate to high T2 signal of lymphomatous masses.

A major weakness of CT as a staging tool is that it provides no information on the presence or absence of *bone marrow* infiltration, which by definition indicates stage IV disease, and places the patient in a worse prognostic group than hepatic, pulmonary, or osseous disease. This is of course partly circumvented by bone marrow biopsy, but if infiltration is patchy, sampling errors can occur.[95,96] MRI is extremely sensitive in the detection of bone marrow disease, affected areas having low signal intensity on T1-weighted sequences and high STIR signal. Newer, fast-STIR and echo-planar imaging (EPI) sequences appear to be more specific for infiltration.[97] Although false-negative studies are seen, usually with microscopic infiltration (<5%) or with low-grade lymphomas, deposits as small as 3 to 5 mm can be identified. MRI can result in upstaging in as many as 33% of patients with negative unilateral iliac crest biopsies.[95,96,98,99] Patients with a positive MRI study appear to have a poorer prognosis, regardless of bone marrow biopsy findings.[100] Immunoscintigraphy with technetium-99m–labeled monoclonal antibodies can also depict bone marrow disease,[101] but there is now more interest in the use of FDG-PET, which to date has shown high sensitivity and specificity.[102,103] As with MRI, a small number of false-negative scans occur with low-grade lymphoma, often PET-negative elsewhere, or with microscopic infiltration. FDG-PET can result in change of stage twice as often as bone marrow biopsy.

Despite the apparent accuracy of these techniques in the detection of bone marrow infiltration, their precise role in the staging of patients with lymphoma is uncertain, given the obvious need to examine bone marrow cytology.

Lymphoma in the Immunocompromised

The WHO classification recognizes four broad groupings associated with an increased incidence of lymphoma and lymphoproliferative disorders[104]:

- Primary immunodeficiency syndromes
- Infection with the human immunodeficiency virus (HIV)
- Iatrogenic immunosuppression after solid organ or bone marrow allografts
- Iatrogenic immunosuppression from methotrexate (usually for autoimmune disorders)

All of these groups have a markedly increased incidence of lymphoma, which share common imaging features.

Lymphomas Associated with HIV

Lymphoma is the first AIDS-defining illness in up to 5% of HIV patients. Various types are seen such as BL and DLBCL (especially in the CNS), some occurring almost exclusively in the HIV population (e.g., primary effusion lymphoma and plasmablastic lymphoma of the oral cavity). The incidence of HD is also increased up to eight-fold.[104]

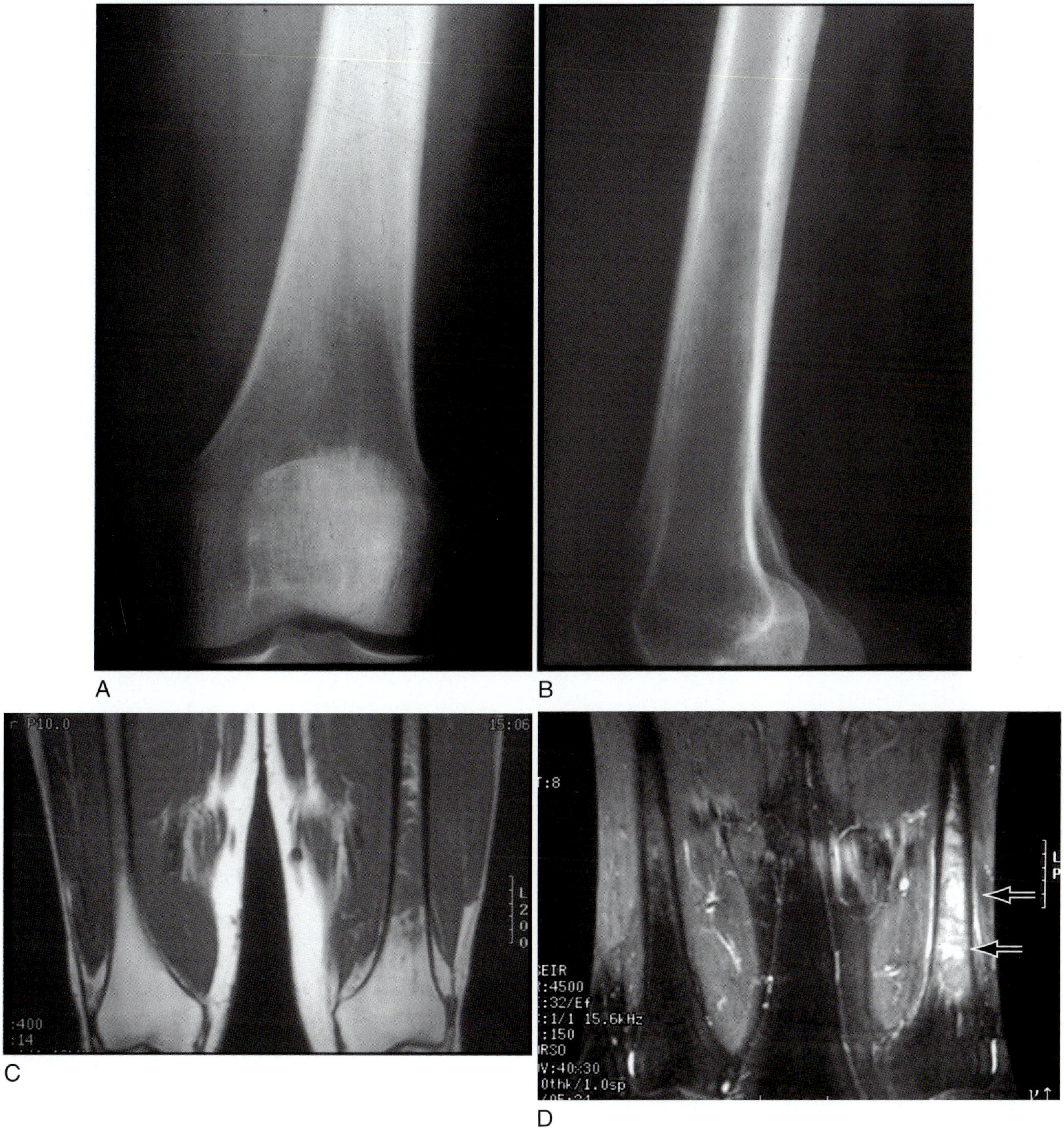

Figure 10–22. Frontal and lateral radiographs of the left femur of a patient with primary NHL of bone showing subtle lytic permeative destruction **(A,B)**. Coronal T1-weighted **(C)** and STIR sequences clearly depict the extent of lymphomatous involvement of the bone marrow (*arrowed*) **(D)**.

Continued

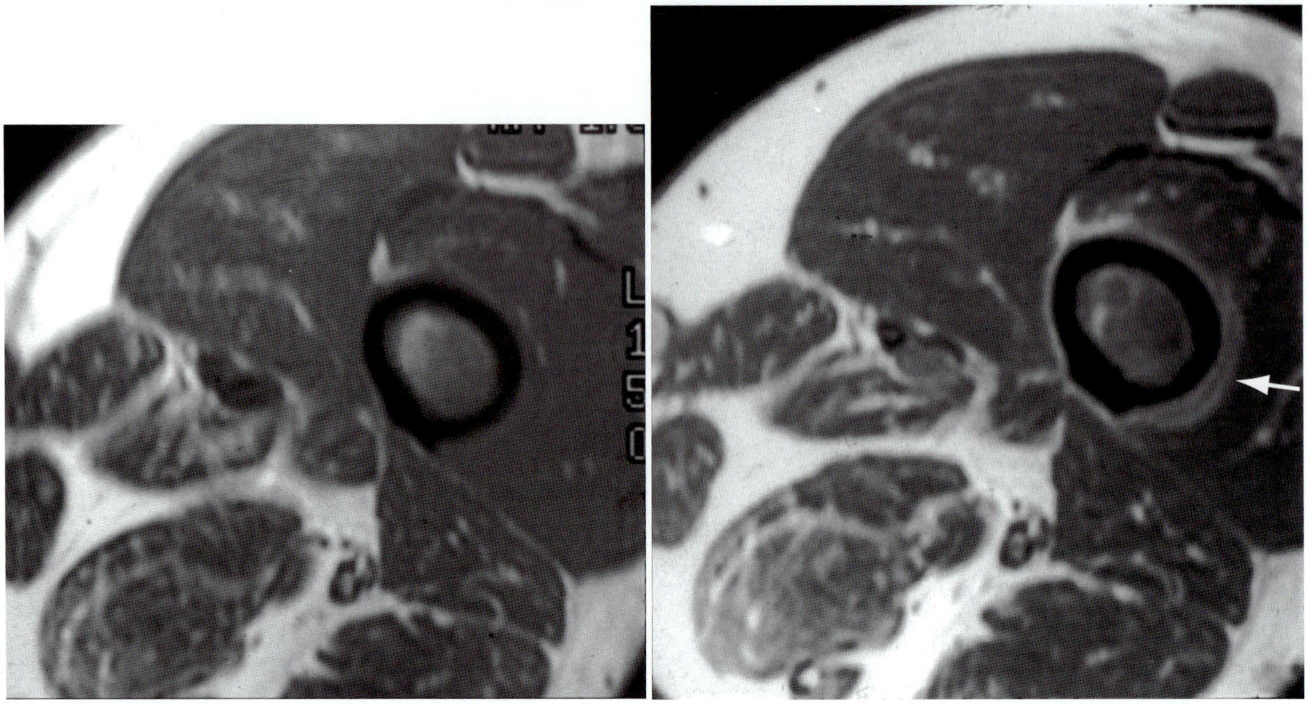

E F

Figure 10–22, cont'd Axial T1-weighted images pre- **(E)** and post-intravenous **(F)** gadolinium showing cortical thinning and periosteal enhancement secondary to lymphomatous infiltration (*arrowed*).

Most have a marked propensity to involve extranodal sites, especially the gastrointestinal tract, CNS (less frequent with the advent of highly active antiretroviral therapy), liver, and bone marrow. Multiple sites of extranodal involvement are seen in over 75% of cases,[105] and peripheral lymph node enlargement is seen in only 30% at presentation. Most tumors are aggressive, with advanced stage and bulky disease at presentation.

In the chest, NHL is usually extranodal; pleural effusion and lung disease are common, with nodules, acinar, and interstitial opacity being described. Hilar and mediastinal nodal enlargement are generally mild. There is a wide differential diagnosis, and in one study the presence of cavitation and nodal necrosis predicted for mycobacterial infection rather than lymphoma.[106]

Within the abdomen, the gastrointestinal tract, liver, kidneys, adrenal glands, and lower genitourinary tract are commonly involved. Mesenteric and retroperitoneal nodal enlargement is less common than in immunocompetent patients, but there are no apparent differences in the CT features of patients with or without AIDS, at least in relation to the small bowel.[107]

Regarding PCNSL, certain features such as rim enhancement and multifocality are seen more often than in the immunocompetent population. This can cause confusion with cerebral toxoplasmosis, though the location of PCNSL in the deep white matter is suggestive.[108] Quantitative FDG-PET uptake can help in the differentiation of PCNSL, toxoplasmosis, and progressive multifocal leucoencephalopathy (PML).[109]

Post-Transplant Lymphoproliferative Disorders (PTLD)

These occur in 2% to 4% of solid organ transplant recipients, depending on the type of transplant, the lowest frequency being seen in renal transplant recipients (1%) and the highest in heart–lung or liver–bowel allografts (5%). In all cases, extranodal disease is disproportionately more common. In patients receiving azathioprine, the allograft itself and the CNS are often involved, whereas in patients who have received cyclosporin A, the gastrointestinal tract is affected more often. Multiple segments of bowel can be affected, and disease can often be recognized within renal transplants. The bone marrow, liver, and lung are also often affected, as are the tonsils.[110,111]

Imaging and Prognostication

In the last few years, there has been increasing emphasis on the role of imaging in prognostication in patients with lymphoma. CT gives limited information inasmuch as it can identify bulky disease and extranodal disease. As indicated above, there is experimental work demonstrating that high-grade tumors tend to be more heterogeneous than low-grade ones of equivalent size.[33] With multidetector CT, it is now possible to measure perfusion and permeability of lymphomatous masses, and preliminary data suggest that these parameters can be related to grade and activity. Furthermore, they may provide an early measure of response to chemotherapy.[112] The association of a positive bone marrow at MRI with a poorer prognosis has been discussed above.[100] Rehn et al.[39] demonstrated that the type of signal abnormality at MRI could be correlated with tumor grade, high-grade tumors tending to have heterogeneous high T2 signal. They developed an inhomogeneity index, which for their patient population, was a better prognostic indicator than serum LDH or tumor size.[40] However, the amount of information provided by conventional cross-sectional imaging is limited compared to that provided by functional studies, in particular FDG-PET (see Chapter 11).

POST-TREATMENT EVALUATION

Imaging is extremely important in monitoring response to treatment, screening for relapse, and evaluating disease extent at the time of relapse. However, there is little consensus on how often imaging should be obtained during or after treatment. Most centers increasingly favor interim CT scans after two or three cycles of chemotherapy so that poor responders can be offered second-line therapy before significant toxicity has accrued from ineffective therapy, and it seems sensible to limit such scans to the areas affected at the time of initial staging. This is an area where functional imaging has undoubted advantages over conventional cross-sectional imaging, since it can identify changes in cell viability well before significant changes have occurred in tumor volume as assessed with CT and MRI. FDG-PET and Ga^{67} scanning both have much greater positive and negative predictive value than CT or even MRI after a few cycles of chemotherapy. The value of gallium scanning is limited by its lower sensitivity and by the significant proportion of non–gallium-avid tumors, whereas FDG-PET scans performed after one to three cycles of chemotherapy appear to predict eventual outcome in NHL more accurately than scans at the end of treatment and conventional imaging, especially with diffuse histologies.[113–115] In one study, all patients with a positive PET scan relapsed, and under 50% would have been predicted by conventional imaging.[116] There is some evidence that this applies to HD as well as NHL.[117]

Achievement of a complete remission following treatment is the most important factor for prolonged survival in both HD and NHL. Thus, final evaluation of response at or within a month of completion of therapy is critical, though there is little evidence on the optimal timing of such scans. Given the speed of modern CT scanners, most centers now scan the chest, abdomen, and pelvis after completion of therapy. Although in the past it has been argued that routine administration of intravenous contrast medium is unnecessary for follow-up scans, in practice, multislice technology allows the acquisition of scans with optimal vascular and parenchymal enhancement throughout the neck, chest, abdomen, and pelvis, facilitating assessment of nodal and extranodal disease. Where there is intrathoracic disease, the chest radiograph is useful in assessing response early on, but changes due to radiotherapy, rebound thymic hyperplasia and thymic cyst formation often make the mediastinum difficult to assess. A CT scan therefore remains crucial in the monitoring of response to treatment for mediastinal disease, especially when the chest radiograph is indeterminate.[118] In patients with intra-abdominal disease, serial CT is essential in monitoring response.

Response Criteria

International standardized response criteria are vital for clinical research, facilitating data interpretation and comparison of therapies. The recent consensus meeting on response criteria in NHL opted for consistency with the Cotswold criteria already in use for HD.[119,120] Key features from the imaging standpoint include the choice of 1.5-cm maximum transverse diameter as the cut-off for normal lymph node size, and a new definition of complete response (unconfirmed) (CR_u) after treatment, where there is a residual mass over 1.5 cm that has diminished in size by more than 75% of the sum of the products of the diameters. Altering the threshold for calling a lymph node normal or enlarged changes the CR rate, though not the overall response rate. Recognition of response with CT depends on changes in size alone, and changes in attenuation are rarely helpful. Modern CT scanners permit accurate reproducible measurements of well-defined nodal masses provided scan parameters are optimized, facilitating accurate measurement of marker lesions. However, there is significant interobserver variation, which is even more pronounced with irregular masses or when there is poor lesion-to-background contrast, and ideally a single observer should measure all marker lesions.[121]

MRI can demonstrate changes in signal intensity, which reflects alterations in the relative amounts of viable tumor, fibrosis, and necrosis. A reduction in the amount of T2 signal indicates response, whereas persistent high T2 signal suggests that there is residual disease.[16,56] (Fig. 10–23). Rahmouni et al.[122] documented four different signal patterns, and found that a change from an "active" to an "inactive" pattern could occur independently of changes in tumor size. A persistent heterogeneous high T2 pattern tended to indicate residual active disease, but false-positive studies were seen because of necrosis and inflammation, especially within the first 6 months, when it is most critical to know whether the patient is responding to treatment. In the chest, it may not be possible to differentiate residual disease from rebound hyperplasia. MRI of the bone marrow can also be difficult to interpret because of reconversion, particularly when G-CSF has been administered and early on after radiotherapy. There is some evidence that SPIO particles facilitate differentiation of normo- or hyper-cellular marrow from persistent infiltration.[123]

In certain situations, other modalities are the method of choice for evaluating response, such as endoscopic ultrasound in gastric MALT lymphoma.[124]

Residual Masses

Though nodal masses can resolve completely after successful treatment, to leave a normal-appearing lymph node, often a residual mass of sterilized fibrous tissue can persist in both HD and NHL. Such masses can be seen at CT in 20% to 50% of patients with NHL and at least 20% of those with HD, being more frequent when there is bulky disease at presentation. Differentiating between residual disease and fibrosis is one of the greatest challenges facing the oncologic radiologist. It is generally not possible to make this distinction with CT, since fibrous tissue has similar attenuation values to that of active tumor—hence the extremely low specificity and positive predictive value of CT after

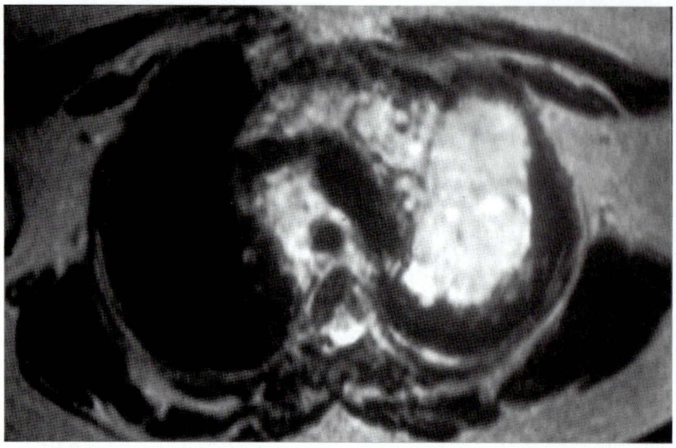

A

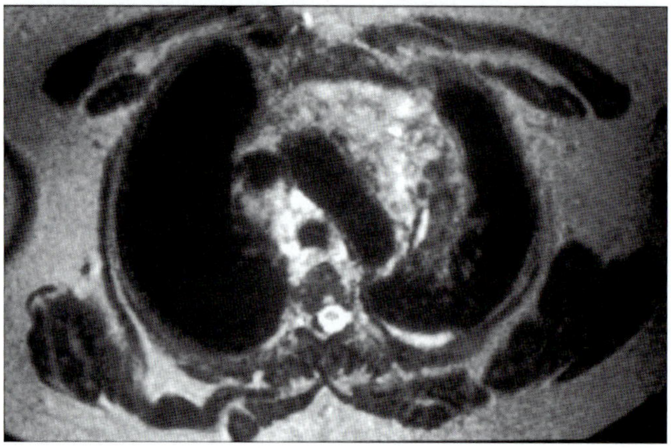

B

Figure 10–23. Axial T2-weighted MR scans of the thorax. Pre- **(A)** and post-therapy **(B)** in a patient with mediastinal LBCL (*arrowed*). The mass has diminished in size, but there is still considerable high T2 signal indicating the presence of active residual disease.

treatment in every series published. Despite this, until very recently, serial CT performed every 2 or 3 months to assess stability has been the commonest method of follow-up. Image-guided core biopsy can be extremely helpful when such masses are accessible,[125,126] but there is always the problem of sampling error.

As discussed above, serial MRI can be used to document response to treatment. One group has demonstrated that low T2-signal intensity of mediastinal masses of HD at presentation predicts for a residual mass, presumably because it reflects the presence of fibrous tissue, which would not be expected to respond to chemotherapy.[127] However, false-positive examinations occur during and after treatment, and microscopic foci of viable tumor account for the relatively low sensitivity of the technique.[16,128] There is limited evidence that enhancement of residual masses after intravenous gadolinium is less marked for patients in remission than in those with persistent disease.[129]

It is in the assessment of the residual mass that functional imaging indubitably performs much better than cross-sectional imaging. This is discussed in detail in Chapter 11. There is now a wealth of evidence that Ga^{67} and FDG-PET have much higher positive and negative predictive values for residual disease, both during and at completion of treatment.[130–135] Problems with Ga^{67} include limited sensitivity for small masses especially below the diaphragm, a significant number of non–gallium-avid lymphomas and false-positive studies. There have been few studies directly comparing Ga^{67} and FDG-PET, but the latter appears more sensitive,[136] and can predict for early relapse even in the absence of a residual mass at CT.[133] Of even more interest is the use of combined PET-CT scanners, since small foci of activity within residual masses can be accurately anatomically localized, facilitating image-guided biopsy.

Follow-up

Strategies for follow-up with imaging will vary between institutions and depending on whether or not there is a residual mass. For patients in CR or CR_u (i.e., where there is a Ga(67) or FDG-PET negative residual mass), it has been argued that routine imaging is desirable to detect asymptomatic early relapse, so that salvage therapy can be offered. However, it may take some time before there is an appreciable change in the size of a residual mass at CT. There is other evidence that CT rarely detects relapse in patients before they become symptomatic. In one series of patients with NHL who attained CR, only two of 36 relapses were diagnosed before patients were symptomatic—and only one was identified by imaging alone.[137] Twenty-five percent of relapses were in new sites alone, whereas the previous site was involved in the remainder. In another series of patients with treated intermediate and high-grade NHL, only 17% of relapses were detected by routine CT (13%) or laboratory tests (4%) alone.[138] Radford et al. found that 86% of relapses in a cohort of patients with HD were detected as a result of investigation of new symptoms rather than by routine follow-up studies.[139] It might be anticipated that surveillance FDG-PET scans would be more sensitive than CT and there is the added advantage of a lower radiation dose (9 mSv vs. 30 mSv), but there is as yet little evidence for this in the literature. Nonetheless, where relapse is suspected, the development of a positive scan is highly suggestive.

SUMMARY

CT is now firmly established as the single imaging modality of choice for initial staging and monitoring of treatment in patients with malignant lymphoma. Some of the problems previously cited, such as the detection of visceral involvement and recognition of disease in minimally enlarged lymph nodes have been at least partially overcome by improvements in scan technology. Nonetheless, there are areas where CT still performs poorly despite technical advances, particularly in the recognition of disease in normal-sized lymph nodes and evaluation of the residual mass. In some instances, MRI fulfils a useful problem-solving role, for example, in the evaluation of the pelvic viscera, and it is the method of choice for staging and follow-up of CNS, head and neck, and musculoskeletal lymphoma. However, in recent years the emphasis on imaging has shifted away from straightforward staging and evaluation of response toward early prognostication and functional assessment of response early on during the course of treatment, and it is in these areas that PET, and particularly PET-CT, holds such great promise.

References

1. Mackenzie R and Dixon AK. Measuring the effects of imaging: an evaluative framework. Clin Radiol 1995;50: 513–18.
2. Fineberg HV, Bauman R, and Sosman M. Computerized cranial tomography: effect on diagnostic and therapeutic plans. JAMA 1977;238:224–7.
3. Goldin J and Sayre JW. A guide to clinical epidemiology for radiologists: Part II. Statistical analysis. Clin Radiol 1996;51:317–24.
4. Begg CB and McNeil BJ. Assessment of radiologic tests: control of bias and other design considerations. Radiology 1988;167:565–9.
5. Fineberg HV, Wittenberg J, Ferrucci JT, et al. The clinical value of body computed tomography over time and technologic change. Am J Roentgenol 1983;141:1067–72.
6. Pombo P, Rodriguez E, Caruncho MV, et al. CT attenuation values and enhancing characteristics of thoracoabdominal lymphomatous adenopathies. J Comput Assist Tomogr 1994;18:59–62.
7. Carroll BA. Ultrasound of lymphoma. Semin Ultrasound 1982;III:114–22.
8. Munker R, Stengel A, Stabler A, et al. Diagnostic accuracy of ultrasound and computed tomography in the staging of Hodgkin's disease. Verification by laparotomy in 100 cases. Cancer 1995;76:1460–6.
9. Clouse ME, Harrison DA, Grassi CJ, et al. Lymphangiography, ultrasonography, and computed tomography in Hodgkin's disease and non-Hodgkin's lymphoma. J Comput Tomogr 1985;9:1–8.
10. Magnusson A, Erikson B, and Hemmingsson A. Investigation of retroperitoneal lymph nodes in Hodgkin's disease. Ups J Med Sci 1984;89:205–12.
11. Steinkamp HJ, Wissgott C, Rademaker J, et al. Current status of power Doppler and color Doppler sonography in the differential diagnosis of lymph node lesions. Eur Radiol 2002;12:1785–93.
12. Neumann CH, Robert NJ, Rosenthal D, et al. Clinical value of ultrasonography for the management of non-Hodgkin lymphoma patients as compared with abdominal computed tomography. J Comput Assist Tomogr 1983;7:666–9.
13. Reznek RH and Husband JE. The radiology of lymphoma. Curr Imaging 1990;2:9–17.
14. Lee JK, Heiken JP, Ling D, et al. Magnetic resonance imaging of abdominal and pelvic lymphadenopathy. Radiology 1984;153:181–8.
15. Dooms GC, Hricak H, Crooks LE, et al. Magnetic resonance imaging of the lymph nodes: comparison with CT. Radiology 1984;153:719–28.
16. Hill M, Cunningham D, MacVicar D, et al. Role of magnetic resonance imaging in predicting relapse in residual masses after treatment of lymphoma. J Clin Oncol 1993;11:2273–8.
17. Nyman R, Rhen S, Ericsson A, et al. An attempt to characterize malignant lymphoma in spleen, liver and lymph nodes with magnetic resonance imaging. Acta Radiol 1987; 28:527–33.
18. Weissleder R, Elizondo G, Wittenberg J, et al. Ultrasmall superparamagnetic iron oxide: an intravenous contrast agent for assessing lymph nodes with MR imaging. Radiology 1990;175:494–8.
19. Bellin MF, Roy C, Kinkel K, et al. Lymph node metastases: safety and effectiveness of MR imaging with ultrasmall superparamagnetic iron oxide particles—initial clinical experience. Radiology 1998;207:799–808.
20. Moog F, Bangerter M, Diederichs CG, et al. Lymphoma: role of whole-body 2-deoxy-2-[F-18]fluoro-D-glucose (FDG) PET in nodal staging. Radiology 1997;203:795–800.
21. Wirth A, Seymour JF, Hicks RJ, et al. Fluorine-18 fluorodeoxyglucose positron emission tomography, galliym-67 scintigraphy, and conventional staging for Hodgkin's disease and non-Hodgkin's lymphoma. Am J Med 2002;112:262–8.
22. Kostakoglu L, Leonard JP, Kuji I, et al. Comparison of fluorine-18 fluorodeoxyglucose positron emission tomography and Ga-67 scintigraphy in evaluation of lymphoma. Cancer 2002;94:879–88.
23. Filly R, Bland N, and Castellino RA. Radiographic distribution of intrathoracic disease in previously untreated patients with Hodgkin's disease and non-Hodgkin's lymphoma. Radiology 1976;120:277–81.
24. Castellino RA, Blank N, Hoppe RT, et al. Hodgkin disease: contributions of chest CT in the initial staging evaluation. Radiology 1986;160:603–5.
25. Castellino RA, Hilton S, O'Brien JP, et al. Non-Hodgkin lymphoma: contribution of chest CT in the initial staging evaluation. Radiology 1996;199:129–32.
26. Apter S, Avigdor A, Gayer G, et al. Calcification in lymphoma occurring before therapy: CT features and clinical correlation. Am J Roentgenol 2002;178:935–8.
27. Hopper KD, Diehl LF, Cole BA, et al. The significance of necrotic mediastinal lymph nodes on CT in patients with newly diagnosed Hodgkin disease. Am J Roentgenol 1990;155:267–70.
28. Heron CW, Husband JE, and Williams MP. Hodgkin disease: CT of the thymus. Radiology 1988;167:647–51.
29. Wernecke K, Vassallo P, Rutsch F, et al. Thymic involvement in Hodgkin disease: CT and sonographic findings. Radiology 1991;181:375–83.
30. Shaffer K, Smith D, Kirn D, et al. Primary mediastinal large-B-cell lymphoma: radiologic findings at presentation. Am J Roentgenol 1996;167:425–30.
31. Spiers AS, Husband JE, and MacVicar AD. Treated thymic lymphoma: comparison of MR imaging with CT. Radiology 1997;203:369–76.
32. Rodriguez M, Rehn SM, Nyman RS, et al. CT in malignancy grading and prognostic prediction of non-Hodgkin's lymphoma. Acta Radiol 1999;40:191–7.
33. Rostock RA, Siegelman SS, Lenhard RE, et al. Thoracic CT scanning for mediastinal Hodgkin's disease: results and therapeutic implications. Int J Radiat Oncol Biol Phsy 1983;9:1451–7.
34. Levis A, Davini O, Garabello D, et al. Role of thoracic CT in the treatment plan of Hodgkin's disease. Haematologica 1990;75:64–8.
35. North LB, Fuller LM, Hagemeister FB, et al. Importance of initial mediastinal adenopathy in Hodgkin disease. Am J Roentgenol 1982;138:229–35.
36. Gallagher CJ, White FE, Tucker AK, et al. The role of computed tomography in the detection of intrathoracic lymphoma. Br J Cancer 1984;49:621–9.
37. Khoury MB, Godwin JD, Halvorsen R, et al. Role of chest CT in non-Hodgkin lymphoma. Radiology 1986;158:659–62.
38. Hopper KD, Diehl LF, Lesar M, et al. Hodgkin disease: clinical utility of CT in initial staging and treatment. Radiology 1988;169:17–22.
39. Rehn SM, Nyman RS, Glimelius BL, et al. Non-Hodgkin lymphoma: predicting prognostic grade with MR imaging. Radiology 1990;176:249–53.
40. Rehn S, Sperber GO, Nyman R, et al. Quantification of inhomogeneities in malignancy grading of non-Hodgkin lymphoma with MR imaging. Acta Radiol 1993;34:3–9.
41. Lee JK, Stanley RJ, Sagel SS, et al. Accuracy of computed tomography in detecting intra-abdominal and pelvic adenopathy in lymphoma. Am J Roentgenol 1978;131: 311–15.

42. Best JJ, Blackledge G, Forbes WS, et al. Computed tomography of abdomen in staging and clinical management of lymphoma. BMJ 1978;2:1675–7.
43. Earl HM, Sutcliffe SB, Fry IK, et al. Computerised tomographic (CT) abdominal scanning in Hodgkin's disease. Clin Radiol 1980;31:149–53.
44. Marglin S and Castellino R. Lymphographic accuracy in 632 consecutive, previously untreated cases of Hodgkin disease and non-Hodgkin lymphoma. Radiology 1981;140: 351–3.
45. Castellino RA, Hoppe RT, Blank N, et al. Computed tomography, lymphography, and staging laparotomy: correlations in initial staging of Hodgkin disease. Am J Roentgenol 1984;143:37–41.
46. Enig B, Bjerregaard JB, Hjollund ME, et al. Detection of neoplastic lymph nodes in Hodgkin's disease and non-Hodgkin lymphoma. Comparison between tomography and lymphography. Acta Radiol Oncol 1985;24:491–5.
47. Strijk P. Lymphography and abdominal computed tomography in the staging of non-Hodgkin lymphoma. With an analysis of discrepancies. Acta Radiol 1987;28:263–9.
48. Pond GD, Castellino RA, Horning S, et al. Non-Hodgkin lymphoma: influence of lymphography, CT, and bone marrow biopsy on staging and management. Radiology 1989;170:159–64.
49. Stomper PC, Cholewinski SP, Park J, et al. Abdominal staging of thoracic Hodgkin disease: CT-lymphangiographic-Ga-67 scanning correlation. Radiology 1993;187:381–6.
50. Libson E, Polliack A, and Bloom RA. Value of lymphangiography in the staging of Hodgkin lymphoma. Radiology 1994;193:757–9.
51. Moskovic E, Fernando I, Blake P, et al. Lymphography—current role in oncology. Br J Radiol 1991;64:422–7.
52. Castellino RA, Marglin S, and Blank N. Hodgkin disease, the non Hodgkin lymphomas, and the leukemias in the retroperitoneum. Semin Roentgenol 1980;15:288–301.
53. Kadin MD, Glatstein EJ, and Dorfman RF. Clinicopathologic studies in 117 untreated patients subject to laparotomy for the staging of Hodgkin's disease. Cancer 1980;27: 1277–94.
54. Urba WJ and Longo DL. Hodgkin's disease. N Engl J Med 1992;326:678–87.
55. Yang ZG, Min PQ, Sone S, et al. Tuberculosis versus lymphomas in the abdominal lymph nodes: evaluation with contrast-enhanced CT. Am J Roentgenol 1999;172:619–23.
56. Greco A, Jelliffe AM, Maher EJ, et al. MR imaging of lymphomas: impact on therapy. J Comput Assist Tomogr 1988;12:785–91.
57. Shipp M, Harrington D, Anderson J, et al. Development of a predictive model for aggressive lymphoma: the International NHL prognostic factors project. N Engl J Med 1993; 329:987–94.
58. Moog F, Bangerter M, Diederichs CG, et al. Extranodal malignant lymphoma: detection with FDG PET versus CT. Radiology 1998;206:475–81.
59. Cobby M, Whipp E, Bullimore J, et al. CT appearances of relapse of lymphoma in the lung. Clin Radiol 1990;41:232–8.
60. Eisner MD, Kaplan LD, Herndier B, et al. The pulmonary manifestations of AIDS-related non-Hodgkin's lymphoma. Chest 1996;110:729–36.
61. Lewis ER, Caskey CI, and Fishman EK. Lymphoma of the lung: CT findings in 31 patients. Am J Roentgenol 1991;156:711–14.
62 Jackson SA, Tung KT, and Mead GM. Multiple cavitating pulmonary lesions in non-Hodgkin's lymphoma. Clin Radiol 1994;49:883–5.
63. Cordier JF, Chailleux E, Lauque D, et al. Primary pulmonary lymphomas. A clinical study of 70 cases in nonimmunocompromised patients. Chest 1993;103:201–8.
64. Murray KA, Chor PJ, and Turner JF Jr. Intrathoracic lymphoproliferative disorders and lymphoma. Curr Probl Diagn Radiol 1996;25:78–106.
65. Ooi GC, Ho JC, Khong PL, et al. Computed tomography characteristics of advanced primary pulmonary lymphoepithelioma-like carcinoma. Eur Radiol 2003;13:522–6.
66. Edinburgh KJ, Jasmer RM, Huang L, et al. Multiple pulmonary nodules in AIDS: usefulness of CT in distinguishing among potential causes. Radiology 2000;214:427–32.
67. Heussel CP, Kauzzar H-U, Heussel GE, et al. Pneumonia in febrile neutropenic patients and in bone marrow and blood stem cell transplant recipients: use of high resolution CT. J Clin Oncol 1999;17:796–805.
68. Celikoglu F, Teirstein AS, Krellenstein DJ, et al. Pleural effusion in non-Hodgkin's lymphoma. Chest 1992;101:1357–60.
69. Tesoro-Tess JD, Biasi S, Balzarini L, et al. Heart involvement in lymphomas. The value of magnetic resonance imaging and two-dimensional echocardiography at disease presentation. Cancer 1993;72:2484–90.
70. Bergin CJ, Healy MV, Zincone GE, et al. MR evaluation of chest wall involvement in malignant lymphoma. J Comput Assist Tomogr 1990;14:928–32.
71. Carlsen SE, Bergin CJ, and Hoppe RT. MR imaging to detect chest wall and pleural involvement in patients with lymphoma: effect on radiation therapy planning. Am J Roentgenol 1993;160:1191–5.
72. Sabate JM, Gomez A, Torrubia S, et al. Lymphoma of the breast: clinical and radiologic features with pathologic correlation in 28 patients. Breast J 2002;8:294–304.
73. Kadin MD, Glatstein EJ, and Dorfman RF. Clinicopathologic studies in 117 untreated patients subject to laparotomy for the staging of Hodgkin's disease. Cancer 1980;27:1277–94.
74. Castellino RA, Goffinet DR, Blank N, et al. The role of radiography in the staging of non-Hodgkin's lymphoma with laparotomy correlation. Radiology 1974;110:329–38.
75. Weissleder R, Elizondo G, Stark DD, et al. The diagnosis of splenic lymphoma by MR imaging: value of superparamagnetic iron oxide. Am J Roentgenol 1989;152:175–80.
76. Harisinghani MG, Saini S, Weissleder R, et al. Splenic imaging with ultrasmall superparamagnetic iron oxide ferumoxtran-10 (AMI-7227): preliminary observations. J Comput Assist Tomogr 2001;25:770–6.
77. Rini JN, Manalili EY, Hoffman MA, et al. F-18 FDG versus Ga-67 for detecting splenic involvement in Hodgkin's disease. Clin Nucl Med 2002;27:572–7.
78. Megibow AJ, Balthazar EJ, Naidich DP, et al. Computed tomography of gastrointestinal lymphoma. Am J Roentgenol 1983;141:541–7.
79. Rohatiner A, d'Amore F, Coiffier B, et al. Report on a workshop convened to discuss the pathological and staging classifications of gastrointestinal tract lymphoma. Ann Oncol 1994;5:397–400.
80. Kessar P, Norton A, Rohatiner AZ, et al. CT appearances of mucosa-associated lymphoid tissue (MALT) lymphoma. Eur Radiol 1999;9:693–6.
81. Fujishima H and Chijiiwa Y. Endoscopic ultrasonographic staging of primary gastric lymphoma. Abdom Imaging 1996;21:192–4.
82. Vorbeck F, Osterreicher C, Puspok A, et al. Comparison of spiral computed tomography with water-filling of the stomach and endosonography for gastric lymphoma of mucosa-associated lymphoid tissue type. Digestion 2002;65:196–9.
83. Raderer M, Vorbeck F, Formanek M, et al. Importance of extensive staging in patients with mucosa-associated lymphoid tissue (MALT)-type lymphoma. Br J Cancer 2000;83:454–7.

84. Van Beers B, Lalonde L, Soyer P, et al. Dynamic CT in pancreatic lymphoma. J Comput Assist Tomogr 1993;17:94–7.
85. Prayer L, Schurawitzki H, Mallek R, et al. CT in pancreatic involvement of non-Hodgkin lymphoma. Acta Radiol 1992;33:123–7.
86. Vincent JM, Morrison ID, Armstrong P, et al. Computed tomography of diffuse, non-metastatic enlargement of the adrenal glands in patients with malignant disease. Clin Radiol 1994;49:456–60.
87. Thurnher S, Hricak H, Carroll PR, et al. Imaging the testis: comparison between MR imaging and US. Radiology 1988;167:631–6.
88. Kim YS, Koh BH, Cho OK, et al. MR imaging of primary uterine lymphoma. Abdom Imaging 1997;22:441–4.
89. Ferrozzi F, Tognini G, Bova D, et al. Non-Hodgkin lymphomas of the ovaries: MR findings. J Comput Assist Tomogr 2000;24:416–20.
90. Zimmerman RA. Central nervous system lymphoma. Radiol Clin North Am 1990;28:697–721.
91. Chamberlain MC, Sandy AD, and Press GA. Leptomeningeal metastasis: a comparison of gadolinium-enhanced MR and contrast-enhanced CT of the brain. Neurology 1990;40:435–8.
92. Yousem DM, Patrone PM, and Grossman RI. Leptomeningeal metastases: MR evaluation. J Comput Assist Tomogr 1990;14:255–61.
93. Moog F, Kotzerke J, and Reske SN. FDG PET can replace bone scintigraphy in primary staging of malignant lymphoma. J Nucl Med 1999;40:1407–13.
94. Stroszczynski C, Oellinger J, Hosten N, et al. Staging and monitoring of malignant lymphoma of the bone: comparison of ^{67}Ga scintigraphy and MRI. J Nucl Med 1999;40:387–93.
95. Linden A, Zankovich R, Theissen P, et al. Malignant lymphoma: bone marrow imaging versus biopsy. Radiology 1989;173:335–9.
96. Döhner H, Guckel F, Knauf W, et al. Magnetic resonance imaging of bone marrow in lymphoproliferative disorders: correlation with bone marrow biopsy. Br J Haematol 1989;73:12–7.
97. Yasumoto M, Nonomura Y, Yoshimura R, et al. MR detection of iliac bone marrow involvement by malignant lymphoma with various MR sequences including diffusion-weighted echo-planar imaging. Skeletal Radiol 2002;31:263–9.
98. Hoane BR, Shields AF, Porter BA, et al. Detection of lymphomatous bone marrow involvement with magnetic resonance imaging. Blood 1991;78:728–38.
99. Shields AF, Porter BA, Churchley S, et al. The detection of bone marrow involvement by lymphoma using magnetic resonance imaging. J Clin Oncol 1987;5:225–30.
100. Tsunoda S, Takagi S, Tanaka O, et al. Clinical and prognostic significance of femoral marrow magnetic resonance imaging in patients with malignant lymphoma. Blood 1997;89:286–90.
101. Altehoefer C, Blum U, Bathmann J, et al. Comparative diagnostic accuracy of magnetic resonance imaging and immunoscintigraphy for detection of bone marrow involvement in patients with malignant lymphoma. J Clin Oncol 1997;15:1754–60.
102. Moog F, Bangerter M, Kotzerke J, et al. 18-F-fluorodeoxyglucose-positron emission tomography as a new approach to detect lymphomatous bone marrow. J Clin Oncol 1998;16:603–9.
103. Carr R, Barrington SF, Madan B, et al. Detection of lymphoma in bone marrow by whole-body positron emission tomography. Blood 1998;91:3340–6.
104. World Health Organization Classification of Tumours. Pathology and Genetics. Tumours of Haematopoietic and Lymphoid Tissues. Lyon: IARC Press, 2001.
105. Radin DR, Esplin JA, Levine AM, et al. AIDS-related non-Hodgkin's lymphoma: abdominal CT findings in 112 patients. Am J Roentgenol 1993;160:1133–9.
106. Jasmer RM, Gotway MB, Creasman JM, et al. Clinical and radiographic predictors of the etiology of computed tomography-diagnosed intrathoracic lymphadenopathy in HIV-infected patients. J AIDS 2002;31:291–8.
107. Balthazar EJ, Noordhoorn M, Megibow AJ, et al. CT of small-bowel lymphoma in immunocompetent patients and patients with AIDS: comparison of findings. Am J Roentgenol 1997;168:675–80.
108. Cordoliani YS, Derosier C, Pharaboz C, et al. Primary cerebral lymphoma in patients with AIDS: MR findings in 17 cases. Am J Roentgenol 1992;159:841–7.
109. O'Doherty MJ, Barrington SF, Campbell M, et al. PET scanning and the human immunodeficiency virus-positive patient. J Nucl Med 1997;38:1575–83.
110. Lee DA, Hartman RP, Trenkner SW, et al. Lymphomas in solid organ transplantation. Abdom Imaging 1998;23:553–7.
111. Pickhardt PJ and Siegel MJ. Abdominal manifestations of posttransplantation lymphoproliferative disorder. Am J Roentgenol 1998;171:1007–13.
112. Dugdale PE, Miles KA, Bunce I, et al. CT measurement of perfusion and permeability within lymphoma masses and its ability to assess grade, activity and chemotherapeutic response. J Comput Assist Tomogr 1999;23:540–7.
113. Mikhaeel NG, Timothy AR, O'Doherty MJ, et al. 8-FDG-PET as a prognostic indicator in the treatment of aggressive non-Hodgkin's lymphoma-comparison with CT. Leuk Lymphoma 2000;39:543–53.
114. Romer W, Hanauske AR, Ziegler S, et al. Positron emission tomography in non-Hodgkin's lymphoma: assessment of chemotherapy with fluorodeoxyglucose. Blood 1998;91:4464–71.
115. Spaepen K, Stroobants S, Dupont P, et al. Early restaging positron emission tomography with ^{18}-fluorodeoxyglucose predicts outcome in patients with aggressive non-Hodgkin's lymphoma. Ann Oncol 2002;13:1356–63.
116. Spaepen K, Stroobants S, Dupont P, et al. Prognostic value of positron emission tomography (PET) with fluorine-18 fluorodeoxyglucose ([18F]FDG) after first-line chemotherapy in non-Hodgkin's lymphoma: is [18F]FDG-PET a valid alternative to conventional diagnostic methods? J Clin Oncol 2001;19:414–19.
117. Kostakoglu L, Coleman M, Leonard JP, et al. PET predicts prognosis after 1 cycle of chemotherapy in aggressive lymphoma and Hodgkin's disease. J Nucl Med 2002;43:1018–27.
118. Heron CW, Husband JE, Williams MP, et al. The value of thoracic computed tomography in the detection of recurrent Hodgkin's disease. Br J Radiol 1988;61:567–72.
119. Cheson BD, Horning SJ, Coiffier B, et al. Report of an international workshop to standardize response criteria for non-Hodgkin's lymphomas. NCI Sponsored International Working Group. J Clin Oncol 1999;17:1244.
120. Lister TA, Crowther D, Sutcliffe S, et al. Report of a committee convened to discuss the evaluation and staging of patients with Hodgkin's disease: Cotswolds meeting. J Clin Oncol 1989;7:1630–6.
121. Hopper KD, Kasales CJ, Van Slyke MA, et al. Analysis of interobserver and intraobserver variability in CT tumor measurements. Am J Roentgenol 1996;167:851–4.
122. Rahmouni A, Tempany C, Jones R, et al. Lymphoma: monitoring tumor size and signal intensity with MR imaging. Radiology 1993;188:445–51.

123. Daldrup-Link HE, Rummeny EJ, Ihssen B, et al. Iron-oxide–enhanced MR imaging of bone marrow in patients with non-Hodgkin's lymphoma: differentiation between tumor infiltration and hypercellular bone marrow. Eur Radiol 2002;12:1557–66.
124. Sackmann M, Morgner A, Rudolph B, et al. Regression of gastric MALT lymphoma after eradication of Helicobacter pylori is predicted by endosonographic staging. MALT Lymphoma Study Group. Gastroenterology 1997;113:1087–90.
125. Pappa VI, Hussain HK, Reznek RH, et al. Role of image-guided core-needle biopsy in the management of patients with lymphoma. J Clin Oncol 1996;14:2427–30.
126. Ben Yehuda D, Polliack A, Okon E, et al. Image-guided core-needle biopsy in malignant lymphoma: experience with 100 patients that suggests the technique is reliable. J Clin Oncol 1996;14:2431–4.
127. Nyman RS, Rehn SM, Glimelius BL, et al. Residual mediastinal masses in Hodgkin disease: prediction of size with MR imaging. Radiology 1989;170:435–40.
128. Rodriguez M. Computed tomography, magnetic resonance imaging and positron emission tomography in non-Hodgkin's lymphoma. Acta Radiol Suppl 1998;417:1–36.
129. Rahmouni A, Divine M, Lepage E, et al. Mediastinal lymphoma:quantitative changes in gadolinium enhancement at MR imaging after treatment. Radiology 2001;219:621–8.
130. Kaplan WD, Jochelson MS, Herman TS, et al. Galliym-67 imaging: a predictor of residual tumor viability and clinical outcome in patients with diffuse large-cell lymphoma. J Clin Oncol 1990;8:1966–70.
131. Front D, Ben Haim S, Israel O, et al. Lymphoma: predictive value of Ga-67 scintigraphy after treatment. Radiology 1992;182:359–63.
132. Jerusalem G, Beguin Y, Fassotte MF, et al. Whole-body positron emission tomography using 18F-fluorodeoxyglucose for posttreatment evaluation in Hodgkin's disease and non-Hodgkin's lymphoma has higher diagnostic and prognostic value than classical computed tomography scan imaging. Blood 1999;94:429–33.
133. Naumann R, Vaic A, Beuthien-Baumann B, et al. Prognostic value of positron emission tomography in the evaluation of post-treatment residual mass in patients with Hodgkin's disease and non-Hodgkin's lymphoma. Br J Haematol 2001;115:793–800.
134. Weihrauch MR, Re D, Scheidhauer K, et al. Thoracic positron emission tomography using 18F-fluorodeoxyglucose for the evaluation of residual mediastinal Hodgkin disease. Blood 2001;98:2930–4.
135. de Wit M, Bumann D, Beyer W, et al. Whole-body positron emission tomography (PET) for diagnosis of residual mass in patients with lymphoma. Ann Oncol 1997;8(Suppl 1):57–60.
136. Van Den Bosche B, Lambert B, De Winter F, et al. 18FDG PET versus high-dose 67Ga scintigraphy for restaging and treatment follow-up of lymphoma patients. Nucl Med Commun 2002;23:1079–83.
137. Weeks JC, Yeap BY, Canellos GP, et al. Value of follow-up procedures in patients with large-cell lymphoma who achieve a complete remission. J Clin Oncol 1991; 9:1196–1203.
138. Elis A, Blickstein D, Klein O, et al. Detection of relapse in non-Hodgkin's lymphoma: role of routine follow-up studies. Am J Hematol 2002;69:41–4.
139. Radford JA, Eardley A, Woodman C, et al. Follow up policy after treatment for Hodgkin's disease: too many clinic visits and routine tests? A review of hospital records. BMJ 1997;314:343–6.
140. Tart RP, Mukherji SK, Avino AJ, et al. Facial lymph nodes: normal and abnormal CT appearance. Radiology 1993:188:695–700.
141. van den Brekel MW, Stel HV, Castelijns JA, et al. Cervical lymph node metastasis; assessment of radiologic criteria. Radiology 1990;177:379–84.
142. Glazer GM, Gross BH, Quint LE, et al. Normal mediastinal lymph nodes: number and size according to American Thoracic Society mapping. Am J Roentgenol 1985;144:261–5.
143. Callen PN, Korobkin M, Isherwood I. Computed tomographic evaluation of the retrocrural prevertebral space. Am J Roentgenol 1977;129:907–10.
144. Dorfman RE, Alpern MB, Gross BH, et al. Upper abdominal lymph nodes: criteria for normal size determined with CT. Radiology 1991;180:319–22.
145. Vinnicombe SJ, Norman AR, Nicolson V, et al. Normal pelvic lymph nodes: evaluation with CT after bipedal lymphangiography. Radiology 1995;194:349–55.

11

Nuclear Medicine

Guy Jerusalem, M.D., Ph.D.
Roland Hustinx, M.D., Ph.D.

POSITRON EMISSION TOMOGRAPHY USING ^{18}F-FLUORODEOXYGLUCOSE

Major advances have been made in the development and application of imaging techniques in oncology. Positron emission tomography (PET) is a unique form of diagnostic imaging that observes in vivo biologic changes using radiopharmaceuticals that closely mimic endogenous molecules. The most widely used radiotracer in oncology at this time is the glucose analogue ^{18}F-fluorodeoxyglucose (^{18}F-FDG). It can be efficiently radiolabeled by an automated method and its longer half-life (110 minutes compared with 20 minutes for carbon-11, for example) provides an opportunity for off-site preparation avoiding the need for an on-site cyclotron. Increased glycolysis is one of the most distinctive biochemical features of malignant cells because of the inefficient metabolism of glucose in malignant tumors. It results from the amplification of the glucose transporter proteins at the tumor cell surface, as well as from increased activity of various key enzymes, including hexokinase. Like glucose, ^{18}F-FDG is transported into cells by a glucose transporter protein and rapidly converted into ^{18}F-FDG-6-phosphate. As the latter is not a substrate for glucose-6-phosphate isomerase, it is biochemically trapped in metabolizing tissues.[1] Patients are studied in the fasting state for at least 6 hours prior to ^{18}F-FDG PET in order to minimize blood insulin levels and glucose utilization of normal tissues. ^{18}F-FDG PET is now routinely used in oncology.[2] Most of this chapter will focus on ^{18}F-FDG PET because it has become the imaging technique of choice in Nuclear Medicine. Although it has been proven to be superior to 67-gallium (^{67}Ga) scintigraphy, the limitations of ^{18}F-FDG PET have to be pointed out.[3] ^{18}F-FDG PET is not a tumor-specific agent. As for other imaging modalities, it is important to be aware of normal variants and benign diseases that may mimic more serious pathology. Physiological uptake of ^{18}F-FDG may be observed in the skeletal muscles after exercise or under tension, in the brown fat, in the myocardium, in the brain, in the urinary tract and in parts of the gastrointestinal tract (especially the stomach and caecum). Routine use of oral muscle relaxants such as benzodiazepines 1 hour before ^{18}F-FDG injection may decrease ^{18}F-FDG uptake in the muscles. Intravenous hydration and furosemide may be given to minimize interfering urinary activity in the kidney, ureter, and bladder. Thymic hyperplasia after treatment and reactive myeloid hyperplasia in bone marrow can mimic tumor infiltration. All acute infectious or inflammatory processes may also simulate malignant diseases. In fact, a high ^{18}F-FDG uptake is observed in neutrophils and macrophages. Increased ^{18}F-FDG uptake has been described, for example, in abscesses, active tuberculosis, fungal infections, sarcoidosis, and pancreatitis. Consequently, PET scans need to be interpreted in conjunction with a pertinent clinical history to help minimize the number of false-positive studies. Appropriate selection, referral and timing of scans in defined clinical situations, along with the knowledge of the potential pitfalls, will further lead to a reduction in the interpretation errors. Fusion PET/CT images will probably also contribute to a higher specificity. False-negative PET findings are related as for other imaging techniques to the spatial resolution of the method. Furthermore, uptake of ^{18}F-FDG is related to both the grade and proliferative activity of the tumor. Lower ^{18}F-FDG uptake is more frequently observed in low-grade, slowly proliferating tumors than in poorly differentiated, rapidly growing tumors. Brain lesions may remain undetected by whole-body PET because of high ^{18}F-FDG uptake in the normal brain. However, if clinically indicated, a PET scan of the brain can be performed under special technical conditions.

STAGING IN HD AND NHL BY ^{18}F-FDG PET

Methodologic problems are inherent to all imaging studies in patients suffering from lymphoma because a biopsy is only realized in a small number of lymphoma locations (Table 11–1). A biopsy is performed to obtain the diagnosis and to determine the histologic subtype of lymphoma. For ethical reasons, further biopsies of previously unknown lesions detected by ^{18}F-FDG PET are only performed when the result would influence staging and treatment. However, in the absence of a histologic proof (gold standard), the calculation of sensitivity and specificity is not possible. Most studies use a standard of reference. They examine the concordance between routine staging procedures (clinical examination, computed tomography, and/or other conventional imaging techniques is the standard of reference) and ^{18}F-FDG PET. Positive findings at both standard of reference and ^{18}F-FDG PET are regarded as actual locations of disease. Negative findings at both methods are regarded as true negative (no involvement by lymphoma). In case of discrepancy, response to treatment and follow-up data are used to assess the precision of the patient's original evaluation. However, this approach heavily biases results in favor of the least specific test, deceptively making it appear to be more accurate.[4]

Staging According to Sites of Disease

Lymph Node Staging

Several studies indicated good performances of PET for lymph node staging (Fig. 11–1).[5–8] ^{18}F-FDG PET detected sometimes additional lymphoma locations not shown by

Table 11–1. Role of ^{18}F-FDG PET in Staging

Confirmed Data
^{18}F-FDG PET is complementary but does not replace conventional staging techniques. Change in staging and treatment is observed in some patients.
Controversial Issue
A bone marrow biopsy has to be done in our opinion because ^{18}F-FDG PET has low sensitivity and specificity in the detection of bone marrow involvement in our experience.
Potential Indications
A baseline ^{18}F-FDG PET study may improve its specificity in the response evaluation during or after treatment. When an abnormal ^{18}F-FDG uptake is seen outside of the initially involved sites, infectious or inflammatory lesions have to be excluded.
^{18}F-FDG PET images may allow a better definition of the radiation fields.

^{18}F-FDG, ^{18}F-fluorodeoxyglucose; PET, positron emission tomography.

conventional staging procedures. ^{18}F-FDG PET should be considered as complementary sources of diagnostic information in lymph node staging.

Extranodal Disease

^{18}F-FDG PET may provide additional information about extranodal lymphoma locations.[9] It has better accuracy than CT for the detection of spleen involvement.[10] Detection of bone marrow involvement by ^{18}F-FDG PET is a controversial issue.[11] Diffuse bone marrow uptake can be observed by ^{18}F-FDG PET in patients with Hodgkin's disease (HD) at diagnosis related to reactive myeloid hyperplasia characteristic of some HD patients. Diffusely increased uptake is usually observed in reactive bone marrow, particularly following chemotherapy and growth factor (e.g., GCSF) administration. However, diffuse bone marrow ^{18}F-FDG uptake can also be caused by bone marrow involvement by malignancies such as lymphomas.[12] Some studies suggested that ^{18}F-FDG PET can correctly assess marrow disease status[13] and can provide additional information,[14] but more recent studies reported disappointing results and concluded that ^{18}F-FDG PET cannot replace bone marrow biopsy independently of the histologic subtype, because it missed bone marrow infiltration in many patients.[11,15,16] ^{18}F-FDG PET can replace bone scintigraphy in the initial staging of HD and non-Hodgkin's lymphoma (NHL).[17] ^{18}F-FDG PET can yield additional information complementary to endoscopy and CT in some patients for the evaluation of gastric high-grade NHL.[18] However, it is not useful for staging or follow-up of gastric NHL of the mucosa-associated lymphoid tissue (MALT) type.[19] Malignant lymphoma should be considered in the differential diagnosis of brain tumors showing high ^{18}F-FDG uptake.[20] The accumulation of ^{18}F-FDG in primary central nervous system (CNS) lymphoma is similar to that seen in anaplastic gliomas and is significantly more important than in low-grade astrocytomas.[21] ^{18}F-FDG PET may help to differentiate lymphoma from non-malignant infectious lesions in patients with AIDS.[22–24] High ^{18}F-FDG uptake most likely represents a malignant process that should be biopsied for confirmation rather than treated presumptively as infectious.[22]

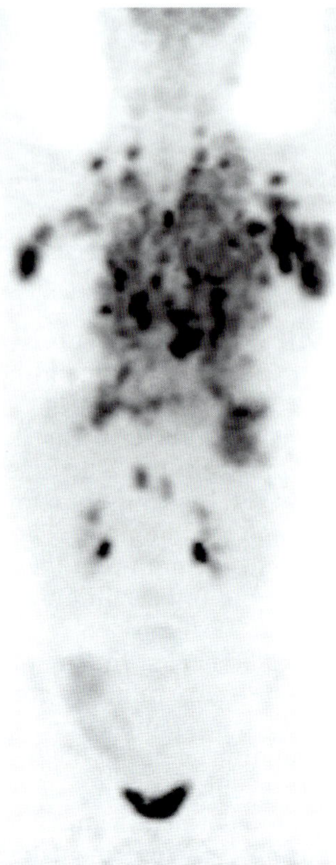

Figure 11–1. High-grade non-Hodgkin's lymphoma at initial diagnosis (3D projection image). There is massive mediastinal involvement as well as bilateral axillary lymph node infiltration. Note the extremely high metabolic activity of the lesions.

Overall Results in Staging and Cost-Effectiveness

The ability of PET to detect disease not suspected from conventional staging procedures has been demonstrated. Some patients have their staging changed,[8,25] and sometimes this will lead to change of treatment.[25] Only large trials incorporating PET evaluation at initial staging would be able to evaluate whether PET can refine prognostic indices and stratification for treatment. PET may have a major role for better defining the treatment of patients with HD, in particular when short-course chemotherapy is combined with involved field radiotherapy (Fig. 11–2). One of the main arguments against the widespread use of PET is its high costs (Fig. 11–2). However, PET might reduce the costs of diagnostic work-up in lymphoma patients by replacing other imaging procedures. Hoh et al.[6] found that ^{18}F-FDG PET may be an accurate and cost-effective method for staging or restaging HD and NHL. Accurate staging was performed in 17 of 18 patients using a ^{18}F-FDG PET-based staging algorithm compared to 15 of 18 patients in the conventional staging algorithm. The total management costs of ^{18}F-FDG PET–based staging algorithm were calculated to be almost half compared to the conventional staging

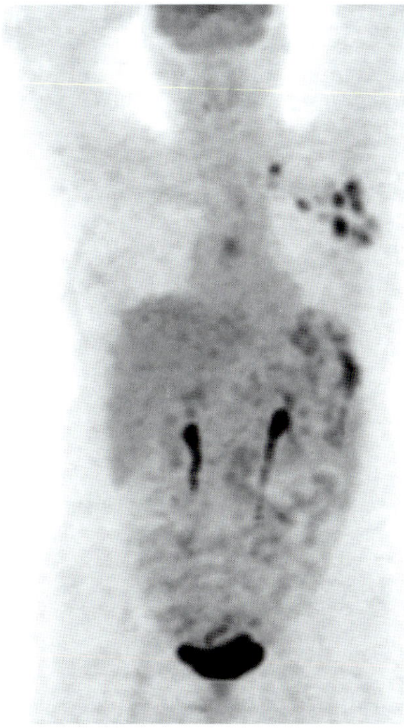

Figure 11–2. Initial evaluation of a patient with Hodgkin's disease (3D projection image). Hypermetabolic nodes are clearly seen in the left axilla and supraclavicular region, as well as in the subcarinal area.

algorithm. In the ^{18}F-FDG PET algorithm, additional diagnostic procedures were required in only two patients to resolve undetermined PET findings. However, not all studies indicated a cost saving by using ^{18}F-FDG PET. Klose et al.[26] found that PET upstaged 4 of 22 patients resulting in correct patient staging of 81.8% for CT and 100% for PET. This resulted in an incremental cost-effectiveness ratio (additional costs per additionally correctly staged patient) of 3,133 euros for PET versus CT.

Other important studies comparing staging based on PET to staging based on conventional imaging techniques will be discussed in the next section.

Results in Histologic Subtypes

Hodgkin's Disease

Although some small, single-institution studies have shown major impact of PET on staging and treatment, only large multicenter trials are able to evaluate the real impact. The results reported by various investigators are influenced by sometimes major methodologic problems. Only in few patients it has been proven by biopsy that the additional sites identified by PET contain disease or that those areas negative on PET, but positive on CT, are devoid of disease. However, one can definitively conclude that PET is useful for staging HD when it is performed in addition to conventional staging procedures. Most authors reported an upstaging or down-staging based on PET (Table 11–2). Although PET does not replace conventional staging techniques, it adds useful information.[27] Several studies indicate that PET failed to detect some lesions[28–31] or showed false-positive results.[28] Down-staging patients because of CT-

Table 11–2. Modification of Staging Based on PET in Hodgkin's Disease

Authors	Number of Cases
Bangerter et al.[28]	6/44 (14%)
Weidmann et al.[29]	3/20 (15%)
Partridge et al.[119]	21/44 (48%)
Jerusalem et al.[30]	7/33 (21%)
Hueltenschmidt et al.[78]	10/25 (40%)
Menzel et al.[120]	6/28 (21%)
Weihrauch et al.[31]	4/22 (18%)

PET, positron emission tomography.

positive and ^{18}F-FDG PET-negative lesions should be performed carefully, and only after a biopsy of the questionable site proved the absence of disease.[31] In the future, PET may be used for the planning of radiation fields. PET images could be registered with radiotherapy-planning CT images, allowing potentially better field arrangements and dose distributions.

Non-Hodgkin's Lymphoma

Correlation Between ^{18}F-FDG Uptake and Histologic Grade

CT and ^{67}Ga scintigraphy have extensively been used for tumor staging but cannot discriminate tumor grade. Rodriguez et al.[32] found that ^{18}F-FDG PET can predict the malignancy grade in NHL. In a study of 23 patients, ^{18}F-FDG uptake discriminated between high-grade and low-grade NHL, whereas 3 transformed low-grade NHL cases behaved in an intermediate manner. They conclude that tumor grading by ^{18}F-FDG PET may have clinical importance on a limited but clearly defined patient population with insufficient histologic data when a biopsy is difficult to obtain. Lapela et al.[33] also observed that a high ^{18}F-FDG accumulation in tumors is associated with a high histologic degree of malignancy as defined by the International Working Formulation or by the Kiel classification. However, not all studies indicated a good correlation between ^{18}F-FDG uptake and histologic grade. Newman et al.[5] studied 16 patients (only 3 at initial diagnosis) and found no difference in uptake between histologic grades. Standard uptake values (SUVs) did not vary significantly between cases of low- and intermediate-grade NHL, ranging from 2.4 to 18.7 in low-grade lymphoma, and from 4.3 to 12.8 in intermediate-grade disease. The highest absolute SUV was obtained in a patient with low-grade NHL. Separate lesions within the same patient were often associated with substantial differences in SUV. Nevertheless, previous treatment may have an impact on the results found in this study.

Correlation Between ^{18}F-FDG Uptake and Proliferative Activity

NHL with a high mitotic count and a high KI-67 labeling index tend to show an important accumulation of ^{18}F-FDG and high glucose metabolism.[34] On the other hand, a low KI-67 labeling index and low ^{18}F-FDG uptake are observed in patients with low-grade NHL. Lapela et al.[33] showed that a high S-fraction as measured by flow cytometry was associated with high ^{18}F-FDG uptake. However, in some patients ^{18}F-FDG uptake correlated poorly with the S-phase fraction.[35] Tumors are heterogeneous not only macroscopically (partially necrotic high-grade tumors), but also at a microscopic and at a metabolic level, whereas only the average metabolic activity will be measured by ^{18}F-FDG PET.

Correlation Between ^{18}F-FDG Uptake and Prognosis

^{18}F-FDG uptake before treatment may be useful for predicting response to therapy and prognosis.[36] The lowest tumor-to-normal tissue contrast ratio (TCR) was observed in a patient with low-grade, small lymphocytic lymphoma. A high TCR was observed in a patient with high-grade, immunoblastic lymphoma and in three intermediate-grade patients with poor prognosis in whom remission was never achieved. However, in some intermediate-grade NHL patients in complete remission, the TCR was not always lower than those of the poor prognosis patients. In the absence of other studies that confirm these results observed in a limited number of patients (n = 21),^{18}F-FDG PET is not routinely used as a prognostic factor before treatment.

Furthermore, Koga et al.[37] showed different levels of ^{18}F-FDG accumulation according to tumor location within the same patient suffering from untreated intermediate-grade NHL. Although CT showed multiple bulky bilateral submandibular, deep cervical, supraclavicular, axillary, hilar, mesenteric, and para-aortic lymph nodes, ^{18}F-FDG PET showed only a high accumulation of the radiotracer in the bilateral submandibular and deep cervical region. Bone marrow involvement was only detected by bone marrow biopsy. An immunohistochemical analysis demonstrated a high glucose transporter 1 (GLUT-1) expression in the right cervical lymph node that was biopsied. On the other hand, a negative GLUT-1 expression was observed in the bone marrow specimen. This case suggests that the differential ^{18}F-FDG accumulation may be associated with the degree of GLUT-1 expression in patients with lymphoma.

Diffuse Large B-Cell Lymphoma

Most PET studies included patients with HD and NHL of various histologic subtypes. Their results were discussed in the "Staging According to Sites of Disease" section. Staging has less impact on treatment in large B-cell lymphoma (LBCL) than in HD because polychemotherapy is indicated for all patients. Among the five factors of the International Prognostic Index, only stage of disease (one or two vs. three or four) and the number of extranodal sites (zero or one vs. two or more) can be influenced by more accurate staging. Radiotherapy is not used in most patients. However, it was important to show that ^{18}F-FDG PET identified LBCL correctly before using it for therapy monitoring. The group from Liège[38] showed that ^{18}F-FDG PET is an efficient, noninvasive method for staging and restaging aggressive NHL, but bone marrow biopsy remains to be performed in addition to PET. Most of the 53 patients suffered from LBCL. The results suggested that ^{18}F-FDG PET is more sensitive than physical examination, and CT for the detection of lymph nodes infiltrated by NHL. PET identified 39 clinically undetected lymph node areas, whereas clinical examination showed only 9 additional lesions not seen by ^{18}F-FDG PET. ^{18}F-FDG PET identified 21 thoracic and abdominopelvic lymph node regions not seen by CT, whereas CT showed only 5 areas not illustrated by ^{18}F-FDG PET. ^{18}F-FDG PET was as effective as CT for the detection of extranodal disease excluding bone marrow. Six lesions were only identified by ^{18}F-FDG PET, and 7 lesions were only shown by CT. ^{18}F-FDG PET missed known bone marrow infiltration in 5 patients. Elstrom et al.[16] found that ^{18}F-FDG PET detected disease in at least one site in all 51 patients with LBCL. Unfortunately, this study gives no information about the lesions that were missed by ^{18}F-FDG PET or those only shown by ^{18}F-FDG PET.

Peripheral T-Cell Lymphoma

Elstrom et al.[16] observed that only 2 of 5 patients suffering from peripheral T-cell lymphoma had ^{18}F-FDG uptake in at least one site of documented disease.

Enteropathy-Type T-Cell Lymphoma

Hoffmann et al.[39] imaged four patients suffering from enteropathy-type T-cell lymphoma (ETCL) before chemotherapy. All four patients showed markedly elevated intestinal ^{18}F-FDG uptake, with a maximal SUV of 6.4 to 8. In three cases, additional intestinal sites were seen and one of these patients had an additional hot spot in the lung. They also studied 12 patients suffering from coeliac disease (CD). SUVs in patients with ETCL were remarkably higher than in patients suffering from CD, irrespective of the activity of CD at the time of imaging.

Follicular and Small Lymphocytic NHL

Preliminary results indicate that the sensitivity of ^{18}F-FDG PET may be insufficient for low-grade NHL,[35] but other studies reported that ^{18}F-FDG PET can correctly identify sites of disease in low-grade NHL.[5,7,40] The first study including a high number of patients with low-grade NHL undergoing staging by ^{18}F-FDG PET was reported by Jerusalem et al.[41] The most important finding was that ^{18}F-FDG PET, when combined with a bone marrow biopsy, identified more lesions, and gave complementary information to conventional procedures for the staging of follicular NHL. ^{18}F-FDG PET detected 40% more abnormal lymph node areas than conventional staging in follicular lymphoma but was inappropriate for the staging of small lymphocytic lymphoma where it detected less than 58% of abnormal lymph node areas. This implies that ^{18}F-FDG PET may be useful for monitoring therapy results in follicular lymphoma. The total number of abnormal lymph node areas detected by ^{18}F-FDG PET for the whole group of patients was higher compared to conventional staging for peripheral (34% more lymph node areas detected) and thoracic (39% more) lymph node areas, but not for abdominal or pelvic lymph nodes (26% fewer areas detected). The optimal detection of abdominal or pelvic lymph nodes might be improved by attenuation correction not performed in this study. Except for bone marrow involvement, ^{18}F-FDG PET was as effective as standard procedures for the detection of other extranodal localizations. However, a few localizations were detected only by ^{18}F-FDG PET and a few others only by conventional procedures. ^{18}F-FDG PET identified more cases of splenic or hepatic involvement but CT showed more cases of pleural or lung involvement. Blum et al.[42] confirmed that ^{18}F-FDG PET may contribute to the management of patients with low-grade follicular NHL. ^{18}F-FDG PET was performed for staging at initial diagnosis (n = 12), for restaging at confirmed progression (n = 12), for possible progression (n = 21), or as part of routine clinical surveillance (n = 4). Treatment was changed according to ^{18}F-FDG PET at initial presentation because of modification of the radiation fields (n = 5) and/or modification of the treatment modality (chemotherapy used instead or in combination with radiotherapy; n = 3) in 6 of 12 patients. Ten of the 37 patients who underwent restaging ^{18}F-FDG PET also had their management influenced by the results. Although the authors found a high impact on patient management suggesting routine use of ^{18}F-FDG PET in follicular NHL, some shortcomings must be pointed out. Indeed, the analysis was retrospective, and there was a potential pre-test bias, as these patients underwent ^{18}F-FDG PET for clinical rather than for research purposes. More importantly, only a few lesions were biopsied. Finally, Elstrom et al.[16] reported that ^{18}F-FDG PET detected disease in at least one site in 41 of 42 patients with follicular NHL. The single case of undetected follicular NHL consisted of an ileal tumor shown only by endoscopic biopsy. Tumor volume may explain some false-negative ^{18}F-FDG PET studies. The two cases of low-grade cutaneous B-cell lymphoma were also not detected by ^{18}F-FDG PET in this study.

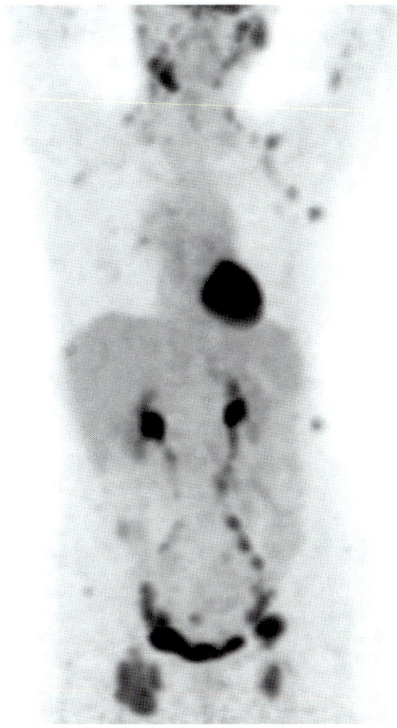

Figure 11–3. Whole-body FDG-PET study (3D projection image) showing multifocal recurrent non-Hodgkin's lymphoma (mantle cell). There is multiple nodal, bony, cutaneous and subcutaneous involvement.

Extranodal B-Cell Lymphoma of the Mucosa-Associated Lymphoid Tissue Type

Hoffmann et al.[19] observed no ^{18}F-FDG uptake in either extranodal or nodal sites of documented lymphoma involvement in all 10 patients included in their study. Nine patients had low-grade lymphomas (5 cases of gastric lymphoma, 2 patients with lymphoma arising in the lung, 1 parotid, and 1 lachrymal gland lymphoma), while 1 patient had a high-grade gastric lymphoma arising from a low-grade background. They concluded that ^{18}F-FDG PET is not useful for staging and follow-up of MALT-type lymphoma.

Nodal Marginal Zone Lymphoma

In a small study of six patients, five ^{18}F-FDG PET scans were positive, depicting all radiologically verified sites of lymphoma involvement, and identifying additional sites of disease. One patient with cervical lymph node involvement had a negative ^{18}F-FDG PET scan.[43]

Mantle Cell Lymphoma

The number of patients who underwent ^{18}F-FDG PET with this diagnosis is too small to assess the utility of ^{18}F-FDG PET. Elstrom et al.[16] detected disease in at least one site in all seven patients with mantle cell lymphoma (MCL) (Fig. 11–3). In contrast, Jerusalem et al.[44] reported a case of false-negative ^{18}F-FDG PET in MCL.

Plasmacytoma and Multiple Myeloma

Durie et al.[45] found that a negative ^{18}F-FDG PET reliably predicts stable monoclonal gammapathy of undetermined significance (MGUS). Myeloma has developed in only 1 of 14 MGUS patients at 8 months. Conversely, all 16 previously untreated patients with active myeloma had focal or diffusely positive ^{18}F-FDG PET findings. ^{18}F-FDG PET has the potential to detect the early phase of bone marrow involvement in patients with extramedullary plasmacytoma,[46] and may therefore be useful for staging at initial presentation.[47] Schirrmeister et al.[48] studied 15 patients with plasmacytoma. ^{18}F-FDG PET detected 20 (10 confirmed) further plasmacytoma lesions, negative on standard staging methods, in four patients, changing the diagnosis from plasmacytoma to multiple myeloma. Consequently, a potentially curative local therapy was changed to a palliative systemic therapy. ^{18}F-FDG PET was false negative in one patient, and indeterminate in another. The same group showed that ^{18}F-FDG PET is highly accurate in detecting multiple myeloma.[49] It revealed a greater extent of disease than routine radiographs. However, other causes than active disease can be associated with diffuse bone marrow uptake of the radiotracer. The authors suggest that PET should not be used routinely in all patients with multiple myeloma, but only in selected situations such as the control of therapy in patients with nonsecretory myeloma when determination of paraprotein levels fails to reflect the activity of disease. ^{18}F-FDG PET may also be useful in the follow-up after transplantation procedures, so that focal sites of relapse may receive earlier local treatment.[47]

RESPONSE EVALUATION DURING OR AFTER TREATMENT BY ^{18}F-FDG PET

The limitations of conventional radiologic procedures for response evaluation are very well known (Table 11–3). Tumor volume reduction based on radiologic criteria is a late sign of effective therapy. Residual masses may be

Table 11–3. Role of ^{18}F-FDG PET in Response Assessment

Confirmed Data

^{18}F-FDG PET is the best noninvasive imaging technique:
For distinguishing responders from nonresponders to reinduction chemotherapy before high-dose chemotherapy.
For the end of treatment evaluation (in particular, in the presence of a residual mass).
Positive findings on PET do not necessarily represent residual disease:
Infectious or inflammatory lesions can accumulate the radiotracer.
A negative PET cannot exclude minimal residual disease:
Do not stop a treatment only based on a negative PET!

Controversial Issue

The best timing of PET:
We suggest waiting at least 1 month after the last day of chemotherapy (whenever possible) because of the risk of a temporarily reduced metabolic activity!
We suggest waiting at least 3 months after radiotherapy (whenever possible) because of the risk of radiotherapy-induced inflammation, but earlier response assessment is possible in most patients (characteristic ^{18}F-FDG uptake pattern after radiotherapy).

Perspectives

Early treatment evaluation:
Persistent tumoral ^{18}F-FDG uptake after a few cycles of chemotherapy indicates a high risk of treatment failure.
Further studies are warranted before using ^{18}F-FDG PET routinely in this indication (best timing?).

^{18}F-FDG, ^{18}F-fluorodeoxyglucose; PET, positron emission tomography.

Table 11–4. Shortcomings of ^{18}F-FDG PET in Response Evaluation: Documented Causes of False-Positive PET Studies

Second primary[51,55,80]
Rebound thymic hyperplasia[67,76,78,121,122]
Histiocytic reaction[76,123]
Benign follicular lymph node hyperplasia[51]
Unspecific lymphadenitis[74]
Pneumonia[65]
Inflammatory lung process[78]
Pleural inflammation[73]
Radiotherapy induced pneumonitis[29,69]
Toxoplasmosis[124]
Tuberculosis[51]
Epitheloid cell granuloma[125]
Eosinophilic granuloma[126]
Erythema nodosum[127]
Thyroid adenoma[78]
Fracture at site of lymphoma infiltration before treatment[65]
Fistula[128]
Granulation tissue[129]
Nonviable scar tissue[72]

^{18}F-FDG, ^{18}F-fluorodeoxyglucose; PET, positron emission tomography.

present at the end of treatment, even in patients responding very well, with normalization of all clinical and biological abnormalities. Unfortunately, there are no reliable radiographic parameters for CT or MRI that permit differentiation between malignant and fibrotic or necrotic tissue. ^{18}F-FDG PET is a functional imaging technique in which the uptake of glucose is related to tumor viability. It has the advantage of functional tissue characterization that is largely independent of morphologic criteria. ^{18}F-FDG PET is now the imaging technique of choice for determining chemosensitivity before high-dose chemotherapy followed by autologous stem cell transplantation (ASCT) and for end of treatment evaluation in lymphoma patients. Promising results have also been reported in early response assessment. However, it is important to take into account the shortcomings of ^{18}F-FDG PET for appropriate utilization of PET findings in the patient management. The spatial resolution of current ^{18}F-FDG PET instrumentation is approximately 5 to 8 mm. Radiotracer uptake in structures less than twice the spatial resolution of the tomograph is underestimated (i.e., partial volume effect). There is also a risk of temporarily reduced metabolic activity soon after chemotherapy. Although the best timing for end of treatment evaluation remains unknown, most investigators suggest waiting at least 1 month after the last day of chemotherapy. Even if the spatial resolution of ^{18}F-FDG PET improves in the future, it cannot exclude minimal residual disease.[50] Consequently, it is not possible to decide to stop a treatment based only on a negative ^{18}F-FDG PET. The insecurities regarding the potential of a residual vital tumor tissue not detected by ^{18}F-FDG PET may be overcome by repeated imaging at time intervals.[51] Positive findings on PET as with all other imaging modalities do not necessarily represent residual disease. Physiologic uptake can be misinterpreted in particular by an inexperienced observer. A learning curve when PET is first introduced at a center may have an impact on the false-positive rate. Meticulous evaluation of PET images is mandatory to avoid false-positive PET findings associated with muscular tension or normal intestinal structures. Documented causes of false-positive PET studies in response assessment of lymphoma patients are shown in Table 11–4.

Early Response Evaluation

Romer et al.[52] reported a rapid decrease of ^{18}F-FDG uptake by tumoral tissue as early as 7 days after chemotherapy for NHL, illustrating the potential role of PET in response evaluation (Fig. 11–4). Early recognition of the ineffectiveness of chemotherapy could allow a more rapid initiation of salvage treatments potentially improving the outcome. Early response evaluation by ^{18}F-FDG PET ("interim PET") after one, a few cycles, or at mid-treatment can predict response, progression-free survival (PFS), and overall survival (OS) in lymphoma patients[53–58] (Table 11–5). Excepting two studies with a mixed patient population,[53,54] all other studies[55–58] included only patients suffering from NHL. All studies used dedicated PET systems except one[53] that used a dual-head coincidence camera. The predictive value of interim ^{18}F-FDG PET is independent of conven-

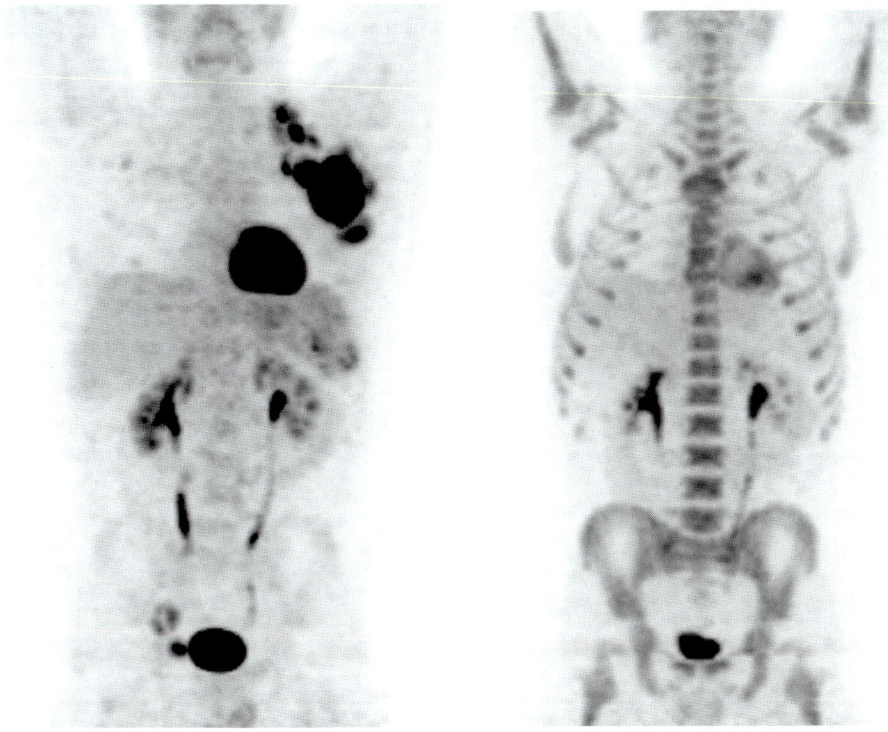

A B

Figure 11–4. High-grade non-Hodgkin's lymphoma in a 23-year-old man. **A:** Hypermetabolic lesions in the left axilla (3D projection image), in the supraclavicular region, in the right inguinocrural area, as well as splenic involvement. **B:** Result of two courses of chemotherapy. There is a complete metabolic response and a high bone marrow uptake, as seen usually in these circumstances.

tional prognostic factors determined before treatment.[58] The interim ^{18}F-FDG PET after two cycles has also clearly better test characteristics (better positive predictive value, negative predictive value, and interobserver agreement) than ^{67}Ga scintigraphy.[55] The best moment (optimal sensitivity and prediction of PFS) to perform ^{18}F-FDG PET remains unknown. Kostakoglu et al.[53] reported that the ^{18}F-FDG PET results obtained after the first cycle correlated better with PFS than ^{18}F-FDG PET findings obtained after completion of chemotherapy. The positive predictive value (PPV) of interim PET in selected studies is 91% (81/89) (Table 11–5), compared to 85% (118/139) for all studies in end-of-treatment evaluations reported in Table 11–6. On the other hand, the negative predictive value (NPV) is 79% (84/106) for interim PET (Table 11–5) and 90% (353/395) for end-of-treatment evaluations (Table 11–6). Most studies are oversimplified by defining only two categories of patients, either with or without residual ^{18}F-FDG uptake within areas initially involved by lymphoma. Mikhaeel et al.[56] described a third group of patients with minimal residual uptake on interim PET defined as low-grade uptake, just above the background, in only one focus. No relapse was observed in all four patients in this group. Consequently, the authors analyzed these patients and the five patients with a negative PET as a group. Semiquantitative studies are probably more appropriate but methodological problems remain to be resolved. In particular, a pronounced decrease of ^{18}F-FDG uptake may be influenced by rapid tumor shrinkage resulting in partial volume effect. Different imaging times over multiple bed positions may also influence SUV analysis because ^{18}F-FDG uptake does not reach a plateau in the 3-hour post-injection time. Torizuka et al.[54] measured, in addition to visual analysis (results included in Table 11–5), the SUV of the tumor demonstrating the highest ^{18}F-FDG uptake at the baseline study and the SUV of the same tumor after one or two cycles of therapy. Using

Table 11–5. Early Response Assessment

Author	NHL	HD	NHL + HD	Number of Cycles Before Evaluation	Follow-up (months)	Positive Predictive Value	Negative Predictive Value
Kostakoglu et al., 2002[53]	17	13	30	1	19	87% (13/15)	87% (13/15)
Torizuka et al., 2004[54]	17	3	20	1–2	24	87% (14/16)	50% (2/4)
Zijlstra et al., 2003[55]	26	0	26	2	25	75% (9/12)	67% (9/14)
Mikhaeel et al., 2000[56]	23	0	23	2–4	30	87% (7/8)	100% (15/15)
Jerusalem et al., 2000[57]	28	0	28	3 (2–5)	17	100% (5/5)	67% (14/21)
Spaepen et al., 2002[58]	70	0	70	3–4	36	100% (33/33)	84% (31/37)
Overall	**181**	**16**	**197**			**91% (81/89)**	**79% (84/106)**

HD, Hodgkin's disease; NHL, non-Hodgkin's lymphoma.

Table 11–6. Predictive Value of Whole-Body ^{18}F-FDG PET for Post-Treatment Evaluation

Authors	Number of Patients			Median Follow-up (months)	Positive Predictive Value	Negative Predictive Value
	HD	NHL	HD + NHL			
Mixed Population						
De Wit et al., 1997[65]	17	17	34	14	70% (12/17)	100% (17/17)
Jerusalem et al., 1999[50]	19	35	54	23	100% (6/6)	83% (40/48)
Zinzani et al., 1999[66]	13	31	44	20	100% (13/13)	97% (30/31)
Bangerter et al., 1999[67]	14	22	36	31	56% (5/9)	93% (25/27)
Mikhaeel et al., 2000[68]	15	17	32	38	89% (8/9)	91% (21/23)
Overall	**78**	**122**	**200**		**81% (44/54)**	**91% (133/146)**
HD						
De Wit et al., 2001[73]	33			26	67% (10/15)	100% (18/18)
Dittmann et al., 2001[74]	26			6	87% (7/8)	94% (17/18)
Spaepen et al., 2001[75]	60			32	100% (5/5)	91% (50/55)
Weihrauch et al., 2001[76]	29			28	60% (6/10)	84% (16/19)
Guay et al., 2003[77]	48			16	92% (11/12)	92% (33/36)
Overall	**196**				**78% (39/50)**	**92% (134/146)**
NHL						
Spaepen et al., 2001[79]		93		21	100% (26/26)	84% (56/67)
Mikhaeel et al., 2000[56]		45		30	100% (9/9)	83% (30/36)
Overall		**138**			**100% (35/35)**	**83% (86/103)**
All studies	*274*	*260*	*534*		*85% (118/139)*	*90% (353/395)*

^{18}F-FDG, ^{18}F-fluorodeoxyglucose; HD, Hodgkin's disease; NHL, non-Hodgkin's lymphoma; PET, positron emission tomography.

60% reduction as a cut-off value, the responders were clearly separated from the nonresponders, with the exception of one nonresponder. The probability that PET remains positive depends on the sensitivity of the tomograph (smallest lesion that can be detected), the biology of the tumor (more rapid response in aggressive tumors), the tumor mass at diagnosis (tumor shrinkage below the detection level, later in larger tumors), the drugs used (impact of monoclonal antibodies such as rituximab), the dose–response of chemotherapy (more rapid regression if higher doses), and the interval between the last day of chemotherapy and ^{18}F-FDG PET (risk of temporarily reduced metabolic activity early after chemotherapy). Furthermore, a transient increase in inflammatory cells may result in overestimation of the fraction of viable cancer cells, as shown in a tumor mouse model.[59] Although the data are promising, they remain preliminary. We estimate that it is not yet indicated to change routinely the treatment strategy based on residual ^{18}F-FDG uptake in PET studies realized after one or a few cycles of chemotherapy. However, further studies determining the role of interim PET in patient management are clearly indicated based on these encouraging results.

Evaluation of Chemosensitivity Before High-Dose Chemotherapy

^{18}F-FDG PET is able to differentiate between responders and nonresponders at an earlier time point than conventional CT or MRI. Several studies indicate that ^{18}F-FDG PET is now the imaging technique of choice for this indication. Patients with a negative ^{18}F-FDG PET after induction or reinduction chemotherapy have a better prognosis and are good candidates for high-dose chemotherapy followed by ASCT. However, even some patients with residual ^{18}F-FDG uptake will have a good outcome after this treatment, and it is questionable if clinicians will cancel high-dose chemotherapy followed by ASCT only because ^{18}F-FDG PET remains positive after induction or reinduction treatment. No standard alternative treatment with curative intent is available at this time. An important challenge for the future is the development of successful treatment strategies for chemorefractory patients identified by ^{18}F-FDG PET.

Becherer et al.[60] studied 16 patients (10 NHL, 6 HD) after induction or reinduction chemotherapy. They found in PET-negative patients an overall and relapse-free 1-year survival rate of 100% compared to 55% and 18%, respectively, in PET-positive patients. Cremerius et al.[61] reported that 6 of 7 patients (NHL) who did not achieve at least a partial metabolic response (PMR) after complete induction chemotherapy before ASCT developed lymphoma progression, while 10 of 15 patients (NHL) with complete metabolic response or PMR remained in continuous remission. Filmont et al.[62] found that PET findings 2 to 5 weeks after initiation of salvage chemotherapy were strongly correlated with disease-free survival in 20 patients (6 HD, 14 NHL). Seven of 8 patients with a negative ^{18}F-FDG PET remained in CR, whereas 11 of 12 patients with a positive ^{18}F-FDG PET relapsed after ASCT. Finally, the study reported by Spaepen et al.[63] confirmed the important prognostic role of ^{18}F-FDG PET in the pre-transplantation evaluation of patients with NHL allowing the selection of chemosensitive patients for high-dose chemotherapy followed by ASCT. Twenty-five of 30 patients with a negative ^{18}F-FDG PET after reinduction chemotherapy remained in CR compared to only 4 of 30 patients with a positive ^{18}F-FDG PET.

Evaluation After Completion of Chemotherapy and/or Radiotherapy

Incomplete regression of a lymphomatous mass after chemotherapy and/or radiotherapy constitutes a major diagnostic problem. Residual masses are more frequently observed in patients with an aggressive NHL and a large tumor mass at diagnosis or those with scleronodular HD. ^{67}Ga scintigraphy has become a standard procedure for the post-treatment evaluation of patients with lymphoma.[64] However, despite the important role of ^{67}Ga scintigraphy in lymphoma imaging, ^{18}F-FDG PET is now considered the imaging technique of choice for the end-of-treatment assessment for patients suffering from lymphoma. A positive PET scan after treatment is related in most patients to residual tumor cells accumulating the radiotracer. However, it is prudent to correlate PET findings with clinical data, other imaging modalities and/or a biopsy before starting salvage therapy. In particular, when abnormal ^{18}F-FDG uptake is seen outside the initially involved sites, infectious or inflammatory lesions have to be excluded. On the other hand, a negative ^{18}F-FDG PET study cannot exclude minimal residual disease leading later to a clinical relapse. Table 11–6 summarizes the PPV and NPV of whole-body PET at the end-of-treatment evaluation as reported in selected papers written in English. In a mixed population of 200 patients (HD: 78, NHL: 122),[50,65–68] the PPV was 81% and the NPV is 91%. Three papers[69–71] were not included because only the region of interest (residual mass) instead of the whole-body was studied by PET. Naumann et al.[72] reported details about the accuracy of PET according to uptake inside or outside of residual masses, but unfortunately not for the overall evaluation, explaining why this study is not included in Table 11–6. They observed a low PPV (30%) in 58 patients (43 HD, 15 NHL). Finally, Mikosch et al.[51] reported data in a large patient population (44 HD, 49 NHL), but some patients had repeated ^{18}F-FDG PET studies (121 studies in 93 patients) owing to recurrent disease or partial remission. Interestingly, they observed a PPV of 79% and a NPV of 92%, comparable to the values found in the mixed patient population at the end of treatment (Table 11–6). In a selected group of 192 patients suffering from HD,[73–77] the PPV is 78% and the NPV is 92%. The paper written by Hueltenschmidt et al.[78] reporting a PPV of 86% (18/21) and a NPV of 96% (15/16) was not included in the analysis because some patients underwent PET several times, and accuracy of PET was not unambiguously verified in all patients. Finally, the PPV is 100% (36/36) and the NPV is 83% (86/103) in a selected group of patients with NHL.[56,79] In the update of our results presented at the American Society of Clinical Oncology (ASCO) meeting in 2003,[80] we found a PPV of 33% (1/3) and a NPV of 94% (34/36) in HD, compared with a PPV of 85% (11/13) and a NPV of 79% (44/56) in NHL. The accuracy was comparable in HD (35/39: 90%) and in NHL (55/69: 80%). We explained the differences observed in our experience according to the histologic subtypes by the better prognosis of HD. Give that relapse is a rare event in HD, the impact of a false-positive PET on the PPV is more important in HD than in NHL. On the other hand, because PET cannot exclude minimal residual disease, and the risk of relapse is more important in NHL, the NPV is lower in NHL than in HD. Several factors can explain major differences between the results reported for PPV and NPV. Patient populations are not only small but most times very heterogeneous. The natural history of low-grade and high-grade NHL is very different, but all patients are analyzed together in some studies. The predictive value of relapse depends also on the initial prognostic factors of patients. The PPV is higher and the NPV is lower in the high-risk patients. Cremerius et al.[70] found a NPV of 90% in patients with a moderate risk compared to 50% to 67% in high-risk patients. PET is only clinically useful if relapse is not definitively known before the patient undergoes the imaging study. Inclusion of patients with known or suspected relapse will improve the PPV. Short follow-up will be in favor of a better NPV. In the update of our results, we found a NPV of only 80%, but follow-up periods were up to 8 years for some patients. We suggested reporting 6-month and 1-year PFS data in order to allow better comparisons between studies. Only two studies discussed the problem of questionable findings.[70,72] In fact, in our practice PET is not always positive or negative, but is sometimes suggestive of residual tumor. Both studies[70,72] reported that accuracy is better if questionable lesions are analyzed as negative findings. However, from a clinical point of view, sensitivity (detection of residual disease allowing earlier salvage therapy) is probably more important than accuracy. In our center, we favor an initial higher-sensitivity interpretation of PET. In order to improve specificity, we correlate our findings a second time with clinical information and other imaging modalities, as well as encourage, whenever possible, a multidisciplinary interpretation.

Response Evaluation After Radioimmunotherapy

Torizuka et al.[81] examined 14 patients with NHL treated by ^{131}I-anti-B1 (CD20) radioimmunotherapy (RIT). They assessed the tumor metabolic response by ^{18}F-FDG PET at 30 to 70 days after RIT in eight patients, and 5 to 7 days after RIT in six patients. They found that the metabolic data obtained 1 to 2 months after RIT correlate well with the ultimate best response of NHL to RIT, whereas early PET data after RIT did not appear to be consistently useful for early prediction of response. Further studies are clearly warranted before using ^{18}F-FDG PET routinely for monitoring response to RIT.

ROUTINE FOLLOW-UP OF ASYMPTOMATIC PATIENTS BY ^{18}F-FDG PET

Patients with a high risk of recurrence and an excellent chance of salvage should be observed closely. Good clinical judgment and a careful history and physical examination are the most important components of monitoring patients after treatment. Routine imaging studies are generally not performed. Relapse of lymphoma is usually identified as a result of investigation of symptoms.[82,83] There are no data available about the role of PET in the routine follow-up of patients suffering from NHL. Preliminary data have been presented by Jerusalem et al. showing that PET is able to detect preclinical relapse in patients with HD.[84] They performed ^{18}F-FDG PET every 4 to 6 months for 2 to 3 years after the end of polychemotherapy and/or radiotherapy in 36 patients. All five patients presenting residual tumor (n = 1) or relapse (n = 4) were correctly identified until 9 months before confirmation by biopsy (n = 4) or by conventional imaging techniques (n = 1). Unfortunately, false-positive ^{18}F-FDG PET studies incorrectly suggested possible relapse in 6 other patients, but conventional imaging techniques and a confirmatory PET some months later were always negative. Rebound thymic hyperplasia was observed in 19% of all PET studies. Further studies determining the impact of PET on outcome and a cost-benefit analysis are warranted before using PET routinely in the follow-up of patients with HD.

USE OF ^{18}F-FDG PET IN CHILDHOOD LYMPHOMA

There are only preliminary data available on the clinical utility and impact on management in childhood lymphoma.[85–87] The role of PET in imaging childhood and adult lymphomas is likely similar. However, a prospective multicenter PET study should be realized to analyze systematically the value of PET in staging and restaging children and adolescents, especially to indicate the role of PET in exclusion of vital tumor in residual masses.

^{67}GA SCINTIGRAPHY

^{67}Ga scintigraphy was the functional imaging technique of choice for the prediction of response early in the course of treatment, and for the assessment of response after treatment in lymphoma before the introduction of ^{18}F-FDG PET into the routine practice of oncology. Unfortunately, using ^{67}Ga scintigraphy as a lymphoma-seeking agent is associated with many drawbacks. Its sensitivity for staging lymphoma varies with localization,[88–98] and the size[89,92,99] and cell type.[89,90,93,95,96,99–104] ^{67}Ga scintigraphy is more effective for evaluating masses in the mediastinum than in the abdomen owing to physiologic abdominal uptake. However, nonspecific uptake in hilar regions[105–108] and in the thymus of young patients with thymic rebound after chemotherapy[109,110] can lead to false-positive studies. The sensitivity of ^{67}Ga is disappointing in tumors smaller than 1.5 to 2 cm.[111] Moreover,[67] a scintigraphy should always be performed before treatment to determine if the individual patient has a gallium-avid lymphoma.[112] Low sensitivity for ^{67}Ga scintigraphy is found by most authors in low-grade NHL. ^{67}Ga scintigraphy is considered to be more inconvenient than ^{18}F-FDG PET because the scanner must be performed several days after the administration of ^{67}Ga, whereas a PET study can be performed 1 hour after the injection of ^{18}F-FDG. ^{18}F-FDG PET also results in lower radiation exposure. Finally, studies that directly compared ^{67}Ga scintigraphy and ^{18}F-FDG PET found that PET provides higher-quality images and appears to be more sensitive for detecting nodal and extranodal sites of disease.[113–118]

THE USE OF ^{18}F-FDG PET IN LYMPHOMA PATIENTS: CONCLUSIONS AND PERSPECTIVES

^{18}F-FDG PET is now routinely used for staging and response evaluation in patients with HD and NHL. Its clinical impact on staging and management of patients has been shown. However, positive findings on PET, as with all other imaging techniques, do not necessarily represent disease, and a biopsy is the only true diagnostic test. As sampling errors may be a limitation of biopsy, in particular in residual masses, PET may be useful to direct the biopsy, if PET is positive. PET should be used within a multidisciplinary team. It is important to correlate the ^{18}F-FDG PET findings with the clinical data and the results of other conventional imaging methods. If necessary, repeated imaging at time interval has to be considered. False-positive PET studies may become negative. On the other hand, minimal residual disease may become detectable. One can speculate that fusion PET/CT images will improve specificity. New radiotracers such as ^{18}F-fluorothymidine may be useful for response assessment in the future.

References

1. Gallagher BM, Fowler JS, Gutterson NI, et al. Metabolic trapping as a principle of radiopharmaceutical design: some factors responsible for the biodistribution of [18F] 2-deoxy-2-fluoro-D-glucose. J Nucl Med 1978;19:1154–61.
2. Jerusalem G, Hustinx R, Beguin Y, et al. PET scan imaging in oncology. Eur J Cancer 2003;39:1525–34.
3. Jerusalem G, Hustinx R, Beguin Y, et al. The value of positron emission tomography (PET) imaging in disease staging and therapy assessment. Ann Oncol 2002;13 Suppl 4:227–34.
4. Segall GM. FDG PET imaging in patients with lymphoma: a clinical perspective. J Nucl Med 2001;42:609–10.
5. Newman JS, Francis IR, Kaminski MS, et al. Imaging of lymphoma with PET with 2-[F-18]-fluoro-2-deoxy-D-glucose: correlation with CT. Radiology 1994;190:111–6.
6. Hoh CK, Glaspy J, Rosen P, et al. Whole-body FDG-PET imaging for staging of Hodgkin's disease and lymphoma. J Nucl Med 1997;38:343–8.
7. Moog F, Bangerter M, Diederichs CG, et al. Lymphoma: role of whole-body 2-deoxy-2-[F-18]fluoro-D-glucose (FDG) PET in nodal staging. Radiology 1997;203:795–800.
8. Jerusalem G, Warland V, Najjar F, et al. Whole-body 18F-FDG PET for the evaluation of patients with Hodgkin's disease and non-Hodgkin's lymphoma. Nucl Med Commun 1999;20:13–20.
9. Moog F, Bangerter M, Diederichs CG, et al. Extranodal malignant lymphoma: detection with FDG PET versus CT. Radiology 1998;206:475–81.
10. Rini JN, Leonidas JC, Tomas MB, et al. 18F-FDG PET versus CT for evaluating the spleen during initial staging of lymphoma. J Nucl Med 2003;44:1072–4.
11. Kostakoglu L and Goldsmith SJ. Fluorine-18 fluorodeoxyglucose positron emission tomography in the staging and follow-up of lymphoma: is it time to shift gears? Eur J Nucl Med 2000;27:1564–78.
12. Chiang SB, Rebenstock A, Guan L, et al. Diffuse bone marrow involvement of Hodgkin lymphoma mimics hematopoietic cytokine-mediated FDG uptake on FDG PET imaging. Clin Nucl Med 2003;28:674–6.
13. Carr R, Barrington SF, Madan B, et al. Detection of lymphoma in bone marrow by whole-body positron emission tomography. Blood 1998;91:3340–6.

14. Moog F, Bangerter M, Kotzerke J, et al. 18-F-fluorodeoxyglucose-positron emission tomography as a new approach to detect lymphomatous bone marrow. J Clin Oncol 1998;16:603–9.
15. Jerusalem G, Silvestre RM, Beguin Y, et al. Does 18F-FDG PET replace bone marrow biopsy (BMB) in patients with Hodgkin's disease (HD) or non-Hodgkin's lymphoma (NHL). Blood 2002;100:768a [Abstract 3039].
16. Elstrom R, Guan L, Baker G, et al. Utility of FDG-PET scanning in lymphoma by WHO classification. Blood 2003;101:3875–6.
17. Moog F, Kotzerke J, and Reske SN. FDG PET can replace bone scintigraphy in primary staging of malignant lymphoma. J Nucl Med 1999;40:1407–13.
18. Rodriguez M, Ahlstrom H, Sundin A, et al. [18F] FDG PET in gastric non-Hodgkin's lymphoma. Acta Oncol 1997;36:577–84.
19. Hoffmann M, Kletter K, Diemling M, et al. Positron emission tomography with fluorine-18-2-fluoro-2-deoxy-D-glucose (F18-FDG) does not visualize extranodal B-cell lymphoma of the mucosa-associated lymphoid tissue (MALT)-type. Ann Oncol 1999;10:1185–9.
20. Kuwabara Y, Ichiya Y, Otsuka M, et al. High [18F]FDG uptake in primary cerebral lymphoma: a PET study. J Comput Assist Tomogr 1988;12:47–8.
21. Rosenfeld SS, Hoffman JM, Coleman RE, et al. Studies of primary central nervous system lymphoma with fluorine-18-fluorodeoxyglucose positron emission tomography. J Nucl Med 1992;33:532–6.
22. Hoffman JM, Waskin HA, Schifter T, et al. FDG-PET in differentiating lymphoma from nonmalignant central nervous system lesions in patients with AIDS. J Nucl Med 1993;34:567–75.
23. Pierce MA, Johnson MD, Maciunas RJ, et al. Evaluating contrast-enhancing brain lesions in patients with AIDS by using positron emission tomography. Ann Intern Med 1995;123:594–8.
24. Heald AE, Hoffman JM, Bartlett JA, et al. Differentiation of central nervous system lesions in AIDS patients using positron emission tomography (PET). Int J STD AIDS 1996;7:337–46.
25. Buchmann I, Reinhardt M, Elsner K, et al. 2-(fluorine-18)fluoro-2-deoxy-D-glucose positron emission tomography in the detection and staging of malignant lymphoma. A bicenter trial. Cancer 2001;91:889–99.
26. Klose T, Leidl R, Buchmann I, et al. Primary staging of lymphomas: cost-effectiveness of FDG-PET versus computed tomography. Eur J Nucl Med 2000;27:1457–64.
27. Jerusalem G and Beguin Y. Does positron emission tomography have a role in routine clinical practice in patients with Hodgkin's disease ? Clin Lymphoma 2002;3:125–6.
28. Bangerter M, Moog F, Buchmann I, et al. Whole-body 2-[18F]-fluoro-2-deoxy-D-glucose positron emission tomography (FDG-PET) for accurate staging of Hodgkin's disease. Ann Oncol 1998;9:1117–22.
29. Weidmann E, Baican B, Hertel A, et al. Positron emission tomography (PET) for staging and evaluation of response to treatment in patients with Hodgkin's disease. Leuk Lymph 1999;34:545–51.
30. Jerusalem G, Beguin Y, Fassotte MF, et al. Whole-body positron emission tomography using 18F-fluorodeoxyglucose compared to standard procedures for staging patients with Hodgkin's disease. Haematologica 2001;86:266–73.
31. Weihrauch MR, Re D, Bischoff S, et al. Whole-body positron emission tomography using 18F-fluorodeoxyglucose for initial staging of patients with Hodgkin's disease. Ann Hematol 2002;81:20–5.
32. Rodriguez M, Rehn S, Ahlstrom H, et al. Predicting malignancy grade with PET in non-Hodgkin's lymphoma. J Nucl Med 1995;36:1790–6.
33. Lapela M, Leskinen S, Minn HR, et al. Increased glucose metabolism in untreated non-Hodgkin's lymphoma: a study with positron emission tomography and fluorine-18-fluorodeoxyglucose. Blood 1995;86:3522–7.
34. Okada J, Yoshikawa K, Itami M, et al. Positron emission tomography using fluorine-18-fluorodeoxyglucose in malignant lymphoma: a comparison with proliferative activity. J Nucl Med 1992;33:325–9.
35. Leskinen-Kallio S, Ruotsalainen U, Nagren K, et al. Uptake of carbon-11-methionine and fluorodeoxyglucose in non-Hodgkin's lymphoma: a PET study. J Nucl Med 1991; 32:1211–8.
36. Okada J, Yoshikawa K, Imazeki K, et al. The use of FDG-PET in the detection and management of malignant lymphoma: correlation of uptake with prognosis. J Nucl Med 1991;32:686–91.
37. Koga H, Matsuo Y, Sasaki M, et al. Differential FDG accumulation associated with GLUT–1 expression in a patient with lymphoma. Ann Nucl Med 2003;17:327–31.
38. Najjar F, Jerusalem G, Paulus P, et al. Intérêt clinique de la tomographie à émission de positons dans la détection et le bilan d'extension des lymphomes non Hodgkiniens de malignité intermédiaire ou élevée. Médecine nucléaire Imagerie fonctionnelle et métabolique 1999; 23:281–90.
39. Hoffmann M, Vogelsang H, Kletter K, et al. 18F-fluoro-deoxy-glucose positron emission tomography (18F-FDG-PET) for assessment of enteropathy-type T cell lymphoma. Gut 2003;52:347–51.
40. Stumpe KD, Urbinelli M, Steinert HC, et al. Whole-body positron emission tomography using fluorodeoxyglucose for staging of lymphoma: effectiveness and comparison with computed tomography. Eur J Nucl Med 1998;25:721–8.
41. Jerusalem G, Beguin Y, Najjar F, et al. Positron emission tomography (PET) with ^{18}F-Fluorodeoxyglucose (^{18}F-FDG) for the staging of low grade non-Hodgkin's lymphoma (NHL). Ann Oncol 2001;12:825–30.
42. Blum RH, Seymour JF, Wirth A, et al. Frequent impact of [18F]fluorodeoxyglucose positron emission tomography on the staging and management of patients with indolent non-Hodgkin's lymphoma. Clin Lymphoma 2003; 4:43–9.
43. Hoffmann M, Kletter K, Becherer A, et al. 18F-fluorodeoxyglucose positron emission tomography (18F-FDG-PET) for staging and follow-up of marginal zone B-cell lymphoma. Oncology 2003;64:336–40.
44. Jerusalem G and Beguin Y. Positron emission tomography in non-Hodgkin's lymphoma (NHL): relationship between tracer uptake and pathological findings, including preliminary experience in the staging of low-grade NHL. Clin Lymphoma 2002;3:56–61.
45. Durie BG, Waxman AD, D'Agnolo A, et al. Whole-body ^{18}F-FDG PET identifies high-risk myeloma. J Nucl Med 2002;43:1457–63.
46. Kato T, Tsukamoto E, Nishioka T, et al. Early detection of bone marrow involvement in extramedullary plasmacytoma by whole-body F-18 FDG positron emission tomography. Clin Nucl Med 2000;25:870–3.
47. Orchard K, Barrington S, Buscombe J, et al. Fluorodeoxyglucose positron emission tomography imaging for the detection of occult disease in multiple myeloma. Br J Haematol 2002;117:133–5.
48. Schirrmeister H, Buck AK, Bergmann L, et al. Positron emission tomography (PET) for staging of solitary plasmacytoma. Cancer Biother Radiopharm 2003;18:841–5.

49. Schirrmeister H, Bommer M, Buck AK, et al. Initial results in the assessment of multiple myeloma using 18F-FDG PET. Eur J Nucl Med Mol Imaging 2002;29:361–6.
50. Jerusalem G, Beguin Y, Fassotte MF, et al. Whole-body positron emission tomography using 18F-fluorodeoxyglucose for posttreatment evaluation in Hodgkin's disease and non-Hodgkin's lymphoma has higher diagnostic and prognostic value than classical computed tomography scan imaging. Blood 1999;94:429–33.
51. Mikosch P, Gallowitsch HJ, Zinke-Cerwenka W, et al. Accuracy of whole-body 18F-FDG-PET for restaging malignant lymphoma. Acta Med Austriaca 2003;30:41–7.
52. Romer W, Hanauske AR, Ziegler S, et al. Positron emission tomography in non-Hodgkin's lymphoma: assessment of chemotherapy with fluorodeoxyglucose. Blood 1998; 91:4464–71.
53. Kostakoglu L, Coleman M, Leonard JP, et al. PET predicts prognosis after 1 cycle of chemotherapy in aggressive lymphoma and Hodgkin's disease. J Nucl Med 2002; 43:1018–27.
54. Torizuka T, Nakamura F, Kanno T, et al. Early therapy monitoring with FDG-PET in aggressive non-Hodgkin's lymphoma and Hodgkin's lymphoma. Eur J Nucl Med Mol Imaging 2004;31:22–8.
55. Zijlstra JM, Hoekstra OS, Raijmakers PG, et al. 18FDG positron emission tomography versus 67Ga scintigraphy as prognostic test during chemotherapy for non-Hodgkin's lymphoma. Br J Haematol 2003;123:454–62.
56. Mikhaeel NG, Timothy AR, O'Doherty MJ, et al. 18-FDG-PET as a prognostic indicator in the treatment of aggressive non-Hodgkin's lymphoma—comparison with CT. Leuk Lymphoma 2000;39:543–53.
57. Jerusalem G, Beguin Y, Fassotte MF, et al. Persistent tumor 18F-FDG uptake after a few cycles of polychemotherapy is predictive of treatment failure in non-Hodgkin's lymphoma. Haematologica 2000;85:613–18.
58. Spaepen K, Stroobants S, Dupont P, et al. Early restaging positron emission tomography with [18]—fluorodeoxyglucose predicts outcome in patients with aggressive non- Hodgkin's lymphoma. Ann Oncol 2002;13:1356–63.
59. Spaepen K, Stroobants S, Dupont P, et al. [[18]]FDG PET monitoring of tumour response to chemotherapy: does [[18]]FDG uptake correlate with the viable tumour cell fraction? Eur J Nucl Med Mol Imaging 2003;30:682–8.
60. Becherer A, Mitterbauer M, Jaeger U, et al. Positron emission tomography with [18F]2-fluoro-D-2-deoxyglucose (FDG-PET) predicts relapse of malignant lymphoma after high-dose therapy with stem cell transplantation. Leukemia 2002;16:260–7.
61. Cremerius U, Fabry U, Wildberger JE, et al. Pre-transplant positron emission tomography (PET) using fluorine-18-fluoro-deoxyglucose (FDG) predicts outcome in patients treated with high-dose chemotherapy and autologous stem cell transplantation for non-Hodgkin's lymphoma. Bone Marrow Transplant 2002;30:103–11.
62. Filmont JE, Czernin J, Yap C, et al. Value of F-18 fluorodeoxyglucose positron emission tomography for predicting the clinical outcome of patients with aggressive lymphoma prior to and after autologous stem-cell transplantation. Chest 2003;124:608–13.
63. Spaepen K, Stroobants S, Dupont P, et al. Prognostic value of pretransplantation positron emission tomography using fluorine 18-fluorodeoxyglucose in patients with aggressive lymphoma treated with high-dose chemotherapy and stem cell transplantation. Blood 2003;102:53–9.
64. Israel O, Front D, Lam M, et al. Gallium 67 imaging in monitoring lymphoma response to treatment. Cancer 1988; 61:2439–43.
65. de Wit M, Bumann D, Beyer W, et al. Whole-body positron emission tomography (PET) for diagnosis of residual mass in patients with lymphoma. Ann Oncol 1997;8 Suppl.1: S57–S60.
66. Zinzani PL, Magagnoli M, Chierichetti F, et al. The role of positron emission tomography (PET) in the management of lymphoma patients. Ann Oncol 1999;10:1181–4.
67. Bangerter M, Moog F, Griesshammer M, et al. Role of whole body FDG-PET imaging in predicting relapse of malignant lymphoma in patients with residual masses after treatment. Radiography 1999;5:155–63.
68. Mikhaeel NG, Timothy AR, Hain SF, et al. 18-FDG-PET for the assessment of residual masses on CT following treatment of lymphomas. Ann Oncol 2000;11:S147–S150.
69. Cremerius U, Fabry U, Neuerburg J, et al. Positron emission tomography with 18F-FDG to detect residual disease after therapy for malignant lymphoma. Nucl Med Commun 1998;19:1055–63.
70. Cremerius U, Fabry U, Kroll U, et al. Clinical value of FDG PET for therapy monitoring of malignant lymphoma—results of a retrospective study in 72 patients. Nuklearmedizin 1999;38:24–30.
71. Maisey NR, Hill ME, Webb A, et al. Are 18fluorodeoxyglucose positron emission tomography and magnetic resonance imaging useful in the prediction of relapse in lymphoma residual masses? Eur J Cancer 2000;36:200–6.
72. Naumann R, Vaic A, Beuthien-Baumann B, et al. Prognostic value of positron emission tomography in the evaluation of post-treatment residual mass in patients with Hodgkin's disease and non-Hodgkin's lymphoma. Br J Haematol 2001;115:793–800.
73. de Wit M, Bohuslavizki KH, Buchert R, et al. 18FDG-PET following treatment as valid predictor for disease-free survival in Hodgkin's lymphoma. Ann Oncol 2001;12: 29–37.
74. Dittmann H, Sokler M, Kollmannsberger C, et al. Comparison of 18FDG-PET with CT scans in the evaluation of patients with residual and recurrent Hodgkin's lymphoma. Oncol Rep 2001;8:1393–9.
75. Spaepen K, Stroobants S, Dupont P, et al. Can positron emission tomography with [18F]-fluorodeoxyglucose after first-line treatment distinguish Hodgkin's disease patients who need additional therapy from others in whom additional therapy would mean avoidable toxicity? Br J Haematol 2001;115:272–8.
76. Weihrauch MR, Re D, Scheidhauer K, et al. Thoracic positron emission tomography using ^{18}F-fluorodeoxyglucose for the evaluation of residual mediastinal Hodgkin disease. Blood 2001;98:2930–4.
77. Guay C, Lepine M, Verreault J, et al. Prognostic value of PET using 18F-FDG in Hodgkin's disease for posttreatment evaluation. J Nucl Med 2003;44:1225–31.
78. Hueltenschmidt B, Sautter-Bihl ML, Lang O, et al. Whole body positron emission tomography in the treatment of Hodgkin disease. Cancer 2001;91:302–10.
79. Spaepen K, Stroobants S, Dupont P, et al. Prognostic value of positron emission tomography (PET) with fluorine-18 fluorodeoxyglucose ([18F]FDG) after first-line chemotherapy in non- Hodgkin's lymphoma: is [18F]FDG-PET a valid alternative to conventional diagnostic methods? J Clin Oncol 2001;19:414–9.
80. Jerusalem G, Warland V, Beguin Y, et al. Accuracy of end of treatment 18F-FDG PET for predicting relapse in patients with Hodgkin's disease (Hd) and non-Hodgkin's lymphoma (Nhl). Proc Am Soc Clin Oncol 2003;22:572 [Abstract 2299].
81. Torizuka T, Zasadny KR, Kison PV, et al. Metabolic response of non-Hodgkin's lymphoma to 131I-anti-B1 radioim-

munotherapy: evaluation with FDG PET. J Nucl Med 2000;41:999–1005.
82. Weeks JC, Yeap BY, Canellos GP, et al. Value of follow-up procedures in patients with large-cell lymphoma who achieve a complete remission. J Clin Oncol 1991; 9:1196–1203.
83. Radford JA, Eardley A, Woodman C, et al. Follow up policy after treatment for Hodgkin's disease: too many clinic visits and routine tests? A review of hospital records. BMJ 1997;314:343–6.
84. Jerusalem G, Beguin Y, Fassotte MF, et al. Early detection of relapse by whole-body positron emission tomography (PET) in the follow-up of patients with Hodgkin's disease (HD). Ann Oncol 2003;14:123–30.
85. Montravers F, McNamara D, Landman-Parker J, et al. [18]FDG in childhood lymphoma: clinical utility and impact on management. Eur J Nucl Med Mol Imaging 2002;29:1155–65.
86. Wickmann L, Luders H, and Dorffel W. 18-FDG-PET-findings in children and adolescents with Hodgkin's disease: retrospective evaluation of the correlation to other imaging procedures in initial staging and to the predictive value of follow up examinations. Klin Padiatr 2003;215: 146–50.
87. Depas G, De Barsy C, Jerusalem G, et al. 18F-FDG PET in children with lymphomas. Eur J Nucl Med Mol Imaging 2005;32:31–8.
88. Adler S, Parthasarathy KL, Bakshi SP, et al. Gallium-67-citrate scanning for the localization and staging of lymphomas. J Nucl Med 1975;16:255–60.
89. Levi JA, O'Connell MJ, Murphy WL, et al. Role of 67gallium citrate scanning in the management of non-Hodgkin's lymphoma. Cancer 1975;36:1690–1741.
90. Horn NL, Ray GR, and Kriss JP. Gallium-67 citrate scanning in Hodgkin's disease and non-Hodgkin's lymphoma. Cancer 1976;37:250–7.
91. Seabold JE, Votaw ML, Keyes JW, Jr, et al. Gallium citrate Ga 67 scanning: clinical usefulness in lymphoma patients. Arch Intern Med 1976;136:1370–4.
92. McCaffrey JA, Rudders RA, Kahn PC, et al. Clinical usefulness of 67gallium scanning in the malignant lymphomas. Am J Med 1976;60:523–30.
93. Brown ML, O'Donnell JB, Thrall JH, et al. Gallium-67 scintigraphy in untreated and treated non–Hodgkin lymphomas. J Nucl Med 1978;19:875–9.
94. King DJ, Dawson AA, and McDonald AF. Gallium scanning in lymphoma. Clin Radiol 1980;31:729–32.
95. Longo DL, Schilsky RL, Blei L, et al. Gallium-67 scanning: limited usefulness in staging patients with non-Hodgkin's lymphoma. Am J Med 1980;68:695–700.
96. Waxman AD, Eller D, Ashook G, et al. Comparison of gallium-67-citrate and thallium-201 scintigraphy in peripheral and intrathoracic lymphoma. J Nucl Med 1996; 37:46–50.
97. Hussain R, Christie DR, Gebski V, et al. The role of the gallium scan in primary extranodal lymphoma. J Nucl Med 1998;39:95–8.
98. Delcambre C, Reman O, Henry-Amar M, et al. Clinical relevance of gallium-67 scintigraphy in lymphoma before and after therapy. Eur J Nucl Med 2000;27: 176–84.
99. Andrews GA, Hubner KF, and Greenlaw RH. Ga-67 citrate imaging in malignant lymphoma: final report of cooperative group. J Nucl Med 1978;19:1013–9.
100. Becker WS, Behr TM, Cumme F, et al. 67Ga citrate versus 99mTc-labeled LL2-Fab' (anti-CD22) fragments in the staging of B-cell non-Hodgkin's lymphoma. Cancer Res 1995;55:5771s–73s.
101. Ben Haim S, Bar-Shalom R, Israel O, et al. Utility of gallium-67 scintigraphy in low-grade non-Hodgkin's lymphoma. J Clin Oncol 1996;14:1936–42.
102. Gallamini A, Biggi A, Fruttero A, et al. Revisiting the prognostic role of gallium scintigraphy in low-grade non-Hodgkin's lymphoma. Eur J Nucl Med 1997;24:1499–1506.
103. Roach PJ, Cooper RA, Arthur CK, et al. Comparison of thallium-201 and gallium-67 scintigraphy in the evaluation of non-Hodgkin's lymphoma. Aust N Z J Med 1998;28:33–8.
104. Mansberg R, Wadhwa SS, and Mansberg V. Tl–201 and Ga-67 scintigraphy in non-Hodgkin's lymphoma. Clin Nucl Med 1999;24:239–42.
105. Champion PE, Groshar D, Hooper HR, et al. Does gallium uptake in the pulmonary hila predict involvement by non-Hodgkin's lymphoma? Nucl Med Commun 1992;13: 730–7.
106. Even-Sapir E, Bar-Shalom R, Israel O, et al. Single-photon emission computed tomography quantitation of gallium citrate uptake for the differentiation of lymphoma from benign hilar uptake. J Clin Oncol 1995;13:942–6.
107. Bar-Shalom R, Israel O, Haim N, et al. Diffuse lung uptake of Ga-67 after treatment of lymphoma: is it of clinical importance? Radiology 1996;199:473–6.
108. Frohlich DE, Chen JL, Neuberg D, et al. When is hilar uptake of 67Ga-citrate indicative of residual disease after CHOP chemotherapy? J Nucl Med 2000;41:269–74.
109. Peylan-Ramu N, Haddy TB, Jones E, et al. High frequency of benign mediastinal uptake of gallium-67 after completion of chemotherapy in children with high-grade non-Hodgkin's lymphoma. J Clin Oncol 1989;7:1800–6.
110. Drossman SR, Schiff RG, Kronfeld GD, et al. Lymphoma of the mediastinum and neck: evaluation with Ga-67 imaging and CT correlation. Radiology 1990;174:171–5.
111. Bekerman C, Hoffer PB, and Bitran JD. The role of gallium-67 in the clinical evaluation of cancer. Semin Nucl Med 1984;14:296–323.
112. Front D and Israel O. The role of Ga-67 scintigraphy in evaluating the results of therapy of lymphoma patients. Semin Nucl Med 1995;25:60–71.
113. Kostakoglu L, Leonard JP, Kuji I, et al. Comparison of fluorine-18 fluorodeoxyglucose positron emission tomography and Ga-67 scintigraphy in evaluation of lymphoma. Cancer 2002;94:879–88.
114. Sasaki M, Kuwabara Y, Koga H, et al. Clinical impact of whole body FDG-PET on the staging and therapeutic decision making for malignant lymphoma. Ann Nucl Med 2002;16:337–45.
115. Shen YY, Kao A, and Yen RF. Comparison of 18F-fluoro-2-deoxyglucose positron emission tomography and gallium-67 citrate scintigraphy for detecting malignant lymphoma. Oncol Rep 2002;9:321–5.
116. Wirth A, Seymour JF, Hicks RJ, et al. Fluorine-18 fluorodeoxyglucose positron emission tomography, gallium-67 scintigraphy, and conventional staging for Hodgkin's disease and non-Hodgkin's lymphoma. Am J Med 2002;112:262–8.
117. Van Den Bossche B, Lambert B, De Winter F, et al. 18FDG PET versus high-dose 67Ga scintigraphy for restaging and treatment follow-up of lymphoma patients. Nucl Med Commun 2002;23:1079–83.
118. Bar-Shalom R, Yefremov N, Haim N, et al. Camera-based FDG PET and 67Ga SPECT in evaluation of lymphoma: comparative study. Radiology 2003;227:353–60.
119. Partridge S, Timothy AR, and O'Doherty MJ. 2-fluorine-18-fluoro-2-deoxy-D-glucose positron emission tomography in the pretreatement staging of Hodgkin's disease: influence on patient management in a single institution. Ann Oncol 2000;11:1273–9.

120. Menzel C, Dobert N, Mitrou P, et al. Positron emission tomography for the staging of Hodgkin's lymphoma—increasing the body of evidence in favor of the method. Acta Oncol 2002;41:430–6.
121. Glatz S, Kotzerke J, Moog F, et al. Vortauschung eines mediastinalen Non-Hodgkin-Lymphomrezidivs durch diffuse Thymushyperplasie im 18F-FDG-PET. Fortschr Rontgenstr 1996;165:309–10.
122. Weinblatt ME, Zanzi I, Belakhlef A, et al. False-positive FDG-PET imaging of the thymus of a child with Hodgkin's disease. J Nucl Med 1997;38:888–90.
123. Yoon SN, Park CH, Kim MK, et al. False-positive F-18 FDG gamma camera positron emission tomographic imaging resulting from inflammation of an anterior mediastinal mass in a patient with non-Hodgkin's lymphoma. Clin Nucl Med 2001;26:461–2.
124. Sandherr M, von Schilling C, Link T, et al. Pitfalls in imaging Hodgkin's disease with computed tomography and positron emission tomography using fluorine-18-fluorodeoxyglucose. Ann Oncol 2001;12:719–22.
125. Bomanji JB, Syed R, Brock C, et al. Challenging cases and diagnostic dilemmas: case 2. Pitfalls of positron emission tomography for assessing residual mediastinal mass after chemotherapy for Hodgkin's disease. J Clin Oncol 2002;20:3347–9.
126. Naumann R, Beuthien-Baumann B, Fischer R, et al. Simultaneous occurence of Hodgkin's lymphoma and eosinophilic granuloma—a potential pitfall in PET imaging. Clin Lymphoma 2002;3:121–4.
127. Cheong KA, Rodgers NG, Kirkwood ID. Erythema nodosum associated with diffuse, large B-cell non-Hodgkin lymphoma detected by FDG PET. Clin Nucl Med 2003;28:652–4.
128. Becherer A, Mitterbauer M, Jaeger U, et al. Positron emission tomography with [18F]2-fluoro-D-2-deoxyglucose (FDG-PET) predicts relapse of malignant lymphoma after high-dose therapy with stem cell transplantation. Leukemia 2002;16:260–7.
129. Lorenzen J, de Wit M, Buchert R, et al. Granulation tissue: pitfall in therapy control with F-18-FDG PET after chemotherapy. Nuklearmedizin 1999;38:333–6.

12

Principles, Indications, and Techniques of Radiation Therapy of Lymphomas

Joachim Yahalom, M.D.

Ionizing radiation is a highly effective modality for the treatment of both Hodgkin's lymphoma (HL) and non-Hodgkin's lymphoma (NHL). The dramatic effects of radiation alone in reducing large lesions and even eliminating HL lesions were reported more than 100 years ago, soon after the discovery of x-rays by Wilhelm Conrad Roentgen. Yet, during the first half of the 20th century, when all lymphomas remained incurable, radiation was used mostly for palliation and responses were brief due to technical constraints and/or poor methods of delivering radiation. As x-ray technology improved in the 1940s and the concept of irradiating beyond the involved area was adopted, patients with early-stage HL and NHL could be cured with radiation alone—the only effective curative modality for lymphomas that was available until the late 1960s.

Prior to the advent of effective chemotherapy, attempts were made to cure even advanced HL and NHL by maximizing the use of radiation alone. Optimizing the selection of patients and tailoring the radiation fields was associated with aggressive staging efforts that included using staging laparotomy for HL and even NHL. Moreover, the dependency on radiation therapy (RT) as the primary modality required wide extension of the radiation field as well as raising the dose to normal tissue tolerance levels. While this mega-radiotherapy led to the cure of many patients, it was also associated with late development of complications, and increased the mortality of cured patients beyond what is expected of the normal population. This was the price of successfully pioneering radiation therapy as a curative modality prior to the availability of effective chemotherapy.

The emergence of more effective and less toxic chemotherapy over the last 30 years led to considerable changes in the use of RT in the management of lymphomas. First, in several types of NHL and in classical HL, chemotherapy has become the primary modality with radiotherapy used for consolidation and reduction of relapse risk. Yet, in some lymphomas, mostly in early-stage low-grade lymphomas where chemotherapy is less effective, radiation alone remained the standard of care.

Radiation alone is currently the treatment of choice for early-stage follicular lymphoma; mucosa-associated lymphoid tissue (MALT) lymphoma and lymphocyte-predominant HL. The role of RT as consolidation following chemotherapy is well established in early-stage "classic" HL, in advanced-stage HL following programs of brief chemotherapy or following incomplete response. Radiotherapy also plays an important role in high-dose therapy programs for salvage of HL and NHL.

Finally, radiotherapy is an excellent palliative modality that provides long-term local control and clinical benefit even for advanced-stage lymphomas such as mantle cell lymphoma, small lymphocytic lymphoma, advanced-stage MALT lymphoma, and follicular lymphoma. These specific types of lymphoma are highly sensitive to radiation, and very low doses may be adequate for local control. The indications for using radiotherapy for treating lymphomas are summarized in Table 12–1.

INDICATIONS FOR RADIOTHERAPY

Hodgkin's Lymphoma

It is important to distinguish between the two well-defined entities of HL: classical HL and the less common nodular lymphocyte predominant Hodgkin's lymphoma (LPHL). The radiation approach to each entity is different. Most patients with LPHL are potentially treated with radiation alone, whereas combined modality therapy is the standard approach for the majority of patients with classical HL.

Lymphocyte-Predominant Hodgkin's Lymphoma

Most (>75%) patients with LPHL present at an early stage; the disease is commonly limited to one peripheral site (neck, axilla, or groin), and involvement of the mediastinum is extremely rare. The treatment recommendations for LPHL differ markedly from those for classic HL. The American National Comprehensive Cancer Network (NCCN) guidelines,[1] the German Hodgkin's Lymphoma Study Group (GHSG),[2] and the European Organization for Research and Treatment of Cancer (EORTC) currently recommend *involved-field radiation alone* as the treatment of choice for early-stage LPHL. It should be emphasized that even if regional radiation fields are selected, the uninvolved mediastinum should not be irradiated, thus avoiding the site most prone for radiation-related short- and long-term side effects. Although there has not been a study that compared extended-field RT (commonly used in the past) with involved field RT, retrospective data suggest that involved-field is adequate.[3] The radiation dose recommended is between 30 to 36 Gy with an optional additional boost of 4 Gy to a (rare) bulky site.

Table 12–1. Indications for Radiotherapy in Treatment of Lymphomas

Radiation Alone, Potentially Curative

Hodgkin's lymphoma, lymphocyte predominance
Stages I–II
Hodgkin's lymphoma, classical[a]
Stages IA–IIA (nonbulky)
Follicular lymphoma
Stages I–II
Stage III (rarely used)
Extranodal marginal zone (MALT) lymphoma
Stages IE–IIE
Nodal marginal zone lymphoma
Stages I–II
Mycosis fungoides
Stages IA, IB, IIA
Anaplastic large-cell lymphoma of skin
Stage IE

Radiation as Part of Potentially Curative Combined Modality Program

Hodgkin's lymphoma, classic
Stages I–II (favorable and unfavorable)
Hodgkin's lymphoma
Advanced stage[b]
Diffuse large B-cell lymphoma
Stages I–II
Primary mediastinal lymphoma
Stages I–II
Peripheral T-cell lymphoma
Stages I–II
Extranodal NK/T-cell lymphoma, nasal type
Primary central nervous system lymphoma
In high-dose therapy programs for Hodgkin's lymphoma, diffuse large B-cell lymphoma, follicular lymphoma, and mantle cell lymphoma

Radiation Effective for Palliation and Local Control

Highly sensitive
Follicular lymphoma
Mantle cell lymphoma
Small lymphocytic lymphoma/chronic lymphocytic leukemia
Marginal zone lymphoma
Mycosis fungoides
Moderately sensitive
Diffuse large-cell lymphoma

[a] Combined modality is treatment of choice.
[b] For bulky sites, incomplete response, and as part of brief chemotherapy program (e.g., Stanford V).

CLASSICAL HODGKIN'S LYMPHOMA

Early Stage (Favorable and Unfavorable): The New Role of Radiation Therapy

Over the last 20 years, the treatment of early-stage classical HL has drastically changed. Combined modality therapy consisting of short-course chemotherapy (most often doxorubicin, bleomycin, vinblastine, dacarbazine [ABVD]) consolidated by reduced-dose radiation carefully directed only to the involved lymph node(s) site successfully replaced radiation alone as treatment of choice.[1,2,4] While no longer the primary treatment, radiotherapy limited to smaller volumes, administered to a reduced dose with improved targeting achieved with new imaging technology and supported by modern delivery systems, remains an important component of effective treatment programs for HL.

Table 12–2. Studies Comparing Radiation Therapy Alone to Combined Modality Therapy in Favorable Patients

Study	Treatment Regimens	FFTF or RFS	OS (years)
GHSG HD7[8]	EF	75%	94% (5)
(617 patients)	ABVD (2) + EF	91%	94%
		p < 0.001	NS
SWOG #9133[7]	STLI	81%	96% (3)
(326 patients)	AV (3) + STLI	94%	98%
		p < 0.001	NS
EORTC/GELA H7F[9]	STLI	81%	95% (5)
(333 patients)	EBVP (6) + IFRT	90%	98%
		p = 0.0001	NS
EORTC/GELA H8F[10]	STLI	80%	95% (4)
(543 patients)	MOPP/ABV (3) + IFRT	99%	99%
		p < 0.0001	p < 0.02

COPP, cyclophosphamide, oncovin, procarbazine, prednisone; EBVP, epirubicin, bleomycin, vinblastine, prednisone; EF, extended field; EFRT, extended-field radiotherapy; EORTC, European Organization for Research and Treatment of Cancer; FFTF, freedom-from-treatment failure; IFRT, involved-field radiotherapy; GELA, Groupe d'etude des lymphomes de l'adulte; MOPP, mechlorethamine, vincristine, procarbazine, prednisone; NS, not significant; OS, overall survival; RFS, relapse-free survival; STLI, subtotal lymphoid irradiation.

The "old" (1950s to 1980s) treatment strategy for HL maximized the use of radical radiotherapy, since it was considered the optimal curative modality in early-stage HL. Even in later years, radiation fields remained extensive in order to reduce the need for the less effective (as compared to ABVD) and relatively toxic chemotherapy combination of that time—mechloroethamine, vincristine, procarbazine, prednisone (MOPP).

Over the last 5 decades, radiotherapy alone cured most early-stage patients. As an example, long-term follow-up of 392 pathologically staged patients without large mediastinal adenopathy treated by the Harvard group demonstrated 10- and 20-year freedom-from-treatment failure rates of 84% and 82%, respectively. The 10- and 20-year overall survival rates were 92% and 82%, respectively. The Harvard group documented, like many others, the late increase in the incidence of second solid tumors as the main cause for decrease in survival rate after 10 years.[5,6]

The lesson from the "radiotherapy period" in HL should not be limited to the increasing awareness of long-term risks associated with the use of large-field radiotherapy. We should appreciate that radiotherapy alone as a "single agent" was (and still is) a highly effective tool in curing HL. Yet, radiotherapy should be adapted to its new role as consolidating treatment using a low dose and a smaller field in order to maximize cure, while reducing the toxicity of either prolonged or potentially toxic regimens of chemotherapy. The development of this concept is described below.

The improved efficacy of combining doxorubicin-based chemotherapy with traditional large-field radiotherapy compared to the same radiotherapy alone was shown in the German Hodgkin's Lymphoma Study Group (GHSG) HD7 study and Southwest Oncology Group (SWOG) #9133 of favorable patients.[7,8] Patients on the combined modality arm had a significantly better freedom-from-treatment failure (FFTF). Overall survival remained the same, probably reflecting good salvage or a still too short follow-up period (Table 12–2).

The EORTC/GELA H7F and H8F trials significantly reduced the irradiated volume in the combined modality arm to include only the site of the originally involved nodes (involved field) as opposed to treatment of all lymph node sites (and the spleen) on the radiation-alone arm. Still, the combined modality arm yielded significantly better relapse-free survival rate than radiation alone (Table 12–2).[9,10]

The studies summarized in Table 12–3 show that when combined with chemotherapy, involved field radiation is as effective as a combination of the same chemotherapy followed by extended field radiation.

The studies shown in Table 12–3 clearly indicate that reducing the radiation field has not detracted from the excellent FFTF or relapse-free survival rates (84% to 95%) or overall survival (92% to 94%) in patients with favorable[11] or unfavorable (GHSG,[12] EORTC/GELA,[13] and Milan[11]) early-stage HL. The detailed analysis of the GHSG H8 study demonstrated that a smaller radiation field was associated with a reduction in acute side effects and a trend for a lower risk of second malignancies (2.8% vs. 4.5%) that may possibly strengthen with more time of follow-up.[12]

Table 12–3. Studies Comparing Involved-Field Radiation with Extended Radiation in Combined Modality Programs for Favorable and Unfavorable Early-Stage Hodgkin's Lymphoma

Study	Treatment Regimens	FFTF or RFS	OS (Years)
Milan[11]	ABVD (4) + STLI	97%	93% (5)
(133 patients)	ABVD (4) + IFRT	94%	94%
		NS	NS
GHSG HD8[12]	COPP/ABVD (4) + EFRT	86%	91% (5)
(1064 patients)	COPP/ABVD (4) + IFRT	84%	92%
		NS	NS
EORTC/GELA	MOPP/ABV (6) + IFRT	94%	90% (4)
H8U[13]	MOPP/ABV (4) + IFRT	95%	95%
(995 patients)	MOPP/ABV (4) + STLI	96%	93%
		NS	NS

ABV, doxorubicin, bleomycin, vinblastine; COPP, cyclophosphamide, oncovin, procarbazine, and prednisone; EBVP, epirubicin, bleomycin, vinblastine, prednisone; EF, extended field; EFRT, extended-field radiotherapy; EORTC, European Organization for Research and Treatment of Cancer; FFTF, freedom-from-treatment failure; IFRT, involved-field radiotherapy; GELA, Groupe d'etude des lymphomes de l'adulte; MOPP, mechlorethamine, vincristine, procarbazine, prednisone; NS, not significant; OS, overall survival; RFS, relapse-free survival; STLI, subtotal lymphoid irradiation.

Combined modality therapy allows not only for a drastic restriction of the irradiated volume, it also permits a meaningful reduction (by up to 50%) in the effective prescribed radiation dose. The GHSG studies of combined modality therapy in unfavorable early-stage patients indicated that disease control with 20 Gy was as effective as with 40 Gy, provided that bulky disease sites were irradiated to 40 Gy.[14] The recently completed GHSG study HD10 for favorable patients randomized patients to either 20 Gy involved-field radiation therapy (IFRT) or 30 Gy IFRT following a short course (two or four cycles) of ABVD.[15] At a median follow-up of 24 months, the overall results are excellent (FFTF of 97%), with no difference between the four arms. The GHSG study of unfavorable patients (HD11) with similar radiotherapy dose design and 24-month FFTF of 90%, also suggests that radiation dose reduction is safe.[16] More mature and detailed results are expected soon. The EORTC/GELA current trial for favorable patients H9F is evaluating EBVP X6 to complete response (CR) followed by either IFRT of 36 Gy or IFRT of 20 Gy. The third arm of patients with CR after six cycles of EBVP and no radiation, was closed early due to an excessive number of relapses. The combined modality arms remained open until the study has been ended.

Conversion from large multisite radiation fields to a smaller and better-defined radiation field allowed also for accurate conformal radiation therapy. The large fields of the past limited the radiation technique to two simple opposed anterior and posterior fields. The conversion to smaller and better defined radiation volumes allowed the utilization of more conformal radiation therapy, based on better imaging, computerized planning programs, and when indicated, advanced tools such as intensity modulated radiotherapy (IMRT). Modern breakthroughs in radiotherapy technology can now be implemented in HL to increase accuracy even further and avoid irradiation of normal organs, and thus improve the therapeutic ratio.

Chemotherapy Alone for Early-Stage Hodgkin's Lymphoma?

The standard treatment for early-stage favorable and unfavorable classical HL recommended by the large European HL groups and by the U.S. National Comprehensive Cancer Network (NCCN) is chemotherapy followed by involved-field radiotherapy.[1] Yet, the idea of eliminating radiotherapy from the treatment program in all stages of HL has been advocated by some.[17,18] Some recent studies addressing this issue are reviewed here.

Two prospective randomized studies evaluated MOPP chemotherapy in early-stage HL alone as an alternative to the "standard" of that time—subtotal lymphoid irradiation (STLI).[19,20] The National Cancer Institute (NCI) study showed that in nonbulky patients, MOPP chemotherapy was at least as effective as STLI.[20] The Italian study, on the other hand, demonstrated that while freedom-from-progression was similar in both treatment groups, the overall survival of the irradiated patients was significantly ($p < 0.001$) better (93% vs. 56%) compared to the MOPP treated group.[19] The inferior survival was the result of the poor response to salvage of the MOPP treated group. The toxicity profile of MOPP and the above conflicting results hindered its consideration for primary treatment of early-stage HL.

When the above MOPP studies were reported, doxorubicin-containing regimens such as ABVD have already demonstrated a lower toxicity profile and superior efficacy compared to MOPP in both advanced- and early-stage HL.[21,22] The EORTC conducted a randomized trial in unfavorable early-stage HL comparing a combination of MOPP and mantle field irradiation to ABVD with the same radiation.[22] At 10 years, failure-free survival was better in the ABVD/RT-treated patients compared to the MOPP/RT group (88% vs. 77%, $p < 0.0001$). There was no difference in overall survival.

The next step was to evaluate the efficacy of ABVD (or similar combinations) alone, omitting radiation if a CR has been obtained at the end of the chemotherapy program. The following studies have recently been published or reported at meetings.

Children Cancer Group #5942

The children Cancer Study Group[23] tested the role of radiation therapy in young patients (<21 years) who attained a CR with risk-adapted chemotherapy (mostly COPP/ABV, four to six cycles). They enrolled 829 patients in the study (68% were early stage). A total of 501 patients who achieved a CR were then randomized to receive either low-dose (21 Gy) involved-field radiotherapy (IFRT) or no further treatment. The accrual was stopped earlier than planned because of a significantly higher number of relapses in the no-radiotherapy arm.

The 3-year event-free survival (EFS) with an intent-to-treat analysis was 92% for patients randomized to receive RT and 87% for those randomized to no further treatment ($p = 0.057$). Since 30 patients switched their treatment after randomization, an analysis "as treated" was performed, and showed a 3-year EFS of 93% for those who received radiation and only 85% for those who were only observed ($p = 0.0024$). At this early analysis, no survival difference was detected.

Tata Memorial Hospital Trial

This is a large prospectively randomized study from the main cancer center in Mumbay, India of 251 patients with HL (55% early stage) who received six cycles of ABVD chemotherapy.[24] Of those, only 179 patients (71%) who achieved a CR were randomized to either IFRT of 30 Gy (+10 Gy boost to bulky sites) or to no further therapy.

At a median follow-up of 63 months, the 8-year event-free survival and overall survival were significantly better for the patients who received consolidation with IFRT compared to those who received ABVD alone (EFS, 88% vs. 76%, $p = 0.01$; overall survival [OS], 100% vs. 89%, $p = 0.002$). Most relapses in the ABVD alone arm were early and systemic, whereas in the ABVD + RT arm, the relapses were late and localized.

National Cancer Institute of Canada/Eastern Cooperative Oncology Group Trial HD-6

This intergroup study included 405 patients with nonbulky stages I and II patients.[25] They were randomized to either receive "standard therapy," namely, subtotal nodal irradiation (STNI) for favorable patients, and ABVD (two cycles) followed by STNI for unfavorable (B, elevated ESR, three or more sites, age ≥40, mixed cellularity histology) patients, or to the experimental arm that consisted of six or four cycles (if CR was attained after two cycles) of ABVD and no RT.

At a median follow-up of 4.2 years, progression-free survival (PFS) with ABVD alone was significantly inferior ($p = 0.006$; HR = 2.6; 5-year PFS estimates 87% vs. 93%). At this early point, no survival difference had been detected. Although the "standard" arm that included RT alone for favorable patients is no longer considered the standard of care, the inferior performance of ABVD alone compared to "standard therapy" in nonbulky early-stage patients cannot be ignored.

EORTC/GELA H9F

This is a large ongoing trial in favorable early-stage patients with classic HL.[26] All patients receive 6 cycles of EBVP (epirubicin, bleomycin, vinblastine, and prednisone). Only patients who achieve a CR are randomized to either IFRT of 36 Gy, IFRT of 20 Gy, or to no radiation. In 2003, the EORTC/GELA groups closed the no RT arm due to an excessive number of relapses in this group. The study remained open for randomization on the two combined modality arms and is awaiting analysis.

Memorial Sloan-Kettering Cancer Center Trial

The Memorial Sloan-Kettering (MSK) trial included 152 patients with nonbulky early-stage HL.[27] Patients were randomized up-front to either received ABDV X6 alone or ABVD X6 followed by radiotherapy. At 60 months, CR duration and freedom from progression (FFP), for ABVD+RT versus ABVD alone are 91% versus 87% ($p = 0.61$), and 86% versus 81% ($p = 0.61$), respectively. Overall survival was 97% with ABVD + RT versus 90% with ABVD alone ($p = 0.08$). Although the differences between the outcome of the two treatment groups were not statistically significant, the study was not powered to detect differences between the treatment strategies that were smaller than 20%, due to the small number of patients and events. The superior overall survival ($p = 0.08$) of the ABVD+RT group is also difficult to explain, and is possibly a result of the small size of this trial.

Advanced-Stage Hodgkin's Lymphoma

Although the role of consolidation radiotherapy after induction chemotherapy remains controversial,[28] irradiation is often added in patients with advanced-stage HL who present with bulky disease or remain in uncertain complete remission after chemotherapy. Retrospective studies have demonstrated that adding low-dose radiotherapy to all initial disease sites after chemotherapy-induced complete response decreases the relapse rate by ~25% and significantly improves overall survival. Interpretation of the impact of radiation in prospective studies has been controversial.[29,30] However, a Southwest Oncology Group (SWOG) randomized study of 278 patients with stage III or IV Hodgkin's disease suggested that the addition of low-dose irradiation to all sites of initial disease after a complete response to MOP-BAP (mechlorethamine, Oncovin [vincristine], prednisone, bleomycin, Adriamycin [doxorubicin], and procarbazine) chemotherapy improves remission duration in patients with advanced-stage disease.[31] An intention-to-treat analysis showed that the advantage of combined modality therapy was limited to patients with nodular sclerosis. No survival differences were observed. A meta-analysis of several randomized studies demonstrated that the addition of radiotherapy to chemotherapy reduces the rate of relapse, but did not show survival benefit for combined modality therapy compared to chemotherapy alone.[32]

Recently, EORTC reported the results of a randomized study that evaluated the role of IFRT in patients with stage III/IV Hodgkin's disease who obtained a CR after MOPP/ABV.[33] Patients received six or eight cycles of MOPP/ABV chemotherapy (number of cycles depended on the response). Patients who did not receive a CR (40% of patients) were not randomized to receive chemotherapy and received IFRT. Of the 418 patients who reached a CR, 85 patients were not randomized to receive treatment for various reasons. A total of 161 patients were randomized to receive no RT and 172 patients were randomized to receive IFRT. The authors concluded that IFRT does not improve the treatment results in patients with Stage III/IV Hodgkin's disease who reached a CR after six to eight courses of MOPP/ABV chemotherapy. The 5-year overall survival rates were 91 and 85 percent, respectively ($p = 0.07$). The data indicated that in comparison with chemotherapy alone, there were more cases of leukemia second tumors on the CR combined modality, but surprisingly, not on the partial response (PR) combined modality arm. In partial responders after six cycles of MOPP/ABV, the addition of IFRT yielded overall survival and event-free survival rates that were similar to those obtained in CR to chemotherapy patients. Among the 250 patients in partial remission after chemotherapy, the 5-year event-free and overall survival rates were 79% and 87%, respectively. The EORTC study has several limitations that detract from its applicability to many advanced-stage patients. First, a relatively small fraction of patients were determined to be in CR, and thus eligible for randomization on the study. The regimen of MOPP/ABV X 6-8 is quite toxic, and this regimen is no longer used in North America.[34] Second, only few patients with bulky disease were randomized on the EORTC study. Lastly, the claim that added RT caused more secondary malignancies on the combined modality has not been evident in patients with PR receiving even higher doses of RT to multiple areas after MOPP/ABV.

The only randomized study questioning the role of consolidation RT after CR to ABVD X 6 (the most common regimen currently used for advance-stage HL) was performed at Tata medical center in India.[24] The study included patients of all stages, but almost half were Stage III or IV. A subgroup analysis of the advanced-stage patients showed a statistically significant improvement of both 8-year event-free survival and 8-year overall survival with added RT compared to ABVD alone (EFS 78% vs. 59%; $p < 0.03$ and OS 100% vs. 80%; $p < 0.006$).

When advanced-stage HL is treated with the new highly effective and less toxic treatment program of Stanford V, it is imperative to follow the brief chemotherapy program with involved field radiotherapy to sites originally larger than 5 cm or to a clinically involved spleen.[35] When radiotherapy was fully or partially omitted on this program, the results were inferior.[36]

In summary, patients in CR after full-dose chemotherapy programs like MOPP/ABV may not need RT consolidation. Yet, patients with bulky disease, or incomplete or uncertain CR, or patients treated in brief chemotherapy programs will benefit from involved field RT to originally bulky or residual disease.

SALVAGE PROGRAMS FOR REFRACTORY AND RELAPSED HODGKIN'S LYMPHOMA

High-dose therapy supported by autologous stem cell transplantation (ASCT) has become a standard salvage treatment for patients who relapsed or remained refractory to chemotherapy or to combined modality therapy. Many of the patients who enter these programs have not received prior radiotherapy or relapsed at sites outside the original radiation field. These patients could benefit from integrating radiotherapy into the salvage regimen.

Poen and colleagues from Stanford analyzed the efficacy and toxicity of adding cytoreductive (pre-transplant; $n = 18$) or consolidative (post-transplant; $n = 6$) RT to 24 of 100 patients receiving high-dose therapy.[37] This study showed that most (69%) relapses after ASCT occurred in sites known to be involved immediately before transplantation. When these sites were irradiated prior to transplantation, no in-field failures occurred. While only a trend in favor of IF-RT could be shown for the entire group of transplanted patients, for patients with Stages I to III freedom from relapse was significantly improved. Limiting the analysis to patients who received no prior RT also resulted in a significant advantage to IF-RT. Fatal toxicity in this series was not influenced significantly by IF-RT.

At the Memorial Sloan Kettering Cancer Center (MSKCC), we developed a program that integrated RT into the high-dose regimen for salvage of HD. We schedule accelerated hyperfractionated irradiation (b.i.d. fractions of 1.8 Gy each) to start after the completion of re-induction chemotherapy and stem cell collection and prior to the high-dose chemotherapy and stem cell transplantation. Patients who have not been previously irradiated received involved field RT (18 Gy in 5 days) to sites of initially bulky (>5 cm) disease and/or residual clinical abnormalities followed by total lymphoid irradiation (TLI) of 18 Gy (1.8 Gy per fraction, b.i.d.) within an additional 5 days. Patients who had prior RT received only involved-field RT (when feasible) to a maximal dose of 36 Gy. This treatment strategy has been in place since 1985, with over 350 patients treated thus far. The first-generation program demonstrated the feasibility and efficacy of the high-dose combined modality regimen resulting in an event-free survival of 47% for the patients receiving TLI followed by cyclophosphamide-etoposide chemotherapy.[38] The recent report of the second-generation, two-step, high-dose chemoradiotherapy program indicated that after a median follow-up of 34 months, the intent-to-treat event free survival and overall survival were 58% and 88%, respectively. For patients who underwent transplantation, the event-free survival was 68%.[39] Treatment-related mortality was 3%, with no treatment-related mortality over the last 8 years. The results of this treatment program in refractory patients were similar to those of relapsed patients.[40] Both groups showed favorable event-free survival and overall survival compared to most recently reported series. Most failures in this salvage program occurred in either nonirradiated extranodal sites or in nodal sites that could not be further irradiated. Although the pattern of failure may suggest that the extensive use of nodal irradiation in our program contributed to its overall success, randomized cooperative group studies would be needed to determine whether integrating RT, such as TLI and/or IFRT contributes to the success of a salvage program of HL.

Follicular Lymphoma

Approximately 20% of patients with low-grade follicular lymphomas present in localized stages (I and II). The standard treatment for these patients is regional or involved-field radiotherapy.[41] Results from large series of patients with Stage I and II indolent lymphomas who were treated with radiotherapy alone are summarized in Table 12–4. It should be noted that in past series, no clear distinction was made between early stages of follicular lymphomas and the less frequent, currently recognized low-grade histologies of marginal zone and small lymphocytic lymphoma. The report of patients with Stage I and II low-grade follicular lymphoma from Stanford with long-term follow-up indicated that a substantial number of patients in this category have, indeed, been "cured" by radiotherapy.[42] The median follow-up was 7.7 years, and observation has maintained for up to 31 years. The median survival after radiotherapy was 14 years. The actuarial survival rates at 5, 10, 15, and 20 years were 82%, 64%, 44%, and 35%, respectively. Freedom from relapse (FFR) at 5, 10, 15, and 20 years was 55%, 44%, 40%, and 37%, respectively. Only 5 of 47 patients who reached 10 years without a relapse developed a late recurrence. There was no significant FFR difference between Stage I and Stage II, or between nodal or extranodal disease. The survival of patients irradiated after the age of 60 years was significantly shorter than the survival of younger patients, but the decrease of survival in this age group was strongly affected by death from other causes.

Most relapses in early-stage patients occur in unirradiated sites during the first 5 to 6 years following therapy.[44] In the Stanford series, administration of radiotherapy to nodal sites on both sides of the diaphragm was associated with a significantly better FFR compared with more localized treatment, but did not translate into a clear survival benefit.[42] Similar experience was reported from M.D. Anderson Cancer Center.[45] In the absence of a clear survival benefit for total lymphoid irradiation in this setting, the common involvement of mesenteric nodes that may require whole abdominal irradiation, and in consideration of the fact that almost half of the patients will eventually require chemotherapy for relapse, we currently employ involved- or regional-field irradiation for these patients.

The optimal radiation dose for indolent lymphoma has not been determined in a prospective study. However, most current radiotherapy series for Stage I and II indolent lymphomas usually employ 30 to 40 Gy, and in-field recurrences have been uncommon. Data from the Princess Margaret Hospital showed in-field disease control in 78% of patients treated with doses of less than 25 Gy and 91% control with doses greater than 25 Gy.[46] At M.D. Anderson, excellent local control was achieved with 30 Gy to lesions smaller than 3 cm.[45] Fuks and Kaplan correlated relapse rates in regional areas of follicular lymphoma with the radiation dose delivered to these sites, and showed 63% relapse in areas receiving less than 27.5 Gy, 27% relapse with a dose range of 30 to 35 Gy, and 12% and 6% relapse rates for 40 Gy and 44 Gy, respectively.[47] We currently recommend 30 to 36 Gy (in 1.8-Gy daily fractions) to involved sites (40 Gy, if bulky) and 24 to 36 Gy to uninvolved adjacent sites.

Several prospective randomized trials failed to demonstrate that the use of radiation followed by chemotherapy was superior to radiation alone in early-stage indolent lymphoma. Most studies used combinations of cyclophosphamide, vincristine, and prednisone (CVP),[48] chlorambucil, and/or cyclophosphamide, daunorubicin, vincristine (Oncovin), and prednisone combination (CHOP).[49] Based on these studies, adjuvant chemotherapy has no role in the treatment of early-stage indolent lymphomas.

Radiotherapy is rarely used in Stage III disease. Yet, the reported experience with radiation therapy is quite encouraging.[50] Several investigators treated patients with extensive irradiation fields that included mantle field, Waldeyer's ring, and the whole abdomen and pelvis, and were termed *comprehensive lymphatic irradiation.* Radiation doses ranged from 20 to 40 Gy. The long-term results are summarized in Table 12–5.

The limited reported experience with RT alone in these series is encouraging, with a 10-year relapse-free survival of 39% to 45%. Most relapses after 5 years have been transformations to a more aggressive histology, and salvage chemotherapy was well tolerated.[54] Favorable prognostic factors in Stage III disease treated with comprehensive lymphatic irradiation include fewer than five sites of involvement, absence of bulky disease, and B symptoms. At M.D. Anderson, comprehensive lymphatic irradiation of Stages I to III FL even resulted in reversal of FL abnormal molecular markers in the bone marrow and/or peripheral blood of almost half of the patients.[55] Other studies explored com-

Table 12–4. Radiotherapy Alone for Stages I and II Indolent Lymphomas

Reference	Patients (*n*)	Stage	Relapse-Free Survival, % (years)	Overall Survival, % (years)
Vaughn et al.[43]	208	I	47 (10)	64 (10)
Suttcliffe et al.[44]	190	I–II	53 (12)	58 (12)
MacManus[42]	177	I–II	44 (15)	40 (15)

Table 12–5. Results of Comprehensive Lymphatic Irradiation in Stage III Indolent Lymphomas

Reference	Patients (*n*)	Median Follow-up (years)	Relapse-Free Survival, % (years)	Overall Survival, % (years)
Paryani et al.[51,52]	61	9.6	39 (10)	48 (10)
Jacobs et al.[53]	34	9.6	40 (15)	28 (15)
Mendenhall and Lynch[54]	11	25	45 (10)	49 (10)

bined modality therapy in Stage III indolent lymphomas. A small randomized study from Stanford found no advantage in survival or FFR to adding CVP chemotherapy to total lymphoid irradiation.[51,52] A study from Mexico City suggested that CVP combined with involved-field radiotherapy or with total lymphoid irradiation was better than CVP alone.[56] The 7-year relapse-free survival rate was 66%, 71%, and 33%, respectively, and this advantage has also translated into a survival benefit. A study from M.D. Anderson Cancer Center of combined modality therapy in Stage III disease yielded results that were similar to those obtained with comprehensive lymphatic irradiation. Although comprehensive lymphatic irradiation is a long, complex, and potentially toxic therapy for patients with an indolent disease, it should be considered for physiologically fit patients, particularly since no alternative strategy has been shown to be curative for disease in this stage.

The rare histology of nodal marginal zone lymphoma in early stage is treated like FL with IFRT alone.

Extranodal Marginal Zone Lymphoma of MALT Lymphoma

The most common organ involved with MALT lymphoma is the stomach. Gastric MALT lymphoma (GML) is often associated with the presence of *Helicobacter pylori* in the stomach, and the antibiotic eradication of this pathogen leads to regression of GML in many patients. Yet, approximately 30% to 50% of patients with *H. pylori*–positive GML will show persistent or progressing lymphoma even after eradication of *H. pylori* with antibiotic therapy, and even in complete responders, almost 15% will relapse within 3 years, suggesting that about half of patients with GML will eventually be considered for additional therapies.[57] Most of those will still have disease limited to the stomach. In these patients and in those who present with no evidence of *H. pylori* infection, involved-field radiation therapy with relatively low radiation dose is the treatment of choice.[41]

Several institutions reported excellent results using involved-field radiotherapy of the stomach in *H. pylori*–independent GML patients who either failed antibiotic therapy or had no evidence for *H. pylori* infection.[58–61] The recent update of the Memorial Sloan-Kettering Cancer Center experience included 51 patients with GML (Stage I-39; Stage II-10; Stage IV-2) who were either *H. pylori*-negative (30) or remained with persistent lymphoma after antibiotic therapies and adequate observation (21).[62] All patients were treated with radiation to the stomach and peri-gastric nodes; the median total dose was 30 Gy in 4 weeks. All patients had regular follow-up endoscopic evaluations and biopsies. Ninety-six percent (49/51) of the patients obtained a biopsy-proven complete response. Of three patients who relapsed, two were salvaged. Three patients died of other malignancies, all second tumors developed outside the radiation field. At a median follow-up of 4 years, FFTF, OS, and cause-specific survival were 89%, 83%, and 100%, respectively. Treatment was well tolerated, with no significant acute or chronic side effects. The experience from Toronto and Boston using the same radiation approach was equally successful,[63–65] supporting the approach that modest dose involved-field radiotherapy is the treatment of choice for patients with persistent GML who have exhausted the antibiotic therapy approach, or are unlikely to respond to it (*H. pylori*–negative patients).[66,67] The treatment techniques for treatment of gastric lymphoma have been recently published.[68]

MALT lymphomas have also been described in various nongastric sites, such as salivary glands, skin, orbit, conjunctiva, lung, thyroid, larynx, breast, kidney, liver, bladder, prostate, urethra, small intestine, rectum, and pancreas, and even in the intracranial dura.[67]

The optimal management of nongastric MALT lymphomas has not yet been clearly established. Retrospective series included patients treated with surgery, radiotherapy and chemotherapy, alone or in combination. Marginal-zone lymphomas are exquisitely sensitive to relatively low doses of radiation. Specifically, ML in sites such as salivary glands, ocular, conjunctiva, thyroid, bladder, and breast have been successfully eradicated with involved-field RT encompassing the involved organ alone with a dose of 24 Gy to 36 Gy.[63,65] Even unusual sites (such as larynx, base of skull, urethra, prostate) that are not easily amenable to surgery have been well controlled by involved-field RT.

Radiation Therapy for Relapsed and Refractory Low-Grade Lymphomas

While chemotherapy and antibody therapy are the primary treatments of advanced-stage low-grade lymphomas, the very high sensitivity of these lymphomas to radiation should not be ignored. Even extremely low doses of radiation can provide long-standing local control and effective palliation. Several European groups showed that patients with low-grade lymphoma and persistent or relapsed disease following several regimens of chemotherapy responded to only two treatments of 2 Gy each (a total of 4 Gy). Using this schedule, a Dutch group reported an overall response rate of 92% in 109 patients (304 symptomatic sites), most with FL; and a complete response rate of 61%.[69,70] The 2-year actuarial freedom from local progression (FFLP) rate was 56%. Similarly, a French team reported an objective response of 81% of the sites, with 57% attaining a complete remission. The 2-year actuarial FFLP rate was 56%.[71]

Mantle Cell Lymphoma

While mantle cell lymphoma (MCL) presents in Stage IV in most patients, and is treated primarily with chemotherapy, its exquisite sensitivity to radiation should not be ignored. A British Columbia Cancer Center study indicated that patients with MCL Stages I and II, benefited significantly from localized RT alone or combined with chemotherapy. The 5-year PFS was 68% for those receiving RT compared to 11% in patients not receiving RT (p = 0.002), and the 6-year overall survival was 71% and 25%, respectively (p = 0.13).[72] At MSKCC, we used low-dose RT for local control and palliation of 38 sites in 21 patients previously treated with chemotherapy. Local control with radiation was obtained in all sites, and a complete response was achieved in 64% of the sites. Ninety-four percent of symptomatic patients obtained pain control with RT. Local progression occurred in 34% of patients at a median time to progression of 10 months. Since only low-dose radiation is required (15 to 30 Gy) in MCL, large nodal sites may be treated with only minor side effects and without jeopardizing other future therapeutic options.

Diffuse Large B-Cell Lymphoma

Early Stage

In the past, radiation alone was considered an appropriate treatment for patients with localized (Stages I and II) diffuse large B-cell lymphoma (DLBCL). Young patients with low-bulk Stage I DLBCL obtained 10-year survival of 87%, but other patients have relapsed in a rate higher than 50%.

Until the 1980s, the majority of patients with early-stage aggressive lymphoma were treated with radiotherapy alone.[44] In clinically staged patients, the use of regional or extended field irradiation for Stage I disease resulted in a cure rate of approximately 50%. The survival of similarly treated Stage II patients was only 20%.[73] Most of the relapses in patients treated with radiotherapy alone were extranodal or occurred outside the irradiated field. More restrictive selection of patients (Stage I only), using staging laparotomy, and treatment with extensive fields of radiation yielded a 10-year relapse-free survival rate of 90% to 100%.[74] Still, even staging laparotomy and total lymphoid irradiation yielded unsatisfactory survival rates of 35% to 55% in patients with pathologic Stage II disease.[75]

The advent of effective chemotherapy for aggressive NHL, and the impracticality of staging laparotomy in relatively old patients with potentially progressive disease, made radiotherapy alone obsolete for most patients with early-stage aggressive lymphoma. Several randomized studies indicated that adjuvant chemotherapy following involved- or extended-field radiotherapy results in significantly better relapse-free survival rates than treatment with radiation alone in early-stage aggressive lymphoma. In some studies, the improved relapse-free survival has translated into a survival advantage.[76] Most studies showed an advantage to combined modality using CVP chemotherapy (without doxorubicin).[48,77] In a randomized study from MSKCC, patients with Stage I were randomly assigned to receive either regional radiation therapy alone or radiation therapy followed by the commonly used CHOP regimen. The MSKCC study showed that in patients with aggressive NHL, the 7-year actuarial relapse-free survival rate for combined modality therapy was 86% compared with 20% for radiotherapy alone (p = 0.004). The corresponding actuarial survival rates were 92% and 47%, respectively (p = 0.08).[49]

Some studies suggested that when chemotherapy is combined with involved-field radiotherapy, less than the standard six cycles of chemotherapy may be required for patients with good prognosis, early-stage NHL (see Table 12–6). At the NCI, 49 patients with Stage I or IE large-cell lymphoma were treated with four cycles of cyclophosphamide, etoposide, doxorubicin, nitrogen mustard, vincristine, procarbazine, high-dose methotrexate, and prednisone (ProMace-MOPP) in reduced doses followed by involved-field radiotherapy to a dose of 40 Gy.[78] Forty-seven of 49 patients achieved a complete response, and all 47 patients remained free of disease with a median follow-up of 4 years. A similar prospective study in Vancouver treated 308 patients with aggressive lymphoma with three cycles of doxorubicin-containing chemotherapy followed by involved-field radiation therapy to a dose of 30 (10 fractions) to 35 (20 fractions) Gy. These patients achieved an 81% progression-free survival, and 80% survival with a median at 5 years and 74% and 63% at 10 years.[79]

The question of whether the addition of radiotherapy improves the relapse-free survival rate and overall survival rate in patients with early-stage aggressive lymphoma who attained a complete response with chemotherapy was controversial until recently.[83] Two small, nonrandomized studies suggested that treatment with chemotherapy alone may yield results comparable to those obtained with combined modality therapy.[81] At M.D. Anderson Cancer Center, patients with Stage I and II achieved a 10-year relapse-free survival rate of 83% and 65%, respectively.[84] At the Univer-

Table 12–6. Combined Modality Programs for Early-Stage Aggressive Lymphomas

Reference	Regimen	Patients (*n*)	Stage	Relapse-Free Survival, %	Overall Survival, %
Kaminsky et al.[80]	CHOP-EFRT	48	I	90	80
			II	70	68
Jones et al.[81]	CHOP-IFRT	17	I–II	87	93
Stewart et al.[82]	CHOP-3–IFRT	78	I–II	84	85
Longo et al.[78]	ProMACE–MOPP-4–IFRT	49	I	100	100
Shenkier et al.[79]	CHOP or CHOP-like x3–4 + IFRT	308	I–II	81	80

CHOP, cyclosphamide, doxorubicin, vincristine, prednisone; EFRT, extended-field radiotherapy; IFRT, involved-field radiotherapy; pro-MACE–MOPP, methotrexate, adriamycin, cyclophosamide, etoposide, mechloroethamine, oncovin, procarbazine, prednisone.

Table 12–7. Role of Radiotherapy in Stages I and II Aggressive Lymphomas: Randomized Studies

	Progression-Free Survival, %			
Reference	Patients (*n*)	CHOP, %	CHOP-RT, %	p value
Horning et al.[87]	345	39	54	0.06
Miller et al.[88]	401	66	77	0.01

CHOP, cyclophosphamide, doxorubicin, vincristine, prednisone.

sity of Arizona, selected patients with Stage I and II disease treated with CHOP alone attained a relapse-free survival rate of 75%.[85]

Adjuvant radiation therapy has become the standard of care in early-stage aggressive NHL following the analysis of two large randomized studies by the ECOG and SWOG.[86] These studies are summarized in Table 12–7. The ECOG study involved patients with bulky or extranodal Stage I and Stage II intermediate grade NHL (according to the Working Formulation).[87] All patients received eight cycles of CHOP chemotherapy. Patients who attained only a partial response following chemotherapy received involved-field radiotherapy to 40 Gy, and 28% converted to complete-response status. Patients in complete response (61%) following chemotherapy alone were randomly assigned either to receive radiotherapy of 30 Gy to site pre-treatment involvement or to observation alone. The recent 15-year update showed a statistically significant advantage to the adjuvant radiotherapy arm. The patients who received adjuvant radiotherapy attained a better failure-free survival rate than those receiving CHOP alone (54% vs. 39%; P = 0.06).[87] Overall survival that included all causes of death in this aging population was better in the irradiated group (60% vs. 44%), but the difference was not statistically significant. Cause-specific survival was not reported.

The SWOG study enrolled patients with Stage I and nonbulky Stage II aggressive NHL. The patients were randomly assigned to receive either eight cycles of CHOP chemotherapy alone, or three cycles of CHOP followed by an involved field of 40 Gy (with an optional boost of up to 55 Gy). At a median follow-up of 4 years, the progression-free survival rate was significantly greater for the short-course CHOP plus radiotherapy group: 77% compared with 66% in the group receiving eight cycles of CHOP with no radiotherapy. The combined modality treatment also resulted in a superior overall survival rate (87% vs. 75%; P = 0.01). Additionally, reversible toxicity occurring during therapy also favored the combined modality arm.[88] Recent analysis is of the SWOG data suggested that patients with early-stage, modified high IPI had inferior survival, and may require more than three cycles of chemotherapy.[89]

The results of both randomized studies confirm the importance of adjuvant radiation therapy to the involved field in patients who attained a complete response following short (three cycles) or long (eight cycles) chemotherapy. A relatively low dose of 30 Gy was adequate for patients who attained a complete response in the ECOG study (using eight cycles of CHOP), while a higher dose (40 to 55 Gy) was used in the short chemotherapy arm of the SWOG study. We currently advocate consolidation with a dose of 30 to 36 Gy for patients who have attained an unquestionable complete response following three to six cycles of chemotherapy. This is based on our (and others') excellent local control data with dose range.[90,91] Yet, other groups have advocated doses in the range of 39 to 51 Gy for disease larger than 3.5 cm.[92] We advise a higher dose (40 to 50 Gy) for uncertain complete responses. For evaluating response, we recommend obtaining a positron emission tomography-computed tomography (PET-CT) scan prior to and following chemotherapy, since a positive PET scan following chemotherapy may indicate an incomplete response that mandates a more aggressive approach.

Advanced Stage

The standard treatment for patients with advanced-stage (III or IV) aggressive lymphoma is combination chemotherapy, and R-CHOP is the most commonly used combination.[89] In North America, radiation therapy as consolidation to even bulky sites or incomplete responders is rarely being considered, although supported by retrospective studies.[93] Surprisingly, the data regarding the irrelevance of radiotherapy in these situations are scanty and/or indirect, at best.[94]

Unfortunately, while the superiority of combined modality over chemotherapy alone has been established for early stages, the concept and feasibility have not been tested in trials for advanced-stage NHL in the United States. It is of interest that recent randomized studies from other countries suggest that radiotherapy, particularly if administered to areas of originally bulky disease, may significantly improve the relapse-free survival and overall survival of patients who attained a CR with chemotherapy.[95–98]

Investigators from Mexico City conducted two consecutive randomized studies with a similar design. In the first study, 218 patients with Stage IV diffuse large-cell lymphoma were included. Following chemotherapy, 155 patients (71%) achieved a complete response. Of the complete responders, 88 patients (56%) originally presented with bulky disease (>10 cm) and therefore were prospectively randomized to observation or to receive involved-field radiotherapy to a dose of 40 to 50 Gy. At 5 years, 72% of 43 patients randomized to receive radiotherapy were alive and disease-free as compared with only 35% of the 45 patients who were not irradiated ($p < 0.01$). Most of the relapses occurred in the original site. Overall survival was also improved for the irradiated patients (81% vs. 55%; $p < 0.01$).[95] In the more recent study, 341 patients with aggressive DLCL and presence of nodal bulky disease (tumor mass >10 cm) in pathologic proven complete response after intensive chemotherapy were randomized to received either radiotherapy (involved fields, 40 Gy) or not. The 5-year EFS and OS in radiated patients were 82% and 87%, respectively. Both EFS and OS were significantly better to the control group: EFS, 55% ($p < 0.001$) and OS, 66% ($p < 0.01$), respectively. Radiotherapy was well tolerated, acute toxicity was mild and until now late toxicity did not appear.[98]

In Milan, 97 patients with Stages III-IV diffuse, large-cell lymphoma that were in CR after chemotherapy were either observed or received consolidation radiotherapy. At 5 years, patients with bulky disease (≥10 cm) who received radiotherapy had a significantly longer time to relapse and a better overall survival ($p = 0.05$) compared with patients who were not irradiated. A multivariate analysis showed that the use of radiotherapy was an independent favorable prognostic factor for relapse ($p = 0.001$) and survival ($p = 0.05$).[96]

In Paris, patients with NHL who underwent high-dose chemotherapy with stem-cell transplantation as up-front treatment or treatment for relapse and received post-transplantation radiotherapy, had a better event-free survival compared with patients who had not received radiotherapy ($p = 0.02$ in multivariate analysis). Other studies have also supported the use of consolidation radiotherapy after high-dose chemotherapy and bone marrow transplantation.[97]

These data support the notion that although intermediate-grade NHL is a systemic disease, and all stages should primarily be treated with chemotherapy. Yet, radiotherapy for bulky or residual disease may improve the outcome of the treatment program. While more studies should address the potential benefit of radiation therapy in advanced-stage disease, the above data provide an adequate basis to justify the combined modality approach in selected cases.

Primary Mediastinal Lymphoma

In most patients, the disease is bulky and limited to the mediastinum. Consolidation with involved field radiotherapy of the mediastinum after a complete or uncertain or partial response with chemotherapy is a standard approach in most centers.[99,100] Several large retrospective studies indicated the superiority of combined modality approach in primary mediastinal lymphoma over chemotherapy alone.[101] Yet, prospective randomized studies evaluating the contribution of RT in mediastinal lymphoma have not been reported.

The radiation therapy considerations in treating T-cell lymphomas of the skin (including mycosis fungoides) are discussed in Chapter 26 and in treating primary CNS lymphoma in Chapter 17C.

RADIATION FIELDS: PRINCIPLES AND DESIGN

In the past, radiation-field design attempted to include multiple involved and uninvolved lymph node sites. The large fields known as "mantle," "inverted Y," and "total lymphoid irradiation" (TLI) were synonymous with the radiation treatment of HL and NHL. These fields should rarely be used nowadays. The involved field, or its slightly larger version—the regional field, encompasses a significantly smaller, but adequate volume when radiotherapy is used as consolidation after chemotherapy in HL and in DLBCL. Even when radiation is used as the only treatment (e.g., early-stage follicular, marginal zone, and lymphocyte-predominant HL), the field should be limited to the involved site or to the involved sites and immediately adjacent lymph node groups. Further, even more limited radiation fields restricted to the originally involved lymph node are currently under study by several European groups.

The many terminologies given to radiation field variations in HL and NHL caused significant confusion and difficulties in comparing treatment programs. While the final determination of the field may vary from patient to patient, and depends on many clinical, anatomic, and normal tissue tolerance considerations, general definitions and guidelines are available and should be followed.[4]

The following are definitions of types of radiation fields used in HL and NHL.

Involved Field

This field is limited to the site of the clinically involved lymph node *group* (Fig. 12–1). For extranodal sites, the field includes the organ alone (if no evidence for lymph node involvement). The "grouping" of lymph nodes is not clearly defined and involved-field borders for common presentation of HL will be discussed below.

Regional Field

This field includes the involved lymph node group field *plus* at least one adjacent clinically uninvolved group (Fig. 12–2). For extranodal disease, it includes the involved organ plus the clinically uninvolved lymph nodes region.

Extended Field

This field includes *multiple* involved and uninvolved lymph node groups. If the multiple sites are limited to one side of the diaphragm, the upper field is called the *mantle* field (Fig. 12–3A). The extended field that includes all lymph node sites below the diaphragm (with or without the spleen) is called *inverted Y*, after its shape (Fig. 12–3B).

When radiation treatment includes all lymph nodes on both sides of the diaphragm, these large fields are combined, the resulting field is called *total lymphoid irradiation (TLI)* or *total nodal irradiation (TNI)*; if the pelvic lymph nodes are excluded, the field is called *subtotal lymphoid irradiation (STLI)* (Fig. 12–4).

Involved Lymph Node(s) Field

This is the most limited radiation field that has just recently been introduced. The clinical treated volume (CTV) includes only the originally involved lymph node(s) volume (pre-chemotherapy) with the addition of a 1-cm margin to create planned treatment volume (Fig. 12–5).

Considerations in Designing Involved-Field Radiotherapy

While it is understood that the involved field should address an area smaller than the classical extended fields of mantle or inverted Y, it is not entirely clear how small the field should remain. Should only the area of the enlarged lymph node (with margins) be irradiated? Should a region of lymph nodes be addressed? And if yes, what are the borders of this region? Many use the lymph node region diagram that was adopted for staging purposes at the Rye symposium (1966) to define a region of lymph nodes.[102] However, this diagram was not developed for individual radiation field design, and strangely enough the chart distinguishes between a mediastinal and a hilar region, has a

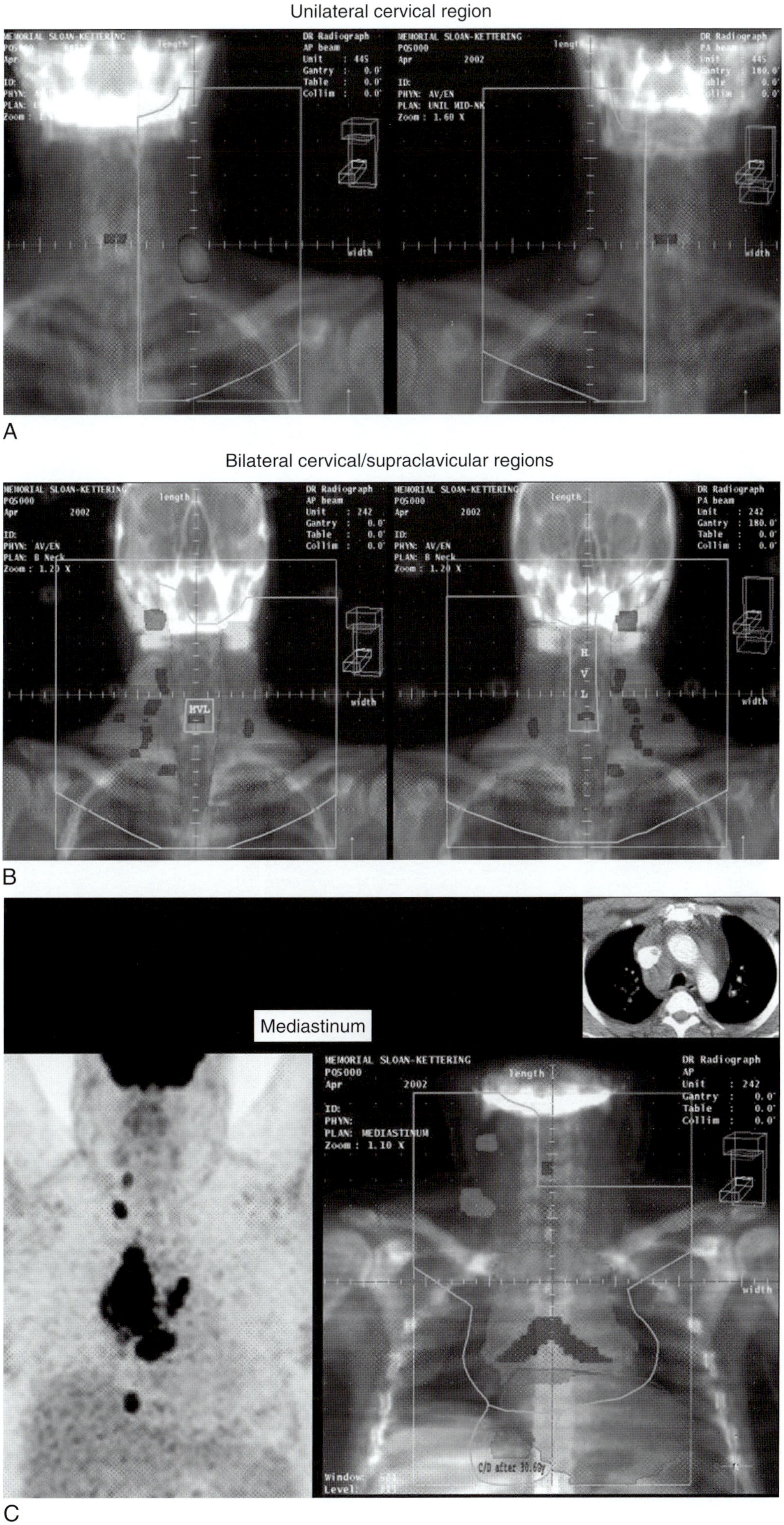

Figure 12–1. Involved field radiotherapy. **A:** Stage I HL involving the right neck. **B:** Stage II HL involving the right neck and the left lower neck. **C:** Stage IIX HL with involvement of the right neck, bulky mediastinum, right hilum, and right cardiophrenic area. (See color insert.)

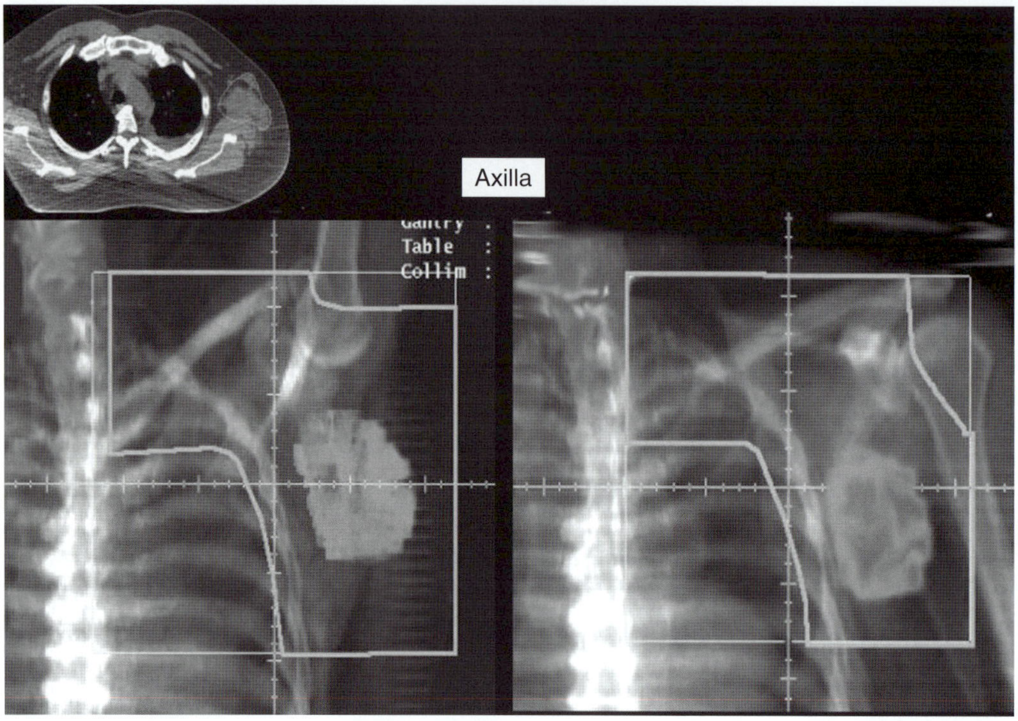

Figure 12–2. Regional field radiotherapy. Stage I HL involving the left axilla. (See color insert.)

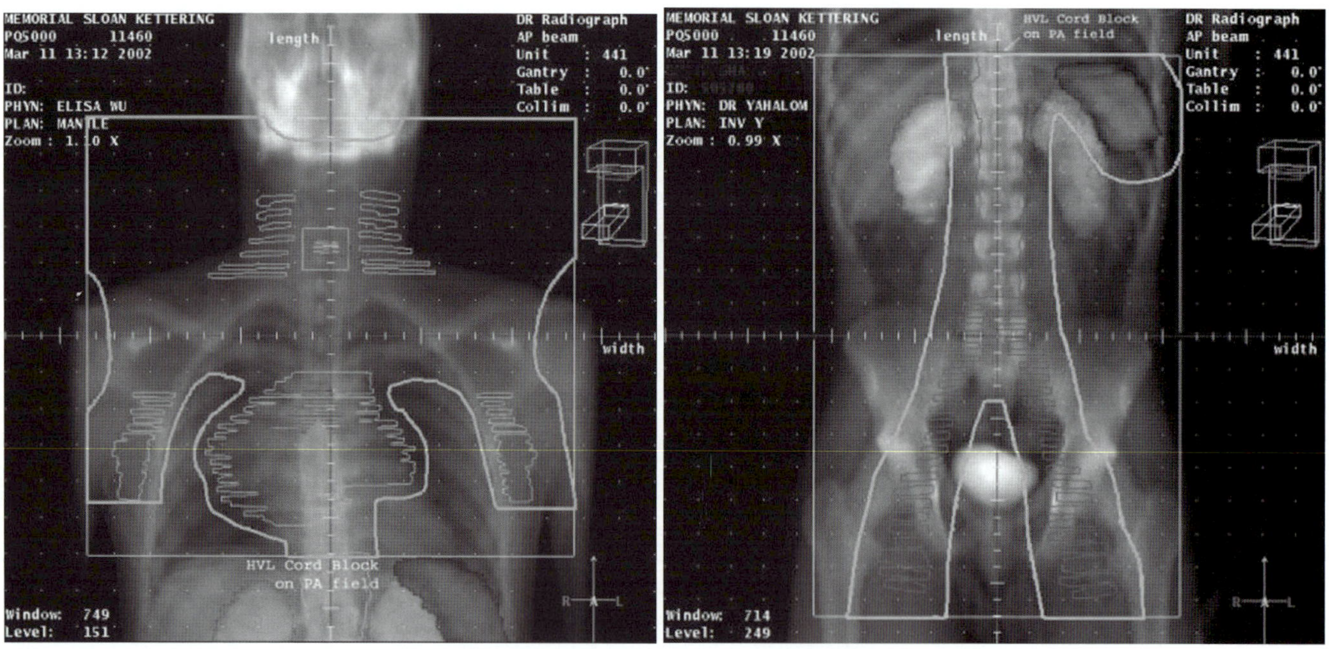

A B

Figure 12–3. Extended field. **A:** Mantle field. **B:** Inverted Y. (See color insert.)

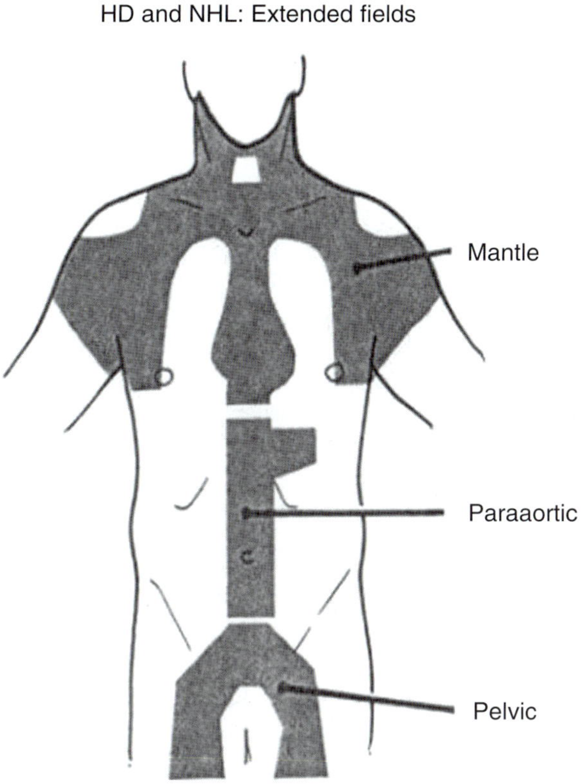

Figure 12–4. Total lymphoid irradiation.

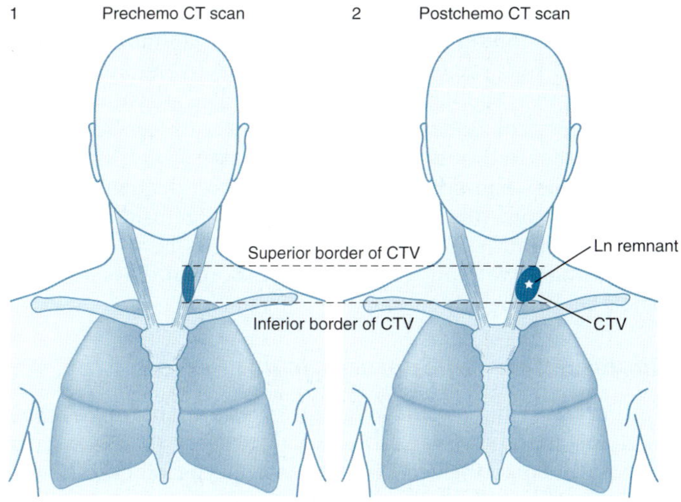

Figure 12–5. Initially involved lymph node field.

separate infra-clavicular lymph region, and does not provide borders of the individual sites. Other questions relate to the change in size (or complete resolution) of the lymph node after chemotherapy. Should the pre-chemotherapy volume be irradiated? Or should we spare the tissues (such as lung) that are no longer involved by the disease by irradiating the post-chemotherapy residual abnormality alone?

There are no definitive answers to the above questions and it is often the individual clinical situation that affects the field design. At the same time, uniform general guidelines are important for assuring a high standard of treatment, and are essential for collaborative group studies.

Suggested Guidelines for Delineating the Involved Field to Nodal Sites

1. IFRT is treatment of a region, not of an individual lymph node.
2. The main involved-field nodal regions are neck (unilateral), mediastinum (including the hilar regions bilaterally), axilla (including the supraclavicular and infraclavicular lymph nodes), spleen, para-aortic lymph nodes, and inguinal (including the femoral and iliac nodes).
3. In general, the fields include the involved pre-chemotherapy sites and volume, with an important exception that involves the transverse diameter of the mediastinal and para-aortic lymph nodes. For the field width of these sites, it is recommended to use the reduced post-chemotherapy diameter. In these areas, the regression of the lymph nodes is easily depicted by computed tomography (CT) imaging and the critical normal tissue is saved by reducing the irradiated volume.
4. The supraclavicular lymph nodes are considered part of the cervical region and if involved alone or with other cervical nodes, the whole neck is unilaterally treated. Only if the supraclavicular involvement is an extension of mediastinal disease and the other neck areas are not involved (based on CT imaging with contrast and gallium/PET imaging, when appropriate) the upper neck (above the larynx) is spared. This is to avoid irradiating the salivary glands when the risk for the area is low.
5. All borders should be easy to outline (most are bony landmarks) and plan on a two-dimensional standard simulation unit. CT data are required for outlining the mediastinal and para-aortic region, and will also help in designing the axillary field.
6. Pre-chemotherapy and post-chemotherapy information (both CT and PET) regarding lymph node localization and size is critical, and should be available at the time of planning the field.

Involved Field Guidelines for Common Nodal Sites

Unilateral Cervical/Supraclavicular Region

Involvement at any cervical level with or without involvement of the supraclavicular (SCL) nodes.

Arms position: akimbo or at sides. Upper border: 1 to 2 cm above the lower tip of the mastoid process and midpoint through the chin. Lower border: 2 cm below the bottom of the clavicle. Lateral border: To include the medial 2/3 of the clavicle. Medial border: (1) If the supraclavicular nodes are not involved, the border is placed at the ipsilateral transverse processes, except when medial nodes close to the vertebral bodies are seen on the initial staging neck CT scan. For medial nodes, the entire vertebral body is included. (2) When the supraclavicular nodes are involved, the border should be placed at the contra-lateral transverse processes. For Stage I patients, the larynx and vertebral bodies above the larynx can be blocked (assuming no medial cervical nodes). Blocks: A posterior cervical cord block is required only if cord dose exceeds 40 Gy. Mid-neck calculations should be performed to determine the maximum cord dose, especially when the central axis is in the mediastinum. A laryngeal block should be used unless lymph nodes were present in that location. In that case, the block should be added at 20 Gy (Fig. 12–1A).

Bilateral Cervical/Supraclavicular Region

Both cervical and supraclavicular regions should be treated as described above regardless of the extent of disease on each side. Posterior cervical cord and larynx blocks should be used as described above. Use a posterior mouth block if treating the patient supine to block the upper field divergence through the mouth (Fig. 12–1B).

Mediastinum

Involvement of the mediastinum and/or the hilar nodes: In HL, this field includes also the medial SCL nodes even if not clinically involved. In NHL, the volume is limited to the mediastinum.

Arms position: akimbo or at sides. The arms-up position is optional if the axillary nodes are involved. Upper border: C5–C6 interspace. If supraclavicular nodes were also involved, the upper border should be placed at the top of the larynx, and the lateral border should be adjusted as described in the section on treating neck nodes. Lower border: The lower of (1) 5 cm below the carina or (2) 2 cm below the pre-chemotherapy inferior border. Lateral border: The post-chemotherapy volume with 1.5-cm margin. Hilar area: To be included with 1-cm margin unless initially involved, whereas the margin should be 1.5 cm.

Mediastinum with Involvement of Cervical Nodes

When both cervical regions are involved, the field is a mantle without the axilla using the guidelines described above. If only one cervical chain is involved, the vertebral bodies, contralateral upper neck, and larynx can be blocked as previously described. Because of the increased dose to the neck (the isocenter is in the upper mediastinum), the neck above the lower border of the larynx should be shielded at 30.6 Gy. If paracardiac nodes are involved, the whole heart should be treated to 14.4 Gy, and the initially involved nodes should be treated to 30.6 Gy (Fig. 12–1C).

Axillary Region

The ipsilateral axillary, infraclavicular, and supraclavicular areas are treated when the axilla is involved. Whenever possible, use CT-based planning for this region. Arms akimbo or arms up. Upper Border: C5–C6 interspace. Lower border: The lower of the two of (1) the tip of the scapula, or (2) 2 cm below the lowest axillary node. Medial border: Ipsilateral cervical transverse process. Include the vertebral bodies only if the SCL are involved. Lateral border: Flash axilla.

Spleen

The spleen is treated only if abnormal imaging was suggestive of involvement. The *post-chemotherapy* volume is treated with 1.5-cm margins.

Abdomen (Para-aortic Nodes)

Upper border: Top of T11 and at least 2 cm above pre-chemotherapy volume. Lower border: Bottom of L4 and at least 2 cm below pre-chemotherapy volume. Lateral borders: The edge of the transverse processes and at least 2 cm from the post-chemotherapy volume.

Inguinal/Femoral/External Iliac Region

These ipsilateral lymph node groups are treated together if any of the nodes are involved.

Upper border: Middle of the sacro-iliac joint. Lower border: 5 cm below the lesser trochanter. Lateral border: The greater trochanter and 2 cm lateral to initially involved nodes. Medial border: Medial border of the obturator foramen with at least 2 cm medial to involved nodes. If common iliac nodes are involved, the field should extend to the L4–L5 inter-space and at least 2 cm above the initially involved nodal border.

INVOLVED FIELDS IN RADIOTHERAPY OF EXTRANODAL SITES

In most cases, the whole involved organ is the target, and draining lymph nodes are not included unless involved. The optimal plan is 3D-conformal and CT-simulation based. The margins for the planned treatment volume depend on quality of imaging and reliability of immobilization, and most importantly, should account for organ motion during respiration. Typically, organs in the head and neck require margins of 1 cm and organs in the mediastinum, abdomen and pelvis require margins of 2 cm.

NEW ASPECTS OF RADIATION FIELD DESIGN AND DELIVERY

As the notion of treating large areas of involved and uninvolved areas has changed in favor of treating only the involved lymph node group or extranodal organ, new options of more conformal radiotherapy have opened up. The old extensive radiation fields such as mantle or inverted Y included multiple sites at various depths (from the body surface), and each site had various limitations of access and tolerance of normal tissue. The only way to include these sites in a single radiation field (and thus avoid overlaps and gaps when radiation fields were matched) was to treat the whole field from only two opposed directions, anterior and posterior. This technique assured the inclusion of most lymph nodes in one field, yet it also resulted in exposure of large volumes of normal organs (e.g., heart, lungs, breasts, and spinal cord) to the full prescribed radiation dose.

The radiotherapy of the involved field alone as practiced today avoids this shortcoming in most cases by allowing the use of three-dimensional conformal radiotherapy (3-D conformal radiation therapy [CRT]). For example, 3-D CRT of an anterior mediastinal mass could avoid radiation of the spine and much of the heart and lung tissue located behind the mass.

The change in the lymphoma radiotherapy paradigm coincided with substantial improvement in imaging and treatment planning technology that has revolutionized the field of radiotherapy over the last 15 years. The integration of fast high-resolution computerized tomography into the simulation and planning systems of radiation oncology has changed how treatment volumes and relationship to normal critical structures are determined and planned. In the recent past, tumor volume determinations were made with fluoroscopy-based simulators that produced less than optimal chest x-ray films that obviously resulted in a need to include wide "safety margins" that detracted from accuracy and sparing of critical organs. The most modern simulators are in fact high-resolution computed tomography (CT) scanners with capabilities and software that allow accurate conformal treatment planning with detailed information on the dose-volume delivered to normal structures in each individual optional plan and the homogeneity of dose delivered to the target. More recently, these simulators are integrated also with a PET scanner that provides additional tumor volume information for consideration during radiation planning.

Intensity modulated radiotherapy (IMRT) is the most advanced planning and radiation delivery mode and is mainly used for small volume cancers that require high radiation doses (e.g., prostate and head neck cancers) or are adjacent to critical organs. IMRT allows for accurately enveloping the tumor with either a homogenous radiation dose ("sculpting") or delivering higher doses to predetermined areas in the tumor volume ("painting"). The end result of this new modality is highly accurate treatment with maximal sparing of normal tissues. In the radiotherapy of lymphoma, there are several clinical situations where IMRT provides a benefit: treatment of very large or complicated tumor volumes in the mediastinum (Fig. 12–6 A–C) and abdomen, head and neck lymphomas. IMRT also allows re-irradiation of sites prior to high-dose salvage programs that otherwise will be prohibited by normal tissue tolerance, particularly of the spinal cord (Fig. 12–7 A–E).[103]

SIDE EFFECTS AND COMPLICATIONS OF RADIOTHERAPY

Side effects of radiotherapy depend on the irradiated volume, dose administered, and technique employed. They are also influenced by the extent and type of prior chemotherapy, if any, and by the patient's age. Most of the information that we use today to estimate risk of radiotherapy is derived from strategies that used radiation alone. The field size and configuration, doses, and technology have all drastically changed over the last decade. Thus, it is probably misleading to judge current radiotherapy for lymphomas and inform patients solely on the basis of various past practices of using radiotherapy alone in treating lymphomas.

It is of interest that most of the data of long-term complications associated with radiotherapy and particularly second solid tumors and coronary heart disease were reported from databases of HL patients treated more than 25 years ago. We have very little information on NHL patients treated with combined modality or with radiation alone and their potential long-term complications. The difference between the two diseases with regard to increased risk reported may be a result of differences in age group treated, length of follow-up, and smaller volumes of RT fields used in NHL. It is also important to note that we have very limited long-term follow-up data on patients with HL or NHL that were treated with chemotherapy alone. Yet, increased incidence of lung cancer following treatment with chemotherapy alone was reported for both HL and NHL.[104–106]

Acute Effects

Radiation, in general, may cause fatigue and areas of the irradiated skin may develop mild sun-exposure–like dermatitis. The acute side effects of irradiating the full neck include mouth dryness, change in taste, and pharyngitis. These side effects are usually mild and transient. The main potential side effects of subdiaphragmatic irradiation are loss of appetite, nausea, and increased bowel movements. These reactions are usually mild and can be minimized with standard antiemetic medications.

Irradiation of more than one field, particularly after chemotherapy, can cause myelosuppression, which may necessitate short treatment interruption, and very rarely, administration of G-colony stimulating factor (G-CSF).

Early Side Effects

Lhermitte's Sign

Less than 5% of patients may note an electric shock sensation radiating down the backs of both legs when the head is flexed (Lhermitte's sign) 6 weeks to 3 months after mantle-field radiotherapy. Possibly secondary to transient demyelinization of the spinal cord, Lhermitte's sign resolves spontaneously after a few months, and is not associated with late or permanent spinal cord damage.

Pneumonitis and Pericarditis

During the same period, radiation pneumonitis and/or acute pericarditis may occur in less than 5% of patients; these side effects occur more often in those who have extensive mediastinal disease. Both inflammatory processes have become rare with modern radiation techniques.

Late Side Effects

Subclinical Hypothyroidism

Irradiation of the neck and/or upper mediastinum can induce subclinical hypothyroidism in about one-third of patients. This condition is detected by elevation of thyroid-stimulating hormone (TSH). Thyroid replacement with levothyroxine (T4) is recommended, even in asymptomatic patients, to prevent overt hypothyroidism and decrease the risk of benign thyroid nodules.

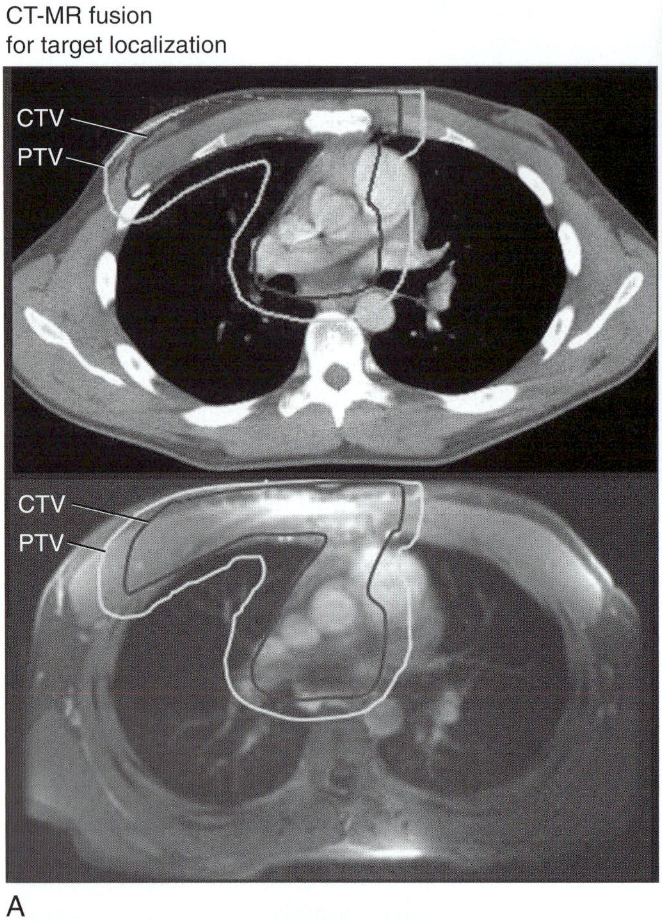

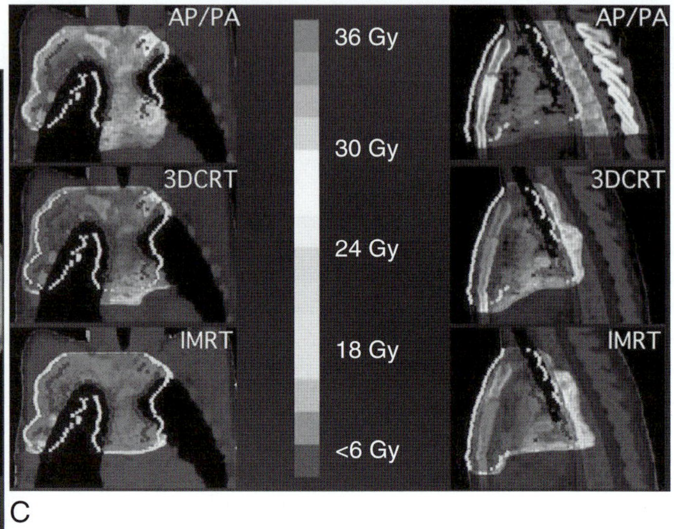

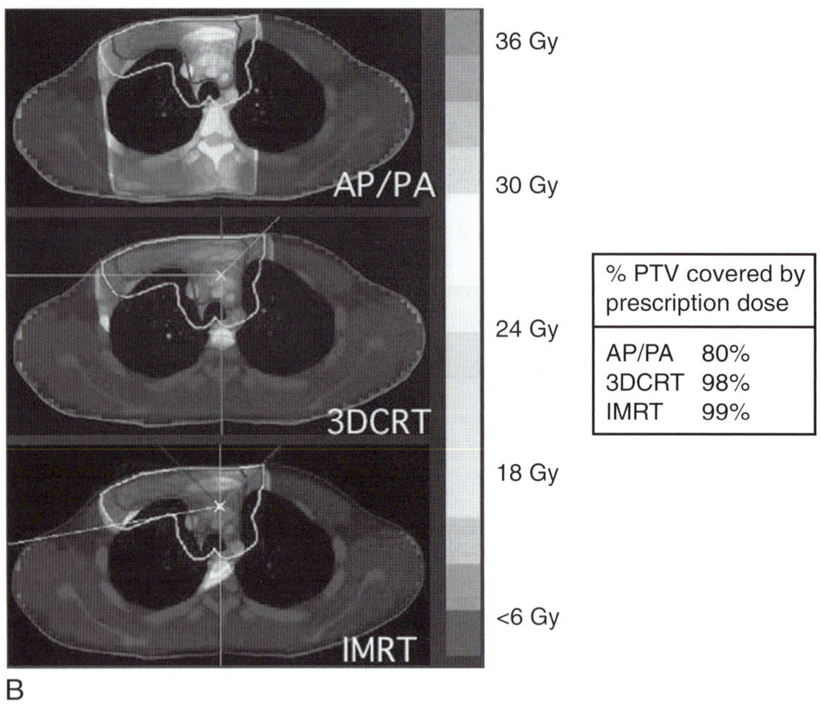

Figure 12–6. (A–C): Intensity-modulated radiation therapy for extensive HL involving the mediastinum and the chest wall. (See color insert.)

Infertility

Only irradiation of the pelvic field may have deleterious effects on fertility. In most patients, this problem can be avoided by appropriate gonadal shielding. In females, the ovaries can be moved into a shielded area laterally or inferomedially near the uterine cervix. Irradiation outside of the pelvis does not increase the risk of sterility.

Secondary Malignancies

Hodgkin's disease patients who were cured with radiotherapy and/or chemotherapy have an increased risk of secondary solid tumors (most commonly, lung, breast, and stomach cancers, as well as melanoma), and NHL 10 or more years after treatment. Unlike MOPP and similar chemotherapy combinations or etoposide, radiotherapy for Hodgkin's disease is not leukemogenic.

Lung Cancer

Patients who are smokers should be strongly encouraged to quit the habit because the increase in lung cancer that occurs after irradiation or chemotherapy has been detected mostly in smokers.

Breast Cancer

For women whose HD was successfully treated at a young age, the main long-term concern is the increased risk of breast cancer.[107] During the last decade, multiple studies have documented and characterized the risk of breast cancer after HD, and have established the following fact that the increase in breast cancer risk is undoubtedly associated with the use of radiation.[108–110] The magnitude of the risk is not completely clear, and different methods of risk reporting and data are found in the literature with relative risk ratios from 2 to 450.[107,111] Unfortunately, relative risk (RR), absolute risk and actuarial risks are often cited without

COMPARISON OF TREATMENT PLANS

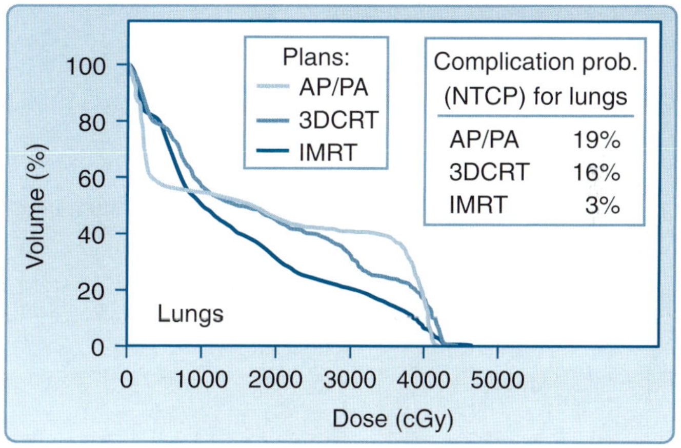

A

Relapsed NSHD after ABVD+36 Gy mantle RT

Post-induction chemotherapy CT

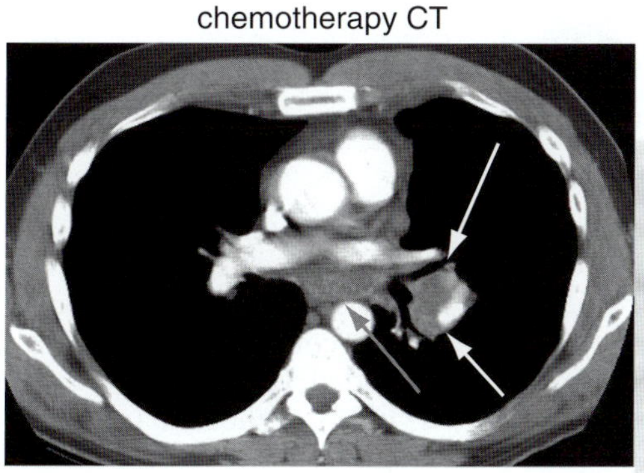

B

Post-chemotherapy PET

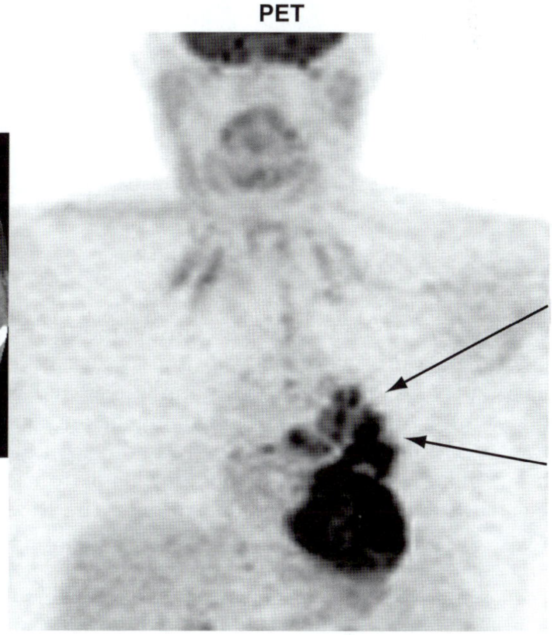

C

Figure 12–7. **(A–E):** Reirradiation of a relapsed mediastinal mass using intensity-modulated radiation therapy to avoid the spinal cord. (See color insert.)

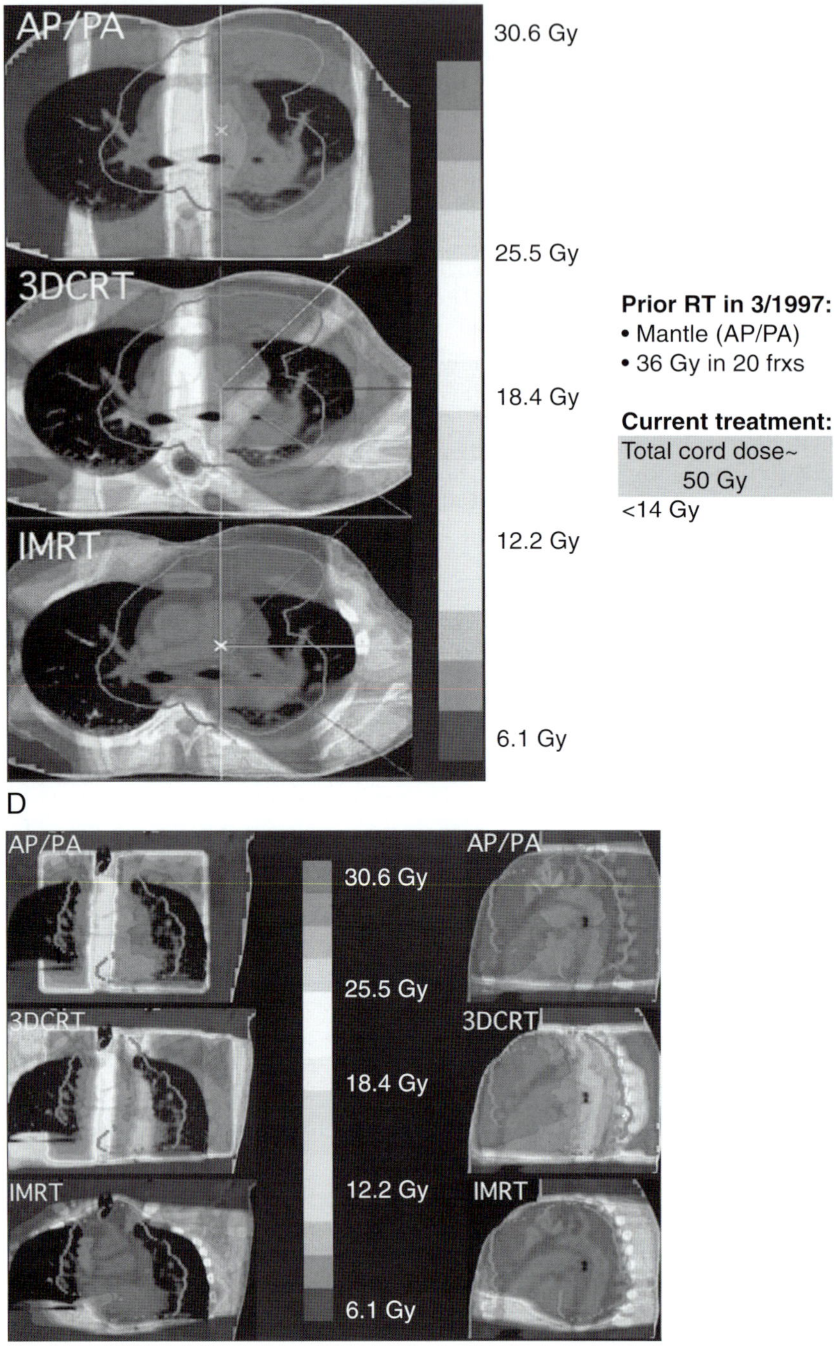

Figure 12–7, cont'd

detailing specifics that could have influenced the findings (i.e., length of follow-up for the group and for the individuals; age group, age-incidence, and actuarial risk of the malignancy in an untreated population; and quality of follow-up, which may result in event over-estimation).[109] In the largest long-term follow-up study of second neoplasms in survivors of HD, which included data from 16 cancer registries of more than 35,000 patients, the RR for breast cancer in women was 2, and the absolute excess risk was 10.5.[107]

The increase in breast cancer risk is inversely related to the patient's age at Hodgkin's disease treatment; no increased risk has been found in women irradiated after 30 years of age. It is also inversely related to the radiation dose to the breast and the volume of breast tissue exposed.[108,109] In a recent study, Travis and colleagues from 13 centers in seven countries reported a large case-control study that included 105 women who developed breast cancer within a cohort of more than 3,800 1-year female survivors of HD diagnosed at age 30 or less.[109] Unique to this study is the use of patients who received a very low radiation dose (less than 4 Gy) or no radiation to the breast area where breast cancer developed. This approach allowed isolating treatment factors and analyzing the radiation dose- and chemotherapy dose-risk relationships. For all patients who received RT alone (≥4 Gy), the RR of breast cancer is 3.2, and increases to 8 in the highest radiation-dose group. The results reported by Travis et al. clearly demonstrate the influence of radiation dose on the risk of breast cancer. Within the range of doses to which the breast was exposed in past years, more radiation translates into a higher risk of developing breast cancer. This information, as well as data from earlier publications showing a significantly lower risk of second tumors when radiation was reduced from 40 Gy to 20 Gy[112,113] support the notion that "lower is better," as long as the radiation dose used augments the HL cure rate.

Radiotherapy alone had been the standard treatment and primary curative modality for HL through the 1970s and early 1980s. Irradiating all lymph node regions, regardless of clinical involvement with HL, had been standard practice, and relatively high doses (over 40 Gy) had been used. Consequently, a substantial amount of breast tissue was exposed to either the full prescribed dose or to an attenuated dose (at field margins or under the lung shields) in almost all women irradiated for HL. Most breast exposure in the "mantle" area, resulted from the radiation of the axillae (65% of tumors in this study developed in the outer part of the breast[109]), and to a lesser extent from wide mediastinal and hilar irradiation. Approximately two-thirds of women with early-stage HL do not require radiation of the axillae, and additional protection to the upper and medial aspects of the breast could be provided by further reducing field size using careful CT-based planning that usually allows for smaller mediastinal volumes, especially post-chemotherapy. During the last decade, reduction in field size has been the most important change in radiation therapy of HL. Reduction in the volume of exposed breast tissue together with dose reduction (from over 40 Gy to a dose in the range of 20 to 30 Gy) is likely to dramatically change the long-term risk profile of young male and female patients cured of HL. Emerging data from trials using smaller fields and lower doses support the expectation that the modern application of "miniradiotherapy" will be associated with a significantly lower risk of breast cancer as well as other solid tumors and cardiac sequelae.[12,113–115] Yet, longer follow-up of studies that employ smaller fields and lower doses is necessary.

Breast cancer is curable in its early stages, and early detection has a significant impact on survival. Breast examination should be part of the routine follow-up for women cured of Hodgkin's disease, and routine mammography should begin about 8 years after treatment.

Coronary Artery Disease

An increased risk of coronary artery disease has recently been reported among patients who have received mediastinal irradiation. To reduce this hazard, patients should be monitored and advised about other established coronary disease risk factors, such as smoking, hyperlipidemia, hypertension, and poor dietary and exercise habits. There are data supporting the notion that reduced fields and lower doses to the mediastinum have reduced the risk of heart disease in irradiated patients.[114,116]

Effects on Bone and Muscle Growth

In children, high-dose irradiation will affect bone and muscle growth and may result in deformities. Current treatment programs for pediatric Hodgkin's disease are chemotherapy based; radiotherapy is limited to low doses.

SUMMARY

Radiation therapy is an invaluable tool for the curative treatment of HL and many types of NHL. Radiotherapy can also provide important palliation for many patients who failed chemotherapy. Like most cancer treatments, radiation may have long-term side effects, particularly second solid tumors. These risks are related to the volume of normal tissue irradiated and to the radiation dose delivered. The use of radiotherapy has drastically changed since the early 1980s; the radiation fields are markedly smaller, the doses are lower, and improved technology of planning and delivery improved the identification of the appropriate target and the precision of delivery, resulting in reduced short and long-term risks to normal structures. When used intelligently, radiation can reduce the amount of chemotherapy and length of treatment, and its optimal integration in treatment programs for lymphomas should continue to be pursued.

References

1. Hoppe RT, et al. NCCN physician guidelines: Hodgkin disease 2005 vol. 1. National Comprehensive Cancer Network. Available at: www.nccn.org. Accessed Sept. 2005.
2. Diehl V, Thomas RK, and Re D. Part II: Hodgkin's lymphoma—diagnosis and treatment. Lancet Oncol 2004;5:19–26.
3. Schlembach PJ, Wilder RB, Jones D, et al. Radiotherapy alone for lymphocyte-predominant Hodgkin's disease. Cancer J 2002;8:377–83.
4. Yahalom J and Mauch P. The involved field is back: issues in delineating the radiation field in Hodgkin's disease. Ann Oncol 2002;13(Suppl 1):79–83.
5. Ng AK, Bernardo MP, Weller E, et al. Long-term survival and competing causes of death in patients with early-stage Hodgkin's disease treated at age 50 or younger. J Clin Oncol 2002;20:2101–8.
6. Ng AK and Mauch PM. Controversies in early-stage Hodgkin's disease. Oncology (Huntingt) 2002;16:588–95, 598; discussion 600, 605, 609–18.
7. Press OW, LeBlanc M, Lichter AS, et al. Phase III randomized intergroup trial of subtotal lymphoid irradiation versus doxorubicin, vinblastine, and subtotal lymphoid irradiation for stage IA to IIA Hodgkin's disease. J Clin Oncol 2001;19:4238–44.
8. Sieber M, Franklin J, Tesch H, et al. Two cycles ABVD plus extended field radiotherapy is superior to radiothearpy alone in early stage Hodgkin's disease: results of the German Hodgkin's Lymphoma Study Group (GHSG) Trial HD7. Blood 2002;100:Abstract 341.
9. Carde P, Noordijk E, and Hagenbeek A. Superiority of EBVP chemotherapy in combination with involved field irradiation over subtotal nodal irradiation in favorable clinical stage I–II Hodgkin's disease: The EORTC-GPMC H7F randomized trial. Proc ASCO 1997;16:13.
10. Hagenbeek A, Eghbali H, Ferme C, et al. Three cycles of MOPP/ABV hybrid and involved-field irradiation is more effective than subtotal nodal irradiation in favorable supradiaphragmatic clinical stages I–II Hodgkin's disease: preliminary results of the EORTC-GELA H9-F randomized trial in 543 patients. Blood 2000;96:Abstract 575.
11. Bonadonna G, Bonfante V, Viviani S, et al. ABVD plus subtotal nodal versus involved-field radiotherapy in early-stage

Hodgkin's disease: long-term results. J Clin Oncol 2004; 22:2835–41.
12. Engert A, Schiller P, Josting A, et al. Involved-field radiotherapy is equally effective and less toxic compared with extended-field radiotherapy after four cycles of chemotherapy in patients with early-stage unfavorable Hodgkin's lymphoma: results of the HD8 trial of the German Hodgkin's Lymphoma Study Group. J Clin Oncol 2003;21:3601–8.
13. Ferme C, Eghbali H, Hagenbeek A, et al. MOPP/ABV hybrid and irradiation in unfavorable supradiaphragmatic clinical stages I–II Hodgkin's disease: comparison of three treatment modalities. Preliminary results of the EORTC-GELA H8-U randomized trial in 995 patients. Blood 2000;96:Abstract 576.
14. Loeffler M, Diehl V, Pfreundschuh M, et al. Dose–response relationship of complementary radiotherapy following four cycles of combination chemotherapy in intermediate-stage Hodgkin's disease. J Clin Oncol 1997;15:2275–87.
15. Diehl V, Brillant C, Engert A, et al. Reduction of combined modality treatment intensity in early stage Hodgkin's lymphoma: interim analysis of the HD 10 trial of the GHSG. Blood 2004;104:Abstract 1307.
16. Diehl V, Brillant C, Engert A, et al. Intensification of chemotherapy and concomitant reduction of radiotherapy dose in intermediate stage Hodgkin's lymphoma: results of the fourth interim analysis of the HD 11 trial of the GHSG. Blood 2004;104:Abstract 1308.
17. DeVita VT Jr. Hodgkin's disease—clinical trials and travails. N Engl J Med 2003;348:2375–6.
18. Longo DL. Radiation therapy in the treatment of Hodgkin's disease—do you see what I see? J Natl Cancer Inst 2003; 95:928–9.
19. Biti GP, Cimino G, Cartoni C, et al. Extended-field radiotherapy is superior to MOPP chemotherapy for the treatment of pathologic stage I–IIA Hodgkin's disease: eight-year update of an Italian prospective randomized study. J Clin Oncol 1992;10:378–82.
20. Longo DL, Glatstein E, Duffey PL, et al. Radiation therapy versus combination chemotherapy in the treatment of early-stage Hodgkin's disease: seven-year results of a prospective randomized trial. J Clin Oncol 1991;9:906–17.
21. Canellos GP, Anderson JR, Propert KJ, et al. Chemotherapy of advanced Hodgkin's disease with MOPP, ABVD, or MOPP alternating with ABVD. N Engl J Med 1992;327:1478–84.
22. Carde P, Hagenbeek A, Hayat M, et al. Clinical staging versus laparotomy and combined modality with MOPP versus ABVD in early-stage Hodgkin's disease: the H6 twin randomized trials from the European Organization for Research and Treatment of Cancer Lymphoma Cooperative Group. J Clin Oncol 1993;11:2258–72.
23. Nachman JB, Sposto R, Herzog P, et al. Randomized comparison of low-dose involved-field radiotherapy and no radiotherapy for children with Hodgkin's disease who achieve a complete response to chemotherapy. J Clin Oncol 2002;20:3765–71.
24. Laskar S, Gupta T, Vimal S, et al. Consolidation radiation after complete remission in Hodgkin's disease following six cycles of doxorubicin, bleomycin, vinblastine, and dacarbazine chemotherapy: is there a need? J Clin Oncol 2004;22:62–8.
25. Meyer R, Gospodarowicz M, Connors JM, et al. A randomized phase III comparison of single-modality ABVD with a strategy that includes radiation therapy in patients with early-stage Hodgkin's disease: The HD-6 rial of the National Cancer Institute of Canada Clinical Trials Group (Eastern Cooperative). Blood 2003;102:Abstract 81.
26. Diehl V, Stein H, Hummel M, et al. Hodgkin's lymphoma: biology and treatment strategies for primary, refractory, and relapsed disease. Hematology (Am Soc Hematol Educ Program) 2003;225–47.
27. Straus DJ, Portlock CS, Qin J, et al. Results of a prospective randomized clinical trial of doxorubicin, bleomycin, vinblastine, and dacarbazine (ABVD) followed by radiation therapy (RT) versus ABVD alone for stages I, II, and IIIA nonbulky Hodgkin disease. Blood 2004;104:3483–9.
28. Prosnitz LR, Wu JJ, Yahalom J. The case for adjuvant radiation therapy in advanced Hodgkin's disease. Cancer Invest 1996;14:361–70.
29. Yahalom J, Ryu J, Straus DJ, et al. Impact of adjuvant radiation on the patterns and rate of relapse in advanced-stage Hodgkin's disease treated with alternating chemotherapy combinations. J Clin Oncol 1991;9:2193–201.
30. Brizel DM, Winer EP, Prosnitz LR, et al. Improved survival in advanced Hodgkin's disease with the use of combined modality therapy [see comments]. Int J Radiat Oncol Biol Phys 1990;19:535–42.
31. Fabian C, Mansfield C, Dahlberg S, et al. Low-dose involved field radiation after chemotherapy in advanced Hodgkin's disease. Ann Intern Med 1994;120:903–12.
32. Loeffler M, Brosteanu O, Hasenclever D, et al. Meta-analysis of chemotherapy versus combined modality treatment trials in Hodgkin's disease. International Database on Hodgkin's Disease Overview Study Group [see comments]. J Clin Oncol 1998;16:818–29.
33. Aleman BM, Raemaekers JM, Tirelli U, et al. Involved-field radiotherapy for advanced Hodgkin's lymphoma. N Engl J Med 2003;348:2396–406.
34. Duggan DB, Petroni GR, Johnson JL, et al. Randomized comparison of ABVD and MOPP/ABV hybrid for the treatment of advanced Hodgkin's disease: report of an intergroup trial. J Clin Oncol 2003;21:607–14.
35. Horning SJ, Hoppe RT, Breslin S, et al. Stanford V and radiotherapy for locally extensive and advanced Hodgkin's disease: mature results of a prospective clinical trial. J Clin Oncol 2002;20:630–7.
36. Chisesi T, Federico M, Levis A, et al. ABVD versus stanford V versus MEC in unfavourable Hodgkin's lymphoma: results of a randomised trial. Ann Oncol 2002;13[Suppl 1]:102–6.
37. Poen JC, Hoppe RT, and Horning SJ. High-dose therapy and autologous bone marrow transplantation for relapsed/refractory Hodgkin's disease: the impact of involved field radiotherapy on patterns of failure and survival [see comments]. Int J Radiat Oncol Biol Phys 1996;36:3–12.
38. Yahalom J, Gulati SC, Toia M, et al. Accelerated hyperfractionated total-lymphoid irradiation, high-dose chemotherapy, and autologous bone marrow transplantation for refractory and relapsing patients with Hodgkin's disease. J Clin Oncol 1993;11:1062–70.
39. Moskowitz CH, Nimer SD, Zelenetz AD, et al. A 2-step comprehensive high-dose chemoradiotherapy second-line program for relapsed and refractory Hodgkin disease: analysis by intent to treat and development of a prognostic model. Blood 2001;97:616–23.
40. Moskowitz CH, Kewalramani T, Nimer SD, et al. Effectiveness of high dose chemoradiotherapy and autologous stem cell transplantation for patients with biopsy-proven primary refractory Hodgkin's disease. Br J Haematol 2004;124: 645–52.
41. Zelenetz AD. NCCN Physician Guidelines: Non-Hodgkin Lymphoma. Nat Comp Cancer Net 2004;2(4):286–294. Available at: www.nccn.org.
42. Mac Manus MP and Hoppe RT. Is radiotherapy curative for stage I and II low-grade follicular lymphoma? Results of a long-term follow-up study of patients treated at Stanford University. J Clin Oncol 1996;14:1282–90.

43. Vaughan Hudson B, Vaughan Hudson G, MacLennan KA, et al. Clinical stage 1 non-Hodgkin's lymphoma: long-term follow-up of patients treated by the British National Lymphoma Investigation with radiotherapy alone as initial therapy. Br J Cancer 1994;69:1088–93.
44. Sutcliffe SB, Gospodarowicz MK, Bush RS, et al. Role of radiation therapy in localized non-Hodgkin's lymphoma. Radiother Oncol 1985;4:211–23.
45. Wilder RB, Jones D, Tucker SL, et al. Long-term results with radiotherapy for Stage I–II follicular lymphomas. Int J Radiat Oncol Biol Phys 2001;51:1219–27.
46. Bush RS, Gospodarowicz M, Sturgeon J, et al. Radiation therapy of localized non-Hodgkin's lymphoma. Cancer Treat Rep 1977;61:1129–36.
47. Fuks Z and Kaplan H. Recurrence rates following radiation therapy of nodular and diffuse malignant lymphomas. Radiology 1973;108:675–9.
48. Nissen NI, Ersboll J, Hansen HS, et al. A randomized study of radiotherapy versus radiotherapy plus chemotherapy in stage I–II non-Hodgkin's lymphomas. Cancer 1983;52:1–7.
49. Yahalom J, Varsos G, Fuks Z, et al. Adjuvant cyclophosphamide, doxorubicin, vincristine, and prednisone chemotherapy after radiation therapy in stage I low-grade and intermediate-grade non-Hodgkin lymphoma. Results of a prospective randomized study. Cancer 1993;71:2342–50.
50. Yahalom J. Radiation therapy for stage III follicular lymphoma—often ignored, but still effective. Int J Radiat Oncol Biol Phys 2001;49:1–2.
51. Paryani SB, Hoppe RT, Cox RS, et al. The role of radiation therapy in the management of stage III follicular lymphomas. J Clin Oncol 1984;2:841–8.
52. Murtha AD, Rupnow BA, Hansosn J, et al. Long-term follow-up of patients with Stage III follicular lymphoma treated with primary radiotherapy at Stanford University. Int J Radiat Oncol Biol Phys 2001;49:3–15.
53. Jacobs JP, Murray KJ, Schultz CJ, et al. Central lymphatic irradiation for stage III nodular malignant lymphoma: long-term results. J Clin Oncol 1993;11:233–8.
54. Mendenhall NP and Lynch JW Jr. The low-grade lymphomas. Semin Radiat Oncol 1995;5:254–66.
55. Ha CS, Cabanillas F, Lee MS, et al. Serial determination of the bcl-2 gene in the bone marrow and peripheral blood after central lymphatic irradiation for stages I–III follicular lymphoma: a preliminary report. Clin Cancer Res 1997;3: 215–9.
56. Aviles A, Diaz-Maqueo JC, Sanchez E, et al. Long-term results in patients with low-grade nodular non-Hodgkin's lymphoma. A randomized trial comparing chemotherapy plus radiotherapy with chemotherapy alone. Acta Oncol 1991;30:329–33.
57. Bertoni F, Conconi A, Capella C, et al. Molecular follow-up in gastric mucosa-associated lymphoid tissue lymphomas: early analysis of the LY03 cooperative trial. Blood 2002; 99:2541–4.
58. Fisher RI, Dahlberg S, Nathwani BN, et al. A clinical analysis of two indolent lymphoma entities: mantle cell lymphoma and marginal zone lymphoma (including the mucosa-associated lymphoid tissue and monocytoid B-cell subcategories): a Southwest Oncology Group study. Blood 1995;85:1075–82.
59. Coiffier B and Salles G. Does surgery belong to medical history for gastric lymphomas? Ann Oncol 1997;8:419–21.
60. Wotherspoon AC, Doglioni C, and Isaacson PG. Low-grade gastric B-cell lymphoma of mucosa-associated lymphoid tissue (MALT): a multifocal disease. Histopathology 1992; 20:29–34.
61. Schechter NR, Portlock CS, and Yahalom J. Treatment of mucosa-associated lymphoid tissue lymphoma of the stomach with radiation alone. J Clin Oncol 1998;16: 1916–21.
62. Yahalom J, Portlock CSP, Gonzales M, et al. H. pylori-independent MALT lymphoma of the stomach: excellent outcome with radiation alone. Blood 2002;100:160a.
63. Tsang RW, Gospodarowicz MK, Pintilie M, et al. Stage I and II MALT lymphoma: results of treatment with radiotherapy. Int J Radiat Oncol Biol Phys 2001;50:1258–64.
64. Fung CY, Grossbard ML, Linggood RM, et al. Mucosa-associated lymphoid tissue lymphoma of the stomach: long-term outcome after local treatment. Cancer 1999;85:9–17.
65. Hitchcock S, Ng AK, Fisher DC, et al. Treatment outcome of mucosa-associated lymphoid tissue/marginal zone non-Hodgkin's lymphoma. Int J Radiat Oncol Biol Phys 2002;52:1058–66.
66. Gospodarowicz MK, Pintilie M, Tsang R, et al. Primary gastric lymphoma: brief overview of the recent Princess Margaret Hospital experience. Recent Results Cancer Res 2000; 156:108–15.
67. Yahalom J. MALT lymphomas: a radiation oncology viewpoint. Ann Hematol 2001;80:B100–5.
68. Della Bianca C, Hunt M, Furhang E, et al. Radiation treatment planning techniques for lymphoma of the stomach. Int J Radiat Oncol Biol Phys 2005;62:745–51.
69. Haas RL, Poortmans P, de Jong D, et al. High response rates and lasting remissions after low-dose involved field radiotherapy in indolent lymphomas. J Clin Oncol 2003;21:2474–80.
70. Haas RL and Girinsky T. HOVON 47/EORTC 20013: chlorambucil vs 2 × 2 Gy involved field radiotherapy in stage III/IV previously untreated follicular lymphoma patients. Ann Hematol 2003;82:458–62.
71. Girinsky T, Guillot-Vals D, Koscielny S, et al. A high and sustained response rate in refractory or relapsing low-grade lymphoma masses after low-dose radiation: analysis of predictive parameters of response to treatment. Int J Radiat Oncol Biol Phys 2001;51:148–55.
72. Leitch HA, Gascoyne RD, Chhanabhai M, et al. Limited-stage mantle-cell lymphoma. Ann Oncol 2003;14:1555–61.
73. Yahalom J. Radiation therapy in the treatment of lymphoma. Curr Opin Oncol 1999;11:370–4.
74. Levitt SH, Lee CK, Bloomfield CD, et al. The role of radiation therapy in the treatment of early stage large cell lymphoma. Hematol Oncol 1985;3:33–7.
75. Hallahan DE, Farah R, Vokes EE, et al. The patterns of failure in patients with pathological stage I and II diffuse histiocytic lymphoma treated with radiation therapy alone. Int J Radiat Oncol Biol Phys 1989;17:767–71.
76. Carde P, Burgers JM, van Glabbeke M, et al. Combined radiotherapy-chemotherapy for early stages non-Hodgkin's lymphoma: the 1975–1980 EORTC controlled lymphoma trial. Radiother Oncol 1984;2:301–12.
77. Monfardini S, Banfi A, Bonadonna G, et al. Improved five year survival after combined radiotherapy-chemotherapy for stage I–II non-Hodgkin's lymphoma. Int J Radiat Oncol Biol Phys 1980;6:125–34.
78. Longo DL, Glatstein E, Duffey PL, et al. Treatment of localized aggressive lymphomas with combination chemotherapy followed by involved-field radiation therapy. J Clin Oncol 1989;7:1295–302.
79. Shenkier TN, Voss N, Fairey R, et al. Brief chemotherapy and involved-region irradiation for limited-stage diffuse large-cell lymphoma: an 18-year experience from the British Columbia Cancer Agency. J Clin Oncol 2002;20:197–204.
80. Kaminski MS, Coleman CN, Colby TV, et al. Factors predicting survival in adults with stage I and II large-cell lymphoma treated with primary radiation therapy. Ann Intern Med 1986;104:747–56.

81. Jones SE, Miller TP, and Connors JM. Long-term follow-up and analysis for prognostic factors for patients with limited-stage diffuse large-cell lymphoma treated with initial chemotherapy with or without adjuvant radiotherapy. J Clin Oncol 1989;7:1186–91.
82. Stewart DA, Vose JM, Weisenburger DD, et al. The role of high-dose therapy and autologous hematopoietic stem cell transplantation for mantle cell lymphoma. Ann Oncol 1995;6:263–6.
83. Longo DL. Combined modality therapy for localized aggressive lymphoma: enough or too much? J Clin Oncol 1989;7:1179–81.
84. Cabanillas F, Bodey GP, and Freireich EJ. Management with chemotherapy only of stage I and II malignant lymphoma of aggressive histologic types. Cancer 1980;46:2356–9.
85. Miller TP and Jones SE. Initial chemotherapy for clinically localized lymphomas of unfavorable histology. Blood 1983;62:413–8.
86. Miller TP. The limits of limited stage lymphoma. J Clin Oncol 2004;22:2982–4.
87. Horning SJ, Weller E, Kim K, et al. Chemotherapy with or without radiotherapy in limited-stage diffuse aggressive non-Hodgkin's lymphoma: Eastern Cooperative Oncology Group study 1484. J Clin Oncol 2004;22:3032–8.
88. Miller TP, Dahlberg S, Cassady JR, et al. Chemotherapy alone compared with chemotherapy plus radiotherapy for localized intermediate- and high-grade non-Hodgkin's lymphoma. N Engl J Med 1998;339:21–6.
89. Fisher RI, Miller TP, O'Connor OA. Diffuse aggressive lymphoma. Hematology (Am Soc Hematol Educ Program) 2004;221–36.
90. Kamath SS, Marcus RB Jr, Lynch JW, et al. The impact of radiotherapy dose and other treatment-related and clinical factors on in-field control in stage I and II non-Hodgkin's lymphoma. Int J Radiat Oncol Biol Phys 1999;44:563–8.
91. Roy I and Yahalom J. Excellent local control with involved-field radiotherapy following CHOP chemotherapy: analysis of 145 patients with early-stage intermediate-grade non-Hodgkin's lymphoma. Int J Radiat Oncol Biol Phys 2001;51:562a–3a.
92. Wilder RB, Tucker SL, Ha CS, et al. Dose–response analysis for radiotherapy delivered to patients with intermediate-grade and large-cell immunoblastic lymphomas that have completely responded to CHOP-based induction chemotherapy. Int J Radiat Oncol Biol Phys 2001;49:17–22.
93. Schlembach PJ, Wilder RB, Tucker SL, et al. Impact of involved field radiotherapy after CHOP-based chemotherapy on stage III–IV, intermediate grade and large-cell immunoblastic lymphomas. Int J Radiat Oncol Biol Phys 2000;48:1107–10.
94. Shipp MA, Klatt MM, Yeap B, et al. Patterns of relapse in large-cell lymphoma patients with bulk disease. implications for the use of adjuvant radiation therapy. J Clin Oncol 1989;7:613–8.
95. Aviles A, Delgado S, Nambo MJ, et al. Adjuvant radiotherapy to sites of previous bulky disease in patients stage IV diffuse large cell lymphoma. Int J Radiat Oncol Biol Phys 1994;30:799–803.
96. Ferreri AJ, Dell'Oro S, Reni M, et al. Consolidation radiotherapy to bulky or semibulky lesions in the management of stage III–IV diffuse large B cell lymphomas. Oncology 2000;58:219–26.
97. Fouillard L, Laporte JP, Labopin M, et al. Autologous stem-cell transplantation for non-Hodgkin's lymphomas: the role of graft purging and radiotherapy posttransplantation—results of a retrospective analysis on 120 patients autografted in a single institution. J Clin Oncol 1998;16:2803–16.
98. Aviles A, Fernandezb R, Perez F, et al. Adjuvant radiotherapy in stage IV diffuse large cell lymphoma improves outcome. Leuk Lymphoma 2004;45:1385–9.
99. Aviles A, Garcia EL, Fernandez R, et al. Combined therapy in the treatment of primary mediastinal B-cell lymphoma: conventional versus escalated chemotherapy. Ann Hematol 2002;81:368–73.
100. Zinzani PL, Martelli M, Bertini M, et al. Induction chemotherapy strategies for primary mediastinal large B-cell lymphoma with sclerosis: a retrospective multinational study on 426 previously untreated patients. Haematologica 2002;87:1258–64.
101. Todeschini G, Secchi S, Morra E, et al. Primary mediastinal large B-cell lymphoma (PMLBCL): long-term results from a retrospective multicentre Italian experience in 138 patients treated with CHOP or MACOP-B/VACOP-B. Br J Cancer 2004;90:372–6.
102. Kaplan HS and Rosenberg SA. The treatment of Hodgkin's disease. Med Clin North Am 1966;50:1591–610.
103. Goodman KA, Toner S, Hunt M, et al. Intensity modulated radiation therapy in the treatment of lymphoma involving the mediastinum. Int J Radiat Oncol Biol Phys 2005;62:198–206.
104. Andre M, Mounier N, Leleu X, et al. Second cancers and late toxicities after treatment of aggressive non-Hodgkin lymphoma with the ACVBP regimen: a GELA cohort study on 2837 patients. Blood 2004;103:1222–8.
105. Travis LB, Gospodarowicz M, Curtis RE, et al. Lung cancer following chemotherapy and radiotherapy for Hodgkin's disease. J Natl Cancer Inst 2002;94:182–92.
106. Travis LB, Curtis RE, Glimelius B, et al. Second cancers among long-term survivors of non-Hodgkin's lymphoma. J Natl Cancer Inst 1993;85:1932–7.
107. Dores GM, Metayer C, Curtis RE, et al. Second malignant neoplasms among long-term survivors of Hodgkin's disease: a population-based evaluation over 25 years. J Clin Oncol 2002;20:3484–94.
108. van Leeuwen FE, Klokman WJ, Stovall M, et al. Roles of radiation dose, chemotherapy, and hormonal factors in breast cancer following Hodgkin's disease. J Natl Cancer Inst 2003;95:971–80.
109. Travis LB, Hill D, Dores GM, et al. Breast cancer following radiotherapy and chemotherapy among young women with Hodgkin's disease. JAMA 2003;289.
110. Yahalom J. Breast cancer after Hodgkin disease: hope for a safer cure. JAMA 2003;290:529–31.
111. Bhatia S, Robison LL, Oberlin O, et al. Breast cancer and other second neoplasms after childhood Hodgkin's disease [see comments]. N Engl J Med 1996;334:745–51.
112. Doria R, Holford T, Farber LR, et al. Second solid malignancies after combined modality therapy for Hodgkin's disease. J Clin Oncol 1995;13:2016–22.
113. Salloum E, Doria R, Schubert W, et al. Second solid tumors in patients with Hodgkin's disease cured after radiation or chemotherapy plus adjuvant low-dose radiation. J Clin Oncol 1996;14:2435–43.
114. Salloum E, Tanoue LT, Wackers FJ, et al. Assessment of cardiac and pulmonary function in adult patients with Hodgkin's disease treated with ABVD or MOPP/ABVD plus adjuvant low-dose mediastinal irradiation. Cancer Invest 1999;17:171–80.
115. Chronowski GM, Wilder RB, Tucker SL, et al. Analysis of in-field control and late toxicity for adults with early-stage Hodgkin's disease treated with chemotherapy followed by radiotherapy. Int J Radiat Oncol Biol Phys 2003;55:36–43.
116. Hancock SL, Tucker MA, and Hoppe RT. Factors affecting late mortality from heart disease after treatment of Hodgkin's disease. JAMA 1993;270:1949–55.

Principles of Treatment

Wyndham H. Wilson, M.D., Ph.D.

The fundamental genetic changes leading to neoplasia involve deregulation of cellular proliferation and death, events that are controlled in large measure by cell cycle checkpoints and by the induction and suppression of apoptosis. Evidence also suggests that abnormalities in these pathways may determine the sensitivity of tumor cells, compared with normal cells, to the cytotoxic effects of irradiation and chemotherapy.[1–3] Understanding the regulation of these pathways and their impact on the efficacy of treatment lies at the frontier of cancer therapy. However, clinical strategies that take advantage of the abnormalities that occur in the regulation of the cell cycle and apoptosis are just beginning, but have an increasingly important role in the design of therapeutic approaches. The classic principles of chemotherapy, including pharmacology, drug resistance, and tumor cell kinetics, continue to form the foundation of treatment strategies. This chapter discusses the classic principles of chemotherapy within the context of the new tumor biology and attempts to provide the reader with a general understanding of current directions in the development of novel treatment strategies for non-Hodgkin's lymphomas.

KINETIC BASIS OF LYMPHOMA TREATMENT

Some 30 years ago, Skipper and associates made a number of fundamental observations regarding the kinetic features of tumor cell growth and the effect of chemotherapy on a rodent leukemia L1210 model system.[4] From these observations, they hypothesized the importance of tumor volume, growth fraction, and the first-order kinetics of chemotherapy cell kill for therapeutic outcome. These concepts have become classic principles of chemotherapy and continue to guide treatment strategies. The clinician must remember, however, that the Skipper model was based on a rapidly proliferating tumor that does not accurately reflect the slower growth and heterogeneity of human tumors. Moreover, recent discoveries in tumor molecular biology clearly demonstrate that malignant cells have numerous abnormalities in cell cycle control that independently affect drug sensitivity.

One of the basic observations that emerged from this model was that the survival of mice inoculated with L1210 cells was inversely proportional to the tumor cell inoculum. In this model system, a single tumor cell was capable of causing death, and the time interval between inoculation and death was proportional to the inoculum. This interval could be calculated from knowledge of the tumor doubling time and inoculum size. These observations formed the basis for the concept of tumor cell kinetics. When the effect of chemotherapy was investigated in this system, the fraction of tumor cells undergoing DNA replication, termed the "growth fraction," greatly influenced drug sensitivity, a finding that likely reflected the greater sensitivity of tumor cells in the DNA synthetic (S) phase of the cell cycle to many classes of chemotherapeutic agents. As a hypothesis of tumor cell sensitivity, however, the principle of growth fraction was a great oversimplification.

Clinically, tumors are heterogeneous. Tumor masses within the same patient vary owing to diverse factors such as blood flow, tissue hypoxia, and mutations that determine tumor biology and drug resistance. Moreover, the growth fraction of tumor cells is dynamic, decreasing as tumors grow and increasing as tumor cells are killed by cytoreductive treatment. The growth fraction also does not affect the cytotoxicity of all chemotherapy drugs equally. Although most drugs are more cytotoxic to cells undergoing DNA synthesis, some agents such as BCNU do not show this selectivity. Thus, the growth fraction should be included among those factors that contribute to the sensitivity of tumor cells to therapy but alone is not predictive of a therapeutic response. The low-grade lymphomas are a good example of the limitations of this principle. It has been proposed that the low-growth fraction of indolent (low-grade) lymphomas may explain the incurability of these tumors with chemotherapy. However, most low-grade lymphomas are sensitive to chemotherapy, so tumor growth fraction alone cannot explain the low cure rate.

Skipper also observed that the number of tumor cells killed by a cycle of chemotherapy depends on first-order kinetics; that is, in the rapidly growing L1210 leukemia cells, a given drug dose killed a constant fraction of cells, independent of cell number.[5] Of course, the sensitivity of the tumor to the chemotherapy directly affects the fraction of cells killed, and in practice this sensitivity changes over multiple courses of chemotherapy. As previously pointed out, when the number of tumor cells decrease, the growth fraction increases, and this may increase tumor sensitivity. However, the tendency of chemotherapy to select out a resistant cell population after repeated courses may in fact have the opposite effect, namely the emergence of a population much less susceptible to the drugs. The fraction of cells killed can be affected by other factors that change with chemotherapy, including tumor perfusion and oxygenation, decreased host resistance to drug side effects, and the proliferation of tumor in sanctuary sites such as the central nervous system. When applied clinically, the fractional cell kill concept suggests that surgical resection of tumor, if of sufficient degree, would be beneficial to the therapeutic outcome. Although this may be true in selected patients with Burkitt's lymphomas in whom an abdominal tumor can be essentially completely resected, as a general rule, surgery does not increase the cure rate of lymphomas.[6]

A corollary of the fractional cell kill hypothesis is the important relationship of drug concentration (or dose) and response (or cell kill). For some but not all drugs, a relatively linear relationship exists between cell kill and dose. This applies particularly to alkylating agents. For other drugs (chiefly the antimetabolites) that depend on cell exposure to drug during vulnerable phases of the cell cycle, the duration of exposure may be more important than drug concentration. Clinically, high-dose therapy with stem cell support takes maximal advantage of the drug concentration–response relationship. Alkylating agents and epipodophyllotoxins are the preferred drugs for this approach because of their relatively linear dose response and favorable therapeutic index.[7]

Although these classical principles do not adequately explain many features of the tumor cell response to chemotherapy, they have had practical application for the design of chemotherapy regimens. The modulation of drug sensitivity by increasing tumor growth fraction has been tested in the treatment of acute myelogenous leukemia. Clinical trials designed to increase tumor response by administering mitogenic agents such as granulocyte-macrophage colony-stimulating factor (GM-CSF) before and during chemotherapy are currently being tested in acute myelogenous leukemia in cooperative group trials, and similar approaches could be tested in lymphomas once the appropriate growth factors are identified.[8] The concept of fractional cell kill has been exploited by chemotherapy regimens that deliver intensive doses of chemotherapy over multiple cycles. This latter approach still remains an important principle for the development of new chemotherapies for lymphomas and has led to the successful use of high-dose chemotherapy with stem cell rescue in relapsed intermediate-grade lymphomas. However, treatment regimens that incorporate modestly intensified therapy, such as the third-generation regimens, have shown no clear benefit over standard therapy such as CHOP (cyclophosphamide, hydroxydaunomycin, Oncovin, prednisone) in the low- and intermediate-grade lymphomas.[9] For this reason, scientifically as opposed to empirically derived treatment approaches should be explored.

DOSE INTENSITY AND DOSE DENSITY

Dose intensity, defined as the dose per unit time, has long been considered to be important for the treatment of lymphomas. Indeed, in animal models, a nonlinear relation between drug dose and tumor cell kill has been demonstrated such that doubling drug doses may increase cell kill by up to 10-fold and reductions of as little as 20% may decrease the cure rate by 50%. Since fractional cell kill is rarely, if ever, 100%, it is not surprising that dose intensity would be important to the clinical outcome. In aggressive B-cell lymphomas, the importance of dose intensity was suggested by an analysis performed by Kwak and coworkers.[10] In this study of CHOP, M-BACOD (methotrexate, bleomycin, Adriamycin [doxorubicin], cyclophosphamide, Oncovin, dexamethasone), and MACOP-B (methotrexate, cyclophosphamide, Oncovin, prednisone, bleomycin) chemotherapy in 115 previously untreated diffuse large-cell lymphomas, the most important predictor of survival was a relative dose intensity (RDI) of doxorubicin greater than 75% of full dose in CHOP. A recent study comparing differences in outcome between young and elderly patients also found that the doxorubicin RDI significantly affected outcome.[11]

Although this and other studies suggest that dose intensity is important, randomized trials comparing regimens that differ in dose intensity have had variable results. In one study, 238 patients with untreated advanced-stage aggressive non-Hodgkin's lymphoma were randomized to receive either standard or escalated BACOP (bleomycin, Adriamycin [doxorubicin], cyclophosphamide, Oncovin [vincristine], prednisone) chemotherapy in which the RDI of doxorubicin was 80% and 108%, respectively.[12] However, the 28% difference in RDI of doxorubicin did not affect the response and survival rates. A randomized trial comparing CHOP (first-generation regimen) to m-BACOD, ProMACE/cytaBOM (prednisone, methotrexate [with leucovorin rescue], Adriamycin, cyclophosphamide, etoposide/cytarabin, bleomycin, Oncovin), and MACOP-B (second- and third-generation regimens) reached similar conclusions.[9] Although the drugs in these regimens were delivered at significantly different RDIs (Table 13–1), the outcomes for all four regimens were similar. Results from randomized studies employing high-dose treatment have been variable. A recent randomized study of high-dose therapy with autologous stem cell rescue versus CHOP in untreated aggressive lymphoma showed a benefit for the high-dose arm, particularly for high-risk patients.[13] High-dose treatment was also found to be superior in a trial where patients in complete remission with standard therapy were randomized to stop or to receive high-dose consolidation.[14]

Table 13–1. Comparative Delivered Dose Intensity of Selected Chemotherapy Regimens ($mg/m^2/week$)[a]

Drug	CHOP[21]	m-BACOD[103]	Pro-MACE-CytaBOM[104]	MACOP-B[21]	Range of Dose Intensity
Cyclophosphamide	221	152.9	173.7	155	1.4
Doxorubicin	14.8	11.2	6.6	22	3.3
Vincristine	0.36[b]	0.28	0.40	0.54[b]	1.9
Methotrexate		73.6	34.9	93.2	2.7
Bleomycin		1.1	1.41	2.08	1.9
Cytarabine			82.6		
Etoposide			32.7		

Note: See text for chemotherapy abbreviations.
[a] Delivered dose intensity from three different clinical trials.
[b] Adjusted to ideal m^2 of 1.7.

In contrast, high-dose treatment did not benefit patients with slow responses to CHOP chemotherapy who were randomized to complete CHOP or to undergo high-dose therapy.[15]

These disparate results appear to challenge the concept of dose intensity, but this conclusion should be interpreted with caution. It is important to recall that dose intensity combines dose rate and dose density, each with a different theoretical benefit. Unfortunately, dose intensity is often misinterpreted as equivalent to drug exposure. Dose rate, however, is not equivalent to drug exposure because of variable pharmacokinetics, which can result in over 10-fold variations in drug area under the curve (AUC).[16] Another important variable is dose–response, which is dependent on the drug class and the individual tumor cell. Microarray studies in lymphomas clearly illustrate widely variable mechanisms of resistance, which clinically translate into differences in dose–response.[17,18] It is not surprising, given these variables and the absence of controls, that studies of dose intensity have been contradictory. Nevertheless, dose–response is an incontrovertible notion that, in the absence of a known optimum dose rate, mandates that a maximum safe dose be administered. Such an approach has been adopted by Wilson et al. in the dose-adjusted EPOCH regimen, where doses are adjusted based on the pharmacodynamics of the administered agents.[16]

Dose density presents a third variable that may be particularly important for rapidly cycling cells. The randomized trials that have assessed the benefit of dose intensity have generally focused on increased drug doses and not on shorter dosing intervals. Delays in drug administration may allow the tumor cells to repair cellular damage and lead to regrowth of surviving tumor in the rest period between cycles. Long delays may ultimately allow the selection and outgrowth of drug-resistant clones. Because the minimal interval between chemotherapy cycles is largely dependent on the rate of hematopoietic recovery, recombinant colony–stimulating factors, such as granulocyte-colony stimulating factor (G-CSF) and granulocyte-macrophage stimulating factor (GM-CSF), allow the more rapid administration of chemotherapy cycles.[19,20] This concept was unsuccessful with the MACOP-B regimen where, unlike other regimens for intermediate-grade lymphomas, chemotherapy was given every week for 12 weeks.[21] However, preliminary results from a randomized study of CHOP for 14 versus 21 days in patients over 60 years with aggressive lymphomas suggested benefit for dose density.[22]

CLASSICAL DRUG RESISTANCE

Because non-Hodgkin's lymphomas typically present with disseminated disease, chemotherapy is the mainstay of treatment, and drug resistance becomes the primary barrier to cure. In 1979, Goldie and Coldman proposed a hypothesis to explain the development of resistance to cytotoxic agents by cancer cells.[23] The hypothesis was based on the observation that resistance of *Escherichia coli* to infection by bacteriophage occurs through the preferential expansion of bacterial clones that have undergone mutation to a resistant phenotype.[24] By extrapolation, Goldie and Coldman predicted that the emergence of drug resistance in human tumors would correlate with the underlying spontaneous mutation rate of specific drug-resistance genes. The emergence of resistant cells may be further hastened by the genomic instability of tumor cells that, in part, results from mutations in the cell cycle regulatory genes such as the p53 tumor suppressor oncogene and may be further increased by exposure to mutagens such as chemotherapy and irradiation.[25] Under the selective pressure of chemotherapy treatment, resistant clones eventually predominate in the tumor.

The Goldie–Coldman hypothesis provides a rationale for some of the principles already established through empiric observation. In patients with large tumor burdens, there is a high probability that tumor cells resistant to any single cytotoxic drug already exist at the time of initial treatment, providing an explanation for the inverse relationship between tumor cell number and curability, and for the greater efficacy of combination chemotherapy compared with single agents. Unfortunately, combination chemotherapy has not been able to overcome resistance in most cases of clinical cancer treatment. One factor is that the probability of resistance to two classes of drugs is greater than the simple product of the mutation rate conferring resistance to each drug alone. Although a unique mutation may be responsible for resistance to a specific drug, and that drug alone, it is unlikely to be the primary clinical cause of drug resistance. Emerging evidence, however, suggests the Goldie–Coldman hypothesis is incorrect. Instead, it is more likely that the resistance observed in vivo is conferred by a high apoptotic threshold, which makes the tumor cells insensitive to multiple agents. In lymphoid malignancies, for example, over-expression of bcl-2 NK-Kappa B and p53, all of which inhibit apoptosis, are associated with drug resistance.[18,26–30]

It used to be thought that a major clinical mechanism of pleiotropic drug resistance was conferred by the multidrug resistance gene (MDR1).[31,32] MDR confers resistance to a broad spectrum of cytotoxic agents derived from natural products, including anthracyclines, epipodophyllotoxins, vinca alkaloids, taxanes, and some camptothecin derivatives (Table 13–2). The product of this gene, the p-glycoprotein (Pgp), functions as a membrane efflux pump that, when over-expressed, decreases intracellular drug levels. In normal cells, Pgp probably functions to eliminate natural environmental toxins that are encountered.[33] Trial designs to overcome MDR-1 comprised some of the earliest paradigms for drug resistance reversal strategies. However, these clinical trials failed to demonstrate the importance of MDR-1 in the clinical outcome of lymphomas.[34]

Once damage has occurred to vital proteins or DNA, or both, the cell can undergo repair, thereby reversing the cytotoxic effects. The desired effect of cytotoxic therapy, of course, is death of the neoplastic cell, an event accomplished through either cellular necrosis or active cell death (Fig. 13–1). Recent evidence suggests that the cellular apparatus that controls the cell cycle is an essential component of the final common pathways through which cytotoxic agents exert their lethal effects.[2,35,36] If this proves to be correct, deregulation at any number of steps in this pathway could lead to drug resistance. Among the most common oncogene or tumor suppressor gene mutations found in lymphoid neoplasms are those that occur in cell cycle control genes, further highlighting the central importance of these pathways in the basic biology of neoplasia.

Table 13–2. Dose, Toxicity, and Mechanism of Resistance of Major Antineoplastic Agents for Lymphomas

Class	Dose[a] (mg/m^2)	Dose Frequency	Acute Toxicity			Other Toxicity	Mechanism of Drug Resistance
			Leukocyte	Platelet	Nausea and Vomiting		
Tubulin Binding Agents							
Paclitaxel	130–250 IV	q 3 wk	Marked	Moderate	Mild	Anaphylactoid response, sensory neuropathy, alopecia	Transport, tubulin mutants
Vincristine	1–1.4 IV	q wk	Mild	Mild	Mild	Distal neuropathy, inappropriate ADH	Transport, tubulin mutants
Vinblastine	6 IV	q wk	Marked	Moderate–marked	Mild	Mucositis	Transport, tubulin mutants
Topoisomerase II Inhibitors							
Etoposide	100–200 IV	q 3–4 wk	Moderate	Mild	Mild	Mucositis	Transport, target modulation
Mitoxantrone	12–14 IV	q 3–4 wk	Marked	Moderate	Mild	Cholestasis, cardiac	Transport, target modulation
Doxorubicin	25–75 IV	q 3–4 wk	Marked	Marked	Moderate	Alopecia, cardiomyopathy	Transport, target modulation
Idarubicin	10–15 IV	q 3–4 wk	Marked	Marked	Moderate	Alopecia, mucositis, cardiomyopathy	Transport, target modulation
Antimetabolites							
Methotrexate	100–400 IV	q 3–4 wk	Moderate–marked	Moderate	Mild	Stomatitis	↓ Polyglutamation, transport ↑ DHFR
Cytarabine (cytosinearabinoside)	300–4000 IV	q 3–4 wk	Marked	Marked	Moderate	Cholestasis, mucositis, neurotoxicity	↓ Activation, ? transport
Deoxycoformycin	4 IV	q 1–2 wk	Mild	Mild	Mild	Neurotoxicity (at high doses), conjunctivitis	Not known, ?↑ adenosine deaminase

2-Chloro-2′-deoxyadenosine	4 IV	qd × 7	Mild	Moderate	Mild	Immune suppression	Not known
Fludarabine	20–25 IV	qd × 5	Moderate–marked	Mild	Mild	Neurotoxicity, stomatitis, hepatitis	↓ Activation
Alkylating Agents							
Cyclophosphamide	350–1500 IV	q 3–4 wk	Marked	Mild	Moderate	Cystitis, pulmonary fibrosis, water retention	↑ Metabolic detoxification, repair of DNA
Ifosfamide	1000 IV	qd × 5 with mesna	Moderate–marked	Moderate	Mild	Nephrotoxicity, cystitis, neurotoxicity	↑ Metabolic detoxification, repair of DNA
Mechlorethamine	6 IV	q 2–4 wk	Marked	Moderate	Moderate	Leukemia	Detoxification, repair of DNA
Chlorambucil	1–3 PO	qd	Moderate	Moderate	Mild	Leukemia	Detoxification, repair of DNA
Dacarbazine	150 IV	qd × 5	Mild	Mild	Marked	Flulike syndrome, venoocclusive	Detoxification, repair of DNA by guanine alkyl transferase
Procarbazine	100 PO	qd × 7–14 d	Moderate	Moderate	Mild	Sensitivity to amines, sterility, leukemia	
CCNU	100–150 PO	q 4 wk	Marked	Marked	Moderate	Leukemia, pulmonary fibrosis, renal failure	
Miscellaneous							
Bleomycin	5–10 IV	q 2–4 wk	Rare	Rare	Mild	Skin, pulmonary fibrosis, fever, hypersensitivity reactions	Metabolism repair
Cisplatin	50–100 IV	q 3–4 wk	Mild	Moderate	Severe	Renal failure, Mg^{2+} wasting, peripheral neuropathy, anemia	Transport, detoxification, repair of DNA

[a] Doses per cycle are typical of those used in combination regimens, but appropriate modification must be made depending on other drugs used, organ dysfunction, and other considerations.
ADH, antidiuretic hormone; DHFR, dihydrofolate reductase.

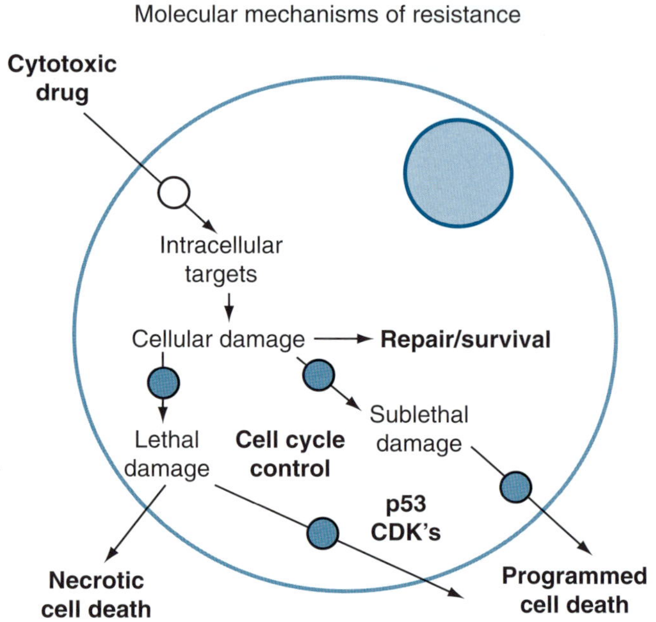

Figure 13–1. Drug resistance mechanisms. MDR, multidrug resistance; apoptosis (programmed cell death).

Although the clinical significance of these mutations with respect to drug resistance is not established, they are among the most important candidates for investigation.

PROGRAMMED CELL DEATH AND CELL CYCLE CONTROL IN LYMPHOMAS

Like normal tissues, tumors are composed of mixtures of cells, some of which are undergoing replication, while others are resting and still others are undergoing active cell death. The death of malignant cells, like their normal counterparts, may occur by necrosis or by apoptosis, an active mechanism of cell death characterized by cleavage of cellular DNA into nucleosome-sized fragments (DNA ladder), chromatin condensation, and nuclear fragmentation.[35] Two main pathways for apoptosis, termed the intrinsic (innate pathway) and extrinsic pathways, have been identified (Fig. 13–2). In the extrinsic pathway, signals from stimulated death receptors on the cell surface activate caspases, which function as the ultimate effectors and lead to the biochemical and morphologic changes of apoptosis. In contrast, the intrinsic pathway is activated by endogenous molecules and

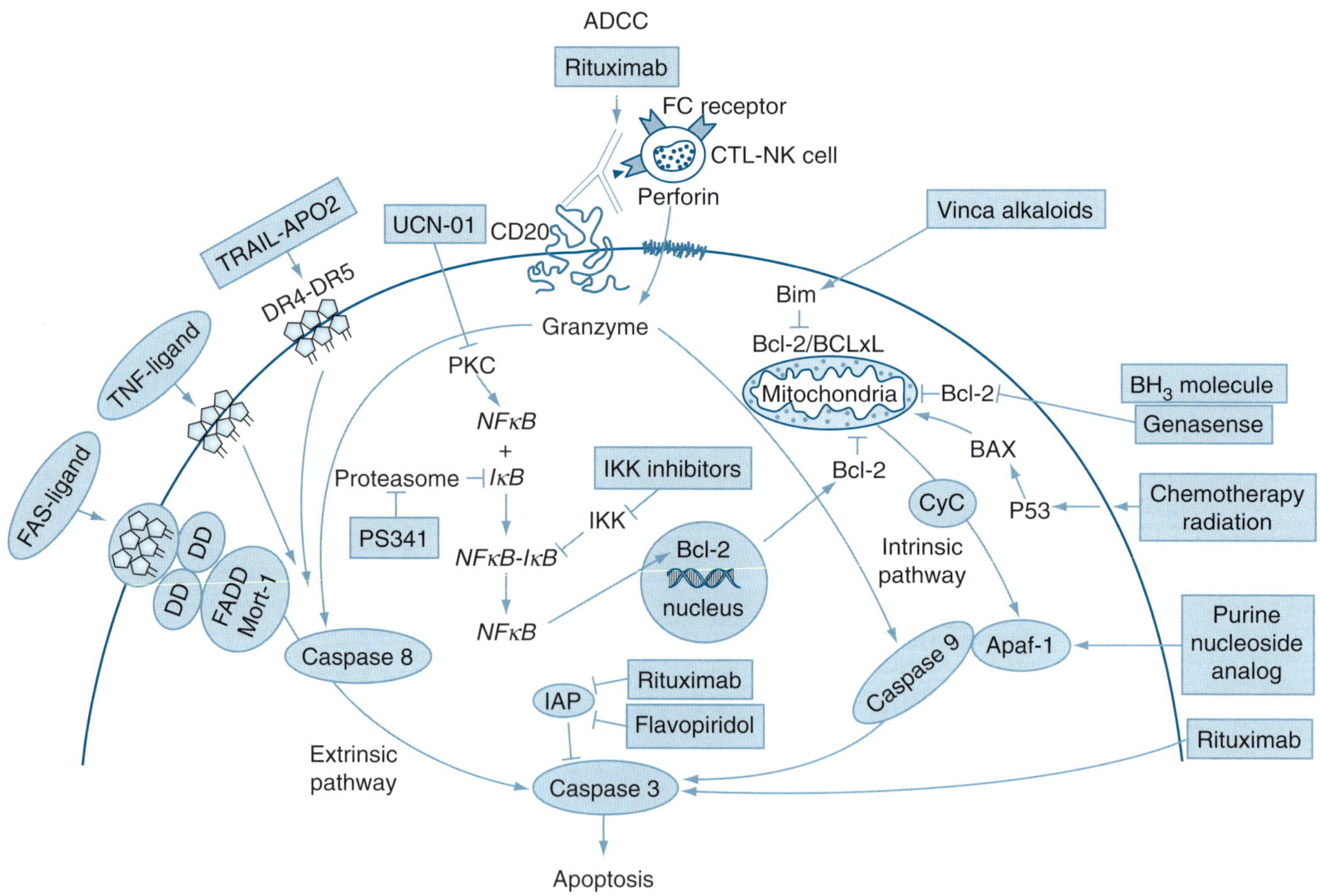

Figure 13–2. Potential apoptotic mechanisms of drug(s) (shown in boxes) action are summarized. The extrinsic and intrinsic apoptosis pathways that lead to the activation of effector cysteine proteases (caspases) ultimately leading to apoptosis are summarized. Also depicted is the antigen-dependent cellular cytotoxicity (ADCC) pathway for rituximab. *Arrows* (↓) represent positive regulation and *bars* (⊥) represent negative regulation. (See text for details.)

is dependent on mitochondrial release of cytochrome c into the cytosol, which in turn activates terminal caspases and cellular death.

The process of apoptosis can be triggered through multiple pathways, including exposure to cytotoxic agents, the loss of essential growth factors, exposure to negative regulators such as tumor necrosis factor and transforming growth factor-β, and the loss or induction of specific genes such as c-myc and p53 (Figure 13–2).[35,37,38] Other events suppress apoptosis, such as the addition of growth factors and the induction or suppression of specific genes and viral proteins.[39] Although pathways leading to apoptosis are present in many tumor cells, some of the triggering pathways may be disrupted and absent, and experimental evidence suggests that disruption of these pathways increases the resistance of cancer cells to cytotoxic agents.[40,41]

Apoptosis plays a central role in the normal biology of lymphocytes and in the process of clonal deletion (Figure 13–2).[42] Hence, it is not unexpected that the induction of apoptosis is particularly important in the biology of lymphomas. At least two genes (BCL-2 and p53) that can affect apoptosis have been found to be either abnormal or deregulated in lymphomas.[26,41,43] Translocations of BCL-2, located on chromosome 18, to the immunoglobulin (Ig) heavy-chain locus on chromosome 14 (t[14;18]) is present in as many as 85% of follicular lymphomas.[44,45] This translocation results in elevated levels of the BCL-2 protein product and prolongs cell survival by blocking apoptosis.[37,44] Although BCL-2 gene rearrangements are infrequent (approximately 10%) in aggressive lymphomas, increased BCL-2 expression is commonly observed, suggesting it plays a role in these tumors as well.[46,47] Viral genes such as Epstein–Barr virus LMP-1, frequently present in Burkitt's lymphomas, can induce expression of BCL-2 and protect cells from apoptosis. Recently, a second protein, called "BAX," has been identified that blocks the apoptosis-repressor activity of BCL-2.[48] The BAX protein, which shares significant homology with BCL-2, is in equilibrium between homodimerization with itself and heterodimerization with BCL-2, and it is this ratio that appears to regulate BCL-2 function. When over-expressed, BAX accelerates apoptosis following a death signal, such as withdrawal of an essential growth factor. The apoptosis-repressor activity of BCL-2 affects drug sensitivity. In vitro, cells that express increased levels of BCL-2 are resistant to radiation- and chemotherapy-induced apoptosis. For example, a high level of BCL-2 expression in leukemias correlated with resistance to several apoptosis-inducing cytotoxic agents, including doxorubicin, methotrexate, and cytarabine.[49] There are at least 20 members of the BCL-2 family that have been identified in mammalian species to date, and include proteins with antiapoptotic effects, such as BCL-2, Bcl-X_L, Bcl-W, Mcl-1, Boo/Diva, and Al/Bff-1, and others such as Bax, Bcl-X_s, Bad, Hrk, Bim, Bik, Blk, APR/Noxa and Bcl-G_s, which have pro-apoptotic properties.

The NFκB transcription factor also plays an important role in apoptosis, and has been linked to multiple lymphoma types including DLBCL and CLL17.[50] Normally, NFκB is sequestered and bound to IκB, and cannot enter the nucleus to increase expression of antiapoptotic genes like BCL-2 and IAPs (inhibitor of apoptotic proteins) (Figure 13–2). In response to a death stimulus, TNF family receptors can trigger NFκB activation through interaction with TRAF family proteins, which phosphorylate IκB. Elevated levels of NFκB are found in CLL, possibly related to stimulation of CD40, a TNF family receptor, by the CD40 ligand, which is found on 15% to 30% of B-CLL.[50,51]

The p53 tumor suppressor gene plays an important role in apoptosis as well. P53 controls the cellular responses to DNA damage by arresting cells in G_1 of the cell cycle so that repair of DNA damage may occur before the cell proceeds through DNA synthesis and mitosis; if essential repairs are not possible, p53 may trigger apoptosis.[25] For example, p53 expression increases in cells exposed to DNA-damaging agents and in prostate epithelial cells undergoing apoptosis following male hormone depletion.[35] Thus, p53 monitors the fidelity of DNA and reduces the inherent mutability of the genome. The importance of p53 mutations in the development of the malignant phenotype is suggested by the presence of p53 mutations in most types of cancers, including chronic lymphocytic leukemias (CLLs) and lymphomas.[41,52] Mutant p53 has been detected in tumor biopsy specimens from as many as 15% of CLL patients and 33% of non-Hodgkin's lymphoma patients, and in even higher proportions in biopsy specimens from heavily pretreated patients.[41]

Mutations in the p53 gene are associated with elevated levels of mutant p53 protein that inactivate wild-type p53 and cause profound biologic effects. Because the normal function of wild-type p53 is to arrest cells in G_1 to allow DNA repair and to promote apoptosis, inhibition of these activities by mutant p53 can lead to genomic instability and a hypermutable state.[25,49] In vitro, this is reflected by cellular resistance to both radiation therapy and chemotherapy. Moreover, in a drug-resistant human lung cancer cell in which both alleles of p53 were deleted, chemosensitivity could be restored by transfer of the wild-type p53 gene into the cells.[53] The hypermutable state that may result from inhibition of normal p53 theoretically could promote the rapid emergence of resistant clones.

Another molecular abnormality found in mantle cell lymphoma results in the deregulation of the G_1 cell cycle checkpoint.[54–56] Most mantle cell lymphomas have a reciprocal 11;14 translocation involving chromosome 11q13, which carries the BCL1 gene, and the Ig heavy-chain locus on chromosome 14q32, resulting in over-expression of BCL1. The product of BCL1, cyclin D1, belongs to a class of proteins (i.e., cyclins) that initiate mitosis.[57] Although the significance of cyclin D1 in mantle cell lymphomas is not clearly understood, its over-expression would appear to overcome an early G_1 checkpoint.

There is sufficient evidence to warrant the development of clinical strategies to overcome the deregulation of apoptosis and cell cycle control. Drugs and therapeutic peptides could be identified that reverse the deregulation of these pathways. A number of potential targets for therapeutic intervention exist, including inhibition of BCL-2 expression or protein activity; up-regulation of neutralizing proteins such as mdm-2 or BAX that inhibit p53 or BCL-2, respectively; suppression of mutant p53 or increased normal p53 expression, or both; and suppression of other oncogenes such as c-myc. Specific therapeutic approaches, some of which are under active investigation, include development of idiotype vaccines, which can kill in a BCL-2 independent manner, and BCL-2 antisense oligonucleotides, which can inhibit BLC-2 epxression.[58–60]

MICROARRAY ANALYSES OF LYMPHOMA

The future of therapeutics lies in the identification of the important oncogenic pathways and the development of targeted agents. Molecular profiling of messenger RNA (mRNA) gene expression represents a powerful new tool for understanding pathways of lymphomagenesis and more accurately identifying lymphoma subtypes. Importantly, the molecular profile of a tumor biopsy is influenced not only by its unique genetic composition but also by its microenvironment, which is comprised of multiple cell types.

Microarray profiling has produced important insights into pathways of lymphomagenesis and potential causes of treatment failure in DLBCL.[17,18] Genes associated with cellular proliferation distinguished DLBCL from more indolent lymphoma subtypes, a finding that corresponds to the known variation in tumor proliferation index as measured by MIB-1/Ki-67 antibodies.[26] The proliferation signature genes are a diverse group and included cell-cycle control and checkpoint genes, DNA synthesis, and replication genes, as well as the Ki-67 gene, which has been associated with a poor outcome with CHOP-based treatments.[26] It may be possible to take therapeutic advantage of the high tumor proliferation rate. In vitro, agents such as doxorubicin and etoposide are schedule dependent and more toxic to rapidly dividing cells. The dose-adjusted EPOCH regimen, which employs an infusional schedule, takes advantage of this phenomena and was equally effective in DLBCL with high or low tumor proliferation.[61]

Genes that distinguished germinal center (GC) B cells from other stages of B-cell differentiation are differentially expressed in the DLBCL cases, and have been used to subdivided cases into those derived from a germinal center B cell, termed a GC B cell–like (GCB), and an activated post-germinal center B cell, termed activated B cell–like (ABC) DLBCL.[17,62] Genes associated with GCB DLBCL include known markers of germinal center differentiation such as CD10 and the bcl-6 gene, which may be translocated or mutated in DLBCL.[63] In contrast, most genes that defined ABC DLBCL are not expressed by normal GC B cells, but instead are induced during in vitro activation of peripheral B cells, such as the IRF4 (MUM-1) gene that is transiently induced during normal lymphocyte activation, and is necessary for antigen receptor–driven B-cell proliferation.[64,65] Recent evidence suggests rituximab may partially overcome the resistance associated with BCL-2 and/or the ABC subtype. In studies by Wilson et al. and Mounier et al., rituximab increased the sensitivity of BCL-2–positive DLBCL to the effects of DA-EPOCH and CHOP chemotherapy, respectively, suggesting biological specificity for the benefit of rituximab.[16,66]

If this new taxonomy defines true DLBCL subtypes, one would also predict that it should have clinical prognostic value and could guide therapeutic development. An analysis revealed a statistically significant difference in overall survival at 5 years of 59% in GCB and 31% in ABC subtypes of DLBCL, indicating that they have different clinical outcomes (Fig. 13–3).[17,62] Importantly, the prognostic outcome of these two subgroups is independent of the International Prognostic Index (IPI), indicating that molecular profiling identifies different features that influence survival. These results led to a larger study by Rosenwald et al. in which samples from 240 patients with DLBCL were analyzed by molecular profiling and for the presence of genomic abnormalities.[18] Using a supervised approach of the gene expression profiles from these cases, a molecular prognostic predictor was developed for DLBCL (Fig. 13–3).[18] The final model combined four expression signatures that were defined by the GCB signature (favorable), MHC class II signature (favorable), lymph-node signature (favorable) and the proliferation signature (unfavorable) (Fig. 13–3). Another study by Shipp et al. undertook a similar goal to develop an outcome predictor using a different array chip that contained 6817 genes.[67] In this study of 58 patients, three of the outcome predictor genes in this model, NOR1, PDE4B, and PKC-β, appear to play a role in chemotherapy response and cellular proliferation.[68–70]

Mantle cell lymphoma (MCL), while relatively uncommon, is both aggressive and incurable with a median survival of 3 to 4 years.[71] To help gain insights into its pathogenesis with an aim of identifying new therapeutic targets and of predicting survival outcome, a study of 101 cases was undertaken.[56] A supervised approach to discover genes associated with survival found that 58% of the predictor genes were associated with cellular proliferation, with higher expression of this signature being associated with worse overall survival. By using a quantitative measure of tumor cell proliferation, a predictive model was developed that subdivided patients into quartiles with median survival times of 0.8, 2.3, 3.3, and 6.7 years. To further elucidate molecular mechanisms of survival, a search for oncogenic events that might explain the variable proliferation was undertaken. In some of the more proliferative MCL cases, there were higher levels of cyclin D1 mRNA due to the preferential expression of a more stable isoform, and more common deletions of the INK4a/ARF locus, which encodes the p16INK4a and p14ARF tumor suppressors.[56,72]

By elucidating pertinent pathways of lymphomagenesis, molecular profiling may identify clinically useful targets, including those for therapeutic development. Shipp et al. highlighted the potential importance of PKC-β as a therapeutic target in DLBCL.[67] Molecular profiling in DLBCL also revealed a high expression of NF-κB target genes in the ABC but not GCB DLBCL subtypes.[18,27] NF-κB signaling interferes with apoptotic cell death triggered by chemotherapeutic agents, and its inhibition in ABC-like DLBCL cell lines was cytotoxic, whereas GCB-like cell lines were unaffected.[27] NF-κB is also constitutively activated in mantle cell lymphoma and its inhibition leads to cell cycle arrest and apoptosis.[73] Bortezomib, a proteasome inhibitor, acts to down-regulate the NF-κB pathway and may enhance the cytotoxicity of chemotherapy in ABC DLBCL and mantle cell lymphomas.[74] Clinical trials are in progress to evaluate bortezomib in these settings. Recent evidence suggests that rituximab may partially overcome the resistance associated with bcl-2 expressing DLBCL, which is likely a surrogate marker for the ABC subtype of DLBCL.[16,66]

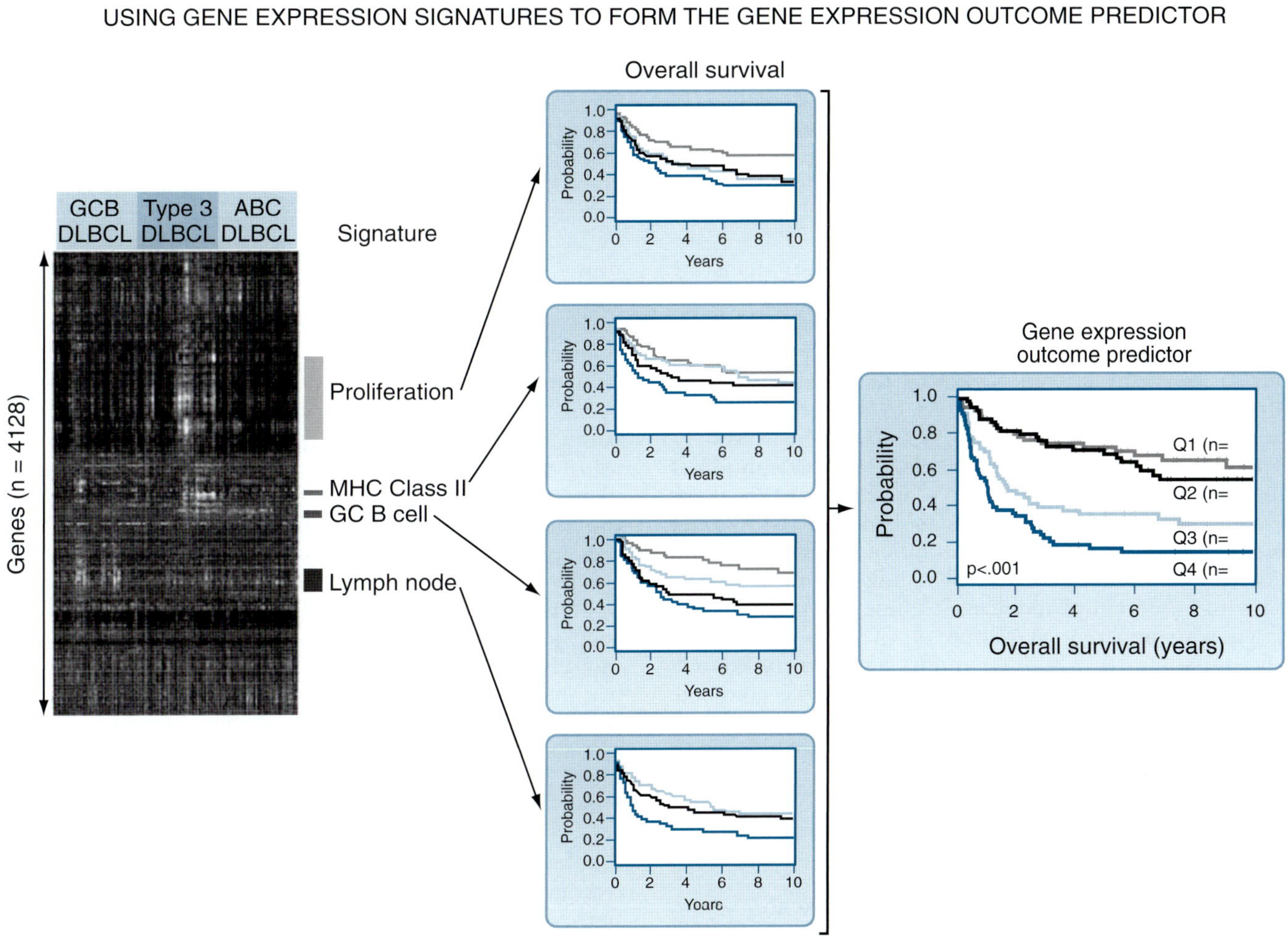

Figure 13–3. Diagnosis of DLBCL subtypes by gene expression and development of a molecular outcome predictor in previously untreated patients with DLBCL following chemotherapy. **A:** The expression levels of 27 genes from the subgroup predictor in 274 DLBCL samples are shown according to the scale at the **left**. Six named genes that showed increased expression in either the ABC or GCB subgroups are shown at the **right**. The likelihood that a DLBCL sample belongs to the ABC or GCB subgroup is shown on **top** and arranged by probability. **B:** Kaplan–Meier estimates of overall survival are shown according to GCB or ABC DLBCL subtype. **C:** Kaplan–Meier estimates of overall survival according to the molecular outcome predictor are shown for each quartile.

NEW DIRECTIONS FOR ANTILYMPHOMA THERAPY

Although the pace for identification of new agents for treating lymphomas has been slow, strategies for drug discovery are changing. At the National Cancer Institute (NCI), human cell line screens have replaced traditional murine leukemias as the primary discovery tool, and although lymphomas are not part of the primary panel, active new drugs identified in the primary 60-cell line panel are then screened against a set of acquired immunodeficiency syndrome–related lymphoma cell lines to expedite the recognition of agents active in this set of neoplasms.[75,76] The emphasis of NCI screening has shifted from synthetic chemicals to natural products, and a series of novel structures with unique sites of action have shown sufficient preclinical activity to warrant preclinical evaluation. The NCI screening approach has been supplemented by the development of computer-based programs that allow recognition of patterns of cell line response that reflect drug interactions with specific molecular targets, identify specific mechanisms of drug action, and provide clues to mechanisms of drug resistance.[77] In this way, the initial screening information, derived from responses of the primary 60 cell lines, provides important leads that determine NCI's interest in further compound evaluation and development.

Complementary to the NCI discovery effort, biotechnology companies have targeted specific molecular processes as the foundation for their drug discovery strategy. These targets include tyrosine kinases that transduce growth signals and regulate cell cycle progression, and proteins that control apoptosis and other important pathways in growth, differentiation, and cell death.[78] To simplify the process of finding lead compounds that interact with these targets, companies have developed automated processes for detecting interactions of a target protein, peptide or nucleic acid sequence with large libraries of randomly generated peptides, oligonucleotides, or synthetic chemicals.[79,80] The lead ligand thus identified then becomes the object of rational chemical design to enhance its binding to the target and to incorporate desirable pharmacologic features such as stability, solubility, and a favorable toxicologic profile. The success of approaches directed at a specific molecular target obviously depends on the wisdom of the initial choice of a suitable target, a choice that may be based on compelling logic but may prove elusive or unimportant in practice. In addition to the complexity of finding new molecules that interact with these targets, these efforts must successfully refine lead compounds so that they have requisite pharmacologic properties and are able to pass the cell membrane and persist as active agents in the living host.

A number of drugs with novel therapeutic targets are under development for lymphoid malignancies (Table 13–3).[81] Flavopiridol is a semisynthetic flavonoid derived from rohitukine, an alkaloid isolated from a plant indigenous to India. Initial studies showed that flavopiridol can induce cell cycle arrest either in G1 by cdk2 inhibition or in G2/M by cdk1 inhibition.[82,83] UCN-01 (7-hydroxystaurosporine) is a potent inhibitor of Ca2+ and phospholipid-dependent protein kinase C (PKC), an important regulator of signal transduction.[84] Studies in leukemic T-cell lines have demonstrated irreversible inhibition of cell growth and evidence of internucleosomal DNA fragmentation consistent with induction of apoptosis.[85] These observations correlated with apparent activation of CDKs 1 and 2, and suggest that targets in addition to PKC must be considered. As a single agent, UCN-01 produced a durable complete remission in a patient with a refractory anaplastic T-cell lymphoma, and induced a complete remission with chemotherapy in a refractory large B-cell lymphoma.[86,87] Bryostatin, another protein kinase inhibitor, is a natural product isolated from the marine bryozoan *Bugula neritina*. Of potential clinical interest is the in vitro observation that it can induce differentiation of refractory B-CLL cells to a hairy-cell phenotype, rendering them susceptible to 2-chlorodeoxyadenosine.[88,89] Depsipeptide, a bicyclic peptide produced by *Chromoabacterium violaceum*, was first identified by Ueda et al. through screening natural products for antitumor activity in myc-expressing tumor cells.[90] Mechanistically, depsipeptide inhibits cell cycle progression at the Go–G1 interface (Fig. 13–2), and blocks p21 protein signal transduction, although it is not known if these actions explain its cytotoxic activity. Cell cycle arrest possibly occurs through inhibition of the ras signal transduction pathway, and in vitro depsipeptide induces reversion of ras-transformed tumor cells to a normal morphology and regulates c-myc mRNA. One recent report also suggested that this agent might act via inhibition of the DNA histone deacetylase enzyme.[91] In vitro, CLL cells demonstrate sensitivity to depsipeptide, through apoptosis, indicating that it should be tested in this disease. Proteasome inhibitors, such as bortezomib, are attractive targets for therapeutic intervention because of the importance of the ubiquitin proteasome pathways in the degradation and regulation of protein action. The proteasome has numerous protein targets, such as p53, p21, p27, and plays a key role in a broad array of cellular processes including cell cycle regulation, cell death, gene expression, and NF-κB activation[92] (Fig. 13–2). Dipeptide boronic acid analogues have been developed that inhibit the chymotryptic activity of the proteasome with effects on tumor cell growth and apoptosis. Bortizomib represents a class of novel proteasome inhibitors, which selectively inhibits the proteasome with a K_ii of 6nM and has a wide range of activity against multiple tumor cell lines. There is increasing evidence that proteasome inhibitors may have a potential role in the therapy of patients with CLL. Proteasome inhibition has been shown to induce apoptosis of CLL lymphocytes without affecting normal lymphocytes, and can sensitize chemo- and radio-resistant CLL cells to apoptosis.

Table 13–3. Drugs with Novel Mechanisms of Action

Agent	Potential Mechanisms of Action
Flavopiridol	Inhibits cyclin D1, CDK1,2,4 Cell cycle arrest in G1 or G2 phase of cell cycle Induces apoptosis by caspase 3 activation Down regulates BCL-2 and Mcl-1 Potential antiangiogenesis
Depsipeptide	Inhibits DNA histone deacetylase enzyme Inhibits cell cycle progression in G0–G1 Induces apoptosis through effects on BCL-2/Bax ratio
Bryostatin 1	Induces differentiation of CLL cells to hairy-cell phenotype Inhibits protein kinase C Induces apoptosis
UCN-01 (7 Hydrox-staurosporine)	Nonspecific protein kinase C inhibitor Inhibits cyclin dependent kinase and induces G1 and G2 cell cycle arrest Synergistic effects with purine analogs (e.g., fludarabine)
PS-341 (bortezomib)	Inhibits degradation of proteins important in cell cycle progression such as cyclin A, B, D, E, and cyclin-dependent kinase inhibitors (CDKI) Inhibits NFκB activation
Genasense	Reduces BCL-2 and its inhibition on apoptosis

Lymphoid malignancies express a number of antigens that are promising targets for monoclonal-based therapy (Table 13–4). Development of monoclonal antibodies has been largely accomplished by the empiric method of immunizing mice against human tumor cells and screening the hybridomas for antibodies of interest. Because murine antibodies have a short half-life and induce a human anti-mouse antibody (HAMA) immune response, they are usually chimeric or humanized when used as therapeutic reagents. Presently, several monoclonal antibodies have received FDA approval and are used in CLL, including rituximab and alemtuzumab. Monoclonal antibodies may be engineered to combine the antibody with a toxin (immunotoxins) or a radioactive isotope (radioimmunoconjugates), or to contain a second specificity (bi-specific antibodies). For example, it is possible to conjugate an antibody with specificity to B-cell lymphomas with an antibody against CD3, which binds to and activates normal T cells, in order to enhance T-cell mediated lysis of the lymphoma cell. One such example of a bispecific antibody contains anti-CD3 and anti-CD19 specificity. Monoclonal antibodies raised

Table 13–4. Monoclonal Antibody-Based Drugs

Target Antigen and Primary Cell Type	Function	Unlabeled	Radioisotope Based	Toxin Based
CD19: B cells	Activation	B4 (murine)	None	B-4 (Ricin)
CD20: B cells	Proliferation/ differentiation	Rituximab (chimeric)	^{31}I-tositumomab ^{90}Y-ibritumomab tiuxetan	None
CD22: B cells	Activation	Epratuzumab (humanized) LL2 (murine)	LL2 ^{31}Iodine, LL2 ^{90}Yttrium	BL-22 (Pseudomonas)
CD52: B and T cells	Unknown	Alemtuzumab (humanized)	None	None
1D10 HLA DR β chain: B cells	Activation	Apolizumab (humanized)	None	None
Lym-1 HLA DR10: B cells	Activation	None	^{31}Iodine ^{67}Copper	None
Tac (CD25 α subunit): B and T cells	Activation	Zenapax (humanized)	None	LMB-2 (Pseudomonas)

against the immunoglobulin idiotype on a B-cell lymphoma represents another therapeutic strategy, which was first reported in 1982 by Levy, et al.[93] More recently, idiotype vaccines have been used to induce an polyclonal host antibody response against the malignant clone, and has shown promise as an effective treatment for minimal residual disease in follicular lymphomas.

Rituximab is the first monoclonal antibody to receive Food and Drug Administration approval. It is a chimeric monoclonal antibody directed against the normal CD20 antigen, which is found on over 95% of B-cell malignancies. Increasingly evident are the synergistic effects of rituximab and chemotherapy, suggesting that it sensitizes lymphoma cells to the apoptotic effects of chemotherapy by directly acting on tumor cells.[94] Alemtuzumab (Campath) is a humanized monoclonal antibody targeted against the CD52 antigen present on the surface of normal neutrophils and lymphocytes as well as most B- and T-cell lymphomas. Clinical activity has been demonstrated in low-grade lymphomas and CLL, including in patients with purine analog refractory disease.[95] Ongoing studies are assessing its activity in combination with chemotherapy in aggressive T-cell lymphomas.

There are many monoclonal antibodies under development. Epratuzumab is a humanized IgG1 monoclonal antibody directed against the CD22 antigen present on both normal and malignant B cells with a distribution similar to CD20. Epratuzumab is currently under evaluation in patients with rituximab-refractory indolent lymphomas and in combination with rituximab in follicular lymphomas.[96,97] Apolizumab is a humanized monoclonal antibody against the 1D10 antigen, a variant of the HLA-DR beta chain, which is neither shed nor down-modulated on antibody binding. The 1D10 antigen is present on normal human cells, including dendritic cells, macrophages, and some activated T cells, and is expressed on 50% to 70% of lymphomas and leukemias.[98]

Monoclonal antibodies have been conjugated to toxins to form immunotoxins. One such immunotoxin, BL22, targets the CD22 antigen found on normal B cells and B-cell malignancies. In a Phase I study of 16 cladarabine refractory patients with hairy-cell leukemia, 11 patients achieved complete responses, highlighting the potential of this approach.[99]

Radioimmunoconjugates provide monoclonal antibody targeted delivery of radioactive particles to tumor cells. ^{131}Iodine (^{131}I) is a commonly used radioisotope since it is readily available, relatively inexpensive, and easily conjugated to a monoclonal antibody. The gamma particles emitted by ^{131}I can be used for both imaging and therapy, but have the drawbacks of releasing free ^{131}I and ^{131}I-tyrosine into the blood and present a potential health hazard to caregivers. The beta-emitter, ^{90}Yttrium (^{90}Y), has emerged as an attractive alternative to ^{131}I, based on its higher energy and longer path length, which may be more effective in tumors with larger diameters. It also has a short half-life and remains conjugated, even after endocytosis, providing a safer profile for outpatient use. Clinically, radioimmunoconjugates have been developed with murine monoclonal antibodies against CD20 conjugated with ^{131}I (tositumomab or Bexxar®) and ^{90}Y (ibritumomab tiuxetan or Zevalin®). Both drugs have shown responses rates in relapsed lymphoma of 65% to 80%, but are likely to be less effective and more toxic in CLL because of bone marrow involvement and the leukemic phase.[100,101]

PROTOCOL DESIGN

Historically, combination chemotherapy empirically evolved out of a need for more effective treatments than were produced by single agents. The development of combination chemotherapy regimens has been largely empiric, particularly for the non-Hodgkin's lymphomas. More recently, however, strategies based on pharmacologic considerations such as pharmacodynamic dosing, dose density and the use of targeted agents are increasingly incorporated into the design of new regimens.

When developing a new chemotherapy regimen, several basic principles should be followed. First and foremost, drugs with the best single-agent activity should be chosen, and attention must be paid to both potential synergism and antagonism. Selection of drugs with nonoverlapping toxicities will allow the administration of higher doses with less toxicity. The choice of dose, rate, and route of drug administration (e.g., oral, or intravenous bolus or infusion) should be based on the pharmacokinetics and schedule dependency of the drugs in question. Experimental modeling of administration schedules (e.g., bolus or continuous infusion), timing of administration, and pharmacodynamics are important.

An important area of research in clinical treatment involves the modulation of the apoptotic threshold. Altering drug schedule to take advantage of increased apoptotic sensitivity during S-phase and modulation of cell cycle checkpoints may significantly affect drug sensitivity. Biologically oriented therapies (such as immunotherapy with lymphokine-activated cells, natural killer cells and cytotoxic T cells, free antibodies, immunotoxins, vaccines, cytokines, and other proteins such as TNF and TGF-β) are in various stages of clinical evaluation. Agents such as rituximab and UCN-01, for example, can sensitize lymphomas to cytotoxic agents and may have value in combination with drugs.[87,102] Ultimately, however, treatment regimens are judged by results, and since so many variables impact on the outcome of chemotherapy, it must be recognized that there still remains a large element of empiricism in protocol design.

References

1. Alenzi FQ, Wyse RK, and Altamimi WG. Apoptosis as a tool for therapeutic agents in haematological diseases. Expert Opin Biol Ther 2004;4:407–20.
2. Lowe SW, Schmitt EM, Smith SW, et al. p53 is required for radiation-induced apoptosis in mouse thymocytes. Nature 1993;362:847–9.
3. Debatin KM, Stahnke K, and Fulda S. Apoptosis in hematological disorders. Semin Cancer Biol 2003;13:149–58.
4. Skipper HE, Schabel FM Jr, and Wilcox WS. Experimental evaluation of potential anticancer agents. Xiii. On the criteria and kinetics associated with "curability" of experimental leukemia. Cancer Chemother Rep 1964;35:1–111.
5. Schabel FM Jr and Simpson-Herren L. Some variables in experimental tumor systems which complicate interpretation of data from in vivo kinetic and pharmacologic studies with anticancer drugs. Antibiot Chemother 1978;23: 113–27.
6. Magrath IT, Lwanga S, Carswell W, et al. Surgical reduction of tumour bulk in management of abdominal Burkitt's lymphoma. Br Med J 1974;2:308–12.
7. Frei E, 3rd, Teicher BA, Holden SA, et al. Preclinical studies and clinical correlation of the effect of alkylating dose. Cancer Res 1988;48:6417–23.
8. Aglietta M, De Felice L, Stacchini A, et al. In vivo effect of granulocyte-macrophage colony-stimulating factor on the kinetics of human acute myeloid leukemia cells. Leukemia 1991;5:979–84.
9. Fisher RI, Gaynor ER, Dahlberg S, et al. Comparison of a standard regimen (CHOP) with three intensive chemotherapy regimens for advanced non-Hodgkin's lymphoma. N Engl J Med 1993;328:1002–6.
10. Kwak LW, Halpern J, Olshen RA, et al. Prognostic significance of actual dose intensity in diffuse large-cell lymphoma: results of a tree-structured survival analysis. J Clin Oncol 1990;8:963–77.
11. Lee KW, Kim DY, Yun T, et al. Doxorubicin-based chemotherapy for diffuse large B-cell lymphoma in elderly patients: comparison of treatment outcomes between young and elderly patients and the significance of doxorubicin dosage. Cancer 2003;98:2651–6.
12. Meyer RM, Quirt IC, Skillings JR, et al. Escalated as compared with standard doses of doxorubicin in BACOP therapy for patients with non-Hodgkin's lymphoma. N Engl J Med 1993;329:1770–6.
13. Milpied N, Deconinck E, Gaillard F, et al. Initial treatment of aggressive lymphoma with high-dose chemotherapy and autologous stem-cell support. N Engl J Med 2004; 350:1287–95.
14. Haioun C, Lepage E, Gisselbrecht C, et al. Survival benefit of high-dose therapy in poor-risk aggressive non-Hodgkin's lymphoma: final analysis of the prospective LNH87-2 protocol—a groupe d'Etude des lymphomes de l'Adulte study. J Clin Oncol 2000;18:3025–30.
15. Verdonck LF, van Putten WL, Hagenbeek A, et al. Comparison of CHOP chemotherapy with autologous bone marrow transplantation for slowly responding patients with aggressive non-Hodgkin's lymphoma. N Engl J Med 1995;332: 1045–51.
16. Wilson WH, Pittaluga S, Gutierrez M, et al. Dose-adjusted EPOCH-rituximab in untreated diffuse large B-cell lymphoma: benefit of rituximab appears restricted to tumors harboring anti-apoptotic mechanisms. Proc Am Soc Hematol 2003;102.
17. Alizadeh AA, Eisen MB, Davis RE, et al. Distinct types of diffuse large B-cell lymphoma identified by gene expression profiling. Nature 2000;403:503–11.
18. Rosenwald A, Wright G, Chan WC, et al. The use of molecular profiling to predict survival after chemotherapy for diffuse large B-cell lymphoma. N Engl J Med 2002; 346:1937–47.
19. Ema H, Suda T, Sakamoto S, et al. Effects of the in vivo administration of recombinant human granulocyte colony-stimulating factor following cytotoxic chemotherapy on granulocytic precursors in patients with malignant lymphoma. Jpn J Cancer Res 1989;80:577–82.
20. Gerhartz HH, Engelhard M, Meusers P, et al. Randomized, double-blind, placebo-controlled, phase III study of recombinant human granulocyte-macrophage colony-stimulating factor as adjunct to induction treatment of high-grade malignant non-Hodgkin's lymphomas. Blood 1993;82:2329–39.
21. Cooper IA, Wolf MM, Robertson TI, et al. Randomized comparison of MACOP-B with CHOP in patients with intermediate-grade non-Hodgkin's lymphoma. The Australian and New Zealand Lymphoma Group. J Clin Oncol 1994;12:769–78.
22. Pfreundschuh M, Truemper TL, Kloess M, et al. 2-weekly vs. 3-weekly CHOP with and without etoposide in for patients >60 years of age with aggressive non-Hodgkin's lymphoma (NHL): Results of the completed NHL-B-2 trial of the DSHNHL. Blood 2002;99:Abstract 3060.
23. Goldie JH and Coldman AJ. A mathematic model for relating the drug sensitivity of tumors to their spontaneous mutation rate. Cancer Treat Rep 1979;63:1727–33.
24. Luria S and Delbruck M. Mutations of bacteria from virus sensitivity to virus resistance. Genetics 1943;28:491–511.
25. Harris CC and Hollstein M. Clinical implications of the p53 tumor-suppressor gene. N Engl J Med 1993;329:1318–27.
26. Wilson WH, Teruya-Feldstein J, Fest T, et al. Relationship of p53, bcl-2, and tumor proliferation to clinical drug resistance in non-Hodgkin's lymphomas. Blood 1997;89:601–9.
27. Davis RE, Brown KD, Siebenlist U, et al. Constitutive nuclear factor kappaB activity is required for survival of activated B cell-like diffuse large B cell lymphoma cells. J Exp Med 2001;194:1861–74.
28. Gascoyne RD, Adomat SA, Krajewski S, et al. Prognostic significance of Bcl-2 protein expression and Bcl-2 gene rearrangement in diffuse aggressive non-Hodgkin's lymphoma. Blood 1997;90:244–51.
29. Ichikawa A, Kinoshita T, Watanabe T, et al. Mutations of the p53 gene as a prognostic factor in aggressive B-cell lymphoma. N Engl J Med 1997;337:529–34.

30. Hermine O, Haioun C, Lepage E, et al. Prognostic significance of bcl-2 protein expression in aggressive non-Hodgkin's lymphoma. Groupe d'Etude des Lymphomes de l'Adulte (GELA). Blood 1996;87:265–72.
31. Gros P, Ben Neriah YB, Croop JM, et al. Isolation and expression of a complementary DNA that confers multidrug resistance. Nature 1986;323:728–31.
32. Gros P, Croop J, Housman D. Mammalian multidrug resistance gene: complete cDNA sequence indicates strong homology to bacterial transport proteins. Cell 1986; 47:371–80.
33. Fojo AT, Ueda K, Slamon DJ, et al. Expression of a multidrug-resistance gene in human tumors and tissues. Proc Natl Acad Sci U S A 1987;84:265–9.
34. Wilson WH, Bates SE, Fojo A, et al. Controlled trial of dexverapamil, a modulator of multidrug resistance, in lymphomas refractory to EPOCH chemotherapy. J Clin Oncol 1995;13:1995–2004.
35. Sachs L and Lotem J. Control of programmed cell death in normal and leukemic cells: new implications for therapy. Blood 1993;82:15–21.
36. Solary E, Bertrand R, Kohn KW, et al. Differential induction of apoptosis in undifferentiated and differentiated HL-60 cells by DNA topoisomerase I and II inhibitors. Blood 1993;81:1359–68.
37. Hockenbery D, Nunez G, Milliman C, et al. Bcl-2 is an inner mitochondrial membrane protein that blocks programmed cell death. Nature 1990;348:334–6.
38. Clarke AR, Purdie CA, Harrison DJ, et al. Thymocyte apoptosis induced by p53-dependent and independent pathways. Nature 1993;362:849–52.
39. Dancescu M, Rubio-Trujillo M, Biron G, et al. Interleukin 4 protects chronic lymphocytic leukemic B cells from death by apoptosis and upregulates Bcl-2 expression. J Exp Med 1992;176:1319–26.
40. Walton MI, Whysong D, O'Connor PM, et al. Constitutive expression of human Bcl-2 modulates nitrogen mustard and camptothecin induced apoptosis. Cancer Res 1993;53:1853–61.
41. Gaidano G, Ballerini P, Gong JZ, et al. p53 mutations in human lymphoid malignancies: association with Burkitt lymphoma and chronic lymphocytic leukemia. Proc Natl Acad Sci U S A 1991;88:5413–7.
42. Arends MJ and Wyllie AH. Apoptosis: mechanisms and roles in pathology. Int Rev Exp Pathol 1991;32:223–54.
43. Zutter M, Hockenbery D, Silverman GA, et al. Immunolocalization of the Bcl-2 protein within hematopoietic neoplasms. Blood 1991;78:1062–8.
44. Tsujimoto Y, Gorham J, Cossman J, et al. The t(14;18) chromosome translocations involved in B-cell neoplasms result from mistakes in VDJ joining. Science 1985;229: 1390–3.
45. Yunis JJ, Frizzera G, Oken MM, et al. Multiple recurrent genomic defects in follicular lymphoma. A possible model for cancer. N Engl J Med 1987;316:79–84.
46. Kondo E, Nakamura S, Onoue H, et al. Detection of bcl-2 protein and bcl-2 messenger RNA in normal and neoplastic lymphoid tissues by immunohistochemistry and in situ hybridization. Blood 1992;80:2044–51.
47. Pezzella F, Tse AG, Cordell JL, et al. Expression of the bcl-2 oncogene protein is not specific for the 14;18 chromosomal translocation. Am J Pathol 1990;137:225–32.
48. Oltvai ZN, Milliman CL, and Korsmeyer SJ. Bcl-2 heterodimerizes in vivo with a conserved homolog, Bax, that accelerates programmed cell death. Cell 1993;74:609–19.
49. Lotem J and Sachs L. Regulation by bcl-2, c-myc, and p53 of susceptibility to induction of apoptosis by heat shock and cancer chemotherapy compounds in differentiation-competent and -defective myeloid leukemic cells. Cell Growth Differ 1993;4:41–7.
50. Furman RR, Asgary Z, Mascarenhas JO, et al. Modulation of NF-kappa B activity and apoptosis in chronic lymphocytic leukemia B cells. J Immunol 2000;164:2200–6.
51. Zapata JM, Krajewska M, Krajewski S, et al. TNFR-associated factor family protein expression in normal tissues and lymphoid malignancies. J Immunol 2000;165:5084–96.
52. Farrugia MM, Duan LJ, Reis MD, et al. Alterations of the p53 tumor suppressor gene in diffuse large cell lymphomas with translocations of the c-MYC and BCL-2 proto-oncogenes. Blood 1994;83:191–8.
53. Fujiwara T, Grimm EA, Mukhopadhyay T, et al. Induction of chemosensitivity in human lung cancer cells in vivo by adenovirus-mediated transfer of the wild-type p53 gene. Cancer Res 1994;54:2287–91.
54. Yatabe Y, Nakamura S, Seto M, et al. Clinicopathologic study of PRAD1/cyclin D1 overexpressing lymphoma with special reference to mantle cell lymphoma. A distinct molecular pathologic entity. Am J Surg Pathol 1996;20:1110–22.
55. Bigoni R, Negrini M, Veronese ML, et al. Characterization of t(11;14) translocation in mantle cell lymphoma by fluorescent in situ hybridization. Oncogene 1996;13:797–802.
56. Rosenwald A, Wright G, Wiestner A, et al. The proliferation gene expression signature is a quantitative integrator of oncogenic events that predicts survival in mantle cell lymphoma. Cancer Cell 2003;3:185–97.
57. O'Connor PM, Ferris DK, Pagano M, et al. G2 delay induced by nitrogen mustard in human cells affects cyclin A/cdk2 and cyclin B1/cdc2-kinase complexes differently. J Biol Chem 1993;268:8298–308.
58. Waters JS, Webb A, Cunningham D, et al. Phase I clinical and pharmacokinetic study of bcl-2 antisense oligonucleotide therapy in patients with non-Hodgkin's lymphoma. J Clin Oncol 2000;18:1812–23.
59. Gutierrez-Puente Y, Zapata-Benavides P, Tari AM, et al. Bcl-2–related antisense therapy. Semin Oncol 2002;29:71–6.
60. Baskar S, Kobrin CB, and Kwak LW. Autologous lymphoma vaccines induce human T cell responses against multiple, unique epitopes. J Clin Invest 2004;113:1498–510.
61. Wilson WH, Grossbard ML, Pittaluga S, et al. Dose-adjusted EPOCH chemotherapy for untreated large B-cell lymphomas: a pharmacodynamic approach with high efficacy. Blood 2002;99:2685–93.
62. Wiestner A and Staudt, LM. Towards a molecular diagnosis and targeted therapy of lymphoid malignancies. Semin Hematol 2003;40:296–307.
63. Dalla-Favera R, Migliazza A, Chang CC, et al. Molecular pathogenesis of B cell malignancy: the role of BCL-6. Curr Top Microbiol Immunol 1999;246:257–63; discussion 263–5.
64. Matsuyama T, Grossman A, Mittrucker HW, et al. Molecular cloning of LSIRF, a lymphoid-specific member of the interferon regulatory factor family that binds the interferon-stimulated response element (ISRE). Nucleic Acids Res 1995;23:2127–36.
65. Mittrucker HW, Matsuyama T, Grossman A, et al. Requirement for the transcription factor LSIRF/IRF4 for mature B and T lymphocyte function. Science 1997;275:540–3.
66. Mounier N, Briere J, Gisselbrecht C, et al. Rituximab plus CHOP (R-CHOP) overcomes bcl-2–associated resistance to chemotherapy in elderly patients with diffuse large B-cell lymphoma (DLBCL). Blood 2003;101:4279–84.
67. Shipp MA, Ross KN, Tamayo P, et al. Diffuse large B-cell lymphoma outcome prediction by gene-expression profiling and supervised machine learning. Nat Med 2002;8:68–74.
68. Brenner C and Kroemer G. Apoptosis. Mitochondria—the death signal integrators. Science 2000;289:1150–1.

69. Manning CD, Burman M, Christensen SB, et al. Suppression of human inflammatory cell function by subtype-selective PDE4 inhibitors correlates with inhibition of PDE4A and PDE4B. Br J Pharmacol 1999;128:1393–8.
70. Leitges M, Schmedt C, Guinamard R, et al. Immunodeficiency in protein kinase cbeta-deficient mice. Science 1996;273:788–91.
71. Barista I, Romaguera JE, and Cabanillas F. Mantle-cell lymphoma. Lancet Oncol 2001;2:141–8.
72. Fang NY, Greiner TC, Weisenburger DD, et al. Oligonucleotide microarrays demonstrate the highest frequency of ATM mutations in the mantle cell subtype of lymphoma. Proc Natl Acad Sci U S A 2003;100:5372–7.
73. Pham LV, Tamayo AT, Yoshimura LC, et al. Inhibition of constitutive NF-kappa B activation in mantle cell lymphoma B cells leads to induction of cell cycle arrest and apoptosis. J Immunol 2003;171:88–95.
74. Adams J. Proteasome inhibition in cancer: development of PS-341. Semin Oncol 2001;28:613–9.
75. Monga M, Sausville EA. Developmental therapeutics program at the NCI: molecular target and drug discovery process. Leukemia 2002;16:520–6.
76. Rabow AA, Shoemaker RH, Sausville EA, et al. Mining the National Cancer Institute's tumor-screening database: identification of compounds with similar cellular activities. J Med Chem 2002;45:818–40.
77. Zaharevitz DW, Holbeck SL, Bowerman C, et al. COMPARE: a web accessible tool for investigating mechanisms of cell growth inhibition. J Mol Graph Model 2002;20:297–303.
78. Powis G and Kozikowski A. Growth factor and oncogene signalling pathways as targets for rational anticancer drug development. Clin Biochem 1991;24:385–97.
79. Ohlmeyer MH, Swanson RN, Dillard LW, et al. Complex synthetic chemical libraries indexed with molecular tags. Proc Natl Acad Sci U S A 1993;90:10922–6.
80. DeWitt SH, Kiely JS, Stankovic CJ, et al. "Diversomers": an approach to nonpeptide, nonoligomeric chemical diversity. Proc Natl Acad Sci U S A 1993;90:6909–13.
81. Senderowicz AM and Sausville EA. Preclinical and clinical development of cyclin-dependent kinase modulators. J Natl Cancer Inst 2000;92:376–87.
82. Melillo G, Sausville EA, Cloud K, et al. Flavopiridol, a protein kinase inhibitor, down-regulates hypoxic induction of vascular endothelial growth factor expression in human monocytes. Cancer Res 1999;59:5433–7.
83. Byrd JC, Shinn C, Waselenko JK, et al. Flavopiridol induces apoptosis in chronic lymphocytic leukemia cells via activation of caspase-3 without evidence of bcl-2 modulation or dependence on functional p53. Blood 1998;92:3804–16.
84. Seynaeve CM, Kazanietz MG, Blumberg PM, et al. Differential inhibition of protein kinase C isozymes by UCN-01, a staurosporine analogue. Mol Pharmacol 1994;45:1207–14.
85. Yamauchi T, Keating MJ, and Plunkett W. UCN-01 (7-hydroxystaurosporine) inhibits DNA repair and increases cytotoxicity in normal lymphocytes and chronic lymphocytic leukemia lymphocytes. Mol Cancer Ther 2002;1: 287–94.
86. Sausville EA, Arbuck SG, Messmann R, et al. Phase I trial of 72-hour continuous infusion UCN-01 in patients with refractory neoplasms. J Clin Oncol 2001;19:2319–33.
87. Wilson WH, Sorbara L, Figg WD, et al. Modulation of clinical drug resistance in a B cell lymphoma patient by the protein kinase inhibitor 7-hydroxystaurosporine: presentation of a novel therapeutic paradigm. Clin Cancer Res 2000;6:415–21.
88. Varterasian ML, Mohammad RM, Shurafa MS, et al. Phase II trial of bryostatin 1 in patients with relapsed low-grade non-Hodgkin's lymphoma and chronic lymphocytic leukemia. Clin Cancer Res 2000;6:825–8.
89. Varterasian ML, Mohammad RM, Eilender DS, et al. Phase I study of bryostatin 1 in patients with relapsed non-Hodgkin's lymphoma and chronic lymphocytic leukemia. J Clin Oncol 1998;16:56–62.
90. Ueda H, Nakajima H, Hori Y, et al. FR901228, a novel antitumor bicyclic depsipeptide produced by Chromobacterium violaceum No. 968. I. Taxonomy, fermentation, isolation, physico-chemical and biological properties, and antitumor activity. J Antibiot (Tokyo) 1994;47:301–10.
91. Nakajima H, Kim YB, Terano H, et al. FR901228, a potent antitumor antibiotic, is a novel histone deacetylase inhibitor. Exp Cell Res 1998;241:126–33.
92. Adams J, Palombella VJ, and Elliott PJ. Proteasome inhibition: a new strategy in cancer treatment. Invest New Drugs 2000;18:109–21.
93. Miller RA, Maloney DG, Warnke R, et al. Treatment of B-cell lymphoma with monoclonal anti-idiotype antibody. N Engl J Med 1982;306:517–22.
94. Reed JC, Kitada S, Kim Y, et al. Modulating apoptosis pathways in low-grade B-cell malignancies using biological response modifiers. Semin Oncol 2002;29:10–24.
95. Osterborg A, Dyer MJ, Bunjes D, et al. Phase II multicenter study of human CD52 antibody in previously treated chronic lymphocytic leukemia. European Study Group of CAMPATH-1H Treatment in Chronic Lymphocytic Leukemia. J Clin Oncol 1997;15:1567–74.
96. Leonard JP, Coleman M, Ketas JC, et al. Phase I/II trial of epratuzumab (humanized anti-CD22 antibody) in indolent non-Hodgkin's lymphoma. J Clin Oncol 2003;21: 3051–9.
97. Furman RR, Coleman M, and Leonard JP. Epratuzumab in Non-Hodgkin's lymphomas. Curr Treat Options Oncol 2004;5:283–8.
98. Shi JD, Bullock C, Hall WC, et al. In vivo pharmacodynamic effects of Hu1D10 (remitogen), a humanized antibody reactive against a polymorphic determinant of HLA-DR expressed on B cells. Leuk Lymphoma 2002;43:1303–12.
99. Kreitman RJ, Wilson WH, Bergeron K, et al. Efficacy of the anti-CD22 recombinant immunotoxin BL22 in chemotherapy-resistant hairy-cell leukemia. N Engl J Med 2001;345:241–7.
100. Kaminski MS, Zelenetz AD, Press OW, et al. Pivotal study of iodine I 131 tositumomab for chemotherapy-refractory low-grade or transformed low-grade B-cell non-Hodgkin's lymphomas. J Clin Oncol 2001;19:3918–28.
101. Gordon LI, Witzig TE, Wiseman GA, et al. Yttrium 90 ibritumomab tiuxetan radioimmunotherapy for relapsed or refractory low-grade non-Hodgkin's lymphoma. Semin Oncol 2002;29:87–92.
102. Wilson WH, Gutierrez M, O'Connor P, et al. The role of rituximab and chemotherapy in aggressive B-cell lymphoma: a preliminary report of dose-adjusted EPOCH-R. Semin Oncol 2002;29:41–7.
103. Dana BW, Dahlberg S, Miller TP, et al. m-BACOD treatment for intermediate- and high-grade malignant lymphomas: a Southwest Oncology Group phase II trial. J Clin Oncol 1990;8:1155–62.
104. Longo DL, DeVita VT Jr, Duffey PL, et al. Superiority of ProMACE-CytaBOM over ProMACE-MOPP in the treatment of advanced diffuse aggressive lymphoma: results of a prospective randomized trial. J Clin Oncol 1991;9:25–38.

14

Allogeneic Stem Cell Transplantation for Non-Hodgkin's and Hodgkin's Lymphoma

Rifca Le Dieu, M.B.B.S.
John G. Gribben, M.D.

Hematopoietic stem cell transplantation (SCT) has become the treatment of choice for patients with relapsed aggressive non-Hodgkin's lymphoma (NHL) and Hodgkin's lymphoma (HL). To date, most patients have been treated with autologous stem cells, and are currently using peripheral blood stem cells mobilized by chemotherapy and recombinant growth factors. Attempts are underway to determine whether SCT has a role to play in the management of patients who present with poor prognostic features and who have less chance of being cured using standard dose chemotherapy. The role of SCT in the management of patients with indolent NHLs remains more controversial, although increasing numbers of patients with advanced stage follicular lymphoma, mantle cell lymphoma, and chronic lymphocytic leukemia are now undergoing SCT. There is increasing concern regarding long-term toxicity of autologous SCT, especially the higher-than-expected long-term risk of development of myelodysplastic syndrome. This has led to renewed interest in the role of allogeneic SCT for patients with NHL, although the major problem here has been the high treatment-related mortality (TRM) associated with the high-dose therapy (HDT) used in conventional conditioning as well as graft-versus-host disease (GVHD). A potential advantage of allogeneic SCT is the potential to exploit a graft-versus-lymphoma (GVL) effect, and many studies are underway exploring the use of reduced intensity conditioning regimens, steps to control disease progression and manipulate donor cells to maximize T-cell responsiveness against lymphoma.

The role of allogeneic SCT in the management of patients with HL is even more controversial. Conventional allogeneic SCT has been associated with high TRM and high probability of relapse, likely due to the very high-risk patients who are considered candidates for this approach. There is, however, evidence of a graft versus Hodgkin's lymphoma effect, and the lower mortality associated with reduced intensity conditioning regimens has led to some increased interest in the use of allogeneic SCT in this disease setting as well.

ALLOGENEIC SCT FOR NON-HODGKIN'S LYMPHOMA

NHLs are a diverse group of disorders with widely differing natural histories. Despite this, most of the published studies of allogeneic SCT in NHL have been relatively small single-institution studies that included a variety of lymphoid malignancies. The results of the larger studies are outlined in Table 14–1. Most patients had advanced disease at the time of transplant,[1–4] but some studies have included patients in first or later remission, usually patients with more aggressive disease.[1–9] Regimens containing total-body irradiation (TBI) have been used most commonly for conditioning, but some studies have used Busulphan or Carmustine (BCNU)-containing regimens,[10] particularly for patients who have already received dose-limiting radiation therapy or who failed previous TBI containing regimens and autologous SCT.[11]

SCT IN AGGRESSIVE NON-HODGKIN'S LYMPHOMA

Hematopoietic SCT has been established as the treatment of choice for patients in the first sensitive relapse of diffuse large B-cell lymphoma (DLBCL)[12]; a number of studies performed in the 1980s established that when patients no longer respond to standard dosage of chemotherapy (resistant relapse), they have little chance of cure with dose escalation to HDT. Of note, high-risk patients appear to benefit most from high-dose therapy and patients with low-risk disease at relapse do not appear to benefit from autologous SCT compared to salvage chemotherapy.[13] To attempt to extrapolate from these studies, a number of studies have addressed the role of HDT and autologous SCT as front-line therapy for patients with poor prognosis DLBCL, but these studies yielded conflicting results.[14–16] Whereas some investigators suggest that HDT may be indicated for patients with increased risk features as presentation, it remains unknown whether the addition of rituximab to CHOP-like regimens would achieve results similar to those seen using HDT and autologous SCT. It is not yet clear precisely which "high-risk" features should be used in consideration of which patients are suitable for SCT as front-line therapy. Among 330 patients in sequential GELA trials who received high-dose CHOP and consolidation autologous SCT, adverse factors for outcome after SCT included marrow involvement, more than one extranodal site, histologic subtype, and dose intensity.[17] These features are, of course, similar to those that would have made patients eligible to consider

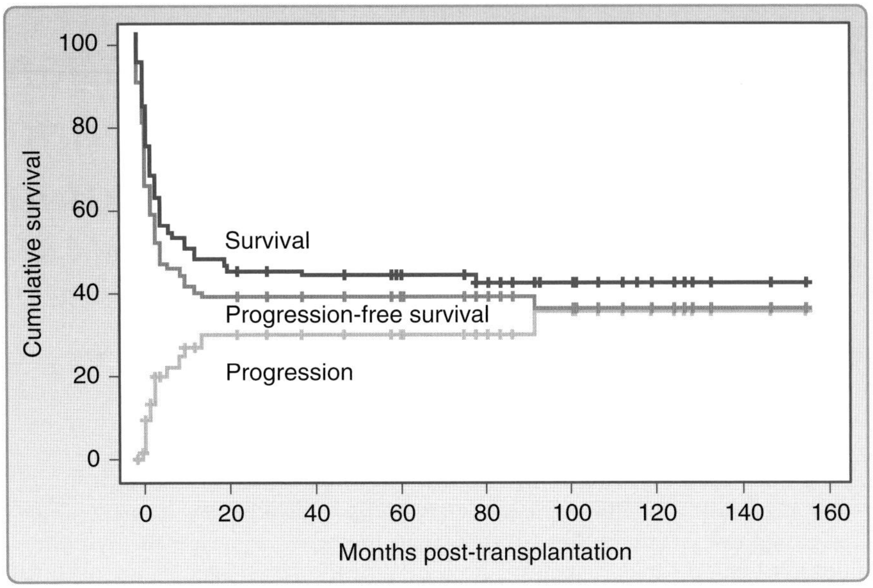

Figure 14–1. Outcome after allogeneic stem cell transplant for aggressive lymphoma. From Dhedin N, Giraudier S, Gaulard P et al. Allogeneic bone marrow transplantation in aggressive non-Hodgkin's lymphoma (excluding Burkitt and lymphoblastic lymphoma): a series of 73 patients from the SEGM database. Societ Francaise de Greffe de Moelle. Br J Haematol 1999;107:154–61, with permission.[9]

Table 14–1. Trials of Allogeneic Stem Cell Transplantation in Non-Hodgkin's Lymphoma

Patients (*n*)	Disease Status	Conditioning Regimen	TRM	OS	Reference
20	13 Primary Refractory 7 Relapses	Cy/TBI	40%	20%	1
17	5 Primary refractory 12 Relapsed	Cy/TBI	53%	18%	2
64	14 First relase 50 Refractory	37 TBI based 27 non-TBI	44%	10% to 65% at 2 years dependent on histology	3
22	All chemosensitive	18 CT/TBI	5%	59% at 40 months	4
25	9 CR1 9 Later CR 7 Active disease	24 CT/TBI 1 BEAM	20%	52%	5
21	3 CR1 3 Later CR 9 Primary refractory 6 Relapsed	16 VP16/CY/TBI 4 CT/TBI 1 BU/Mel/CY	48%	38% at 1 year	7
37	7 CR1 10 PR1 3 Rel 1 17 refractory	Ara-C/Cy/TBI	35%	45% at 5 years	8
73	14 CR1 11 Later CR 21 Responding relapse 27 Refractory	64 TBI 9 Bu	44%	41% at 5 years 76% for patients in CR	9
30	3 CR2 10 Responding relapse 17 Refractory	BEAM	40%	48% at 2 years	10
26	5 Early 21 Late	CBV	62%	26% at 2 years	11

TRM: transplant-related mortality; OS: overall survival; CR: complete remission; CR1: first complete remission; CR2: second complete remission; PR1: first partial remission; rel 1: first relapse; TBI: total body irradiation; Cy: cyclophosphamide; BEAM: carmustine, etoposide, cytarabine, melphelan; VP16: etoposide; Bu: busulphan; Mel: melphelan; Ara-C: cytarabine; CBV: cyclophosphamide.

transplantation, and in particular, patients at very high risk of relapse after autologous SCT are often considered for allogeneic SCT. What then is the role of allogeneic SCT in this disease setting?

Allogeneic SCT has been examined in a number of Phase I and Phase II studies in patients with DLBCL and more aggressive histologies.[2,7,10,11,18,19] A major problem with allogeneic SCT has been the high TRM and morbidity of the procedure, as well as continued relapse of disease in the aggressive lymphomas (Fig. 14–1). Most of these studies have been in young patients with advanced disease. Studies of allogeneic SCT in first remission have usually been performed in patients with Burkitt's lymphoma (BL) or lymphoblastic lymphoma (LL).[20,21]

Comparison of the outcome after allogeneic compared to autologous SCT has been difficult because of the difference in clinical characteristics of patients who undergo these types of procedures. A case-controlled study of patients reported to the European Bone Marrow Transplant Registry (EBMTR) investigated the relative roles and efficacy of allogeneic versus autologous SCT by matching 101 allogeneic with 101 autologous SCT patients. These were matched from the 938 autologous patients and 122 allogeneic patients who underwent SCT and who were reported to the registry at that time.[22] Progression-free survival (PFS) was similar in both types of transplants (49% allogeneic SCT, and 46% autologous SCT), and there was a lower, but not statistically significant, incidence of relapse and progression after allogeneic SCT (23%) compared to autologous SCT (38%) (Fig. 14–2). In LL, allogeneic SCT was associated with a decreased incidence of relapse (24% vs. 48%; pp = 0.035), but PFS was not significantly different since patients who underwent allogeneic SCT had a higher procedure-related mortality (24% allogeneic vs. 10% autologous SCT; p = 0.06). A significantly lower relapse/progression rate was observed in patients with chronic GVHD (cGVHD) compared with those patients without (0% cGVHD vs. 35% no cGVHD; p = 0.02). This study suggested that autologous and allogeneic SCT are comparable for DLBCL, and that in LL a GVL effect may account for the lower relapse rate for patients undergoing allogeneic SCT.

Overall the role of allogeneic SCT in the aggressive lymphomas is controversial. The procedure is associated with high TRM, and where possible autologous SCT should be offered as the treatment of choice. Only a fraction of the most advanced patients, in whom autologous SCT has no role to play, may be salvaged by the use of allogeneic SCT when a suitable donor is available.

Reduced-intensity conditioning (RIC) regimens have been used to increase the upper age limit at which patients can undergo allogeneic SCT, and have been shown to decrease the TRM of allogeneic SCT. This procedure is dependent upon a GVL effect and for aggressive disease, nonmyeloablative regimens are indicated only for patients with minimal disease, as the RIC regimens are unable to control the tumor before the generation of a GVL effect and the lack of ability to control rapidly proliferating disease.[23]

ROLE OF SCT IN INDOLENT LYMPHOMAS

Although HDT and SCT have become established as the treatment of choice for patients with relapsed aggressive lymphomas, this approach remains more controversial in patients with indolent lymphomas, and to date there is only a single prospective randomized trial that addresses this issue in patients with follicular lymphoma (FL).[24] In this study, 140 patients with relapsed FL were registered, but only 89 patients with chemosensitive disease were randomized to receive either three further cycles of chemotherapy (n = 24), or HDT and autologous SCT using unpurged (n = 33) or purged (n = 32) stem cells. With a 69-month median follow-up, the patients who received HDT had improved PFS (p = 0.0009) and overall survival (OS) (p = 0.026), although there was no benefit of purging.[24]

Autologous SCT has also been used more commonly than allogeneic SCT in the management of patients with follicular lymphoma. Long-term disease-free survival (DFS) has been observed in patients with indolent lymphomas after allogeneic SCT,[25–30] and there has been a trend towards increasing use of allogeneic SCT in the management of this disease as outlined in Table 14–2.

In a report of the International Bone Marrow Transplant Registry (IBMTR), results are described for 904 patients with FL.[31] Among these patients, 176 patients underwent allogeneic SCT, 131 patients underwent autologous SCT using purged stem cells, and 597 used unpurged autologous stem cells. The TRM in these three groups was 30%, 14%, and 8%, respectively; disease recurrence in 21%, 43%, and 58%, and 5-year OS was 51%, 62%, and 55%, respectively (Fig. 14–3). The use of TBI-containing regimens was asso-

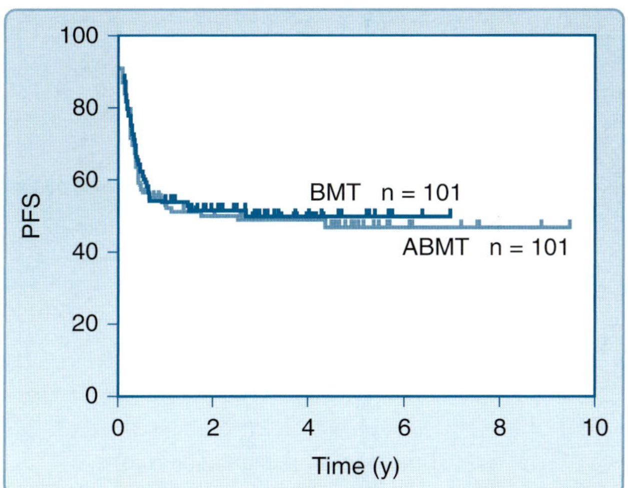

Figure 14–2. Outcome after allogeneic compared to autologous stem cell transplant in a matched pair registry analysis. (From Chopra R, Goldstone AH, Pearce R, et al. Autologous versus allogeneic bone marrow transplantation for non-Hodgkin's lymphoma: a case-controlled analysis of the European Bone Marrow Transplant Group Registry data. J Clin Oncol 1992;10:1690–5,[22] with permission.)

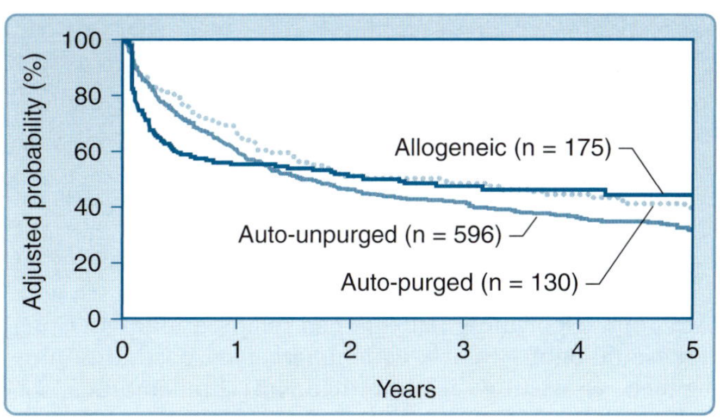

Figure 14–3. Outcome after allogeneic and autologous stem cell transplant for indolent lymphoma. (From van Besien K, Loberiza FR Jr, Bajorunaite R, et al. Comparison of autologous and allogeneic hematopoietic stem cell transplantation for follicular lymphoma. Blood 2003;102:3521–9,[31] with permission.)

Table 14–2. Allogeneic Stem Cell Transplantation in Indolent Lymphomas

Histology	Patients (*n*)	Median Age (range)	Status	Conditioning Regimen	Outcome	TRM	Reference
FL	10	36 (23 to 45)	2 Sensitive 8 Refractory	8 Cy/TBI	80% PFS	20%	25
FL 6 SLL 4	10	43 (31 to 550)	3 Sensitive 8 Refractory	Cy/TBI	68% PFS at 2 yrs	30%	26
FL 13 SLL 2	15	47 (30 to 57)	12 Sensitive (3 later CR) 3 Refractory	Cy/TBI +/- other	39% PFS at 3 years	33%	27
FL 93 SLL 20	113	38 (15 to 61)	66 Sensitive 39 Refractory	TBI 93 Non-TBI 20	49% PFS at 3 years	40%	28
FL 16 CLL 10	26	42 (20 to 52)	6 Induction failure 5 Sensitive 2 Refractory 7 Untested	24 Cy/TBI	54% PFS	30%	29
FL 29	29	42 (20 to 53)	5 Induction failure 18 Sensitive relapse 6 Resistant relapse	27 Cy/TBI	53% PFS at 5 years	24%	30

carmustine, etoposide
TRM: transplant-related mortality, FL: follicular lymphoma, SLL: small lymphocytic lymphoma, CLL: chronic lymphocytic lymphoma, CR: complete remission, Cy: cyclophosphamide, TBI: total body irradiation, PFS: progression-free survival.

ciated with increased TRM but decreased risk of relapse. The use of allogeneic SCT was associated with increased TRM, but significantly lower risk of disease recurrence in keeping with a GVL effect in this disease. Trends suggest that outcomes are improving, and this is highly likely to continue with the increased use of RIC regimens since the time these registry data were collated. Further steps that decrease the TRM after allogeneic SCT are therefore likely to result in improved outcome in these diseases, with resulting improvement in outcome after allogeneic compared with autologous SCT, although long-term follow-up will be required to confirm this.

REDUCED-INTENSITY CONDITIONING REGIMENS FOR INDOLENT NON-HODGKIN'S LYMPHOMA

As discussed above, there is increased use of RIC regimens in the indolent lymphomas, as outlined in Table 14–3.[32–41] The first report was from the M.D. Anderson Cancer Center, and although at that time the follow-up was very short, this report demonstrated the feasibility of this approach and that it could induce remission in chemoresistant patients.[32] Since that time a number of studies have clearly demonstrated evidence of a GVL effect that can be exploited in indolent lymphomas, particularly FL and SLL/CLL.[33–41]

The impact of the addition of Alemtuzumab to RIC for patients with lymphoma has also reported.[36–38,41] In the largest series, 88 patients with lymphoma, including 41 with indolent, 37 with aggressive, and 10 patients with MCL, and 31 of these patients had relapsed following previous autologous SCT.[37] Patients received a conditioning regimen consisting of Alemtuzumab, Fludarabine, and Melphelan, and received short-course cyclosporin as GVHD prophylaxis. The source of stem cells was from human leukocyte antigen (HLA)–matched siblings in 65 patients, and from matched unrelated donors in 23 patients. The use of this conditioning regimen was associated with a low incidence of GVHD, and the TRM was decreased in patients with indolent compared to aggressive lymphomas. The 3-year PFS was 65% for patients with indolent lymphoma, 50% for patients with MCL, and 34% for aggressive lymphoma (p = 0.002) (Fig. 14–4). Donor lymphocyte infusion (DLI) was given to 36 patients, 21 for relapsed or persistent disease, and 15 for persistence of mixed chimerism. The use of DLI to treat relapse after allogeneic SCT is solely dependent on the existence of a GVL effect. In seven patients with FL and SLL who had relapsed after prior allogeneic SCT, six patients responded with four in CR maintained for 43 to 89 months.

Patients with very poor outcome are those who have relapsed after previous autologous SCT. The outcome fol-

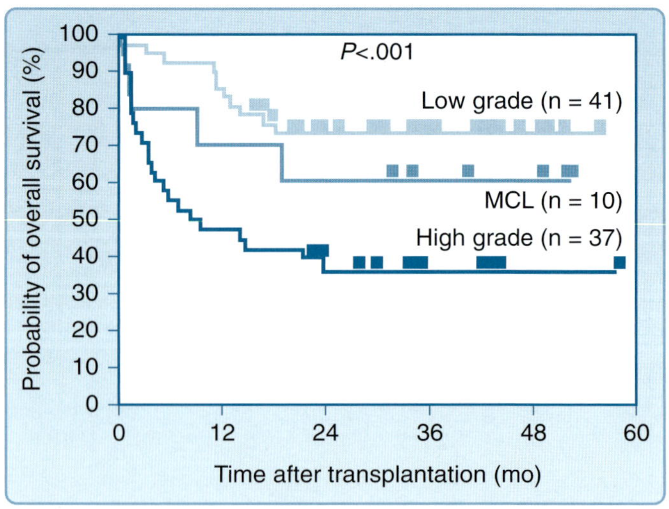

Figure 14–4. Outcome after allogeneic stem cell transplant for non-Hodgkin's lymphoma following reduced intensity conditioning. (From Morris E, Thomson K, Craddock C, et al. Outcomes after alemtuzumab-containing reduced-intensity allogeneic transplantation regimen for relapsed and refractory non-Hodgkin lymphoma. Blood 2004;104:3865–71,[37] with permission.)

Table 14–3. Reduced-Intensity Conditioning Allogeneic Stem Cell Transplantation in Lymphoma

Patients (*n*)	Prior Treatments Median (range)	Conditioning	GVHD	Graft Failure	Outcome	Reference
15	3 (2 to 7)	Cyclo/Flu Cisplt/Flu/Cyt	Acute 47%	4	8 CR 2 with aGVHD 4 with cGVHD	32
23	3 (2 to 6)	Flu/Bu/ATG	Acute 34%	0%	PFS 40% at 37 months	33
20	2 (1 to 5)	Cyclo/Flu/ Rituximab	Acute 20% Chronic 64%	0	PFS 84% at 2 years	34
13	3 (1 to 7)	200 cGY TBI	Acute 54% Chronic 62%	1	7 CR 2 PR 2 died PD 1 died TRM	35
44	3 (0 to 6)	Flu/Mel/ Alemtuzumab	Acute 16% Chronic 2%	1	22 CR 11 PR 3 progression	36
88	4 (2 to 6)	Flu/Mel/ Alemtuzumab	Acute 30%	4	OS indolent 73% 3 years OS aggressive 34% 3 years	37
65	2 (1 to 6) 11% Prior autografts	BEAM/ Alemtuzumab	Acute 17% Chronic 17%	3	PFS 69% at 2 years	38
17	3 (1 to 8)	Flu/Cyclo/ Rituximab		0	7 CR 2 PR	39
77	3 (0 to 8)	Various	Acute 34% Chronic 58%	0	TRM 18% PFS 56% at 2 years OS 72% at 2 years	40
47	62% Prior autografts	Flu/Mel/ Alemtuzumab	Acute 23% Chronic 6%	2	OS 75.5% at 1 year PFS 61.5% at 1 year	41
188	3 48% Prior autografts	Various	Acute 37% Chronic 17%	3	TRM 25.5% OS 50% at 2 years	67

GVHD: graft versus host disease, Cyclo: cyclophosphamide, Flu: fludarabine, Cisplt: cisplatin, Cyt: cytarabine, Bu: busulphan, ATG: anti-thymocyte globulin, TBI: total body irradiation, Mel: melphelan, BEAM: carmustine, etoposide, cytarabine, melphelan, CR: complete remission, aGVHD: acute graft versus host disease, cGVHD: chronic graft versus host disease, PFS: progression-free survival, PR: partial remission, PD: progressive disease, TRM: transplant-related mortality, OS: overall survival.

lowing myeloablative allogeneic SCT of 114 such patients has been reported from the IBMTR.[42] At 3 years, the TRM was 22%, and the probability of disease progression was 52%. The use of TBI-conditioning regimens and achievement of CR at the time of allogeneic SCT were associated with improved outcome. The use of RIC regimens appears to be associated with improved outcome. In 20 such patients, there was only one TRM from fungal infection, and the 3-year PFS an excellent 95%.[43]

ALLOGENEIC SCT IN MANTLE CELL LYMPHOMA

Patients with mantle cell lymphoma (MCL) have particularly poor outcome and SCT is being increasingly examined in these patients. In studies from the M.D. Anderson Cancer Center, 33 patients with MCL were treated with hyper-CVAD followed by HDT therapy using cytoxan and total-body irradiation and autologous SCT. At a median follow-up of 49 months, overall survival was 77%, but DFS was already decreased to 43%.[44] The results following RIC regimens from the same center have been reported for 18 patients, 5 of whom failed previous autologous SCT.[45] Patients were treated with fludarabine and cytoxan (13 patients), or fludarabine, cisplatin, and cytarabine (5 patients). Tacrolimus and methotrexate were used as post-transplant immunosuppressive therapy. No patient died within 100 days, and the EFS at a median follow-up of 26 months was very encouraging at 82%. Only three patients had relapsed, and one of these had responded to DLI. Results from the Fred Hutchinson Cancer Research Center have also been reported for RIC allogeneic SCT for 33 patients with relapsed and refractory MCL, including 14 patients who had failed previous autologous SCT.[46] Sixteen patients received HLA-matched sibling allogeneic stem cells, and 17 HLA-matched unrelated donor stem cells. Seventy-five percent of patients achieved CR, TRM was 24%, and disease progression occurred in 9%. Overall survival at 2 years was 65%, with DFS of 60% (Fig. 14–5). Although follow-up is short, these results are suggestive that a GVL effect can be exploited in this disease resulting in better disease control and a decreased likelihood of relapse after allogeneic SCT.

ALLOGENEIC SCT IN T-CELL NON-HODGKIN'S LYMPHOMA

Patients with T-cell lymphomas generally have poor outcome, but relatively few studies to date have examined the role of SCT in the management of these diseases. A national survey in Finland outlined their experience of autologous SCT in 37 patients, 14 with peripheral T-cell lymphoma (PCTL), 14 with anaplastic large-cell lymphoma (ALCL), and 9 others.[47] Eighteen of these patients

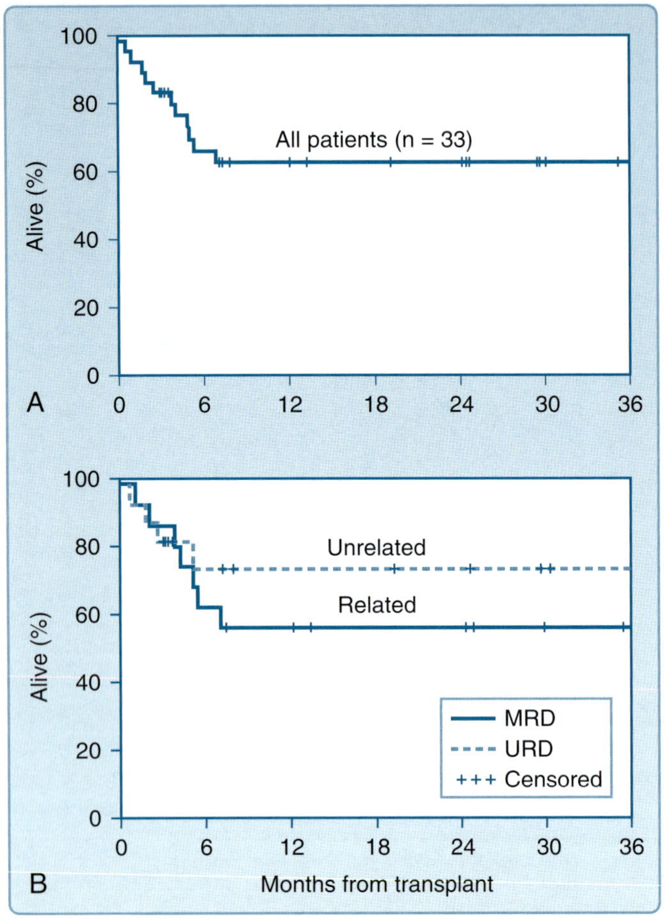

Figure 14–5. Outcome after allogeneic stem cell transplant for mantle cell lymphoma. (From Maris MB, Sandmaier BM, Storer BE, et al. Allogeneic hematopoietic cell transplantation after fludarabine and 2 Gy total body irradiation for relapsed and refractory mantle cell lymphoma. Blood 2004;104:3535–42,[46] with permission.)

were treated in first complete or partial remission. The TRM was 11%. With a median follow-up of only 2 years, 16 of these patients had relapsed, and the 5-year estimated OS was 54%. The outcome was better for patients with ALCL compared to other histologies. Two recent studies examined the role of allogeneic SCT in the management of these diseases. In a pilot Phase II study to examine feasibility, 17 patients with relapsed and refractory PCTL underwent allogeneic SCT followed by a RIC regimen using thiotepa, cytoxan, and fludarabine, and post-transplant immunosuppression using cyclosporin A and short-course methotrexate.[48] Eight of these patients had failed previous autologous SCT. One patient died of sepsis in the setting of acute GVHD (aGVHD), and two patients had progressive disease. The remaining 14 patients remain alive with 12 in CR (Fig. 14–6). These findings are highly suggestive of a GVL effect that can be exploited in this disease setting as well. A second study reported the outcome in three patients with refractory cutaneous T-cell lymphoma, and RIC regimen with HLA-matched sibling donor SCT.[49] Although all three patients relapsed, this occurred in the setting of immunosuppression for GVHD, and all patients had disease response with removal of immunosuppressive therapy, again suggestive of a GCL effect in this disease.

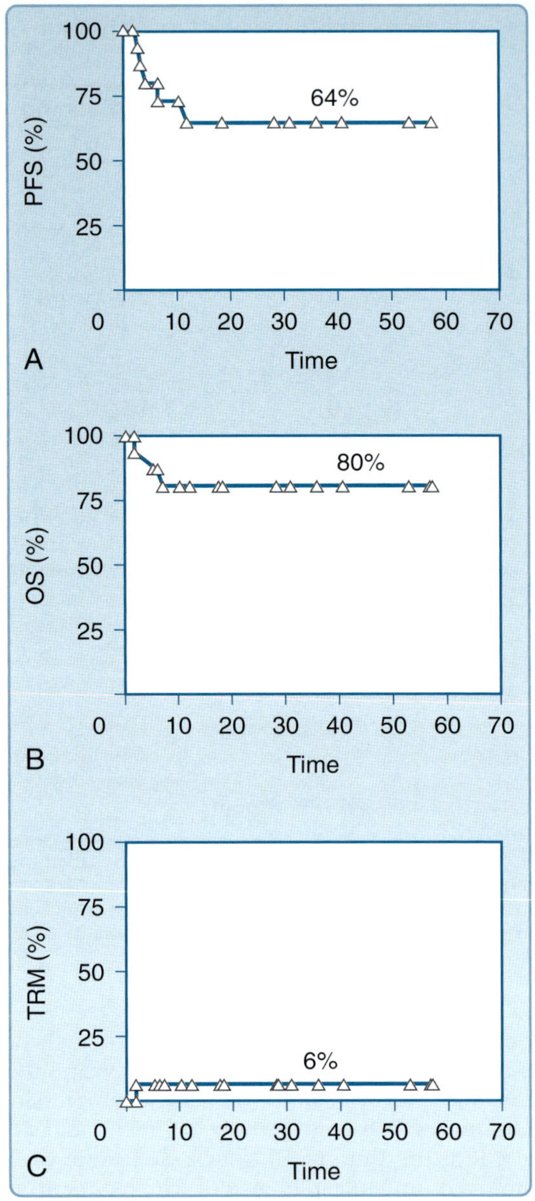

Figure 14–6. Outcome after allogeneic stem cell transplant for T-cell lymphoma. (From Corradini P, Dodero A, Zallio F, et al. Graft-versus-lymphoma effect in relapsed peripheral T-cell non-Hodgkin's lymphomas after reduced-intensity conditioning followed by allogeneic transplantation of hematopoietic cells. J Clin Oncol 2004;22:2172–6,[48] with permission.)

ALLOGENEIC TRANSPLANTATION IN HODGKIN'S LYMPHOMA

The outcome for patients with HL has improved dramatically over the last 50 years. About 80% of patients in all anatomic stages and of all histologic subtypes can now expect to be cured with modern treatment strategies.[50] In spite of this, 30% of patients with advanced disease will have disease progression; one-third of these are due to induction failure while two-thirds relapse after achieving CR. Of those patients who relapse, 40% to 45% occur within 12 months of completing initial therapy, and outcome in this group is poor with conventional salvage chemotherapy alone. The use of autologous SCT may lead to long-term

Table 14–4. Trials of Allogeneic Stem Cell Transplantation in Hodgkin's Disease

Patients (*n*)	Treatment-Related Mortality	Outcome	Reference
53	43%	PFS 27% at 10 years	52
53	53%	PFS 26% at 5 years	53
8	63%	2 CCR at 3 years+	54
8	50%	1 CCR at 2 years+	55
100	61%	PFS 15% at 3 years	59
45	31%	PFS 15% at 4 years	60
167	52%	OS 25% ay 4 years	61

PFS: progression-free survival, CCR: continuous complete remission, OS: overall survival.

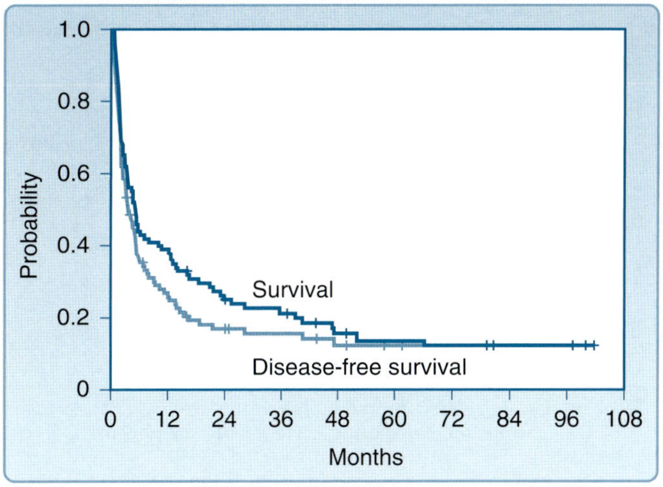

Figure 14–7. Outcome after allogeneic stem cell transplant for Hodgkin's lymphoma. From Gajewski JL, Phillips GL, Sobocinski KA et al. Bone marrow transplants from HLA-identical siblings in advanced Hodgkin's disease. J Clin Oncol 1996;14:572–8.

DFS,[51] presumably due to the effect of chemotherapy dose intensification. However, there is a continuing risk of relapse, and secondary AML/MDS for up to 12 years post-autograft.[52]

Allogeneic SCT has not been used extensively in HL, but has been evaluated in a number of Phase I and Phase II studies, often with small numbers of patients.[53–57] In theory, it should be more effective than ASCT as it provides a stem cell source free of contaminating tumor cells, and adds immunologic attack against the malignant cells, but these advantages are offset by the increased toxicity of the procedure.[58] In addition, as most published series contain few patients as outlined in Table 14–4, there is little information on allogeneic SCT in HL patients. Results after conventional allogeneic SCT for HL are shown in Fig. 14–7. Two registry-based retrospective analyses on allogeneic SCT in HL were published in 1996. The first analyzed the results of 100 HLA-matched sibling allografts in advanced HL reported to the IBMTR between 1982 and 1992.[59] The 3-year OS and DFS were 21% and 15%, respectively, with a 3-year probability of relapse of 65%. The 100-day probability of aGVHD was 35%, and the 3-year probability of cGVHD was 45%. These poor results must be viewed in the context that all patients had advanced disease with 89% not in remission at the time of transplant, 50% had poor performance status, and 27% had active infection in the week before transplant. In the 1200 patients with HL reported to the EBMTR, only 45 underwent allogeneic SCT.[60] The outcome in these patients was compared to 45 patients who underwent autologous SCT, and who were matched for sex, age at time of diagnosis and at transplantation, stage of disease at diagnosis, bone marrow involvement at diagnosis and at transplantation, year of transplantation, disease status at time of transplantation, and conditioning regimen with or without TBI. No difference in 4-year actuarial probability of survival, PFS, and relapse and nonrelapse mortality was found between allogeneic and autologous SCT, although the TRM at 4 years was significantly higher for allogeneic SCT patients, suggesting no advantage of allogeneic SCT from HLA-matched sibling allograft over autologous SCT. This analysis was updated in 2003,[61] in which 1185 allogeneic transplants for lymphoma (as first transplant) reported between 1982 and 1998 were compared with 14,687 autologous procedures performed over the same period. In this analysis, 167 patients with HL received allogeneic SCT. Actuarial OS at 4 years was 24.7% for HL, lower than any other lymphoma type, with the poor outcome due to high procedure-related mortality of 51.7%. Matched analysis showed that overall survival was better in the autologous group; relapse rate, although better in the allogeneic group for most types of lymphoma, was worse in HL.

These data are not encouraging for routine use of allogeneic SCT in HL. Its application is limited by HLA-matched donor availability and the high TRM. This may be related to characteristics of the disease itself or to the poor prognosis of the patients selected.[59,60] Results might potentially be better if allogeneic SCT was performed earlier in the course of the disease, although there is natural reluctance to subject patients to this approach because of the high morbidity and mortality of the procedure. Currently, allogeneic transplantation should be limited to those in whom autologous SCT is precluded, such as in patients who fail to mobilize stem cells, and those with hypoplastic, fibrotic, or tumor-involved marrow.

As in other malignancies, there is increased interest in the use of allogeneic SCT with the advent of RIC regimens. This is of particular importance in a disease setting such as HL where the TRM of allogeneic SCT has been so high. What then is the evidence that there is a graft versus Hodgkin's (GVH) effect that can be exploited in this disease? In an early study, there was a suggestion that patients who underwent syngeneic stem cell transplant had earlier relapse than those who have an allogeneic stem cell transplant, although these results were not statistically significant.[54] The rate of relapse has been suggested to be lower after allogeneic SCT compared to autologous SCT.[52,53]

Table 14–5. Trials of Reduced-Conditioning Intensity Allogeneic Stem Cell Transplantation in Hodgkin's Disease

Patients (*n*)	Status	Conditioning	TRM	Outcome	Reference
10	Sensitive 8 Resistant 2	Flu/Mel/Alemtuzumab	0%	OS 73%, PFS 71% at 1 year	36
12	NS	Flu/Mel/Alemtuzumab	20%	OS 53%, PFS 50% at 14 months	62
40	Sensitive 26 Resistant 14	Flu/Cy/+/-ATG 14 Flu/Mel 26	22%	OS 39%, PFS 21% at 18 months OS 73%, PFS 37%	63
10	Sensitive 6 Resistant 4	BEAM	10%	7 in CCR at 1 year	66
52	Sensitive 28 Resistant 19	Various	17%	OS 56%, PFS 42% at 2 years	67

TRM: transplant-related mortality, NS: not stated, Flu: fludarabine, Mel: melphelan, Cy: cyclophosphamide, ATG: anti-thymocyte globulin, BEAM: carmustine, etoposide, cytarabine, melphelan, OS: overall survival, PFS: progression-free survival, CCR: continuous complete remission.

Several studies have also suggested that there may be a lower relapse rate in patients who develop aGVHD.[59,60] Perhaps the strongest data for a GVH effect are reports of relapsed HL responding to donor lymphocyte infusions after allogeneic SCT.[62,63] More data are required, but it does seem clear that a GVH effect does exist, although this is certainly not as potent as that seen in CML.[64]

Several small series of relapsed HD patients treated with RIC allogeneic SCT have been reported as outlined in Table 14–5.[33,35,36,62,63,65–69] In general, the patients included have been heavily pre-treated, with many having failed previous autologous SCT. In these heavily pre-treated patients, even with RIC regimens there is a high transplant-related mortality rate, partly due to the fact that the majority of these patients of patients were allografted with resistant disease. Conditioning regimens vary but most contain fludarabine and the United Kingdom studies have largely included the anti–T-cell monoclonal antibody Alemtuzumab to prevent development of GVHD. Acute and chronic GVHD is still a problem with incidences ranging from 0% to 75% (with the lowest incidence found in the study using Alemtuzumab), but TRM is lower than that observed in conventional allografts.

The largest series examined outcome in 52 patients with relapsed HL.[67] In this registry study, there was a wide variety in conditioning regimens, but most included fludarabine. The 2-year TRM was 17.3% with a 2-year overall survival of 56.3%, and PFS of 42%. Of note, the patients with HL had a better outcome than those patients with aggressive NHL or MCL.

A study by Carella et al. in 2000 examined the strategy of performing autologous SCT in 10 patients with relapsed disease to induce a minimal disease state followed by RIC allogeneic SCT.[70] Patients received HDT with carmustine, etoposide, cytarabine, and melphelan (BEAM) followed by re-infusion of stem cells. At a median of 61 days post-engraftment, patients were given fludarabine with cyclophosphamide daily for 3 days and non-T-cell–depleted allogeneic stem cells were subsequently infused. Seven patients were still alive at a median of 1 year post, five of whom were in complete remission. Six patients developed acute GVHD (3 of Grade 3), and one had chronic GVHD.

The results of RIC certainly appear better than those with conventional allografting, but this approach is still associated with significant morbidity and mortality from GVHD, and long-term follow-up of these patients is still not available. Nonetheless, RIC allogeneic SCT appears to be a useful treatment modality in relapsed HD post-autograft. Further studies are required to assess the optimal regimen, appropriate timing for this type of transplant, and mechanisms to reduce the toxicity of GVHD.

In summary, conventional allogeneic transplantation has a limited role to play in the management of Hodgkin's disease in view of the high toxicity involved. There is increasing evidence, however, for a GVH effect, and new nonmyeloablative regimens with subsequent donor lymphocyte infusions are showing impressive response rates with lower mortality, considering the heavily pre-treated patients upon whom this technique has been used. For the technique to be more widely used, it seems likely that additional steps will be required after allogeneic SCT to prevent disease progression. Studies examining the role of such autologous followed by RIC allogeneic SCT and/or addition of anti-CD30 monoclonal antibodies are currently under investigation.

References

1. Appelbaum FR, Thomas ED, Buckner CD, et al. Treatment of non-Hodgkin's lymphoma with chemoradiotherapy and allogenic marrow transplantation. Hematol Oncol 1983;1: 149–57.
2. Phillips GL, Herzig RH, Lazarus HM, et al. High-dose chemotherapy, fractionated total-body irradiation, and allogeneic marrow transplantation for malignant lymphoma. J Clin Oncol 1986;4:480–8.
3. van Besien KW, Mehra RC, Giralt SA, et al. Allogeneic bone marrow transplantation for poor-prognosis lymphoma: response, toxicity and survival depend on disease histology. Am J Med 1996;100:299–307.
4. Soiffer RJ, Freedman AS, Neuberg D, et al. CD6+ T cell-depleted allogeneic bone marrow transplantation for non-Hodgkin's lymphoma. Bone Marrow Transplant 1998;21: 1177–81.
5. Ernst P, Maraninchi D, Jacobsen N, et al. Marrow transplantation for non-Hodgkin's lymphoma: a multi-centre study from the European Co-operative Bone Marrow Transplant Group. Bone Marrow Transplant 1986;1:81–6.
6. Nademanee AP, Forman SJ, Schmidt GM, et al. Allogeneic bone marrow transplantation for high risk non-Hodgkin's lymphoma during first complete remission. Blut 1987;55: 11–8.

7. Shepherd JD, Barnett MJ, Connors JM, et al. Allogeneic bone marrow transplantation for poor-prognosis non-Hodgkin's lymphoma. Bone Marrow Transplant 1993;12:591–6.
8. Juckett M, Rowlings P, Hessner M, et al. T cell–depleted allogeneic bone marrow transplantation for high-risk non-Hodgkin's lymphoma: clinical and molecular follow-up. Bone Marrow Transplant 1998;21:893–9.
9. Dhedin N, Giraudier S, Gaulard P, et al. Allogeneic bone marrow transplantation in aggressive non-Hodgkin's lymphoma (excluding Burkitt and lymphoblastic lymphoma): a series of 73 patients from the SFGM database. Societ Francaise de Greffe de Moelle. Br J Haematol 1999;107: 154–61.
10. Przepiorka D, van Besien K, Khouri I, et al. Carmustine, etoposide, cytarabine and melphalan as a preparative regimen for allogeneic transplantation for high-risk malignant lymphoma. Ann Oncol 1999;10:527–32.
11. Demirer T, Weaver CH, Buckner CD, et al. High-dose cyclophosphamide, carmustine, and etoposide followed by allogeneic bone marrow transplantation in patients with lymphoid malignancies who had received prior dose-limiting radiation therapy. J Clin Oncol 1995;13:596–602.
12. Philip T, Guglielmi C, Hagenbeek A, et al. Autologous bone marrow transplantion as compared with salvage chemotherapy in relapses of chemotherapy-sensitive non-Hodgkin's lymphoma. New Engl J Med 1995;333:1540–45.
13. Blay J, Gomez F, Sebban C, et al. The International Prognostic Index correlates to survival in patients with aggressive lymphoma in relapse: analysis of the PARMA trial. Blood 1998;15:3562–8.
14. Gianni AM, Bregni M, Sienna S, et al. High-dose chemotherapy and autolgous bone marrow trasnplantation compare with MACOP-B in aggressive B-cell lymphoma. N Engl J Med 1997;336:1290–7.
15. Santini G, Salvagno L, Leon P, et al. VACOP-B versus VACOP-B plus autologous bone marrow transplantation for advanced diffuse non-Hodgkin's lymphoma: results of a prospective randomized trial by the non-Hodgkin's Lymphoma Cooperative Study Group. J Clin Oncol 1998;16:2796–802.
16. Milpied N, Deconinck E, Gaillard F, et al. Initial treatment of aggressive lymphoma with high-dose chemotherapy and autologous stem-cell support. N Engl J Med 2004;350: 1287–95.
17. Mounier N, Gisselbrecht C, Briere J, et al. Prognostic factors in patients with aggressive non-Hodgkin's lymphoma treated by front-line autotransplantation after complete remission: a cohort study by the Groupe d'Etude des Lymphomes de l'Adulte. J Clin Oncol 2004;22:2826–34.
18. Appelbaum FR, Sullivan KM, Buckner CD, et al. Treatment of malignant lymphoma in 100 patients with chemotherapy, total body irradiation, and marrow transplantation. J Clin Oncol 1987;5:1340–7.
19. van Besien K, Thall P, Korbling M, et al. Allogeneic transplantation for recurrent or refractory non-Hodgkin's lymphoma with poor prognostic features after conditioning with thiotepa, busulfan, and cyclophosphamide: experience in 44 consecutive patients. Biol Blood Marrow Transplant 1997;3: 150–6.
20. De Witte T, Awwad B, Boezeman J, et al. Role of allogenic bone marrow transplantation in adolescent or adult patients with acute lymphoblastic leukaemia or lymphoblastic lymphoma in first remission. Bone Marrow Transplant 1994;14: 767–74.
21. Troussard X, Leblond V, Kuentz M, et al. Allogeneic bone marrow transplantation in adults with Burkitt's lymphoma or acute lymphoblastic leukemia in first complete remission. J Clin Oncol 1990;8:809–12.
22. Chopra R, Goldstone AH, Pearce R, et al. Autologous versus allogeneic bone marrow transplantation for non-Hodgkin's lymphoma: a case-controlled analysis of the European Bone Marrow Transplant Group Registry data. J Clin Oncol 1992; 10:1690–5.
23. Maloney DG. Graft-vs.-lymphoma effect in various histologies of non-Hodgkin's lymphoma. Leuk Lymphoma 2003; 44(Suppl 3):S99–105.
24. Schouten HC, Qian W, Kvaloy S, et al. High-dose therapy improves progression-free survival and survival in relapsed follicular non-Hodgkin's lymphoma: results from the randomized European CUP trial. J Clin Oncol 2003;21:3918–27.
25. van Besien KW, Khouri IF, Giralt SA, et al. Allogeneic bone marrow transplantation for refractory and recurrent low-grade lymphoma: the case for aggressive management. J Clin Oncol 1995;13:1096–102.
26. Verdonck LF, Dekker AW, Lokhorst HM, et al. Allogeneic versus autologous bone marrow transplantation for refractory and recurrent low-grade non-Hodgkin's lymphoma. Blood 1997;90:4201–5.
27. Mandigers CM, Raemaekers JM, Schattenberg AV, et al. Allogeneic bone marrow transplantation with T-cell–depleted marrow grafts for patients with poor-risk relapsed low-grade non-Hodgkin's lymphoma. Br J Haematol 1998;100: 198–206.
28. van Besien K, Sobocinski KA, Rowlings PA, et al. Allogeneic bone marrow transplantation for low-grade lymphoma. Blood 1998;92:1832–6.
29. Toze CL, Shepherd JD, Connors JM, et al. Allogeneic bone marrow transplantation for low-grade lymphoma and chronic lymphocytic leukemia. Bone Marrow Transplant 2000;25: 605–12.
30. Toze CL, Barnett MJ, Connors JM, et al. Long-term disease-free survival of patients with advanced follicular lymphoma after allogeneic bone marrow transplantation. Br J Haematol 2004;127:311–21.
31. van Besien K, Loberiza FR Jr, Bajorunaite R, et al. Comparison of autologous and allogeneic hematopoietic stem cell transplantation for follicular lymphoma. Blood 2003;102: 3521–9.
32. Khouri IF, Keating M, Korbling M, et al. Transplant-lite: induction of graft-versus-malignancy using fludarabine-based nonablative chemotherapy and allogeneic blood progenitor-cell transplantation as treatment for lymphoid malignancies. J Clin Oncol 1998;16:2817–24.
33. Nagler A, Slavin S, Varadi G, et al. Allogeneic peripheral blood stem cell transplantation using a fludarabine-based low intensity conditioning regimen for malignant lymphoma. Bone Marrow Transplant 2000;25:1021–8.
34. Khouri IF, Saliba RM, Giralt SA, et al. Nonablative allogeneic hematopoietic transplantation as adoptive immunotherapy for indolent lymphoma: low incidence of toxicity, acute graft-versus-host disease, and treatment-related mortality. Blood 2001;98:3595–9.
35. McSweeney PA, Niederwieser D, Shizuru JA, et al. Hematopoietic cell transplantation in older patients with hematologic malignancies: replacing high-dose cytotoxic therapy with graft-versus-tumor effects. Blood 2001;97:3390–400.
36. Kottaridis PD, Milligan DW, Chopra R, et al. In vivo CAMPATH-1H prevents graft-versus-host disease following nonmyeloablative stem cell transplantation. Blood 2000;96: 2419–25.
37. Morris E, Thomson K, Craddock C, et al. Outcomes after alemtuzumab-containing reduced-intensity allogeneic transplantation regimen for relapsed and refractory non-Hodgkin lymphoma. Blood 2004;104:3865–71.
38. Faulkner RD, Craddock C, Byrne JL, et al. BEAM-alemtuzumab reduced-intensity allogeneic stem cell transplantation for lymphoproliferative diseases: GVHD, toxicity, and survival in 65 patients. Blood 2004;103:428–34.

39. Khouri IF, Lee MS, Saliba RM, et al. Nonablative allogeneic stem cell transplantation for chronic lymphocytic leukemia: impact of rituximab on immunomodulation and survival. Exp Hematol 2004;32:28–35.
40. Dreger P, Brand R, Hansz J, et al. Treatment-related mortality and graft-versus-leukemia activity after allogeneic stem cell transplantation for chronic lymphocytic leukemia using intensity-reduced conditioning. Leukemia 2003;17: 841–8.
41. Chakraverty R, Peggs K, Chopra R, et al. Limiting transplantation-related mortality following unrelated donor stem cell transplantation by using a nonmyeloablative conditioning regimen. Blood 2002;99:1071–8.
42. Freytes CO, Loberiza FR, Rizzo JD, et al. Myeloablative allogeneic hematopoietic stem cell transplantation in patients who relapse after autologous stem cell transplantation for lymphoma: a report of the international bone marrow transplant registry. Blood 2004;104:3797–803.
43. Escalon MP, Champlin RE, Saliba RM, et al. Nonmyeloablative allogeneic hematopoietic transplantation: a promising salvage therapy for patients with non-Hodgkin's lymphoma whose disease has failed a prior autologous transplantation. J Clin Oncol 2004;22:2419–23.
44. Khouri IF, Saliba RM, Okoroji GJ, Acholonu SA, Champlin RE. Long-term follow-up of autologous stem cell transplantation in patients with diffuse mantle cell lymphoma in first disease remission: the prognostic value of beta2-microglobulin and the tumor score. Cancer 2003;98:2630–5.
45. Khouri IF, Lee MS, Saliba RM, et al. Nonablative allogeneic stem-cell transplantation for advanced/recurrent mantle-cell lymphoma. J Clin Oncol 2003;21:4407–12.
46. Maris MB, Sandmaier BM, Storer BE, et al. Allogeneic hematopoietic cell transplantation after fludarabine and 2 Gy total body irradiation for relapsed and refractory mantle cell lymphoma. Blood 2004;104:3535–42.
47. Jantunen E, Wiklund T, Juvonen E, et al. Autologous stem cell transplantation in adult patients with peripheral T-cell lymphoma: a nation-wide survey. Bone Marrow Transplant 2004; 33:405–10.
48. Corradini P, Dodero A, Zallio F, et al. Graft-versus-lymphoma effect in relapsed peripheral T-cell non-Hodgkin's lymphomas after reduced-intensity conditioning followed by allogeneic transplantation of hematopoietic cells. J Clin Oncol 2004;22: 2172–6.
49. Herbert KE, Spencer A, Grigg A, et al. Graft-versus-lymphoma effect in refractory cutaneous T-cell lymphoma after reduced-intensity HLA-matched sibling allogeneic stem cell transplantation. Bone Marrow Transplant 2004;34:521–5.
50. Re D, Thomas RK, Behringer K, et al. From Hodgkin's disease to Hodgkin lymphoma: biological insights and therapeutic potential. Blood 2005;105:4553–60.
51. Diehl V, Stein H, Hummel M, et al. Hodgkin's lymphoma: biology and treatment strategies for primary, refractory, and relapsed disease. Hematology (Am Soc Hematol Educ Program) 2003:225–47.
52. Akpek G, Ambinder RF, Piantadosi S, et al. Long-term results of blood and marrow transplantation for Hodgkin's lymphoma. J Clin Oncol 2001;19:4314–21.
53. Anderson JE, Litzow MR, Appelbaum FR, et al. Allogeneic, syngeneic, and autologous marrow transplantation for Hodgkin's disease: the 21-year Seattle experience. J Clin Oncol 1993;11:2342–50.
54. Appelbaum FR, Sullivan KM, Thomas ED, et al. Allogeneic marrow transplantation in the treatment of MOPP-resistant Hodgkin's disease. J Clin Oncol 1985;3:1490–4.
55. Phillips GL, Reece DE, Barnett MJ, et al. Allogeneic marrow transplantation for refractory Hodgkin's disease. J Clin Oncol 1989;7:1039–45.
56. Dann EJ, Daugherty CK, Larson RA. Allogeneic bone marrow transplantation for relapsed and refractory Hodgkin's disease and non-Hodgkin's lymphoma. Bone Marrow Transplant 1997;20:369–74.
57. Lundberg JH, Hansen RM, Chitambar CR, et al. Allogeneic bone marrow transplantation for relapsed and refractory lymphoma using genotypically HLA-identical and alternative donors. J Clin Oncol 1991;9:1848–59.
58. Sureda A and Schmitz N. Role of allogeneic stem cell transplantation in relapsed or refractory Hodgkin's disease. Ann Oncol 2002;13 Suppl 1:128–32.
59. Gajewski JL, Phillips GL, Sobocinski KA, et al. Bone marrow transplants from HLA-identical siblings in advanced Hodgkin's disease. J Clin Oncol 1996;14:572–8.
60. Milpied N, Fielding AK, Pearce RM, et al. Allogeneic bone marrow transplant is not better than autologous transplant for patients with relapsed Hodgkin's disease. European Group for Blood and Bone Marrow Transplantation. J Clin Oncol 1996; 14:1291–6.
61. Peniket AJ, Ruiz de Elvira MC, Taghipour G, et al. An EBMT registry matched study of allogeneic stem cell transplants for lymphoma: allogeneic transplantation is associated with a lower relapse rate but a higher procedure-related mortality rate than autologous transplantation. Bone Marrow Transplant 2003;31:667–78.
62. Branson K, Chopra R, Kottaridis PD, et al. Role of nonmyeloablative allogeneic stem-cell transplantation after failure of autologous transplantation in patients with lymphoproliferative malignancies. J Clin Oncol 2002;20:4022–31.
63. Anderlini P, Saliba R, Acholonu S, et al. Reduced-intensity allogeneic stem cell transplantation in relapsed and refractory Hodgkin's disease: low transplant-related mortality and impact of intensity of conditioning regimen. Bone Marrow Transplant 2005;35:943–51.
64. Kolb HJ and Holler E. Adoptive immunotherapy with donor lymphocyte transfusions. Curr Opin Oncol 1997;9: 139–45.
65. Anderlini P, Giralt S, Andersson B, et al. Allogeneic stem cell transplantation with fludarabine-based, less intensive conditioning regimens as adoptive immunotherapy in advanced Hodgkin's disease. Bone Marrow Transplant 2000;26:615–20.
66. Cooney JP, Stiff PJ, Toor AA, et al. BEAM allogeneic transplantation for patients with Hodgkin's disease who relapse after autologous transplantation is safe and effective. Biol Blood Marrow Transplant 2003;9:177–82.
67. Robinson SP, Goldstone AH, Mackinnon S, et al. Chemoresistant or aggressive lymphoma predicts for a poor outcome following reduced-intensity allogeneic progenitor cell transplantation: an analysis from the Lymphoma Working Party of the European Group for Blood and Bone Marrow Transplantation. Blood 2002;100:4310–6.
68. Dey BR, McAfee S, Sackstein R, et al. Successful allogeneic stem cell transplantation with nonmyeloablative conditioning in patients with relapsed hematologic malignancy following autologous stem cell transplantation. Biol Blood Marrow Transplant 2001;7:604–12.
69. Michallet M, Bilger K, Garban F, et al. Allogeneic hematopoietic stem-cell transplantation after nonmyeloablative preparative regimens: impact of pretransplantation and posttransplantation factors on outcome. J Clin Oncol 2001; 19:3340–9.
70. Carella AM, Cavaliere M, Lerma E, et al. Autografting followed by nonmyeloablative immunosuppressive chemotherapy and allogeneic peripheral-blood hematopoietic stem-cell transplantation as treatment of resistant Hodgkin's disease and non-Hodgkin's lymphoma. J Clin Oncol 2000;18: 3918–24.

15

Biological Therapy of Non-Hodgkin's Lymphomas

Andrew Zelenetz, M.D., Ph.D.

The designation "biological therapy" is applied to a wide range of therapies including biological response modifiers, nonspecific immunotherapy, targeted therapy with monoclonal antibodies, and vaccination. An exhaustive overview of the biological therapy of non-Hodgkin's lymphoma (NHL) is beyond the scope of this chapter. Rather, this chapter will review some of the established biological therapies that have had an impact on clinical care as well as potentially emerging therapies in preclinical and clinical development.

Interferons are a group of glycoproteins produced as a defense to viral infection. They have antiproliferative and immunomodulatory effects and were investigated as potential anticancer therapy.[1] Clinical development of interferon-α in NHL followed the demonstration of activity in the preclinical murine model.[2] Single-agent activity was demonstrated in a number of Phase II studies. Phase III trials have yielded variable results with respect to overall survival. The role of interferon in the treatment of lymphoma is discussed.

Cytokines modulate immune responses by altering the activity of target cells. A number of *interleukins* have been examined for their ability to treat lymphoma as single agents, and in combination with other treatments, particularly *monoclonal antibodies*.

The promise of antibodies as "magic bullets" for therapy was introduced by Paul Ehrlich more than 100 years ago.[3] This dream grew closer to fruition in 1975 with the report by Kohler and Milstein[4] of the ability to generate monoclonal antibodies of defined specificity. However, it was not until 1997 with the approval of rituximab that this promise was fulfilled. Subsequently, other antibodies and antibody conjugates have been approved for the therapy of lymphoid malignancies. This chapter will detail the role of antibodies in the management of NHL.

Monoclonal antibodies are directed against a single epitope and therefore are subject to failure by mutation of the target. This was a limitation of anti-idiotypic monoclonal antibodies pioneered by Levy and Miller for the treatment of follicular NHL.[5] This limitation can potentially be overcome by *vaccination* with the antigenic target and the subsequent generation of a polyclonal immune response. Furthermore, whole-cell vaccine approaches have been tested in which the specific antigen remains undefined. This chapter will discuss some of the potentials and limitations of vaccines for NHL as they complete late-stage clinical trials.

NONSPECIFIC IMMUNOTHERAPY

Interferon-α

Interferon-α (INF-α) has a number of biological effects including the inhibition of tumor cell growth by mechanisms that are not well understood. The role of INF-α in the treatment of NHL was first investigated in a preclinical model of the AKR/J mouse. This mouse carries the AK virus, which leads to the spontaneous development of thymic lymphoblastic lymphomas. AKR/J mice treated with INF-α prevented the development of lymphoma, but did not result in regression of established tumors.[2] In this model, chemotherapy plus INF-α was superior to either chemotherapy alone or INF-α alone at preventing tumor growth.[6] Based on the preclinical prevention of tumor growth, INF-α was evaluated in humans. INF-α was shown to have single-agent activity in indolent NHL in a number of clinical trials; however, complete responses were uncommon, and response durations were relatively short.[7–13] Nonetheless, these trials demonstrated that INF-α was an active agent in the management of indolent NHL, and the preclinical observation of synergy (or additive effects) with chemotherapy led to the evaluation of integrating INF-α into conventional chemotherapy regimens.[14,15] Over the past 2 decades, a large number of trials have sought to determine what role, if any, INF-α has in the management of NHL. The results of numerous randomized clinical trials have been contradictory, with some trials showing a benefit in failure-free and/or overall survival and others showing no benefit at all.[16–23] These trials differed significantly in design; critical variables included intensity of chemotherapy, INF-α combined with chemotherapy, INF-α as maintenance, and INF-α both in combination and as maintenance.

To critically assess the role of interferon in the management of follicular NHL, Rohatiner and collaborators from various cooperative groups undertook a meta-analysis of 10 Phase III randomized trials that included a total of 1922 patients with untreated follicular lymphoma and that evaluated the role of INF-α. The addition of INF-α to chemotherapy did not alter the response rate. However, there was a significant survival benefit in the meta-analysis, although there were substantial differences between studies (Fig. 15–1A). The adjusted overall survival is shown in Fig. 15–1B. Interestingly, there is no apparent benefit in the first 3 years; only after 3 years do the survival curves diverge, favoring the patients treated with INF-α. One study from

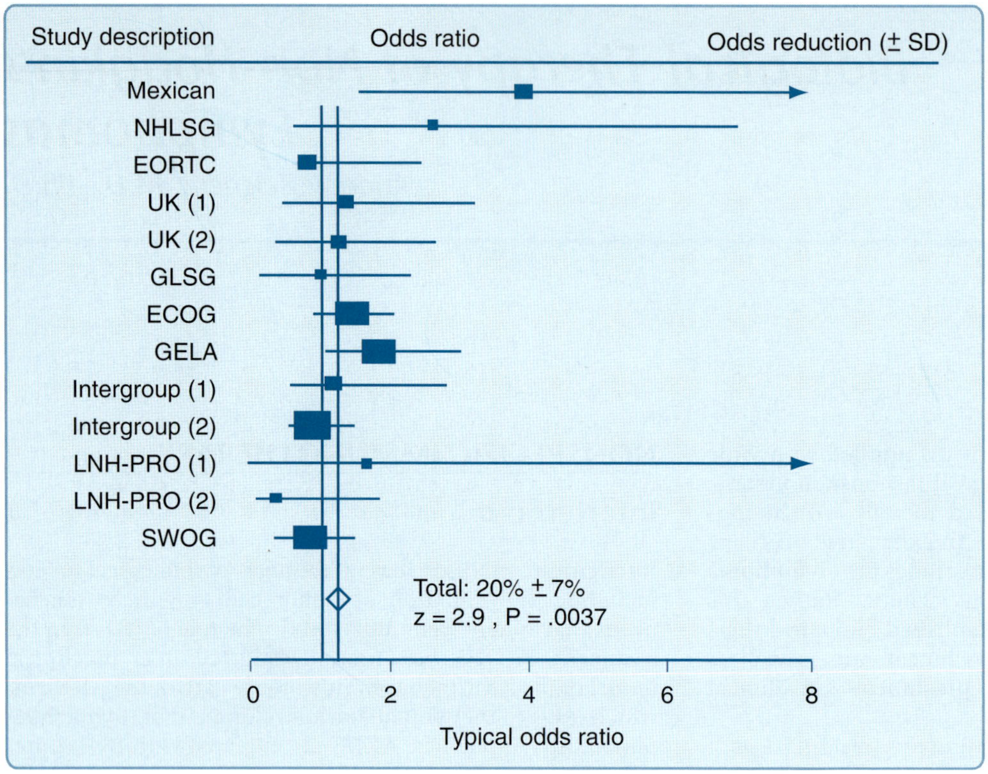

A

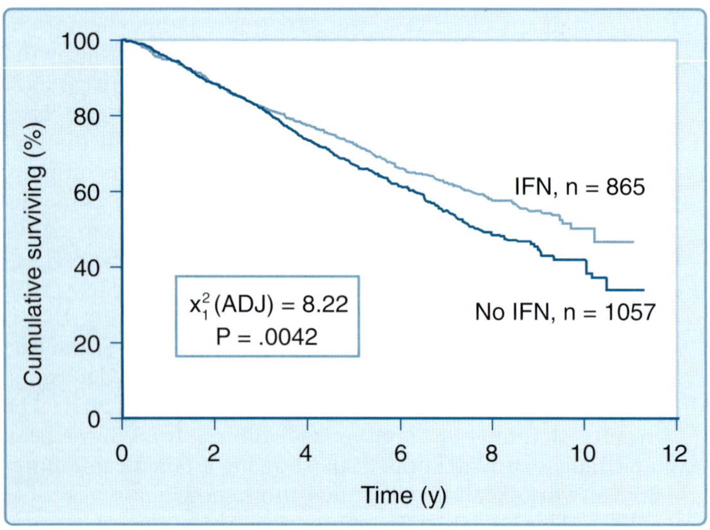

B

Figure 15–1. Meta-analysis of randomized trials evaluating the role of INF-α in the treatment of follicular lymphoma on overall survival. (From Rohatiner AZ, Gregory WM, Peterson B, et al. Meta-analysis to evaluate the role of interferon in follicular lymphoma. J Clin Oncol 2005;23:2215–23,268 with permission.)

Mexico[24] was a significant outlier with a much greater impact on survival; however, when this study was excluded there was still a significant impact on survival for the inclusion of INF-α. The meta-analysis examined these data to explain the underlying heterogeneity in outcome. Survival advantage was associated with administrations of INF-α as a component of relatively intensive initial therapy, administration of ≥5 million units per dose, a cumulative dose of ≥36 million units per month, and INF-α combined with chemotherapy rather than used as maintenance. The use of INF-α as maintenance or in combination with alkylator therapy (single agent or cyclophosphamide, vincristine, prednisone [CVP]) was not associated with a survival benefit. In this analysis, INF-α was associated with a prolongation of remission duration regardless of the nature of the chemotherapy regimen, INF-α dose, or administration with chemotherapy or as maintenance. However, given the toxicity of INF-α, its use should be with regimens shown to prolong survival rather than simply to improve remission duration.

A pegylated form of INF-α has been developed for the treatment of hepatitis C infection.[25] The pegylation of the interferon alters the pharmacokinetics significantly, prolonging the half-life, and thus reducing the frequency of administration; in addition, the toxicity is significantly ameliorated. The role of pegylated INF-α in the treatment of lymphoma is under investigation, but results have not been published.

An alternative approach in the use of INF-α in the treatment of NHL is to combine it with other biological therapy. One approach that has been explored is the combination of INF-α with rituximab (see Bioimmunotherapy section).

Interleukins

Interleukin-2

Interleukins are intercellular signaling molecules that can modulate immune response. Interleukin-2 (T-cell growth factor, IL-2) is capable of inducing T- and NK-cell proliferation thereby potentiating innate antitumor activity of these cells. It exerts its function by binding to the IL-2 receptor (IL-2R), which is composed of three chains: CD25 [IL-2α, Tac], CD122 [IL-2Rβ], and CD132 [IL-2Rγ]. The IL-2Rβ and IL-2γ chains are shared with other interleukin receptors. The affinity of IL-2 for the IL-2R depends on the combination of receptor subunits involved: the low-affinity receptor is comprised of Tac and IL-2Rγ, the medium-affinity receptor is composed of IL-2Rβ and IL-2Rγ, the pseudo–high-affinity receptor is composed of Tac, IL-2β, and the high-affinity receptor is composed of all three subunits.[26] Tac is normally expressed by a population of CD4+ immunoregulatory cells; however, expression is also seen in some lymphomas, including ATLL (HTLV-1-associated), CTCL, HCL, Hodgkin's disease (HD), and some other B-cell lymphomas.[27] In the 1980s, Rosenberg and colleagues at the National Institutes of Health described the ability of lymphokine-activated killer cells (LAK) generated by treatment with IL-2 to eradicate tumors in murine model systems and for human LAK cells to kill autologous tumors.[28,29] They investigated the use of high-dose IL-2 and LAK cells in patients with NHL, and reported four responses among 19 patients with relapsed and refractory NHL; the responses were seen in patients with follicular lymphoma.[30] Although this was a demonstration of clinical activity, toxicity precluded further evaluation of this approach. A single-agent study by the Groupe d'Etude des Lymphomes de l'Adulte (GELA) evaluated the efficacy of continuous infusion (CI) IL-2 in patients with relapsed and refractory NHL.[31] Sixty-one patients were treated, and Grade 4 toxicity was seen in 29 patients with discontinuation of therapy in 12. The most common toxicities were cardiac, renal, vascular leak, and thrombocytopenia. Despite toxicity, responses were seen in 11 patients, with the greatest activity in patients with mycosis fungoides (five of seven patients responded). Although these data supported clinical activity of IL-2 with or without LAK, the toxicity was formidable and alternative approaches to the use of IL-2 were investigated. VanBesien and colleagues tested the hypothesis that IL-2 would be best used in the setting of minimal residual disease such as that seen following high-dose therapy with autologous stem cell transplant.[32,33] Patients with disease responding to second-line chemotherapy consisting of ifosfamide and etoposide were infused with peripheral blood progenitor cells (PBPCs) that had been incubated in vitro with IL-2 for 18 to 24 hours and then reinfused on day 0. Starting 24 hours after the administration of the IL-2 stimulated PBPCs, IL-2 was administered by continuous infusion with 1 mIU/m^2/day for a planned 21 days followed by a 1-week rest. Maintenance IL-2 consisted of two 5-day courses of IL-2 4 mIU/m^2 twice daily separated by 48 hours; this 12-day treatment was repeated approximately monthly for a total of four cycles. Sixty patients underwent transplantation, and 56 patients received IL-2 stimulated PBPCs; toxicity of this infusion was mild. The 21-day course of CI IL-2 was completed in only 30% of patients, with 60% receiving half or less of the planned dose because of subjective intolerance and fever. Forty-two patients started maintenance IL-2, and only 28 received the planned four cycles, but only four patients received the planned dose of therapy; dose reduction occurred in 35 patients secondary to toxicity. In the 60 patients proceeding to high-dose therapy with autologous stem cell rescue (HDT/ASCT), the estimated 3-year progression-free survival (PFS) and overall survival (OS) were 59% and 44%, respectively; this is not substantially different than would have been expected without the IL-2. There was no correlation between PFS and the cumulative dose of either post-ASCT IL-2 or maintenance IL-2. Thus, IL-2 did not appear to have a favorable impact on minimal residual disease when used in this manner. Thus, single-agent IL-2 does not have an established role in the treatment of NHL. The ability of IL-2 to increase antibody-dependent cell-mediated cytotoxicity (ADCC) provides a sound rationale for the study of combination therapy of IL-2 with monoclonal antibody (see Bioimmunotherapy section). An engineered fusion protein of IL-2 and diphtheria toxin, dentileukin difitox, is approved for therapy and is discussed below (see Immunotoxins section).

Interleukin-12

Interleukin-12 (IL-12) binds to the IL-12 receptor (IL-12R), which is composed to two subunits, β1 and β2; the high-affinity β1/β2 receptors are expressed on T cells, NK cells, and dendritic cells. IL-12 acts to induce interferon-γ (INF-γ) production, activate cytotoxic T cells and NK cells, and inhibit angiogenesis. In preclinical models, IL-12 has been shown to induce antitumor response including a preclinical Burkitt's lymphoma (BL) model.[34] In a Phase I trial of IL-12 in patients with cutaneous T-cell lymphoma (CTCL), five of nine patients responded, including two complete remissions.[35] Younes and colleagues at M.D. Anderson Cancer Center (MDACC) conducted a Phase II study of IL-12 in NHL and HD.[36] Six of 29 patients with NHL had a major response, whereas none of the 10 patients with HD responded. Responses were seen in 3 of 14 patients with diffuse large B-cell lymphoma (DLBCL), and 3 of 11 patients with follicular lymphoma (FL). The most prominent side effect was flu-like symptoms, and reversible Grade 3 hepatotoxicity was seen in three patients. Treatment with IL-12 significantly increased circulating CD8+ cells, but did not affect CD4+ cells, vascular endothelial growth factor, basic fibroblast growth factor, or INF-γ levels in the blood.

IL-12 has also been studied in the post-transplant setting to address minimal residual disease.[37] Robertson and colleagues treated 12 patients with hematologic malignancies (8 with NHL) in a Phase I study with IL-12 beginning at a median of 66 days post-HDT/ASCT. Patients received 30, 100, or 250 ng/kg once as an inpatient, and then, after a 2-week rest, for 5 days every 3 weeks as an outpatient. Common toxicity included fever, chills, asthenia, nausea, vomiting and transaminitis. Transient thrombocytopenia and neutropenia were also seen. This study demonstrated that IL-12 can be given safely following HDT/ASCT, but additional studies are necessary to evaluate if it can reduce recurrence and prolong survival.

These results suggest that IL-12 deserves further evaluation in the management of NHL. Some preliminary data are available about combination approaches (see Bioimmunotherapy section).

Using Cytokines to General Antitumor Effector Cells

Negrin and colleagues at Stanford University Medical School have identified a cytokine-induced killer (CIK) cells are highly effective cytotoxic antitumor effector cells that have enhanced cytotoxicity and more rapid proliferation than LAK cells.[38] These cells can be generated from aphaeresis products of patients undergoing HDT/ASCT by priming the cells with an 18- to 24-hour incubation with INF-γ, followed by treatment with IL-2 and the anti-CD3 antibody OKT3; the resulting cells are CD56+ and CD3+.[39] A Phase I study of escalating CIK doses has been conducted in patients with HD and NHL relapsed following HDT/ASCT. Groups of three patients were treated with 1 × 109, 5 × 109, and 1 × 1010 CIKs. Toxicity was minimal, and there were no partial responses in these very refractory patients.[40] The CIKs generated in this manner appear to be more effective and less toxic than LAKs, as they do not require IL-2 administration after administration of the cells; therefore, this approach of using cytokines to generate effector cells warrants further study.

MONOCLONAL ANTIBODIES

The ability to produce monoclonal antibodies of defined specificity provided the possibility of targeting tumor cells for therapeutic purposes. Both B and T cells express a variety of potential cell surface targets: immune receptors, lineage-restricted antigens, and targets for induction of apoptosis. T and B cells express a clone-specific cell surface immune receptor: the cell surface immunoglobulin on the B-cell and the T-cell receptor on T cells (see Fig. 15–2). The exquisite tumor specificity of the immune receptors represents both a benefit in that only the tumor will be targeted and a obstacle in that each patient requires a custom therapy. An alternative to targeting a tumor-specific antigen is to target lineage-restricted antigens. There are a number of well-characterized lineage-restricted antigens for both B cells (e.g., CD19, CD20, CD22, CD37) and T cells (e.g., CD3, CD4, CD8, CD30, CD52). Although both normal and tumor cells are targeted, the constant generation of new B and T cells allows for the replenishment of nonmalignant lymphocytes. Finally, some tumors express receptors that bind apoptosis-inducing ligands such as FAS or the Tumor Necrosis Factor–Related Apoptosis-Inducing Ligand (TRAIL) receptor. Antibodies with agonistic activity against these receptors can potentially induce tumor regressions. A large number of monoclonal antibodies have been developed for the treatment of NHL, and an exhaustive review is beyond the scope of this chapter. The material herein will focus on the most clinically significant antibodies or targets that have provided meaningful insight into the promise and pitfalls of monoclonal antibody therapy (Table 15–1).

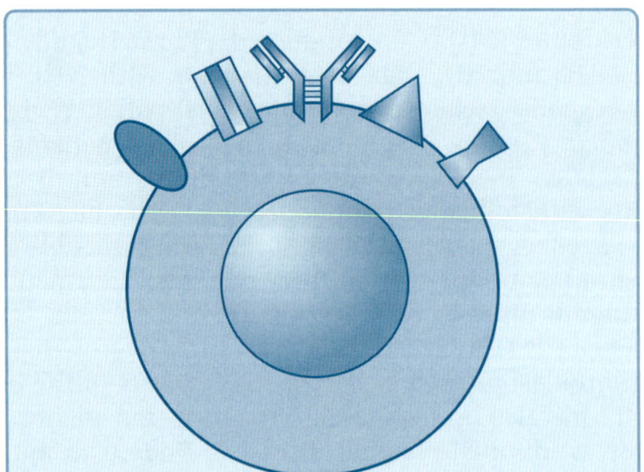

T cells	B cells
TCR, CD3, CD4 CD25, CD30, CD52	sIg, CD19, CD20 CD22, CD52, HLA-DR, CD37

Figure 15–2. Targets for immunotherapy on B and T cells.

Table 15–1. A Selection of Lineage Restricted Antibodies Evaluated in Clinical Trials

Antibody	Target	Approved/ Investigational
Rituximab	CD20	Approved
Epratuzumab	CD22	Investigational
Hu-anti-TAC	CD25	Investigational
MDX-060	CD30	Investigational
SGN-30	CD30	Investigational
Alemtuzumab	CD52w	Approved
Galiximab	CD80	Investigational
Hu1D10	Anti-HLA class II	Investigational

Note: The antibodies above the line react with high restricted antigens found either on a single lineage (CD20, CD22) or particular states of cellular activation (CD25, CD30). The antibodies below the line are not restricted to a single lineage of cells, but are relative to restrictions in the expression.

Mechanisms of Action of Monoclonal Antibodies

Targeting of the monoclonal antibody to the tumor is achieved through the specificity of the immunoglobulin variable region. However, the constant region (Fc) of the antibody is critical in determining host response. The Fc region controls antibody catabolism. Administration of antibodies with nonhuman Fc regions tend to have much shorter serum half-lives, necessitating the administration of high doses of antibody to achieve effective concentrations. A variety of approaches can be taken to alter the Fc region of monoclonal antibodies. Chimeric antibodies have a human Fc region with a nonhuman variable region and are derived by molecular cloning. These antibodies often have prolonged serum half-lives, and have dramatically reduced, but not eliminated, human antichimeric antibody (HACA) responses. Humanized antibodies refer to those antibodies, which in addition to the Fc portion of the antibody being derived from human sequences, the complementarity-determining regions (CDRs) of the variable regions are molecularly grafted with human sequences. Finally, fully human monoclonal antibodies can be derived from genetically modified mice that express human immunoglobulin genes[41,42] or human combinatorial libraries.[43]

In addition to control of catabolism and antigenicity, the Fc portion of an antibody controls complement-dependent cytotoxicity (CDC) and recruitment of effector cells for ADCC (Fig. 15–3).[44]

CDC involves the binding of C1q to the antibody bound to the tumor cell. This triggers a proteolytic cascade culminating in the formation of the membrane attack complex and cell lysis. Alternatively, effector cells (neutrophils, macrophages, and NK cells) expressing complement receptors can bind and mediate phagocytosis or tumor lysis. The sensitivity of cells to CDC is regulated by the tumor cell expression of CD46, CD55, and CD59. CD59 inhibits the binding of the membrane attack complex to the tumor cell, thereby reducing the ability of complement to mediate tumor kill.[45] CD55—also referred to as decay-accelerating factor—acts to prevent the formation of, and accelerate the decay of, C3 convertases, thereby protecting cells form complement-mediated lysis.[46] CD46 sets a barrier to complement activation by limiting the formation and activation of C3 convertases. Expression of these inhibitors of complement-mediated lysis by tumor cells renders them insensitive to complement.[47]

ADCC is mediated by effector cells that express Fc receptors (FcR), including neutrophils, monocytes, macrophages, and NK-cells. There are two activating FcRs, FcγRI (CD64), and FcγRIII (CD16), and one inhibitory FcγRII (CD32).[48] Allelic polymorphisms of FcγRII and FcγRIII differ in the ability to bind Fc regions, and can influence the response to monoclonal antibodies.[49–52] Another important factor in the ability of an antibody to induce ADCC is the immunoglobulin isotype; IgG1 is superior to IgG4 in mediating ADCC.

Another action of monoclonal antibodies is to directly induce apoptosis. In some cases, the antibodies mimic apoptosis-inducing ligands. For example, an antibody, HGS-ETR1, to the TRAIL-receptor 1, mimics the binding of TRAIL to the receptor and induces cell death in a number of tumor cell lines including NHL.[53] Some antibodies can bind and induce apoptosis through less well-defined pathways, such as the binding of CD20. Yet another mechanism is to alter the microenvironment, such as altering angiogenesis with bevacizumab (antivascular endothelial growth

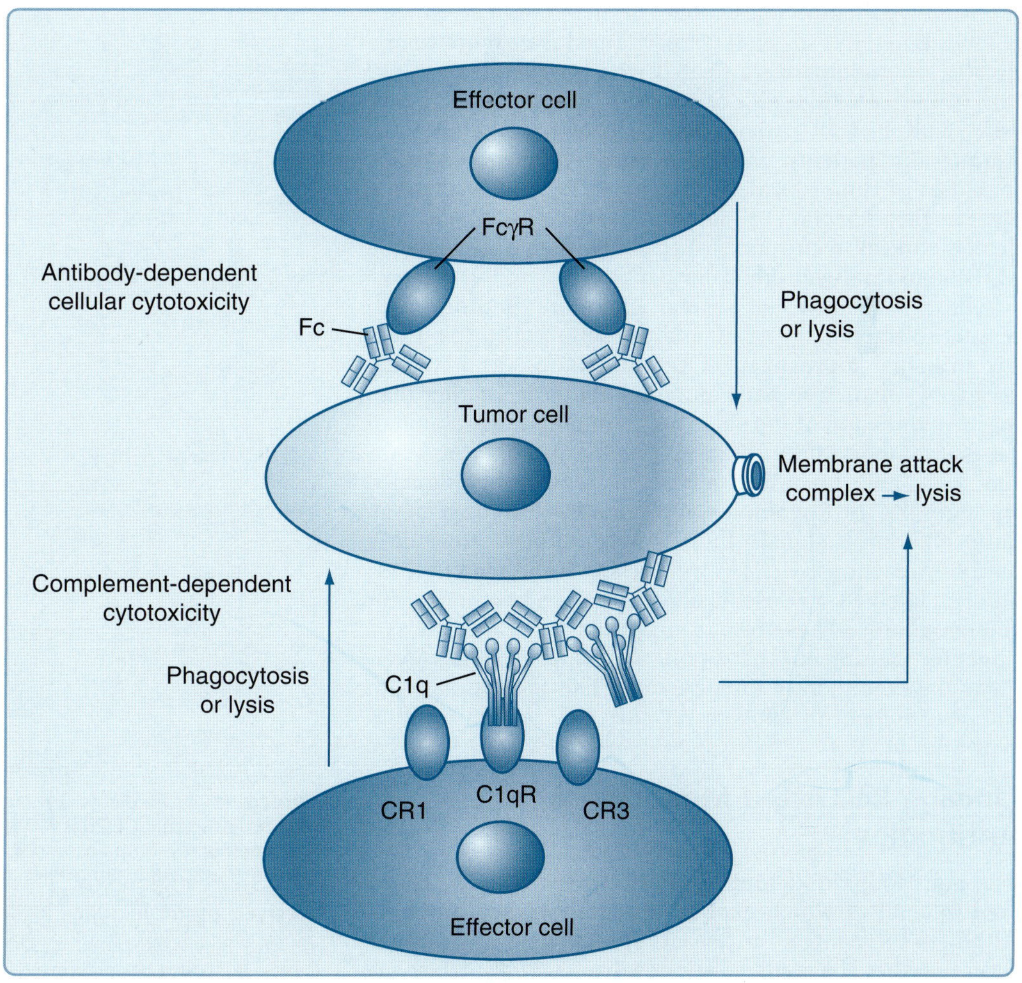

Figure 15–3. Role of antibodies in CDC and ADCC. (From Carter P. Improving the efficacy of antibody-based cancer therapies. Nat Rev Cancer 2001;1:118–29,[44] with permission.)

factor). Although there are ongoing studies of bevacizumab in lymphoma, results have not been reported.

Another approach to the use of monoclonal antibodies is to take advantage of tumor targeting to carry tumorocidal compounds to the tumor. Because lymphomas are highly sensitive to radiation therapy, there has been extensive exploration of the use of radioummunoconjugates for lymphoma therapy. Two agents, yttrium 90-ibritumomab tiuxetan and iodine I131 tositumomab, have been approved for clinical use in follicular NHL (see Radioimmunotherapy section). Drug immunoconjugates have also been evaluated in lymphomas, including antibodies carrying ricin,[54,55] and pseudomonas endotoxins[56] have been evaluated in clinical trials. A variant of this approach is to construct antibodies with dual specificities including the tumor and an effector cell.

Anti-Idiotypic Monoclonal Antibodies

The B-cell receptor complex is made of a variety of invariant components as well as the clone specific surface immunoglobulin (sIg) molecule. The clonotypic sIg can be isolated and purified by traditional means of fusion of the lymphoma or with molecular techniques.[57] Levy and colleagues pioneered the use of murine monoclonal antibodies directed against the sIg, referred to as anti-idiotypic monoclonal antibodies. The work established an important proof of principle that unmodified monoclonal antibodies can demonstrate antitumor activity.[58] In a series of trials (anti-idiotypic antibodies alone or in combination with chlorambucil, INF-α, or IL-2) performed over more than a decade, 45 patients were treated with an overall response rate (ORR) of 66% and a complete remission (CR) rate of 18%, with 13% of patients having prolonged remissions. Among the patients with prolonged response, sensitive measures of tumor burden (clonotypic PCR, flow cytometry for the detection of idiotype-positive cells) did not detect clinical recurrence, suggesting that anti-idiotypic MAbs could induce tumor dormancy.

These trials revealed several important findings with respect to the biology of FL and the action of MAbs. First, the principal mechanism of tumor failure was antigenic escape by ongoing somatic mutation of the sIg[59] rather than loss of expression of the sIg,[60] suggesting that expression of the sIg is important for tumor survival. Anti-idiotypic MAbs that were able to induce remission consistently signaled through the BCR complex, presumably resulting in an antiproliferative signal. Interestingly, human antimouse antibody reactions (HAMA) were relatively blunted in these studies, likely as a consequence of prior chemotherapy for the lymphoma. These results suggested that the sIg was a target for therapy but that a polyvalent approach may overcome the limitation of tumor escape. This is a rationale for the development of idiotype vaccines (see section on Idiotype Vaccines).

Lineage-Restricted Monoclonal Antibodies

The non-Hodgkin's lymphomas are derived from B, T, and NK cells, all of which express lineage-restricted antigens. Although these targets are far less specific than the immune receptor, they have the distinct advantage that they are expressed universally. The suitability to any target for antibody therapy will depend on both the target and the antibody. For example, treatment with an immunotoxin that requires internalization, a target that rapidly internalizes (modulates) the antigen–antibody complex off the surface, would be preferable. In contrast, unmodified antibodies that do not have a strong direct biological effect (i.e., signaling with induction of apoptosis) require the activation of complement and the recruitment of effector cells; therefore, a stable nonmodulating membrane target would be preferable. In all cases, significant shedding of the target antigen into the circulation can impair tumor targeting.[61]

A number of unmodified antibodies targeted to lineage-restricted antigens have been evaluated in clinical trials, often with limited activity. However, CD20 has proven to be an excellent target for treatment with unmodified antibodies and conjugated.

CD20 as Target for Immunotherapy

CD20 (Fig. 15–4) is expressed in a lineage and developmentally restricted manner, initially appearing in the pre-B-

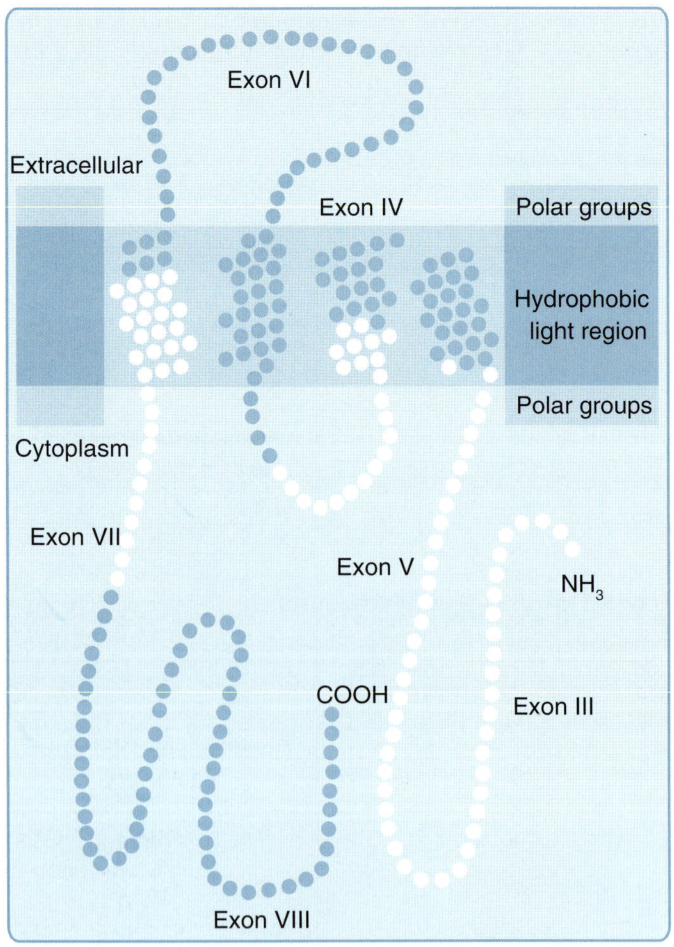

Figure 15–4. Predicted structure of CD20. Experimental evidence demonstrates that CD20 is a Type II transmembrane protein with four transmembrane domains and a single extracellular domain to which all the therapeutic antibodies bind. The diagnostic antibody, L26, binds to the intracellular domain. (From Mason DY, Comans-Bitter WM, Cordell JL, et al. Antibody L26 recognizes an intracellular epitope on the B-cell–associated CD20 antigen. Am J Pathol 1990; 136: 1215–22,[65] with permission.)

cell stage of B-cell ontogeny and disappearing on differentiation to the plasma cell.[62,63] It is a 33-kD, Type III, tetraspan-transmembrane phosphoprotein with a 44–amino acid extracellular domain.[64,65] CD20 acts as a calcium channel localized to lipid rafts.[66,67] Nonetheless, the specific function of CD20 is unknown, and knockout of CD20 in the mouse has no impact on B-cell development or function.[68] Furthermore, other functions such as tissue localization, signal transduction, proliferation, affinity maturation, and T-cell–dependent antibody responses are not impacted in the CD20–/– mice.[69]

CD20 is generally not shed into the serum, although there is a report of circulating CD20 in patients with CLL.[70] Binding of anti-CD20 antibody to CD20 does not result in modulation of the antigen from the cell surface.[71–74] There have been conflicting reports regarding the regulation of CD20 expression. Recombinant IL-4 has been reported to result in down-regulation of CD20 expression in nonstimulated and preactivated normal B cell, whereas IL-1, IL-2, IL-3, IL-6, INF-α, INF-γ, GM-CSF, TGF-β, TNF-α, and lymphotoxin had no effect.[75] In another study, CLL cells were found to increase CD20 expression in response to IL-4, TNF-α, and GM-CSF, whereas TGF-β, G-CSF, IL-2, IL-2, and IL-3 had no effect.[76] In another study of CLL cells, INF-α treatment increased the expression of CD20.[77] Low-dose external beam radiation has been shown to increase the expression of CD20 in vitro.[78] The lack of a consistent pattern of activity may reflect difference in responsiveness at different stages of B-cell development; alternatively, these could be the result of methodologic differences. Nonetheless, these data make it difficult to predict the utility of combined cytokine and anti-CD20 therapy.

Biological Effects of Anti-CD20 Antibodies

The B1 antigen (CD20) was identified as the target of a monoclonal antibody derived from immunization of mice with human B-cell lymphoma. The anti-B1 antibody identified a cell surface protein uniquely found on B cells that was expressed nearly universally on B-cell lymphomas.[79,80] Anti-B1 combined with complement proved to be effective in purging bone marrow of tumor cells for high-dose therapy and autologous stem cell transplant.[81,82] Press and colleagues[83] in Seattle evaluated the clinical activity of another murine anti-CD20 antibody 1F5 as well as anti-B1. In a proof-of-concept experiment, four patients were treated with 1F5 in which penetration of the antibody into tumor tissue was seen; in the two patients receiving the highest doses in this study, transient responses were observed.[83] The anti-B1 antibody (tositumomab) was shown to have clinical activity in a randomized trial versus ^{131}I-anti-B1 (iodine I131 tositumomab) (see section on Radioimmunotherapy).[84]

Rituximab was developed and specifically engineered for treatment of B-cell NHL.[85] The immunoglobulin heavy- and light-chain genes were cloned from the murine anti-CD20 antibody 2B8 into an expression vector containing the human constant regions from the IgG1 isotype of the heavy chain and the kappa light chain.[86] The chimeric antibody, C2B8 (rituximab), was able to mediate CDC and ADCC and deplete B cells in macaque cynomologous monkeys. This antibody was approved for clinical use in 1997 based on activity as a single agent in patients with relapsed and refractory indolent lymphoma.[87,88] The clinical activity is reviewed in depth below.

The anti-CD20 antibodies—IF5, tositumomab, and rituximab—differ in several of their biological activities. Rituximab appears to be superior to fixing complement. This has recently been related to the segregation of CD20 into specialized membrane structures call lipid rafts.[89–91] Both 1F5 and rituximab, which fix complement very effectively, were associated with the redistribution of CD20 into lipid rafts. In contrast, tositumomab, a poor activator of complement, failed to translocate CD20 into lipid rafts.[90]

Anti-CD20 antibodies (tositumomab, rituximab, 1F5) induce apoptosis.[92–96] The signaling events associated with apoptosis include activation of SRC-family tyrosine kinases Lck and Fyn, Ca+ flux, and activation of capases. PPI, an inhibitor of SRC family kinases, attenuates apoptosis.[94] However, there is some disagreement regarding the ability of the various anti-CD20 antibodies to induce apoptosis. In one report, rituximab was a more potent inducer of apoptosis than 1F5 or anti-B1,[94] whereas others have reported greater apoptosis with anti-B1.[95,96] Interestingly, two groups found that the F(ab')$_2$ fragment of anti-B1, but not 1F5, was able to induce apoptosis.[95,96] The F(ab')$_2$ fragment of anti-B1, but not 1F5, was also able to induce tumor regression in xenografts.[96]

New Anti-CD20 Antibodies

Based on an increased understanding of the biological effects of anti-CD20 antibodies, new anti-CD20 antibodies have been developed.[97,98] Rituximab is a chimeric antibody with the variable regions entirely derived from the murine variable region of the parent antibody 2B8. Although human antichimeric antibody (HACA) responses have not been a major issue in patients with lymphoma, it has emerged as a problem in other indications such as systemic lupus erythematosus.[99] To minimize the immune response to the antibody, Stein and colleagues humanized the murine A20 anti-CD20 antibody by CDR-grafting.[97] The resulting antibody IMMU-106 (hA20) is comparable to rituximab in both binding affinity and apparent dissociation constants. Similar activity to rituximab was also seen in antiproliferative effects on cell lines, and in SCID mice xenografts of the Raji lymphoma cell line. The F(ab')$_2$ fragments of IMMU-206 and rituximab were inactive in the xenograft model, demonstrating that both of these antibodies require the Fc region for their biological activity.[97] Other than the humanization, it is not clear if IMMU-206 would have clinical advantage over rituximab, given comparable preclinical characterization.

Teeling and colleagues took another approach to the development of new anti-CD20 antibodies.[98] They immunized human immunoglobulin transgenic mice with cells transfected with human CD20. They isolated several fully human antibodies: 11B8 is a Type II antibody that, like anti-B1, does not cause CD20 to segregate into lipid rafts; and 2F2 and 7D8, which are Type I antibodies like rituximab that segregate CD20 into lipid rafts. The two Type I antibodies, 2F2 and 7D8, were very potent in CDC, with the ability to lyse rituximab-resistant target in vitro. Both of these antibodies had substantially slower off rates compared to rituximab; the slower off rate was associated with the enhancement of CDC. It is hypothesized that the dramatic improvement in CDC will have clinical utility with possible activity in patients resistant to rituximab.

These drugs address the perceived limitations of rituximab, the approved unmodified antibody for the treatment of B-cell NHL. However, clinical trials are necessary to determine if these new unmodified anti-CD20 antibodies are more effective than rituximab, or have activity in situations where rituximab is not optimal.

Mechanism of Activity of Rituximab

As reviewed above, there is evidence that rituximab has multiple potential mechanisms of action including CDC, ADCC, and direct induction of apoptosis. Although these activities have been demonstrated in various ways, the dominant mechanism in vivo remains controversial.

The role of ADCC was evaluated in a murine model in which the FcR was knocked out.[100] Mice deficient for the activating FcγRIII receptor are unable to induce ADCC, since the effector cells cannot bind to the antibody coated tumor cells. In the FcγRIII–/– growth of a human lymphoma, the xenograft was not inhibited by rituximab. In mice deficient for the inhibitory FcγRIIB receptor, the antitumor effect of unmodified antibodies was exaggerated. Additional evidence for the role of ADCC in the activity of rituximab in vivo comes from the study of polymorphisms of the Fc receptors. The FcγRIII receptor is polymorphic with either a valine or phenylalanine at position 158. The 158V allotype has a higher affinity for IgG1.[101] Catron and colleagues reported that patients with follicular lymphoma who were homozygous for FcγRIII-158V had higher response rates to a standard 4-week course of rituximab at 2 and 12 months after treatment.[49] Weng and Levy confirmed the findings with respect to the FcγRIII-158 polymorphism, and also reported that homozygosity of the FcγRIIa-131 H allotype was also associated with superior response compared to the H/R or R/R allotypes.[50] Similar, although slightly variant results, were reported by Treon and colleagues at the Dana Farber Cancer Institute (DFCI) for patients with Waldenström's macroglobulinemia (WM) treated with rituximab.[102] In addition to the FcγRIIIA 158 polymorphism, they also analyzed the FcγRIIIA 48 polymorphism. Unlike the results reported above, both the 158 V/V and 158 V/F were associated with a better response to rituximab; however, at a median follow-up of 13 months, there was no difference in time to progression (TTP). The position 48 polymorphism did not independently determine response. Taken as a whole, these results provide compelling evidence for the central role of ADCC in vivo.

Several lines of evidence support a role for complement in the action of rituximab in vivo. Golay and colleagues found that the ability of rituximab to mediate CDC was highly variable among various cell lines and fresh tumor specimens.[103] There was a strong correlation between expression of CD55 and CD59 in the cell lines and tumor specimens and resistance to CDC. Blocking CD55 and CD59 with specific antibodies increased CDC. Similar findings were reported by Harjunpaa and colleagues; neutralization of CD55 and CD59 in lymphoma cell lines enhanced CDC.[104] Patients with paroxysmal nocturnal hemoglobinuria (PNH) do not express glycosylphosphatidylinositol (GPI) anchored proteins, including CD55 and CD59, as a consequence of mutation of PIGA. A B-cell line derived from a patient with PNH was more sensitive to rituximab plus complement than the isogenic cell line that had been transfected with PIGA to restore CD55 and CD59 expression.[105] In contrast, in a study from Stanford University Medical School, Weng and Levy reported that expression of inhibitors of complement mediated lysis, CD46, CD55, and CD59, on pre-treatment tumor cells did not predict resistance to rituximab.[106] Manches and colleagues examined rituximab-induced killing in 28 fresh lymphoma samples (FL, 7; small lymphocytic lymphoma [SLL], 7; DLBLC, 7; mantle cell lymphoma [MCL], 7).[107] They found little variation in ADCC and induction of apoptosis, but did identify differences in CDC that were related to CD20 antigen density and complement regulatory proteins. FL was highly sensitive to CDC; moderately sensitive to DLBLC and MCL; and resistant to SLL. They concluded that CDC is an important determinant of rituximab in vivo, but the study did not show a direct relationship between CDC on a given sample and in vivo response. The relative importance of ADCC versus CDC for the in vivo activity of rituximab remains uncertain.

Single-Agent Immunotherapy with Rituximab

Indolent NHL

The development of the chimeric monoclonal antibody rituximab (C2B8) altered the therapy of indolent lymphoma.[86] In the early Phase I single-dose, dose-escalation trials, tumor regressions were seen (two partial response [PR] and four minor responses in 15 patients).[87] A subsequent study of 4-week doses identified a biologically effective dose of 375 mg/m^2, again with clinical responses that were particularly frequent in patients with indolent lymphoma.[108] The subsequent "pivotal" study was a Phase II design that included 166 patients with relapsed and refractory indolent lymphoma treated with 4-week doses of rituximab.[88] The overall response rate was 48%, and the median time to progression was 13 months. The overall response rate was higher in patients with follicular lymphoma (60%) than in the patients with SLL (International Working Formulation [IWF] A) (12%). Based on these data, the U.S. Food and Drug Administration (FDA) approved the clinical use of rituximab for patients with relapsed and recurrent follicular lymphoma. A subsequent Phase II study at the same dose and schedule demonstrated that patients initially responding to rituximab could be retreated at the time of progression, but the response rate was only 40%.[109] These data ushered in the era of immunotherapy that has fundamentally altered the treatment of B-cell NHL. Although these data demonstrate that rituximab has substantial activity, they do not inform us as to the optimal use of this agent.

Rituximab has been used to treat newly diagnosed indolent lymphoma with response rates ranging form 52% to 73%, with a PFS of about 12 months.[110–112] Building on the single-agent activity in indolent lymphomas, investigators from the Sarah Cannon Cancer Center evaluated planned re-treatment with 4-week courses of rituximab at 6-month intervals.[113] This study demonstrated a 34-month PFS and an increasing CR rate with time. However, the Phase II study design made it difficult to ascertain whether either of these observations was superior to a single 4-week course. The Swiss Group for Clinical Cancer Research (SAKK)[114] examined the role of extended dosing in a randomized trial. Patients were treated with a standard 4-week course of rituximab followed by randomization to observation or prolonged therapy given as one dose of rituximab every 8 weeks for four doses; patients with progression after the initial rituximab were excluded from the randomization. A total of 185 patients were enrolled; the ORR to the rituximab was 67% in chemotherapy-naive patients and 46% in previously treated patients. A total of 151 patients were eligible for randomization. At a median follow-up of 35 months, the median event-free survival (EFS) favored the prolonged therapy group (23 months vs. 12 months, $p = 0.02$) with a larger benefit in the chemonaive subset (36 months vs. 19 months, $p = 0.004$). Interestingly, the CR rate was identical in both treatment groups, suggesting that achievement of CR did not require additional rituximab. IgM plasma levels decreased for a significantly longer time after prolonged treatment, but this was not associated with an increased infectious risk. These data support that EFS can be extended with maintenance or prolonged rituximab.

A randomized Phase II study was conducted to determine if maintenance rituximab (4-week doses every 6 months) was superior to re-treatment with 4-week doses of rituximab at disease progression.[115] Patients (n = 114) were treated with rituximab and randomized (n = 90) if they had stable or responding disease. The endpoint of the study was the duration of rituximab benefit, which was the same between the two arms: maintenance, 31 months, versus re-treatment groups, 27 months. However, this randomized Phase II does not have sufficient power to make definitive conclusions, and the Eastern Cooperative Oncology Group (ECOG) is conducting a large Phase III study (RESORT) to address the question of maintenance versus re-treatment at progression.

Waldenström's Macroglobulinemia

Byrd and colleagues reported responses in three of seven patients (43%) with symptomatic WM treated with 4 or 8 weeks of rituximab at the 375 mg/m^2 dose with a median duration of 6.6 months.[116] Confirmation of single-agent activity was reported by Treon and colleagues in a larger retrospective study of 30 patients, as there were PR in 27% and MR in 33% of patients; however, most patients had improvements in hemoglobin and platelet counts.[117] Importantly, it has been observed that some patients with WM experience an increase in their monoclonal IgM during treatment with rituximab.[118] Dimopoulos and colleagues reported on a prospective trial in 27 patients with newly diagnosed and relapsed WM; the overall ORR was 44%, with an ORR of 40% in treatment naive and 50% in previously treated patients.[119] There have been two reports of an extended dosing schedule with four additional doses given 3 months after the first. This was not associated with a higher ORR (35%), but there may be a benefit in remission durability.[120,121] A prognostic factor analysis identified an IgM level of ≤4 g/dL and albumin ≥3.5 g/dL as independent factors associated with a better response to rituximab. Patients with zero, one, or two adverse factors had TTP of more than 40, 11, and 3.6 months, respectively.

DLBCL and Mantle Cell Lymphoma

The GELA demonstrated that rituximab had modest single-agent activity, with a 37% overall response rate in patients with relapsed and refractory DLBCL and MCL.[122] Although response durations were short, this established that rituximab had activity in DLBCL and that further evaluation was warranted. These studies led to the evaluation of chemoimmunotherapy for the treatment of DLBCL resulting in a new standard (see DLBCL: Advanced Stage).

Pan and colleagues at Memorial Sloan-Kettering Cancer Center (MSKCC), reported on single-agent activity of rituximab in patients with DLBCL who had failed autologous stem cell transplant.[123] Seventeen patients with DLBCL (n = 13) and MCL (n = 4) were treated with single-agent rituximab in patients with disease progression following HDT/ASCT, with an ORR and CR of 53% and 23%, respectively. The median PFS for responders was 13 months. In a more detailed analysis, Kewalramani and colleagues analyzed the natural history of NHL failing HDT/ASCT.[124] The median survival was 7.7 months, but was significantly longer in patients treated with rituximab versus those treated with chemotherapy (28.6 months vs. 4.1 months).

A European intergroup conducted a study of single-agent rituximab in patients with newly diagnosed and recurrent MCL.[125] In a total of 74 patients (34 untreated, 40 relapsed), the overall response rate was 38%, which was unaffected by prior treatment. The median duration of response was 1.2 years. These results were similar to a small pilot trial using 8 consecutive weeks of treatment, and some patients were treated at a higher dose.[122] Thus, neither the longer treatment duration nor the higher dose appeared to be important for the single-agent activity in MCL.

The SAKK conducted a study to determine if prolonged dosing of rituximab could improve the outcome of patients with untreated and relapsed mantle cell lymphoma treated with single-agent rituximab.[126] All patients received 4-week doses of rituximab at the standard dose of 375 mg/m^2. Patients with stable or responding disease were randomized to observation versus rituximab given at a dose of 375 mg/m^2 every 8 weeks for an additional four doses. A total of 104 patients were treated on this trial, with a response rate of 27%. After the induction therapy, polymerase chain reaction amplification of the t(11;14) translocation breakpoint became negative in the peripheral blood of 4 of 20 informative patients, and only 1 of 14 informative bone marrows. Sixty-one patients were randomized (stable or responding disease), and there was no difference in outcome (EFS, RD, OS) between the prolonged therapy group and the observation group. These data demonstrate modest single-agent activity for rituximab in MCL.

Rituximab Combined with Chemotherapy

Synergy between rituximab and chemotherapy has been demonstrated in vitro. Reports of synergy include doxorubicin, cisplatinum, fludarabine, fenretinide (4-HPR), gemcitabine, vinorelbine, prednisone, bendamustine, and paclitaxel.[127–134] The mechanism underlying chemosensitization by rituximab has been investigated.[130,134,135] Ghetie and colleagues reported that synergy was much more active with rituximab homodimers, which resulted in cross-linking of CD20 on the cell surface. Jazirehi and colleagues at UCLA reported that rituximab downregulated the expression of anti-apoptotic proteins in the BCL2 family ($Bcl-X_L$ and Bcl-2). They have reported that the down-regulation of $Bcl-X_L$ is by inhibiting the NK-κB signaling pathway, thereby resulting in chemosensitization. However, it remains to be demonstrated that these mechanisms are important in the clinical activity of rituximab. Demonstrating synergistic combination in vivo is often very difficulty. At a minimum, to establish that rituximab is synergistic in a clinically meaningful way, it would be necessary to demonstrate superior outcome for the combination of chemotherapy and rituximab (C+R) when compared to the sequence of chemotherapy followed by rituximab (C→?R). A number of trials with this design have been conducted and are reviewed below. In general, evidence that is supportive of a synergistic rather than additive impact of rituximab on chemotherapy has been lacking.

Indolent Lymphoma

Phase II studies have suggested that rituximab can add to the clinical benefit of combination chemotherapy in patients with indolent lymphoma. For example, compared to historical controls rituximab improved the EFS with single-agent fludarabine as well as CHOP.[136,137] However, small trial sizes and potential selection biases make definitive conclusions impossible to draw. A series of randomized studies has been undertaken to address this question in untreated and relapsed indolent lymphoma.

The German Low-Grade Lymphoma Study Group (GLSG) examined the impact of adding rituximab to the FCM (fludarabine, cyclophosphamide, mitroxantrone) regimen in patients with relapsed or refractory FL and MCL.[138] A total of 147 patients were randomized and 128 were evaluable. In the FL patients, the ORR (94% vs. 70%) favored the R-FCM arms. In the FL patient subgroup, there was a benefit in median PFS for the R-FCM patients (not reached at 3 years) versus FCM (21 months, $p = 0.0139$). At 2 years, the estimated OS was 90% in R-FCM as compared with 70% on the FCM arm ($p = 0.0943$). Thus, in rituximab-naive patients with recurrent disease, rituximab adds a palliative benefit to chemotherapy (no impact on OS) in patients with FL.

A multicenter study in England examined the addition of rituximab to CVP chemotherapy.[139] The chemotherapy was a modified CVP with a low dose of cyclophosphamide (750 mg/m^2) and prednisone (40 mg/m^2). Patients treated with R-CVP had significantly improved OR and CR rates as well as time-to-treatment failures (TTF). However, the study had an unusual definition of time to treatment failure, as patients with less than a PR after four cycles were considered treatment failures. This had a disproportionate impact on the chemotherapy arm. Therefore, the TTP is a more reliable comparison in this trial. TTP for R-CVP and CVP was 32 months and 15 months ($p < 0.0001$). Although the results in the control arm seem to be suboptimal, this was a study with about 50% of patients with high-risk disease according to the Follicular Lymphoma International Prognostic Index (FLIPI). Thus, cross-trial comparisons must be made carefully and should take into account the differences in study populations.

The rationale for the combination of rituximab with chemotherapy has been the suggestion of synergy in vitro with various chemotherapeutic agents, including doxorubicin; this provided the rationale for the R-CHOP regimen.[137] The GLSG conducted a randomized trial of CHOP versus R-CHOP in FL.[140] The study has a second randomization evaluating two doses of interferon alpha in patients over 60 years of age and evaluating HDT/ASCT versus interferon alpha in patients ≤60 years of age. Preliminary results have demonstrated that R-CHOP has superior OR and CR rates. In this study, 606 patients were randomized. However, at the time of presentation, only 394 patients were evaluable. R-CHOP provided only a modest increase in OR and CR rates. However, R-CHOP significantly increased the median TTF ($p < 0.0007$). At a median follow-up of 3 years, the TTF was not reached in the R-CHOP arm and was 2–6 years in the CHOP arm. However, the analysis is complicated by the second randomization, and further follow-up is necessary to determine if there is a survival benefit.

Zinzani and colleagues conducted a comparison of fludarabine and mitroxantrone (FM) with or without rituximab to CHOP with or without rituximab in patients with newly diagnosed FL.[141] Patients ($n = 140$) were initially randomized to receive FM versus CHOP. Patients in molecular CR for the t(14;18) translocation were observed. Patients with a molecular positive CR or a PR irrespective of the molecular status received rituximab. FM produced a superior CR (molecular positive or negative) of 68% versus 42% ($p = 0.003$); the molecular negative CR was 39% versus 19% ($p = 0.001$). Ninety-five patients received rituximab, and 58% were converted to molecular remissions. This clearly demonstrates the potential for rituximab to address minimal residual disease. There was no difference in PFS or OS among the various treatment groups, although the follow-up of 19 months is very short for a study in FL.

These randomized trials indicate that rituximab added to chemotherapy can improve OR, CR, and EFS or PFS, but the impact on OS is not yet clear. This is in contrast to the data presented above for DLBCL. The long natural history of FL confounds the survival endpoints in these studies. If the data ultimately demonstrate a survival advantage, there will be no controversy regarding the inclusion of rituximab in up-front treatment. However, if the benefit is only on PFS or EFS and not OS, then the timing of the use of rituximab may become crucial. Since patients develop resistance to rituximab, its use early in the course may compromise the later effectiveness of the drug. Thus, additional follow-up of the chemo-immunotherapy trials is essential.

Waldenström's Macroglobulinemia

R-CHOP has also been evaluated in the treatment of patients with WM.[142] In this retrospective study of 13 patients, 7 had refractory disease, 3 had relapsed disease, and 3 were untreated; 6 patients had received prior rituximab. Three patients achieved an uncertain complete remission (CRu), and 8 patients achieved a PR. The median

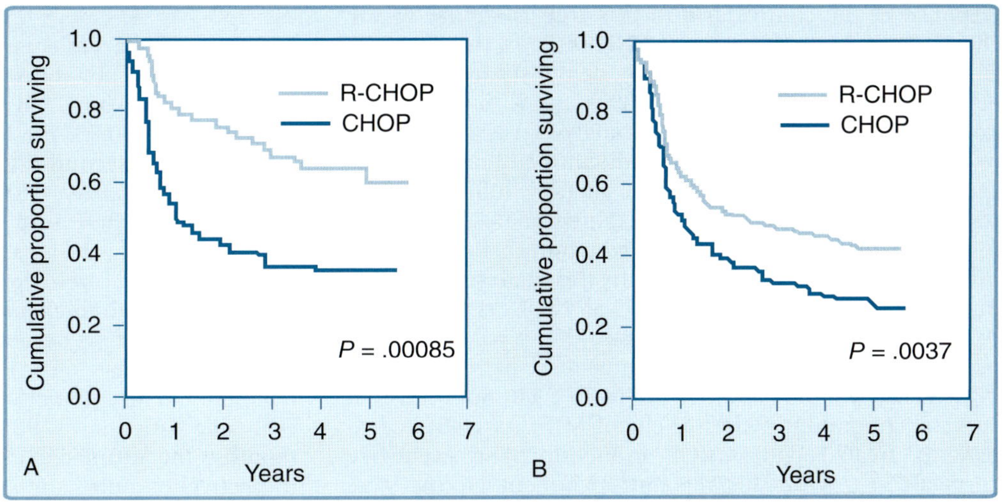

Figure 15–5. R-CHOP versus CHOP in patients aged 60 to 80 years with DLBLC, EFS by age-adjusted IPI. (From Feugier P, Van Hoof A, Sebban C, et al. Long-term results of the R-CHOP Study in the treatment of elderly patients with diffuse large B-cell lymphoma: a study by the Groupe d'Etude des Lymphomes de l'Adulte. J Clin Oncol 2005;23:4117–26,[148] with permission.)

hematocrit rose from 30.5% to 39.3% (p = 0.001); the median IgM monoclonal spike fell from 5230 mg/dL to 1690 mg/dL (p = 0.001); and the median serum viscosity fell from 2.9 cp to 1.6 cp (p = 0.01). The durability of response could not be assessed in this small study because the median follow-up was only 9 months. Nonetheless, the improvement in the laboratory parameter is dramatic, and suggests that the combination is very active. A prospective trial is warranted.

DLBCL: Advanced Stage

The combination of single-agent activity without overlapping toxicity provided rationale for the combination of rituximab with conventional chemotherapy. A multicenter Phase II study of rituximab (day 1 of each cycle) and CHOP (day 3 of each cycle) for patients with untreated DLBCL was conducted to evaluate safety and efficacy.[143] Thirty-three patients were treated with six cycles of R-CHOP at 21-day intervals, and the principal toxicities were infusional reactions during the first dose of rituximab and the expected toxicities of CHOP. The addition of the rituximab did not appear to augment the toxicity of the chemotherapy. The overall response rate was 94%, with 61% complete responders. At the time of publication, the follow-up was short (26 months), and the median time to progression had not been reached. Among 13 patients who had a t(14;18) translocation identified by the polymerase chain reaction (PCR) at baseline, 11 had molecular remission at the end of therapy. The efficacy was felt to be at least as good as that expected for patients treated with CHOP. Based on these favorable Phase II results, several randomized studies were conducted to see if rituximab enhanced the efficacy of CHOP chemotherapy.[144–146]

In its LNH 98.5, the GELA compared eight cycles of conventional CHOP chemotherapy to eight cycles of the combination of rituximab (day 1 of each cycle) with CHOP (day 1 of each cycle) for patients aged 60 to 80 years.[144] The addition of rituximab to the CHOP chemotherapy resulted in significant improvement in complete response (76% vs. 53%, p = 0.005), as well as 5-year event-free (47% vs. 29%; $p < 0.00001$) and overall survival (58% vs. 45%, p = 0.0073).[147] The benefit has been durable with increased separation of the Kaplan–Meier survival curves with increasing length of follow-up.[148] The relative benefit of the chemoimmunotherapy was greater in the patients with low- and low-intermediate risk disease determined by the age-adjusted IPI; nonetheless, even among the poor-risk patients there was a significant improvement in the outcome (Fig. 15–5).

The ECOG 4494 study examined a very similar patient population (aged ≥ 60 years), although the dosing of the rituximab was different (Fig. 15–6).[145] Two doses of rituximab were administered before Cycle 1, and one dose of rituximab was administered before Cycles 3, 5, and 7 (if necessary). Treatment was given for six to eight cycles, those in a complete response after four cycles received six cycles, and all other patients received eight. In addition to posing the question regarding the role of adding rituximab to CHOP, it evaluated the impact of maintenance rituximab (MR) administered for four doses every 6 months for 2 years. Interpretation of the trial results was complicated by the 2x2 trial design, since it was based on the erroneous assumption that there was no interaction between the randomizations. The overall response rate was unaffected by the second randomization. In contrast to the GELA LNH 98.5 trial, there was no difference in the response rate between the R-CHOP and CHOP (79% vs. 76%). The

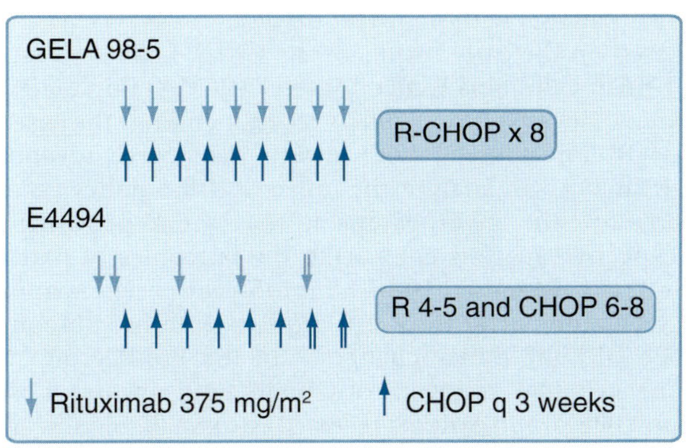

Figure 15–6. Comparison of the schedule for the chemoimmunotherapy arms therapy in the GELA 98-5 and ECOG 4494 trials comparing R-CHOP to CHOP for patients.

response of the control arm in this trial is similar to the chemo-immunotherapy arm of LNH 98.5. In the pair-wise analysis of induction, R-CHOP demonstrated a small benefit at 3 years in event-free (53% vs. 46%, $p = 0.04$) but not overall survival. However, this analysis was complicated by the interaction between the induction and maintenance therapies. Because the induction therapy influenced the results of the maintenance, a weighted analysis was performed to elucidate the effect of induction therapy without influence from the maintenance. In this analysis, R-CHOP improved 3-year, event-free survival (52% vs. 39%, $p = 0.003$) and overall survival (67% vs. 58%, $p = 0.05$). In the pairwise analysis evaluating maintenance, patients receiving MR had a significant increase in TTF, but not in overall survival. Importantly, the benefit of MR was restricted to patients treated with CHOP induction. The event-free survivals at 2 years for the four treatment groups were R-CHOP, 77%; R-CHOP+MR, 79%; CHOP, 47%; and CHOP+MR, 74%. Thus, the E4494 trial confirmed the benefit of R-CHOP for patients over the age of 60 years, and demonstrated that in DLBCL, MR has no added benefit to induction therapy with chemo-immunotherapy.

Both the GELA LNH 98.5 and ECOG 4494 studies focused on patients 60 years of age and older. Two additional studies have examined the benefit of chemo-immunotherapy for DLBCL in younger patients.[146,149] The Mint trial was an international multicenter study for patients with untreated DLBCL aged 18 to 60 years with low-risk disease (IPI 0 or 1, Stages II–IV, and Stage I with bulk). Patients were randomized to receive six cycles of a CHOP-like regimen, or the same chemotherapy plus rituximab of 375 mg/m^2 on days 1, 22, 43, 64, 85, and 106. Radiotherapy was planned to sites of initial bulk and/or extranodal involvement.[146] CHOP-like chemotherapy included CHOEP (44%), CHOP (48%), MACOP-B (4%), and PMitCEBO (prednisolone, mitoxantrone, cyclophosphamide, etoposide, bleomycin, vincristine)[150] (4%). The use of these regimens was balanced in the chemotherapy (CHEMO) alone and rituximab plus chemotherapy (R-CHEMO) arms. Like the GELA study, the R-CHEMO arm had a higher CR (86% vs. 68%, $p < 0.0001$). This was associated with an improvement in the estimated 2-year EF (76% vs. 60%, $p < 0.0001$) and overall survival (94% vs. 87%, $p < 0.001$). This study supports the use of rituximab plus anthracycline-based chemotherapy in the initial management of young patients with very favorable DLBCL; however, it does not directly address patients with poor-risk disease.

Based on the early results of the GELA LNH 98.5 study, the British Columbia Cancer Agency (BCCA) implemented a policy on March 1, 2001, recommending the use of R-CHOP for patients with newly diagnosed advanced-stage DLBCL. To analyze the impact of that policy recommendation, the investigators at the BCCA performed a retrospective analysis comparing the outcomes of patients with newly diagnosed DLBCL for a 3-year period spanning the 18 months prior to (Pre-R) and 18 months subsequent to (Post-R) the policy change.[149] In the Pre-R group, 9% of the patients received rituximab, and in the Post-R group, 85% of the patients received rituximab. Significantly more patients received radiation therapy in the Pre-R group compared to the Post-R (25% vs. 15%, $p = 0.04$). For the entire population, the Post-R group had a superior estimated 2-year PFS (71% vs. 52%, $p = 0.00009$) and OS (77% vs. 53%, $p = 0.0001$) compared to the Pre-R group. However, in the patients under 60 years, the 2-year estimated EFS was not statistically significant (70% post-R vs. 60% pre-R, $p = 0.18$). In this subset, the OS was superior (87% post-R vs. 69% pre-R, $p = 0.018$), but this may reflect differences in second-line therapy in patients treated in different time spans. Although these results confirm the efficacy of R-CHOP in a community setting, they raise a question about the management of younger patients. Clearly, a more careful prospective evaluation of the role adding rituximab to chemotherapy for young patients with poor-risk DLBLC is necessary.

Rituximab has also been added to the DA-EPOCH regimen.[151] The complete response rate (CR/CRu) of the 61 evaluable patients was 92%. At the median follow-up of 22 months, the estimated PFS and OS were 79% and 84%, respectively, quite similar to the historical control.[152] However, in a subset analysis based on the expression of BCL2 as judged by immunohistochemistry, there was an improved outcome in patients whose tumors expressed the BCL2 gene product if they were treated with DA-EPOCH-R compared to DA-EPOCH. Additions of rituximab did not improve the outcome in patients whose tumors did not express BCL2 protein. Analysis of GELA LNH 98.5 also demonstrated a benefit for the addition of rituximab among the patients expressing BCL2 (Fig. 15–7).[153] An analysis of E4494 did not find this relationship between BCL2 protein expression and benefit with rituximab. In E4494, the lack of BCL6 expression was associated with a poorer outcome for patients receiving CHOP (without maintenance), which was not seen in patients receiving rituximab.[154] It is possible that in these studies, BCL2 expression or lack of BCL6 expression is a surrogate for another distinguishing feature such as nongerminal center lymphomas.[155] Based on these data, it is premature to use the expression of BCL2 protein or the lack of expression of BCL6 protein to select patients for treatment with chemotherapy alone versus chemo-immunotherapy.

DLBCL: Relapse

The curative potential of HDT/ASCT is restricted to relapsed chemosensitive patients.[156] Thus, the effectiveness of the second-line regimen is of paramount importance. To be suitable as pretransplant therapy, a second-line regimen should have the following features: effective cytoreduction, low incidence of nonhematologic toxicity, brief duration of therapy, and ability to mobilize peripheral blood progenitor cells.[157–160] Numerous second-line regimens have been evaluated for the treatment of relapsed and refractory NHL.[161–167] The ICE (ifosfamide, carboplatin, etoposide) regimen was developed to minimize the nonhematologic toxicity associated with second-line therapy.[161] Rituximab has been added to the ICE regimen,[165] improving the CR rate compared to a historical control, and has provided a trend to improve long-term outcome. However, this was in a group of rituximab-naive patients; the effectiveness in patients already failing chemo-immunotherapy is unknown. This is being addressed in the ongoing Collaborative Trial in Relapse Aggressive Lymphoma (CORAL) study, which compares the R-ICE chemotherapy to R-DHAP chemotherapy with a second randomization to post-HDT/ASCT rituximab or observation.

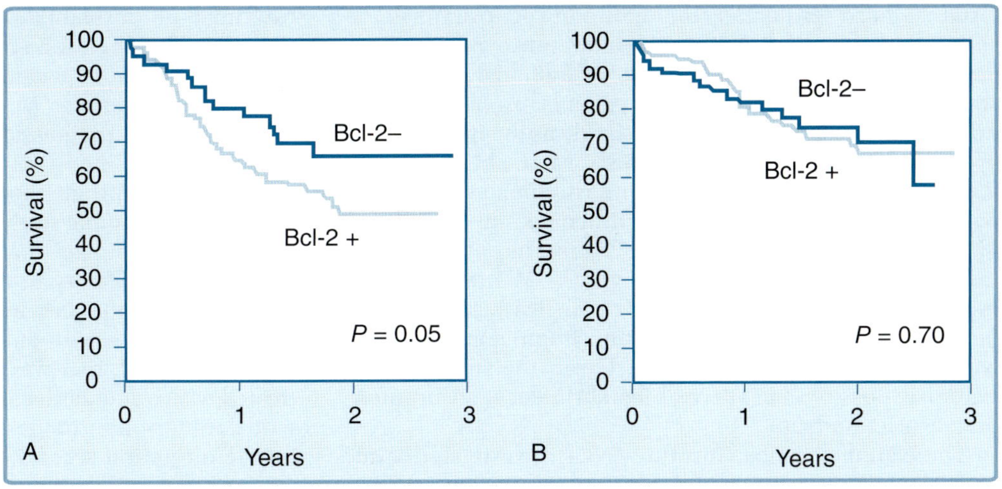

Figure 15–7. Rituximab can overcome the adverse effect of Bel-2 expression in DLBCL. (From Mounier N, Briere J, Gisselbrecht C, et al. Rituximab plus CHOP (R-CHOP) overcomes bcl-2–associated resistance to chemotherapy in elderly patients with diffuse large B-cell lymphoma (DLBCL). Blood 2003;101:4279–84,[153] with permission.)

Investigators at Stanford University Medical School have evaluated the role of rituximab administered as an adjuvant (two 4-week courses at day 42 and day 180) following HDT/ASCT in NHL.[168] This study included various histologies including DLBCL (71%, n = 25), MCL (9%, n = 3), and other B-cell lymphomas (20%, n = 7). In a subset analysis restricted to the patients with relapsed (n = 13) or refractory (n = 8) DLBCL, the 2-year estimated EFS and OS were 81% and 85%, respectively. These are very intriguing results, but interpretation is limited because the patients were rituximab naive; thus, the impact of prior rituximab is unknown. Similar results have been reported for adjuvant rituximab after both autologous and allogeneic stem cell transplant.[169] This approach is being tested in an ongoing ECOG trial comparing adjuvant rituximab to observation.

DLBCL: Early Stage

The Southwest Oncology Group (SWOG) has presented results of a pilot study investigating the role of chemo-immunotherapy with R-CHOP for three cycles followed by involved-field radiotherapy (IFRT).[170] Patients with one or more risk factors according to a modified IPI were eligible. Early results suggest an improvement in PFS, but not OS, compared to historical controls at 2 years. Outside the setting of a clinical trial, the evidence would support the use of R-CHOPx3 and IFRT for patients with limited-stage disease with risk factors. For patients with very limited-stage disease (Clinical Stage [CS] I, no risk factors), CHOPx3 and IFRT have excellent results. In practice, very limited-stage patients are not likely to be distinguished from limited-stage patients, and therefore the addition of rituximab to the CHOP would be appropriate given that there is no trial evidence to support this approach. However, definitive evidence of superiority of this approach requires a randomized comparison of chemo-immunotherapy versus chemo-immunotherapy and IFRT. For patients with bulky disease, treatment with regimens appropriate for aggressive lymphoma should be used. Because of the lack of vindesine in the United States, the ACVBP (doxorubicin, cyclophosphamide, vindesine, bleomycin, prednisone) regimen cannot be used.

Mantle Cell Lymphoma

The MDACC group built on their experience with the alternating hyper-CVAD (cyclophosphamide, etoposide, doxorubicin, dexamethasone) and MA (methotrexate cytarabine) with the addition of rituximab. Rituximab was added to both of the alternating regimens that were administered for a total of six to eight cycles (hyper-CVAD and MA are counted as separate cycles).[171] Ninety-seven patients were treated, and the CR/CRu rate after six cycles was 87%. The estimated 3-year EFS and OS were 67% and 81%, respectively. Despite these encouraging results, the survival curve has no plateau, and there is a steady relapse rate over time, suggesting that the R-hyper-CVAD/R-MA regimen alone was not curative. The toxicity of the regimen was significant with five deaths on study (5%), and four patients subsequently developing myelodysplasia syndrome (MDS) with three deaths.

Investigators at the DFCI tested the addition of rituximab to CHOP chemotherapy.[172] Forty patients were treated in this trial with an overall response rate of 96% (CR 48%). The median PFS was 16.6 months, or no different than historical controls. Twenty-five of the patients had a t(11;14) translocation breakpoint that was amplifiable by the PCR. Nine of 25 patients who had informative PCR achieved a molecular remission. The median PFS was the same in patients who achieved a molecular remission as those who did not.

The GLSG undertook a large randomized Phase III study of CHOP with or without rituximab for patients with untreated mantle cell lymphoma.[173] There was a secondary randomization that was stratified by age: patients over 60 years were randomized to two doses of adjuvant interferon alpha, and the younger patients were randomized to adjuvant HDT/ASCT or interferon alpha. A total of 122 patients were randomized: CHOP, n = 60; and R-CHOP, n = 62. Analyzed according to initial randomization, R-CHOP was significantly superior to CHOP in overall response rate (94% vs. 75%; p = 0.0054) and complete remission rate (34% vs. 7%; p = 0.00024). There was also a significant benefit in the median TTF (21 vs. 14 months, p = 0.0131). Despite the improvement in TTF, there was no advantage to the chemo-immunotherapy arm in PFS or OS.

GLSG also evaluated the addition of rituximab to FCM (fludarabine, cyclophosphamide, mitroxantrone) for patients with relapsed and refractory follicular lymphoma and mantle cell lymphoma (24 patients in each arm).[138] Addition of rituximab did not significantly improve the overall response rate (FCM-R 58% vs. FCM 46%, p = 0.282), but there were 29% CRs with rituximab versus none without. Although there was no difference in the median PFS (FCM-R 8 months vs. FCM 4 months, p = 0.3887), there was a difference in median OS (FCM-R not reached vs. FCM 11 months, p = 0.0042). It is unclear why the treatment could result in a significant improvement of OS without an improvement in PFS. Given the small sample size, it is possible the survival benefit reflects an unintentional selection bias.

The National Cancer Institute (NCI) investigators evaluated DA-EPOCH-R with idiotype vaccination in patients with untreated MCL.[174] Twenty-six patients were treated with DA-EPOCH-R with an overall response rate of 100% (complete response 92%). Interestingly, the proliferation signature that had been identified to be important in the outcome of patients with MCL treated with CHOP-based regimens[175,176] was not predictive of outcome with DA-EPOCH-R. The mechanism by which this regimen would overcome the proliferation signature is unknown. The impact of the idiotype vaccination on outcome is unknown. The DA-EPOCH-R regimen profoundly impacted on humoral responses, although T-cell responses to the Id-KLH/GM-CSF vaccine were seen.

Bioimmunotherapy with Rituximab

Combination with Interferon-α

Among the immunomodulatory effects of INF-α is the enhancement of antibody-dependent, cell-mediated cytotoxicity.[177,178] As mentioned above, based on the murine model, ADCC is thought to be central to the activity of rituximab.[100] Based on the rationale that both INF-α and rituximab have independent activity in indolent lymphoma, Davis and colleagues reported the results of a Phase II trial combining rituximab and interferon in 38 patients with indolent B-cell lymphoma.[179] Patients were to be treated with INF-α at a dose of 2.5 million or 5 million units three times weekly for 12 weeks (ideal 36 doses, mean actually delivered was 31). Starting on week 5, the patients received rituximab on the standard schedule of 375 mg/m^2/week for 4 weeks. The overall response rate was 45%, not different than the result expected with single-agent rituximab.[88] However, in contrast to the pivotal study in which the median time to progression of responders was 13 months, with the combined INF-α and rituximab therapy, the median time to progression of responders was 25.2 months. However, the sample size was too small to conclude that the combination resulted in a superior outcome; a randomized trial will be necessary to answer this question. The Nordic Lymphoma Group has investigated the addition of interferon to patients with suboptimal responses to rituximab. Patients with FL that was untreated or in first relapse were treated with a standard 4-week course of rituximab. Patients with a minor or partial response were randomly assigned to interferon with a second course of rituximab to rituximab alone. A report of preliminary results suggests an improvement in response to the combined therapy, although final results of this study have not been published.[180] There is no information regarding the durability of response.

Combination with Interleukin-2

Interleukin-2 has several biological activities (Table 15–2) that could potentiate the effectiveness of monoclonal antibodies, including enhancing ADCC and independent antitumor activity.[181] In a report by Friedberg and colleagues, low-dose IL-2 was given to 20 patients with refractory and relapsed FL for 56 days with rituximab (375 mg/m^2), given on days 15, 22, 29, and 36.[182] The IL-2 increased circulating CD8+ and CD56+ cells in all evaluable patients. The overall response rate and response duration were 55% and 13 months, respectively, very similar to the single-agent activity of rituximab.

Gluck and colleagues conducted another evaluation of IL-2 and rituximab; the hypothesis was that the expansion of NK cells would augment ADCC.[183] Rituximab was given at a dose of 375 mg/m^2 weekly for 4 weeks. Two IL-2 schedules were evaluated: daily (MTD 6 MIU) or thrice weekly (MTD 14 MIU). The dose-limiting toxicities were asthenia and reversible transaminase elevations. Of patients treated at the MTD, five of nine patients on the daily schedule showed a response and four of five patients on the three-times-per-week schedule responded, with a median TTP of 14.9 and 16.1 months, respectively. The biological effect as measured by NK cell levels was greater on the three-times-

Table 15–2. Potentially Beneficial Effects of Cytokines for Non-Hodgkin's Lymphoma

INF-α	INF-γ	IL-12	IL-2
Enhanced cell-mediated cytotoxicity	Enhanced cell-mediated cytotoxicity	Enhanced cell-mediated cytotoxicity	Enhanced cell-mediated cytotoxicity
Inhibition of IL-4 and IL5 production	Inhibition of IL-4 and IL5 production	Induction of INF-γ production	Induction of INF-γ production
Inhibition of tumor cell growth	Primes dendritic cells for IL-12 production	Primes dendritic cells for cytokine production	Enhances expression of IL-12 receptors
Enhanced MHC class I protein expression	Enhanced MHC class II protein expression	Inhibition of IL-4 and IL-5 production	Prevents Stat 4 dephosphorylation during chronic IL-12 administration

From Rook AH, Kuzel TM, Olsen EA. Cytokine therapy of cutaneous T-cell lymphoma: interferons, interleukin-12, and interleukin-2. Hematol Oncol Clin North Am 2003;17:1435–48, ix,[181] with permission.

per-week schedule. ADCC activity was increased and maintained after IL-2 therapy in responder patients and those with stable disease. Thus, the data are not clear if there is a benefit. However, the results from the Gluck study justify continued evaluation of IL-2 in combination with rituximab in a larger patient population.

Combination with Interleukin-12

IL-12 also can potentiate the ADCC, and induces the production of INF-γ, which can exert an anti-angiogenic effect (Table 15–2). Ansell and colleagues at the Mayo Clinic conducted a Phase I study of the combination of a standard 4-week course of rituximab with twice weekly IL-12 given at escalating doses of 30 ng/kg to 500 ng/kg in patients with B-cell NHL.[184] Dose-limiting toxicities were flu-like symptoms and liver function abnormalities. At IL-2 doses above 100 ng/mL, both INF-γ and IP-10 levels were increased above baseline. Responses were seen in 29 of 43 patients, with 11 CRs; CRs were more common at doses greater than or equal to 300 ng/mL. Unlike the IL-2 study above, both the ORR and CR rate were higher than expected, and the combination deserves additional evaluation. NK cell lytic activity was not increased in patients receiving the combination of IL-12 and rituximab except at the 300 ng/kg dose. This combination requires further evaluation.[185]

Combination with Thalidomide

Kaufman and colleagues in Vienna reported a novel combination of rituximab and thalidomide for the treatment of MCL.[186] The rationale was based on the anecdotal observation of disease stabilization induced by thalidomide in a patient with refractory MCL. Sixteen patients with mantle cell lymphoma relapsing (n = 15) or progressing (n = 1) following anthracycline-containing therapy were treated with rituximab 375 mg/m^2 four times weekly and thalidomide 200 mg po daily for 14 days, and then increased to 400 mg po daily, which was continued until progression or relapse. Thirteen of 16 patients had an objective response to the combination, with CR/CRu in five and PR in eight. Disease in both nodal and extranodal sites responded to treatment. The median PFS was 20.4 months, which was superior to the prior course of therapy in which the median PFS was 12.7 months. The basis for this activity is uncertain. It may be a consequent alteration in the tumor microenvironment induced by thalidomide.[187] An alternative explanation is the thalidomide has an immunomodulatory effect that potentiates NK- and LAK-mediating killing.[188] This combination deserves further study.

Epratuzumab

CD22

The B-cell antigen CD22 is a 135-kD B-cell antigen; it is a sialoglycoprotein that is widely expressed as a cytoplasmic protein, but is a surface protein in late stages of B-cell ontogeny, and expression is lost on differentiation to the plasma cell.[189] Two isoforms, α and β, are expressed that arise from alternative splicing (Fig. 15–8); the β isoform is more commonly expressed. The intracellular domain has immunoreceptor tyrosine–based motifs (ITIMs) that are phosphorylated with activation of the B-cell receptor (BCR). The ITIM can bind the SHP-1 tyrosine phosphatase, which inhibits BCR signaling. CD22 has two functions. First, it acts as an adhesion molecule with specificity for sialic acid in the α2,6-linkage, which has a role in controlling homing to the bone marrow. Second, CD22 is a negative regulator of BCR signaling. In mice in which CD22 has been knocked out, there is an augmented immune response, heightened calcium fluxes, and cell proliferation obtained at lower antigen concentrations, B-cell signaling is hyperresponsive, peritoneal B-1 cell population is expanded, and autoantibody titers are increased.[190] CD22 internalizes rapidly after binding to ligand or anti-CD22 antibodies, and even undergoes constitutive internalization on unstimulated B cells.[191]

CD22 expression in lymphoid organs is in follicular mantle and marginal zone B cells with general sparing of the germinal center.[192] CD22 expression on malignant B cell varies from 60% to 85%, depending on a number of variable including lymphoma subtype, antibody used, tissue preservation, and detection by flow versus flow cytometry.[193] Anti-CD22 monoclonal antibodies can block CD22-ligand interactions, which induce cell death in BL cell lines.[194] Tumor reductions have been seen in xenograft models with unmodified, radiolabeled, and toxin-conjugated antibodies.[195–198]

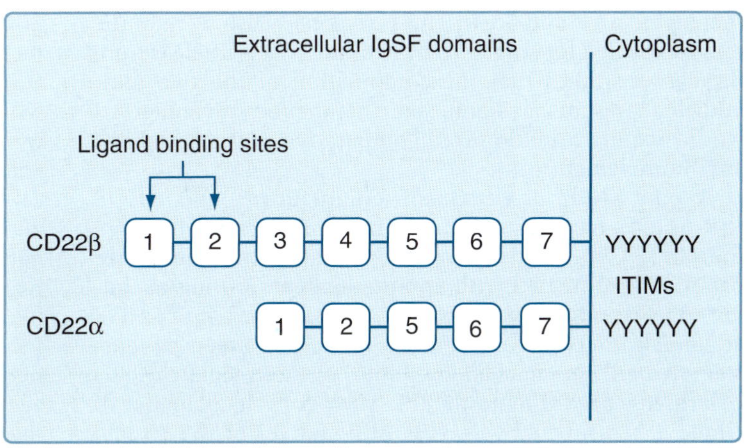

Figure 15–8. Structure of CD22. (Modified from Cesano A, Gayko U. CD22 as a target of passive immunotherapy. Semin Oncol 2003;30:253–7,[189] with permission.)

Clinical Results with Epratuzumab

The lineage restriction and the preclinical activity suggested that the anti-CD22 antibody, epratuzumab, had potential antilymphoma agent in the clinic. Leonard and his colleagues at Weill Cornell Medical Center conducted a Phase I/II study of epratuzumab using a 4-week dose escalation schedule in patients with refractory indolent and aggressive lymphoma.[199,200] Fifty-five patients with indolent NHL (FL 40, SLL [IWF] 13, marginal zone lymphoma 1, acute lymphoblastic leukemia [ALL] 1) were treated with escalating doses of epratuzumab ranging from 120 mg/m^2 to 1000 mg/m^2, and the toxicity was mild. The most common toxicities were nausea, fatigue, back pain, and anemia; Grade 3 or 4 toxicity was uncommon, and no human anti-human antibody was seen. B-cell (75%) but not T-cell depletion was seen, which persisted for up to 9 months. The bulk of patients (n = 25) were treated at the 360 mg/m^2 and 480 mg/m^2 doses. Eight of 51 evaluable patients had a response (3 CR and 6 PR). All the responders were patients with FL; the median TTP for responders was 20 months. A cohort of 56 patients with aggressive NHL (DLBCL 35, MCL 9, MZL 4, FL 8) had similar toxicity. In this group, there were five responders among the 52 evaluable patients all of whom had DLBCL. This Phase I/II experience demonstrated that the unmodified anti-CD22 antibody had single-agent activity in NHL.

Based on preclinical data suggesting an additive benefit, rituximab and epratuzumab have been tested in combination and presented as preliminary results.[201,202] In the study by Leonard and colleagues, epratuzumab was given at a dose of 360 mg/m^2 followed by rituximab at a dose of 375 mg/m^2 weekly for 4 weeks. Twenty-one patients were treated with FL (n = 15), MZL (n = 1), and DLBCL (n = 5). The combination was well tolerated and similar to antibody monotherapy. Nineteen patients were evaluable for response: DLBCL two of three (CR 1, PR 1); indolent NHL 8 of 16 (CR 4, CRu 3, PR 1). Although the ORR was similar to monotherapy, the quality of the responses was better than expected. The study by Strauss and colleagues was a multicenter European study for patients with relapsed/refractory NHL. The dosing was the same as the Leonard study, and treatment was well tolerated. Sixty-five patients were enrolled with indolent lymphoma (n = 45, 36 FL) and aggressive lymphoma (n = 20, 13 DLBCL). Of the 35 evaluable patients with indolent lymphoma, 20 responded, with 8 CR/CRu and 12 PR. Among the 13 patients with DLBCL, there were 3 PR and 3 CR. These responses also were in the range expected for single-agent rituximab. It is unclear from these two studies that the combination of the two antibodies represents a significant therapeutic advantage; it would require a randomized comparative trial to establish any improvement.

A pilot study of rituximab, epratuzumab, and CHOP (ER-CHOP) has been conducted in a collaboration between the Mayo Clinic and Stanford University.[203] In this study, patients were treated with epratuzumab at 360 mg/m^2 followed by rituximab at 375 mg/m^2, and standard dose CHOP at 3-week intervals for six to eight cycles. Fifteen patients were treated. Patients had low (46%) or intermediate (46%) risk disease according to the IPI. The per cycle incidence of Grade 4 neutropenia was 31%, although 13 of the 15 had at least one episode of Grade 4 neutropenia. There were 14 evaluable patients for response, with 7 CR and 5 PR. The regimen appeared to be associated with greater than expected toxicity, but only a randomized comparison with R-CHOP could evaluate if there is a benefit to the addition of epratuzumab.

T-Cell Lymphoma

There is limited experience using monoclonal antibodies for T-cell lymphoma. There is limited experience using antibodies directed at CD3, CD4, and CD5, but the toxicity proved to be significant. For example, Bertram and colleagues evaluated a murine anti-CD5 antibody T101 for the treatment of T-cell lymphoma.[204] Eight patients with CTCL and 5 patients with other T-cell lymphoma were treated with 1 to 500 mg administered weekly. There was one CR (peripheral T-cell lymphoma) and one PR (CLTCL). However, there was significant toxicity associated with the administration of the antibody, including superventricular arrhythmia, blood pressure instability, shortness of breath, pruritus, hives, and flushing. HAMA developed in three patients. With this murine monoclonal antibody, toxicity outweighed the benefit, precluding further clinical development.

Waldman and his colleagues at the NCI used the murine anti-CD25 antibody to treat patients with HTLV-1–associated ATLL.[205] CD25 is not expressed on normal resting T cells, and provides a more targeted therapy than some other T-cell–restricted antigens. As a result, the antibody infusions were well tolerated, and normal T cells were not depleted from the peripheral blood. Nineteen patients were treated with PR in four patients and CR in two. However, the effectiveness was limited by development of HAMA and the short half-life of infused antibodies.[27] Humanized anti-Tac (HAT) antibodies have been derived from an $IgG_1\kappa$ and are more effective in ADCC; they are currently in clinical trials.

Alemtuzumab is a humanized anti-CD52 monoclonal antibody that has been approved for the treatment of relapsed and refractory CLL.[206] CD52 is a GPI-anchored glycoprotein that is highly expressed on both B and T cells, including many lymphoid malignancies. Enblad and colleagues conducted a pilot study of alemtuzumab for patients with relapsed or refractory peripheral T-cell lymphoma.[207] Fourteen heavily pretreated patients were enrolled and treated with 3 mg on day 1, 10 mg on day 3, and then 30 mg three times per week for up to 12 weeks. Patients received a median of 6 weeks of therapy. Toxicity was similar to other trials with this antibody; infusion reactions with chills were common, and hypotension and dyspnea were less common. There was significant hematologic toxicity with pancytopenia in four patients. Infectious complications were also common with CMV reactivation in six patients, one patient died of miliary tuberculosis, one patient died of a generalized herpes zoster infection, and two patients developed pulmonary aspergillosis. Overall, five patients responded to treatment, with three CR and two PR. Although there was some clinical activity, there were five treatment-related deaths; further development of this agent for peripheral T-cell lymphoma would require effective means of controlling the infectious complications.

RADIOIMMUNOTHERAPY

Most subtypes of NHL are sensitive to radiation therapy, and particularly MCL and FL. The systemic nature of these diseases limits the role of external beam radiation therapy to the uncommon cases of localized disease or use in a palliative mode. Total body irradiation is commonly used in the context of HDT/ASCT, but toxicity limits its use without stem cell support. Radioimmunoconjugates offer an alternative approach to the delivery of radiation in which radiation is targeted by the specificity of a monoclonal antibody.[208] One of the potential benefits of radioimmunotherapy (RIT) over unmodified antibodies is the cross-fire effect (Fig. 15–9). The nuclear decay of the radioisotope delivers radiation to nearby cells that may have not been targeted as a result of antigen variation or limitation of diffusion into the tumor. However, it is the cross fire that is also a potential source of toxicity because normal cells adjacent to the tumor will receive radiation. This is particularly a problem in the bone marrow; for this reason, most studies limit the extent of bone marrow involvement to less than 25% of the intratrebecular space.

Two anti-CD20 radioimmunotherapy agents have been approved by the FDA: 90Y-ibritumomab tiuxetan and iodine I131 tositumomab. In Phase II studies, both agents have demonstrated activity in patients with relapsed and refractory indolent lymphoma, rituximab-refractory, and transformed lymphoma with ORR (40% to 84%) and TTP of 8 to 16 months.[208–214] For a subset of, the remissions following RIT can be very durable.[215] Toxicity of the treatment is largely hematological. The risk of secondary leukemia is similar to other patients with multiple recurrent indolent lymphoma.[216]

Indolent Lymphoma

Single-Agent Anti-CD20 RIT

Two randomized studies have been conducted to demonstrate superiority over unlabeled antibody. A comparison of the murine antibody tositumomab was compared to iodine I131 tositumomab to determine if the radioisotope contributed to the efficacy of the drug.[84] Seventy-eight patients were randomized. ORR significantly favored the radiolabeled antibody compared to the unlabeled antibody: 55% versus 19% ($p = 0.002$). Median response duration (not reached vs. 28.1 months) and TTP (6.3 months vs. 5.3 months, $p = 0.031$) favored the radiolabeled antibody. Patients with disease progression after tositumomab could cross over to the iodine I131 tositumomab arm. Following cross over to RIT, the ORR (68% vs. 16%, $p = 0.002$), median response durations (12.6 vs. 7.6 months, $p = 0.001$), and median TTP (12.4 vs. 5.5 months, $p = 0.01$) were superior to results with prior unlabeled antibody response. This trial clearly demonstrates that the radioisotope adds efficacy to the treatment.

In the second randomized trial, rituximab was compared to 90Y-ibritumomab tiuxetan to determine if the radioantibody was superior to the chimeric unlabeled antibody.[217] The primary endpoint was ORR, and it was underpowered to identify differences in PFS. A total of 143 patients were randomized to rituximab alone (70) or RIT (73). The OR and CR rates favored the RIT arm: 80% versus 56% ($p = 0.002$), and 30% versus 16% ($p = 0.04$). TTP was not different between arms, but durable responses of 6 months or greater were seen more often following RIT than rituximab (64% vs. 47%, $p = 0.03$). These data support the conclusion that RIT provides superior responses, but larger randomized trials are needed to demonstrate if there are benefits in EFS and OS.

RIT as Initial Therapy

Kaminski and colleagues at the University of Michigan conducted a recent provocative study of iodine I131 tositumomab as initial therapy for FL demonstrated high response (OR 95%, CR 75%).[218] With PCR for the t(14;18) translocation, 80% of the informative patients had molecular remissions. Median PFS was 6.1 years. Toxicity was principally hematological and readily reversible. These results suggest that in selected patients, a single course of RIT can have substantial long-term benefit.

RIT for Minimal Residual Disease Following Chemotherapy

RIT could provide radiation to all sites of disease without the toxicity and technical difficulty of TBI. SWOG conducted a pilot study, S9911, to evaluate the safety and efficacy of adjuvant iodine I131 tositumomab following a

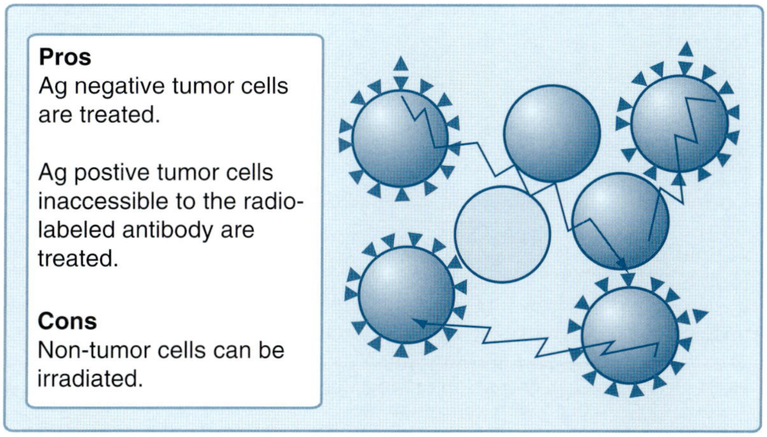

Figure 15–9. The cross-fire effect. (From Zelenetz AD. Radioimmunotherapy for lymphoma. Curr Opin Oncol 1999;11:375–80,[208] with permission.)

course of six cycles of CHOP chemotherapy.[219] Toxicity was primarily hematological and was more severe during the chemotherapy than during the RIT. ORR was 90%. The final response after RIT improved in 57% of the patients who had less than a CR to CHOP. The estimated 2-year EFS and OS were 81% and 97%, respectively. This trial established the feasibility of sequential chemotherapy and RIT. It is currently being evaluated in a Phase III comparison to rituximab and CHOP chemotherapy (SWOG S0016).

Mantle Cell Lymphoma

MCL is sensitive to radiation; however, the role of external beam is limited in the management of the disease because of the systemic nature of the disease. Radioimmunotherapy is a means of providing systemic radiation therapy to multiple sites of disease. Preliminary results of two trials have been presented. Untreated patients with MCL were treated with sequential radioimmunotherapy (RIT) with iodine I131 tositumomab (65 to 75 cGy, whole body) followed by conventional CHOP chemotherapy.[220] There was an overall response rate to the RIT of 83% (CR 50%), and the chemotherapy improved the CR to 90%. Investigators at MDACC treated a group of 15 patients with relapsed and refractory MCL with 90Y-ibritumomab tiuxetan (0.3 to 0.4 mCi 90Y/kg).[221] There was an overall response rate of 33% (all CR/CRu). These trials are very preliminary, and response durations are not available, although they suggest that conventional dose RIT has activity in both untreated and relapsed/refractory disease.

At the Fred Hutchinson Cancer Research Center (FHCRC), the role of high-dose RIT with stem cell support for MCL was investigated.[222] The systemic distribution of disease with extensive bone marrow and peripheral blood involvement raised the concern that the dosimetry of RIT in MCL would be different that other tumors. In 25 patients with MCL treated with high-dose RIT, the biodistribution and dosimetry were similar to other histologies.[223] Sixteen patients were treated with iodine I131 tositumomab at a dose calibrated to deliver 20 to 25 Gy to normal organs, followed 10 days later by high-dose etoposide (30 to 60 mg/kg) and cyclophosphamide (60 to 100 mg/kg). Patients then had autologous stem cell reinfused. At 3 years, the PFS and OS were 61% and 91%, respectively, in a population that had a median of three prior treatment and seven patients with chemorefractory disease. Substitution of high-dose RIT is a promising approach, but larger controlled studies are necessary to validate these findings.

T-Cell Lymphoma

Waldman and his colleagues at the NCI have pioneered the development of radiolabeled anti-CD25 therapy. Eighteen patients with ATLL were treated with ^{90}Y-labeled anti-CD25; the first nine patients were dose escalated, and the remainder were treated at a uniform 10-mCi dose; responding patients could receive up to eight additional doses.[224] Sixteen patients were evaluable for response, with a PR in 7 and CR in 2. The remissions were more durable than a previous trial using unmodified anti-CD25. Toxicity was largely hematological. To improve the tumor to blood dosing radiation, they have explored the role of pretargeting (see Future Directions).

Future Directions

RIT directed at other targets has been evaluated clinically including CD19, CD21, CD22, and HLA-DR.[225–228] The radiolabeled Lym-1 and epratuzumab have shown significant clinical activity, and further development is ongoing. A variety of radioisotopes other than yttrium-90 and iodine-131 have been evaluated, and some have potential clinical advantages in particular clinical situations. For example, alpha-particle emitters have the ability to kill cells with the energy from a single disintegration; combined with the extremely short path length for energy discharge, alpha emitters are potential isotopes to address minimal residual disease.[229] Other isotopes have been evaluated (Table 15–3) including beta emitters, alpha emitters, and auger emitters.[230–232] Although some of these alternative radionuclides have superior properties in comparison to iodine-131 and yttrium-90, some have limited availability and are quite expensive. However, trials evaluating these alternatives are ongoing.

Table 15–3. Radioisotopes Potentially Useful in Lymphoma Radioimmunotherapy

Radionuclide	Therapeutic Emission	Imaging Emission	Residualizing	Availability
Iodine-131	β	γ	No	Excellent
Yttrium-90	β	None	Yes	Excellent
Copper-67	β	γ	Yes	Fair
Lutetium-177	β	γ	Yes	Fair
Rhenium-186	β	γ	No	Excellent
Rhenium-188	β	None	No	Excellent
Copper-64	Positron	Positron	Yes	Fair
Bismuth-213	α	γ	Unknown	Fair
Actinium-225	α,β	γ	Unknown	Fair
Iodine-125	Auger	None	No	Fair
Iodine-123	Auger	γ	No	Excellent
Indium-111	Auger	γ	Yes	Excellent

From DeNardo GL. Concepts in radioimmunotherapy and immunotherapy: radioimmunotherapy from a lym-1 perspective. Semin Oncol 2005;32:S27–35,[228] with permission.

One of the limitations of using conventional radioimmunoconjugates is the relatively low ratio of dose to tumor relative to some normal organs. One approach to address this problem has been the development of pretargeting strategies. Another approach is to administer streptavidin conjugated antibodies followed by a clearing agent; then the radioisotope bound to biotin is administered, which can then target to tumor, nonbound radio-biotin is rapidly cleared.[233] This approach has been evaluated both preclinically and clinically with demonstration of favorable dosimetry with improved tumor to normal organ ratios.[233–236] Another approach to pretargeting is the use of bispecific monoclonal antibodies (bsMAb) that recognize targets and a peptide that can be radiolabeled.[237] Sharkey and colleagues coupled the Fab' of the humanized anti-CD20 antibody hA20 to the Fab' of a murine antibody directed against the peptide histamine-succinyl-glycine (HSG). Animals treated with the bsMAb were followed 48 hours later by administration of radiolabeled HSG, and compared to animals treated with a directly conjugated antibody. At 3 hours, the tumor:blood ratios for the pretargeted were similar to the best ratio achieved by the directly conjugated antibodies (which occurred at day 7). However, after 1 day, the pretargeting approach was 10-fold higher than the directly conjugated antibody. The animals also had a superior response compared to the directly conjugated antibody. These pretargeted approaches are potentially very effective, and further clinical development is ongoing.

ENGINEERED T CELLS

Incubation of peripheral blood lymphocytes with cytokines can induce nonspecific cytotoxic antitumor effector cells such as LAK or CIK cells (see Nonspecific Immunotherapy section above). Another approach that has been used to expand autoreactive T cells is ex vivo expansion with beads doubly coated with anti-CD3 and anti-CD28 to provide a potent proliferative response.[238] A Phase I study has been completed with cells using this approach in patients with relapsed/refractory NHL undergoing HDT/ASCT.[239] Of 36 patients enrolled, 22 proceeded to HDT/ASCT and 17 received the ex vivo expanded T cells. Patients received escalating doses of T cells. Toxicity included fever and infusion reactions, as well as an episode of CHF at dose level 3. One Grade 3 CNS neurotoxicity occurred at dose level 2. Five patients developed a delayed lymphocytosis, and 10 patients had a relative lymphocytosis. In vivo, there was restoration of INF-γ secretion following intracellular stimulation with PMA (phorbol myristate acetate) and ionomycin but incomplete restoration of PHA (phytohemagglutinin) responsiveness. In this small study, it was impossible to determine if the infusion of these cells altered the clinical outcome. The technology of the ex vivo expansion has been optimized, and by varying the culture conditions (specifically the ratio of anti-CD28 to anti-CD3), antigen-specific T cells can be expanded.[240] These cells are currently being evaluated in clinical trials in patients with CLL.

Another approach to using T cells therapeutically is to engineer cytotoxic cells to recognize a specific antigen. Brentjens and colleagues at MSKCC have reported on the transduction of T cells with a chimeric antigen receptor capable of binding to CD19 on B cells, and the subsequent in vitro expansion of T cells with IL-15 and CD80 stimulation.[241] These transduced T cells can kill tumors in a murine model system. Furthermore, the transduced T cells from a patient with CLL can lyse autologous CLL cells in vitro. This approach will be evaluated in clinical trials in CLL and NHL.

Investigators from the City of Hope Medical Center (COH) and the FHCRC have used a similar approach, transducing T cells with a chimeric antigen receptor recognizing CD20.[242,243] Following cloning and ex vivo expansion, the engineered T cells expressed INF-γ in response to binding to CD20. These cells can be expanded in the presence of lymphoma and IL-2. The cells can lyse fresh tumors from patients with FL, SLL, splenic marginal zone lymphoma (SMZL), CLL, and DLBCL. Phase I clinical trials have been initiated using these engineered T cells.

Bispecific Antibodies

Conventional monoclonal antibodies target tumors by the specificity of the variable region, and activate effector mechanism via the Fc domains (Fig. 15–3). Bispecific antibodies combine two targeting domains, one for the tumor, and a second for some form of effector. Bispecific antibodies have been derived by chemical coupling the Fab' fragments from two antibodies or by somatic cell methods, and therefore have been a challenge to manufacture on a clinical scale. Newer molecular techniques have become available to engineer bispecific single-chain antibodies that may have some manufacturing advantages.[244] There have been limited clinical trials with bispecific antibodies in lymphoid malignancies; however, some preliminary data are available.

Hartmann and colleagues in Germany have studied a bispecific antibody, HRS-3/A9, in HD that recognizes CD30 on the tumor cell and CD16 (FcγRIIIA) on effector cells.[245–247] In the initial Phase I trial, patients received up to 64 mg/m^2, which was the maximum dose because of limited availability of HRS-3/A9. The treatment was well tolerated, although the development of HAMA antibodies was seen in 9 of 15 patients, and 4 patients developed allergic reactions precluding continued therapy. Nonetheless, two responses were seen among the 15 patients treated. In a subsequent trial, patients were treated with either a CI for 4 days or an every-other-day bolus schedule. In responding patients, re-treatment was attempted after 4 weeks, and in patients with stable disease, a second course was given after IL-2 treatment and followed by GM-CSF. Sixteen patients were treated with 1 CR and 3 PR; three responses occurred in patients receiving the bispecific antibody by CI. Two of the responses occurred after the first cycle of therapy. Five patients with stable disease (SD) after one cycle received cytokines plus HRS-3/A9, and two additional patients responded. The IL-2 significantly increased NK cell levels in all five patients treated. A larger study would be needed to confirm that CI and cytokines are important in the activity of HRS-3/A9. The major hurdle to further study has been the manufacture of the bsMAb.

Another trial of a bsMAb in HD was conducted by Borchmann and colleagues using the bispecific antibody H22xKi-4.[248] The bsMAb was derived from chemical coupling of Fab' fragments of the anti-CD30 antibody Ki-4 and the humanized anti-CD64 (FcγRI) antibody. The resulting bsMAb binds to tumor cells and monocytes, neutrophils, and macrophages. Toxicity in this Phase I study included mild hypotension, tachycardia, fatigue, and fever. Ten patients were treated with escalating doses (1 to 20 mg/m^2) every other day for four doses; four responses were seen, three PR and one CR. Further investigation is ongoing with this bsMAb.

Manzke and colleagues conducted a Phase I study of a CD3xCD19 bsMAb for indolent lymphoma.[249] The rationale was to recruit T cells and activate them in situ with an anti-CD28 antibody. In this pilot study, both the bsMAb and the anti-CD28 antibody were injected into a single site at increasing doses (30 μg to 1600 μg). Toxicity included injection-site erythema, particularly at the higher dose levels. HAMA developed in 5 of the 10 patients, and 2 patients had a locoregional response. Elevation of serum TNFα at 2 or 3 days post-therapy suggested activation of CD4-positive T cells. This study provided proof of concept that targeting T cells is possible.

Other combinations of targets have been explored preclinically, including CD64xCD19 and CD64xCD37.[250] Despite the provocative preclinical and clinical data, bsMAb has important practical limitations as a consequence of immunogenicity and manufacture. However, practical development will certainly depend on successful development of molecular bsMAbs that can address these important limitations.

Immunotoxins and Ligand Toxins

Arming antibodies with toxins is another approach to increasing antibody potency. Several immunotoxins have been investigated. Anti-B4 (anti-CD19)–blocked ricin was originally evaluated for treatment of B-cell NHL. Although early-phase clinical trials suggested some activity, a randomized Phase III trial for minimal residual disease following HDT/ASCT was negative, and further clinical development has been halted.[54,251] Other evaluated immunotoxins—H65-RTA (ricin A) against CD5, RFB4-deglycosylated ricin A directed against CD25, and anti-Tac(Fv)-PE38 (pseudomonas endotoxin) against CD25—have all shown some clinical activity, but are associated with vascular leak syndrome, and limited by anti-immunotoxin antibodies.[55,56,252]

One of the most clinically active immunotoxins to date has been BL22, a recombinant immunotoxin containing an anti-CD22 variable domain fused to truncated pseudomonas endotoxin.[253] Thirty-one patients with B-cell lymphoma were enrolled in a dose escalation trial, 16 of whom had chemoresistant hairy cell leukemia (HCL). To diminish the inflammatory adverse effects, patients treated with ≥40 μg/kg of BL22 were given infliximab (anti-TNFα) and rofecoxib. Patients were treated at 3-week intervals if they did not have neutralizing antibodies. Among the 16 patients with HCL, 11 had a CR and 2 had a PR. Three patients relapsed from CR at 7, 8, and 12 months, and were reinduced into CR with BL22. Two patients developed reversible hemolytic uremic syndrome. Other toxicities included transient hypoalbuminemia and transaminases elevations. HA22, an engineered derivative of BL22 with increased cytotoxicity, has increased antitumor activity without increased toxicity in xenograft models and is a candidate for clinical development.[254]

An alternative to targeting toxins to tumor cells is to integrate the toxin into a receptor ligand that binds with relative selectively to tumor cells. One such molecule is denileukin difitox, which is approved for the treatment of CTCL. The drug is a recombinant fusion toxin in which the native receptor-binding domain of diphtheria toxin has been replaced by human IL-2.[255] In the Phase I study, the dose-limiting toxicity was reversible transaminase elevations; other toxicities included rash, nausea, chest tightness, fever, and creatinine elevation. Half of the patients developed an antibody response to the drug. Three of 18 patients had a clinical response that led to further clinical development. Olsen and colleagues reported the results of a Phase III trial of denileukin difitox in patients with CTCL who had been previously treated.[256] The randomization was between 9 and 18 μg/kg/day for 5 days, every 3 weeks for up to eight cycles. Seventy-one patients were treated, with an ORR of 30% (PR 20%, CR 10%). The median response duration was 6.9 months, and there was no difference between the doses. The predominant adverse events included flu-like symptoms, infusion reactions, and vascular leak. Transient elevation of transaminase and hypoalbunemia was common. This established the clinical activity of denileukin difitox in CLCL, for which it is currently approved for clinical use. Other tumors express CD25, and the activity of the drug is being investigated in NHL and CLL.[257]

Immunotoxins have shown activity, although toxicity is significant, and neutralizing antibodies are common. Further improvement in the technology is needed to improve efficacy and reduce toxicity.

IDIOTYPE VACCINES

One of the limitations of passive immunotherapy with MAb is the potential for resistance because of antigenic drift. Active immunotherapy with vaccines could provide a polyclonal antitumor humoral response, and the potential for a cellular immune response as well. The most tumor-specific antigen available in B- and T-cell lymphoma is the immunoglobulin receptor. As discussed above, the idiotype protein can be isolated from tumor B cells by rescue fusion. This protein can be used for vaccination after conjugation to a foreign protein such as keyhole limpet hemocyanin (KLH). Recently, there is preclinical evidence that the TCR can also be used as an immunogen when conjugated to KLH for T-cell lymphoma.[258] Other approaches to lymphoma vaccination are being explored, including whole-cell vaccines and heat shock proteins, but these have not undergone clinical investigation.[259,260]

Levy and colleagues at Stanford University Medical School have pioneered the use of the B-cell idiotype for NHL.[261] Initially, the idiotype protein was isolated by rescue fusion to a nonsecretory myeloma cell, although more recently a variety of recombinant methods have been used, including naked DNA.[262] The general strategy with protein-based vaccines has been to conjugate the idiotype protein to KLH (Id-KLH) in order to present the self-epitopes in the context of a foreign protein to break tolerance. The Id-KLH is administered to the patient after cytoreduction with chemotherapy with an immune adjuvant; over the years, a number of different immune adjuvants have been used.[261] Forty-one patients were treated and long-term follow-up has been presented.[263] Twenty patients developed an idiotype-specific immune response. The median follow-up after last chemotherapy was 5.3 years. The overall survival of patients generating an anti-Id response was significantly greater than the patients who did not generate an immune response. However, experience has demonstrated that successful vaccination is not simply measured by the potency of the vaccine, but that the chemotherapy used plays a vital role.[263] Levy and colleagues evaluated a cytoreductive regimen of CVP alternating with fludarabine, followed by the same Id-KLH vaccine that they had previously shown to be effective in patients cytoreduced with CVP; in this trial, the inclusion of the fludarabine ablated the immune response (Levy R, Stanford University Medical School, personal communication, 2000). In a trial of Id-KLH vaccine for MCL following cytoreduction with dose-adjusted EPOCH-R, Wilson and colleagues found that the intensive chemotherapy significantly reduced the development of immune response to the KLH component of the vaccine, and humoral anti-Id responses were impaired.[174] However, anti-idiotype T-cell responses were seen in this trial. The trial was not designed to evaluate the clinical impact of the vaccination on outcome.

These data demonstrate that patients treated with Id-KLH can respond to the vaccine, and those who generate an immune response have a superior outcome compared to matched historical controls or immune nonresponders. However, this outcome may not be the result of the vaccination, but rather the ability to generate an immune response may be a powerful selection for patients who are destined to do well. To address this important concern, randomized Phase III clinical trials are necessary to assess if Id-KLH vaccination has an impact on clinical outcome. Several Phase III studies are being conducted to evaluate idiotype vaccination. Genitope (Redwood City, CA) has completed accrual to the pivotal Phase III study of a recombinant Id-KLH vaccine for patients with FL. In this trial, patients underwent tumor cytoreduction with CVP chemotherapy, and responding patients (CR or PR) were randomized to receive Id-KLH or a KLH placebo vaccine. Results are expected in late 2005 or 2006. A second trial of Id-KLH vaccine sponsored by the NCI is slightly different in that patients undergo cytoreduction with a novel chemotherapy regimen, PACE (prednisone, doxorubicin, cyclophosphamide, etoposide), and only patients in a CR are randomized to receive the Id-KLH vaccine versus placebo. The accrual to this study is ongoing. Fravrille (San Diego, CA) is currently conducting a Phase III study of an Id-KLH vaccine in which the idiotype immunoglobulin heavy- and light-chain genes are first cloned into baculovirus, and the protein is produced following the infection insect cells. In this trial, patients undergo cytoreduction with rituximab, and patients are then randomized to receive Id-KLH vaccine or placebo. This trial is interesting in that B cells are depleted by the rituximab cytoreduction. This may lead to enhanced cellular immunity, initially followed by humoral immunity after B-cell recovery. Accrual to this study is ongoing. The outcome of these trials will determine the role of Id-KLH vaccination in NHL.

CPG OLIGONUCLEOTIDES

Immunostimulatory sequences (ISSs) are short oligonucleotides containing unmethylated CpG dinucleotides that have multiple effects on the immune system, including induction of INFα, INF-β, TNFα, and IL-12, which can augment NK activity.[264,265] Friedberg and colleagues conducted a trial of rituximab with CpG oligonucleotide 1018 ISS based on the hypothesis that the oligonucleotide would enhance ADCC.[266] Rituximab was administered weeks 1 through 4, and the oligonucleotide during weeks 2 through 5. Using RT-PCR analysis, INF-α/β–inducible genes showed an oligonucleotide dose-related increase in expression. Six of 19 patients had a clinical response, which is what would be expected from rituximab alone. Nonetheless, the ability to identify biological response suggests that further evaluation of CpG oligonucleotides in a more favorable patient population is warranted.

Human B cells detect CpG motifs via the toll receptor 9 (TLR9). Jahrdorfer and colleagues evaluated responses of prior NHL tumor cells to CpG oligonucleotides.[267] Most B-cell malignancies respond by up-regulating expression of co-stimulatory molecules (CD40, CD54 [ICAM-1], CD80 [B7-1], CD86 [B7-2]), antigen-presentation molecules (MHC I and MHC II), and CD20, and by proliferation. In vitro, the strongest effects were seen in CLL and MZL; however, FL, SLL, MCL, and DLBCL also showed a response. The variability observed may have important implications on the role of CpG oligonucleotides in different subtypes of NHL.

SUMMARY

Biological therapy of lymphoma has become a clinically important component of care. Although rituximab is currently the most widely used form of biotherapy, this review has identified a number of emerging areas of investigation that are likely to be important in clinical management of patients. RIT is a highly active therapy that is underutilized in routine practice. A new generation of anti-CD20 antibodies has the potential to improve on the activity of rituximab. The bsMAbs have interesting clinical activity, but a number of technical hurdles need to be addressed before they can be produced and used safely on a clinical scale. ISSs, IMIDs, and cytokines may have potential for augmenting the clinical activity of MAbs; combination studies are ongoing in the clinic. Given the wealth of exciting biological therapies, new strategies have to evolve to rapidly evaluate these agents in clinical trials. The current low rates of accrual of patients with lymphoma in clinical trials will hamper the evaluation of these new agents and prevent their timely evaluation.

References

1. Tossing G. New developments in interferon therapy. Eur J Med Res 2001;6:47–65.
2. Gresser I, Maury C, Tovey M. Interferon and murine leukemia. VII. Therapeutic effect of interferon preparations after diagnosis of lymphoma in AKR mice. Int J Cancer 1976;17:647–51.
3. Ehrlich P. The partial function of cells. (Nobel Prize address given on 11 December 1908 at Stockholm). Int Arch Allergy Appl Immunol 1954;5:67–86.

4. Kohler G, Milstein C. Continuous cultures of fused cells secreting antibody of predefined specificity. Nature 1975; 256:495–7.
5. Levy R, Miller RA. Therapy of lymphoma directed at idiotypes. J Natl Cancer Inst Monogr 1990:61–8.
6. Gresser I, Maury C, Tovey M. Efficacy of combined interferon cyclophosphamide therapy after diagnosis of lymphoma in AKR mice. Eur J Cancer 1978;14:97–9.
7. Gutterman JU, Blumenschein GR, Alexanian R, et al. Leukocyte interferon-induced tumor regression in human metastatic breast cancer, multiple myeloma, and malignant lymphoma. Ann Intern Med 1980;93:399–406.
8. Louie AC, Gallagher JG, Sikora K, et al. Follow-up observations on the effect of human leukocyte interferon in non-Hodgkin's lymphoma. Blood 1981;58:712–8.
9. Foon KA, Sherwin SA, Abrams PG, et al. Treatment of advanced non-Hodgkin's lymphoma with recombinant leukocyte A interferon. N Engl J Med 1984;311:1148–52.
10. Quesada JR, Hawkins M, Horning S, et al. Collaborative phase I–II study of recombinant DNA-produced leukocyte interferon (clone A) in metastatic breast cancer, malignant lymphoma, and multiple myeloma. Am J Med 1984;77: 427–32.
11. Horning SJ, Merigan TC, Krown SE, et al. Human interferon alpha in malignant lymphoma and Hodgkin's disease. Results of the American Cancer Society trial. Cancer 1985;56: 1305–10.
12. O'Connell MJ, Colgan JP, Oken MM, et al. Clinical trial of recombinant leukocyte A interferon as initial therapy for favorable histology non-Hodgkin's lymphomas and chronic lymphocytic leukemia. An Eastern Cooperative Oncology Group pilot study. J Clin Oncol 1986;4:128–36.
13. Wagstaff J, Loynds P, Crowther D. A phase II study of human rDNA alpha-2 interferon in patients with low grade non-Hodgkin's lymphoma. Cancer Chemother Pharmacol 1986;18:54–8.
14. Rohatiner AZ, Richards MA, Barnett MJ, et al. Chlorambucil and interferon for low grade non-Hodgkin's lymphoma. Br J Cancer 1987;55:225–6.
15. Chisesi T, Capnist G, Vespignani M, et al. Interferon alfa-2b and chlorambucil in the treatment of non-Hodgkin's lymphoma. Invest New Drugs 1987;5(Suppl):S35–40.
16. Solal-Celigny P, Lepage E, Brousse N, et al. Recombinant interferon alfa-2b combined with a regimen containing doxorubicin in patients with advanced follicular lymphoma. Groupe d'Etude des Lymphomes de l'Adulte. N Engl J Med 1993;329:1608–14.
17. Peterson BA, Petroni GR, Oken MM, et al. Cyclophosphamide versus cyclophosphamide plus interferon alfa-2b in follicular low-grade lymphomas: an intergroup phase III trial (CALGB 8691 and EST 7486). Proc Am Soc Clin Oncol 1997;16:14a(Abstr 48).
18. Chisesi T, Congiu M, Contu A, et al. Randomized study of chlorambucil (CB) compared to interferon (alfa-2b) combined with CB in low-grade non-Hodgkin's lymphoma: an interim report of a randomized study. Non-Hodgkin's Lymphoma Cooperative Study Group. Eur J Cancer 1991; 27(Suppl 4):S31–3.
19. Arranz R, Garcia-Alfonso P, Sobrino P, et al. Role of interferon alfa-2b in the induction and maintenance treatment of low-grade non-Hodgkin's lymphoma: results from a prospective, multicenter trial with double randomization. J Clin Oncol 1998;16:1538–46.
20. Solal-Celigny P, Lepage E, Brousse N, et al. Doxorubicin-containing regimen with or without interferon alfa-2b for advanced follicular lymphomas: final analysis of survival and toxicity in the Groupe d'Etude des Lymphomes Folliculaires 86 Trial. J Clin Oncol 1998;16:2332–8.
21. Rohatiner A, Radford J, Deakin D, et al. A randomized controlled trial to evaluate the role of interferon as initial and maintenance therapy in patients with follicular lymphoma. Br J Cancer 2001;85:29–35.
22. Smalley RV, Weller E, Hawkins MJ, et al. Final analysis of the ECOG I-COPA trial (E6484) in patients with non-Hodgkin's lymphoma treated with interferon alfa (IFN-alpha2a) plus an anthracycline-based induction regimen. Leukemia 2001;15: 1118–22.
23. Baldini L, Brugiatelli M, Luminari S, et al. Treatment of indolent B-cell nonfollicular lymphomas: final results of the LL01 randomized trial of the Gruppo Italiano per lo Studio dei Linfomi. J Clin Oncol 2003;21:1459–65.
24. Aviles A, Neri N, Huerta-Guzman J, et al. Interferon alpha 2b as maintenance therapy improves outcome in follicular lymphoma. Leuk Lymphoma 2004;45:2247–51.
25. Shiffman ML. Pegylated interferons: what role will they play in the treatment of chronic hepatitis C? Curr Gastroenterol Rep 2001;3:30–7.
26. Waldmann TA. The interleukin-2 receptor. J Biol Chem 1991;266:2681–4.
27. Foss FM, Waldmann TA. Interleukin-2 receptor–directed therapies for cutaneous lymphomas. Hematol Oncol Clin North Am 2003;17:1449–58.
28. Eberlein TJ, Rosenstein M, Rosenberg SA. Regression of a disseminated syngeneic solid tumor by systemic transfer of lymphoid cells expanded in interleukin 2. J Exp Med 1982; 156:385–97.
29. Rosenberg SA, Eberlein TJ, Grimm EA, et al. Development of long-term cell lines and lymphoid clones reactive against murine and human tumors: a new approach to the adoptive immunotherapy of cancer. Surgery 1982;92: 328–36.
30. Weber JS, Yang JC, Topalian SL, et al. The use of interleukin-2 and lymphokine-activated killer cells for the treatment of patients with non-Hodgkin's lymphoma. J Clin Oncol 1992;10:33–40.
31. Gisselbrecht C, Maraninchi D, Pico JL, et al. Interleukin-2 treatment in lymphoma: a Phase II multicenter study. Blood 1994;83:2081–5.
32. van Besien K, Margolin K, Champlin R, et al. Activity of interleukin-2 in non-Hodgkin's lymphoma following transplantation of interleukin-2–activated autologous bone marrow or stem cells. Cancer J Sci Am 1997;3(Suppl 1):S54–8.
33. Van Besien K, Mehra R, Wadehra N, et al. Phase II study of autologous transplantation with interleukin-2-incubated peripheral blood stem cells and posttransplantation interleukin-2 in relapsed or refractory non-Hodgkin lymphoma. Biol Blood Marrow Transplant 2004;10:386–94.
34. Colombo MP and Trinchieri G. Interleukin-12 in anti-tumor immunity and immunotherapy. Cytokine Growth Factor Rev 2002;13:155–68.
35. Rook AH, Wood GS, Yoo EK, et al. Interleukin-12 therapy of cutaneous T-cell lymphoma induces lesion regression and cytotoxic T-cell responses. Blood 1999;94:902–8.
36. Younes A, Pro B, Robertson MJ, et al. Phase II clinical trial of interleukin-12 in patients with relapsed and refractory non-Hodgkin's lymphoma and Hodgkin's disease. Clin Cancer Res 2004;10:5432–8.
37. Robertson MJ, Pelloso D, Abonour R, et al. Interleukin 12 immunotherapy after autologous stem cell transplantation for hematologic malignancies. Clin Cancer Res 2002;8: 3383–93.
38. Schmidt-Wolf IG, Lefterova P, Mehta BA, et al. Phenotypic characterization and identification of effector cells involved in tumor cell recognition of cytokine-induced killer cells. Exp Hematol 1993;21:1673–9.

39. Alvarnas JC, Linn YC, Hope EG, et al. Expansion of cytotoxic CD3+ CD56+ cells from peripheral blood progenitor cells of patients undergoing autologous hematopoietic cell transplantation. Biol Blood Marrow Transplant 2001;7: 216–22.
40. Leemhuis T, Wells S, Scheffold C, et al. A phase I trial of autologous cytokine-induced killer cells for the treatment of relapsed Hodgkin disease and non-Hodgkin lymphoma. Biol Blood Marrow Transplant 2005;11:181–7.
41. Mendez MJ, Green LL, Corvalan JR, et al. Functional transplant of megabase human immunoglobulin loci recapitulates human antibody response in mice. Nat Genet 1997;15: 146–56.
42. Ishida I, Tomizuka K, Yoshida H, et al. Production of human monoclonal and polyclonal antibodies in TransChromo animals. Cloning Stem Cells 2002;4:91–102.
43. Rauchenberger R, Borges E, Thomassen-Wolf E, et al. Human combinatorial Fab library yielding specific and functional antibodies against the human fibroblast growth factor receptor 3. J Biol Chem 2003;278:38194–205.
44. Carter P. Improving the efficacy of antibody-based cancer therapies. Nat Rev Cancer 2001;1:118–29.
45. Venneker GT, Asghar SS. CD59: a molecule involved in antigen presentation as well as downregulation of membrane attack complex. Exp Clin Immunogenet 1992;9:33–47.
46. Kinoshita T, Medof ME, Silber R, et al. Distribution of decay-accelerating factor in the peripheral blood of normal individuals and patients with paroxysmal nocturnal hemoglobinuria. J Exp Med 1985;162:75–92.
47. Jurianz K, Ziegler S, Garcia-Schuler H, et al. Complement resistance of tumor cells: basal and induced mechanisms. Mol Immunol 1999;36:929–39.
48. Ravetch JV, Bolland S. IgG Fc receptors. Annu Rev Immunol 2001;19:275–90.
49. Cartron G, Dacheux L, Salles G, et al. Therapeutic activity of humanized anti-CD20 monoclonal antibody and polymorphism in IgG Fc receptor FcgammaRIIIa gene. Blood 2002;99:754–8.
50. Weng WK, Levy R. Two immunoglobulin G fragment C receptor polymorphisms independently predict response to rituximab in patients with follicular lymphoma. J Clin Oncol 2003;21:3940–7.
51. Tax WJ, Tamboer WP, Jacobs CW, et al. Role of polymorphic Fc receptor Fc gammaRIIa in cytokine release and adverse effects of murine IgG1 anti-CD3/T cell receptor antibody (WT31). Transplantation 1997;63:106–12.
52. Louis E, El Ghoul Z, Vermeire S, et al. Association between polymorphism in IgG Fc receptor IIIa coding gene and biological response to infliximab in Crohn's disease. Aliment Pharmacol Ther 2004;19:511–9.
53. Pukac L, Kanakaraj P, Humphreys R, et al. HGS-ETR1, a fully human TRAIL-receptor 1 monoclonal antibody, induces cell death in multiple tumour types in vitro and in vivo. Br J Cancer 2005;92:1430–41.
54. Grossbard ML, Freedman AS, Ritz J, et al. Serotherapy of B-cell neoplasms with anti-B4-blocked ricin: a phase I trial of daily bolus infusion. Blood 1992;79:576–85.
55. Engert A, Diehl V, Schnell R, et al. A Phase-I study of an anti-CD25 ricin A-chain immunotoxin (RFT5-SMPT-dgA) in patients with refractory Hodgkin's lymphoma. Blood 1997; 89:403–10.
56. Kreitman RJ, Wilson WH, White JD, et al. Phase I trial of recombinant immunotoxin anti-Tac(Fv)-PE38 (LMB-2) in patients with hematologic malignancies. J Clin Oncol 2000;18:1622–36.
57. Press OW, Leonard JP, Coiffier B, et al. Immunotherapy of non-Hodgkin's lymphomas. Hematology (Am Soc Hematol Educ Program) 2001:221–40.
58. Davis TA, Maloney DG, Czerwinski DK, et al. Anti-idiotype antibodies can induce long-term complete remissions in non-Hodgkin's lymphoma without eradicating the malignant clone. Blood 1998;92:1184–90.
59. Cleary ML, Meeker TC, Levy S, et al. Clustering of extensive somatic mutations in the variable region of an immunoglobulin heavy chain gene from a human B cell lymphoma. Cell 1986;44:97–106.
60. Levy R, Levy S, Brown SL, et al. Anti-idiotype antibodies reveal the existence of somatic mutation in human B cell lymphoma. Monogr Allergy 1987;22:194–203.
61. Nadler LM, Stashenko P, Hardy R, et al. Serotherapy of a patient with a monoclonal antibody directed against a human lymphoma-associated antigen. Cancer Res 1980;40: 3147–54.
62. Kehrl JH, Riva A, Wilson GL, et al. Molecular mechanisms regulating CD19, CD20 and CD22 gene expression. Immunol Today 1994;15:432–6.
63. Tedder TF, Engel P. CD20: a regulator of cell-cycle progression of B lymphocytes. Immunol Today 1994;15:450–4.
64. Stamenkovic I and Seed B. Analysis of two cDNA clones encoding the B lymphocyte antigen CD20 (B1, Bp35), a type III integral membrane protein. J Exp Med 1988;167: 1975–80.
65. Mason DY, Comans-Bitter WM, Cordell JL, et al. Antibody L26 recognizes an intracellular epitope on the B-cell–associated CD20 antigen. Am J Pathol 1990;136:1215–22.
66. Bubien JK, Zhou LJ, Bell PD, et al. Transfection of the CD20 cell surface molecule into ectopic cell types generates a Ca2+ conductance found constitutively in B lymphocytes. J Cell Biol 1993;121:1121–32.
67. Li H, Ayer LM, Polyak MJ, et al. The CD20 calcium channel is localized to microvilli and constitutively associated with membrane rafts: antibody binding increases the affinity of the association through an epitope-dependent cross-linking-independent mechanism. J Biol Chem 2004;279:19893–901.
68. O'Keefe TL, Williams GT, Davies SL, et al. Mice carrying a CD20 gene disruption. Immunogenetics 1998;48:125–32.
69. Uchida J, Lee Y, Hasegawa M, et al. Mouse CD20 expression and function. Int Immunol 2004;16:119–29.
70. Manshouri T, Do KA, Wang X, et al. Circulating CD20 is detectable in the plasma of patients with chronic lymphocytic leukemia and is of prognostic significance. Blood 2003;101:2507–13.
71. Press OW, Appelbaum F, Ledbetter JA, et al. Monoclonal antibody 1F5 (anti-CD20) serotherapy of human B cell lymphomas. Blood 1987;69:584–91.
72. Press OW, Farr AG, Borroz KI, et al. Endocytosis and degradation of monoclonal antibodies targeting human B-cell malignancies. Cancer Res 1989;49:4906–12.
73. Press OW, Howell-Clark J, Anderson S, et al. Retention of B-cell-specific monoclonal antibodies by human lymphoma cells. Blood 1994;83:1390–7.
74. Vervoordeldonk SF, Merle PA, van Leeuwen EF, et al. Preclinical studies with radiolabeled monoclonal antibodies for treatment of patients with B-cell malignancies. Cancer 1994;73:1006–11.
75. Dancescu M, Wu C, Rubio M, et al. IL-4 induces conformational change of CD20 antigen via a protein kinase C-independent pathway. Antagonistic effect of anti-CD40 monoclonal antibody. J Immunol 1992;148:2411–6.
76. Venugopal P, Sivaraman S, Huang XK, et al. Effects of cytokines on CD20 antigen expression on tumor cells from patients with chronic lymphocytic leukemia. Leuk Res 2000;24:411–5.
77. Sivaraman S, Venugopal P, Ranganathan R, et al. Effect of interferon-alpha on CD20 antigen expression of B-cell

chronic lymphocytic leukemia. Cytokines Cell Mol Ther 2000;6:81–7.
78. Kunala S, Macklis RM. Ionizing radiation induces CD20 surface expression on human B cells. Int J Cancer 2001;96:178–81.
79. Stashenko P, Nadler LM, Hardy R, et al. Characterization of a human B lymphocyte-specific antigen. J Immunol 1980; 125:1678–85.
80. Nadler LM, Ritz J, Hardy R, et al. A unique cell surface antigen identifying lymphoid malignancies of B cell origin. J Clin Invest 1981;67:134–40.
81. Nadler LM, Takvorian T, Botnick L, et al. Anti-B1 monoclonal antibody and complement treatment in autologous bone-marrow transplantation for relapsed B-cell non-Hodgkin's lymphoma. Lancet 1984;2:427–31.
82. Bast RC, Jr., De Fabritiis P, Lipton J, et al. Elimination of malignant clonogenic cells from human bone marrow using multiple monoclonal antibodies and complement. Cancer Res 1985;45:499–503.
83. Johnson TA, Press OW. Therapy of B-cell lymphomas with monoclonal antibodies and radioimmunoconjugates: the Seattle experience. Ann Hematol 2000;79:175–82.
84. Davis TA, Kaminski MS, Leonard JP, et al. The radioisotope contributes significantly to the activity of radioimmunotherapy. Clin Cancer Res 2004;10:7792–8.
85. Grillo-Lopez AJ, White CA, Varns C, et al. Overview of the clinical development of rituximab: first monoclonal antibody approved for the treatment of lymphoma. Semin Oncol 1999;26:66–73.
86. Reff ME, Carner K, Chambers KS, et al. Depletion of B cells in vivo by a chimeric mouse human monoclonal antibody to CD20. Blood 1994;83:435–45.
87. Maloney DG, Liles TM, Czerwinski DK, et al. Phase I clinical trial using escalating single-dose infusion of chimeric anti-CD20 monoclonal antibody (IDEC-C2B8) in patients with recurrent B-cell lymphoma. Blood 1994;84: 2457–66.
88. McLaughlin P, Grillo-Lopez AJ, Link BK, et al. Rituximab chimeric anti-CD20 monoclonal antibody therapy for relapsed indolent lymphoma: half of patients respond to a four-dose treatment program. J Clin Oncol 1998;16: 2825–33.
89. Borisch B, Semac I, Soltermann A, et al. Anti-CD20 treatments and the lymphocyte membrane: pathology for therapy. Verh Dtsch Ges Pathol 2001;85:161–6.
90. Cragg MS, Morgan SM, Chan HT, et al. Complement-mediated lysis by anti-CD20 mAb correlates with segregation into lipid rafts. Blood 2003;101:1045–52.
91. Semac I, Palomba C, Kulangara K, et al. Anti-CD20 therapeutic antibody rituximab modifies the functional organization of rafts/microdomains of B lymphoma cells. Cancer Res 2003;63:534–40.
92. Shan D, Ledbetter JA, Press OW. Apoptosis of malignant human B cells by ligation of CD20 with monoclonal antibodies. Blood 1998;91:1644–52.
93. Hofmeister JK, Cooney D, Coggeshall KM. Clustered CD20 induced apoptosis: src-family kinase, the proximal regulator of tyrosine phosphorylation, calcium influx, and caspase 3-dependent apoptosis. Blood Cells Mol Dis 2000; 26:133–43.
94. Shan D, Ledbetter JA, Press OW. Signaling events involved in anti-CD20–induced apoptosis of malignant human B cells. Cancer Immunol Immunother 2000;48: 673–83.
95. Cardarelli PM, Quinn M, Buckman D, et al. Binding to CD20 by anti-B1 antibody or F(ab')(2) is sufficient for induction of apoptosis in B-cell lines. Cancer Immunol Immunother 2002;51:15–24.
96. Cragg MS, Glennie MJ. Antibody specificity controls in vivo effector mechanisms of anti-CD20 reagents. Blood 2004;103: 2738–43.
97. Stein R, Qu Z, Chen S, et al. Characterization of a new humanized anti-CD20 monoclonal antibody, IMMU-106, and Its use in combination with the humanized anti-CD22 antibody, epratuzumab, for the therapy of non-Hodgkin's lymphoma. Clin Cancer Res 2004;10:2868–78.
98. Teeling JL, French RR, Cragg MS, et al. Characterization of new human CD20 monoclonal antibodies with potent cytolytic activity against non-Hodgkin lymphomas. Blood 2004;104:1793–800.
99. Looney RJ, Anolik JH, Campbell D, et al. B cell depletion as a novel treatment for systemic lupus erythematosus: a phase I/II dose-escalation trial of rituximab. Arthritis Rheum 2004;50:2580–9.
100. Clynes RA, Towers TL, Presta LG, et al. Inhibitory Fc receptors modulate in vivo cytoxicity against tumor targets. Nat Med 2000;6:443–6.
101. Koene HR, Kleijer M, Algra J, et al. Fc gammaRIIIa-158V/F polymorphism influences the binding of IgG by natural killer cell Fc gammaRIIIa, independently of the Fc gammaRIIIa-48L/R/H phenotype. Blood 1997;90:1109–14.
102. Treon SP, Hansen M, Branagan AR, et al. Polymorphisms in FcgammaRIIIA (CD16) receptor expression are associated with clinical response to rituximab in Waldenstrom's macroglobulinemia. J Clin Oncol 2005;23:474–81.
103. Golay J, Zaffaroni L, Vaccari T, et al. Biologic response of B lymphoma cells to anti-CD20 monoclonal antibody rituximab in vitro: CD55 and CD59 regulate complement-mediated cell lysis. Blood 2000;95:3900–8.
104. Harjunpaa A, Junnikkala S, Meri S. Rituximab (anti-CD20) therapy of B-cell lymphomas: direct complement killing is superior to cellular effector mechanisms. Scand J Immunol 2000;51:634–41.
105. Nagajothi N, Matsui WH, Mukhina GL, et al. Enhanced cytotoxicity of rituximab following genetic and biochemical disruption of glycosylphosphatidylinositol anchored proteins. Leuk Lymphoma 2004;45:795–9.
106. Weng WK, Levy R. Expression of complement inhibitors CD46, CD55, and CD59 on tumor cells does not predict clinical outcome after rituximab treatment in follicular non-Hodgkin lymphoma. Blood 2001;98:1352–7.
107. Manches O, Lui G, Chaperot L, et al. In vitro mechanisms of action of rituximab on primary non-Hodgkin lymphomas. Blood 2003;101:949–54.
108. Maloney DG, Grillo-Lopez AJ, Bodkin DJ, et al. IDEC-C2B8: results of a phase I multiple-dose trial in patients with relapsed non-Hodgkin's lymphoma. J Clin Oncol 1997;15: 3266–74.
109. Davis TA, Grillo-Lopez AJ, White CA, et al. Rituximab anti-CD20 monoclonal antibody therapy in non-Hodgkin's lymphoma: safety and efficacy of re-treatment. J Clin Oncol 2000;18:3135–43.
110. Hainsworth JD, Burris HA 3rd, Morrissey LH, et al. Rituximab monoclonal antibody as initial systemic therapy for patients with low-grade non-Hodgkin lymphoma. Blood 2000;95:3052–6.
111. Colombat P, Salles G, Brousse N, et al. Rituximab (anti-CD20 monoclonal antibody) as single first-line therapy for patients with follicular lymphoma with a low tumor burden: clinical and molecular evaluation. Blood 2001;97: 101–6.
112. Witzig TE, Vukov AM, Habermann TM, et al. Rituximab therapy for patients with newly diagnosed, advanced-stage, follicular grade I non-Hodgkin's lymphoma: a phase II trial in the North Central Cancer Treatment Group. J Clin Oncol 2005;23:1103–8.

113. Hainsworth JD, Litchy S, Burris HA 3rd, et al. Rituximab as first-line and maintenance therapy for patients with indolent non-Hodgkin's lymphoma. J Clin Oncol 2002;20:4261–7.
114. Ghielmini M, Schmitz SF, Cogliatti SB, et al. Prolonged treatment with rituximab in patients with follicular lymphoma significantly increases event-free survival and response duration compared with the standard weekly x 4 schedule. Blood 2004;103:4416–23.
115. Hainsworth JD, Litchy S, Shaffer DW, et al. Maximizing therapeutic benefit of rituximab: maintenance therapy versus re-treatment at progression in patients with indolent non-Hodgkin's lymphoma—a randomized phase II trial of the Minnie Pearl Cancer Research Network. J Clin Oncol 2005; 23:1088–95.
116. Byrd JC, White CA, Link B, et al. Rituximab therapy in Waldenstrom's macroglobulinemia: preliminary evidence of clinical activity. Ann Oncol 1999;10:1525–7.
117. Treon SP, Agus DB, Link B, et al. CD20-directed antibody-mediated immunotherapy induces responses and facilitates hematologic recovery in patients with Waldenstrom's macroglobulinemia. J Immunother 2001;24:272–9.
118. Treon SP, Branagan AR, Hunter Z, et al. Paradoxical increases in serum IgM and viscosity levels following rituximab in Waldenstrom's macroglobulinemia. Ann Oncol 2004;15: 1481–3.
119. Dimopoulos MA, Zervas C, Zomas A, et al. Treatment of Waldenstrom's macroglobulinemia with rituximab. J Clin Oncol 2002;20:2327–33.
120. Dimopoulos MA, Zervas C, Zomas A, et al. Extended rituximab therapy for previously untreated patients with Waldenstrom's macroglobulinemia. Clin Lymphoma 2002;3:163–6.
121. Treon SP, Emmanouilides C, Kimby E, et al. Extended rituximab therapy in Waldenstrom's macroglobulinemia. Ann Oncol 2005;16:132–8.
122. Coiffier B, Haioun C, Ketterer N, et al. Rituximab (anti-CD20 monoclonal antibody) for the treatment of patients with relapsing or refractory aggressive lymphoma: a multicenter phase II study. Blood 1998;92:1927–32.
123. Pan D, Moskowitz CH, Zelenetz AD, et al. Rituximab for aggressive non-Hodgkin's lymphomas relapsing after or refractory to autologous stem cell transplantation. Cancer J 2002;8:371–6.
124. Kewalramani T, Nimer SD, Zelenetz AD, et al. Progressive disease following autologous transplantation in patients with chemosensitive relapsed or primary refractory Hodgkin's disease or aggressive non-Hodgkin's lymphoma. Bone Marrow Transplant 2003;32:673–9.
125. Foran JM, Rohatiner AZ, Cunningham D, et al. European phase II study of rituximab (chimeric anti-CD20 monoclonal antibody) for patients with newly diagnosed mantle-cell lymphoma and previously treated mantle-cell lymphoma, immunocytoma, and small B-cell lymphocytic lymphoma. J Clin Oncol 2000;18:317–24.
126. Ghielmini M, Schmitz SF, Cogliatti S, et al. Effect of single-agent rituximab given at the standard schedule or as prolonged treatment in patients with mantle cell lymphoma: a study of the Swiss Group for Clinical Cancer Research (SAKK). J Clin Oncol 2005;23:705–11.
127. Demidem A, Lam T, Alas S, et al. Chimeric anti-CD20 (IDEC-C2B8) monoclonal antibody sensitizes a B cell lymphoma cell line to cell killing by cytotoxic drugs. Cancer Biother Radiopharm 1997;12:177–86.
128. Alas S, Bonavida B, Emmanouilides C. Potentiation of fludarabine cytotoxicity on non-Hodgkin's lymphoma by pentoxifylline and rituximab. Anticancer Res 2000;20: 2961–6.
129. Shan D, Gopal AK, Press OW. Synergistic effects of the fenretinide (4-HPR) and anti-CD20 monoclonal antibodies on apoptosis induction of malignant human B cells. Clin Cancer Res 2001;7:2490–5.
130. Ghetie MA, Bright H, Vitetta ES. Homodimers but not monomers of Rituxan (chimeric anti-CD20) induce apoptosis in human B-lymphoma cells and synergize with a chemotherapeutic agent and an immunotoxin. Blood 2001;97:1392–8.
131. Emmanouilides C, Jazirehi AR, Bonavida B. Rituximab-mediated sensitization of B-non-Hodgkin's lymphoma (NHL) to cytotoxicity induced by paclitaxel, gemcitabine, and vinorelbine. Cancer Biother Radiopharm 2002;17: 621–30.
132. Rose AL, Smith BE, Maloney DG. Glucocorticoids and rituximab in vitro: synergistic direct antiproliferative and apoptotic effects. Blood 2002;100:1765–1773.
133. Rummel MJ, Chow KU, Hoelzer D, et al. In vitro studies with bendamustine: enhanced activity in combination with rituximab. Semin Oncol 2002;29:12–14.
134. Jazirehi AR, Gan XH, De Vos S, et al. Rituximab (anti-CD20) selectively modifies Bcl-xL and apoptosis protease activating factor-1 (Apaf–1) expression and sensitizes human non-Hodgkin's lymphoma B cell lines to paclitaxel-induced apoptosis. Mol Cancer Ther 2003;2:1183–93.
135. Jazirehi AR, Huerta-Yepez S, Cheng G, et al. Rituximab (chimeric anti-CD20 monoclonal antibody) inhibits the constitutive nuclear factor-{kappa}B signaling pathway in non-Hodgkin's lymphoma B-cell lines: role in sensitization to chemotherapeutic drug-induced apoptosis. Cancer Res 2005;65:264–76.
136. Czuczman MS, Grillo-Lopez AJ, White CA, et al. Treatment of patients with low-grade B-cell lymphoma with the combination of chimeric anti-CD20 monoclonal antibody and CHOP chemotherapy. J Clin Oncol 1999;17:268–76.
137. Czuczman MS, Weaver R, Alkuzweny B, et al. Prolonged clinical and molecular remission in patients with low-grade or follicular non-Hodgkin's lymphoma treated with rituximab plus CHOP chemotherapy: 9-year follow-up. J Clin Oncol 2004;22:4711–6.
138. Forstpointner R, Dreyling M, Repp R, et al. The addition of rituximab to a combination of fludarabine, cyclophosphamide, mitoxantrone (FCM) significantly increases the response rate and prolongs survival as compared with FCM alone in patients with relapsed and refractory follicular and mantle cell lymphomas: results of a prospective randomized study of the German Low-Grade Lymphoma Study Group. Blood 2004;104:3064–71.
139. Marcus R, Imrie K, Belch A, et al. CVP chemotherapy plus rituximab compared with CVP as first-line treatment for advanced follicular lymphoma. Blood 2005;105: 1417–23.
140. Hiddemann W, Dreyling MH, Forstpointner R, et al. Combined immuno-chemotherapy (R-CHOP) significantly improves time to treatment failure in first line therapy of follicular lymphoma results of a prospective randomized trial of the German Low Grade Lymphoma Study Group (GLSG). Blood 2003;102:Abstract 352.
141. Zinzani PL, Pulsoni A, Perrotti A, et al. Fludarabine plus mitoxantrone with and without rituximab versus CHOP with and without rituximab as front-line treatment for patients with follicular lymphoma. J Clin Oncol 2004;22: 2654–61.
142. Treon SP, Hunter Z, Barnagan AR. CHOP plus rituximab therapy in Waldenstrom's macroglobulinemia. Clin Lymphoma 2005;5:273–7.
143. Vose JM, Link BK, Grossbard ML, et al. Phase II study of rituximab in combination with CHOP chemotherapy in patients with previously untreated, aggressive non-Hodgkin's lymphoma. J Clin Oncol 2001;19:389–97.

144. Coiffier B, Lepage E, Briere J, et al. CHOP chemotherapy plus rituximab compared with CHOP alone in elderly patients with diffuse large-B-cell lymphoma. N Engl J Med 2002; 346:235–42.
145. Habermann TM, Weller E, Morrison VA, et al. Rituximab-CHOP versus CHOP with or without maintenance rituximab in patients 60 years of age or older with diffuse large B-cell lymphoma (DLBCL): an update. Blood 2004;104:Abstract 127.
146. Pfreundschuh M, Truemper L, Gill D, et al. First analysis of the completed mabthera international (MInT) trial in young patients with low-risk diffuse large B-cell lymphoma (DLBCL): addition of rituximab to a CHOP-like regimen significantly improves outcome of all patients with the identification of a very favorable subgroup with IPI = O and no bulky disease. Blood 2004;104:Abstract 157.
147. Coiffier B, Feugier P, Sebban C, et al. Long-term results of the GELA study, R-CHOP vs. CHOP in elderly patients with diffuse large B-cell lymphoma. Blood 2004;104:Abstract 1383.
148. Feugier P, Van Hoof A, Sebban C, et al. Long-term results of the R-CHOP study in the treatment of elderly patients with diffuse large B-cell lymphoma: a study by the Groupe d'Etude des Lymphomes de l'Adulte. J Clin Oncol 2005;23:4117–26.
149. Sehn LH, Donaldson J, Chhanabhai M, et al. Introduction of combined CHOP-rituximab therapy dramatically improved outcome of diffuse large B-cell lymphoma (DLBC) in British Columbia (BC). Blood 2003;102:Abstract 88.
150. Hoskin PJ. Weekly chemotherapy using PMitCEBO in the palliation of recurrent non-Hodgkin's lymphoma. Acta Oncol 1997;36:573–6.
151. Wilson WH, Pittaluga S, Gutierrez M, et al. Dose-adjusted EPOCH-rituximab in untreated diffuse large B-cell lymphoma: benefit of rituximab appears restricted to tumors harboring anti-apoptotic mechanisms. Blood 2003;102: Abstract 356.
152. Wilson WH, Grossbard ML, Pittaluga S, et al. Dose-adjusted EPOCH chemotherapy for untreated large B-cell lymphomas: a pharmacodynamic approach with high efficacy. Blood 2002;99:2685–93.
153. Mounier N, Briere J, Gisselbrecht C, et al. Rituximab plus CHOP (R-CHOP) overcomes bcl-2–associated resistance to chemotherapy in elderly patients with diffuse large B-cell lymphoma (DLBCL). Blood 2003;101:4279–84.
154. Winter JN, Weller E, Horning SJ, et al. Rituximab (R) alters the prognostic indicator profile in diffuse aggressive non-Hodgkin lymphomas. Blood 2003;102:Abstract 345.
155. Hans CP, Weisenburger DD, Greiner TC, et al. Confirmation of the molecular classification of diffuse large B-cell lymphoma by immunohistochemistry using a tissue microarray. Blood 2004;103:275–82.
156. Philip T, Armitage JO, Spitzer G, et al. High-dose therapy and autologous bone marrow transplantation after failure of conventional chemotherapy in adults with intermediate-grade or high-grade non-Hodgkin's lymphoma. N Engl J Med 1987;316:1493–8.
157. Velasquez WS, Cabanillas F, Salvador P, et al. Effective salvage therapy for lymphoma with cisplatin in combination with high-dose Ara-C and dexamethasone (DHAP). Blood 1988;71:117–22.
158. Velasquez WS, McLaughlin P, Tucker S, et al. ESHAP—an effective chemotherapy regimen in refractory and relapsing lymphoma: a 4-year follow-up study. J Clin Oncol 1994; 12:1169–76.
159. Colwill R, Crump M, Couture F, et al. Mini-BEAM as salvage therapy for relapsed or refractory Hodgkin's disease before intensive therapy and autologous bone marrow transplantation. J Clin Oncol 1995;13:396–402.
160. Girouard C, Dufresne J, Imrie K, et al. Salvage chemotherapy with mini-BEAM for relapsed or refractory non-Hodgkin's lymphoma prior to autologous bone marrow transplantation. Ann Oncol 1997;8:675–80.
161. Moskowitz CH, Bertino JR, Glassman JR, et al. Ifosfamide, carboplatin, and etoposide: a highly effective cytoreduction and peripheral-blood progenitor-cell mobilization regimen for transplant-eligible patients with non-Hodgkin's lymphoma. J Clin Oncol 1999;17:3776–85.
162. Magagnoli M, Sarina B, Balzarotti M, et al. Mobilizing potential of ifosfamide/vinorelbine-based chemotherapy in pretreated malignant lymphoma. Bone Marrow Transplant 2001;28:923–7.
163. Mayer J, Vasova I, Koristek Z, et al. Ifosfamide- and etoposide-based chemotherapy as salvage and mobilizing regimens for poor prognosis lymphoma. Eur J Haematol 2001; 64(Suppl):21–27.
164. Watts MJ, Ings SJ, Leverett D, et al. ESHAP and G-CSF is a superior blood stem cell mobilizing regimen compared to cyclophosphamide 1.5 g m(-2) and G-CSF for pre-treated lymphoma patients: a matched pairs analysis of 78 patients. Br J Cancer 2000;82:278–82.
165. Kewalramani T, Zelenetz AD, Nimer SD, et al. Rituximab and ICE as second-line therapy before autologous stem cell transplantation for relapsed or primary refractory diffuse large B-cell lymphoma. Blood 2004;103:3684–8.
166. Pavone V, Gaudio F, Guarini A, et al. Mobilization of peripheral blood stem cells with high-dose cyclophosphamide or the DHAP regimen plus G-CSF in non-Hodgkin's lymphoma. Bone Marrow Transplant 2002;29:285–90.
167. Zelenetz AD, Hamlin P, Kewalramani T, et al. Ifosfamide, carboplatin, etoposide (ICE)-based second-line chemotherapy for the management of relapsed and refractory aggressive non-Hodgkin's lymphoma. Ann Oncol 2003;14(Suppl 1:i5–10.
168. Horwitz SM, Negrin RS, Blume KG, et al. Rituximab as adjuvant to high-dose therapy and autologous hematopoietic cell transplantation for aggressive non-Hodgkin lymphoma. Blood 2004;103:777–83.
169. Shimoni A, Hardan I, Avigdor A, et al. Rituximab reduces relapse risk after allogeneic and autologous stem cell transplantation in patients with high-risk aggressive non-Hodgkin's lymphoma. Br J Haematol 2003;122:457–64.
170. Miller TP, Unger JM, Spier C, et al. Effect of adding rituximab to three cycles of CHOP plus involved-field radiotherapy for limited-stage aggressive diffuse B-cell lymphoma (SWOG-0014). Blood 2004;104:Abstract 158.
171. Romaguera JE, Fayad L, Rodriguez MA, et al. Rituximab plus hyper-CVAD (R-HCVAD) alternating with rituximab plus high-dose methotrexate-cytarabine (R-M/A) in untreated mantle cell lymphoma (MCL): prolonged follow-up confirms high rates of failure-free survival (FFS) and overall survival (OS). Blood 2004;104:Abstract 128.
172. Howard OM, Gribben JG, Neuberg DS, et al. Rituximab and CHOP induction therapy for newly diagnosed mantle-cell lymphoma: molecular complete responses are not predictive of progression-free survival. J Clin Oncol 2002;20:1288–94.
173. Lenz G, Dreyling M, Hoster E, et al. Immunochemotherapy with rituximab and cyclophosphamide, doxorubicin, vincristine, and prednisone significantly improves response and time to treatment failure, but not long-term outcome in patients with previously untreated mantle cell lymphoma: results of a prospective randomized trial of the German Low Grade Lymphoma Study Group (GLSG). J Clin Oncol 2005;23:1984–92.
174. Wilson WH, Neelapu S, Rosenwald A, et al. Idiotype vaccine and dose-adjusted EPOCH-rituximab treatment in untreated mantle cell lymphoma: preliminary report on clinical

outcome and analysis of immune response. Blood 2003; 102:Abstract 358.
175. Rosenwald A, Wright G, Wiestner A, et al. The proliferation gene expression signature is a quantitative integrator of oncogenic events that predicts survival in mantle cell lymphoma. Cancer Cell 2003;3:185–97.
176. Martinez N, Camacho FI, Algara P, et al. The molecular signature of mantle cell lymphoma reveals multiple signals favoring cell survival. Cancer Res 2003;63:8226–32.
177. Herberman RB, Ortaldo JR, Rubinstein M, et al. Augmentation of natural and antibody-dependent cell-mediated cytotoxicity by pure human leukocyte interferon. J Clin Immunol 1981;1:149–53.
178. Ortaldo JR, Pestka S, Slease RB, et al. Augmentation of human K-cell activity with interferon. Scand J Immunol 1980;12:365–9.
179. Davis TA, Maloney DG, Grillo-Lopez AJ, et al. Combination immunotherapy of relapsed or refractory low-grade or follicular non-Hodgkin's lymphoma with rituximab and interferon-alpha-2a. Clin Cancer Res 2000;6:2644–52.
180. Kimby E. Beyond immunochemotherapy: combinations of rituximab with cytokines interferon-alpha2a and granulocyte colony stimulating factor [corrected]. Semin Oncol 2002;29:7–10.
181. Rook AH, Kuzel TM, Olsen EA. Cytokine therapy of cutaneous T-cell lymphoma: interferons, interleukin-12, and interleukin-2. Hematol Oncol Clin North Am 2003;17: 1435–48, ix.
182. Friedberg JW, Neuberg D, Gribben JG, et al. Combination immunotherapy with rituximab and interleukin 2 in patients with relapsed or refractory follicular non-Hodgkin's lymphoma. Br J Haematol 2002;117:828–34.
183. Gluck WL, Hurst D, Yuen A, et al. Phase I studies of interleukin (IL)-2 and rituximab in B-cell non-Hodgkin's lymphoma: IL-2 mediated natural killer cell expansion correlations with clinical response. Clin Cancer Res 2004; 10:2253–64.
184. Ansell SM, Witzig TE, Kurtin PJ, et al. Phase 1 study of interleukin-12 in combination with rituximab in patients with B-cell non-Hodgkin lymphoma. Blood 2002;99: 67–74.
185. Ansell SM. Adding cytokines to monoclonal antibody therapy: does the concurrent administration of interleukin-12 add to the efficacy of rituximab in B-cell non-Hodgkin lymphoma? Leuk Lymphoma 2003;44:1309–15.
186. Kaufmann H, Raderer M, Wohrer S, et al. Antitumor activity of rituximab plus thalidomide in patients with relapsed/refractory mantle cell lymphoma. Blood 2004;104: 2269–71.
187. Hideshima T, Chauhan D, Shima Y, et al. Thalidomide and its analogs overcome drug resistance of human multiple myeloma cells to conventional therapy. Blood 2000;96: 2943–50.
188. Davies FE, Raje N, Hideshima T, et al. Thalidomide and immunomodulatory derivatives augment natural killer cell cytotoxicity in multiple myeloma. Blood 2001;98:210–6.
189. Cesano A, Gayko U. CD22 as a target of passive immunotherapy. Semin Oncol 2003;30:253–7.
190. O'Keefe TL, Williams GT, Davies SL, et al. Hyperresponsive B cells in CD22-deficient mice. Science 1996;274:798–801.
191. Shan D, Press OW. Constitutive endocytosis and degradation of CD22 by human B cells. J Immunol 1995;154: 4466–75.
192. Dorken B, Moldenhauer G, Pezzutto A, et al. HD39 (B3), a B lineage-restricted antigen whose cell surface expression is limited to resting and activated human B lymphocytes. J Immunol 1986;136:4470–9.
193. Pawlak-Byczkowska EJ, Hansen HJ, Dion AS, et al. Two new monoclonal antibodies, EPB-1 and EPB-2, reactive with human lymphoma. Cancer Res 1989;49:4568–77.
194. Tuscano JM, Riva A, Toscano SN, et al. CD22 cross-linking generates B-cell antigen receptor-independent signals that activate the JNK/SAPK signaling cascade. Blood 1999;94: 1382–92.
195. Ghetie MA, Richardson J, Tucker T, et al. Antitumor activity of Fab' and IgG-anti-CD22 immunotoxins in disseminated human B lymphoma grown in mice with severe combined immunodeficiency disease: effect on tumor cells in extranodal sites. Cancer Res 1991;51:5876–80.
196. Mattes MJ, Shih LB, Govindan SV, et al. The advantage of residualizing radiolabels for targeting B-cell lymphomas with a radiolabeled anti-CD22 monoclonal antibody. Int J Cancer 1997;71:429–35.
197. Kreitman RJ, Wang QC, FitzGerald DJ, et al. Complete regression of human B-cell lymphoma xenografts in mice treated with recombinant anti-CD22 immunotoxin RFB4(dsFv)-PE38 at doses tolerated by cynomolgus monkeys. Int J Cancer 1999;81:148–55.
198. Stein R, Govindan SV, Mattes MJ, et al. Targeting human cancer xenografts with monoclonal antibodies labeled using radioiodinated, diethylenetriaminepentaacetic acid-appended peptides. Clin Cancer Res 1999;5:3079s–87s.
199. Leonard JP, Coleman M, Ketas JC, et al. Phase I/II trial of epratuzumab (humanized anti-CD22 antibody) in indolent non-Hodgkin's lymphoma. J Clin Oncol 2003;21:3051–9.
200. Leonard JP, Coleman M, Ketas JC, et al. Epratuzumab, a humanized anti-CD22 antibody, in aggressive non-Hodgkin's lymphoma: phase I/II clinical trial results. Clin Cancer Res 2004;10:5327–34.
201. Leonard JP, Coleman M, Matthews JC, et al. Epratuzumab (anti-CD22) and rituximab (anti-CD20) combination immunotherapy for non-Hodgkin's lymphoma: preliminary response data. J Clin Oncol 2002;20:1060 (2004 ASCO Annual Meeting Proceedings).
202. Strauss SJ, Lister TA, Morschauser F, et al. Multi-centre, phase II study of combination antibody therapy with epratuzumab plus rituximab in relapsed/refractory indolent and aggressive NHL: promising preliminary results. J Clin Oncol 2002;20:6579 (2004 ASCO Annual Meeting Proceedings).
203. Micallef IN, Kahl BS, Gayko U, et al. Initial results of a pilot study of epratuzumab and rituximab in combination with CHOP chemotherapy (ER-CHOP) in previously untreated patients with diffuse large B-cell lymphoma (DLBCL). J Clin Oncol 2002;20:6580 (2004 ASCO Annual Meeting Proceedings).
204. Bertram JH, Gill PS, Levine AM, et al. Monoclonal antibody T101 in T cell malignancies: a clinical, pharmacokinetic, and immunologic correlation. Blood 1986;68:752–61.
205. Waldmann TA, Goldman CK, Bongiovanni KF, et al. Therapy of patients with human T-cell lymphotrophic virus I-induced adult T-cell leukemia with anti-Tac, a monoclonal antibody to the receptor for interleukin-2. Blood 1988;72:1805–16.
206. Ravandi F, O'Brien S. Alemtuzumab. Expert Rev Anticancer Ther 2005;5:39–51.
207. Enblad G, Hagberg H, Erlanson M, et al. A pilot study of alemtuzumab (anti-CD52 monoclonal antibody) therapy for patients with relapsed or chemotherapy-refractory peripheral T-cell lymphomas. Blood 2004;103:2920–4.
208. Zelenetz AD. Radioimmunotherapy for lymphoma. Curr Opin Oncol 1999;11:375–380.
209. Witzig TE, White CA, Wiseman GA, et al. Phase I/II trial of IDEC-Y2B8 radioimmunotherapy for treatment of relapsed or refractory CD20(+) B-cell non-Hodgkin's lymphoma. J Clin Oncol 1999;17:3793–803.

210. Vose JM, Wahl RL, Saleh M, et al. Multicenter phase II study of iodine-131 tositumomab for chemotherapy-relapsed/refractory low-grade and transformed low-grade B-cell non-Hodgkin's lymphomas. J Clin Oncol 2000;18: 1316–23.
211. Kaminski MS, Zelenetz AD, Press OW, et al. Pivotal study of iodine I 131 tositumomab for chemotherapy-refractory low-grade or transformed low-grade B-cell non-Hodgkin's lymphomas. J Clin Oncol 2001;19:3918–28.
212. Witzig TE, Flinn IW, Gordon LI, et al. Treatment with ibritumomab tiuxetan radioimmunotherapy in patients with rituximab-refractory follicular non-Hodgkin's lymphoma. J Clin Oncol 2002;20:3262–9.
213. Zelenetz AD. A clinical and scientific overview of tositumomab and iodine I 131 tositumomab. Semin Oncol 2003;30:22–30.
214. Horning SJ, Younes A, Jain V, et al. Efficacy and safety of tositumomab and iodine-131 tositumomab (Bexxar) in B-cell lymphoma, progressive after rituximab. J Clin Oncol 2005;23:712–9.
215. Gordon LI, Witzig T, Molina A, et al. Yttrium 90-labeled ibritumomab tiuxetan radioimmunotherapy produces high response rates and durable remissions in patients with previously treated B-cell lymphoma. Clin Lymphoma 2004;5:98–101.
216. Bennett JM, Kaminski MS, Leonard JP, et al. Assessment of treatment-related myelodysplastic syndromes and acute myeloid leukemia in patients with non-Hodgkin's lymphoma treated with tositumomab and iodine I 131 tositumomab (BEXXAR(R)). Blood 2005;12:4576–82.
217. Witzig TE, Gordon LI, Cabanillas F, et al. Randomized controlled trial of yttrium-90-labeled ibritumomab tiuxetan radioimmunotherapy versus rituximab immunotherapy for patients with relapsed or refractory low-grade, follicular, or transformed B-cell non-Hodgkin's lymphoma. J Clin Oncol 2002;20:2453–63.
218. Kaminski MS, Tuck M, Estes J, et al. 131I-tositumomab therapy as initial treatment for follicular lymphoma. N Engl J Med 2005;352:441–9.
219. Press OW, Unger JM, Braziel RM, et al. A phase 2 trial of CHOP chemotherapy followed by tositumomab/iodine I 131 tositumomab for previously untreated follicular non-Hodgkin lymphoma: Southwest Oncology Group Protocol S9911. Blood 2003;102:1606–12.
220. Zelenetz AD, Donnelly G, Halaas J, et al. Initial treatment of mantle cell lymphoma with sequential radioimmunotherapy with tositumoamb/iodine I131 I-tositumoamb followed by CHOP chemotherapy results in a high complete remission rate. Blood 2003;102:Abstract 1477.
221. Oki Y, Pro B, Delpassand E, et al. A Phase II study of yttrium 90 (90Y) ibritumomab tiuxetan (Zevalin®) for treatment of patients with relapsed and refractory mantle cell lymphoma (MCL). Blood 2004;104:Abstract 2632.
222. Gopal AK, Rajendran JG, Petersdorf SH, et al. High-dose chemo-radioimmunotherapy with autologous stem cell support for relapsed mantle cell lymphoma. Blood 2002;99: 3158–62.
223. Rajendran J, Gopal A, Durack L, et al. Comparison of radiation dose estimation for myeloablative radioimmunotherapy for relapsed or recurrent mantle cell lymphoma using (131)I tositumomab to that of other types of non-Hodgkin's lymphoma. Cancer Biother Radiopharm 2004;19:738–45.
224. Waldmann TA, White JD, Carrasquillo JA, et al. Radioimmunotherapy of interleukin-2R alpha-expressing adult T-cell leukemia with tttrium-90-labeled anti-Tac. Blood 1995;86: 4063–75.
225. Czuczman MS, Straus DJ, Divgi CR, et al. Phase I dose-escalation trial of iodine 131-labeled monoclonal antibody OKB7 in patients with non-Hodgkin's lymphoma. J Clin Oncol 1993;11:2021–9.
226. Goldenberg DM. The role of radiolabeled antibodies in the treatment of non-Hodgkin's lymphoma: the coming of age of radioimmunotherapy. Crit Rev Oncol Hematol 2001;39: 195–201.
227. Vallera DA, Elson M, Brechbiel MW, et al. Radiotherapy of CD19 expressing Daudi tumors in nude mice with yttrium-90-labeled anti-CD19 antibody. Cancer Biother Radiopharm 2004;19:11–23.
228. DeNardo GL. Concepts in radioimmunotherapy and immunotherapy: radioimmunotherapy from a lym-1 perspective. Semin Oncol 2005;32:S27–35.
229. Zalutsky MR, Bigner DD. Radioimmunotherapy with alpha-particle emitting radioimmunoconjugates. Acta Oncol 1996;35:373–9.
230. Postema EJ, Frielink C, Oyen WJ, et al. Biodistribution of 131I-, 186Re-, 177Lu-, and 88Y-labeled hLL2 (Epratuzumab) in nude mice with CD22-positive lymphoma. Cancer Biother Radiopharm 2003;18:525–33.
231. DeNardo GL, Kennel SJ, Siegel JA, et al. Radiometals as payloads for radioimmunotherapy for lymphoma. Clin Lymphoma 2004;5(Suppl 1):S5–10.
232. Michel RB, Rosario AV, Andrews PM, et al. Therapy of small subcutaneous B-lymphoma xenografts with antibodies conjugated to radionuclides emitting low-energy electrons. Clin Cancer Res 2005;11:777–86.
233. Press OW, Corcoran M, Subbiah K, et al. A comparative evaluation of conventional and pretargeted radioimmunotherapy of CD20-expressing lymphoma xenografts. Blood 2001;98: 2535–43.
234. Zhang M, Yao Z, Garmestani K, et al. Pretargeting radioimmunotherapy of a murine model of adult T-cell leukemia with the alpha-emitting radionuclide, bismuth 213. Blood 2002;100:208–16.
235. Hamblett KJ, Press OW, Meyer DL, et al. Role of biotin-binding affinity in streptavidin-based pretargeted radioimmunotherapy of lymphoma. Bioconjug Chem 2005;16: 131–8.
236. Forero A, Weiden PL, Vose JM, et al. Phase 1 trial of a novel anti-CD20 fusion protein in pretargeted radioimmunotherapy for B-cell non-Hodgkin lymphoma. Blood 2004;104: 227–36.
237. Sharkey RM, Karacay H, Chang CH, et al. Improved therapy of non-Hodgkin's lymphoma xenografts using radionuclides pretargeted with a new anti-CD20 bispecific antibody. Leukemia 2005.%%
238. Garlie NK, LeFever AV, Siebenlist RE, et al. T cells coactivated with immobilized anti-CD3 and anti-CD28 as potential immunotherapy for cancer. J Immunother 1999;22: 336–45.
239. Laport GG, Levine BL, Stadtmauer EA, et al. Adoptive transfer of costimulated T cells induces lymphocytosis in patients with relapsed/refractory non-Hodgkin lymphoma following CD34+-selected hematopoietic cell transplantation. Blood 2003;102:2004–13.
240. Kalamasz D, Long SA, Taniguchi R, et al. Optimization of human T-cell expansion ex vivo using magnetic beads conjugated with anti-CD3 and anti-CD28 antibodies. J Immunother 2004;27:405–18.
241. Brentjens RJ, Latouche JB, Santos E, et al. Eradication of systemic B-cell tumors by genetically targeted human T lymphocytes co-stimulated by CD80 and interleukin-15. Nat Med 2003;9:279–86.
242. Jensen MC, Cooper LJ, Wu AM, et al. Engineered CD20-specific primary human cytotoxic T lymphocytes for targeting B-cell malignancy. Cytotherapy 2003;5:131–8.

243. Wang J, Press OW, Lindgren CG, et al. Cellular immunotherapy for follicular lymphoma using genetically modified CD20-specific CD8+ cytotoxic T lymphocytes. Mol Ther 2004;9:577–86.
244. Kriangkum J, Xu B, Nagata LP, et al. Bispecific and bifunctional single chain recombinant antibodies. Biomol Eng 2001;18:31–40.
245. Hartmann F, Renner C, Jung W, et al. Treatment of refractory Hodgkin's disease with an anti-CD16/CD30 bispecific antibody. Blood 1997;89:2042–7.
246. Hartmann F, Renner C, Jung W, et al. Anti-CD16/CD30 bispecific antibodies as possible treatment for refractory Hodgkin's disease. Leuk Lymphoma 1998;31:385–92.
247. Hartmann F, Renner C, Jung W, et al. Anti-CD16/CD30 bispecific antibody treatment for Hodgkin's disease: role of infusion schedule and costimulation with cytokines. Clin Cancer Res 2001;7:1873–81.
248. Borchmann P, Schnell R, Fuss I, et al. Phase 1 trial of the novel bispecific molecule H22xKi-4 in patients with refractory Hodgkin lymphoma. Blood 2002;100:3101–7.
249. Manzke O, Tesch H, Borchmann P, et al. Locoregional treatment of low-grade B-cell lymphoma with CD3xCD19 bispecific antibodies and CD28 costimulation. I. Clinical phase I evaluation. Int J Cancer 2001;91:508–15.
250. Ely P, Wallace PK, Givan AL, et al. Bispecific-armed, interferon gamma-primed macrophage-mediated phagocytosis of malignant non-Hodgkin's lymphoma. Blood 1996;87: 3813–21.
251. Grossbard ML, Multani PS, Freedman AS, et al. A Phase II study of adjuvant therapy with anti-B4-blocked ricin after autologous bone marrow transplantation for patients with relapsed B-cell non-Hodgkin's lymphoma. Clin Cancer Res 1999;5:2392–8.
252. LeMaistre CF, Rosen S, Frankel A, et al. Phase I trial of H65-RTA immunoconjugate in patients with cutaneous T-cell lymphoma. Blood 1991;78:1173–82.
253. Kreitman RJ, Wilson WH, Bergeron K, et al. Efficacy of the anti-CD22 recombinant immunotoxin BL22 in chemotherapy-resistant hairy-cell leukemia. N Engl J Med 2001;345: 241–7.
254. Bang S, Nagata S, Onda M, et al. HA22 (R490A) is a recombinant immunotoxin with increased antitumor activity without an increase in animal toxicity. Clin Cancer Res 2005;11:1545–50.
255. LeMaistre CF, Meneghetti C, Rosenblum M, et al. Phase I trial of an interleukin-2 (IL-2) fusion toxin (DAB486IL-2) in hematologic malignancies expressing the IL-2 receptor. Blood 1992;79:2547–54.
256. Olsen E, Duvic M, Frankel A, et al. Pivotal phase III trial of two dose levels of denileukin diftitox for the treatment of cutaneous T-cell lymphoma. J Clin Oncol 2001;19:376–88.
257. Eklund JW, Kuzel TM. Denileukin diftitox: a concise clinical review. Expert Rev Anticancer Ther 2005;5:33–8.
258. Lambert SL, Okada CY, Levy R. TCR vaccines against a murine T cell lymphoma: a primary role for antibodies of the IgG2c class in tumor protection. J Immunol 2004;172: 929–36.
259. Arnold D, Faath S, Rammensee H, et al. Cross-priming of minor histocompatibility antigen-specific cytotoxic T cells upon immunization with the heat shock protein gp96. J Exp Med 1995;182:885–9.
260. Bondanza A, Zimmermann VS, Rovere-Querini P, et al. Inhibition of phosphatidylserine recognition heightens the immunogenicity of irradiated lymphoma cells in vivo. J Exp Med 2004;200:1157–65.
261. Timmerman JM, Levy R. The history of the development of vaccines for the treatment of lymphoma. Clin Lymphoma 2000;1:129–39; discussion 140.
262. Timmerman JM, Singh G, Hermanson G, et al. Immunogenicity of a plasmid DNA vaccine encoding chimeric idiotype in patients with B-cell lymphoma. Cancer Res 2002;62:5845–52.
263. Hsu FJ, Caspar CB, Czerwinski D, et al. Tumor-specific idiotype vaccines in the treatment of patients with B-cell lymphoma—long-term results of a clinical trial. Blood 1997;89:3129–35.
264. Krieg AM. CpG motifs in bacterial DNA and their immune effects. Annu Rev Immunol 2002;20:709–60.
265. Krieg AM. CpG motifs: the active ingredient in bacterial extracts? Nat Med 2003;9:831–5.
266. Friedberg JW, Kim H, McCauley M, et al. Combination immunotherapy with a CpG oligonucleotide (1018 ISS) and rituximab in patients with non-Hodgkin lymphoma: increased interferon-alpha/beta-inducible gene expression, without significant toxicity. Blood 2005;105:489–95.
267. Jahrsdorfer B, Muhlenhoff L, Blackwell SE, et al. B-cell lymphomas differ in their responsiveness to CpG oligodeoxynucleotides. Clin Cancer Res 2005;11:1490–9.
268. Rohatiner AZ, Gregory WM, Peterson B, et al. Meta-analysis to evaluate the role of interferon in follicular lymphoma. J Clin Oncol 2005;23:2215–23.

Specific Disorders 3

16

Adult Burkitt's Lymphoma

Kristie A. Blum, M.D.
Gerard Lozanski, M.D.
John C. Byrd, M.D.

First described by Dennis Burkitt as a malignant tumor with a predilection for the jaw in East African children in 1958,[1] Burkitt's lymphoma (BL) is a highly aggressive non-Hodgkin's lymphoma (NHL) that often presents in extranodal sites or as an acute leukemia. Originally thought to represent two different lymphoproliferative disorders, BL was historically classified as a small non-cleaved cell lymphoma[2,3] in patients with a solid tumor or nodal mass, and as L3 acute lymphoblastic leukemia (FAB L3 ALL)[4] in patients with more than 25% bone marrow involvement. However, on the basis of shared molecular and genetic features, the recently adopted World Health Organization (WHO) Classification of Lymphoid Diseases[5] recognizes the lymphoma and leukemic phases of BL as a single entity: a mature B-cell neoplasm, subtype Burkitt's lymphoma/Burkitt cell leukemia. The hallmark of this disease is the over-expression of the oncogene c-Myc, most commonly resulting from translocations of the *c-myc* gene on chromosome 8 and the immunoglobulin heavy chain (*IgH*) gene on chromosome 14, although variant translocations have been described.[6]

GENETIC FEATURES

Eighty percent of BL cases harbor t(8;14), resulting in the juxtaposition of the *c-myc* gene with IgH enhancer elements that drive c-Myc mRNA and protein production.[7] In the remaining 20% of BL cases, translocations occurring between chromosomes 2 and 8, t(2;8)(p12;q24), or chromosomes 8 and 22, t(8;22)(q24;q11), place the *c-myc* gene adjacent to either κ or λ light-chain loci and enhancer elements, respectively.[7–9] As heavy-chain and light-chain loci are specifically active in mature B cells, it is not difficult to understand how *c-myc* transcription is favored in BL harboring t(8;14), t(2;8), or t(8;22).

Three different clinical variants of BL have been described: endemic, sporadic, and immunodeficiency BL. The endemic form is most commonly observed in equatorial Africa, in children ages 4 to 7, with involvement of the jaw, kidneys, liver, mesentery, retroperitoneum, or endocrine glands. Sporadic BL is observed primarily in children and adolescents, although adults can be affected, accounting for 1% to 2% of all adult lymphomas in Western Europe and the United States.[10] The immunodeficiency subtype is frequently observed in the setting of human immunodeficiency virus (HIV) infection, and unlike other HIV-related lymphomas, is frequently noted in patients with CD4 counts exceeding 200 cells/μL.[11]

MORPHOLOGY AND IMMUNOPHENOTYPE

In addition to the different clinical variants of BL, two morphologic variants have been identified: classic BL and atypical or Burkitt's-like lymphoma (BLL).[5,12] Medium-sized cells with abundant, basophilic cytoplasm, often containing lipid vacuoles; round nuclei with clumped chromatin and multiple nucleoli; and a diffuse, monotonous pattern of infiltration are characteristic of classic BL.[10,12] A "starry sky" appearance has been described in this type of NHL due to its abundant proliferative rate, frequent apoptoses, and numerous macrophages containing ingested apoptotic tumor cells (Fig. 16–1A and B). The Burkitt-like variant, a provisional entity in the Revised European-American classification of lymphoid malignancies (REAL classification)[12] and a subcategory of BL in the WHO classification,[5] has greater pleomorphism in nuclear size and shape, with fewer nucleoli than classic BL. In many cases, BLL has features intermediate between diffuse large B-cell lymphoma (DLBCL) and BL, making pathologic diagnosis difficult. This entity has been quite troublesome, with a variety of reviews reporting differing characteristics of BLL, including translocation of t(14:18), lack of *c-myc* rearrangements, more frequent nodal presentations, and poor prognosis.[13,14] However, a recent review of BLL cases in the Southwest Oncology Group using the REAL classification criteria for BLL indicated that BLL can be distinguished from DLBCL by CD10 expression (85% vs. 27%), presence of *c-myc* translocations (80% vs. 0%), lack of t(14;18) (0% vs. 14%), and a high proliferative rate (Ki-67 staining of 88% vs. 53%).[15] Therefore, in accordance with the WHO Classification of Lymphoid Diseases, BLL should contain the translocation t(8;14) or an alternative *c-myc* rearrangement, and a high growth fraction, with Ki-67 staining exceeding 95%.[5]

BL cells express surface IgM, Bcl-6, CD19, CD20, CD22, CD10, and CD79a, and are negative for CD5, CD23, and TdT (Fig. 16–1 and Fig. 16–2). In contrast, precursor B-cell ALL is usually TdT positive and does not express surface immunoglobulin. The expression of Bcl-6 and CD10 suggests a germinal center origin for BL. Sequence analysis of the Ig variable heavy-chain and light-chain genes in BL confirms that the endemic, sporadic, and immunodeficiency-associated variants of BL have all arisen from a germinal center B cell, with evidence of somatic hypermutation.[16–19]

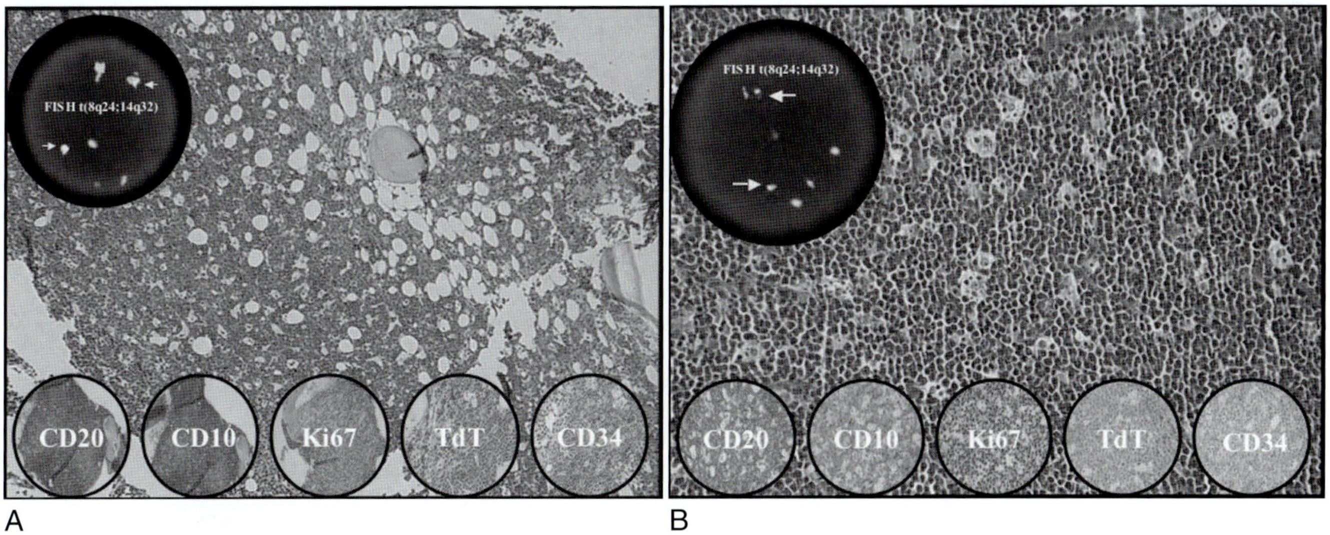

Figure 16–1. Typical morphology of bone marrow with involvement by Burkitt's lymphoma. **(A,B)** Characteristic immunophenotype illustrated by immunohistochemistry: CD20+, CD10+, Ki67+ (100%), TdT– and CD34–. Classical translocation involving cMYC and immunoglobulin heavy-chain genes is illustrated by FISH analysis with probes for 14q32 (IgH), *green*; 8q24 (MYC), *red*; and chromosome 8 centromere probe, *aqua*. Fusion product t (8q24; 14q32) in *yellow* (indicated by *arrows*). (See color insert.)

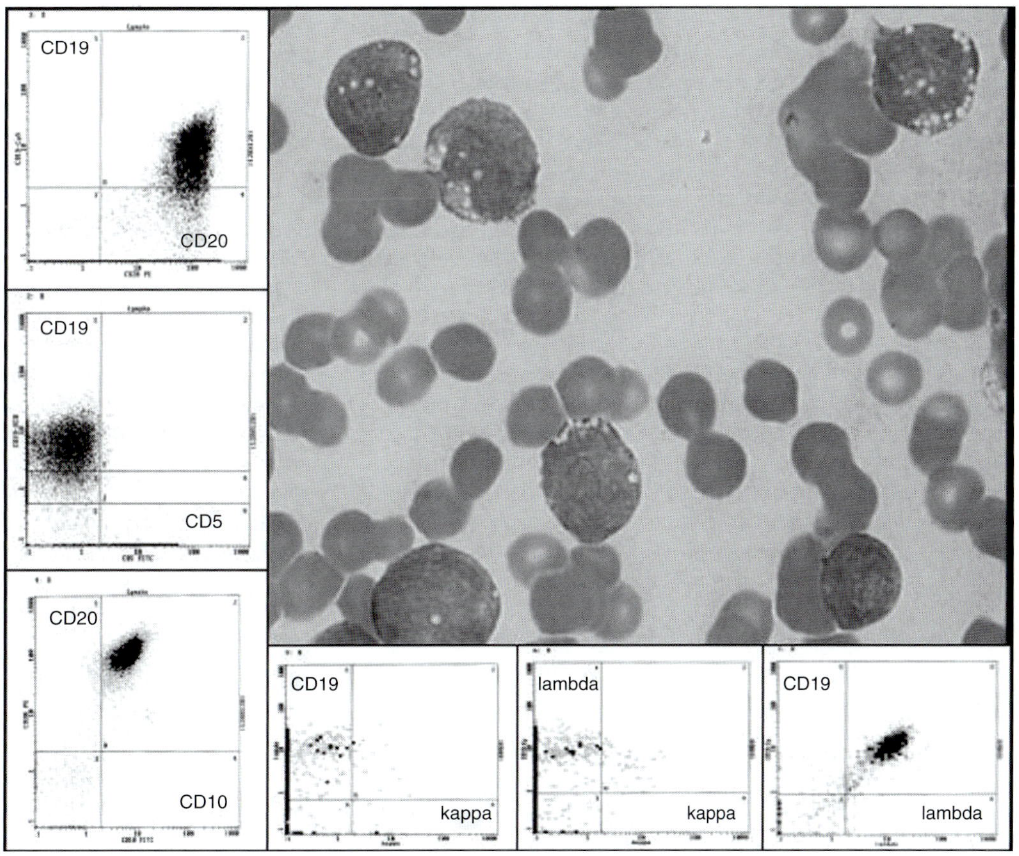

Figure 16–2. Typical morphology of Burkitt's leukemia. Characteristic immunophenotype is illustrated by flow cytometric analysis: CD10+, CD19+, CD20+ (bright), surface immunoglobulin light-chain lambda restricted (bright), and CD5–. (See color insert.)

CLINICAL PRESENTATION

Adult patients with sporadic or immunodeficiency-associated BL typically present with extranodal disease, with the abdomen being the most frequent site of involvement. Symptoms can include abdominal pain, nausea, vomiting, bowel obstruction, gastrointestinal bleeding, or syndromes mimicking acute appendicitis or intussusception. Intra-abdominal presentations usually affect the bowel or intra-abdominal lymph nodes, although kidney, pancreas, liver, spleen, or ovarian involvement can occur. At diagnosis, patients usually have bulky disease and ele-

Table 16–1. St. Jude/Murphy Staging System for Burkitt's Lymphoma

Stage	Description
I	A single tumor (extranodal) or a single anatomic area (nodal) with the exclusion of the mediastinum or abdomen.
II	A single extranodal tumor with regional node involvement.
	Two single extranodal tumors on the same side of the diaphragm with or without regional node involvement.
	Primary gastrointestinal tumor with or without involvement of associated mesenteric nodes only.
	Two or more nodal areas on the same side of the diaphragm.
IIR	Completely resected intra-abdominal disease.
III	Two single extranodal tumors on opposite sides of the diaphragm.
	All primary intrathoracic tumors (mediastinal, pleural, thymic).
	All paraspinal or epidural tumors, regardless of other tumor sites.
	All extensive primary intra-abdominal disease.
	Two or more nodal areas on opposite sides of the diaphragm.
IIIA	Localized, but nonresectable intra-abdominal disease.
IIIB	Widespread multiorgan abdominal disease.
IV	Any of the above with initial central nervous system and/or bone marrow involvement (<25% involvement, >25% is defined as L3 ALL).

vated lactate dehydrogenase and uric acid levels. Bone marrow and central nervous system (CNS) involvement is frequent, affecting 50% to 70% and 20% to 40% of adults, respectively.[20–24]

Due to the frequency of extranodal disease, several staging systems have been used for BL. Adult trials frequently reference the Ann Arbor system, although some authors find this system inadequate due to its inability to fully describe the extent of extranodal involvement. Therefore, some trials, particularly in the pediatric setting, report stage according to the St. Jude or Murphy staging schema (Table 16–1). It is important to note that this staging system recognizes Burkitt's leukemia, or the presence of greater than 25% bone marrow involvement as a separate entity, unlike the current WHO classification.[5] Also, this staging system was developed when surgery was often used for both diagnostic and therapeutic purposes, with the goal of surgery often being complete resection of intra-abdominal disease. Current therapy of BL does not routinely incorporate de-bulking surgery due to the existence of highly effective chemotherapy and a recent retrospective study demonstrating an increased rate of local complications and toxic death and a significantly decreased event-free survival (52% vs. 79%, p = 0.07) with early surgery.[25]

TREATMENT

Historically, treatment of BL mimicked the high-intensity, prolonged regimens used for the treatment of ALL with induction, consolidation, and maintenance phases. Such therapy is generally ineffective for most patients with BL and results in low frequency of cure. The high growth fraction of BL (doubling time of approximately 25 hours) favors re-entry of remaining viable malignant cells into the cell cycle and rapid growth between chemotherapy cycles with subsequent development of resistance. Short duration, intensive regimens that minimize treatment delays and maintain serum drug concentrations over at least 48 to 72 hours have improved outcomes for patients with BL.

Several crucial therapeutic principles in BL were first explored in the pediatric setting. With the knowledge that BL cells are exquisitely sensitive to cyclophosphamide, and that cyclophosphamide has a 6-hour half-life, Murphy et al.[26] piloted the use of fractionated cyclophosphamide (six doses of 300 mg/m^2 every 12 hours) in pediatric patients with BL. Murphy et al. hypothesized that a fractionated administration schedule would ensure exposure of every dividing tumor cell to the active alkylating metabolites of cyclophosphamide. In addition, the Murphy regimen incorporated high-dose methotrexate and cytarabine into alternate cycles of therapy, and shortened treatment intervals in order to prevent emergence of drug resistance.[26] Finally, Murphy's regimen included aggressive intrathecal CNS prophylaxis and eliminated the traditional maintenance phase, with planned treatment completed within 6 months.[26] With the incorporation of fractionated cyclophosphamide, alternation of non–cross-resistant cytotoxic agents between treatment cycles, a shortened duration of therapy, minimal treatment delays, and aggressive CNS prophylaxis, advanced-stage pediatric BL became a curable entity, with 2-year disease-free survivals (DFS) reaching 75% to 89%.[20,26–30] Efforts are now directed at improving these outcomes by incorporating higher doses of methotrexate (up to 5000 mg/m^2), high-dose cytarabine (3000 mg/m^2), and ifosfamide into these pediatric regimens.[20,29–33] Attempts to further reduce therapy in patients with limited-stage disease and without CNS involvement at diagnosis are also underway.[31,32,34]

With frequent involvement of the CNS and the bone marrow, adults were once thought to have a less favorable outcome than pediatric patients with BL; however, several recent studies suggest that treatment with intensive chemotherapy and adequate CNS prophylaxis can be curative even in the setting of advanced-stage disease or immunodeficiency.[20,21,35–37] With high-intensity, brief-duration regimens, 75% to 90% of adults achieve a complete response (CR), with 50% to 84% of patients maintaining these remissions at least 1 year following therapy (Table 16–2).[20,21,23,24,38–40] Several pediatric regimens, modified for

Table 16–2. Common Chemotherapy Regimens Used in Treatment of Burkitt's Lymphoma

Reference	Protocol	Number of Patients Treated	Median Age (Range)	CR	DFS or EFS	OS
Longo et al.[69]	ProMACE-MOPP	17	36 (19–90)	64.7%	61% at 15 years	35% at 15 years
	ProMACE-Cytabom	8		100%	86% at 15 years	88% at 15 years
McMaster et al.[38]	Vanderbilt	20	44.5 (21–69)	85%	60% at 5 years	N/A
Lopez et al.[47]	MD Anderson 81-01 and 84-30	44	32 (17–72)	80%	60% at 5 years	52% at 5 years
Bernstein et al.[39]	Stanford	18	25 (15–75)	78%	71.3% at 1 year	66.8% at 2 years
Divine et al.[48]	ACVBP	52	34	85%	47% at 5 years	53% at 5 years
Divine et al.[23,35]	LMB 81, 84, 86, and 89	51	33	83%	61% at 2 years	66% at 2 years
Hoelzer et al.[36]	BNHL83	24	33 (15–38)	63%	50% at 8 years	49% at 8 years
	BNHL86	35	36 (18–65)	74%	71% at 4 years	51% at 4 years
Todeschini et al.[24]	Modified POG 8617	8	35 (19–64)	100%	75% at 28 months	N/A
Magrath et al.[20,43]	CODOX-M/IVAC	26	25 (18–59)	92.3%	84% at 1 year	N/A
LaCasce et al.[40]	CODOX-M/IVAC	14	47	86%	72% at 21 months	N/A
Mead et al.[22]	CODOX-M/IVAC	52	35 (15–60)	75%	64.6% at 2 years	72.8% at 2 years
Thomas et al.[21]	Hyper-CVAD	26	58 (17–79)	81%	N/A	49% at 3 years
Cabanillas et al.[41]	R-hyper-CVAD	20	52 (27–77)	89%	86% at 1 year	N/A
Lee et al.[44]	CALGB 9251	54	44 (18–71)	80%	50% at 4 years	52% at 4 years

DFS, disease-free survival; EFS, event-free survival; N/A, not available; OS, overall survival.

use in adults, have been quite successful in the treatment of adult BL including the French LMB 81, 84, 86, and 89 regimens, the German Berlin-Frankfurt-Munster (BFM) protocols, and CODOX-M/IVAC.[20,23,30,35,36] Additional protocols, including the Stanford regimen, Hyper-CVAD, and Cancer and Leukemia Group B (CALGB) 9251,[21,39,41,42] have been evaluated primarily in adults, but incorporate many of the chemotherapeutic principles found to be effective in the treatment of pediatric BL. However, comparison of these treatment regimens is difficult in adult BL due to: (1) differences in patient populations among the trials, particularly regarding age; (2) differences in pathology (Burkitt's leukemia or BLL is excluded in some trials); and (3) differences in staging, with several trials employing the St. Jude system, while others use the Ann Arbor system.

In a retrospective review of 65 adults treated according to the pediatric LMB 81, 84, 86, and 89 regimens, 58 (89%) patients achieved a CR with therapy and 3-year overall survival (OS) reached 74%, despite the fact that the majority of patients had advanced-stage disease or evidence of leukemic involvement.[35] Seven of 12 patients who presented with CNS involvement remained disease-free up to 56 months after therapy. These LMB protocols consist of an initial cytoreductive phase using cyclophosphamide and prednisone to rapidly diminish the tumor burden and minimize the risk of tumor lysis, followed by two cycles of induction therapy, and one to two cycles of consolidation therapy. Both methotrexate and cytarabine are included in either the induction or consolidation arms; however, the doses of these agents vary in each protocol (Table 16–3). A prospective study of LMB-89 in adults confirmed the retrospective findings, with a CR rate of 83% and a 2-year OS of 66%.[23]

Based on their success in pediatric BL with the BFM protocols, the German Multicenter Study Group for the treatment of adult ALL (GMALL) developed two protocols, B-NHL 83 and B-NHL 86, for the treatment of adult Burkitt's leukemia.[36] Similar to the LMB trials, these studies also included a cytoreductive phase to minimize the risk of tumor lysis. Following this pre-phase, six cycles of alternating chemotherapy regimens were given, with fractionated cyclophosphamide, methotrexate, and low dose cytarabine in each of these alternating cycles. The B-NHL 86 regimen escalated the dose of methotrexate to 1500 mg/m^2 and added ifosfamide to the B-NHL 83 regimen (Fig. 16–3). Results were comparable to those noted in the French LMB trials, with 4- to 8-year DFS reaching 50% to 71%.[36]

Magrath et al.[20] pioneered the use of the CODOX-M/IVAC regimen in children and adults with BL. This regimen incorporates three cycles of CODOX-M for patients with low-risk disease (a single extranodal site or completely resected intra-abdominal disease and a normal LDH), and four cycles of alternating CODOX-M/IVAC for patients with high-risk disease (Fig. 16–3). CODOX-M/IVAC combines fractionated cyclophosphamide with higher doses of methotrexate (6720 mg/m^2) and cytarabine (2000 mg/m^2) than administered in the LMB and B-NHL trials, with the exception of LMB 86 and 89 where patients received up to 8000 mg/m^2 of methotrexate. CRs were noted in 24 of 26 adult patients treated, with 22 patients alive and disease-free at

Text continued on p. 289

Table 16–3. Comparison of Chemotherapy Regimens for Burkitt's Lymphoma

Reference	Protocol	Duration	Cyclophosphamide[a]	Methotrexate[a]	Cytarabine[a]	Ifosfamide[a]	IT Prophylaxis
Longo et al.[69]	ProMACE-MOPP	6–9 cycles	500–650 mg/m^2 × 1–2 doses	500–3000 mg/m^2	None	None	CNS XRT if BM positive
	ProMACE-Cytabom	6 cycles	650 mg/m^2 × 1 dose	120 mg/m^2	300 mg/m^2	None	CNS XRT if BM positive
McMaster et al.[38]	Vanderbilt	2 cycles	1500 mg/m^2 × 2 doses	200 mg/m^2	None	None	Given at investigator's discretion
Lopez et al.[47]	M.D. Anderson 81-01	15 cycles	1000 mg/m^2 × 1 dose	1000 mg/m^2	20 mg/m^2 q 8 hours × 15 doses	1000 mg/m^2 × 5 doses	IT MTX, ARA-C, and HC
	M.D. Anderson 84-30	9 cycles	1000 mg/m^2 × 1 dose	1000 mg/m^2	500 mg/m^2 × 1 dose and 20 mg/m^2 q 8 hours ×15 doses	None	IT MTX, ARA-C, and HC
Bernstein et al.[39]	Stanford	6–9 cycles	1200 mg/m^2	3000 mg/m^2	None	None	IT MTX
Divine et al.[48]	ACVBP	8 cycles	1200 mg/m^2	3000 mg/m^2 as maintenance for patients with a CR only	For patients in CR only	For patients in CR only	IT MTX and HC
Divine et al.[23,35]	LMB 81, 84, 86, and 89	4–7months	Cytoreduction: 300 mg/m^2 × 1 dose Induction: 500–1000 mg/m^2 × 3 doses Consolidation: None	Cytoreduction: None Induction: 3000–8000 mg/m^2 Consolidation: 3000 mg/m^2	Cytoreduction: None Induction: None Consolidation: 100–3000 mg/m^2 × 4–5 doses	Cytoreduction: None Induction: None Consolidation: None	IT MTX, ARA-C, and HC (CNS XRT only if + CNS disease)

Hoelzer et al.[36]	B-NHL 83	6 cycles	Cytoreduction: 200 mg/m^2 × 5 doses Treatment: 200 mg/m^2 × 5 doses	500 mg/m^2	300 mg/m^2	None	CNS XRT, IT MTX (spinal XRT if + CNS disease)
	B-NHL 86	6 cycles	Cytoreduction: 200 mg/m^2 × 5 doses Treatment: 200 mg/m^2 × 5 doses	1500 mg/m^2	150 mg/m^2 q 12 hours × 8 doses	800 mg/m^2 × 5 doses	CNS XRT, IT MTX, ARA-C, and DEX (spinal XRT if + CNS disease)
Todeschini et al.[24]	Modified POG 8617	6 cycles	300 mg/m^2 q 12 hours × 6 doses	1000 mg/m^2	3000 mg/m^2 q 12 hours × 4 doses	None	IT MTX and ARA-C
Magrath et al.[20,43]	CODOX-M/IVAC	Low risk—3 cycles CODOX-M	800 mg/m^2 × 1 dose + 200 mg/m^2 × 4 doses	6720 mg/m^2	None	None	IT MTX + ARA-C (CNS XRT only if + CNS disease)
		High risk—4 cycles CODOX-M/IVAC	800 mg/m^2 × 1 dose + 200 mg/m^2 × 4 doses	6720 mg/m^2	2000 mg/m^2 q 12 hours × 4 doses	1500 mg/m^2 × 5 doses	IT MTX + ARA-C (CNS XRT only if + CNS disease)
Thomas et al.[21]	Hyper-CVAD	8 cycles	300 mg/m^2 q 12 hours × 6 doses for 4 cycles	1000 mg/m^2 for 4 cycles	3000 mg/m^2 q 12 hours × 4 doses for 4 cycles	None	IT MTX and ARA-C (CNS XRT only if + CNS disease)
Lee et al.[44]	CALGB 9251	6 cycles	Cytoreduction: 200 mg/m^2 × 5 doses Treatment: 200 mg/m^2 × 5 doses	1500 mg/m^2	150 mg/m^2 × 2 doses	800 mg/m^2 × 5 doses	IT MTX, ARA-C, HC, and CNS XRT

[a] All chemotherapy doses are total doses per cycle unless otherwise noted.
ARA-C, cytarabine; BM, bone marrow; CNS-XRT, whole-brain irradiation; DEX, dexamethasone; HC, hydrocortisone; IT, intrathecal; MTX, methotrexate; PRED, prednisolone.

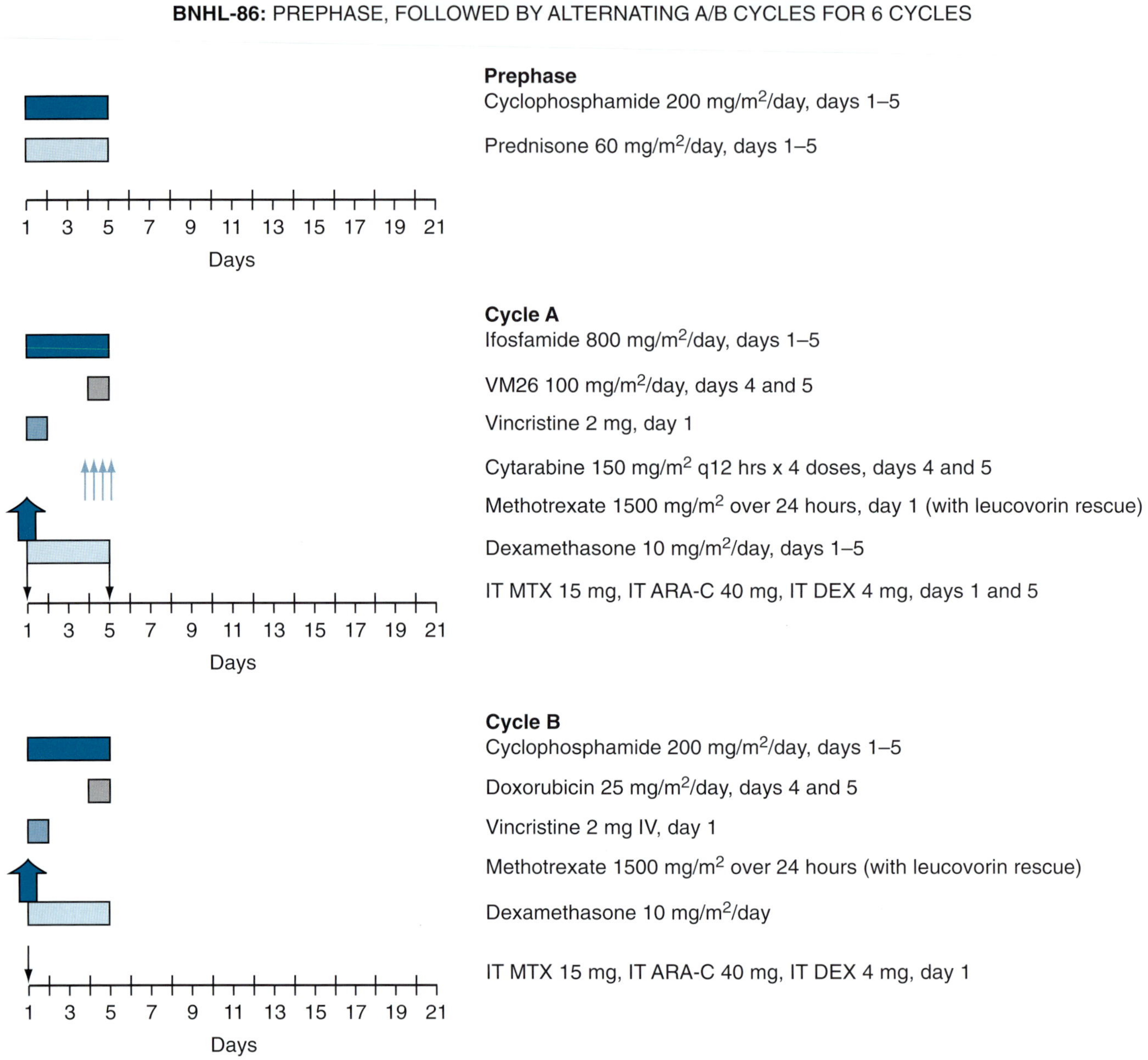

Figure 16–3. Chemotherapy regimens used in the treatment of adult BL 15.

STANFORD REGIMEN

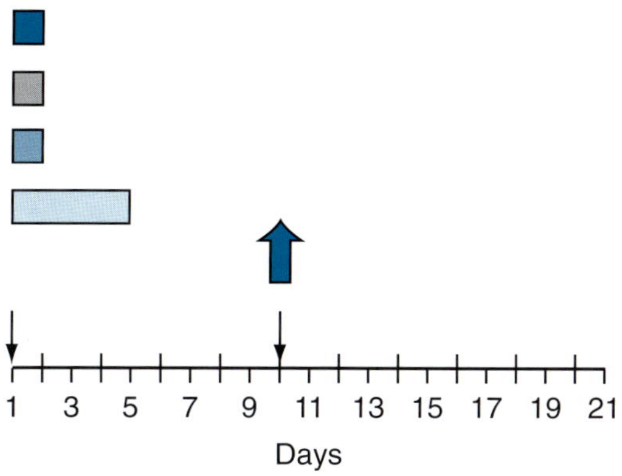

Cyclophosphamide 1200 mg/m^2, day 1

Doxorubicin 40 mg/m^2, day 1

Vincristine 1.4 mg/m^2 (maximum 2 mg), day 1

Prednisone 40 mg/m^2, days 1–5

Methotrexate 3000 mg/m^2 (with leucovorin rescue), day 10

IT Methotrexate 12 mg, days 1 and 10

***CODOX-M/IVAC:** ALTERNATE CODOX-M/IVAC CYCLES FOR 4 CYCLES

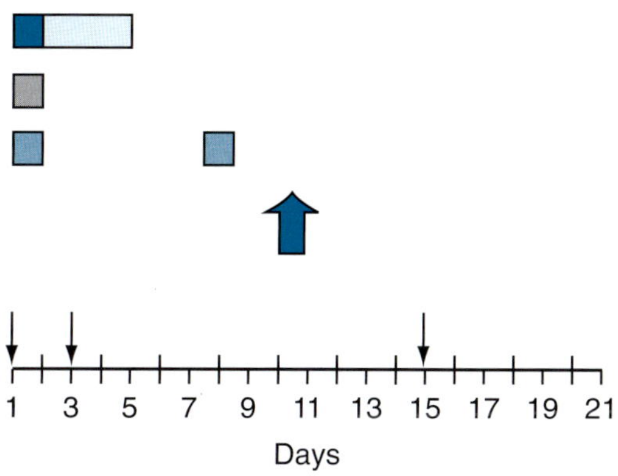

Cyclophosphamide 800 mg/m^2, day 1 and 200 mg/m^2/day, days 2–5

Doxorubicin 40 mg/m^2/day, day 1

Vincristine 1.5 mg/m^2/day, days 1 and 8

Methotrexate 1200 mg/m^2 over 1 h and then 240 mg/m^2/hr for 23 hr (with leucovorin rescue), day 10

IT ARA-C 70 mg, days 1 and 3, IT MTX 12 mg, day 15

CODOX-M*

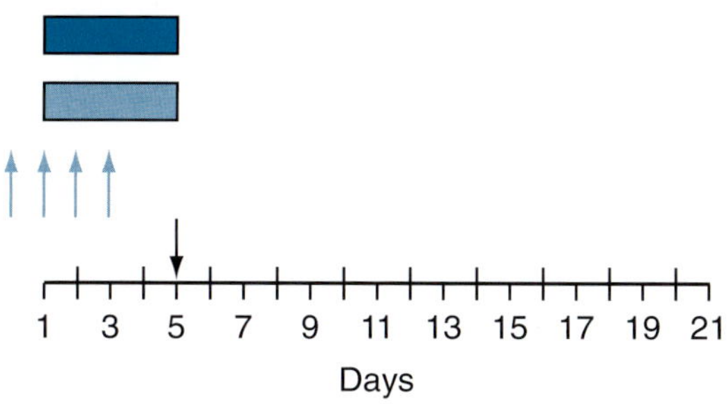

Ifosfamide 1500 mg/m^2/day, days 1–5 (with Mesna)

Etoposide 60 mg/m^2/day, days 1–5

Cytarabine 2 g/m^2 every 12 hours for 4 doses, days 1 and 2

IT MTX 12 mg, day 5

IVAC*

Figure 16–3, cont'd

Continued

CALGB 9251: PREPHASE, FOLLOWED BY ALTERNATING CYCLES 2–7

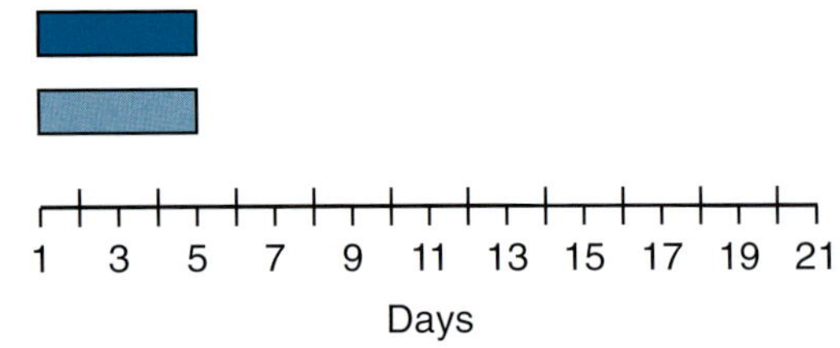

Prephase
Cyclophosphamide 200 mg/m^2/day, days 1–5

Prednisone 60 mg/m^2/day, days 1–5

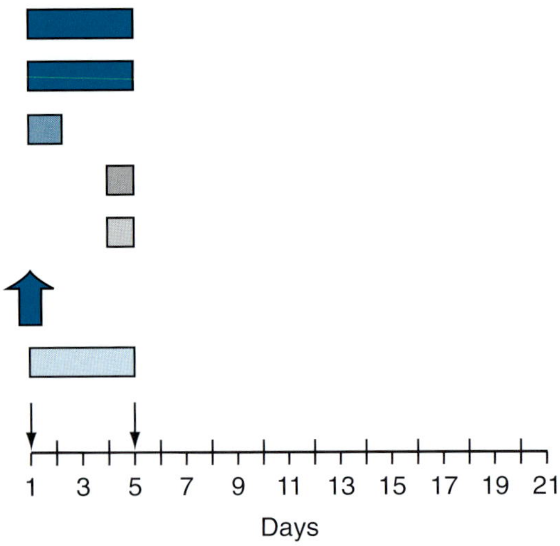

Cycles 2, 4, and 6
Ifosfamide 800 mg/m^2/day, days 1–5

Mesna 200 mg/m^2/day, at 0, 4, and 8 hours after ifosfamide, days 1–5

Vincristine 2 mg, day 1

Etoposide 80 mg/m^2/day, days 4 and 5

Cytarabine 150 mg/m^2/day continuous infusion, days 4 and 5

Methotrexate 150 mg/m^2 over 30 min, then 1.35 g/m^2 over 23.5 hrs, day 1 (with leucovorin rescue)

Dexamethasone 10 mg/m^2/day, days 1–5

IT MTX 15 mg, IT ARA-C 40 mg, IT HC 50 mg, days 1 and 5

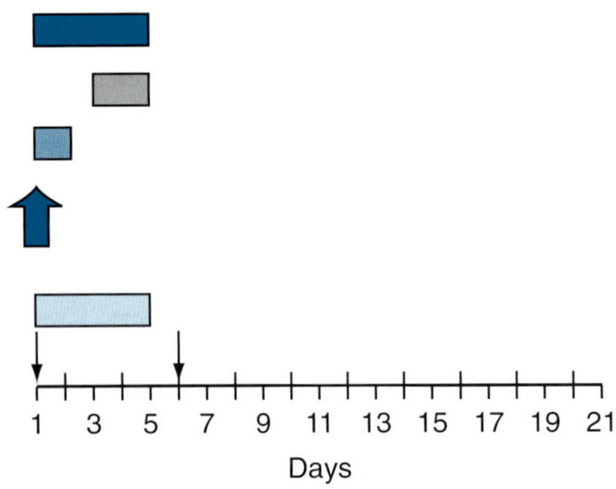

Cycles 3, 5, and 7
Cyclophosphamide 200 mg/m^2/day, days 1–5

Doxorubicin 25 mg/m^2/day, days 4 and 5

Vincristine 2 mg IV, day 1

Methotrexate 150 mg/m^2 over 30 min, then 1.35 g/m^2 over 23.5 hrs, day 1 (with leucovorin rescue)

Dexamethasone 10 mg/m^2/day, days 1–5

IT MTX 15 mg, IT ARA-C 40 mg, IT HC 50 mg, days 1 and 5*
* Cranial irradiation 24 Gy in 12 fractions after cycle 3

Figure 16–3, cont'd

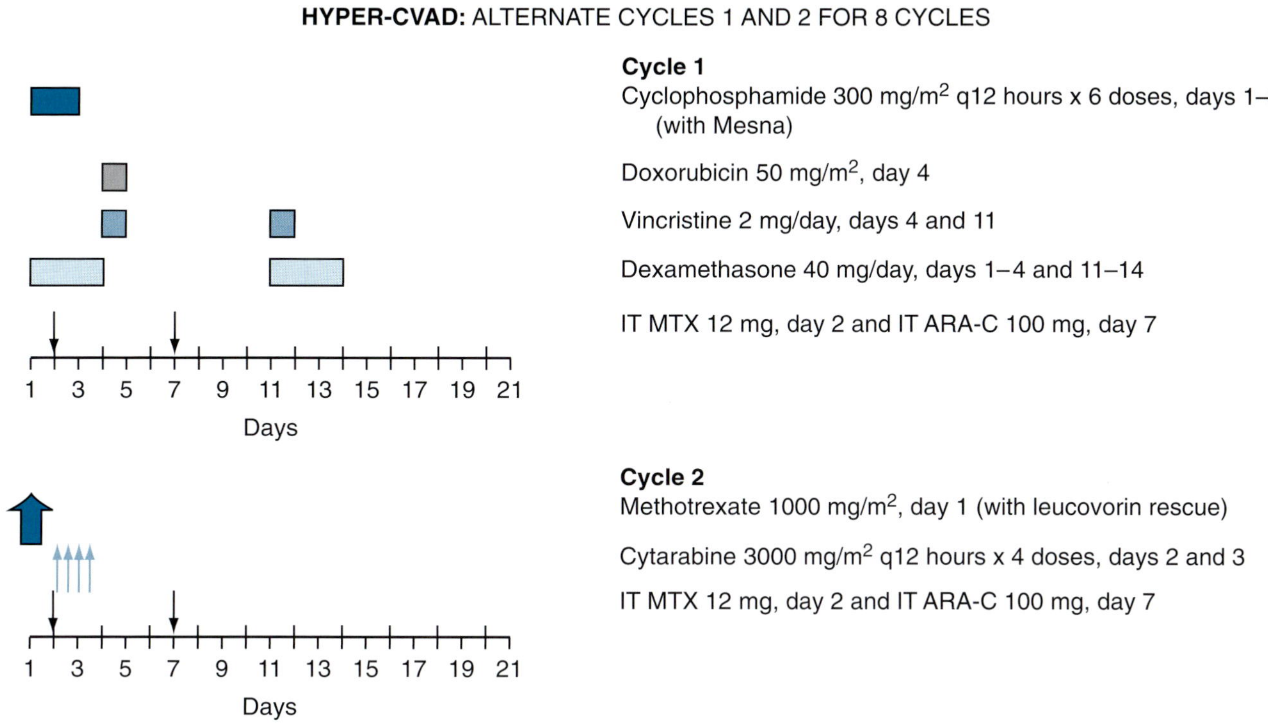

Figure 16–3, cont'd

47 months of follow-up.[43] While the results of this study seem remarkable, it is important to recognize that this study involved a relatively young adult patient population, with a median age of 25, although 70% of patients had advanced-stage disease by both the St. Jude and the Ann Arbor staging systems. A trial using this regimen in Europe reported 2-year event-free survival (EFS) and OS of 64.6% and 72.8%, respectively, in 52 patients with a median age of 35.[22] In 14 patients with a median age of 47, the Magrath regimen produced responses in 86% of patients, with 72% alive and disease free after 21 months of follow-up.[40] In this older group, myelosuppression was universal, and treatment-related deaths were reported in five patients.[22,40]

Other brief-duration, high-intensity regimens that have had success in BL include the Vanderbilt and Stanford regimens. After noting poor outcomes with conventional intermediate-grade lymphoma regimens like BACOP (bleomycin, doxorubicin, cyclophosphamide, vincristine, and prednisone) and COMP (cyclophosphamide, vincristine, methotrexate, and prednisone), McMaster et al.[38] evaluated 20 patients treated with a more aggressive regimen consisting of two intensive inpatient induction courses only. With this regimen containing high-dose cyclophosphamide, 200 mg/m^2 of methotrexate, bleomycin, vincristine, and doxorubicin, CRs were achieved in 85% of patients, and 5-year DFS reached 60%.[38] The Stanford group achieved similar results with a regimen containing high-dose cyclophosphamide (1500 mg/m^2) and mid-cycle high-dose methotrexate (3000 mg/m^2) administered over six to nine cycles (Fig. 16–3).[39] With this regimen, 2-year OS reached 66.8%; however, the best responses were noted in patients with limited stage disease (a single extra-abdominal tumor site or a completely resected intra-abdominal disease), where 2-year OS was 100%, compared to 53.8% in the advanced setting.[39]

Two other regimens have been examined exclusively in adults, namely CALGB 9251 and Hyper-CVAD. The CALGB regimen contains a cytoreductive phase, followed by three cycles each of two different regimens administered every 3 weeks (Fig. 16–3).[44] In 40 evaluable patients, CRs were noted in 80% and 4-year DFS approached 50%. However, severe neurologic toxicity (transverse myelitis, peripheral neuropathy, aphasia, cortical blindness, and dementia) was seen in 10 of 74 patients enrolled in this trial, attributed to the combination of high-dose methotrexate (1500 mg/m^2), triple intrathecal chemotherapy, and whole-brain irradiation (24 Gy) used for CNS prophylaxis. The cranial radiation was subsequently eliminated for patients without bone marrow involvement at presentation and the rate of neurologic events decreased. With the Hyper-CVAD regimen (Fig. 16–3), a modified Murphy regimen used to treat adult Burkitt's leukemia at M.D. Anderson, 81% of patients achieved a CR, and the 3-year OS was 49%.[21] Notably, this study contained a much older population of patients (median age of 58) than reported in other trials. Similar to CALGB findings, patients over the age of 60 had an inferior outcome (3-year OS of 17% vs. 77%), attributable to increased disease progression (32% vs. 3%) and treatment-related toxicity (16% vs. 9%).[21] In the CALGB study, only 32% of patients over 50 were able to complete six to seven cycles of treatment, compared to 79% of younger patients.[44] Mortality (21% vs. 9%), disease progression (32% vs. 3%), and toxicity (16% vs. 9%) were once again noted to be higher in those patients over 50.[44] As demonstrated by the higher rate of relapse in elderly patients with BL, these poor outcomes may not simply be related to treatment-induced toxicity. Thomas et al.[21] noted an increased incidence of complex cytogenetic abnormalities in older patients, including *bcl-2* gene rearrangements, which may contribute to a more aggressive phenotype.

Several investigators have incorporated up-front autologous stem cell transplantation into their treatment regimens for patients with poor prognosis BL. To date none of these studies appear to improve on brief duration, intensive chemotherapy alone for BL. Three-year OS rates of 60% to 72% have been reported following autologous stem cell transplantation in first CR,[45,46] similar to that attained with chemotherapy alone. Treatment-related mortality may exceed that of chemotherapy alone in those patients receiving up-front transplants, as demonstrated by data from the French LMB trials where 54% (7/13) of patients who underwent transplantation in first CR (6 allogeneic and 7 autologous) survived, compared to 89% (40/45 patients) of patients receiving chemotherapy only.[35] Therefore, on the basis of these small studies, there is no role for transplantation in first CR in BL.

CENTRAL NERVOUS SYSTEM PROPHYLAXIS

As CNS involvement is common in BL, CNS prophylaxis is required for the treatment of all adults with BL. Most BL regimens take a combination approach to CNS prophylaxis, relying on the efficacy of high-dose methotrexate, high-dose cytarabine, and intrathecal chemotherapy in the prevention of CNS relapse. Some earlier studies have incorporated whole-brain and occasionally spinal radiation into the prophylaxis regimen; however, there are no data to support that these modalities improve outcomes over combination therapy with intravenous and intrathecal chemotherapy alone. In fact, DFS was higher in BFM-86 despite elimination of the cranial and spinal radiation incorporated in earlier BFM-81 and 83 pediatric trials.[30] In addition, as demonstrated by the CALGB trial,[44] the risk of long-term, severe neurotoxicity is higher with the addition of radiation to intrathecal chemotherapy and high-dose methotrexate. Therefore, currently there is no role for prophylactic cranial or spinal irradiation in the treatment of BL, when CNS prophylaxis is provided by intrathecal chemotherapy coupled with high-dose methotrexate or cytarabine.

TREATMENT OF LIMITED-STAGE BL

Treatment recommendations are difficult in BL due to the lack of multicenter Phase III trials comparing regimens, the small numbers of patients treated on the available Phase II studies, and difficulty extrapolating these trials to clinical practice where elderly patients or patients with a poor performance status may be encountered. Several studies have noted very favorable results in early-stage (Ann Arbor Stages I to III or St. Jude Stages I to II) BL, with CR rates of 100% and 2- to 5-year freedom from progression (FFP) rates of 95% to 100%, compared to CR rates of 57%, and 2- to 5-year FFP rates of 29% to 60% in the advanced setting.[39,47] On the basis of these very encouraging results, three cycles of CODOX-M or the Stanford protocol may be suitable for those patients who present with limited disease. With the Magrath regimen, low-risk patients received three cycles of CODOX-M without alternating IVAC, while in the Stanford series, patients with limited-stage disease received six cycles of therapy rather than nine.[20,39] Two-year EFS of 83% to 100% have been observed with these regimens in low-risk patients.[20,22,39] Therefore, very brief duration regimens may be feasible in early-stage BL.

PROGNOSTIC FEATURES, SALVAGE THERAPY, AND STEM CELL TRANSPLANTATION

While debate is ongoing over the most relevant prognostic factors in BL, several studies have identified advanced age, advanced stage, poor performance status, CNS involvement, bone marrow involvement, anemia, the presence of peripheral blasts or an elevated white blood cell count, and an elevated LDH as indicative of a poor outcome in adult BL.[21,22,47,48] Not all series report bone marrow or CNS involvement as poor prognostic features,[21,36] suggesting that the incorporation of fractionated cyclophosphamide, high-dose methotrexate, cytarabine, or intensive intrathecal chemotherapy into the current treatment regimens may improve outcomes in this historically poor performing group. In addition, in some series, HIV positivity or histologic classification (BL or BLL) have had no impact on survival, confirming that with aggressive therapy, HIV patients with BL and patients with BLL can expect favorable outcomes.[35,47,48]

The majority of patients respond to treatment within 4 to 6 weeks of initiating therapy for BL.[21,39] With the Hyper-CVAD regimen, the median time to CR was 22 days, and 70% of patients achieved a CR within the first 4 weeks of therapy.[21] For those patients who relapse, this generally occurs within the first year of initiating therapy, although relapses have been noted 17 to 55 months after the completion of therapy have been reported.[21–23,35,48] Failure to achieve CR is a particularly poor prognostic sign. All patients who achieve a PR with therapy have been found to relapse and die of progressive disease without additional therapy.[20,39,48] Therefore, patients should be followed very closely for a response, with disease assessed after 6 to 8 weeks of therapy, and alternative therapy rapidly initiated for those patients failing to achieve a CR.

For those patients failing to achieve a CR or relapsing after treatment, the optimal salvage strategy is unknown. Certainly additional therapy with non–cross-reactive agents—particularly cytarabine, ifosfamide, or cisplatin—can be provided, particularly if these agents were not used front-line. However, even with non–cross-resistant chemotherapy, few to no BL patients respond at the time of relapse. Autologous or allogeneic stem cell transplant may represent an alternative strategy in the salvage setting; however, published series addressing high-dose therapy in BL are confounded by both selection bias and absence of detailed pathologic review. In a retrospective review from the European Group for Blood and Marrow Transplantation, 15 patients with BL or BLL in second or greater remission, 14 patients with primary refractory disease, and 10 patients in first partial remission received an autologous stem transplant.[46] Three-year OS was 37% for patients with chemosensitive relapse, and 7% for patients with chemo-refractory disease. In adult patients treated according to the LMB protocols, three patients who received an autologous transplant for refractory disease died.[35] In this same trial, one of two patients treated with an allogeneic transplant, and one patient treated with an autologous transplant at the time of second CR were alive 24 and 59 months following the transplant.[35] In a retrospective review of 89 children treated with autologous bone marrow transplantation for poor prognosis BL, 5-year EFS was 56.6% in patients achieving a PR with first-line therapy and 48.7% for patients with a chemosensitive relapse, compared to patients with primary refractory disease or chemoresistant relapse who all died within a year.[49] Therefore, autologous transplantation may be reasonable in relapsing patients or those who attain a PR after front-line therapy, provided that they remain chemosensitive. The data are less encouraging for those patients with resistant disease. Even less data are available regarding the efficacy of related or unrelated allogeneic transplantation in patients with BL.[35,50,51] From 1982 to 1998, 71 patients with BL were reported to have received allogeneic transplant (63 matched related, 3 matched unrelated, and 4 unmatched related) at the time of first CR (38.5%) or greater (24.6%) relapse.[52] Seventeen percent of patients had chemosensitive disease, while 20% were reported to have chemoresistant disease. As has been seen with autologous transplant, disease status at transplantation (first CR and chemosensitivity) has a significant effect on OS.[52] Interestingly, the presence of acute graft-versus-host disease had no impact on survival.[52] In matched patients treated with an autologous transplant, the relapse rate was equivalent between the allogeneic and autologous arms and OS was superior in the autologous arm. These data call into question the existence of a graft-versus-lymphoma effect in BL.

THERAPY-RELATED TOXICITY

In most trials, the most commonly encountered toxicities have consisted of myelosuppression and infections. With the Vanderbilt and Stanford regimens, leukopenia was reported in 100% and 23.4% of cycles, respectively, with three treatment-related deaths due to either tumor lysis syndrome or sepsis.[38,39] With the LMB, B-NHL 83 and 86, CODOX-M/IVAC, and Hyper-CVAD regimens, neutrophil counts below 500 cells/μL were reported in 81% to 100% of cycles, platelet transfusions were required in 35% to 71%, and severe infections were reported in 19% to 55% of patients.[20,21,35,36] Mucositis, cytarabine-related reactions including cerebellar toxicity, and thrombocytopenia-related hemorrhage have also been commonly reported. In order to minimize some of these toxicities, many regimens incorporate fungal, bacterial, and viral prophylaxis, and administer colony-stimulating factors, although the value of these agents is unknown. All patients receiving Hyper-CVAD received granulocyte colony-stimulating factor (GCSF) at a dose of 10 μg/kg starting 24 hours after chemotherapy and continuing until the total WBC reached 3×10^9/L. With GCSF, the average time to neutrophil recovery was 17 days, and was similar in both the under 60 and the ≥60 age groups.[21] With the Magrath regimen, low-risk and high-risk patients were randomized to receive granulocyte-macrophage colony stimulating factor (GM-CSF).[20] There was no difference in the control and GM-CSF arms with respect to incidence of documented infection, duration of neutropenia, and incidence of fever of unknown origin; however, GM-CSF treated patients did experience delayed platelet recovery.[20] Much less is known about the role of prophylactic antibiotics, antifungals, and antivirals in the treatment of BL, as no randomized studies have evaluated the use of these agents in this setting. Nonetheless, it is the authors' approach to administer GCSF (filgrastrim) in adult patients with BL and to apply aggressive prophylactic measures similar to that recommended for the management of acute leukemia.[53]

TREATMENT OF IMMUNODEFICIENCY-ASSOCIATED BL

HIV-positive patients have been included in several of the previously described chemotherapy trials in BL including the Vanderbilt, M.D. Anderson 81-01 and 84-30, and Hyper-CVAD trials.[37,38,47] Among the 12 HIV-positive patients treated on the M.D. Anderson 81-01 and 84-30 trials, 2 patients died of progressive disease and 4 patients died of secondary infections after successfully completing chemotherapy for BL.[47] Twelve of 13 HIV-positive patients receiving Hyper-CVAD (9 of whom received therapy in conjunction with highly active antiretroviral therapy [HAART]) achieved a CR, with 8 patients remaining in CR a median of 31 months after diagnosis.[37] The median survival was 12 months, and this correlated with the addition of HAART to the treatment regimen. All four patients not receiving HAART in conjunction with chemotherapy died. In a pilot trial combining CODOX-M/IVAC with HAART, three of three patients treated were able to maintain a CD4 count above 200 throughout therapy, and two patients remain disease-free after 35 months of follow-up.[54]

Toxicities in the HIV population consist primarily of myelosuppression. With the Hyper-CVAD regimen, all patients required multiple red cell and platelet transfusions, and 21% required dose modifications due to prolonged myelosuppression.[37] Thirty-five percent of cycles were complicated by fever or infections, including fungal pneumonia, CMV retinitis, and *Xanthomonas maltophilia* sepsis.[37] With CODOX-M/IVAC, HIV-positive patients experienced a longer duration of thrombocytopenia and more frequent culture-positive infections than their non-HIV infected counterparts; however, no differences were noted in the frequency of neutropenia, anemia, sepsis, or mucositis.[55] Therefore, HIV-positive patients with BL can be successfully treated with intensive chemotherapy, but close observation with transfusion support and antibiotic therapy is necessary. The addition of HAART to these regimens may improve outcomes and minimize the risk of opportunistic infections, but further evaluation is needed.

NEW MODALITIES FOR TREATMENT

Despite the improvement in CR, DFS, and OS rates with intensive chemotherapy in BL, novel treatment regimens are needed, particularly for patients with poor prognostic features at diagnosis, patients who fail to attain a complete remission within 1 to 2 months of therapy initiation, and patients who relapse. Several novel targeted therapies active in low-grade and intermediate-grade NHL may also be effective for the treatment of BL. For example, the monoclonal anti-CD20 antibody, rituximab, has had remarkable success as a single agent and in combination with chemotherapy in follicular and DLBCL. With the frequent expression of CD20 in BL, rituximab may also improve outcomes in BL in both the front-line and relapsed settings. Rituximab has recently been incorporated into the Hyper-CVAD regimen (R-Hyper-CVAD), with dosing on days 1 and 11 of cycles 1 and 3 and on days 1 and 8 of cycles 2 and 4.[41] To date, 20 patients have received R-Hyper-CVAD, with CRs reaching 89%, and a 1-year DFS of 86%. These response and early disease-free survival rates compare favorably with those observed with Hyper-CVAD alone, although further follow-up is needed to assess the impact on OS.[21] In addition to the M.D. Anderson group, the CALGB has incorporated rituximab into its latest BL regimen (CALGB 10002), with rituximab administration occurring during each cycle except the cytoreductive phase. This study is currently accruing patients and is expected to take 3 years to complete. Other monoclonal antibodies directed at other common B-cell antigens, namely CD22 and HLA-DR, may also have a future role in the treatment of BL.

Other novel therapies that may have potential benefit, but have not yet been evaluated in BL, include DNA methyltransferase inhibitors, histone deacetylase inhibitors, proteasome inhibitors, and cell cycle regulators. Hypermethylation of DAP-kinase, p16INK4a, and p15INK4B,[56,57] and the interaction of the Myc/Max heterodimers with a histone acetyltransferase[58] in BL suggest that epigenetic modifications are important in BL. While studies are ongoing with the DNA methyltransferase inhibitor decitabine in myeloid malignancies,[59] this agent has not yet been evaluated in NHL. Several histone deacetylase inhibitors including depsipeptide, MS-275, and suberoylanilide hydroxamic acid (SAHA) are currently being evaluated in B-cell malignancies[60–64]; however, their role in BL is unknown. Proteasome inhibition has effectively induced apoptosis in BL cell lines,[65] despite previous demonstrated defects in proteasome-mediated degradation of c-Myc.[66] In severe combined immunodeficiency mice bearing BL tumors, treatment with a proteasome inhibitor (Z-LLF-CHO) can lead to tumor regression.[65] Perhaps other aberrantly expressed proteins, including pro-apoptotic proteins, are affected by the inhibition of the proteasome, explaining the efficacy of proteasome inhibition despite continued c-Myc over-expression. Based on these data, studies with bortezomid are indicated in BL. Flavopiridol, a synthetic flavone capable of directly antagonizing cyclin dependent kinases 1 and 2, may also have activity in rapidly proliferating lymphoma cells.[67] While this agent has not been specifically in BL, responses have been noted in Phase I trials in patients with non-Hodgkin's lymphoma.[68] In the future, therapeutic targeting of c-Myc over-expression in BL through antisense deoxynucleotides or short interfering RNA duplexes targeting c-Myc mRNA may prove to be successful.

In conclusion, a remarkable shift in the therapeutic paradigm of BL has occurred. Once thought to be incurable in adults due to its high proliferative rates, BL has proven to be quite chemosensitive even in patients with CNS or bone marrow involvement at presentation. Important strides continue to be made within the field of BL with the incorporation of several active agents from fractionated cyclophosphamide to high-dose methotrexate into a variety of promising treatment regimens. While the optimal therapeutic strategy for BL is unknown, continued progress in the development of targeted therapies will potentially improve outcomes in this disease.

Acknowledgments

This work was supported in part by the National Cancer Institute (P01 CA95426-01A1), Sidney Kimmel Cancer Research Foundation, Leukemia and Lymphoma Society of America, and D. Warren Brown Foundation. JCB is a clinical scholar of the Leukemia and Lymphoma Society of America.

References

1. Burkitt D. A sarcoma involving the jaws in African children. Br J Surg 1958;46:218–23.
2. Lukes R, Collins R. New approaches to the classification of the lymphomata. Br J Cancer 1975;31:1–28.
3. Non-Hodgkin's lymphoma pathologic classification project. National Cancer Institute sponsored study of classifications of non-Hodgkin's lymphoma: Summary and description of a working formulation for clinical usage. Cancer 1982;49: 2112–35.
4. Bennett J, Catovsky D, Daniel M, et al. Proposed revised criteria for the classification of acute myeloid leukemia: a report of the French-American-British Cooperative Group. Ann Intern Med 1985;103:620–5.
5. Harris N, Jaffe E, Diebold J, et al. World Health Organization classification of neoplastic diseases of the hematopoietic and lymphoid tissues: report of the Clinical Advisory Committee meeting—Airlie House, Virginia, November 1997. J Clin Oncol 1999;17:3835–49.
6. Magrath I. The pathogenesis of Burkitt's lymphoma. Adv Cancer Res 1990;55:133–270.
7. Hecht J, Aster J. Molecular biology of Burkitt's lymphoma. J Clin Oncol 2000;18:3703–21.
8. Neri A, Barriga F, Knowles D, et al. Different regions of the immunoglobulin heavy-chain locus are involved in chromosomal translocations in distinct pathogenetic forms of Burkitt's lymphoma. Proc Natl Acad Sci U S A 1988;85: 2748–52.
9. Gerbitz A, Mautner J, Geltinger C, et al. Deregulation of the proto-oncogene c-myc through t(8;22) translocation in Burkitt's lymphoma. Oncogene 1999;18:1745–53.
10. Diebold J, Jaffe E, Raphael M, et al. Burkitt lymphoma. In: Jaffe E, Harris N, Stein H, et al., eds. Pathology and Genetics of Tumors of Hematopoietic and Lymphoid Tissues. Lyon: IARC Press, 2001:181–4.
11. Davi F, Delecluse H, Guiet P, et al. Burkitt-like lymphomas in AIDS patients: characterization within a series of 103 human immunodeficiency virus–associated non-Hodgkin's lymphomas. J Clin Oncol 1998;16:3788–95.
12. Harris N, Jaffe E, Stein H, et al. A revised European–American classification of lymphoid neoplasms: a proposal from the International Lymphoma Study Group. Blood 1994;84: 1361–92.
13. Yano T, van Krieken JHJM, Magrath I, et al. Histogenetic correlations between subcategories of small noncleaved cell lymphomas. Blood 1992;79:1282–90.
14. Macpherson N, Lesack D, Klasa R, et al. Small noncleaved, non-Burkitt's (Burkitt-like) lymphoma: cytogenetics predict

outcome and reflect clinical presentation. J Clin Oncol 1999;17:1558–67.
15. Braziel R, Arber D, Slovak M, et al. The Burkitt-like lymphomas: a Southwest Oncology Group study delineating phenotypic, genotypic, and clinical features. Blood 2001; 97:3713–20.
16. Chapman C, Zhou J, Gregory C, et al. V_H and V_L gene analysis in sporadic Burkitt's lymphoma shows somatic hypermutation, intraclonal heterogeneity, and a role for antigen selection. Blood 1996;88:3562–8.
17. Chapman C, Mockridge C, Rowe M, et al. Analysis of V_H genes used by neoplastic B cells in endemic Burkitt's lymphoma shows somatic hypermutation and intraclonal heterogeneity. Blood 1995;85:2176–81.
18. Chapman C, Wright D, and Stevenson F. Insight into Burkitt's lymphoma from immunoglobulin variable region gene analysis. Leuk Lymphoma 1998;30:257–67.
19. Elache V, Magnac C, Pritsch O, et al. Complete nucleotide sequence of IgV genes in three cases of Burkitt lymphoma associated with AIDs. Leuk Lymphoma 1996;20:281–90.
20. Magrath I, Adde M, Shad A, et al. Adults and children with small non–cleaved-cell lymphoma have a similar excellent outcome when treated with the same chemotherapy regimen. J Clin Oncol 1996;14:925–34.
21. Thomas D, Cortes J, O'Brien S, et al. Hyper-CVAD program in Burkitt's type adult acute lymphoblastic leukemia. J Clin Oncol 1999;17:2461–70.
22. Mead G, Sydes M, Walewski J, et al. An international evaluation of CODOX-M and CODOX-M alternating with IVAC in adult Burkitt's lymphoma: results of United Kingdom Lymphoma Group LY06 study. Ann Oncol 2002;13:1264–74.
23. Divine M, Cassasus P, Koscielny S, et al. Adult Burkitt lymphoma. A prospective multicenter trial with the LMB protocol. Proc Am Soc Clin Oncol 2000;19:80a.
24. Todeschini G, Tecchio C, Degani D, et al. Eighty-one percent event-free survival in advanced Burkitt's lymphoma/leukemia: no differences in outcome between pediatric and adult patients treated with the same intensive pediatric protocol. Ann Oncol 1997;8:S77–81.
25. Frappaz D, Miron I, Brunat-Mentigny M, et al. Is there still a place for initial surgery in advanced Burkitt's lymphoma (BL)? Proc Am Soc Clin Oncol 1995;14:a.
26. Murphy S, Bowman W, Abromowitch M, et al. Results of treatment of advanced-stage Burkitt's lymphoma and B cell (S Ig+) acute lymphoblastic leukemia with high-dose fractionated cyclophosphamide and coordinated high-dose methotrexate and cytarabine. J Clin Oncol 1986;4:1732–9.
27. Patte C, Phillip T, Rodary C, et al. High survival rate in advanced-stage B-cell lymphomas and leukemias without CNS involvement with a short intensive polychemotherapy: results from the French Pediatric Oncology Society of a randomized trial of 216 children. J Clin Oncol 1991;9: 123–32.
28. Schwenn M, Blattner S, Lynch E, et al. HiC-COM: a 2-month intensive chemotherapy regimen for children with stage III and IV Burkitt's lymphoma and B-cell acute lymphoblastic leukemia. J Clin Oncol 1991;9:133–8.
29. Bowman W, Shuster J, Cook B, et al. Improved survival for children with B-cell acute lymphoblastic leukemia and stage IV small noncleaved-cell lymphoma: a pediatric oncolgy group study. J Clin Oncol 1996;14:1252–61.
30. Reiter A, Schrappe M, Ludwig W-D, et al. Favorable outcome of B-cell acute lymphoblastic leukemia in childhood: a report of three consecutive studies of the BFM group. Blood 1992;90:2471–8.
31. Reiter A, Schrappe M, Parwaresch R, et al. Non-Hodgkin's lymphomas of childhood and adolescence: results of a treatment stratified for biologic subtypes and stage—a report of the Berlin-Frankfurt-Munster Group. J Clin Oncol 1995; 13:359–72.
32. Spreafico F, Massimino M, Luksch R, et al. Intensive, very short-term chemotherapy for advanced Burkitt's lymphoma in children. J Clin Oncol 2002;20:2783–8.
33. Schwenn M, Mahmoud H, Bowman W, et al. The addition of VP-Ifosfamide intensification did not improve event-free survival (EFS) for central nervous system (CNS) negative patients with advanced-stage small noncleaved cell (SNCC) lymphoma or B-cell acute lymphoblastic leukemia (B-ALL): a Pediatric Oncology Group (POG) study. Proc Am Soc Clin Oncol 2001;20:1465a.
34. Patte C, Gerrard M, Auperin A, et al. Results of the randomised international trial FAB LMB 96 for the "intermediate risk" childhood and adolescent B-cell lymphoma: reduced therapy is efficacious. Proc Am Soc Clin Oncol 2003;22: 3198a.
35. Soussain C, Patte C, Ostronoff M, et al. Small noncleaved cell lymphoma and leukemia in adults. A retrospective study of 65 adults treated with the LMB pediatric protocols. Blood 1995;85:664–74.
36. Hoelzer D, Ludwig W-D, Thiel E, et al. Improved outcome in adult B-cell acute lymphoblastic leukemia. Blood 1996; 87:495–508.
37. Cortes J, Thomas D, Rios A, et al. Hyperfractionated cyclophosphamide, vincristine, doxorubicin, and dexamethasone, and highly active antiretroviral therapy for patients with acquired immunodeficiency syndrome-related Burkitt lymphoma/leukemia. Cancer 2002;94:1492–9.
38. McMaster M, Greer J, Greco A, et al. Effective treatment of small-noncleaved-cell lymphoma with high-intensity, brief-duration chemotherapy. J Clin Oncol 1991;9:941–6.
39. Bernstein J, Coleman C, Strickler J, et al. Combined modality therapy for adults with small noncleaved cell lymphoma (Burkitt's and non-Burkitt's types). J Clin Oncol 1986; 4:847–58.
40. LaCasce A, Howard O, Li S, et al. The Magrath regimen is effective in older adults with Burkitt's and Burkitt-like lymphomas. Proc Am Soc Clin Oncol 2002;21:1150a.
41. Cabanillas M, Thomas D, Cortes J, et al. Outcome with hyper-CVAD and rituximab in Burkitt (BL) and Burkitt-like (BLL) leukemia/lymphoma. Proc Am Soc Clin Oncol 2003; 22:2309a.
42. Lee E, Pettoni G, Freter C, et al. Brief duration high intensity chemotherapy for patients with small non-cleaved lymphoma (IWF J) and FAB L3 acute lymphoblastic leukemia in adults: preliminary results of CALGB 9251. Proc Am Soc Clin Oncol 1997;16:a.
43. Adde M, Shad A, Venzon D, et al. Additional chemotherapy agents improve treatment outcome for children and adults with advanced B-cell lymphomas. Semin Oncol 1998;25:33–9.
44. Lee E, Petroni G, Schiffer C, et al. Brief-duration high-intensity chemotherapy for patients with small noncleaved-cell lymphoma or FAB L3 acute lymphocytic leukemia: results of Cancer and Leukemia Group B study 9251. J Clin Oncol 2001;19:4014–22.
45. Nademanee A, Molina A, O'Donnell M, et al. Results of high-dose therapy and autologous bone marrow/stem cell transplantation during remission in poor-risk intermediate- and high-grade lymphoma: International Index high and high-intermediate risk group. Blood 1997;90:3844–52.
46. Sweetenham J, Pearce R, Taghipour G, et al. Adult Burkitt's and Burkitt-like non-Hodgkin's lymphoma—outcome for patients treated with high-dose therapy and autologous stem-cell transplantation in first remission or at relapse: results from the European Group for Blood and Marrow Transplantation. J Clin Oncol 1996;14:2465–72.

47. Lopez T, Hagemeister F, McLaughlin P, et al. Small noncleaved cell lymphoma in adults: superior results for stages I-III disease. J Clin Oncol 1990;8:615–22.
48. Divine M, Lepage E, Briere J, et al. Is the small non-cleaved cell lymphoma histologic subtype a poor prognostic factor in adult patients? A case controlled analysis. J Clin Oncol 1996; 14:240–248.
49. Ladenstein R, Pearce R, Hartmann O, et al. High-dose chemotherapy with autologous bone marrow rescue in children with poor-risk Burkitt's lymphoma: a report from the European Bone Marrow Transplant Registry. Blood 1997; 90:2921–30.
50. Ungkanont A, Mongkonsritrakoon W, Jootar S, et al. Allogeneic stem cell transplantation in a patient with refractory Burkitt's lymphoma using non-myeloablative conditioning regimen. Bone Marrow Transplant 2000;26:1351–4.
51. Grigg A and Seymour J. Graft versus Burkitt's lymphoma effect after allogeneic marrow transplantation. Leuk Lymphoma 2002;43:889–92.
52. Peniket A, Ruiz de Elvira M, Taghipour G, et al. An EBMT registry matched study of allogeneic stem cell transplants for lymphoma: allogeneic transplantation is associated with a lower relapse rate but a higher procedure-related mortality rate than autologous transplantation. Bone Marrow Transplant 2003;31:667–78.
53. Hughes W, Armstron D, Bodey G, et al. 2002 Guidelines for the use of antimicrobial agents in neutropenic patients with cancer. Clin Infect Dis 2002;34:730–51.
54. Lichtman S and Calderon N. Alternating CODOX-M and IVAC in HIV positive patients with Burkitt's lymphoma. Proc Am Soc Clin Oncol 2003;22:2471a.
55. Wang E, Straus D, Teruya-Feldstein J, et al. Intensive chemotherapy with cyclophosphamide, doxorubicin, high-dose methotrexate/ifosfamide, etoposide, and high-dose cytarabine (CODOX-M/IVAC) for human immunodeficiency virus–associated Burkitt lymphoma. Cancer 2003;98:1196– 205.
56. Katzenellenbogen R, Baylin S, and Herman J. Hypermethylation of the DAP-kinase CpG island is a common alteration in B-cell malignancies. Blood 1999;93:4347–53.
57. Klangby U, Okan I, Magnusson K, et al. P16/INK4a and p15/INK4b gene methylation and absence of p16/INK4a mRNA and protein expression in Burkitt's lymphoma. Blood 1998;91:1680–7.
58. McMahon S, Wood M, and Cole M. The essential cofactor TRRAP recruits the histone acetyltransferase hGCN5 to c-Myc. Mol Cell Biol 2000;20:556–62.
59. Issa J, Garcia-Manero G, Giles F, et al. Phase I study of low-dose prolonged exposure schedules of the hypomethylating agent 5-aza-2'-deoxycytidine (Decitabine) in hematopoeitic malignancies. Blood 2003 (prepublished November 6, 2003; DOI 10.1182/blood-2003-03-0687).
60. Aron J, Parthun M, Marcucci G, et al. Depsipeptide (FR901223) induces histone acetylation and inhibition of histone deacetylase in chronic lymphocytic leukemia cells concurrent with activation of caspase 8–mediated apoptosis and down-regulation of c-FLIP protein. Blood 2003;102: 652–8.
61. Byrd J, Shinn C, Ravi R, et al. Depsipeptide (FR901228): A novel therapeutic agent with selective, in vitro activity against human B-cell chronic lymphocytic leukemia cells. Blood 1999;94:1401–8.
62. Bruner R, Marcucci G, Binkley P, et al. Phase I trial of the histone deacetylase inhibitor depsipeptide (FR901228) in fludarabine refractory chronic lymphocytic leukemia. Blood 2002;100:1492a.
63. Ryan Q, Headlee D, Sparreboom A, et al. A phase I trial of an oral histone deacetylase inhibitor, MS-275, in advanced solid tumor and lymphoma patients. Proc Am Soc Clin Oncol 2003;22:802a.
64. Heaney M, O'Connor O, Richon V, et al. Clinical experience with the histone deacetylase inhibitor suberoylanilide hydroxamic acid (SAHA) in heavily pre-treated patients with hematological malignancies. Proc Am Soc Clin Oncol 2003;22: 2321a.
65. Orlowski R, Eswara J, Orlowski M, et al. Novel demonstration of tumor growth delay in a murine model of human Burkitt's lymphoma after treatment with a proteasome inhibitor. Proc Am Soc Clin Oncol 1998; 17:a.
66. Bahram F, von der Lehr N, Cetinkaya C, et al. C-Myc hot spot mutations in lymphomas result in inefficient ubiquitination and decreased proteasome-mediated turnover. Blood 2000; 95:2104–10.
67. Arguello F, Alexander M, Sterry J, et al. Flavopiridol induces apoptosis of normal lymphoid cells, causes immunosuppression, and has potent antitumor activity in vivo against human leukemia and lymphoma xenografts. Blood 1998; 91:2482–90.
68. Senderowicz A, Headlee D, Stinson S, et al. Phase I trial of continuous infusion flavopiridol, a novel cyclin-dependent kinase inhibitor, in patients with refractory neoplasms. J Clin Oncol 1998;16:2986–99.
69. Longo D, Duffey P, Jaffe E, et al. Diffuse small noncleaved-cell, non-Burkitt's lymphoma in adults: a high-grade lymphoma responsive to ProMACE-based combination therapy. J Clin Oncol 1994;12:2153–9.

17

Large-Cell Lymphoma

17A

NODAL, SPLENIC

Jonathan W. Friedberg, M.D.
Richard I. Fisher, M.D.

As a group, diffuse large-cell lymphomas account for approximately one-third of all non-Hodgkin's lymphomas (NHLs), and 75% are of B-cell origin. Approximately one-third of patients present with early-stage disease (Stage I or II), with the remainder having clinically disseminated disease at diagnosis.[1] The natural history of the disease is aggressive, with a median survival of less than 1 year in untreated patients. Considerable improvements in the understanding of the biology of this heterogeneous disease entity should lead to significant therapeutic progress over the next several years.

CLINICAL AND BIOLOGICAL FEATURES AND STAGING

Although diffuse large B-cell lymphoma can occur at any age, it is, in general, a disease of middle-aged and older adults.[2] Unlike indolent lymphomas that are almost always widely disseminated at diagnosis, diffuse large B-cell lymphomas present as early-stage disease in approximately 30% of cases. Because they are potentially curable and because the best, and frequently only, chance of cure resides in the initial therapeutic choice, it is essential that the patient be accurately and completely staged at the time of diagnosis. It is imperative that the expertise of an experienced hematopathologist be sought in every case to establish the diagnosis and to ensure that the patient's lymphoma is accurately classified.

The staging system used for these lymphomas is the Ann Arbor staging system (Table 17–1), which was originally proposed as a staging system for Hodgkin's disease.[3] Although it is used extensively, the four-stage system has limitations when applied to NHL. For example, although the Ann Arbor system clearly separates patients by extent of disease, it does not address the issue of disease bulk. Bulk of disease has both prognostic and therapeutic importance in NHL. For example, patients with Stage II disease that is nonbulky have a better prognosis than do patients with bulky Stage II disease (bulk being defined as a tumor mass >10 cm in diameter in one location or a mediastinal mass greater than one-third of the thoracic diameter). Although patients with and without bulky disease both may be classified as having Stage II disease according to the Ann Arbor system, the optimal therapy for each might be quite different.

Several other pretreatment prognostic factors have been identified for NHL, including patient age, presence or absence of B symptoms, serum lactose dehydrogenase (LDH), tumor size as discussed earlier, number of nodal and extranodal sites of disease, and stage of disease at diagnosis.[4–6] Each of these clinical characteristics has been identified in one or more series of patients with aggressive lymphoma to be of prognostic importance with regard to patient outcome.

The International Non-Hodgkin's Lymphoma Prognostic Factors Project used pretreatment clinical prognostic factors in a sample of several thousand patients with aggressive lymphomas treated with doxorubicin-based combination chemotherapy to develop a predictive model of outcome for aggressive NHL.[6] Five pretreatment characteristics were found to be independently statistically significant: age in years (≤60 versus >60); tumor Stage I or II (localized) versus III or IV (advanced); number of extranodal sites of involvement (≤1 versus >1); patient performance status (0 or 1 versus ≥2); and serum LDH level (normal versus abnormal). With the use of these five pretreatment risk factors, patients could be assigned to one of four risk groups based on the number of presenting risk factors: low (0 or 1); low intermediate (2); high intermediate (3); and high (4 or 5). When patients were analyzed by risk factors, they were found to have very different outcomes with regard to complete response (CR), relapse-free survival (RFS), and overall survival (OS) rates. For example, low-risk patients had an 87% CR rate and an OS rate of 73% at 5 years. This is in contrast with a 44% CR rate and 26% 5-year survival in patients classified in the high-risk group.

It is assumed that prognostic factors are surrogate markers of the biologic heterogeneity of the lymphomas. Their biologic diversity is only beginning to be understood. For example, the expression of the nuclear Ki-67 antigen, which is an index of cell proliferation, appears to identify a subset of patients whose lymphomas exhibit a very virulent course. Miller and colleagues demonstrated that the OS rate of patients with a high Ki-67 proliferative index was significantly reduced compared with patients whose lymphomas had a low proliferative index.[7] One-year survival estimates among 60 patients studied was 82% for those with a low proliferative index versus 18% for those with a high proliferative index. Using a multivariate regression analysis

Table 17–1. Ann Arbor Staging Classification

Stage	Criteria
I	Involvement of a single lymph node region or of a single extranodal organ or site (I_E)
II	Involvement of ≥2 lymph node regions on the same side of the diaphragm, or localized involvement of an extranodal site or organ (II_E) and of ≥1 lymph node regions on the same side of the diaphragm
III	Involvement of lymph node regions on both sides of the diaphragm, which may also be accompanied by localized involvement of an extranodal organ or site (III_E) or spleen (III_S) or both (III_{SE})
IV	Diffuse or disseminated involvement of ≥1 distant extranodal organs with or without associated lymph node involvement

Fever >38°, night sweats, and/or weight loss >10% of body weight in the 6 months preceding admission are defined as systemic symptoms, and denoted by the suffix B. Asymptomatic patients are denoted by the suffix A.

Table 17–2. Pre-Treatment Staging Evaluation

1. History and physical examination
2. Complete blood count and chemistry survey including LDH
3. Chest radiograph
4. CT scan of chest, abdomen, and pelvis
5. Bilateral iliac crest bone marrow biopsies
6. Other, as indicated by results of 1–5 (see text)

incorporating commonly used clinical prognostic features, the authors confirmed the independent effect of proliferation on survival. Based on these data, it thus appears that the Ki-67 monoclonal antibody identifies a group of patients with rapidly fatal NHL for whom currently used chemotherapy regimens appear to be inadequate.

Cytogenetic studies and molecular analysis of protooncogenes and tumor suppressor genes are providing insights into the pathogenesis of diffuse large B-cell NHL. Unlike the case with the indolent lymphomas, no single genetic abnormality has been consistently found to be associated with diffuse large-cell lymphoma, but rearrangement of *bcl*-2 has been observed to occur in 20% to 30% of patients. A high level of *bcl*-2 protein occurs in 25% to 80% of diffuse large B-cell lymphoma depending on the study, and this appears to be associated with worse prognosis.[8,9] The adverse prognosis associated with this marker may be abrogated by the addition of monoclonal antibody therapy to the chemotherapy regimen.[10]

Offit and coworkers have reported on the incidence of rearrangement of the *bcl*-6 gene in patients with diffuse large-cell lymphoma.[11] This gene is known to have structural similarities to a class of transcription factors that participate in the control of cell proliferation and differentiation. The authors studied the incidence of *bcl*-6 gene rearrangement in 102 patients with diffuse large-cell lymphoma. Presence of the rearrangement was found in 23 patients, 19 of whom had extranodal disease. Other studies suggest that up to 70% express bcl-6 protein, consistent with a germinal center origin, independent of bcl-6 gene rearrangement. Rearrangement of *bcl*-6 appeared to correlate with a favorable clinical outcome, with the 3-year freedom from progression being estimated to be 82% as compared with 56% for patients without this rearrangement.

A number of recent studies have attempted to define germinal-center and non-germinal center phenotypes in DLBCL, using markers such as bcl-6, CD10 (germinal center) and MUM1/IRF4 and CD138 (post-germinal center). In some anatomic sites, a germinal center immunophenotype, particularly Bcl-6 expression, has been associated with a better prognosis.[12] The use of microarray to analyze gene expression has demonstrated the significant biologic and karyotypic diversity among diffuse large B-cell lymphomas. Microarray analysis of gene expression by one group has delineated three categories of DLBCL—one with a germinal-center-like signature, one with an activated B-cell signature, and a third, intermediate group.[13] Signatures have been shown to correlate with survival, independent of the clinical factors observed in the International Prognostic Index (IPI), and other known risk factors.[14] A recent study from Stanford University has demonstrated that measurement of the expression of six genes: *LMO2*, *BCL6*, *FN1*, *CCND2*, *SCYA3*, and *BCL2*, by PCR, is sufficient to predict overall survival in diffuse large-B-cell lymphoma,[15] yielding prognostic information similar to that found in the more cumbersome gene array analysis.

Future clinical trials will integrate this biologic prognostic information in eligibility criteria, with the ultimate goal of allowing clinicians to tailor therapy to the individual patient based on pretreatment biological assessment of the patient's prognosis.[16]

A proposed pretreatment staging evaluation is outlined in Table 17–2. As a minimum, all patients should have a (1) complete blood count and chemistry survey, including LDH; (2) chest radiograph and computed tomographic (CT) scan of the thorax; (3) CT scan of the abdomen and pelvis; and (4) iliac crest bone marrow biopsy (bilateral preferred). Because bone marrow involvement with large cells increases the likelihood of lymphomatous involvement of the meninges, many clinicians would recommend that a lumbar puncture be performed in these patients for cytologic and chemical analyses of the cerebrospinal fluid, along with MRI evaluation of the CNS.

In certain situations additional studies may be indicated. For example, patients who have unexplained bone pain or elevation of the alkaline phosphatase level should be evaluated with a bone scan. Plain radiographs of any abnormal area on the bone scan should be obtained to look for lymphomatous involvement of the skeleton. Because there is a high correlation between the involvement of Waldeyer's ring and the involvement of the gastrointestinal tract, the finding of disease in Waldeyer's ring necessitates studies of the gastrointestinal tract to document the presence or absence of disease.

There are two major roles for nuclear scintigraphy in the evaluation of a patient with diffuse large B-cell lymphoma.[17] These functional scans may improve staging at the time of diagnosis, particularly through the detection of otherwise occult abdominal or splenic disease difficult to assess on anatomic imaging. Perhaps more importantly, nuclear scintigraphy may help to characterize a residual mass on anatomic imaging following therapy as either fibrosis or residual active lymphoma. Positron emission tomography (PET) is a novel functional imaging technique that can use a glucose analog [2-fluoro-2-deoxy-D-glucuse (FDG)] radiolabeled with the positron emitter fluorine-18 to evaluate glycolytic activity, which is increased in malignancies, including lymphoma. The data supporting widespread use of this modality for patients with lymphoma remains limited, and largely retrospective.[18] FDG-PET appears to detect disease sites both above and below the diaphragm on staging of lymphoma, and may have particular utility in the evaluation of the spleen.[19] Moreover, persistently positive PET scans during and after chemotherapy have high sensitivity for predicting subsequent relapse; however, a significant false-positive rate mandates corroborative evidence with biopsy or anatomic imaging before proceeding to additional salvage therapy.

TREATMENT

Diffuse large B-cell lymphoma is a systemic disease at the time of diagnosis; therefore, chemotherapy is the mainstay of treatment. Although the standard chemotherapy regimen has not significantly changed over 25 years, the relatively recent incorporation of monoclonal antibody therapy into the standard treatment program represents improvements in overall survival for the majority of patients with this disease.

EARLY-STAGE DISEASE (STAGES I AND II NONBULKY)

History

Historically, irradiation as a sole modality of treatment was the therapy employed in the management of early-stage diffuse large-cell lymphoma. In these patients treated with radiation therapy alone, relapses were observed in nodal sites both within and outside the irradiated field.[20] In addition, relapses occurred in bone marrow and other parenchymal organs, suggesting the presence of microscopic disease in these organs at the time of diagnosis. The size of the irradiated field did not correlate with treatment outcome, suggesting that the use of larger ports would not have contributed to improved treatment outcome.

Radiation therapy as the sole modality of treatment for early-stage aggressive lymphoma is mainly of historical interest. Several series have now shown excellent results with the use of combined modality therapy (chemotherapy and radiation therapy). Hence, standard treatment now consists of chemotherapy alone or, more commonly, radiation therapy in combination with chemotherapy.

Randomized Trials

Four prospective randomized trials have evaluated the role of radiation therapy in patients with early-stage diffuse large B-cell lymphoma. The Southwest Oncology Group (SWOG) Trial randomized 401 Stage I and nonbulky Stage II patients to receive either three cycles of CHOP and involved-field irradiation (40 Gy to 55 Gy) or eight cycles of CHOP alone.[21] The 5-year progression-free survival (77% vs. 64%, p = 0.03) and overall survival (82% vs. 72%, p = 0.02) results favored the CHOP and involved-field radiation therapy treatment arm, although at 5 to 10 years this survival benefit is less apparent, with late disease recurrences observed in the radiation therapy arm. A separate analysis of progression-free and OS was performed using a modified international prognostic index (IPI) consisting of the following risk factors: age more than 60, Stage II disease, and increased LDH. Patients with zero or one risk factor had a higher progression-free and OS compared to patients with two or three risk factors. As a result of this trial, combination chemotherapy and adjuvant RT radiation therapy have become the standard care for patients with Stage I–II diffuse large B-cell lymphoma. Patients with a higher modified IPI or poor prognostic pre-treatment factors have a higher recurrence risk, suggesting that new treatment approaches are needed for these patients.

The Eastern Cooperative Oncology Group (ECOG) randomized 365 patients with bulky Stage I (mediastinal or retroperitoneal involvement or masses greater than 10 cm), Stage IE, and Stage II–IIE disease to eight cycles of CHOP chemotherapy with or without radiation therapy. Patients with no response or progression to chemotherapy were removed from the study. Patients in complete remission were randomized to 30 Gy involved-field radiation therapy or no further treatment.[22] Patients in partial remission received 40 Gy to the site(s) of pretreatment involvement plus radiation to contiguous uninvolved region(s). In patients randomized after complete remission, the 5-year disease-free survival (73% vs. 58%, p = 0.03), freedom from recurrence (73% vs. 58%, p = 0.04), and survival (84% vs. 70, p = 0.06) all favored the patients who received adjuvant involved-field irradiation (58). At 10 years, the disease-free survival continues to favor the addition of radiation therapy (57% vs. 46%, p = 0.04), but the survival differences no longer are statistically significant, similar to the aforementioned SWOG trial. In the patients who achieved a partial remission, 28% converted to a complete remission with the addition of 40-Gy radiation therapy.

The results of two European randomized trials were presented as abstracts at the 2002 American Society of Hematology meetings. Fillet and Bonnet compared CHOP x 4 with CHOP x 4 followed by 40 Gy in 518 patients more than 60 years of age who all had an age-adjusted IPI score of 0.[23] The 5-year event-free (CHOP 69% vs. CHOP + RT 64%) and overall survival (CHOP 78% vs. CHOP + RT 70%) did not differ between the two regimens. Additional follow-up of this study is required before making definitive conclusions. Reyes et al. compared CHOP x 3 followed by 30- to 40-Gy involved-field radiotherapy with the chemotherapy regimen ACVBP (doxorubicin, cyclophosphamide, vindesine, bleomycin, and prednisone), followed by consolidation chemotherapy using methotrexate, ifosfamide, etoposide, and cytarabine in 631 patients with low-risk, localized aggressive lymphoma.[24] Event-free survival (CHOP + RT 74% vs. ACVBP 83%) and OS (CHOP + RT 80% vs. ACVBP 89%) were both significantly better in the chemotherapy alone arm. Unfortunately, a significant number of patients in this study had bulky disease, for whom CHOP x 3 + RT would have been predicted to be inadequate.

Summary: Treatment of Early-Stage Diffuse Large B-Cell Lymphoma

Abbreviated CHOP chemotherapy plus involved-field radiation therapy is excellent therapy for patients with low-risk, nonbulky early-stage diffuse large-cell lymphomas (DLCL). Patients with poor prognostic features, such as advanced stage, tumor bulk, or high LDH, remain at considerable risk for disease progression, and current clinical trials are designed to improve outcome in this group of patients. Of note, the SWOG has completed a Phase II trial evaluating the integration of rituximab into the combined modality program for treatment of early-stage large B-cell lymphoma; results are not available at the time of this writing.

ADVANCED-STAGE DISEASE (STAGES II BULKY, III, AND IV)

History

Investigators at the National Cancer Institute (NCI) were among the first to demonstrate that some patients with advanced-stage disease are curable. Using combination chemotherapy regimens, they were able to achieve complete remissions in 45% of treated patients, with approximately 70% to 80% of these being durable remissions.[25] In the early studies, relapses beyond 2 years after therapy were rare, and therefore a disease-free survival (DFS) of 2 years was tantamount to cure. Based on these observations, subsequent trials focused on achieving higher numbers of CRs, with the assumption being that this would translate into increased numbers of patients cured of their disease.

The CHOP (cyclophosphamide, doxorubicin, vincristine, prednisone) regimen was one of the first combination therapy programs to use doxorubicin. Between 1974 and 1981, the SWOG conducted a series of trials to evaluate CHOP-based regimens in patients with aggressive lymphoma.[26–28] The CR rates for patients with clinical Stage III or IV aggressive histologies of NHL varied from 44% to 61%. The CR rates for patients with diffuse large-cell lymphoma varied from 58% to 62%. Coltman et al. updated these results with up to 14 years of follow-up, demonstrating that CHOP is curative for 32% of patients with advanced diffuse large-cell lymphoma.[29] This analysis provided an important benchmark for future comparison of pilot studies, and demonstrated that patients continue to relapse following CHOP chemotherapy for up to 7 years, thereby challenging the widely held tenet that a 2-year DFS was tantamount to cure. This finding has obvious implications with regard to follow-up of these patients, as well as to the interpretation of study results published after only a short period of follow-up.

With the recognition of the need to improve on the results achieved with the CHOP regimen, new and more complex regimens were developed in the 1970s and 1980s. These regimens are frequently referred to as the second- and third-generation regimens to distinguish them from the earlier regimens such as CHOP. Initial single-institution studies of the second- and third-generation regimens appeared promising, and suggested that the number of patients cured of their disease might be double that which had been achieved with the CHOP regimen. These results were not surprising because many patients treated in the single-institution studies had less advanced-stage disease and were younger than the patients treated in the cooperative group trials of CHOP. More than 40 randomized clinical trials have been reported to identify the best treatment regimen for patients with advanced diffuse aggressive lymphoma. The majority of these trials have not found a significant treatment advantage for any particular regimen.

Two-Arm Randomized Trials

ECOG performed a prospective, randomized trial to compare prospectively standard therapy CHOP with m-BACOD.[30] A total of 392 patients were enrolled, of whom 325 were eligible for the study. Patients with Stages III and IV diffuse mixed or diffuse large-cell lymphoma with no prior treatment were eligible. Eighty-eight (51%) of 174 patients treated with CHOP and 85 (56%) of 151 patients treated with m-BACOD achieved a CR ($p = 0.32$). With a median follow-up of 4 years, 91 patients treated with CHOP and 71 treated with m-BACOD have died. After 2 and 5 years, survival rates were 59% and 48%, respectively, for CHOP, and 62% and 49%, respectively, for m-BACOD. There was no significant difference in OS between the two treatments ($p = 0.49$), and there was no significant difference between the two treatments with respect to time to treatment failure. There also was no difference in CR duration between the CHOP and m-BACOD arms. The two arms did differ with regard to toxicity. Patients treated with m-BACOD had significantly more toxic reactions than did those treated with CHOP. Most notable were the differences between treatment with regard to moderate, severe, and life-threatening pulmonary toxicity (CHOP 3% vs. m-BACOD 23%), infections (CHOP 13% vs. m-BACOD 35%), thrombocytopenia (CHOP 2% vs. m-BACOD 37%), and stomatitis (CHOP 2% vs. m-BACOD 37%). Given this toxicity, CHOP would have to be considered the preferable therapy, given a choice between these two regimens.

The New Zealand Lymphoma Study Group reported results of a prospective, randomized trial comparing the third-generation regimen MACOP-B with the CHOP regimen.[31] A total of 304 patients were enrolled in the study, of whom 236 were eligible. Patients with bulky Stage I and Stages II, III, and IV disease were eligible. Eligible histologies included diffuse small cleaved cell, diffuse mixed small and large-cell, follicular large-cell, diffuse large-cell, and immunoblastic lymphomas. Responding patients received at least six cycles of CHOP or two cycles after achieving a CR. MACOP-B was administered over the prescribed 12-week period. Median age of patients was 54 years for the MACOP-B arm and 53 years for the CHOP arm. A total of 125 patients (53%) were randomized to MACOP-B, and 111 (47%) to CHOP. Sixty-four (51%) of 125 patients treated with MACOP-B achieved a CR, as compared with 65 (59%) of 111 patients treated with CHOP ($p = 0.3$). CR rates for patients with diffuse mixed, diffuse large-cell, and large-cell immunoblastic lymphomas were 54% with MACOP-B and 59% with CHOP. Estimated failure-free survival at 4 years was 44% for MACOP-B and 32% for CHOP. Fifty-two patients on each arm have died. Estimated survival at 4 years was 56% for MACOP-B and 51% for CHOP ($p = 0.69$).

Similar to the ECOG trial, there was a difference in toxicity between the treatment arms. Patients who received MACOP-B experienced significantly more Grade 3 or 4 hematologic toxicity ($p = 0.04$), stomatitis ($p < 0.0001$), and gastrointestinal ulceration ($p = 0.03$) as compared with the CHOP patients.

CHOP versus m-BACOD versus ProMACE = CytaBOM versus MACOP-B

The most definitive study was an intergroup trial conducted by SWOG and ECOG—1138 previously untreated patients with Stages II bulky, III, and IV disease with intermediate- or high-grade histology—were randomized to one of four treatment arms: CHOP, m-BACOD, ProMACE-CytaBOM, or MACOP-B.[32] A total of 899 patients were eligible for the study. Each of the regimens was administered exactly as had been described in the prior Phase II studies. The median age of patients was 54 years, with 25% of the patients aged over 64. With a median follow-up of 49 months, no differences were observed among the four treatment arms with respect to CR or overall response rates: CR rates were 44% for CHOP, 48% for m-BACOD, 56% for ProMACE-CytaBOM, and 51% for MACOP-B. Because assessment of CR is difficult owing to persistent abnormalities on CT scans after treatment, the time to treatment failure, which is a measure of time to progression, relapse, or death from any cause, was analyzed as a more accurate estimate of the fraction of patients cured by the initial therapy. Forty-three percent of all eligible patients were estimated to be alive without disease at 3 years. By treatment arm, 43% on the CHOP arm, 43% on the m-BACOD arm, 44% on the ProMACE-CytaBOM arm, and 40% on the MACOP-B arm are projected to be alive without disease at 3 years ($p = 0.35$). Projected OS at 3 years for all eligible patients was 52%; 49% on the MACOP-B arm, 51% on the m-BACOD arm, 53% on the ProMACE-CytaBOM arm, and 55% on the CHOP arm ($p = 0.90$).

Toxicity observed in this trial was similar to that reported in Phase II trials of the same regimens. Severe toxic reactions were related to granulocytopenia and subsequent infection. Grade 4 or life-threatening toxicity occurred in 31% of patients on the CHOP arm, 54% on the m-BACOD arm, 29% on the ProMACE-CytaBOM arm, and 43% on the MACOP-B arm. The incidence of Grade 5 or fatal toxicity was 1% in the CHOP patients, 3% in the ProMACE-CytaBOM patients, 5% in the m-BACOD patients, and 6% in the MACOP-B patients. The difference in the fatality rates was not statistically different ($p = 0.09$). However, when fatal and life-threatening reactions were combined, significant differences were found between regimens, with CHOP and ProMACE-CytaBOM being less toxic than m-BACOD and MACOP-B ($p = 0.001$).

Hence, in this large prospective, randomized study, once again the efficacy of the CHOP regimen was found to be equivalent to the newer chemotherapy regimens. The toxicity profile as well as cost would also favor the use of CHOP over any of the three regimens with which it was compared.

Summary: Standard Chemotherapy for Disseminated Diffuse Large B-Cell Lymphoma

Based on the available data from randomized, prospective studies, CHOP remains the standard chemotherapy for advanced-stage, diffuse large-cell and immunoblastic lymphoma. With a projected DFS rate of 43%, it is obvious that it is far from ideal therapy, and there is clearly a need for better treatment approaches. We strongly advocate participation in a clinical trial that is, in fact, the best available treatment. Outside of a clinical trial, CHOP-based therapy (currently with monoclonal antibody therapy; see next section) remains standard therapy for these lymphomas. Patients who present with lymphomatous involvement of the meninges should receive a course of intrathecal chemotherapy; many clinicians would also give cranial radiation therapy in addition to the chemotherapy in this situation.

New Therapeutic Approaches

Newer therapeutic approaches include (1) the addition of monoclonal antibody therapy to chemotherapy; (2) dose intensification using standard chemotherapy, and (3) providing autologous stem cell support as rescue from marrow-ablative chemotherapy.

Monoclonal Antibody Therapy

Attempts have been made to improve the response to CHOP by combining it with the monoclonal antibody rituximab. An early study of 33 patients showed a 97% response rate and a 73% complete response rate.[33] The Groupe d'Etude des Lymphomes de l'Adulte (GELA) group randomized 399 previously untreated patients with diffuse large B-cell lymphoma, 60 to 80 years old, to receive either eight cycles of CHOP every 3 weeks or eight cycles of CHOP plus rituximab given on day 1 of each cycle.[34] With a median follow-up of 2 years, the addition of rituximab to the CHOP regimen increased the CR rate (76% vs. 63%, $p = 0.005$), and prolonged both event-free and OS in these patients, without a clinically significant increase in toxicity.

A larger (N = 632) intergroup U.S. study randomized a similar population of patients to CHOP versus CHOP with rituximab given on a different schedule[35] as described in follicular lymphoma.[36] Responding patients then were randomized to receive either rituximab maintenance therapy (4 doses q 6 months × 2 years) or no maintenance. Preliminary results suggest a progression-free survival benefit to the addition of rituximab; however, no OS benefit is yet apparent. There was no clear benefit to rituximab maintenance when rituximab was incorporated into the initial treatment regimen. Using a weighted analysis, an OS benefit was apparent when rituximab was combined with CHOP chemotherapy. Finally, preliminary results from an international trial evaluating the combination of CHOP and rituximab in patients under age 60 analyzed 326 patients.[37] Patients receiving rituximab with chemotherapy had a significantly longer time-to-treatment failure (84% vs. 62.5%) compared with chemotherapy alone.

Based largely on the published results from GELA, CHOP with rituximab therapy (all therapy administered on day 1) has emerged to become the standard initial treatment for advanced-stage diffuse large B-cell lymphoma in the United States. An unplanned subgroup analysis of the GELA trial demonstrated that the benefit of rituximab appeared limited to patients with lymphoma that overexpressed bcl-2 on immunohistochemistry.[10] Ongoing research will better define groups of patients with large-cell lymphoma, if any, who do not benefit from the addition of monoclonal antibody therapy to chemotherapy.

Dose Intensification

The concept of dose intensity may be an important determinant of treatment outcome; simply stated, it argues that increasing the drug dose per unit time will increase its effectiveness. It does appear that treatment-related variables such as the dose intensity of drug delivered play a role in determining outcome. What is not clear is the independence of treatment-related variables from pre-treatment characteristics.

The third-generation regimens focused on the delivery of six to eight active drugs given at the highest possible dose intensity. As noted earlier, this approach did not seem to impact on improved results as compared with older regimens such as CHOP. With the availability of colony-stimulating factors (CSFs), the ability to maximize dose intensity has been improved as compared with dosages that can be delivered without CSF support. Hence, one rational approach to maximizing the efficacy of therapy is to dose-escalate the drugs given in standard regimens with CSF support.

Two recent studies suggest possible benefits to dose intensification strategies. The SWOG conducted a pilot study evaluating dose-intensified CHOP (CHOP-DI: cyclophosphamide 1600 mg/m^2, doxorubicin 65 mg/m^2, and vincristine 1.4 mg/m^2) with filgrastim support, every 14 days for six planned courses.[38] Treatment with CHOP-DI was safely administered in the cooperative group setting, and resulted in survival 14% better compared with historical SWOG controls. Moreover, the NHL-B1 trial from Germany randomized patients to six cycles of CHOP-21, CHOP-14, CHOEP-21 (CHOP plus etoposide 100 mg/m^2 day 1 through day 3), or CHOEP-14 in a 2 × 2 factorial study design.[39] Patients in the 2-week regimens received G-CSF starting from day 4. Patients in this trial also received radiotherapy (36 Gy) to sites of initial bulky disease and extranodal disease. In patients older than age 60, 5-year overall survival rates were 40.6% for CHOP-21, and 53.3% for CHOP-14, suggesting a benefit to intensified therapy in this group of patients.[40] Additional trials incorporating monoclonal antibody therapy into intensified programs are ongoing.

Autologous Stem Cell Transplantation

High-dose chemotherapy with autologous bone marrow support has established itself as effective salvage therapy for selected patients with refractory or relapsed diffuse aggressive lymphoma.[41] Although there has been considerable variability in the selection criteria of these studies, several consistent findings have been observed. The patients who are likely to achieve a complete remission and possible cure are those who responded well to initial therapy, who respond well to salvage therapy pretransplant, and who enter transplant with no or minimal residual disease. Patients progressing on salvage therapy as well as those who responded poorly to initial therapy are unlikely to benefit. A variety of regimens have been used and shown to be effective. However, the role of ASCT as initial therapy for patients judged to be at high risk of treatment failure with conventional therapy remains to be defined, despite several large clinical trials.[42]

In a small, underpowered trial conducted by Gianni and coworkers, 75 patients with poor-risk aggressive NHL were randomized to treatment with MACOP-B or with a novel high-dose chemotherapy regimen requiring hematopoietic progenitor cell autotransplantation.[43] By using a cross-over design, the authors sought to determine not only which was the most effective therapy but also which was the best therapeutic strategy; that is, does upfront versus salvage high-dose therapy result in better overall patient survival? The toxic death rate on the high-dose arm of the study was initially high (16%) but has decreased with modification of the treatment regimen. Thirty-eight patients were randomized to the high-dose therapy, and 37 patients were randomized to MACOP-B. After a median follow-up of 43 months, there is a statistically significant improvement in RFS (93% vs. 68%, $p = 0.05$) and freedom from progression (88% vs. 41%, $p = 0.0001$) in favor of the high-dose therapy arm. OS was not statistically improved, however, being 73% on the high-dose arm versus 62% on the MACOP-B arm. This outcome has not been reproduced in other studies.

GELA reported on a subset of 916 patients treated with the LNH87 protocol.[44] Of these patients, 451 presented with two (n = 318) or three (n = 133) risk factors. After reaching complete remission to induction therapy, 236 of these higher risk patients were assessable for the consolidation phase, with 125 patients in the HDT arm and 111 in the sequential chemotherapy arm. In this retrospectively analyzed subgroup, there was an OS benefit to HDT.

The Italian Cooperative Group compared methotrexate with leucovorin rescue, doxorubicin, cyclophosphamide, vincristine, prednisone, and bleomycin (MACOP-B; arm A) with an abbreviated regimen of MACOP-B (8 weeks) followed by HDT and ASCT (arm B) for intermediate–high-risk/high-risk patients (according to the age-adjusted IPI).[45] From September 1994 to April 1998, 150 patients with aggressive lymphoma were enrolled in the trial. According to the intention-to-treat analysis at a median follow-up of 24 months, 5-year OS probability in arms A and B was 65% and 64%, respectively, demonstrating no benefit to early HDT.

Recently, the GOELAMS group published results of a randomized trial comparing high-dose therapy plus autologous stem-cell support with the standard regimen of cyclophosphamide, doxorubicin, vincristine, and prednisone (CHOP).[46] The estimated event-free survival rate at 5 years was significantly higher among patients who received high-dose therapy than among patients who received CHOP. However, the OS benefit was limited to the subgroup of patients with high intermediate risk defined by the IPI.

Therefore, several studies have now concluded that all patients with aggressive lymphoma *do not* benefit when stem-cell transplantation is incorporated into their initial treatment strategy compared with patients who are treated with conventional strategy of initial chemotherapy followed by stem-cell transplant at first relapse.[47,48] Thus, there seems to be no indication to add autologous stem-cell transplantation (ASCT) to the initial combination chemotherapy treatment for *all* patients with aggressive lymphoma. However, all positive trials have incorporated a standard course of induction therapy (rather than an abbreviated course) prior to consolidative transplantation, and focused on patients with high clinical risk. An international consensus conference reached the conclusion that high-dose therapy and autotransplantation in patients with high-risk IPI scores seemed to provide benefit,[49] and this is the subject of an ongoing intergroup randomized trial in the United States. At the present time, we do not recommend routine use of ASCT as consolidative therapy for newly diagnosed large-cell lymphoma outside a clinical trial.

Summary: Therapy of De Novo Large B-Cell Lymphoma

Most patients with advanced-stage diffuse large B-cell lymphoma are not cured with conventional therapy. Hence, each treating physician must recognize the inadequacy of current therapy and urge all eligible patients to participate in well-designed clinical trials. The best therapy remains to be defined, and therefore the best approach for the patient is an experimental approach designed to improve our ability to cure the disease. If a patient is not eligible or does not wish to participate in a clinical trial, CHOP with rituximab is now the gold standard against which all new therapy must be compared.

THERAPY FOR PROGRESSIVE DISEASE

The initial step in planning salvage chemotherapy is to determine the goal of treatment. Some patients who fail to achieve an initial remission or relapse from complete remission can be cured. This is less likely in elderly patients, those with extensive disease, and those with a poor performance status. In such patients less intensive, palliative systemic treatments, with single agent vincristine, cytarabine, alkylating agents, or anthracyclines might be better pursued. Responses to single agent rituximab occur approximately 30% of the time, and are generally of brief duration.[50] Radiotherapy can also be used to alleviate the symptoms at a particular site of involvement in patients with relapsed diffuse large B-cell lymphoma.

Most younger patients receive second-line combination chemotherapy regimens. These regimens usually incorporate drugs such as cisplatin, ifosfamide, etoposide, and cytarabine, often in combination with rituximab. For example, the Memorial Sloan-Kettering Cancer Center has recently published results of R-ICE chemotherapy (rituximab, ifosfamide, carboplatin, etoposide), in patients with recurrent aggressive non-Hodgkin's lymphoma.[51] The CR rate was 53%, significantly better than the 27% CR rate achieved among 147 similar consecutive historical control patients with DLBCL treated with ICE[52]; the partial response (PR) rate was 25%. This was a very effective cytoreduction and mobilization regimen in patients with NHL, and has become a widely used salvage and stem cell mobilization option for patients eligible for subsequent autologous stem cell transplantation. Progression-free survival rates of patients who underwent transplantation after RICE were marginally better than those of 95 consecutive historical control patients who underwent transplantation after ICE.

An international randomized trial referred to as the Parma, Italy study defined the role of bone marrow transplant in relapsed DLCL.[41] In this trial, 109 patients who had relapsed from complete remission and responded to two cycles of DHAP (dexamethasone, cytarabine, cisplatin) were randomly allocated to high-dose chemotherapy or continued treatment with DHAP. Both groups were to receive involved-field radiotherapy, which is often used as adjunctive therapy in the setting of stem cell transplantation.[53] Bone marrow transplantation was associated with a superior failure-free survival (51% vs. 12% at 5 years) and OS (53% vs. 32% at 5 years). This trial enrolled only young patients at first relapse who remained chemosensitive. Salvage ABMT, as currently used, will result in survival of approximately 50% of all patients who actually receive transplants; however, but only a minority of all patients meet all the strict selection criteria for ideal outcome following transplantation. For these patients, however, high-dose therapy and autologous bone marrow transplantation are the treatments of choice.

Allogeneic bone marrow transplantation has been used less frequently for patients with diffuse large B-cell lymphoma. While occasional patients failing autologous transplantation can have prolonged survival with allogeneic transplantation, overall results have favored autologous transplantation, due to toxicity associated with allogeneic transplantation. Ongoing studies in high-risk patients are evaluating nonmyeloablative allogeneic transplantation.

Acknowledgment

JWF is supported in part by a career development award from the National Cancer Institute (CA 102216-01).

References

1. Armitage JO and Weisenburger DD. New approach to classifying non-Hodgkin's lymphomas: clinical features of the major histologic subtypes. Non-Hodgkin's Lymphoma Classification Project. J Clin Oncol 1998;16:2780–95.
2. Greenlee RT, Hill-Harmon MB, Murray T, et al. Cancer statistics, 2001. CA Cancer J Clin 2001;51:15–36.
3. Carbone PP, Kaplan HS, Musshoff K, et al. Report of the Committee on Hodgkin's Disease Staging Classification. Cancer Res 1971;31:1860–1.
4. Fisher RI, Hubbard SM, DeVita VT, et al. Factors predicting long-term survival in diffuse mixed, histiocytic, or undifferentiated lymphoma. Blood 1981;58:45–51.
5. Fisher RI, DeVita VT Jr, Johnson BL, et al. Prognostic factors for advanced diffuse histiocytic lymphoma following treatment with combination chemotherapy. Am J Med 1977;63:177–82.
6. The International Non-Hodgkin's Lymphoma Prognostic Factors Project. A predictive model for aggressive non-Hodgkin's lymphoma. N Engl J Med 1993;329:987–94.
7. Miller TP, Grogan TM, Dahlberg S, et al. Prognostic significance of the Ki-67–associated proliferative antigen in aggressive non-Hodgkin's lymphomas: a prospective Southwest Oncology Group trial. Blood 1994;83:1460–6.

8. Barrans SL, Carter I, Owen RG, et al. Germinal center phenotype and bcl-2 expression combined with the International Prognostic Index improves patient risk stratification in diffuse large B-cell lymphoma. Blood 2002;99:1136–43.
9. Gascoyne RD, Adomat SA, Krajewski S, et al. Prognostic significance of Bcl-2 protein expression and Bcl-2 gene rearrangement in diffuse aggressive non-Hodgkin's lymphoma. Blood 1997;90:244–51.
10. Mounier N, Briere J, Gisselbrecht C, et al. Rituximab plus CHOP (R-CHOP) overcomes bcl-2–associated resistance to chemotherapy in elderly patients with diffuse large B-cell lymphoma (DLBCL). Blood 2003;101:4279–84.
11. Offit K, LoCoco F, Louie DC, et al. Rearrangement of the bcl-6 gene as a prognostic marker in diffuse large-cell lymphoma. N Engl J Med 1994;331:74–80.
12. Lossos IS, Jones CD, Warnke R, et al. Expression of a single gene, BCL-6, strongly predicts survival in patients with diffuse large B-cell lymphoma. Blood 2001;98:945–51.
13. Rosenwald A, Wright G, Chan WC, et al. The use of molecular profiling to predict survival after chemotherapy for diffuse large B-cell lymphoma. N Engl J Med 2002;346:1937–47.
14. Shipp MA, Ross KN, Tamayo P, et al. Diffuse large B-cell lymphoma outcome prediction by gene-expression profiling and supervised machine learning. Nat Med 2002;8:68–74.
15. Lossos IS, Czerwinski DK, Alizadeh AA, et al. Prediction of survival in diffuse large–B-cell lymphoma based on the expression of six genes. N Engl J Med 2004;350:1828–37.
16. Staudt LM. Molecular diagnosis of the hematologic cancers. N Engl J Med 2003;348:1777–85.
17. Mavromatis BH and Cheson BD. Pre- and post-treatment evaluation of non-Hodgkin's lymphoma. Best Pract Res Clin Haematol 2002;15:429–47.
18. Friedberg JW and Chengazi V. PET scans in the staging of lymphoma: current status. Oncologist 2003;8:438–47.
19. Kostakoglu L, Leonard JP, Kuji I, et al. Comparison of fluorine-18 fluorodeoxyglucose positron emission tomography and Ga-67 scintigraphy in evaluation of lymphoma. Cancer 2002;94:879–88.
20. Hallahan DE, Farah R, Vokes EE, et al. The patterns of failure in patients with pathological Stage I and II diffuse histiocytic lymphoma treated with radiation therapy alone. Int J Radiat Oncol Biol Phys 1989;17:767–771.
21. Miller TP, Dahlberg S, Cassady JR, et al. Chemotherapy alone compared with chemotherapy plus radiotherapy for localized intermediate- and high-grade non-Hodgkin's lymphoma. N Engl J Med 1998;339:21–26.
22. Horning S and Glick J, et al. Final report of E1484: CHOP v CHOP + radiotherapy for limited stage diffuse aggressive lymphoma. Blood 2001;98:724a.
23. Fillet G and Bonnet C. Radiotherapy is unnecessary in elderly patients with localized aggressive non-Hodgkin's lymphoma: results of the GELA LNH 93-4 study. Blood 2002;100:92a.
24. Reyes F, Lepage E, Munck JN, et al. Superiority of chemotherapy alone with the ACVBP regimen over treatment with three cycles of CHOP plus radiotherapy in low risk localized aggressive lymphoma: The LNH93-1 GELA study. Blood 2002;100:93a.
25. DeVita VT, Canellos GP, Chabner B, et al. Advanced diffuse histiocytic lymphoma, a potentially curable disease. Lancet 1975;1:248–50.
26. Jones SE, Grozea PN, Metz EN, et al. Superiority of adriamycin-containing combination chemotherapy in the treatment of diffuse lymphoma: a Southwest Oncology Group study. Cancer 1979;43:417–25.
27. Jones SE, Grozea PN, Metz EN, et al. Improved complete remission rates and survival for patients with large cell lymphoma treated with chemoimmunotherapy: a Southwest Oncology Group Study. Cancer 1983;51:1083–90.
28. Jones SE, Grozea PN, Miller TP, et al. Chemotherapy with cyclophosphamide, doxorubicin, vincristine, and prednisone alone or with levamisole or with levamisole plus bcg for malignant lymphoma: a Southwest Oncology Group Study. J Clin Oncol 1985;3:1318–1324.
29. Coltman CA, Dahlberg S, Jones SE, et al. Southwest Oncology Group studies in diffuse large cell lymphoma: a subset analysis, In Kimura K, ed. Cancer Chemotherapy: Challenges for the Future. Tokyo: Excerpta Medica, 1988:194–202.
30. Gordon LI, Harrington D, Andersen J, et al. Comparison of a second-generation combination chemotherapeutic regimen (m-BACOD) with a standard regimen (CHOP) for advanced diffuse non-Hodgkin's lymphoma. N Engl J Med 1992;327:1342–9.
31. Cooper IA, Wolf MM, Robertson TI, et al. Randomized comparison of MACOP-B and CHOP in patients with intermediate grade non-Hodgkin's lymphoma. J Clin Oncol 1994;12:769–78.
32. Fisher RI, Gaynor ER, Dahlberg S, et al. Comparison of a standard regimen (CHOP) with three intensive chemotherapy regimens for advanced non-Hodgkin's lymphoma. N Engl J Med 1993;328:1002–6.
33. Vose JM, Link BK, Grossbard ML, et al. Phase II study of rituximab in combination with CHOP chemotherapy in patients with previously untreated, aggressive non-Hodgkin's lymphoma. J Clin Oncol 2001;19:389–97.
34. Coiffier B, Lepage E, Briere J, et al. CHOP chemotherapy plus rituximab compared with CHOP alone in elderly patients with diffuse large–B-cell lymphoma. N Engl J Med 2002;346:235–42.
35. Czuczman MS, Grillo-Lopez AJ, White CA, et al. Treatment of patients with low-grade B-cell lymphoma with the combination of chimeric anti-CD20 monoclonal antibody and CHOP chemotherapy. J Clin Oncol 1999;17:268–76.
36. Haberman TM, Weller EA, Morrison VA, et al. Phase III trial of rituximab-CHOP vs. CHOP with a second randomization to maintenance rituximab or observation in patients 60 years of age and older with diffuse large B cell lymphoma. Blood 2003;102:6a.
37. Pfreundschuh MG, Truemper L, Ma D, et al. Randomized intergroup trial of first line treatment of patients <= 60 years with diffuse large B cell non-Hodgkin's lympohma with a CHOP-like regimen with or without the anti-CD20 antibody rituximab—early stopping after the first interim analysis. Proc ASCO 2004;23:556a.
38. Blayney DW, LeBlanc ML, Grogan T, et al. Dose-intense chemotherapy every 2 weeks with dose-intense cyclophosphamide, doxorubicin, vincristine, and prednisone may improve survival in intermediate- and high-grade lymphoma: a Phase II study of the Southwest Oncology Group (SWOG 9349). J Clin Oncol 2003;21:2466–73.
39. Pfreundschuh M, Truemper L, Kloess M, et al. 2-Weekly or 3-weekly CHOP chemotherapy with or without etoposide for the treatment of young patients with good prognosis (normal LDH) aggressive lymphomas: results of the NHL-B1 trial of the DSHNHL. Blood 2004;104(3):626–33.
40. Pfreundschuh M, Truemper L, Kloess M, et al. 2-Weekly or 3-weekly CHOP chemotherapy with or without etoposide for the treatment of elderly patients with aggressive lymphomas: results of the NHL-B2 trial of the DSHNHL. Blood 2004;104:626–33.
41. Philip T, Guglielmi C, Hagenbeek A, et al. Autologous bone marrow transplantation as compared with salvage chemotherapy in relapses of chemotherapy-sensitive non-Hodgkin's lymphoma. N Engl J Med 1995;333:1540–5.
42. Fisher RI. Autologous stem-cell transplantation as a component of initial treatment for poor risk patients with aggressive

non-Hodgkin's lymphoma: resolved issues versus remaining opportunities. J Clin Oncol 2002;20:4411–2.

43. Gianni AM, Bregni M, Siena S, et al. High dose chemotherapy and autologous bone marrow transplantation compared with MACOP-B in aggressive B-cell lymphoma. N Engl J Med 1997;336:1290–7.
44. Haioun C, Lepage E, Gisselbrecht C, et al. Survival benefit of high-dose therapy in poor-risk aggressive non-Hodgkin's lymphoma. Final analysis of the Prospective LNH87-2 Protocol—A Groupe d'Etude des Lymphomes de l'Adulte Study. J Clin Oncol 2000;18:3025–30.
45. Martelli M, Gherlinzoni F, De Renzo A, et al. Early autologous stem-cell transplantation versus conventional chemotherapy as front-line therapy in high-risk, aggressive non-Hodgkin's lymphoma: an Italian multicenter randomized trial. J Clin Oncol 2003;21:1255–62.
46. Milpied N, Deconinck E, Gaillard F, et al. Initial treatment of aggressive lymphoma with high-dose chemotherapy and autologous stem-cell support. N Engl J Med 2004;350:1287–95.
47. Haioun C, Lepage E, Gisselbrecht C, et al. Comparison of autologous bone marrow transplantation with sequential chemotherapy for intermediate-grade and high-grade non-Hodgkin's lymphoma in first complete remission: a study of 464 patients. Groupe d'Etude des Lymphomes de l'Adulte. J Clin Oncol 1994;12:2543–51.
48. Santini G, Salvagno L, Leoni P, et al. VACOP-B versus VACOP-B plus autologous bone marrow transplantation for advanced diffuse non-Hodgkin's lymphoma: results of a prospective randomized trial by the non-Hodgkin's Lymphoma Cooperative Study Group. J Clin Oncol 1998;16:2796–802.
49. Shipp MA, Abeloff MD, Antman KH, et al. International consensus conference on high-dose therapy with hematopoietic stem cell transplantation in aggressive non-Hodgkin's lymphomas: report of the jury. J Clin Oncol 1999;17:423–9.
50. Coiffier B, Haioun C, Ketterer N, et al. Rituximab (anti-CD20 monoclonal antibody) for the treatment of patients with relapsing or refractory aggressive lymphoma: a multicenter Phase II study. Blood 1998;92:1927–32.
51. Kewalramani T, Zelenetz AD, Nimer SD, et al. Rituximab and ICE as second-line therapy before autologous stem cell transplantation for relapsed or primary refractory diffuse large B-cell lymphoma. Blood 2004;103:3684–8.
52. Moskowitz CH, Bertino JR, Glassman JR, et al. Ifosfamide, carboplatin, and etoposide: a highly effective cytoreduction and peripheral-blood progrenitor-cell mobilization regimen for transplant-eligible patients with non-Hodgkin's lymphoma. J Clin Oncol 1999;17:3776–85.
53. Friedberg JW, Neuberg D, Monson E, et al. The impact of external beam radiation therapy prior to autologous bone marrow transplantation in patients with non-Hodgkin's lymphoma. Biol Blood Marrow Transplant 2001;7:446–53.

17B

PRIMARY MEDIASTINAL

Pier Luigi Zinzani, M.D., Ph.D.

Primary mediastinal large B-cell lymphoma (PMLBCL) was first described as a distinct clinicopathologic entity in the 1980s.[1,2] It is an uncommon but not rare entity with a worldwide distribution and has been included in both the Real European American Lymphoma (REAL)[3] and World Health Organization (WHO) classifications.[4] PMLBCL constitutes 5% to 10% of all high-grade non-Hodgkin's lymphoma, and 2% of all cases of lymphoma.[5] It has a characteristic morphologic and immunophenotypic picture showing a diffuse proliferation of large cells with clear cytoplasm, and the presence of variable degrees of sclerosis that causes its typical compartmentalization pattern.

This mediastinal lymphoma must be distinguished from other lymphomas that can present with anterior mediastinal masses, including Hodgkin's disease, nodal-type diffuse large B-cell lymphoma, anaplastic large T/null-cell lymphoma, and thymic MALT (mucosa associated lymphoma tissue) lymphoma. Knowledge of the clinical features, adequate tissue for morphologic analysis, complete immunophenotyping, and assessment of proliferation fraction are all helpful in differential diagnosis.[6–11] Recently, gene expression profiling strongly supported a relation between PMLBCL and Hodgkin's disease: over one-third of the genes that were more highly expressed in PMLBCL than in other diffuse large B-cell lymphoma were also characteristically expressed in Hodgkin's lymphoma cells.[12]

This lymphoma presents with characteristic clinical features that are almost specific. PMLBCL affects younger patients than do other adult lymphomas. The median age is the mid-30s; children and older adults may be affected as well, but the disease is rare in people over age 65. About 60% to 70% of affected individuals are women. The patients show a bulky mediastinal mass often invading adjacent organs and structures (lung, superior vena cava, pleura, pericardium, and the chest wall) producing typical symptoms of cough, chest pain, and dyspnea.[13–17] Bulky mediastinal disease is observed in more than 60% to 70% of the patients, and intrathoracic extension to adjacent organs is present in about 50% of patients. PMLBCL can at times present with superior venacaval compression or obstruction and, for this reason, requires rapid completion of diagnosis and staging. The tumor almost never involves lymph nodes. When it spreads beyond the mediastinum and the pleural cavity, it involves sites not commonly involved with lymphoma, such as the kidneys, adrenals, liver, central nervous system, and ovaries.[18–20] Only 20% of the patients are in stage III–IV at diagnosis, and extranodal spread or bone marrow involvement is rare.

Table 17–3 summarizes the clinical comparison of nodal, diffuse large B-cell lymphoma, PMLBCL and Hodgkin's disease.

STAGING CONCEPTS

Complete staging work-up for PMLBCL is the same as that routinely used for nodal NHL. It includes an accurate physical examination, complete hematologic and biochemical exams, abdomen ultrasonography, total-body computerized tomography, and bone marrow biopsy. Diagnostic tissue sample is obtained by mediastinoscopy, by biopsy of the tumor mass through the supraclavicular fossa, or by anterior mediastinotomy or minithoracotomy. Formal thoracotomy is infrequently required and total excision is rarely an option. Gallium^{67} scanning (^{67}GaSPECT) is a specific tool for discriminating fibrotic and tumor tissue, and therefore its utility in the restaging of mediastinal masses after combined modality therapy.[21,22] In our study,[22] this restaging technique allows identification of a subset of patients with residual radiographic abnormalities who need no further therapy (negative ^{67}GaSPECT) and of poor prognosis

Table 17–3. Comparison of Diffuse Large B-Cell Lymphoma (DLBCL), Primary Mediastinal Large B-Cell Lymphoma (PMLBCL) and Hodgkin's Disease

	Nodal DLBCL	PMLBCL	Hodgkin's Disease
Median age (years)	55	35	Bimodal curve with peaks at ages 15–40
Nodal/extranodal presentation	65%/35%	0%/100%	90%/10%
Sex distribution (M:F)	1.2:1	1:2	1.5:1
Stage I–II/III–IV	40%/60%	80%/20%	55%/45%
Bulky disease	30%	60%–70%	20%/80%

Table 17–4. Studies on Treatment and Outcome of Patients with Primary Mediastinal Large B-Cell Lymphoma Treated with CHOP/CHOP-Like Regimens

Reference	n	Regimen (n)	Local RT	PR %	CR %	FFS % (years)
Jacobson (1988)[15]	30	CHOP/CHOP-like (22), C-MOPP (2)	Yes		80	59 (5)
Haioun (1989)[18]	20	CHOP (4) or variants (16)	Yes	55	45	40 (2)
Kirn (1993)[27]	57	M/m-BACOD (38), CHOP (10), other (9)	Yes	39	53	45 (5)
Lazzarino (1993)[19]	30	CHOP (14), MACOP-B or VACOP-B (16)	Yes		55	38 (3)
Rodriguez (1994)[29]	18	Doxorubicin regimens	Yes	12	67	45 (2)
Cazals-Hatem (1996)[5]	141	Intensive regimens	No	31	48	61 (3)
Lazzarino (1997)[16]	106	Doxorubicin regimens	Yes	42	23	50 (3)
Abou Ellela (1999)[30]	43	CAP-BOB and variants	NR		63	39 (5)
Bieri (1999)[33]	27	Doxorubicin regimens	Yes	15	55	44 (10)
Nguyen (2000)[34]	40	Doxorubicin regimens	Yes	41	41	67 (5)

CR, complete response; FFS, failure-free survival; n, number of patients; PR, partial response; RT, radiation therapy.

patients who do require further treatment (i.e., autologous bone marrow transplantation). ^{18}FDG-PET has a better resolution than gallium scanning, as well as increased sensitivity and a shorter procedure time. ^{18}FDG-PET has demonstrated excellent usefulness in residual masses assessment, considering the elevated tracer uptake that characterizes this lymphoma; it should be used and interpreted in conjunction with the history, physical examination, and CT scans. PMLBCL is always gallium- or PET-positive at diagnosis, and persistent positivity after therapy is a harbinger of relapse. Over 40% of patients have residual radiographic abnormalities in the mediastinum even after successful treatment, so chest radiographs and CT scans are not useful in making therapeutic decisions. In our ongoing study on PMLBCL, patients have been evaluated with ^{18}FDG-PET after 1 month of treatment to analyze the prognostic role of a rapid negativization of PET scan on the outcome.

TREATMENT CONCEPTS

There have been no randomized treatment trials focusing on patients with PMLBCL. However, several series have been reported, and permit some conclusions to be drawn.[15–19,23–36] First, radiation therapy alone is ineffective in this disease. Second, the use of CHOP chemotherapy led to the early impression that the prognosis of patients with PMLBCL was worse than that for the more common diffuse large-cell lymphoma. However, with the application of more aggressive combination chemotherapy programs (third-line generation regimens), it appears that the complete response (CR) rate, disease-free survival, and OS of patients with PMLBCL are at least as good and probably better than those for diffuse large-cell lymphoma. The GELA group used LNH84 and LNH87 in both PMLBCL and diffuse large-cell lymphoma, and found a superior CR rate and superior 3-year OS rate for patients with PMLBCL. Table 17–4 summarizes the results of most series on PMLBCL utilizing CHOP or CHOP-like regimens as first-line treatment. Many groups have empirically delivered radiation therapy to responding patients; it is difficult to assess whether this has improved treatment outcome. In centers that have used both first-generation chemotherapy regimens such as CHOP, and the more aggressive third-generation ones such as MACOP-B, the results have clearly favored the latter. Todeschini et al.[26] used CHOP without achieving a single CR; in contrast, in the 15 patients treated with more aggressive regimens (MACOP-B and m-BACOD), 13 (87%) achieved a CR, and only one of CRs relapsed. Lazzarino et al.[19] treated 30 patients: the CR rate to CHOP was 36%, while that to MACOP-B or VACOP-B was 73%. In the last studies,[22,36] we have utilized MACOP-B regimen in two prospective multicenter trials: in 50 patients[22] and in 89 patients[36] with a CR rate of 86% and 88%, respectively. Figs. 17–1 and 17–2 show the OS and the relapse-free survival

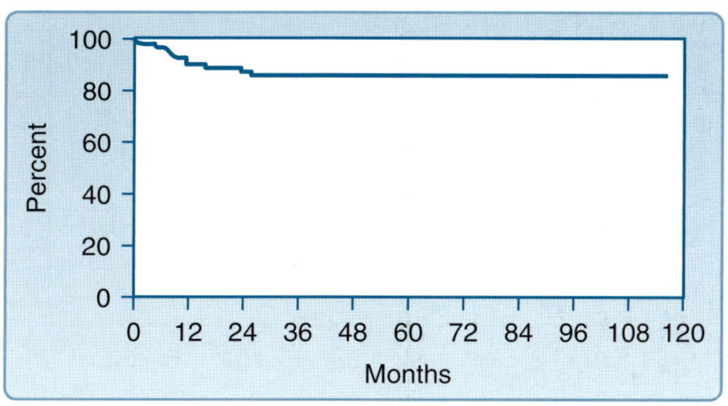

Figure 17–1. Overall survival curve of 89 patients with primary mediastinal large B-cell lymphoma treated with MACOP-B plus mediastinal radiation therapy (with permission by *Haematologica*).

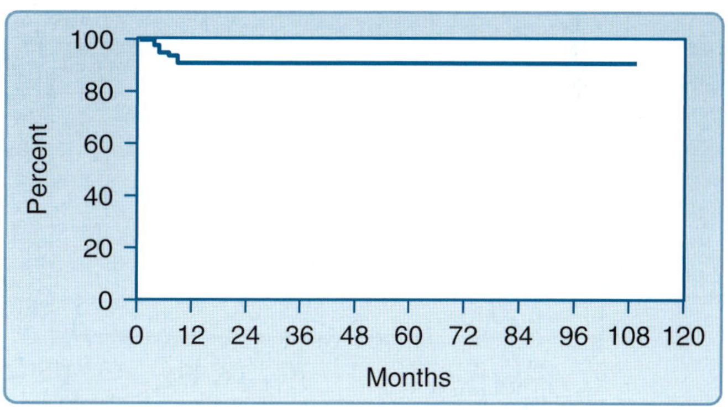

Figure 17–2. Relapse-free survival curve of 78 complete response patients treated with MACOP-B plus mediastinal radiation therapy (with permission by *Haematologica*).

Table 17–5. Studies on Treatment and Outcome of Patients with Primary Mediastinal Large B-Cell Lymphoma Treated with MACOP-B Regimen

Reference	n	Regimen (n)	Local RT	PR %	CR %	FFS % (Years)
Todeschini (1990)[26]	21	CHOP-B (6), MACOP-B (12), m-BACOD (3)	Yes	25	64	52 (3)
Bertini (1991)[25]	18	MACOP-B	Yes	6	89	73 (2)
Falini (1995)[6]	18	MACOP-B (7), F-MACHOP (11)	No	33	61	61 (2)
Zinzani (1996)[17]	22	MACOP-B (20), F-MACHOP (2)	Yes		95	86 (2)
Martelli (1998)[35]	37	F-MACHOP (10), MACOP-B (27)	No	10	90	70 (5)
Zinzani (1999)[22]	50	MACOP-B	Yes		86	93 (8)
Zinzani (2001)[36]	89	MACOP-B	Yes	4	88	91 (9)

CR, complete response; FFS, failure-free survival; n, number of patients; PR, partial response; RT, radiation therapy.

curves of one of these multicenter trials.[36] The results of most series on PMLBCL treated with MACOP-B regimen are reported in Table 17–5.

Fisher et al.[37] have reported that CHOP and intensive third-generation regimens produce equivalent results. This observation may limit discussion about the use of more aggressive protocols for PMLBCL. However, the debate is still open, because it is difficult to compare the advantages of the different types of protocols, and it is also difficult to explain the rather different CR and survival rates reported by different institutions using similar regimens. At the same time, although the value of adjuvant radiation therapy after chemotherapy requires confirmation, it could play an important role in the achievement of long-term progression-free survival, especially in patients with bulky disease at presentation.

Recently, two retrospective studies have reported data concerning the comparison between CHOP and CHOP-like regimens versus MACOP-B and MACOP-B-like regimens as induction chemotherapy in PMLBCL patients.[38,39] Our multinational retrospective study compared the outcomes of 426 patients with PMLBCL after first-generation (CHOP and CHOP-like regimens; 105 patients); third-generation (MACOP-B, VACOP-B, ProMACECytaBOM; 277 patients)[38]; and high-dose chemotherapy strategies (high-dose sequential [HDS], autologous bone marrow transplantation [ABMT]; 44 patients). In all these subgroups, the most patients underwent radiation therapy after chemotherapy. With chemotherapy, CR rates were 49%, 51%, and 53%, with first-generation, third-generation, and high-dose chemotherapy strategies, respectively. The final CR rates, after radiation therapy on the mediastinum, became 61% for CHOP and CHOP-like regimens, 79% for MACOP-B and other regimens, and 75% for HDS/ABMT. Projected 10-year OS rates were 44%, 71%, and 77%, respectively (Fig. 17–3); and projected 10-year progression-free survival rates were 35%, 67%, and 78%, respectively (Fig. 17–4). In addition, after the radiation therapy, 81% of the patients who had already achieved a partial response obtained CR status. Table 17–6 summarizes the outcome after radiotherapy.

Todeschini et al.[39] reported the long-term results from a retrospective multicenter Italian experience in 138 PMLBCL patients treated with CHOP (43 patients) or MACOP-B/VACOP-B (95 patients). CR was 51% in the CHOP group and 80% in MACOP-B/VACOP-B. The addition of radiation therapy on mediastinum mass consolidation improved the outcome irrespectively of the type of chemotherapy.

These two retrospective studies confirm the superiority of the third-generation chemotherapy strategies over first-generation ones. In addition, they highlight the role of radiation therapy for converting cases of PR to CR, and probably also of reinforcing existing CRs.

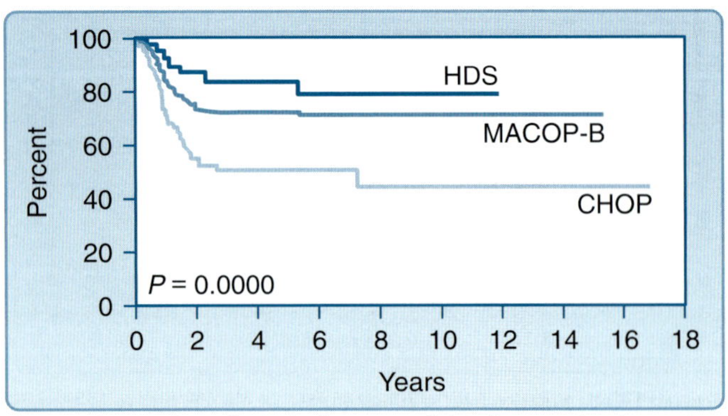

Figure 17–3. Overall survival curves of the three main chemotherapy subgroups (with permission by *Haematologica*).

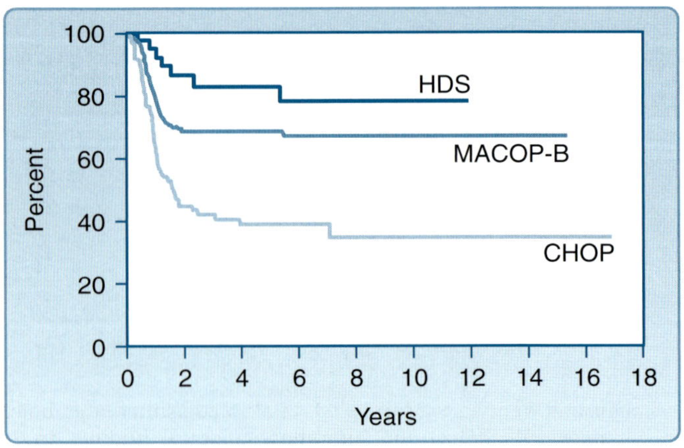

Figure 17–4. Progression-free survival curves of the three main chemotherapy subgroups (with permission by *Haematologica*).

Table 17–6. Therapeutic Outcome with Inclusion of Radiation Therapy

Chemotherapy Subgroup	Patients Who Achieved CR after CHT	Conversions to CR Among Patients Who Received RT While in PR	Global CR After Chemotherapy and RT
First generation	50/105 (49%)	14/21 (67%)	64/105 (61%)
Third generation	142/277 (51%)	76/90 (84%)	218/277 (79%)
High dose	23/44 (53%)	10/13 (77%)	33/44 (75%)
Overall	215/426 (51%)	100/124 (81%)	315/426 (74%)

RT, radiation therapy; CHT, chemotherapy; PR, partial response.
From Hematologica, with permission.

NEW TREATMENTS

The role of high-dose approaches including ABMT and HDS treatment needs to be confirmed because the actual reported data do not prove superiority of high-dose chemotherapy over conventional chemotherapy in Phase II trials.[40–44] In our retrospective study, the encouraging results of the high-dose chemotherapy subgroup of patients are very interesting. However, in view of the low number of patients treated, further studies are needed to assess the validity of using HDS or ABMT in particularly high-risk subsets.

Recently, we started with a front-line treatment including MACOP-B and rituximab; the schedule includes one administration of rituximab every 3 weeks for a total of four doses (at week 1, 4, 7, and 10 of MACOP-B regimen). All patients underwent mediastinal radiation therapy after the combined modality. Concerning the disease evaluation, all patients are submitted to PET and CT scans before the treatment (both), after 4 weeks (only PET scan), after 8 weeks (only CT scan), 1 months after MACOP-B plus rituximab (both), and 3 months after radiation therapy (both). In the future, another important addition to the therapeutic armamentarium will be the inclusion of radioimmunoconjugates in sequential combination with conventional chemotherapy.

REFERENCES

1. Lichtenstein AK, Levine A, Taylor CR, et al. Primary mediastinal lymphoma in adults. Am J Med 1980;68:509–14.
2. Levitt LJ, Aisenberg AC, Harris NL, et al. Primary non-Hodgkin's lymphoma of the mediastinum. Cancer 1982;50:2486–92.
3. Harris NL, Jaffe ES, Stein H, et al. A revised European–American classification of lymphoid neoplasms: a proposal from the International Lymphoma Study Group. Blood 1994;84:1361–92.
4. Jaffe ES, Harris NL, Stein H, et al. World Health Organization Classification of Tumours. Pathology and Genetics of Tumours of Hematopoietic and Lymphoid Tissues. Lyon: IARC Press, 2001.
5. Cazals-Hatem D, Lepage E, Brice P, et al. Primary mediastinal large B-cell lymphoma. A clinicopathologic study of 141 cases compared with 916 nonmediastinal large B-cell lymphomas, a GELA ("Groupe d'Etude des Lymphomes de l'Adulte") study. Am J Surg Pathol 1996;20:877–88.
6. Falini B, Venturi S, Martelli M, et al. Mediastinal large B-cell lymphoma: clinical and immunohistological findings in 18 patients treated with different third-generation regimens. Br J Haematol 1995;89:780–9.
7. Moller P, Lammler B, Eberlein-Gonska M, et al. Primary mediastinal clear cell lymphoma of B-cell type. Virchows Arch A Pathol Anat Histopathol 1986;409:79–92.
8. de Leval L, Ferry JA, Falini B, et al. Expression of bcl-6 and CD10 in primary mediastinal large B-cell lymphoma: evidence for derivation from germinal center B cells? Am J Surg Pathol 2001;25:1277–82.
9. Scarpa A, Bonetti F, and Menestrina F. Mediastinal large cell lymphoma with sclerosis. Genotypic analysis establishes its B nature. Virchows Arch A Pathol Anat Histopathol 1987;412:17–21.
10. Tsang P, Cesarman E, Chadburn A, et al. Molecular characterization of primary mediastinal B cell lymphoma. Am J Pathol 1996;148:2017–25.
11. Joos S, Otano-Joos MI, Ziegler S, et al. Primary mediastinal (thymic) B-cell lymphoma is characterized by gains of chromosomal material including 9p and amplification of the REL gene. Blood 1996;87:1571–8.
12. Rosenwald A, Wright G, Leroy K, et al. Molecular diagnosis of primary mediastinal B cell lymphoma identifies a clinically favorable subgroup of diffuse large B cell lymphoma related to Hodgkin lymphoma. J Exp Med 2003;198;851–62.
13. The Non-Hodgkin's Lymphoma Classification Project. A clinical evaluation of the International Lymphoma Study Group classification of non-Hodgkin's lymphoma. Blood 1997;89:3909–18.
14. Lamarre L, Jacobson J, Aisenberg A, et al. Primary large cell lymphoma of the mediastinum. Am J Surg Pathol 1989; 13:730–9.
15. Jacobson JO, Aisenberg AC, Lamarre L, et al. Mediastinal large cell lymphoma: an uncommon subset of adult lymphoma curable with combined modality therapy. Cancer 1988;62: 1893–8.
16. Lazzarino M, Orlandi E, Paulli M, et al. Treatment outcome and prognostic factors for primary mediastinal (thymic) B-cell lymphoma: a multicenter study of 106 patients. J Clin Oncol 1997;15:1646–53.
17. Zinzani PL, Bendandi M, Frezza G, et al. Primary mediastinal B-cell lymphoma with sclerosis: clinical and therapeutic evaluation of 22 patients. Leuk Lymphoma 1996;21:311–6.
18. Haioun C, Gaulard P, Roudot-Thoraval F, et al. Mediastinal diffuse large B-cell lymphoma with sclerosis: a condition with a poor prognosis. Am J Clin Oncol 1989;12:425–9.
19. Lazzarino M, Orlandi E, Paulli M, et al. Primary mediastinal B-cell lymphoma with sclerosis: an aggressive tumor with distinctive clinical and pathological features. J Clin Oncol 1993;11:2306–13.
20. Bishop P, Wilson W, Pearson D, et al. CNS involvement in primary mediastinal large B-cell lymphoma. J Clin Oncol 1999;17:2479–85.
21. Abrahamsen AF, Lien HH, Aas M, et al. Magnetic resonance imaging and 67gallium scan in mediastinal malignant lymphoma: a prospective pilot study. Ann Oncol 1994;5:433–6.

22. Zinzani PL, Martelli M, Magagnoli M, et al. Treatment and clinical management of primary mediastinal large B-cell lymphoma with sclerosis: MACOP-B regimen and mediastinal radiotherapy monitored by (67) gallium scan in 50 patients. Blood 1999;94:3289–93.
23. Lavabre-Bertrand T, Donadio D, Fegueux N, et al. A study of 15 cases of primary mediastinal lymphoma of B-cell type. Cancer 1992;69:2561–6.
24. Rohatiner AZ, Whelan JS, Ganjoo RK, et al. Mediastinal large-cell lymphoma with sclerosis (MLCLS). Br J Cancer 1994;69:601–4.
25. Bertini M, Orsucci L, Vitolo U, et al. Stage II large B-cell lymphoma with sclerosis treated with MACOP-B. Ann Oncol 1991;2:733–7.
26. Todeschini G, Ambrosetti A, Meneghini V, et al. Mediastinal large–B-cell lymphoma with sclerosis: a clinical study of 21 patients. J Clin Oncol 1990;8:804–8.
27. Kirn D, Mauch P, Shaffer K, et al. Large-cell and immunoblastic lymphoma of the mediastinum: prognostic and pathologic features in 57 patients. J Clin Oncol 1993;11:1336–43.
28. Aisenberg AC. Primary large-cell lymphoma of the mediastinum. J Clin Oncol 1993;11:2291–8.
29. Rodriguez J, Pugh WC, Romaguera JE, et al. Primary mediastinal large cell lymphoma. Haematol Oncol 1994; 12:175–84.
30. Abou-Elella AA, Weisenburger DD, Vose JM, et al. Primary mediastinal large B-cell lymphoma: a clinicopathologic study of 43 patients from the Nebraska lymphoma study group. J Clin Oncol 1999;17:784–90.
31. Perrone T, Frizzera G, and Rosai J. Mediastinal diffuse large-cell lymphoma with sclerosis. A clinicopathologic study of 60 cases. Am J Clin Pathol 1986;10:176–91.
32. Al-Sharabati M, Chittal S, Duga-Neulet I, et al. Primary anterior mediastinal B-cell lymphoma: a clinicopathological and immunohistochemical study of 16 cases. Cancer 1991; 67:2579–83.
33. Bieri S, Roggero E, Zucca E, et al. Primary mediastinal large B-cell lymphoma (PMLCL): the need for prospective controlled clinical trials. Leuk Lymphoma 1999;35:139–46.
34. Nguyen LN, Ha CS, Hess M, et al. The outcome of combined-modality treatments for Stage I and II primary large B-cell lymphoma of the mediastinum. Int J Radiat Oncol Biol Physicians 2000;47:1281–5.
35. Martelli MP, Martelli M, Pescarmona E, et al. MACOP-B and involved field radiation therapy is an effective therapy for primary mediastinal large B-cell lymphoma with sclerosis. Ann Oncol 1998;9:1027–9.
36. Zinzani PL, Martelli M, De Renzo A, et al. Primary mediastinal large B-cell lymphoma with slerosis: a clinical study of 89 patients treated with MACOP-B chemotherapy and radiation therapy. Haematologica 2001;86:187–91.
37. Fisher RI, Gaynor ER, Dahlberg S, et al. Comparison of a standard regimen (CHOP) with three intensive chemotherapy regimens for advanced non-Hodgkin's lymphoma. N Engl J Med 1993;329:1002–6.
38. Zinzani PL, Martelli M, Bertini M, et al. Induction chemotherapy strategies for primary mediastinal large B-cell lymphoma with sclerosis: a retrospective multinational study od 426 previously untreated patients. Haematologica 2002;87:1258–64.
39. Todeschini G, Secchi S, Morra E, et al. Primary mediastinal laerge B-cell lymphoma (PMLBCL): long-term results from a retrospective multicentre Italian experience in 138 patients treated with CHOP or MACOP-B/VACOP-B. Br J Cancer 2004;90:372–6.
40. Nademanee A, Molina A, O'Donnell M, et al. Results of high-dose therapy and autologous bone marrow/stem cell transplantation during remission in poor-risk intermediate and high-grade lymphoma: international index high and high-intermediate risk group. Blood 1997;90:3844–52.
41. Popat U, Przepiork D, Champlin R, et al. High-dose chemotherapy for relapsed and refractory diffuse large B-cell lymphoma: mediastinal localization predicts for a favorable outcome. J Clin Oncol 1998;16:63–9.
42. Sehn LH, Antin JH, Shulman LN, et al. Primary diffuse large B-cell lymphoma of the mediastinum. Outcome following high-dose chemotherapy and autologous hematopoietic cell transplantation. Blood 1998;91:717–23.
43. Aisenberg AC. Primary large cell lymphoma of the mediastinum. Semin Oncol 1999;26:251–8.
44. Van Besien K, Kelta M, Bahaguna P. Primary mediastinal B-cell lymphoma: a review of pathology and management. J Clin Oncol 2001;19:1855–64.

17C

PRIMARY CENTRAL NERVOUS SYSTEM LYMPHOMA

Howard A. Fine M.D.
Jay S. Loeffler M.D.

Primary central nervous system lymphoma (PCNSL) is defined as a non-Hodgkin's lymphoma that is confined to the craniospinal axis without systemic involvement. PCNSL is not to be confused with established systemic lymphoma with secondary spread to the central nervous system (CNS), which occurs in 5% to 29% of patients with systemic lymphoma.[1] Historically, this entity was referred to as "reticulum cell sarcoma," "microglioma," or "perivascular sarcoma," but it has now been well established that the cell of origin is a malignant lymphocyte.[2–5] This chapter discusses the epidemiology, pathology, clinical diagnosis, and results of therapy, as well as the current recommendations and future directions for PCNSL in immunocompetent and immunocompromised patients. Since the publication of our contribution (chapter 21) to the last edition of *The Lymphomas*, increased attention has been drawn to the biology and therapy of this disorder.[6]

EPIDEMIOLOGY

Immunocompromised Patients

In the past, PCNSL was considered a rare tumor, accounting for 1% to 2% of all lymphomas and less than 5% of all primary CNS tumors.[7–9] Although most patients with PCNSL are immunocompetent, patients with both acquired and congenital immunodeficiencies are at significant risk for the development of this tumor. The two congenital immunodeficiency states that are most commonly associated with PCNSL are severe combined immunodeficiency and the Wiskott-Aldrich syndromes.[10,11] PCNSL has also been reported in immunoglobulin A deficiency syndrome.[12] Not all congenital immunodeficiency syndromes, however, are associated with an increased risk of PCNSL. For example, although ataxia-telangiectasia is clearly associated with an increased risk of systemic lymphomas, there have been no reported cases of PCNSL.[13]

Iatrogenic immunodeficiency also predisposes to the development of this tumor. The largest group of these patients consists of organ allograft recipients. In particular, kidney recipients have a significantly increased risk of lymphomas, presumable secondary to chronic iatrogenic immunosuppression. Penn reported that the risk of developing lymphoma in a large group of renal allograft recipients was 350 times that of the immunocompetent population.[14] As many as 50% of these lymphomas were PCNSL. Recent data suggest that cardiac allograft recipients may be at even greater risk for the development of PCNSL.[15] In a series of 182 heart allograft recipients, Weintraub and Warnke reported three cases of PCNSL, a rate that appears higher than that in the renal transplant population.[15] Why this should be true is unclear, although it is possible that this apparent increase in PCNSL in heart transplant patients may reflect a greater degree of immunosuppression currently used in transplant protocols (in particular the use of cyclosporine), compared with regimens used over a decade ago when Penn[14] first reported experience with the kidney allograft recipient.

Other disease conditions, particularly those believed to involve autoimmune mechanisms, such as systemic lupus erythematosus, rheumatoid arthritis, and sarcoidosis, have been associated with the development of PCNSL.[16–18] Whether there is truly an increased risk of PCNSL in this patient population is not known. Furthermore, even if there is an increased risk of the development of this tumor in this patient population, it is difficult to know whether the risk factor is the disease itself or the immunosuppressive therapy (such as glucocorticoids) used to treat many of these patients.

The largest group of immunodeficient patients who are at risk for the development of PCNSL are those infected with the human immunodeficiency virus (HIV). In particular, patients with the diagnosis of acquired immunodeficiency syndrome (AIDS) are at particularly high risk of PCNSL—the reported incidence is 2% to 6%.[19] The marked increase in the incidence of PCNSL as a whole can be largely, although not exclusively, attributed to the outbreak of the AIDS epidemic. A number of years ago, the AIDS Cooperative Group reported the development of eight cases of lymphoma in 55 patients being treated in trials of antiviral drugs (azidothymidine), five of whom developed PCNSL.[20] Although this represented a relatively small patient population, it does suggest a higher than expected number of PCNSL cases. Thus, it appeared probable that as supportive care improved for patients with AIDS, the incidence of PCNSL would continue to rise in this patient population; an assumption that appeared to come true. Now, in the era of highly active retrovival therapy (HAART), the natural history of HIV disease is again changing. The effects, however, on the incidence and behavior of PCNSL in HAART-treated patients remain to be well established.

Immunocompetent Patients

Of just as much concern as the rise of PCNSL in immunocompromised patients is the apparent increase in the incidence of this disease in otherwise normal, immunocompetent patients. In 1988, Eby and coworkers, using data from the National Cancer Institute's Surveillance, Epidemiology, and End Results (SEER) program, compared the incidence of PCNSL from 1973 to 1975 to the incidence from 1982 to 1984.[21] They excluded from their analysis young, never-married men, a group previously believed to be at risk for AIDS. These investigators found that the incidence of PCNSL increased from 2.7 to 7.5 cases per 10 million population from the study period in the 1970s to that in the 1980s. It could be argued that this apparent increase in the incidence of PCNSL is an artifact of the inclusion of undiagnosed AIDS patients and/or better screening techniques (such as computed tomography [CT] scans, magnetic resonance imaging [MRI] scans, and stereotaxic surgery). The fact, however, that the observed increase occurred, for the most part, before the AIDS epidemic and before the advent of these more sensitive screening techniques, argues for a true increase in the incidence of PCNSL. Supportive of these observations, investigators at Memorial Sloan-Kettering Cancer Center in New York have reported a 17-fold increase in PCNSL in the 5 years between 1985 and 1990 compared with the previous 20 years.[22] The etiologic factors responsible for this increase in PCNSL in non-AIDS patients are unknown at this time. Some have speculated that if the incidence of this disease continues to rise at the present rate, it will be the most common primary tumor of the CNS in the new millennium. Before such sweeping conclusions can be drawn, however, it should be realized that not every institution has seen the same dramatic increase in the frequency of this tumor. In our own experience, we have witnessed a three-fold increase in PCNSL in non-AIDS patients from 1987 to 1992 compared with the rate from 1981 to 1986. Since 1992, however, the number of patients diagnosed with PCNSL has remained constant, and PCNSL (in non-AIDS patients) represented only 1.2% of all primary brain tumors undergoing biopsy at our institution. In agreement with this, a recent study using a population-based study of incidence, clinicopathologic features and outcomes of the Alberta Cancer Registry from 1975 to 1996 failed to show the PCNSL was increasing in incidence, at least in Alberta.[23]

BIOLOGY

Immunocompetent Patients

The etiology of the neoplastic lymphocyte clone in immunocompetent patients with PCNSL remains speculative. Several hypotheses concerning the pathophysiology exist, the most simple of which is that the neoplastic transformation occurs in clones of lymphocytes that routinely inhabit the CNS.[24] Alternatively, neoplastic transformation may occur in a systemic population of lymphocytes that possess specific tropism for the CNS (i.e., through expression of specific cell surface adhesion molecules), or develop such a tropism after the transformation events. In support of the latter hypothesis, Bashir and colleagues examined immunophenotypic markers in 18 cases of CNS lymphoma (14 primary and 4 secondary).[25] As had been previously reported, all lymphoma cells were of B-cell origin. Although most tumors were positive for pan–B-cell markers, most CNS lymphoma cells were negative for various B-cell–restricted activation markers such as B5, Blast 2, and BB1. This is in contrast to systemic lymphomas, which are almost always positive for these antigens. There were no significant immunophenotypic differences between primary and secondary CNS lymphomas. The total number of CNS lymphomas examined in this study was small; however, if these data can be confirmed in a larger series, the hypothesis that PCNSL represents a clonal proliferation of lymphoma cells with a predilection for the CNS will be supported. The reason for this is that if PCNSL was the result of transformation of a naturally occurring CNS lymphocyte population, one would expect different phenotypes between primary and secondary CNS lymphomas.

A third hypothesis for the etiology of PCNSL is based on the idea that the CNS is a immunologic sanctuary. Neoplastic lymphocytes may be eradicated systemically by an intact immune system but find relative protection within the CNS. This could explain the curious observation that systemic dissemination of PCNSL is unusual, even in advanced stages of disease. This hypothesis is based on the premise that the CNS has a "privileged" status relative to the immune system. Although this concept is still evolving, the original concept was first proposed many years ago with the discovery of the blood–brain barrier (BBB). The anatomic substrate for the BBB is the continuous sealing of interendothelial spaces by tight junctions and the lack of fenestrations or pores normally found in capillaries in other parts of the body.[26,27] Thus, the BBB effectively limits the movement of macromolecules into or out of the brain parenchyma.[27] Relative to immunologic reactions, these physiologic restraints imparted by the BBB may effectively limit the exposure of foreign antigens within the CNS to the cellular and humoral immune system. This "hiding" of foreign antigen effectively isolates the CNS from the immune system, making the CNS a so-called immunologically privileged site.

Experimental evidence confirming the immunologically privileged status of the CNS comes from experiments in the 1920s by Murphy and Sturm, who demonstrated that mouse sarcoma could survive in rat brain.[28] Alternately, the tumor failed to grow if an autograft of rat splenic tissue was cotransplanted with the mouse sarcoma, demonstrating the animals' immunocompetence to destroy the xenograft if antigen-presenting and effector cells could "see" the foreign antigens in the correct context. Since these initial experiments, many types of incompatible tissue types have been transplanted into animal and human brains with little or no graft rejection.[29,30]

In addition to the growing data demonstrating diminished antigen presentation within the CNS, some investigators have suggested that the BBB may limit the movement of immune effector cells into the CNS. Neither experimental nor clinical evidence supports this conclusion and animal models of autoimmune diseases such as experimental allergic encephalitis (EAE) and clinical disease states such as multiple sclerosis demonstrate the potential ability of immune effector cells to invade the CNS.[31] Thus, the difficulty of the intact immune system to see foreign antigens within the CNS may be the principal determinant of the presumed immunologic privileged status of the CNS. Although much has yet to be learned, these data clearly suggest that some type of immunologic sanctuary for tumor cells may exist within the CNS. Thus, regardless of how and where PCNSL malignant lymphocytes develop, once these cells gain access to the CNS, they appear to proliferate rapidly within the subarachnoid space and disseminate throughout the craniospinal axis without significant impedance from the immune system.

Immunocompromised Patients

As mentioned, the high incidence of PCNSL in the AIDS population resembles that in other immunosuppressed patients, implicating the immune system in the pathogenesis of this disease. There are many biologic similarities between AIDS patients and the congenital or iatrogenic immunosuppressed populations who develop PCNSL. The malignant lymphocytes in these two groups of immunocompromised patients tend to be oligoclonal or polyclonal and usually high-grade (immunoblastic and small non-cleaved) tumors, in contrast with the monoclonal tumors found in PCNSLs of immunocompetent patients, which are often low- to intermediate-grade tumors.[32] Another similarity between these two groups of immunocompromised patients is the tendency for the degree of immunosuppression to be related to the risk of developing PCNSL. For example, the risk of PCNSL in transplant patients is related to the dose and number of immunosuppressive agents as well as the duration of treatment. An analogous situation appears to occur in patients with AIDS, in whom the risk of developing PCNSL increases with declining CD4 lymphocyte counts (and thus more immunosuppression).[33]

Epstein–Barr virus (EBV) appears to play a role in the pathogenesis of PCNSL in the immunosuppressed population. In contrast with immunocompetent patients with PCNSL, immunosuppressed patients with PCNSL consistently have EBV genomic DNA found within their malignant lymphocytes.[34–37] This relationship is intriguing since EBV is known to induce B-lymphocyte proliferation in vitro. Furthermore, there is strong epidemiologic evidence linking EBV to endemic Burkitt's lymphoma.[38,39] It is believed that EBV infects certain B lymphocytes, causing a clonal expansion that in an immunocompetent patient is limited by immune mechanisms, particularly cellular immune responses. In the immunocompromised hosts, the T-lymphocyte population is quantitatively (AIDS) and/or qualitatively (cyclosporine-treated/T-cell depletion for allogeneic bone marrow transplantation) abnormal, allowing EBV-induced B-lymphocyte proliferation to proceed unrestrained. This, along with the possibly decreased immunologic surveillance within the CNS may contribute to the development of PCNSL in this patient population. Consistent with this hypothesis is a report from Memorial Sloan-Kettering Cancer Center that demonstrated that EBV-associated lymphoma occurring after allogeneic bone marrow transplantation was associated with T-cell depletion of the donor marrow.[31] The importance of an intact cellular response was suggested by the observation that five of these transplant patients with EBV-related lymphomas were successfully treated with unirradiated donor leukocytes, achieving either clinical or pathologic complete responses.

CLINICAL AND RADIOGRAPHIC PRESENTATION

Many manuscripts have appeared in the literature reporting the clinical characteristics of small series of patients with either AIDS- or non–AIDS-associated PCNSL. Several years ago we reviewed 40 reports of non–AIDS-associated PCNSL[40–88] and 32 reports of AIDS-associated PCNSL,[13,20,89–118] and synthesized the data for these 1100 patients to determine general clinical characteristics and treatment outcomes in this patient population. Much of the data in this chapter are abstracted from this database.[32]

Immunocompetent and Immunocompromised Patients

The median age of diagnosis of PCNSL is 55 years for immunocompetent patients and 31 years for AIDS patients, although PCNSL has been described in patients of all ages (Table 17–7). A male-to-female ratio of 3:2 is seen in the immunocompetent patients, whereas 90% of AIDS patients are males. This preponderance of male over female AIDS patients with PCNSL almost certainly represents the early epidemiology of the AIDS epidemic. Now, as an increasing

Table 17–7. Patient Characteristics at Diagnosis

Characteristics	Immunocompetent Group	AIDS Group
Total number of patients	792	315
Male/female ratio	442/328 (1.35:1)	118/16 (7.38:1)
Mean age (years)	55.2	30.8
History of opportunistic infection or Kaposi's sarcoma symptoms	Not available	115/143 (80%)
Average duration before diagnosis (months)	2.77	1.81
Types: Neurologic (%)	56.4	51.0
Deficits: Mental status changes (%)	34.6	53.3
Seizures (%)	11.2	26.7
Increased intracranial pressure (%)	32.4	14.2

AIDS, acquired immunodeficiency syndrome.

number of women are being infected with HIV, it is quite likely that we will see an increasing number of immunocompromised women developing PCNSL.

Most patients present with symptoms suggestive of an intracranial mass lesion. As with any primary or metastatic lesion of the CNS, symptoms are related to tumor size and location. However, there are some neurologic symptoms that are more typical of this patient population compared with populations with other intracranial tumors. Since 50% of these lesions develop in the frontal lobes and the lesions are often multifocal, personality changes, headaches, and lethargy are common symptoms. Seizures are less commonly seen in patients with PCNSL than in patients with gliomas, meningiomas, or metastatic disease, probably because these lesions less commonly involve the seizure-prone cerebral cortex at the time of diagnosis. The duration of symptoms is usually only a few weeks or months, but the range can be up to many months.

Patients with AIDS-associated PCNSL can present with clinical signs and symptoms slightly different from those of their immunocompetent counterparts. AIDS patients more often present with an encephalopathic picture, characterized by significant changes in mental status. The global neurologic deficits associated with AIDS-associated PCNSL are probably a result of a number of factors including the multifocal nature of the disease, associated infectious processes such as viral encephalitis and/or toxoplasmosis, and progressive multifocal leukoencephalopathy. It has been demonstrated at autopsy that many AIDS patients with PCNSL have at least one (and often more) additional active pathologic CNS processes.[119]

It can be assumed that most patients with PCNSL have disseminated disease throughout the CNS at the time of diagnosis. Radiographically, however, only 25% of immunocompetent patients and 50% of AIDS patients have multifocal lesions at diagnosis (Table 17–8). When a multifocal radiographic picture is seen in an otherwise healthy person, the diagnosis of systemic metastatic cancer is often entertained. Since the treatment of metastatic cancer is quite different from the treatment of PCNSL in the immunocompetent host (see later), the importance of a histologic diagnosis cannot be overstated.

Ocular involvement by lymphoma is another manifestation of the multifocal nature of PCNSL. The retro-orbital area is the most common site of eye metastases from systemic lymphoma, whereas malignant cells more commonly infiltrate the vitreous, retina, and/or choroid in PCNSL patients.[120–122] Diagnosis is usually made by the demonstration of a pleocytosis within the aqueous humor by slit-lamp examination. The prevalence of ocular involvement in PCNSL at the time of diagnosis remains unclear. Some reports claim it to be as high as 20%; however, our review of the literature suggests that it is found in only 5%, although one must question whether most patients are eventually evaluated for ocular involvement. Although some patients may complain of blurred vision or vitreous floaters, most patients are unaware of ocular involvement. If a deliberate effort to screen patients for ocular involvement is not made, many cases will undoubtedly be missed. Thus, a careful neurophthalmologic examination including the use of slit-lamp examination of the vitreous and indirect ophthalmoscopy for retinal or choroidal disease is recommended for all patients before the initiation of therapy.

Table 17–8. Radiographic Findings at Presentation

Radiographic Finding	Immunocompetent Group	AIDS Group
Angiography	60 avascular, 13 vascular	No data
Brain scan	8 of 8 positive for technetium 99m	No data
CT scan		
Noncontrast	201	67
Hypodense	21 (10.4%)	6 (9.0%)
Iso- or hyperdense	180 (89.6%)	61 (91.0%)
Contrast		
Any enhancement	245 (97.2%)	91 (90.1%)
No enhancement	7 (2.8%)	10 (9.9%)
Pattern of enhancement		
Irregular	86 (45.0%)	25 (39.1%)
Homogeneous	105 (55.0%)	39 (60.9%)
Ring	0 (0.0%)	47 (52.0%) for all enhanced scans
Distribution		
Solitary	290 (72.0%)	87 (48.0%)
Multiple	100 (25.0%)	94 (52.0%)
Diffuse	14 (3.0%)	No data

AIDS, acquired immunodeficiency syndrome.

Whatever the true incidence of ocular involvement by PCNSL, it has been well documented that the disease process occasionally begins in the eye as a nonspecific, unilateral uveitis. The uveitis typically does not respond to conventional therapy and usually becomes bilateral. As many as 80% of patients with ocular lymphoma progress to PCNSL.[121,122] Thus, any patient with ocular lymphoma should undergo enhanced MRI of the brain as part of the initial evaluation.

Rarely, PCNSL can arise from the leptomeninges and spinal cord (<10% of all PCNSL) in isolation of brain disease. PCNSL of the spinal cord presents usually with bilateral lower limb weakness in the absence of back pain. Pain and sensory symptoms can follow, but the cerebrospinal fluid is usually normal. Prognosis is poor, with survival averaging only a few months. Leptomeningeal presentation, like carcinomatous or lymphomatous meningitis, is associated with cranial neuropathies, progressive lumbosacral root syndrome, and often signs and symptoms of increased intracranial pressure. This is in contrast with more common presentations of PCNSL, in which clinical signs or symptoms of leptomeningeal disease (e.g., cranial neuropathies, hydrocephalus, cervical and lumbosacral radiculopathies) are uncommon despite the relatively high incidence of a malignant pleocytosis at presentation. Diagnosis of PCNSL presenting as leptomeningeal disease is established by a meningeal biopsy and/or the finding of malignant lymphocytes within the CNS. These patients often have hydrocephalus with no obvious parenchymal disease. Our experience suggests that these patients have a prognosis as poor as those presenting with spinal cord disease.

Radiographic imaging studies may be suggestive of the diagnosis of PCNSL (see Table 17–8). Angiographic studies have shown that most of these lesions are avascular or hypovascular in nature. Brain scanning with or without single-photon emission computed tomography (SPECT) capabilities using technetium 99m demonstrates increased uptake in almost all patients with PCNSL. These observations are, however, mainly of historical interest, for modern imaging with CT and/or MRI has replaced angiography and nuclear brain scanning. Ninety percent of patients with PCNSL have an isodense or hyperdense lesion on nonenhanced CT scan. This corresponds to an intense signal on the nonenhanced T_1 MRI image. This appearance differs from that of other primary brain tumors (gliomas and meningiomas) and most metastatic lesions, which tend to be hypodense. The hyperdense radiographic appearance of PCNSL probably represents both the close packing of the small lymphocytic cells (which generally have high nuclear-to-cytoplasmic ratios) and the fact that PCNSL tends to have less associated cerebral edema than gliomas and most metastatic tumors.

After the administration of contrast material, more than 90% of PCNSLs enhance on CT and MRI; half of them do so homogeneously. A T_1-weighted MRI scan with gadolinium often demonstrates a greater number of lesions than are seen on CT. The lesions are most often (75%) located adjacent to cortical convexities or ventricular surfaces with indistinct borders and a variable amount of cerebral edema. Thus, an angiographically avascular lesion that is isohyperdense in relation to the normal cortex, enhances homogeneously, and is located adjacent to the ventricular surface is highly suggestive of PCNSL.

A special note should be made concerning those rare PCNSL lesions that do not enhance on CT and/or MRI. DeAngelis reported that 10 of 85 (12%) immunocompetent patients with PCNSL had nonenhancing lesions.[22] This group of patients was not treated with corticosteroids before scanning and had nonenhancing lesions at diagnosis or at relapse. In a few patients with multifocal disease, some lesions enhanced, whereas others did not on the same scan. Nonenhancing tumors cause significant diagnostic problems and present therapeutic implications, suggesting that the tumor resides behind an intact BBB (see Treatment section).

Although AIDS- and non–AIDS-associated PCNSL have similar radiographic findings, there are some important differences. The most important difference is the incidence of radiographic multifocal disease, which is twice as common in AIDS patients compared with their non–AIDS-associated PCNSL counterparts (50% vs. 25%, respectively). Additionally, ring enhancement, a pattern rarely seen in non-AIDS PCNSL patients, is seen in 50% of AIDS patients.

DIAGNOSIS

Immunocompetent Patients

Although the diagnosis of PCNSL usually requires histologic verification, the diagnostic algorithm differs for the immunocompetent versus the AIDS patient (Fig. 17–5A). In the immunocompetent patient who is found to have an intracranial mass with radiographic criteria suggestive of PCNSL (as described previously), a tissue diagnosis should be made immediately. Corticosteroids should be withheld until diagnostic tissue is obtained unless the patient is in immediate danger of herniation. The reason for this is that corticosteroids appear to have significant cytotoxic activity against PCNSL such that two-thirds of patients have some radiographic response to steroids alone, with some patients achieving a complete radiographic remission. Even for patients not experiencing a radiographic complete response, the lymphotoxic effects of corticosteroids can disrupt cellular morphology, making histologic diagnosis from biopsied material impossible. If the patient requires the immediate use of corticosteroids or if PCNSL was not considered and the patient was placed on corticosteroids, repeat CT and/or MRI should be performed before a diagnosis is made. If the tumor is smaller or resolved completely, the diagnosis of PCNSL is quite likely. Nevertheless, non-neoplastic contrast-enhancing lesions such as multiple sclerosis and sarcoidosis can also resolve after corticosteroid administration, and thus a tissue diagnosis should still be obtained. If the lesion has completely resolved on the corticosteroid therapy, the patient should be slowly weaned from the drug and followed closely for recurrence of the abnormality on CT and/or MRI. If it recurs, the patient should have a tissue diagnosis made immediately.

Our recommendation is to try to establish the diagnosis without neurosurgical intervention whenever possible. Therefore, if a lumbar puncture can be safely performed (no evidence of obstruction or increased intracranial pressure), cerebrospinal fluid should be obtained for both routine studies and cytologic examination. Although previous reports have suggested that the incidence of positive cerebrospinal fluid cytologic tests at the diagnosis of PCNSL is small, our review of the literature suggests that a malignant pleocytosis may be found in nearly one-third of all patients. Markers of clonogenicity such as κ and λ light-chain immunohistochemistry and polymerase chain reaction (PCR) amplification of B-cell immunoglobulin gene rearrangement may be helpful in distinguishing between a clonal proliferation of lymphocytes in the cerebrospinal fluid from a reactive pleocytosis.[123–125] Even with these additional studies, however, most patients require a biopsy of the intracranial mass to establish the pathologic diagnosis.

When a tissue diagnosis is required, several neurosurgical techniques are appropriate. The easiest and safest procedure is a stereotactic biopsy. In the hands of an experienced neurosurgeon, stereotactic biopsy can be performed in almost any region of the brain without significant risks. A potential problem with samples obtained from stereotactic biopsies is the small amount of tissue, potentially making it difficult to differentiate lymphoma from inflammatory cells. With the use of immunohistochemical stain-

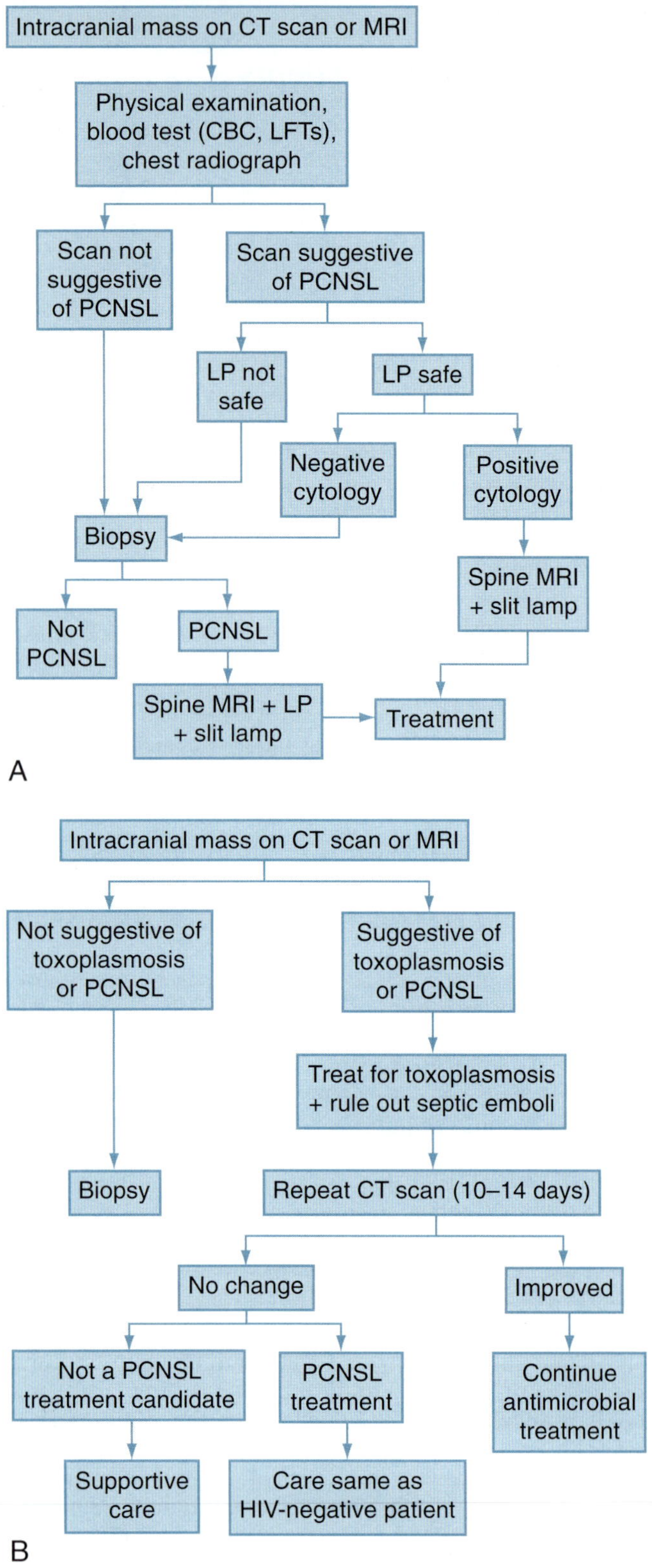

Figure 17–5. Diagnostic algorithms for patients found to have had computed tomographic (CT) or magnetic resonance imaging (MRI) scans demonstrating lesions consistent with primary central nervous system lymphoma. **A:** Diagnostic algorithm for immunocompetent human immunodeficiency virus (HIV) seronegative patients. **B:** Diagnostic algorithm for HIV-seropositive patients. CBC, complete blood count; LFT, liver function test; PCNSL, primary central nervous system lymphoma; LP, lumbar puncture.

ing and molecular analysis (i.e., PCR), however, a definitive diagnosis can usually be made. If a definitive diagnosis cannot be obtained via a stereotactic biopsy, an open biopsy for additional tissue is recommended. No data are available to suggest that an extended craniotomy and major resection of tumor are beneficial to these patients, probably because radiation and chemotherapy offer such an effective means of cytoreduction. For patients who present with both eye and CNS involvement, a histological diagnosis can be made through a vitrectomy and retinal biopsy.

After histologic confirmation of PCNSL, patients should undergo a full evaluation of the craniospinal axis, if this was not done before surgery. This includes examination of the cerebrospinal fluid, enhanced MRI of the spinal axis, and a neurophthalmologic examination as described previously. The extent of staging that is necessary to evaluate the possibility of systemic disease should be kept to a minimum. From our experience, as well as that in the literature, a thorough physical examination, routine blood studies, and a chest radiograph are sufficient for screening for systemic involvement. If these procedures are unrevealing, it is unlikely that more extensive studies (gallium scans, body CT scans, bone marrow aspirate, and biopsy) will disclose an occult systemic lymphoma.

Immunocompromised Patients

The diagnostic decision algorithm in AIDS patients is more difficult because of the higher probability of another CNS abnormality such as toxoplasmosis or multifocal leukoencephalopathy.[19,126] The multiple small, ring-enhancing lesions characteristic of cerebral toxoplasmosis, in particular, can appear identical to PCNSL on CT and/or MRI scans. The decision process is further complicated by the poor survival of AIDS patients with PCNSL (see later), leading many physicians to conclude that these patients should not be subjected to an invasive procedure but rather treated empirically. A reasonable strategy for an AIDS patient with presumed PCNSL (enhancing, periventricular lesion or lesions) is to empirically treat the patient with antitoxoplasmosis drugs, during which time the patient can be evaluated for bacteremia, fungemia, or other sources of septic emboli (Fig. 17–5B). This strategy is probably only valid for patients who have positive serologic tests for toxoplasmosis. For the rare HIV-positive patient who is negative for toxoplasmosis antibodies, the likelihood of cerebral toxoplasmosis is small. Luft and colleagues recently reported a prospective trial using this approach in 49 AIDS patients with enhancing CNS lesions.[127] Thirty-five (71%) of 49 patients responded to clindamycin and pyrimethamine therapy, and 30 (86%) of these had clinical improvement by day 7. Thirty-two (91%) of those with a response improved by day 14. Two of the patients in whom therapy failed underwent a stereotactic biopsy and were found to have PCNSL. Therefore, if an AIDS patient has not improved clinically or radiographically after 10 to 14 days of empiric antitoxoplasmosis therapy, a stereotactic biopsy should be considered.

Since structural imaging studies such as CT and MRI cannot accurately differentiate infectious from malignant cerebral lesions in patients with AIDS, there is a growing interest in evaluating the role of functional imaging such as

SPECT and positron emission tomography (PET) for these patients. Hoffman and associates reported results using [^{18}F]fluoro-2-deoxyglucose (FDG) and PET in 11 AIDS patients with cerebral lesions.[128] FDG-PET was able to accurately differentiate between PCNSL and abnormalities with an infectious cause in all patients. Both qualitative visual inspection of the images and semiquantitative analysis using count ratios were performed and revealed similar results. Thus, it appears from this pilot that FDG-PET may be useful in the management of AIDS patients with CNS lesions since high FDG uptake most likely represents a PCNSL.

We believe that all other non-AIDS immunocompromised patients who present with an enhancing periventricular lesion (or lesions) require a histologic confirmation of PCNSL before any therapy is initiated.

PATHOLOGY

Immunocompetent Patients

Histologically, PCNSL grows in sheets of cells, infiltrating the brain parenchyma between blood vessels in a characteristic vasocentric pattern. Tumor margins are poorly defined and usually extend a substantial distance from the borders of the mass lesion seen on radiographic studies. Neither necrosis nor hemorrhage is a common histologic feature; however, as is true for any large intracerebral mass, necrosis can occasionally be found. In our 792 immunocompetent patients with PCNSL, pathologic examination was available in 539 patients (Table 17–9). When immunophenotyping was performed, almost all PCNSLs were of B-lymphocyte origin. According to the International Working Formulation definitions, 50% of the PCNSLs in immunocompetent patients were large cell, with the next most common histologic type being immunoblastic (18%) (Fig. 17–6) (see also color section). There was an equal distribution of other histologic types. T-cell lymphomas are relatively rare and tend to present with leptomeningeal disease. Although there is a suggestion that the incidence of T-cell PCNSL is rising, many believe this is an artifact owing to the increasing use of newer immunohistochemical stains that might be detecting reactive T lymphocytes. This is an important point since for unclear reasons many PCNSLs are associated with a reactive lymphocytosis.

A recent retrospective review of 33 primary tumor tissue samples from 33 patients with PCNSL suggests that the presence of BCL-6 antigen predicts for a more favorable outcome. Expression of BCL-6 was significantly associated with longer OS ($p = 0.002$; median survival, 101 vs. 14.7 months) While similar findings have been reported in

Table 17–9. Method of Tissue Diagnosis and Histologic Type

	Immunocompetent	AIDS
Positive cerebrospinal fluid cytologic tests	79/255 (31%)	3/13 (23%)
Surgery		
Biopsy (only)	170 (38%)	78 (70%)
Resection	277 (62%)	33 (30%)
Histologic type		
Large cell	268 (50%)	61 (37%)
Immunoblastic	96 (18%)	57 (35%)
Centroblastic	38 (7%)	
Lymphoblastic	37 (7%)	
Lymphocytic	23 (4%)	1
Small non-cleaved	21 (4%)	42 (25%)
Small cleaved	20 (4%)	
Mixed	19 (4%)	3 (2%)
Not otherwise specified	17 (3%)	0
Total	539 patients (68% of all patients)	164 patients (52% of all patients)

AIDS, acquired immunodeficiency syndrome.

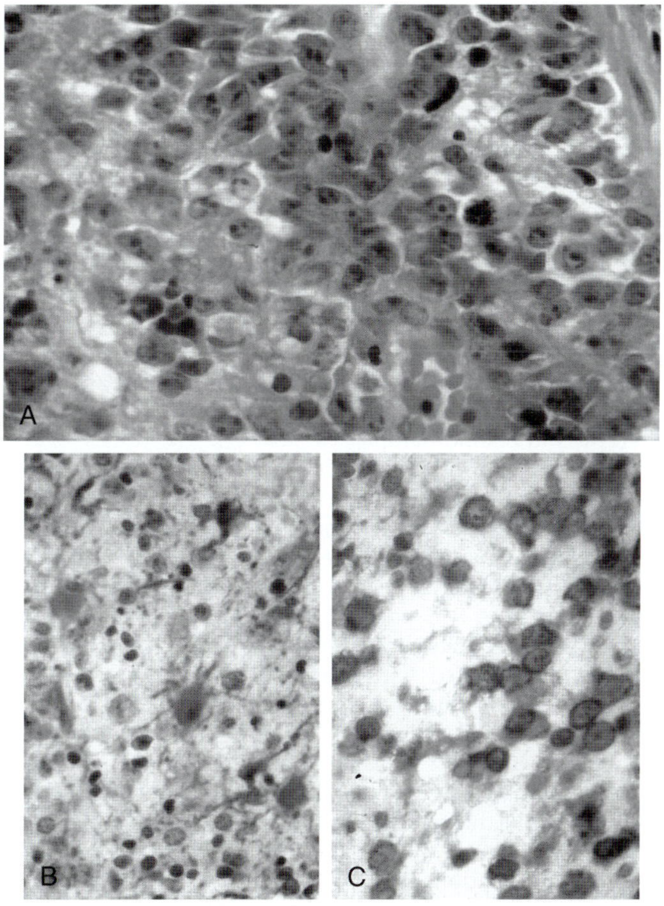

Figure 17–6. Histologic sections of a large-cell primary central nervous system lymphoma. **A:** The tumor is characterized by angiocentricity (tendency to aggregate around small blood vessels), as well as clumped, peripherally located nuclear chromatin, and prominent nucleoli (hematoxylin and eosin, 400). **B:** Glial fibrillary acidic protein (GFAP) immunoperoxidase staining of the tumor. GFAP is a known intermediate filament found exclusively in cells of astrocytic origin. The darkly staining cells with the elongated processes are reactive astrocytes, often found in areas of abnormality within the cerebrum (tumor, infection, ischemia). **C:** Leukocyte common antigen (LCA) immunoperoxidase staining of the tumor. LCA is a protein found on the surface of almost all cells of lymphocytic origin. The darkly staining cells are the tumor cells, proving the lymphocytic nature of this neoplasm. (See also color section.)

patients with systemic diffuse large B-cell lymphomas, this was the first demonstration that BCL-6 expression is associated with better prognosis for patients with PCNSL.[44]

Immunocompromised Patients

There does appear to be a difference between the frequency of specific histologic subtypes in AIDS-associated PCNSL and that in immunocompetent patients. In our review of 315 AIDS patients, pathologic examination was available in 164 patients. Sixty percent of the AIDS patients had a high-grade histologic type (compared with 22% of immunocompetent patients), with large-cell (37%), immunoblastic (35%), and small non-cleaved (25%) the three most predominate subtypes. When reported, almost all AIDS-associated PCNSLs contained EBV genomic DNA, a finding quite rare in immunocompetent patients.

TREATMENT

Immunocompetent Patients

Radiation Therapy

The literature is replete with anecdotal experiences with either surgery, radiation therapy, chemotherapy, or some combination of these. As discussed in the previous section on diagnosis, the only role of surgery in this disease is to establish a diagnosis and to offer ventricular shunting in the rare case of persistent hydrocephalus. Unlike the situation in patients with malignant gliomas, the extent of surgery has little role in prolonging survival or improving the quality of life for patients with PCNSL. The reasons for this are related to the diffuse infiltrative and multifocal nature of PCNSL and the effectiveness of corticosteroids, radiation therapy, and chemotherapy.

Postoperative whole-brain radiation therapy has been the conventional therapy for patients with PCNSL, with median survivals of 8 to 18 months in most series. A review of 308 patients with PCNSL treated with radiation therapy and corticosteroids alone reported only 21 survivors at 5 years.[71]

Early studies documented improved survival of patients with PCNSL treated with surgery and radiation therapy compared with surgery alone. Henry and colleagues reported a median survival of 4.6 months after surgical excision alone and 15.2 months after surgery and radiation therapy.[129] It was also noted that most patients improved neurologically during the first few weeks of therapy, and complete responses were seen in most patients at the completion of radiation therapy. Uncontrolled, retrospective studies suggested that a dose–response relationship existed for PCNSL. This was first reported in 1967 by Sagerman and associates, who noted near-100% treatment failures at doses below 30 Gy, but observed some prolonged survivors at higher doses.[130] Later studies confirmed that the only 2-year survivors were patients treated with doses of whole-brain radiation at or above 45 Gy. Murray and colleagues' analysis of 198 patients included 54 patients who received 50 Gy or greater, with the remainder receiving lower doses.[60] Actuarial survival (life table) at 5 years was 42.3% for patients treated with greater than 50 Gy compared with 12.8% for those receiving lower doses ($p < 0.05$).

Some authors have suggested the use of craniospinal radiation in the initial treatment of patients with PCNSL. This recommendation was based on the relatively high incidence of leptomeningeal dissemination at the time of relapse. There are no convincing data, however, that craniospinal radiation therapy is superior to whole-brain therapy in prolonging disease-free survival. This is because in most patients whose disease recurs in the leptomeninges, it also recurs in the brain at the site of original presentation. Furthermore, craniospinal radiation fields significantly affect large amounts of bone marrow in the vertebral bodies and the pelvis. This can make subsequent administration of systemic chemotherapy more difficult secondary to diminished bone marrow reserve. Therefore, we do not recommend the routine use of spinal axis radiation therapy except in the rare cases of PCNSL presenting as an intramedullary mass.

In the absence of a prospective randomized study, the Radiation Therapy Oncology Group (RTOG) evaluated a high-dose regimen of radiation therapy in a single-arm prospective study conducted from 1983 to 1987.[131] Forty-one immunocompetent patients received 40 Gy to the whole brain and meninges followed by a boost of 20 Gy to the original enhancing tumor volume and a 2-cm margin in all directions. The median survival for the entire group was 11.6 months, with 48% of the patients alive at 1 year and 28% at 2 years. A univariate analysis showed improved survival for patients with a better preradiation Karnofsky performance status (KPS), a lower age, and male sex. Patients with a KPS of 70% or greater survived 21.1 months (median) compared with 5.6 months (median) for KPS of less than 70 ($p = 0.001$). Below the age of 60 years, patients survived a median of 23.1 months compared with 7.6 months for older patients ($p = 0.001$). A multivariate analysis using the Cox regression model indicated that KPS was the most significant prognostic variable ($p < 0.01$). Survival according to sex was also statistically significant ($p < 0.01$), with the median survival for men 19.8 months compared with 6.8 months for women. Although the Cox regression analysis indicated that sex was the second most important prognostic factor, closer inspection showed that the women were older and tended to have a worse KPS. Therefore, the selection of sex in the model may have masked the true prognostic significance of age. In fact, when the investigators excluded sex from the regression model, age became significant ($p < 0.05$). The actuarial survival curves from all subsets showed a continuous downward force of mortality, suggesting that radiation therapy alone was not a curative therapy for patients with PCNSL. Based on these disappointing results, the RTOG concluded that further studies should include some form of chemotherapy.

Careful analysis of patterns of failure after radiation therapy can provide direction for future therapy. Although initial clinical and radiographic responses to radiation therapy are gratifying, failure to achieve durable local control remains the major therapeutic challenge in the treatment of PCNSL. In the recent RTOG study discussed previously, in only 3 of 41 patients did therapy fail outside the nervous system, and in 1 patient it failed in the eye. Overall, therapy failed in 92% of patients within the radiation therapy volume, 83% suffered only local relapse, and 9% had both local and distant failure. Most "in-field" failures, however, were outside the original site of disease. Loeffler and associates reviewed the patterns of failure of 254 patients in the literature, and found documentation of sites of failure in 204.[71] Relapse within the radiation therapy volume occurred in 78% of patients, with only 8% failing outside the CNS.

Since most patients with relapsed PCNSL have received prior high doses of radiation therapy, further conventional radiation therapy cannot be safely administered. However, there is a growing interest in the use of stereotactic radiosurgery for small, focally recurrent PCNSL. Radiosurgery is the delivery of a single dose of highly accurate and precise small-field irradiation using stereotactically directed, highly collimated, narrow beams of radiation. Since 1988, we have treated 20 patients. These lesions generally responded extremely well in a period of only a few weeks. However, in all patients the therapy subsequently failed in new cranial or spinal sites. The median survival from radiosurgery was 9 months. This single-day outpatient procedure is an excellent source of palliation for relapsed PCNSL, but because of the highly infiltrative nature of this disease, it should not be considered as a potentially curative therapy.

Intraocular lymphoma frequently coexists with PCNSL. However, it can also be present even before the diagnosis of PCNSL is established. In such patients, bilateral orbital radiotherapy is required (30 Gy in 15 fractions). In general, the eyes can be included in the WBRT fields by removing the standard eye shielding or treated with opposed lateral separate fields. Since the lens is included in the irradiated volume, all surviving patients will eventually develop cataracts. These can be removed surgically and synthetic lens placed with excellent functional outcome. Recent work, however, suggests that high-dose MTX can penetrate the ocular chambers, and possibly delay or eliminate the need to irradiate.[45]

In summary, even with the use of the highest tolerable doses (60 Gy) of radiation therapy, prolonged disease-free survival is rare when radiation is used alone. Ultimately, in the vast majority of patients, the disease will recur within the radiation therapy volume (whole brain). Why is PCNSL so resistant to radiation therapy when histologically identical local (Stage I, IE) extraneural lymphomas are readily curable? Some have suggested that the microenvironment of the brain alters the radiosensitivity of PCNSL, and others have argued that PCNSL is truly a systemic disease and that CNS "reseeding" occurs, thus preventing any local therapy from being effective. Whatever the explanation, the growing data suggest that surgery and radiation therapy alone are not sufficient to eradicate PCNSL.

Chemotherapy

With both the recognition that radiation therapy alone is not curative of PCNSL and the successful use of chemotherapy in systemic lymphomas, there has come a growing interest in systemic therapy to treat patients with PCNSL. Along with all the difficulties of drug therapy for systemic lymphomas, PCNSL presents several unique challenges to the effective use of chemotherapy. Probably the largest challenge is problematic drug delivery secondary to variable penetration of different chemotherapeutic agents into the brain parenchyma. The limiting factor here is the unique microarchitecture of the cerebral vasculature, the BBB. What makes the BBB unique compared with other vascular beds is the presence of tight junctions between cells rather than the usual fenestrations found between endothelial cells in most other parts of the body.[26] This effectively eliminates any passive diffusion of large water-soluble molecules from the blood to the CNS.[27] In addition, endothelial cells that make up the BBB tend to have few cytoplasmic vacuoles, thus limiting the transfer of material into the CNS through passive endocytosis. Finally, it has been shown that endothelial cells that constitute the BBB have an extraordinary number of mitochondria, suggesting that these cells are quite metabolically active. It has been suggested that this metabolic activity is geared toward keeping potentially toxic substances out of the CNS. Consistent with this hypothesis is the observation that cerebral endothelium expresses high levels of the multidrug-resistant (MDR) p-glycoprotein.[132] Thus, the cerebral endothelium is an effective barrier to the entry of many potentially toxic substances, including chemotherapy.

Despite the limitations of variable drug penetration through the BBB, it has been known for more than a decade that a number of chemotherapeutic agents are capable of inducing responses in patients with recurrent PCNSL (Fig. 17–7 and Fig. 17–8). This is because some lipid-soluble and/or very small-molecular-weight drugs are capable of penetrating the BBB. These include drugs such as the nitrosoureas, methotrexate, cytarabine, procarbazine, and 5-flurouracil. More interesting, however, is the observation that some drugs, such as cyclophosphamide and vincristine, are neither small nor lipid-soluble but still have activity against PCNSL. This probably relates to the fact that in areas of significant tumor burden, the BBB is variably disrupted, thus allowing access to certain drugs not normally capable of crossing an intact BBB. There are two important points, however, about this breakdown of the BBB by PCNSL. First,

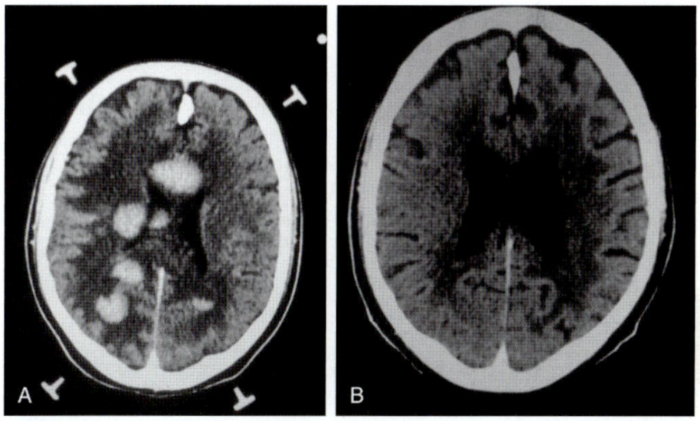

Figure 17–7. **A:** Before therapy. This CT scan is quite suggestive of the diagnosis of primary central nervous system lymphoma because of the brightly enhancing, multifocal, periventricular appearance of these lesions, with less mass effect than might otherwise be expected from other primary brain tumors or metastases. **B:** After chemotherapy. This CT scan of the same patient, obtained after just three cycles of systemic chemotherapy (cyclophosphamide, vincristine, and high-dose methotrexate), demonstrates a complete radiographic response. Of note, the patient no longer required glucocorticoids to control cerebral edema, and was neurologically asymptomatic at the time of this scan.

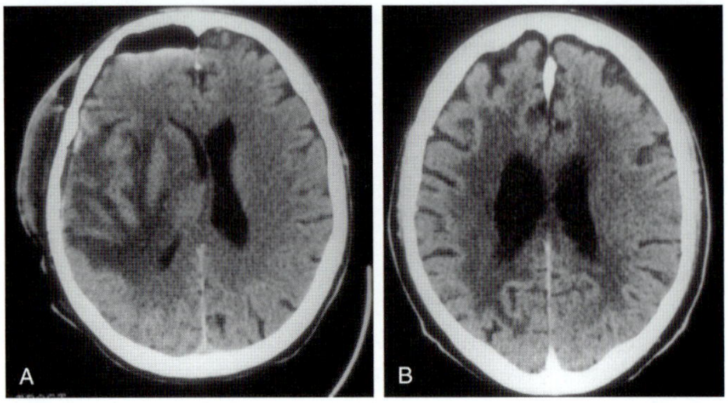

Figure 17–8. **A:** Before therapy. This CT scan reveals a large, heterogeneous mass with a significant amount of edema and mass effect. The radiographic characteristics are most suggestive of a high-grade astrocytoma, although the biopsy revealed a large-cell lymphoma. The patient had significant cognitive and behavioral changes at this point and was hemiparetic. **B:** After chemotherapy. This CT scan of the same patient, obtained after just three cycles of systemic chemotherapy (cyclophosphamide, vincristine, and high-dose methotrexate), demonstrates a complete radiographic response. The patient no longer required glucocorticoids after the second cycle of chemotherapy, and he regained full neurologic function.

the disruption is not absolute, but rather variable, and thus even in the middle of a large tumor, drug delivery is unlikely to be as effective as it would be to a systemic tumor. Furthermore, since some components of the BBB still exist, certain very large, polar molecules (like the anthracyclines) are probably still excluded from the CNS. The second important aspect about the disrupted BBB is that it can be repaired after effective tumor treatment. PET scan data have demonstrated that a water-soluble drug like cyclophosphamide, which normally has only minimal BBB penetration, passes into a PCNSL very well when used before other treatments. As the tumor regresses, however, the BBB repairs itself, making subsequent delivery of cyclophosphamide much less efficient. This is a very important consideration when designing treatment strategies.

The other unique challenge to the use of chemotherapy in the treatment of PCNSL is the potential for serious neurotoxicity. Historical data from the experience with childhood leukemia suggests that methotrexate (possibly the most active agent for PCNSL) is synergistic with cranial radiation for predisposing to long-term neurotoxicity, particulary leukoencephalopathy. It has been suggested that the timing of drug administration relative to cranial radiation is an important factor for the likelihood that the patient will develop this treatment complication. In general, it appears that chemotherapy given before cranial radiation is safer than chemotherapy given after radiation. This appears to be the case from the childhood leukemia experience with methotrexate, and data from Children's Hospital of Boston indicate that children treated with cisplatin before radiation have less sensorineural hearing loss than children treated in the reverse order.[133,134] Thus, for reasons of both improved drug delivery and decreased chances of neurotoxicity, preradiation chemotherapy is probably the optimal way to incorporate drugs into the initial treatment regimen of PCNSL.

The first series of patients treated prospectively with preradiation chemotherapy was reported by Gabbai and coworkers, who used methotrexate 3.5 g/m^2, followed by leucovorin rescue, for three cycles before cranial radiation (Table 17–10).[135] Of the 13 initially reported patients, there were 9 CRs and 4 PRs to the chemotherapy alone. With longer follow-up and an additional 9 patients, the current median survival is more than 27 months. Neuwelt and associates reported the results of a technically difficult protocol whereby patients were treated with the combination of cyclophosphamide 15 to 30 mg/kg intravenously and methotrexate 1.5 g given by intracarotid injection along with mannitol-induced hyperosmotic BBB disruption.[76] In addition, patients were treated with procarbazine 100 to 150 mg/day and dexamethasone (Decadron) 24 mg/day for a total of 14 days. Patients were treated with 5000 cGy whole-brain radiation only at the time of tumor progression. With this regimen, 13 of 16 patients experienced a

Table 17–10. Results of Three Preradiation Chemotherapy Trials

Study	Number of Patients	Median Age (Years)	Chemotherapy	Response	Radiation (cGy)	Median Survival (months)
Gabbai (1989)[135]	13	62	Methotrexate (3.5 g/m^2 × 3)	Complete response: 9/13 (69%) Partial response: 4/13 (31%)	3000 (12/13 patients)	27[a]
Neuwelt (1991)[76]	16	53.7	Blood–brain barrier disruption; cyclophosphamide/ methotrexate % procarbazine	Complete response: 13/16 (81%) Partial response: 3/16 (19%)	5000 (9/16 patients)	44.5
DeAngelis (2002)[47]	31	58	Methotrexate (IV % via Ommaya shunt) % cytarabine	Complete response: 0 Partial response: 17/22 (77%) Stable disease: 5/22	4000 % 1440 boost	42.5

[a]Nine patients added to the original report with longer follow-up.

complete response to chemotherapy. Eventually 6 of the 13 patients relapsed and required radiation therapy. The median survival of the group as a whole was 44.5 months. Treatment was associated with a moderate degree of acute neurologic toxicity, although the authors claim that long-term neurologic toxicity was minimal. A major unresolved question is the need for BBB disruption. Clearly, methotrexate can cross an intact BBB, and some animal data suggest that BBB disruption increases the entry of the drug into normal brain to a much greater extent than into the area of the brain involved by tumor. Thus it is possible that BBB disruption, with its associated risks and difficulties, may not be necessary if the proper drugs are administered correctly. Certainly, one important point demonstrated by the study of Neuwelt and colleagues[76] is the fact that when effective chemotherapy is administered to patients with PCNSL, it may be possible to withhold radiation therapy.

In another prospective series of PCNSL patients, DeAngelis et al. treated 22 newly diagnosed patients with two doses of intravenous methotrexate ($1\,g/m^2$) along with six doses of intrathecal methotrexate (12 mg).[42] After radiation therapy given as 4000 cGy to the whole brain plus a 1440-cGy boost to the tumor, patients were treated with high-dose cytarabine. With this regimen, 17 of 22 patients experienced partial responses to the chemotherapy. The median survival was 42.5 months. It is of interest that DeAngelis et al.[42] observed no complete responses, in contrast to the findings of Gabbai and colleagues. It is likely that the significantly lower doses of methotrexate in the regimen of DeAngelis et al.[42] (a total of 2 vs. $10.5\,g/m^2$ in the study of Gabbai and colleagues[135]) at least partially accounted for this difference. Observing these patients for long-term neurotoxicity will be important given that they were treated with both intravenous and intrathecal methotrexate and cytarabine (the latter a known neurotoxic agent) in combination with cranial irradiation.

O'Brien at al. published the results of a Phase II Trans-Tasman radiation Oncology Group with brief low-dose methotrexate and whole brain radiotherapy.[46] Median survival was 33 months; however, 6 of 44 patients treated developed progressive dementia suggestive of late radiation injury.

The RTOG completed a less encouraging study (protocol 88-06) in which 51 patients were treated with pre-radiation chemotherapy consisting of cyclophosphamide, doxorubicin, vincristine, and dexamethasone followed by 41.4-Gy whole-brain radiation with an 18-Gy boost to the tumor.[136] Overall the median survival was a disappointing 12.8 months. When patients were separated by age, it was found that those older than 60 years of age had much poorer outcomes than those younger than 60 years (2-year survival 30% vs. 62%, respectively). In fact, the survival of patients younger than 60 years of age treated on this protocol was statistically superior to that of a similar group of patients treated on RTOG protocol 83-15, which used the same radiation therapy but no chemotherapy. This trial can be criticized for the choice of the chemotherapy regimen, for although CHOP (cyclophosphamide, hydroxydaunomycin, Oncovin, prednisone) chemotherapy is clearly an effective regimen for systemic high-grade lymphomas, it does not have an optimal pharmacokinetic profile for the treatment of PCNSL. In particular, the use of doxorubicin must be considered suspect given that the anthracyclines are large water-soluble, polar molecules that probably do not penetrate even a disrupted BBB. The toxicity of the regimen is increased and the dose intensity of the effective drugs (i.e., cyclophosphamide) are diminished by the addition of the anthracycline with its associated additional myelosuppression.

The RTOG reported their results of a Phase II study that enrolled 102 patients with PCNSL. Patients were treated with pre-irradiation chemotherapy with five cycles of methotrexate, vincristine, procarbazine, and intraventricular methotrexate. After chemotherapy, all patients went on to receive 45 Gy WBRT. Median progression-free survival was 24 months, and OS was 36.9 months. Age was an important factor predicting for survival, with median survival of 50.4 months for those patients younger than 60 years, and 21.8 months for patients 60 or older ($p < 0.001$).[47] However, 12 patients (15%) experienced severe delayed neurologic toxicity, eight of whom died. In the authors' opinion, the late neurotoxicity was primarily related to the radiotherapy.

A recent study by the New Approaches to Brain Tumor Therapy (NABTT) group utilized high-dose ($8\,g/m^2$) methotrexate with deferred radiotherapy for immunocompetent patients with PCNSL. Twenty-five patients were treated with a complete response rate of 52%, partial response rate of 22%, 4% stable disease, and 22% progession. Median progression-free survival was 12.8 months with a median OS not being reached at 22.8+ months. Toxicity was modest with no Grade 3 or 4 events. These survival results compare favorably to combined modality series, but with substantially reduced toxicity including neurocognitive.[48] Similar results were reported from investigators from the National Neurological Institute in Milan, Italy. Boiardi et al. reported a 38-month disease-free survival period and a 48-month OS period for 14 patients achieving a complete response to the chemotherapy regiment of MBACOD and no radiotherapy.[49]

Deferred radiotherapy may be particularly appealing for elderly patients. These patients are very prone to late radiation injury. Ng et al. recently reported high-dose methotrexate alone for 10 patients with a median age of 72.5 years.[50] Overall response rate was 90% with a median survival of 36 months. None of these patients suffered significant late effects of treatment.

The experience from MSKCC was recently reported. Fifty-two patients were treated with five cycles of high-dose methotrexate, procarbazine, and vincristine. Thirty of these patients went on to receive 45 Gy (20 fractions) of whole-brain radiotherapy. Twenty-two older patients deferred radiotherapy to diminish their risk of late neurotoxicity until recurrence was documented. Of interest, older patients had similar median survival with or without the addition of radiotherapy: 32 versus 33 months, respectively. However, late neurotoxicity was significantly more common in those older patients who received WBRT ($p = 0.00004$).[51]

Not all recent studies of methotrexate only have been positive. The German Cancer Society Neuro-Oncology Working Group's trial NOA-03 involving 37 patients treated with high-dose methotrexate resulted in only a 30% complete response rate and a median disease-free survival for those complete responders of only 13.7 months.[52] It is not clear why these data are so different than the experiences described above.

In conclusion, growing data suggest that preradiation chemotherapy improves the outcome of immunocompetent patients with PCNSL. Many questions still remain, however, including identification of the specific patient population that benefits from chemotherapy, the correct regimen, the need for intrathecal drug administration, and the optimal radiation therapy dose, fractionation, and volume. Indeed, with optimization of the chemotherapy regimen, it remains to be seen whether some patients can be spared cranial radiation altogether, thus lessening the chances of long-term neurotoxicity.

Immunocompromised Patients

Unfortunately, the recent advances made in the treatment of PCNSL in immunocompetent patients have not carried over to severely immunosuppressed patients. In our retrospective review of all cases of PCNSL, the OS of AIDS patients was significantly lower than that seen in immunocompetent patients regardless of treatment (2.6 vs. 18.8 months, respectively) (Table 17–11). Even when matched for similar treatment approaches, such as radiation therapy alone, survival was much worse in the AIDS population (3 vs. 16.6 months). There are several possible explanations for this difference, including the fact that AIDS patients may have intrinsically more radioresistant tumors as reflected by the fact that complete response rates are lower in the AIDS patients than in immunocompetent patients. Certainly, the differences in the biology of these tumors (i.e., EBV-positive, high-grade morphology) are consistent with a possible difference in sensitivity to cytotoxic stimuli. Another possible explanation for decreased responsiveness to radiation therapy and lower OS may be the tendency for AIDS patients to be treated with lower doses of radiation than their immunocompetent counterparts (12% of immunocompetent patients treated over the last 15 years were treated with less than 35 Gy, whereas nearly 56% of AIDS patients were).[32]

Although factors such as differences in the biology of the tumor and treatment approaches may partially account for differences in the poorer survival of AIDS patients with PCNSL, clearly the most important reason is their underlying HIV disease. Levine[33] was the first to point out that the average CD4 lymphocyte count in AIDS patients who develop PCNSL is less than 50 cells/mm^3. Thus, most of these patients are in the terminal phase of their HIV disease. Baumgartner and colleagues reported autopsy results on 21 AIDS patients with PCNSL.[97] Of 13 patients not treated, all had disease disseminated throughout the CNS, with 10 deaths directly attributable to tumor progression. However, an additional eight patients were treated with radiation, and two of them had residual tumor at autopsy. Only one of these patients died from tumor progression, with the remaining patients dying from opportunistic infections. The survival of both groups of patients was similar regardless of treatment. Therefore, it does not appear that eradication of PCNSL in the majority of patients with advanced AIDS is likely to significantly prolong survival. Thus, for quality-of-life reasons, most AIDS patients should be offered at least an accelerated course of treatment (i.e., 30 Gy over 10 fractions to the whole brain). In order to reduce treatment time and the amount of irradiated tissue, some investigators have suggested that radiosurgery should be considered as a primary treatment in AIDS associated PCNSL.[53] Early results suggest very brisk responses both radiographically and clinically to radiosurgery in these patients. However, OS remains extremely poor as described above.

Ultimately, prolonging survival in patients with AIDS-associated PCNSL will require improvements in the treatment of their HIV disease. To that end, a resent review of 111 patients with HIV associated PCNSL in Australia demonstrated significantly improved survival in patients receiving whole brain radiation with HAART compared to those who received radiation alone and no treatment for their HIV disease.[137] Secondary to the poor overall outcome of patients with advanced HIV and PCNSL, and their poor tolerance of systemic chemotherapy, many experts in the field (including these authors) had recommended in the past that HIV-infected patients with PCNSL should for the most part be treated with radiation alone and not chemotherapy. Now that patients are living longer with HAART therapy, yet are still developing PCNSL often while their immunological function is relatively good (high CD4+ cell counts and low viral loads), the role of systemic chemotherapy in the treatment of PCNSL will need to be re-evaluated. Given how well high-dose methotrexate with leucovorin rescue is tolerated by immunocompetent patients, one would tend to believe that it will likewise be well tolerated by otherwise healthy HIV-infected patients on effective HAART therapy. Even if such treatment is well tolerated, however, it is unknown whether the antitumor effectiveness seen in immunocompetent patients with PCNSL will be mirrored in the HIV population given the differences in the biology of the tumors. Nevertheless, it is clear that the time has come to begin to explore such questions.

Table 17–11. Type of Treatment and Survival

Treatment and Survival	Immunocompetent Group	AIDS Group
Treatment		
None	66 (9.6%)	45 (25.9%)
Radiation	450 (65.8%)	115 (66.1%)
Chemotherapy	168 (24.6%)	14 (8.0%)
Total	684[a]	174
Survival (months)		
No therapy	2.69	0.93
Radiation	16.61	2.96
Chemotherapy	29.07	No data
Overall average (months)	18.85	2.61

[a] Treatment data available for 86% of all patients.
AIDS, acquired immunodeficiency syndrome.

CONCLUSION

PCNSL is a disease distinct from other extranodal systemic lymphomas in its biology, clinical presentation, and treatment. PCNSL in the AIDS and immunocompetent host appears to be a different disease entity with respect to clinical and radiographic presentation, histologic type, and response to treatment. Although radiation therapy has historically been the standard of treatment, increasing data suggest that the addition of preradiation chemotherapy may significantly improve outcomes in most immunocompetent hosts. The optimal chemotherapy regimen(s) need to be determined and the role of radiotherapy as part of the initial therapy has been seriously questioned by recent trials. Treatment for AIDS patients with PCNSL has not been as successful and is generally considered palliative. Substantial improvement in the prognosis of these patients awaits advances in the treatment of their underlying HIV and opportunistic infections although preliminary information suggests that the treatment of PCNSL in HIV-infected patients may dramatically change in the coming years with the advent of effective HAART. Participants from Europe, North America, Israel, and Australia held a working group meeting in Lugano, Switzerland in 2002 to exchange the latest scientific information of PCNSL.[54] The working group's mission was to analyze methodologic issues in the design of clinical trials, to reach consensus on treatment recommendations and prognostic factors, to discuss clinical and molecular targets for future studies, and to establish an international collaborative group to conduct laboratory and clinical investigation in PCNSL. It is through such global efforts that more successful outcomes for patients with PCNSL will be achieved.

References

1. Bleyer W and Byrne T. Leptomeningeal cancer in leukemia and solid tumors. Curr Probl Cancer 1988;12:181–238.
2. Hanbery JW and Dugger GS. Perithelial sarcoma of the brain. A clinicopathologic study of thirteen cases. Arch Neurol Psychiatry 1964:74:732–61.
3. Barnett LB and Schwartz E. Cerebral reticulum cell sarcoma after multiple renal transplants. J Neurol Neurosurg Psychiatry 1974;37:966–70.
4. Benedek L and Juba A. Uber das Microgliom. Dtsch Z Nervehnheilk 1941;152:159–63.
5. Schaumburg HH, Plank CR, and Adams RD. The reticulum cell sarcoma-microglioma group of brain tumors. Brain 1972;95:199–212.
6. Lister A, Abrey LE, and Sandlund JT. Central nervous system lymphoma. Hematology (Am Soc Hematol Educ Program) 2002;283–96.
7. Freeman C, Berg JW, and Cutler SJ. Occurrence and prognosis of extranodal lymphomas. Cancer 1972; 29:252–60.
8. Jellinger K, Radaskiewicz TH, and Slowik F. Primary malignant lymphomas of the central nervous system in man. Acta Neuropathol (Berl) 1975;6(suppl):95–102.
9. Zimmerman HM. Malignant lymphomas of the nervous system. Acta Neuropathol (Berl) 1975;6(suppl):69–74.
10. Brand MM and Marinkovich VA. Primary malignant reticulosis of the brain in Wiskott–Aldrich syndrome. Report of a case. Arch Dis Child 1969;44:536–42.
11. Model LM. Primary reticulum cell sarcoma of the brain in Wiskott-Aldrich syndrome. Report of a case. Arch Neurol 1977;34:633–5.
12. Littman P and Wang CC. Reticulum cell sarcoma of the brain: a review of the literature and a study of 19 cases. Cancer 1975;35:1412–20.
13. DeWeese TL, Hazuka MB, Hommel DJ, et al. AIDS-related non-Hodgkin's lymphoma: The outcome and efficacy of radiation therapy. Int J Radiat Oncol Biol Phys 1991;20:803–8.
14. Penn I. Development of cancer as a complication of clinical transplantation. Transplant Proc 1977;9:1121–7.
15. Weintraub J and Warnke RA. Lymphoma in cardiac allotransplant recipients. Clinical and histological features and immunologic phenotypes. Transplantation 1982;33:347–51.
16. Diette KM, Caro WA, and Roenigk HH Jr. Malignant lymphoma presenting with cutaneous granulomas. J Am Acad Dermatol 1984;10:896–902.
17. Good AE, Russo HR, Schnitzer B, et al. Intracranial histiocytic lymphoma with rheumatoid arthritis. J Rheumatol 1978;5:75–8.
18. Lipsmeyer EA. Development of malignant cerebral lymphoma in a patient with systemic lupus erythematosus treated with immunosuppression. Arthritis Rheum 1972;15:183–6.
19. Snider WD, Simpson DM, Nielsen S, et al. Neurological complications of acquired immune deficiency syndrome: analysis of 50 patients. Ann Neurol 1983;14:403–18.
20. Pluda M, Yarchoan R, Jaffe ES, et al. Development of non-Hodgkin lymphoma in a cohort of patients with severe human immunodeficiency virus (HIV) infection on long-term antiretroviral therapy. Ann Intern Med 1990;113:276–82.
21. Eby NL, Grufferman S, Flannelly CM, et al. Increasing incidence of primary brain lymphoma in the U.S. Cancer 1988;62:2461–5.
22. DeAngelis LM. Primary central nervous system lymphoma. PPO Update 1992;6:1–16.
23. Hao D, DiFrancesco LM, Brasher PM, et al. Is primary CNS lymphoma really becoming more common? A population-based study of incidence, clinicopathological features and outcomes in Alberta from 1975–1996. Ann Oncol 1999; 10:65–70.
24. Plotkin SR and Batchelor TT. Primary nervous-system lymphoma. Lancet Oncol 2001;2:354–65.
25. Bashir R, Freedman A, Harris N, et al. Immunophenotypic profile of CNS lymphoma: A review of eighteen cases. J Neurooncol 1989;7:249–54.
26. Reese TS and Karnovsky MJ. Fine structural localization of a blood-brain barrier to exogenous peroxidase. J Cell Biol 1967;37:207–17.
27. Rall DP and Zubrod CG. Mechanisms of drug absorption and excretion: Passage of drugs in and out of the central nervous system. Ann Rev Pharmacol 1962;2:109–16.
28. Murphy JB and Sturm E. Conditions determining the transplantability of tissues in the brain. J Exp Med 1923; 38:183–86.
29. Medawar PB. Immunity to homologous grafted skin. The fate of skin homografts transplanted to the brain, to subcutaneous tissue and to the anterior chamber of the eye. Br J Exp Pathol 1948;29:58–64.
30. Greene HSN. Heterotransplantation of tumours. Ann N Y Acad Sci 1957;69:818–29.
31. Weiner HL and Hauser SL. Neuroimmunology. I. Immunoregulation in neurological disease. Ann Neurol 1982;11: 437–49.
32. Fine HA and Mayer RJ. Primary central nervous system lymphoma. Ann Intern Med 1993;119:1093–104.
33. Levine AM. Acquired immunodeficiency syndrome-related lymphoma. Blood 1992;80:8–20.
34. Hochberg FH, Miller G, and Schooley RT. Central-nervous-system lymphoma related to Epstein–Barr virus. N Engl J Med 1983;309:745–8.
35. Bashir RM, Harris NL, Hochberg FH, et al. Detection of Epstein–Barr virus in CNS lymphomas by in-situ hybridization. N Engl J Med 1989;39:813–7.
36. Ho M, Miller G, Atchison RW, et al. Epstein–Barr virus infections and DNA hybridization studies in posttransplant

lymphoma and lymphoproliferative lesions: The role of primary infection. J Infect Dis 1985;152:876–86.
37. Ho M, Jaffe R, Miller G, et al. The frequency of Epstein–Barr virus infection and associative lymphoproliferative syndrome after transplantation and its manifestations in children. Transplantion 1988;45:719–27.
38. Magrath I. Clinical and pathological features of Burkitt's lymphoma and their relevance to treatment. In: Levine PH, Ablash DV, Pearson GR, et al., eds. Epstein–Barr and Associated Diseases. Boston: Martinus Nijhoff, 1985:631–43.
39. Klein G. Lymphoma development in mice and human: diversity of inhibition is followed by convergent cytogenetic evaluation. Proc Natl Acad Sci U S A 1979;76:2442–6.
40. Hochberg FH and Miller DC. Primary central nervous system lymphoma. J Neurosurg 1988;68:835–53.
41. O'Neill BP and Illig JJ. Primary central nervous system lymphoma. Mayo Clin Proc 1989;64:1005–20.
42. DeAngelis LM, Yahalom J, Thaler HT, et al. Combined modality therapy for primary CNS lymphoma. J Clin Oncol 1992;10:635–43.
43. Neuwelt EA, Frenkel EP, Gumerlock MK, et al. Developments in the diagnosis and treatment of primary CNS lymphoma: a prospective series. Cancer 1986;58:1609–20.
44. Braaten KM, Betensky RA, de Leval L, et al. BCL-6 expression predicts improved survival in patients with primary central nervous system lymphoma. Clin Cancer Res 2003;9:1063–9.
45. Batchelor TT, Kolak G, Ciordia R, et al. High-dose methotrexate for intraocular lymphoma. Clin Cancer Res 2003;9:711–5.
46. O'Brien P, Roos D, Pratt G, et al. Phase II multicenter study of brief single-agent methotrexate followed by irradiation in primary CNS lymphoma. J Clin Oncol 2000;18:519–26.
47. DeAngelis LM, Seiferheld W, Schold SC, et al. Combination chemotherapy and radiotherapy for primary central nervous system lymphoma. Radiation Therapy Oncology Group Study 93-10. J Clin Oncol 2002;20:4643–8.
48. Batchelor T, Carson K, O'Neill A, et al. Treatment of primary CNS lymphoma with methotrexate and deferred radiotherapy: a report of NABTT 96-07. J Clin Oncol 2003;21: 1044–9.
49. Bioardi A, Silvani A, Pozzi A, et al. Chemotherapy is effective as early treatment for primary central nervous system lymphoma. J Neurol 1999;246:31–7.
50. Ng S, Rosenthal MA, Ashley D, et al. High-dose methotrexate for primary CNS lymphoma in the elderly. J Neurooncol 2000;2:40–4.
51. Abrey LE, Yahalom J, and DeAngelis LM. Treatment of primary CNS lymphoma: the next step. J Clin Oncol 2000;18:3144–50.
52. Herrlinger U, Schabet M, Brugger W, et al. German Cancer Society Neuro-Oncology Working Group NOA-03 multicenter trial of single-agent high-dose methotrexate for primary central nervous system lymphoma. Ann Neurol 2002; 51:247–52.
53. Nicolato A, Gerosa MA, Foroni R, et al. Gamma knife radiosurgery in AIDS-related primary central nervous system lymphoma. Stereotact Funct Neurosurg 1995;64:42–55.
54. Ferreri AJ, Abrey LE, Blay JY, et al. Summary statement on primary central nervous system lymphomas from the Eighth International Conference on Malignant Lymphoma, Lugano, Switzerland, June 12 to 15, 2002. J Clin Ooncol 2002; 21:2407–14.
55. Kawakami Y, Tabuchi K, Ohnishi R, et al. Primary central nervous system lymphoma. J Neurosurg 1985;62:522–7.
56. Freeman CR, Shustik C, Brisson ML, et al. I. Primary malignant lymphoma of the central nervous system. Cancer 1986;58:1106–11.
57. Mendenhall NP, Thar TL, Agee OF, et al. Primary lymphoma of the central nervous system: computerized tomography scan characteristics and treatment results for 12 cases. Cancer 1983;52:1993–2000.
58. Gonzalez DG and Schuster-Uitterhoeve AL. Primary non-Hodgkin's lymphoma of the central nervous system. Cancer 1983;51:2048–52.
59. Grant JW, Gallagher PJ, and Jones DB. Primary cerebral lymphoma. Arch Pathol Lab Med 1986;110:897–901.
60. Murray K, Kun L, and Cox J. Primary malignant lymphoma of the central nervous system. J Neurosurg 1986;65: 600–7.
61. Di Marco A, Rosta L, Campostrini F, et al. The role of radiation therapy in the management of primary non-Hodgkin's lymphomas of the central nervous system: clinical study of 10 cases. Tumori 1986;72:565–73.
62. Hobson DE, Anderson BA, Carr I, et al. Primary lymphoma of the central nervous system: Manitoba experience and literature review. Can J Neurol Sci 1986;13:55–61.
63. Bertoncelli C, Zigrossi P, Campanini M, et al. Primary lymphoma of the central nervous system. A clinical and immunohistological study of 8 patients. Haematologica 1987;72:137–42.
64. Pollack IF, Lunsford LD, Flickinger JC, et al. Prognostic factors in the diagnosis and treatment of primary central nervous system lymphoma. Cancer 1989;63:939–47.
65. McLaughlin P, Velasquez WS, Redman JR, et al. Chemotherapy with dexamethasone, high-dose cytarabine, and cisplatin for parenchymal brain lymphomas. J Natl Cancer Inst 1988;80:1408–12.
66. Allegranza A, Mariani C, Giardini R, et al. Primary malignant lymphomas of the central nervous system: a histological and immunohistological study of 12 cases. Histopathology 1984;8:781–91.
67. Stewart DJ, Russell N, Atack EA, et al. Cyclophosphamide, doxorubicin, vincristine, and dexamethasone in primary lymphoma of the brain: a case report. Cancer Treat Rep 1983;67:287–91.
68. Cohen IJ, Vogel R, Matz S, et al. Successful non-neurotoxic therapy [without radiation] of a multi-focal primary brain lymphoma with a methotrexate, vincristine, and BCNU protocol [DEMOB]. Cancer 1986;57:6–11.
69. Vakili ST, Muller J, Shidnia H, et al. Primary lymphoma of the central nervous system: a clinico-pathologic analysis of 26 cases. J Surg Oncol 1986;33:95–102.
70. Schiffer D, Chio A, Giordana MT, et al. Primary lymphomas of the brain: a clinicopathologic review of 37 cases. Tumori 1987;73:585–92.
71. Loeffler JS, Ervin TJ, Mauch P, et al. Primary lymphomas of the central nervous system: Patterns of failure and factors that influence survival. J Clin Oncol 1985;3:490–4.
72. Yasunaga T, Takahashi M, Uozumi H, et al. Radiation therapy of primary malignant lymphoma of the brain. Acta Radiol Oncol 1986;25:23–8.
73. Woodman R, Shin K, and Pineo G. Primary non-Hodgkin's lymphoma of the brain. Medicine (Baltimore) 1985;64: 425–30.
74. Michalski JM, Garcia DM, Kase E, et al. Primary central nervous system lymphoma: analysis of prognostic variables and patterns of treatment failure. Radiology 1990;176: 855–60.
75. Pittman K, Olweny CL, North JB, et al. Primary central nervous system lymphoma. Oncology 1991;48: 184–7.
76. Neuwelt EA, Goldman DL, Dahlborg SA, et al. Primary CNS lymphoma treated with osmotic blood brain barrier disruption: prolonged survival and presentation of cognitive function. J Clin Oncol 1991;9:1580–90.

77. Rampen FH, van Andel JG, Sizoo W, et al. Radiation therapy in primary non-Hodgkin's lymphomas of the CSN. Eur J Cancer 1980;16:177–84.
78. Berry MP and Simpson WJ. Radiation therapy in the management of primary malignant lymphoma of the brain. Int J Radiat Oncol Biol Phys 1981;7:55–9.
79. Spillane JA, Kendall BE, and Moseley IF. Cerebral lymphoma: clinical radiological correlation. J Neurol Neurosurg Psychiatry 1982;45:199–208.
80. Merkel KH and Hansmann ML. Primary non-Hodgkin's lymphomas of the central nervous system. Pathol Res Pract 1986;181:430–3.
81. Watanabe M, Tanaka R, Takeda N, et al. Correlation of computed tomography with the histopathology of the primary malignant lymphoma of the brain. Neuroradiology 1992;34: 36–42.
82. Bogdahn U, Bogdahn S, Mertens HG, et al. Primary non-Hodgkin's lymphomas of the CNS. Acta Neurol Scand 1986;73:602–14.
83. Sagerman RH, Collier CH, and King GA. Radiation therapy of microgliomas. Radiology 1983;149:567–70.
84. Helle TL, Britt RH, and Colby TV. Primary lymphoma of the central nervous system. Clinicopathological study of experience at Stanford. J Neurosurg 1984;60:94–103.
85. Frank G, Ferracini R, Spagnolli F, et al. Primary intracranial lymphomas. Surg Neurol 1985;23:3–8.
86. Spaun E, Midholm S, Pederson NT, et al. Primary malignant lymphoma of the central nervous system. Surg Neurol 1985;24:646–50.
87. Remick SC, Diamond C, Migliozzi JA, et al. Primary central nervous system lymphoma in patients with and without the acquired immune deficiency syndrome. Medicine (Baltimore) 1990;69:345–60.
88. Casadei GP and Gambacorta M. A clinicopathological study of seven cases of primary high-grade malignant non-Hodgkin's lymphoma of the central nervous system. Tumori 1985;71:501–7.
89. So YT, Beckstead JH, and Davis RL. Primary central nervous system lymphoma in acquired immune deficiency syndrome: a clinical and pathological study. Ann Neurol 1986; 20:566–72.
90. Poon T, Matoso I, Tchertkoff V, et al. CT features of primary cerebral lymphoma in AIDS and non-AIDS patients. J Comput Assist Tomogr 1989;13:6–9.
91. Formenti SC, Gill PS, Lean E, et al. Primary central nervous system lymphoma in AIDS. Cancer 1989;63:1101–7.
92. Loureiro C, Gill PS, Meyer PR, et al. Autopsy findings in AIDS-related lymphoma. Cancer 1988;62:735–9.
93. Levine AM, Sullivan-Halley J, Pike MC, et al. Human immunodeficiency virus-related lymphoma. Cancer 1991; 68:2466–72.
94. MacMahon EM, Glass JD, Hayward SD, et al. Epstein–Barr virus in AIDS-related primary central nervous system lymphoma. Lancet 1991;338:969–73.
95. Goldstein JD, Zeifer B, Chao C, et al. CT appearance of primary CNS lymphoma in patients with acquired immunodeficiency syndrome. J Comput Assist Tomogr 1991;15: 39–44.
96. Dina TS. Primary central nervous system lymphoma versus toxoplasmosis in AIDS. Radiology 1991;179:823–8.
97. Baumgartner JE, Rachlin JR, Beckstead JH, et al. Primary central nervous system lymphomas: natural history and response to radiation therapy in 55 patients with acquired immune deficiency syndrome. J Neurosurg 1990; 73:206–11.
98. Chappell ET, Guthrie BL, and Orenstein J. The role of stereotactic biopsy in the management of HIV-related focal brain lesions. Neurosurgery 1992;30:825–9.
99. Goldstein JD, Dickson DW, Moser FG, et al. Primary central nervous system lymphoma in acquired immune deficiency syndrome. Cancer 1991;67:2756–65.
100. Ziegler JL, Beckstead JA, Volberding PA, et al. Non-Hodgkin's lymphoma in 90 homosexual men. N Engl J Med 1984;311: 565–70.
101. DiCarlo EF, Amberson JB, Metroka CE, et al. Malignant lymphomas and the acquired immunodeficiency syndrome. Arch Pathol Lab Med 1986;110:1012–16.
102. Nakhleh RE, Manivel JC, Hurd D, et al. Central nervous system lymphomas. Arch Pathol Lab Med 1989;113:1050–6.
103. Pitlik SD, Fainstein V, Bolivar R, et al. Spectrum of central nervous system complications in homosexual men with acquired immune deficiency syndrome [Letter]. J Infect Dis 1983;148:771–2.
104. Italian Cooperative Group for AIDS-Related Tumors. Malignant lymphomas in patients with or at risk for AIDS in Italy. J Natl Cancer Inst 1988;80:855–60.
105. McArthur JC. Neurologic manifestations of AIDS. Medicine (Baltimore) 1987;66:407–37.
106. Capanna AH, LaMancusa JJ, Erculei F, et al. Primary cerebral lymphoma in two consortial partners afflicted with acquired immune deficiency syndrome. Neurosurgery 1987;21:920–3.
107. Mernick MH, Malamud SC, Haubenstock A, et al. Non-Hodgkin's lymphoma in AIDS: report of 11 cases and literature review. Mt Sinai J Med 1986;53:664–7.
108. Snow RB and Lavyne MH. Intracranial space-occupying lesions in acquired immune deficiency syndrome patients. Neurosurgery 1985;16:148–53.
109. Koppel BS, Wormser GP, Tuchman AJ, et al. Central nervous system involvement in patients with acquired immune deficiency syndrome (AIDS). Acta Neurol Scand 1985;71: 337–53.
110. Gill PS, Levine AM, Meyer PR, et al. Primary central nervous system lymphoma in homosexual men. Clinical, immunologic, and pathologic features. Am J Med 1985;78:742–8.
111. Anders KH, Latta H, Chang BS, et al. Lymphomatoid granulomatosis and malignant lymphoma of the central nervous system in the acquired immunodeficiency syndrome. Hum Pathol 1989;20:326–34.
112. Kaplan MH, Susin M, Pahwa SG, et al. Neoplastic complications of HTLV-III infection. Am J Med 1987;82:389–96.
113. Kalter SP, Riggs SA, Cabanillas F, et al. Aggressive non-Hodgkin's lymphoma in immunocompromised homosexual males. Blood 1985;66:655–9.
114. Lowenthal DA, Straus DJ, Campbell SW, et al. AIDS-related lymphoid neoplasia: the Memorial Hospital experience. Cancer 1988;61:2325–37.
115. Ahmed T, Wormser GP, Stahl RE, et al. Malignant lymphomas in a population at risk for acquired immune deficiency syndrome. Cancer 1987;60:719–23.
116. Knowles DM, Chamulak GA, Subar M, et al. Lymphoid neoplasia associated with the acquired immunodeficiency syndrome (AIDS). Ann Intern Med 1988;108:744–53.
117. Kaplan LD, Abrams DI, Feigal AL, et al. AIDS-associated non-Hodgkin's lymphoma in San Francisco. JAMA 1989;261: 719–24.
118. Song SK, Schwartz IS, and Breakstone BA. Lymphoproliferative disorder of the central nervous system in AIDS. Mt Sinai J Med 1986;53:686–9.
119. Gabuzda DH and Hirsch MS. Neurologic manifestations of infection with human immunodeficiency virus. Clinical features and pathogenesis. Ann Intern Med 1987;107:383–91.
120. Appen RE. Posterior uveitis and primary cerebral reticulum cell sarcoma. Arch Ophthalmol 1975;93:123–4.
121. Char DH, Ljung B-M, Miller T, et al. Primary intraocular lymphoma (ocular reticulum cell sarcoma) diagnosis and management. Ophthalmology 1988;95:625–30.

122. Rockwood EJ, Zakov ZN, and Bay JW. Combined malignant lymphoma of the eye and CNS (reticulum-cell sarcoma). J Neurosurg 61:369–74, 1984.
123. Duggan DB, Ehrlich GD, Davey FP, et al. HTLV-I-induced lymphoma mimicking Hodgkin's disease: Diagnosis by polymerase chain reaction amplification of specific HTLV-1 sequences in tumor DNA. Blood 1988;71:1027–32.
124. Ezrin-Waters C, Klein M, Deck J, et al. Diagnostic importance of immunological markers in lymphoma involving the central nervous system. Ann Neurol 1984;16: 668–72.
125. Jones GR, Mason WH, Fishman LS, et al. Primary central nervous system lymphoma without intracranial mass in a child. Diagnosis by documentation of monoclonality. Cancer 1985;56:2804–8.
126. Anders KH, Guerra WF, Tomiyasu U, et al. The neuropathology of AIDS. Am J Pathol 1986;124:537–58.
127. Luft BJ, Hafner R, Korzun AH, et al. Toxoplasmic encephalitis in patients with the acquired immunodeficiency syndrome: Members of the ACTG 077p/ANRS 009 Study Team. N Engl J Med 1993;329:995–1000.
128. Hoffman JM, Waskin HA, Schifter T, et al. FDG-PET in determining lymphoma from nonmalignant central nervous system lesions in patients with AIDS. J Nucl Med 1993;34: 567–75.
129. Henry JM, Heffner RR, Dillard SH, et al. Primary malignant lymphomas of the central nervous system. Cancer 1974;34: 1293–302.
130. Sagerman RH, Cassady JR, and Chang CH. Radiation therapy for intracranial lymphoma. Radiology 1967;88:552–4.
131. Nelson DF, Martz KL, Bonner H, et al. Non-Hodgkin's lymphoma of the brain: Can high dose, large volume radiation therapy improve survival? Report on a prospective trial by the Radiation Therapy Oncology Group (RTOG): RTOG 83-15. Int J Radiat Oncol Biol Phys 1992;23:9–17.
132. Tatsuta T, Naito M, Oh-hara T, et al. Functional involvement of P-glycoprotein in blood-brain barrier. J Biol Chem 1992; 267:20383–91.
133. Shapiro WR and Young DF. Neurologic complications of antineoplastic therapy. Acta Neurol Scand 1984;70:125–32.
134. Kretschmar CS, Warren MP, Lavally BL, et al. Ototoxicity of pre-radiation cisplatin for children with central nervous system tumors. J Clin Oncol 1990;8:1191–8.
135. Gabbai AA, Hochberg FH, Linggood RM, et al. High-dose methotrexate for non-AIDS primary central system lymphoma. J Neurosurg 1989;70:190–4.
136. Schultz C, Scott CTW, Fisher B, et al. Pre-irradiation chemotherapy (CTX) with cytoxan, adriamycin, vincristine, and decadron (CHOD) for primary central nervous system lymphoma (PCNSL): initial report of Radiation Therapy Oncology Group (RTOG) protocol 88-06. Proc ASCO 1994; 485:174.
137. Newell ME, Hoy JF, Cooper SG, et al. Human immunodeficiency virus-related primary central nervous system lymphoma: factors influencing survival in 111 patients. Cancer 2004;100:2627–36.

Primary Extranodal Non-Hodgkin's Lymphomas

Tamara N. Shenkier, M.D., F.R.C.P.C.
Joseph M. Connors, M.D., F.R.C.P.C.

At least 25% of non-Hodgkin's lymphomas (NHL) arise in tissue other than the lymph nodes, spleen, or the bone marrow.[1–3] They are classified as primary extranodal lymphomas, implying that they arose in the extranodal tissue and that widespread disease is not clinically evident. This distinguishes extranodal presentation with or without lymphadenopathy, that is, Stage I or IIE, from Stage IV disease in which extranodal involvement is part of a disseminated process. For the purpose of this chapter, primary extranodal lymphoma describes lymphoma with either absent or minor nodal involvement with a clinically dominant site of primary involvement to which the treatment must be directed.

Primary extranodal lymphomas have been recorded in virtually every tissue of the body, but certain tissues are much more commonly involved, such as the gastrointestinal (GI) tract and Waldeyer's ring (tonsil, nasopharynx, and base of tongue). Fig. 18–1 demonstrates the distribution of extranodal sites in 723 consecutive cases of localized B-cell non-Hodgkin's lymphoma seen at the British Columbia Cancer Agency (a provincially based tertiary referral center). The factors that determine preferential patterns of spread of lymphoma and the receptiveness of certain tissues or organs to accommodate metastatic growth are unknown. However, chronic inflammatory stimulation from either autoimmune conditions or infectious agents precedes lymphoma in several sites including the thyroid, stomach, intestinal tract, and periorbital soft tissue. The common theme at these sites appears to be chronic antigenic stimulation.

The primary extranodal lymphomas are most usefully classified using the World Health Organization (WHO) scheme, which, in addition to histologic appearance, uses immunophenotype, cytogenetics, and molecular studies to define the distinct NHL entities.[4] Although primary extranodal lymphomas may arise from B or T cells, this chapter addresses only those of B-cell origin. Furthermore, as other chapters in this text specifically discuss lymphomas of the skin and central nervous system (CNS), as well as NHL's arising in the setting of acquired immunosuppression, these topics will not be discussed here.

The natural history and prognosis of extranodal lymphomas largely reflect the frequency with which indolent histologic types constitute a substantial proportion of presentations, conferring a "favorable" prognosis. The majority of such indolent extranodal lymphomas arise from mucosa-associated lymphoid tissue (MALT) and are classified as marginal zone, extranodal, and MALT-type. These typically arise in the gastrointestinal tract, orbit, salivary glands, or lung. In contrast, the more aggressive entities, which are usually diffuse large B-cell lymphoma (DLBCL), more commonly arise from testis, sinus, bone, Waldeyer's ring, and thyroid. The relative frequencies of these pathologic diagnoses and the distribution of these diagnoses at each extranodal site for 723 consecutive patients with localized extranodal NHL seen at the British Columbia Cancer Agency between 1981 and 2003 are shown in Tables 18–1 and 18–2. Since involvement of extranodal sites in patients with disseminated aggressive histology lymphoma is a poor prognostic factor, it is interesting to consider whether localized extranodal DLBCL confers a different prognosis than a presentation of similar stage in a nodal site.[5] At the British Columbia Cancer Agency, we have studied the long-term outcome of 295 patients with localized DLBCL, and have demonstrated that extranodal presentation does not confer a worse prognosis, as shown in Figs. 18–2 and 18–3. If the 27 cases of testicular lymphoma, the one extranodal site that does have a poorer prognosis than others, are excluded, the curves are superimposable.[6]

Modest differences in the proportion of lymphomas that present in an extranodal site have been recorded in different countries: United States 24%, Canada 27%, Israel 36%, Lebanon 44%, Denmark 37%, the Netherlands 41%, Italy 48%, and Hong Kong 29%.[3] The reasons for this variation include variable inclusion of T-cell diseases, different definitions of primary extranodal versus disseminated disease, and genuine differences in the types of lymphomas seen around the world. For example, the lower incidence of follicular lymphoma in Asia and higher frequency of diffuse large B-cell lymphoma in the Middle East undoubtedly affect the frequency of extranodal lymphomas in these regions. The incidence of NHL on the whole has shown a steady increase over the past 60 years. Fig. 18–4 shows a 2% per year rise in incidence in Canada since 1984 for both males and females. The same trend has been demonstrated for gastrointestinal lymphomas, particularly in Europe and Japan.[7–9] It is reasonable to assume that the same is true of NHL's involving other extranodal sites, but specific reliable data addressing this are not available.

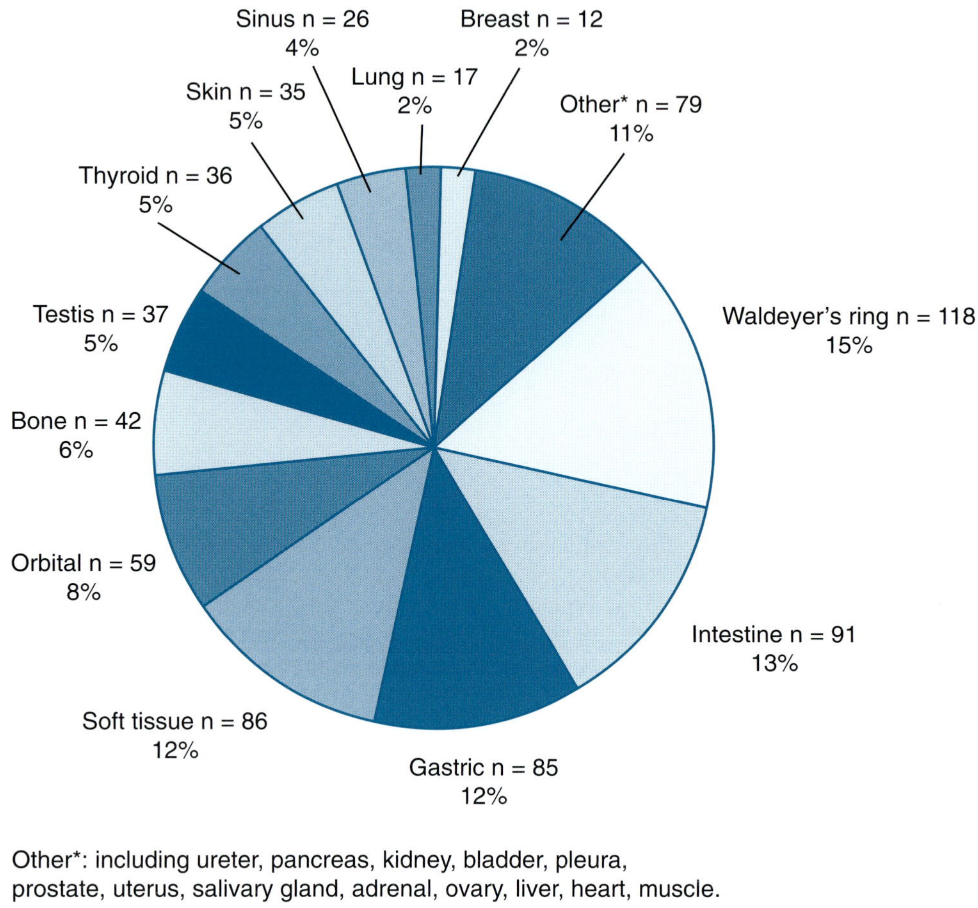

Figure 18–1. Distribution of extranodal sites in 723 consecutive cases of Stage I or II B-cell non-Hodgkin's lymphoma seen at the British Columbia Cancer Agency, 1981–2003.

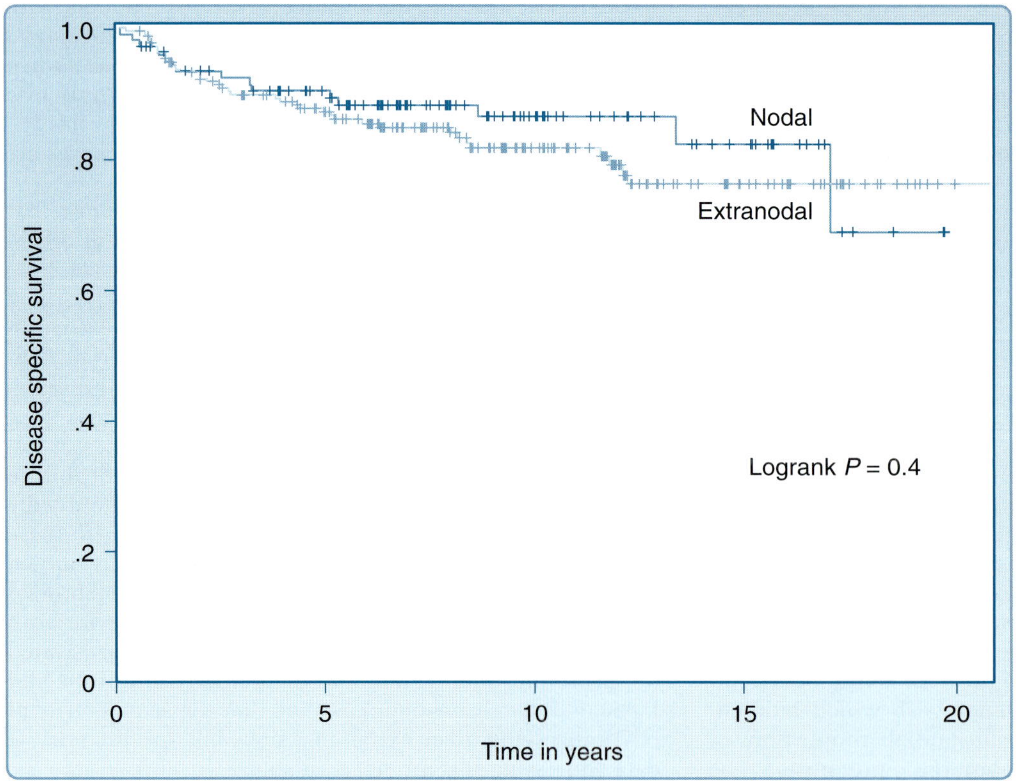

Figure 18–2. Disease-specific survival for 295 patients with localized diffuse large B-cell lymphoma treated with brief chemotherapy and involved-region irradiation: comparison of nodal versus extranodal presentations.

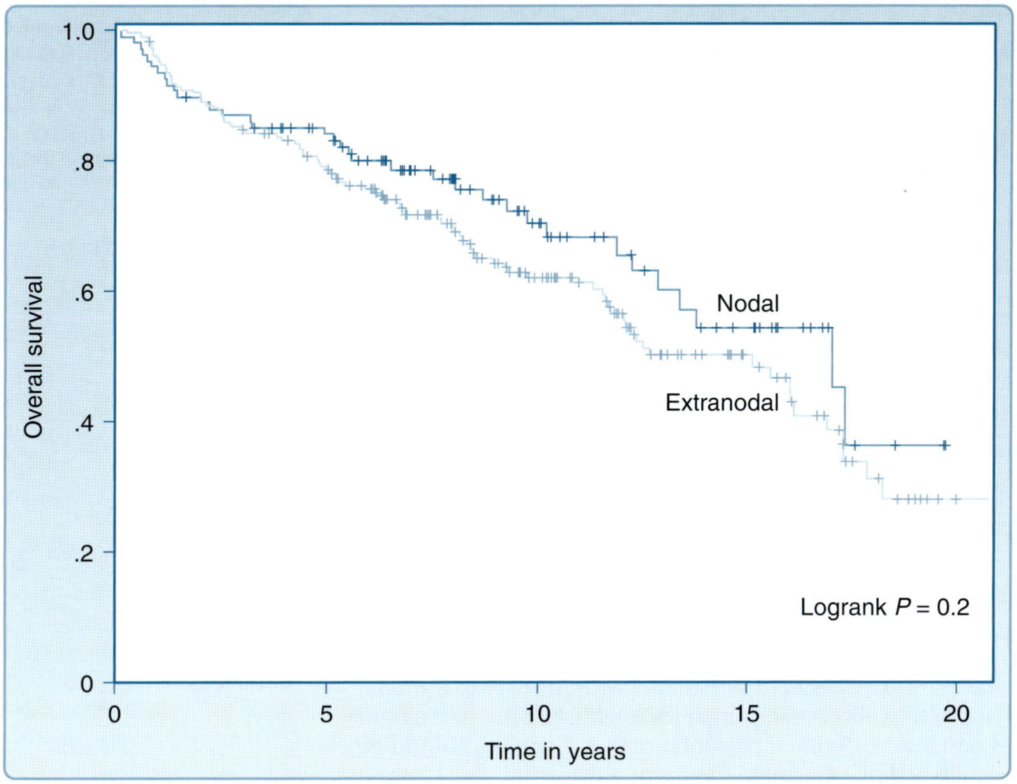

Figure 18–3. Overall survival for 295 patients with localized diffuse large B-cell lymphoma treated with brief chemotherapy and involved-region irradiation: comparison of nodal versus extranodal presentations.

CANCER INCIDENCE OVER TIME
NON-HODGKIN'S LYMPHOMA, ALL AGES, CANADA 1984–2000
AGE-STANDARDIZED INCIDENCE RATE PER 100,000 (CANADA 1991)

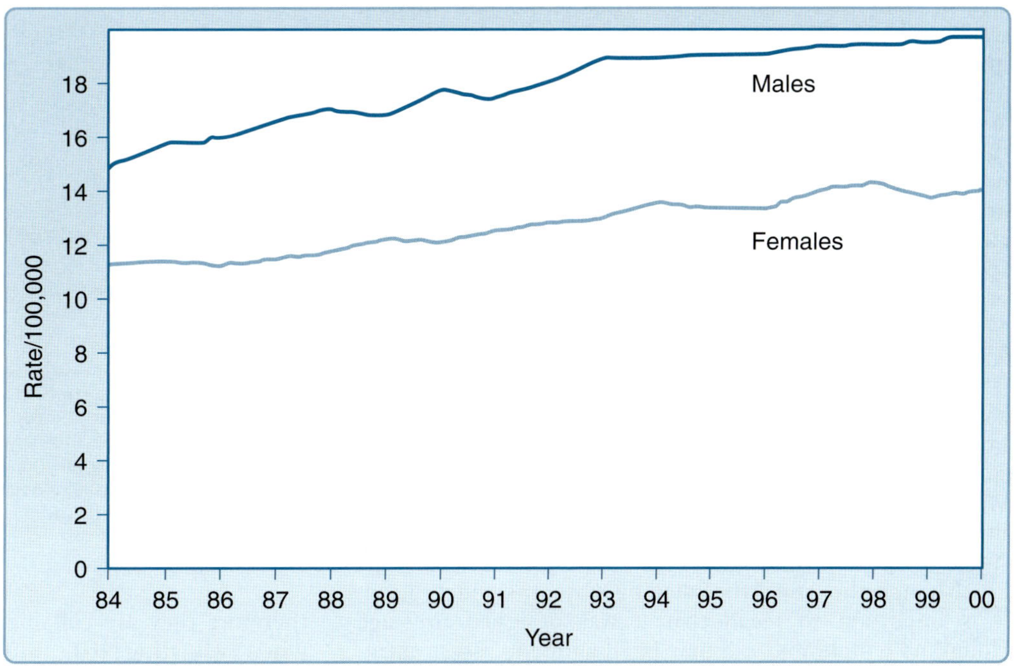

Figure 18–4. Incidence of non-Hodgkin's lymphoma, 1984–2000, Canada.

Table 18–1. Distribution of WHO Diagnoses Seen in 723 Consecutive Patients with Stage I or II B-Cell Extranodal Lymphoma at the British Columbia Cancer Agency, 1981–2003

Pathologic Diagnosis	Number	%
DLBCL	454	63
Marginal zone lymphoma, extranodal, MALT type	133	18
Follicular lymphoma	76	11
Lymphoma, NOS	25	3
Mantle cell lymphoma	17	2
Small lymphocytic lymphoma	9	1
Lymphoplasmacyctic lymphoma	9	1

DLBCL, diffuse large B-cell lymphoma; MALT, mucosa-associated lymphoid tissue; NOS, not otherwise specified.

GENERAL PRINCIPLES

Initial Evaluation

The clinical assessment of patients with primary extranodal lymphoma follows the principles established for assessment of patients with nodal presentations. A diagnosis should be established by excisional biopsy of a whole involved lymph node or by incisional biopsy of the extranodal mass. Core biopsies are less desirable. The diagnostic biopsy should be processed and interpreted by an experienced hematopathologist. The staging workup should include history (searching for constitutional symptoms, localized pain or obstructive symptoms), physical exam, complete blood count, liver and renal function tests, serum protein electropheresis, lactate dehydrogenase (LDH), hepatitis B and C and human immunodeficiency virus serologies, imaging tests, and a bone marrow biopsy. The minimal imaging investigations include a chest radiograph and computed tomography (CT) of the abdomen and pelvis. Additional appropriate imaging tests should be performed to delineate the local extent of extranodal disease and its size, invasiveness and effect on other organs. This usually requires CT or magnetic resonance imaging (MRI) of the local region. Certain sites of extranodal presentation require additional specific tests because of a predilection for simultaneous organ involvement elsewhere. For example, the presence of asymptomatic GI lymphoma should be excluded in patients with primary involvement of oropharyngeal soft tissue. This is best accomplished with contrast studies of the stomach and small bowel, with endoscopy and biopsy added to investigate any suspicious lesion. Those with primarily stomach involvement should have an ENT exam to exclude Waldeyer's ring involvement. Patients with unilateral testicular lymphoma should have a testicular ultrasound to rule out contralateral disease.

Table 18–2. Distribution of WHO Diagnoses at Each Extranodal Site Seen in 709 of 723[a] Consecutive Patients with Stage I or II B-Cell Extranodal Lymphomas at British Columbia Cancer Agency, 1981–2003

	WHO Classification		
Extranodal Site (cases)	*Type*	*n*	%
Waldeyer's ring (118)	DLBCL	76	64
	FL	15	13
	MALT	14	12
	Mantle cell	13	11
Intestine (91)	DLBCL	64	70
	FL	16	17
	MALT	6	7
	Other	5	6
Soft tissue (86)	DLBCL	61	71
	FL	12	14
	MALT	5	6
	Other	8	9
Gastric (85)	DLBCL	51	60
	MALT	30	35
	Other	4	5
Orbital (59)	MALT	36	62
	FL	8	13
	DBLCL	4	7
	LPL	4	7
	SLL	4	7
	Other	3	5
Bone (42)	DLBCL	35	83
	Other	7	17
Testis (37)	DLBCL	34	92
	Other	3	8
Thyroid (36)	DLBCL	32	89
	MALT	4	11
Skin (35)	MALT	17	49
	DLBCL	11	31
	FL	7	20
Sinus (26)	DLBCL	22	86
	Other	4	14
Lung (17)	DLBCL	10	56
	MALT	6	39
	Other	1	6
Breast (12)	DLBCL	8	67
	other	4	33
Other sites combined (65)	DLBCL	44	68
	FL	10	15
	MALT	5	8
	Other	4	6
	Mantle cell	2	3

[a] Assignment to one specific site could not be made in 14 cases due to overlapping involvement of multiple locoregional sites.
DLBCL, diffuse large B-cell lymphoma; FL= follicular lymphoma; LPL = lymphoplasmacytic; MALT = marginal zone lymphoma, extranodal, mucosal-associated lymphoid tissue; SLL= small lymphocytic lymphoma; WHO, World Health Organization.

Although the Ann Arbor staging system is widely used, it is important to recall that it was designed to stage Hodgkin's lymphoma, and may be ill-suited to assess extranodal lymphoma. For example, Waldeyer's ring and Peyer's patches of the small intestine are considered lymphatic tissue. However, most clinicians recognize the unique characteristics of primary lymphoma affecting these organs, and therefore they are classified as extranodal sites of disease when evaluating NHLs. Furthermore, the Ann Arbor system gives little useful guidance for describing the extent of local disease, invasion of adjacent organs and tumor bulk. Despite these limitations this system can be useful if included as part of a pragmatic approach to staging that

Table 18–3. Pragmatic Treatment-Oriented Approach to Staging Non-Hodgkin's Lymphoma

Limited Stage	Advanced Stage
Ann Arbor I, II	Ann Arbor III, IV
and	or
Bulk < 10 cm	Bulk > 10 cm
and	or
no B symptoms	B symptoms

Table 18–4. Proposed Staging System for Gastrointestinal Non-Hodgkin's Lymphomas

Stage I	Tumor confined to gastrointestinal tract without serosal penetration
	Single primary site
	Multiple, noncontiguous lesions
Stage II	Tumor extending into abdomen from primary site—nodal involvement
	II_1 Local (gastric/mesenteric)
	II_2 Distant (para-aortic/para-caval)
Stage II_E	Penetration of serosa to involve adjacent "structures"; enumerate actual site of involvement, such as Stage II_E (pancreas), stage II_E (large intestine)
	Perforation/peritonitis
Stage IV	Disseminated extranodal involvement or a gastrointestinal tract lesion with supradiaphragmatic nodal involvement

From Rohatiner A. Report on a workshop convened to discuss the pathological and staging classifications of gastrointestinal tract lymphoma. Ann Oncol 1994;5:397–400,[10] with permission.

divides patients into two groups, "limited" and "advanced," based on the criteria shown in Table 18–3. Ann Arbor staging of GI lymphomas in particular is unsatisfactory as it does not accurately discriminate minimal from more extensive organ involvement. A specific staging system for GI lymphomas (Table 18–4) has been proposed, but has not been widely adopted.[10]

Although the biology of lymphomas is increasingly being delineated at a molecular level, this has not yet been applied widely to the clinical setting. The Ann Arbor stage supplemented by a measure of bulk, notation of the sites of involvement, and WHO pathologic classification remains the foundation for determining the prognosis and treatment of patients with NHL.

Prognostic Factors

The International Prognostic Index (IPI) can be applied to patients presenting with extranodal lymphoma of both aggressive and indolent histologies.[11] Many series describing specific extranodal sites have applied the IPI, and shown that it has discriminating value in predicting outcome. A modification of the IPI for localized aggressive DLCL has been described for patients presenting with Stages I and II extranodal NHL.[12]

Treatment Principles

In most situations, patients with primary extranodal lymphoma and localized disease are treated with curative intent. A palliative approach is reserved for instances when the condition of the patient or the extent and/or location of the disease indicates that a radical treatment would confer little chance of cure. In addition to the limited extent of the extranodal lymphoma, knowledge of the pathologic type and the extent and pattern of disease is essential to select the appropriate treatment strategy. It is also important to know whether a particular infectious agent, such as *Helicobacter pylori* in gastric MALT marginal zone lymphoma, has been identified because there are several examples where eradication of the infection causes regression of the malignant process. This will be addressed in more detail as specific entities are described later in the chapter.

Apparent confinement of lymphoma to a localized area or within a specific organ might suggest, at first, that treatment such as surgical removal or local irradiation would prove curative. The underlying biology of the lymphomas, however, makes clear why such an approach often fails. The neoplastic cell in lymphomas, the lymphocyte, is inherently capable of circulation throughout the vascular fluids of the body and migration into tissues. It is, therefore, not surprising that neoplasms derived from such circulating cells metastasize early and frequently in the course of the disease. Thus, patients treated with locally effective measures often later develop evidence of lymphoma at distant sites, even though a meticulous staging evaluation at diagnosis revealed no distant disease. The obvious solution is to incorporate systemic treatment into the original treatment plan. This strategy underlies the most successful approaches currently employed for primary extranodal lymphomas.

Cure with surgery is infrequent but a resection of the primary tumor may be very helpful. For example, resection of the segment of bowel involved by lymphoma may relieve obstruction, eliminate risk of perforation, reduce the likelihood of hemorrhage and facilitate subsequent treatment. Orchidectomy establishes the diagnosis in testicular lymphoma and removes bulk tumor from a sanctuary site. However, because effective systemic therapy and radiation are also available, aggressive surgical approaches requiring sacrifice of function (e.g., amputation for bone lymphoma or subtotal gastrectomy for gastric lymphoma) are seldom indicated.

The central principle of radiation therapy is to deliver a curative dose of radiation to a target volume that includes the full extent of disease with appropriate margins while minimizing injury to normal tissue. The correct application of dose and fractionation schedule depends on site, pathologic type and tumor bulk. Indolent lymphomas are more responsive to radiation and doses of 20 to 35 Gy delivered in 10 to 20 fractions over 2 to 4 weeks result in local control rates in excess of 95%. Irradiation alone for patients with aggressive histology lymphoma is not usually successful in achieving long-term control of disease. Series report relapses in as many as 50% in Stage I and 75% of those with

Stage II disease respectively, most of which are at sites distant to the area irradiated.[13–19] However, in the setting of combined modality therapy, excellent local control has been obtained with doses of 30 to 35 Gy delivered in 1.75- to 3-Gy fractions. Furthermore when systemic chemotherapy is combined with irradiation for DLBCL, relapse-free and overall survival are improved over results using irradiation alone. Combined modality treatment with three cycles of CHOP followed by local radiation is an effective treatment for localized nodal or extranodal DLBCL and is equivalent to eight cycles of CHOP.[12,20] With this approach, the progression-free survival of patients is about 80% at 5 years and 75% at 10 years. The specific extranodal site of disease (except in primary CNS lymphoma) does not influence the choice of chemotherapy regimen. The addition of rituximab to CHOP has been shown to improve the survival of patients with advanced-stage or bulky limited-stage DLBCL, both in randomized trials and in population-based studies.[21,22] While this has not been specifically evaluated for limited-stage DLBCL, adding rituximab has been shown to improve progression free and overall survival when added to standard cytotoxic chemotherapy in most B-cell lymphoproliferative conditions, and therefore, addition of rituximab to CHOP should be considered whenever extranodal DLBCL is being treated.[23]

As a general principle, the systemic therapy of indolent B-cell neoplasms of extranodal sites can be summarized as follows: localized lymphoma that has been shown to have an underlying inciting infectious etiology, such as gastric MALToma, should be treated with a course of specific antibiotics. The association between other infectious agents and MALTomas of nongastric sites (conjunctiva, small intestine, skin) is rapidly evolving.[24–30] For such patients, especially when they have no or minimal symptoms, it is reasonable to prescribe a brief course of specific antibiotics according to the inciting agent detected. Localized extranodal indolent histology lymphomas not known to be associated with infectious agents should be treated with involved-field irradiation. For symptomatic patients with localized indolent B-cell neoplasms that cannot be treated with irradiation because of proximity to radiosensitive tissue, a course of systemic therapy is indicated. In addition, patients with symptomatic disease that has relapsed following irradiation or antibiotic therapy should also be considered for such treatment. Useful agents include alkylators, such as chlorambucil or cyclophosphamide, or purine analogues such as fludarabine. Single-agent rituximab also has proven efficacy as do radioimmunoconjugates, but the best role for these newer agents is still being defined.[31–33] Combination therapy with conventional cytotoxic agents and rituximab is also a rapidly evolving field.

Assessment of Response and Follow-up

Assessment of response to treatment for extranodal lymphomas should follow standard principles for lymphoma at any site. The criteria published by the International Working Group on Response Assessment in Lymphomas provide detailed guidance and should be followed.[34] Certain characteristics of extranodal lymphoma, however, make application of these criteria problematic. For example, gastric lymphoma may not be evident on any imaging test, but only detectable by endoscopy, and response can be difficult to quantify. Bone lymphoma may leave an area of sclerosis very similar in extent to that present at diagnosis, and nuclear medicine scans such as technetium bone scan or gallium scan may remain positive months after completion of curative treatment. Initial results with positron emission tomography (PET) appear promising, and this technique may allow more accurate post-treatment assessment of extranodal lymphomas in the future.

Issues that require special consideration during follow-up after treatment of extranodal lymphoma include the following:

- Knowledge of the likelihood of and time to progression. For example, the presence of residual radiologic abnormalities 6 weeks after completion of radiation for orbital MALT lymphoma does not necessarily indicate treatment failure, as the disease may regress slowly. Residual lymphocytic infiltrate and gastric mucosal abnormalities may persist for months to years following eradication of *H. pylori*, and mandates, at a minimum, close follow-up with endoscopic assessment at 3- to 6-month intervals.
- Knowledge of the pattern of relapse. In situations where local relapse is uncommon, such as orbital lymphoma or small bulk Waldeyer's ring lymphoma treated with irradiation, long-term repeated imaging of the presenting site is not indicated, but particular attention to any new more distant adenopathy or persistent gastrointestinal symptoms is warranted. In limited-stage DLBCL, over 50% of relapses occur within 2 to 3 years after the diagnosis, but late relapses continue to occur up to 15 years after diagnosis; therefore, prolonged follow-up is warranted.[20]
- Correlation of certain extranodal primary sites with specific sites of relapse. For example, CNS relapse is seen in higher frequency with sinus and testicular lymphomas; gastrointestinal relapse is more common in patients with Waldeyer's ring lymphoma; and contralateral tissue relapse is more frequent in certain paired organs such as testis, salivary or lacrimal glands, conjunctiva, or lung.
- Subsequent organ or tissue abnormality as a result of prior involvement by lymphoma or as a consequence of treatment, such as hypothyroidism following thyroid irradiation, risk of pathologic fracture secondary to bone lymphoma, or vitamin B12 deficiency as a consequence of resection of the terminal ileum.
- Whether the primary extranodal lesion was resected or remains in situ. If it remains in situ, it will remain the principal focus of local recurrence especially if the disease was bulky at presentation or not irradiated.
- Association of the initial lymphoma with a monoclonal serum paraprotein. Although not generally a common finding, certain extranodal subtypes are reported to be associated with a monoclonal gammopathy even in the absence of bone marrow involvement.[35] Patients with immunoproliferative small intestinal disease (a special subtype of MALT lymphoma) usually have an aberrant alpha heavy chain in the peripheral blood.[36] Primary pulmonary lymphoma is reported to have a paraproteinemia in 30% to 40% of cases.[37,38] In these situations, the monoclonal gammopathy can be a clinically useful marker of response or relapse.

Management of Relapse

Management of relapse of extranodal lymphoma is individualized according to the patient's age, disease-free interval, site and pathology of the relapse, and the patient's overall condition, including consideration of comorbid illnesses and age-related organ dysfunction. Usually, systemic treatment with either cytotoxic chemotherapy or rituximab is necessary. Younger patients with relapsed DLBCL that responds to second-line chemotherapy may be candidates for high-dose consolidation with autologous stem cell transplant. In selected cases of indolent lymphoma recurring with localized non-bulky disease, irradiation alone may offer long-term disease control.

Treatment Complications

The usual early and late treatment complications from irradiation or systemic chemotherapy that develop in patients with nodal lymphomas can also be seen in patients with extranodal presentations. These are discussed in more detail in other chapters. In addition, there are specific complications that arise due to initial organ involvement or therapy directed to specific extranodal tissues. These include the risk of hypothyroidism following irradiation or resection of thyroid lymphomas; the possibility of cataracts or retinal dysfunction following irradiation of the orbit; the risk of hypogonadism after scrotal irradiation for testicular lymphoma; malabsorption or vitamin B12 deficiency as a consequence of resection of the terminal ileum; xerostomia from oropharyngeal or salivary gland irradiation; and osteoporosis and the risk of pathologic fracture after the treatment of bone lymphoma. Being alert to site-specific complications can allow early intervention for the management of these problems and potentially avert significant morbidity.

SITE-SPECIFIC PRIMARY EXTRANODAL LYMPHOMAS

Gastric

The stomach is the most common single site of involvement by extranodal lymphoma.[2] Gastric lymphomas may be either indolent or aggressive in type, and some patients display both types together at diagnosis. The incidence of both gastric and intestinal lymphoma in the United States, Europe, and Japan has been rising over the last 20 years. A portion of this increase may be secondary to improved methods of diagnosis both in procuring and processing the biopsy specimens. However, exposure or susceptibility to other risk factors such as *H. pylori*, ultraviolet light, chemicals, and excessive protein or fat in the diet may also be contributing to this increase.[7–9]

Lymphoma of the stomach typically causes dyspeptic symptoms, especially nausea, mild to moderate epigastric discomfort and, less often, anorexia or early satiety. Detectable hemorrhage is unusual and is a strong signal of higher-grade disease if present. Because the symptoms are chronic, intermittent, and often responsive to antacid remedies, the antecedent history before diagnosis may be long. Fever and night sweats are uncommon, but weight loss is typical, usually as a consequence of the local problem rather than as a manifestation of a constitutional illness. Today most diagnoses of gastric lymphoma are made on the basis of gastroscopic appearance and biopsy, although the occasional patient is still discovered to have gastric lymphoma at the time of resection for ulcer disease or presumed gastric carcinoma. Contrast radiographs and computed tomography are insensitive methods of finding lymphoma in the stomach, but useful to search for involvement of the small intestine or disease elsewhere in the abdomen and pelvis. Endoscopic ultrasound, when available, can delineate the extent of gastric wall and perigastric nodal involvement.[39] Endoscopy usually reveals mild to severe gastritis ranging from focal to diffuse. More than superficial ulceration, frank hemorrhage or perforation, if present, suggests aggressive histology disease. Because the diagnosis rests so frequently on gastroscopic biopsy, such specimens should be as large and deep as possible and should be obtained from each region of the stomach in addition to all abnormal sites. This is necessary so that adequate material is available for examination for presence of *H. pylori*, and determination of the grade and extent of the lymphoma. To complete staging, upper airway and oropharyngeal examination is required as well as all the usual procedures performed for nodal lymphomas.

An overview of several large series reported in literature outlining the demographics, treatment, and outcome for patients with gastric lymphoma is shown in Table 18–5. One series in particular in Japan examined the trends in the clinicopathologic features of gastrointestinal lymphoma over three periods: before MALT lymphoma was recognized as a specific entity (1963–1982); after it was recognized (1983–1992); and after the introduction of *H. pylori* eradication for gastric MALToma (1993–2002).[9] This study reveals an increase in the proportion of patients with low-grade B-cell versus high-grade B-cell disease over time, and a decline in percentage of patients being treated with surgical resection with a reciprocal increase in patients who receive systemic treatments such as antibiotics and/or cytotoxics over time.

Gastric MALT Lymphoma

In at least two-thirds of cases of MALT lymphoma, the disease is localized at diagnosis.[40] The connection between *H. pylori* and gastric disease in general[41] and gastric lymphoma in particular[42–48] is well established. This microorganism may provide the antigenic stimulus for sustaining growth of lymphoma in the stomach, although the exact mechanism by which chronic inflammation develops into frank malignancy is still unclear. Since most patients with *H. pylori* gastritis do not develop lymphoma, additional genetic or environmental factors may play a role. Nevertheless, this spiral gram-negative bacillus can cause a low-grade B-cell mucosa-associated lymphoid tumor (MALT) of the stomach, and is probably responsible for at least some of the higher-grade gastric lymphomas, either by transformation from a low-grade MALT or by induction of de novo large cell disease.

The most important item in the chain of evidence connecting *H. pylori* to gastric lymphoma is directly relevant to clinical practice. Eradication of the organism frequently leads to complete regression of the MALT

Table 18–5. Overview of Recent Series in Literature Outlining Demographics, Histology, Therapy, and Outcome for Patients with Primary Localized Gastrointestinal Lymphoma

Reference Study Type	Number	Median Age (y)	% Male	Histology		Treatment		Outcome		Comments
Tondini (1993)[62]	114	50		Aggressive	70%	Resection	89%	10-y FFP	84%	
Retrospective review	73% gastric			Indolent	30%	Adjuvant	83%	OS	86%	
						chemoRx		10-y FFP		
								(a) Aggressive	79%	
								(b) Indolent	97%	
Nakamura (2003)[9]	342	58	50	(a) MALT	50%	Surgery	52%	5-y OS	77%	
Surgical series				(b) DLBCL		alone				
1963–2002	100% gastric			+MALT	15%					
	90% localized			–MALT	23%			5-y OS		
				(c) FL	6%	Nonsurgical	22%	(a) MALT	87%	
				(d) T cell	6%	Both	24%	(b) DLBC	63%	
Liang (1995)[152]		53	54	Aggressive	65%	Resection	74%	5y DFS	67%	7% of cases
Retrospective series	63% gastric			Indolent	12%	XRT	38%	OS	70%	were T cell
						ChemoRx	88%			
Cortelazzo (1999)[63]	312	61	52	DLBCL	100%	Surgery	77%	5-y FFS	67%	
Retrospective review				(a) +MALT	15%			OS	75%	
1972–1997	100% gastric			(b) –MALT	85%	XRT	9%	5-y OS by IPI		
								Low	90%	
						Adjuvant	80%	Intermediate	63%	
						chemoRx		High	40%	
Ibrahim (1999)[153]	185	54	57	DLBCL	100%	Resection	54%	5-y OS	68%	CMT better than
Retrospective review	82% localized					ChemoRx	79%			single
1982–1999						CMT	48%			modality RX

ChemoRx, chemotherapy, usually with an anthracycline; CMT, combined modality therapy (surgery, chemotherapy, plus/minus irradiation); DFS, disease-free survival; DLBCL, diffuse large B-cell lymphoma; EFS, event-free survival; FFP, freedom from progression; FL, follicular lymphoma; IPI, International Prognostic Index; MALT, mucosa associated lymphoid tissue lymphoma; OS, overall survival; XRT, irradiation; y, years.

lymphoma.[42,44,45,47] Antibiotics can be effective as the sole initial treatment for the disease. The organism can be eradicated in up to 90% of cases, and most symptoms respond promptly; however, the lymphoma may regress slowly. Complete regression is documented about 50% to 70% of the time, and depends on the extent of the primary lesion.[49–51] Cases in which the disease is confined to the mucosa and submucosa are more likely to be associated with the *H. pylori* organism, and are more likely to respond than more locally advanced lesions involving the muscularis mucosa, serosa, or perigastric lymph nodes.[46,50]

It is essential for the patient to have follow-up endoscopic examinations for several reasons. If *H. pylori* is not eradicated, a second course of antibiotics is indicated and may be effective at least 50% of the time. If *H. pylori* has been eliminated, the MALT lymphoma may persist, sometimes in association with large-cell disease.[52] If this is proven with biopsies, treatment appropriate for this higher-grade lymphoma based on stage of disease and condition of the patient is necessary. If the disease is still localized, this usually requires multiagent chemotherapy with three cycles of CHOP plus rituximab followed by involved-region irradiation. A more prolonged course of chemotherapy can also be used and has been shown to be equivalent to combined modality approach.[12] If *H. pylori* is eliminated and no higher grade lymphoma can be found, it is reasonable to continue to follow persistent low-grade MALT lymphoma with serial endoscopies. Gradual regression of the disease has been recorded to take as long as 28 months; however, outside of the setting of a carefully conducted clinical trial, it would be imprudent to wait longer than 6 to 9 months after eradication of *H. pylori* for the MALT lymphoma to resolve. If the disease persists either on gross or microscopic exam, then further antilymphoma treatment should be given. Single-agent chemotherapy with an agent such as chlorambucil or cyclophosphamide or upper abdominal irradiation is effective, but the oral chemotherapy is usually better tolerated. A recent study has established the safety and efficacy of rituximab in both previously treated and untreated extranodal MALT lymphoma.[31] Even after complete histologic remission, polymerase chain reaction (PCR) testing targeted to the immunoglobulin heavy-chain genes can demonstrate evidence of clonality.[51] This molecular evidence of minimal residual disease does not appear to be associated with histologic relapse. However, given the natural history of indolent lymphomas, longer-term follow-up of these patients is necessary before firm recommendations for overall management can be made.

Gastric DLBCL

When aggressive lymphoma is found in the stomach, it is almost always of a diffuse large B-cell type. This can arise de novo or be found on a background of MALT. In either case, treatment must be directed at the aggressive histology disease. Although authorities have debated the necessity of primary surgery (partial gastrectomy) for these patients citing a 25% risk of serious hemorrhage or perforation, most patients can be managed successfully with chemotherapy and irradiation without initial surgical resection.[53–62] The best approach in an era when the diagnosis is being made earlier on the basis of gastroscopy is between the extremes of never or always resecting the disease. Patients who present with or develop significant hemorrhage or actual perforation should undergo partial gastrectomy in addition to planned chemotherapy and irradiation. The rest with gastric DLBCL should be treated with standard multiagent chemotherapy after usual staging is complete. Those with Stage IAE or IIAE disease can switch to upper abdominal irradiation after brief chemotherapy, usually three cycles, with a high expectation of cure. A stage-modified IPI has been shown to be able to stratify patients with Stage I or II disease into excellent (>90% chance of cure) and poorer (<60% chance of cure) risk categories.[20,63] Those with B symptoms, bulky tumors larger than 10 cm or Stage III or IV disease should complete an extended full course of CHOP plus rituximab chemotherapy, reserving irradiation for those with residual disease after completion of the chemotherapy. This latter strategy should cure at least 50% to 60% of those with advanced disease.[21,22] Finally, following completion of treatment, it is reasonable to administer a course of anti *H. pylori* treatment for these patients whether or not the organism was actually demonstrated.

Intestinal Lymphoma

Small bowel lymphomas account for 20% to 40% of primary gastrointestinal lymphomas. In Western populations, 60% to 80% of intestinal lymphomas are of B-cell origin, mostly DLBCL of the distal small intestine, especially the ileocecal region.[64,65] A recent Japanese study also showed that the majority of lesions are of B-cell origin.[66] Follicular, mantle, and marginal cell lymphomas make up approximately 30% of cases, with DLBCL accounting for the majority, and Burkitt's lymphoma accounting for 1% to 2% of cases. A rare type of lymphoma, α chain disease, or immunoproliferative small intestinal disease (IPSID), is now known to be a type of B-cell MALT lymphoma involving the small intestine. This disorder occurs in Mediterranean regions and has been reported to respond to broad-spectrum antibiotics such as tetracycline. Recently researchers have demonstrated an association between *Campylobacter jejuni* and IPSID, a situation analogous to that of *H. pylori* and gastric MALT lymphoma.[24]

Typically, patients with intestinal lymphoma present with symptoms of obstruction, crampy abdominal pain, and weight loss. Gastrointestinal bleeding or perforation is seen less often. The tumors are diagnosed either endoscopically (in the case of upper small bowel involvement) or at the time of resection of the lesion.[67,68]

The majority of patients with intestinal DLBCL have localized disease, and following diagnosis and staging, should be treated with CHOP plus rituximab-type chemotherapy. When the entire tumor has been surgically removed, a brief course of chemotherapy is sufficient, usually three cycles of CHOP plus rituximab. Radiation is not appropriate because the mobility of the intestinal structures would necessitate a whole abdominal technique. Therefore, when residual disease is present, a full course of six to eight cycles of chemotherapy alone should be used. A recent publication has confirmed the efficacy of this approach with over 90% of patients surviving at 2 years.[67]

The treatment for intestinal MALT lymphoma not associated with *C. jejuni* is similar to other types of indolent

B-cell lymphomas. Chemotherapy with alkylators, purine analogues, or rituximab has demonstrated efficacy. If *C. jejuni* is present, it would be reasonable to consider antibiotic treatment best administered within a clinical trial setting. The treatment of intestinal polyposis from mantle cell lymphoma is similar to the management of this condition with or without GI involvement. An overview of several large series reported in the literature outlining the demographics, treatment, and outcome for patients with small intestinal NHL is shown in Table 18–6.

Sinus Lymphoma

The bony sinuses of the face and head include the ethmoid, frontal, sphenoid, and maxillary sinuses. Infrequently, primary NHL can develop in these extranodal sites. The incidence of this disease in North America is less than 3% of all NHLs. When lymphoma develops in one of these sinuses, it frequently involves nearby bone and usually presents with local pain, nasal or upper airway obstruction, rhinorrhea, facial swelling, or epistaxis. If the tumor develops in a periorbital location proptosis, vision loss, or diplopia may be prominent. Over 85% of cases are DLBCL, and typically follow an aggressive course with a strong tendency to cause local destruction, invade across natural anatomic barriers, and metastasize systemically. This disease needs to be distinguished from another virulent head and neck lymphoma, nasal NK/T-cell lymphoma, which is more common in Southeast Asia and etiologically linked to Epstein–Barr virus (and outlined in Chapter 25). Once the diagnosis has been established by biopsy sinus B-cell lymphoma should be rapidly staged, and treatment should then proceed in three phases: systemic, local, and finally prophylactic against spread to the CNS. Systemic treatment should employ CHOP with rituximab. The number of cycles should be appropriate for the stage: brief, usually three cycles, for the majority of patients who present with localized disease; or prolonged, usually six to eight cycles for patients with B symptoms, tumor exceeding 10 cm in greatest diameter, or Stage III or IV disease. The chemotherapy should be followed by involved-region irradiation to a dose of at least 3500 cGy in 15 to 20 fractions for all patients who were treated with brief chemotherapy, and any advanced-stage patients who have residual disease after their full course of chemotherapy. However, careful judgment must be used, and if, because of the size or shape of the field, the irradiation would cause a threat to vision or excessive mucosal toxicity, it would be reasonable to extend the chemotherapy to a full six to eight courses and omit the irradiation, especially if a complete response is achieved.

It is not surprising that invasive lymphoma developing within the porous structure of the bones at the base of the skull and, therefore, next to the brain has a tendency to spread to the CNS.[69,70] Given the rarity of this presentation of lymphoma and the variable natural history that all lymphomas can display, it is also not surprising that estimates of the risk of spread to the CNS ranges from 0% to 50%. The true rate is probably between 20% and 40%, and indicates a high risk of this serious complication. A policy of administering six doses of intrathecal chemotherapy over 3 weeks, alternating between methotrexate and cytarabine, to all patients with paranasal sinus lymphoma, was instituted at the British Columbia Cancer Agency beginning in 1984.[71] Prior to that time, a 50% rate of spread to the CNS was seen, but this has reduced to less than 10%. This is convincing evidence that intrathecal chemotherapy is an essential component of the successful treatment of lymphoma presenting in the paranasal sinuses.

If all three necessary parts of the treatment of lymphoma presenting in the paranasal sinuses are included in the treatment plan, the patient typically receives brief systemic chemotherapy, involved-region irradiation, and intrathecal chemoprophylaxis against spread to the CNS. Most patients treated according to such a plan can be cured. Table 18–7 shows the results of using this approach to treatment for all patients seen at the British Columbia Cancer Agency since 1984.[72] These data verify that with the special addition of intrathecal chemoprophylaxis, a substantial proportion of patients with localized lymphoma of the paranasal sinuses can be cured.

Testicular Lymphoma

Primary testicular lymphoma represents 1% to 2% of all NHLs, and is the most common cause of a neoplastic mass in the testicle of a man over 60 years old. It typically presents as a painless or slightly uncomfortable mass without other urologic symptoms. Histologically, at least 90% of these lymphoma are of diffuse large cell type and of B-cell origin. Patients with lymphoblastic or Burkitt's lymphomas constitute about 3% of all patients with testicular NHL.[6] Eighty percent of cases are localized to the testicle (Stage I), or testicle and pelvic or abdominal lymph nodes (Stage II) at presentation. In the remaining 20%, the testicle is a site of involvement with widespread disease. After the diagnosis has been established by initial orchidectomy, patients should be staged as usual for lymphoma. Any mass in the remaining testis should be characterized by ultrasonography. An otherwise unexplained solid mass should be assumed to be lymphoma. Patients with Stage III or IV disease or B symptoms should be managed similarly to others with advanced-stage aggressive histology disease with an extended course of multiagent chemotherapy. The recent improvement in outcomes with the addition of rituximab to CHOP chemotherapy support the hypothesis that this combination may also be of benefit in the subset of primary DLBCL of the testicle.[21]

Although most patients with localized extranodal DLBCL are suitable candidates for brief chemotherapy and involved-region irradiation, this is not true of testicular lymphoma. A recent large multinational retrospective review of testicular DLBCL has emphasized this and several other special aspects of the management of this condition.[6] For example, even for patients with Stage I or II disease, the outcome seems worse than what has been reported for DLBCL at other sites. Up to 50% of these patients experience a treatment failure. The sites of failure include contralateral testis, CNS (mostly brain parenchyma although leptomeninges can also be involved), and other extranodal sites. The addition of irradiation following completion of chemotherapy in a dose of 2500 cGy in 10 to 15 fractions to the entire scrotum virtually eliminates the risk of contralateral testicular relapse, by dealing with lymphoma present in a privileged site where it may not be affected by

Table 18–6. Overview of Recent Series in Literature Outlining Demographics, Histology, Therapy, and Outcome for Patients with Primary Small Intestinal Lymphoma

Reference Study Type	Number	Median Age (y)	% Male	Histology		Treatment		Outcome		Comments
Domizio (1993)[64] 1950–1993 Retrospective	119	65	66	T cell B cell (a) Aggressive (b) MALT (c) Both (d) Other indolent	34% 66% 62% 20% 11% 7%	Resection (a) Alone (b) Chemo RX (c) XRT (d) CMT	97% 30% 44% 6% 21%	5-y OS (a) Indolent (b) Aggressive B cell T cell	 75% 50% 25%	50% of T-cell NHL were associated with gluten enteropathy Perforation confers poor prognosis
Nakamura (2000)[154] 1962–2002 Retrospective	96 86% Localized	58	67	T cell High-grade B cell MALT Other B cell	13% 50% 28% 9%	Surgery ChemoRX ± XRT CMT	47% 16% 35%	5-y OS	60%	B-cell phenotype associated with better survival
Ibrahim (1999)[153] 1982–1999 Retropsective	66 86% Localized	45	67	DLCL	100%	Any surgery Any chemo Any XRT	80% 94% 15%	5-y OS	58%	Albumin <30 g/L poor prognostic feature
Daum (2003)[67] Prospective Nonrandomized 1995–1999	56	63 (T cell) 57 (B cell)	33 (T cell) 50 (B cell)	T cell B cell	62% 38%	Any surgery CHOP (a) T cell (b) B cell	93% 66% 95%	2-y OS T cell B cell	 28% 94%	Prior celiac disease T cell 66% B cell 5%
Kohno (2003)[66] 1981–2000	143	54	76	T cell B cell (a) DLBCL (b) Burkitt (c) MALT (d) MCL	15% 85% 69% 13% 8% 6%	CHOP	100%	5-y OS B-cell T-cell	 48% 20%	Small bowel = 70% Large bowel = 17% Multiple = 13%

ChemoRx, chemotherapy, usually with an anthracycline; CHOP, cyclophosphamide, doxorubicin, vincristine, prednisone; CMT, combined modality therapy (surgery, chemotherapy, plus/minus irradiation); DFS, disease-free survival; DLBCL, diffuse large B-cell lymphoma; EFS, event-free survival; FFP, freedom from progression; FL, follicular lymphoma; IPI, International Prognostic Index; MALT, mucosa associated lymphoid tissue lymphoma; OS, overall survival; XRT, irradiation; y, years.

Table 18–7. Outcome for 44 Patients with Primary Lymphoma of Paranasal Sinuses Treated with Brief Chemotherapy, Irradiation, and Intrathecal Chemotherapy

		n	%
Gender	Male	26	60
Age (y)	Median	66	
Histologic type			
	Diffuse large B cell	34	77
	Immunoblastic	6	13
	T cell	2	5
	Unclassified	2	5
Stage	IE	21	48
	IIE	23	52
Survival	Overall (5 years)		47
	Disease-specific (5 years)		61

From Laskin J, Savage KJ, Gascoyne RD, et al. Primary paranasal sinus lymphoma: natural history and improved outcome with central nervous system chemoprophylaxis. Cancer 2005, (in press)[71] with permission.

systemic chemotherapy. Such irradiation causes azoospermic infertility and brief acute cutaneous toxicity lasting 2 to 3 weeks. Typically, low normal testosterone levels and potency are maintained. CNS relapse can be seen as an isolated event (8% of cases) or as part of more widespread relapse (13%) in patients presenting with localized testicular lymphoma.[6] In more advanced disease, Stage III or IV, the incidence of subsequent CNS involvement is about 20%. Currently the available evidence shows that intrathecal chemoprophylaxis, intravenous high-dose methotrexate with folinic acid rescue, or prophylactic cranial irradiation does not appear to decrease the incidence of recurrence in the CNS for these patients. Such approaches should be areas of clinical investigation. Finally, because up to 50% of patients with localized testicular lymphoma experience a relapse after a brief course of chemotherapy, a more prolonged course of multiagent chemotherapy with CHOP plus rituximab should be considered.

In summary, following diagnostic inguinal orchidectomy and appropriate staging, all otherwise suitable patients with testicular lymphoma should receive six to eight cycles of CHOP-type chemotherapy with rituximab followed by prophylactic scrotal irradiation. The addition of CNS prophylaxis is appealing in view of the pattern of relapses, but has not been proven to decrease CNS relapses.[6] Finally, because of an unusual continuous pattern of relapse, even beyond 10 years, which seems unique to this site of lymphoma, prolonged follow-up appears warranted.

Waldeyer's Ring

Waldeyer's ring describes the lymphoid tissue of the tonsil, base of tongue, and nasopharynx. Although recent clinical and immunohistochemical data suggest that these tissues should be considered of nodal origin, they are best considered a unique extranodal site because of their distinctive presentation and patterns of relapse. Dysphagia, airway obstruction, Eustachian tube blockage, mass lesion, and neck lymphadenopathy are the common modes of presentation, depending on the principal site of the tumor. Frequently, the lesion may be visible on simple physical exam, and even better visualized by an otolaryngologist using fiber optic equipment. Such assessment is recommended since multiple sites of involvement may be apparent within the tissues of Waldeyer's ring. The lesion itself and any surrounding neck adenopathy should be delineated by CT or MRI imaging. Although surgery (such as tonsillectomy) provides a tissue diagnosis and may de-bulk the primary lesion, resection alone is quite unlikely to be curative. Full staging is mandatory, as 30% of patients with tonsilar lymphoma have advanced disease. Evaluation should include investigation of the GI tract with contrast imaging or endoscopy, given a clear pattern of association between Waldeyer's ring lesions and the GI tract (and vice versa).[73–76]

Most lymphoid tumors (60% to 80%) presenting as localized disease in the region of the oropharynx are diffuse, large B cell. Other histologic types seen in this location include follicular (14%), mantle cell (12%), and MALT lymphomas (9%). Sixty percent of cases present with localized disease. An overview of several large series reported in the literature outlining the demographics, treatment, and outcome for patients with lymphoma involving Waldeyer's ring is shown in Table 18–8.

Treatment of patients with Waldeyer's ring lymphoma should be undertaken in accordance with the histologic subtype and stage of disease. For limited-stage DLBCL, it should consist of three cycles of CHOP plus rituximab followed by local irradiation unless the irradiation would engender too much local toxicity, especially xerostomia. One randomized trial that looked at 316 patients with Stage I Waldeyer's ring, large-cell lymphoma reported a higher relapse rate for patients treated with CHOP or irradiation alone compared to combined modality therapy.[75] Twenty-three percent of patients who received CHOP-like chemotherapy alone relapsed in Waldeyer's ring compared to 5% of those treated with chemotherapy plus irradiation. Patients with bulky (>10 cm) tumors, B symptoms, or Stage III or IV disease should be treated with six to eight cycles of CHOP plus rituximab, with irradiation reserved for those who are left with proven residual disease. Patients with localized, indolent lymphoma of Waldeyer's ring can achieve long-term disease control with irradiation alone. Those with more extensive low-grade lymphoma can be treated with single-agent or combination chemotherapy when symptomatic disease progression occurs.

One of the notable characteristics of Waldeyer's ring lymphoma is its association with GI disease. In a large randomized study already described,[75] roughly 30% to 35% of those who relapsed did so in the GI tract, despite meticulous staging at diagnosis that included gastroscopy with multiple gastric biopsies. The GI tract deserves special attention both in the treatment and follow-up of patients with lymphoma initially presenting in Waldeyer's ring.

Bone

Involvement of the bone by non-Hodgkin's lymphoma is not uncommon in patients with advanced-stage lymphoma, but constitutes only about 5% of lymphomas presenting with localized disease. The presenting symptoms for

Table 18–8. Overview of Series in Literature Outlining Demographics, Histology, Therapy, and Outcome for Patients with Localized Waldeyer's Ring Non-Hodgkin's Lymphoma

Reference Study Type	Number	Median Age (y)	% Male	Histology	Treatment	Outcome	Comments
Aviles (1996)[75] Randomized trial	316	55	50	DLCL 97%	1. IRRT 2. CHOP-type 3. IRRT → CHOP-type	5-y FFS 1. 48% 2. 43% 3. 83% ($p < 0.001$)	30% relapses occurred in GI tract
Krol (2001)[155] Retrospective series	77 (74% localized)	66	48	DLBCL 66% FL 14% MCL 4% SLL 3%	None 7% CMT 6% IRRT 40% ChemoRx 12%	Not reported separately for localized subgroup	T cell 3%
Ezzat (2001)[156] Retrospective review	130	55	67	DLBCL 84%	ChemoRx 45% IRRT 20% CMT 35%	5-y OS 58%	
Harabuchi (1997)[157]	71 (72% localized)	45	50	DLCL 94%	IRRT 49% CMT 51%	5-y DFS 58% OS 68%	T cell 6%
Liang (1997)[158] Retrospective review	47	63	49	DLCL 58% indolent 18%	IRRT 49% CMT 62%	5 y RFS Aggressive 72% Indolent 100% 5-y OS Aggressive 71% Indolent 75%	70% Unknown immuno-phenotype

ChemoRx, chemotherapy, usually with an anthracycline; CHOP-type, cyclophosphamide, doxorubicin, vincristine, prednisone, bleomycin; CMT, combined modality therapy (surgery, chemotherapy, plus/minus irradiation); DFS, disease-free survival; DLBCL, diffuse large B-cell lymphoma; EFS, event-free survival; FFP, freedom from progression; FL, follicular lymphoma; IPI, International Prognostic Index; IRRT, involved region radiotherapy; MALT, mucosa associated lymphoid tissue lymphoma; OS, overall survival; y, years.

lymphoma involving the bone are usually localized bone pain (most commonly in a long bone) and occasionally a palpable mass. The radiologic appearance usually shows lytic or "moth-eaten" radiolucent lesions with a wide transitional zone between the tumor and normal bone and patches of sclerosis. To establish a histologic diagnosis, tissue from the bony lesion or, if present, an associated soft tissue mass, must be obtained. Fine-needle aspiration (FNA) is insufficient for diagnosis as is core biopsy, which frequently shows crush artifact. For an accurate diagnosis, an open biopsy, processed according to lymphoma pathologic protocols, is required. Radical surgery including amputation is not necessary for successful therapy, but surgery to alleviate the risk of impending pathologic fracture is appropriate in the context of continuing combined modality therapy. In over 85% of cases of bone lymphoma, the histologic diagnosis is DLBCL. In addition to the usual staging for lymphoma, an MRI scan of the primary bone lesion is particularly helpful to determine the medullary, cortical, and soft tissue extent of disease and to identify other sites of involvement in the skeleton. An overview of several large series reported in the literature outlining the demographics, treatment, and outcome for patients with primary bone lymphoma is shown in Table 18–9.

The mainstay of therapy for DLBCL of the bone is chemotherapy with or without irradiation. Localized disease should be treated with either brief chemotherapy, usually three cycles of CHOP plus rituximab, followed by involved-region irradiation or more prolonged chemotherapy alone with irradiation reserved for those patients with residual disease. Patients with more advanced disease at presentation should be treated with six to eight cycles of CHOP plus rituximab with irradiation reserved for proven residual disease.

Determining the response to treatment for patients with bone lymphoma can be difficult because the original radiologic abnormalities seldom revert to normal. Nuclear medicine scans with technetium or gallium may remain abnormal due to bone remodeling or fibrosis even in the absence of active lymphoma. Positron emission tomographic scanning may be helpful but has not been sufficiently tested in this situation. A practical approach to this clinical problem is to irradiate the residual bone disease if doing so will not cause excessive toxicity.

One complication of therapy unique to bone lymphoma is pathologic fracture. Patients may experience fracture before or after therapy due to damage from the lymphoma, from irradiation, or because of avascular necrosis following chemotherapy. Risk factors for fracture include extensive involvement of a weight-bearing bone, high-dose irradiation (>50 to 60 Gy), and prior osteoporosis. Orthopedic referral is recommended for either prophylactic fixation or following an acute fracture. The prognosis of this condition appears to be similar to that of DLBCL at other sites. The IPI provides useful prognostic information in primary bone lymphomas.[5,77]

Thyroid

Lymphomas of the thyroid gland constitute 2% to 3 % of all non-Hodgkin's lymphomas and 5% of thyroid malignancies. Women are affected more frequently than men, and the median age of presentation is over 60 years. Patients usually present with a growing mass in the neck causing local obstructive and infiltrative symptoms, such as hoarseness, dysphagia, or dyspnea. Tumors are often locally bulky (5 to 10 cm), and neck adenopathy is common but constitutional symptoms are unusual. Although the incidence of clinically apparent pre-existing Hashimoto's or autoimmune thyroiditis (with or without associated hypothyroidism) ranges from 27% to 100% in reported series, the surrounding thyroid tissue adjacent to the malignant lymphoma almost always shows histologic evidence of autoimmune thyroiditis.[78–80] One population-based study estimated that the risk

Table 18–9. Overview of Recent Series in Literature Outlining Demographics, Histology, Therapy, and Outcome for Patients with Primary Bone Lymphomas

Reference Study Type	Number	Median Age (y)	% Male	Histology by WF (Grade)		Treatment		Outcome		Comments
Baar (1999)[159]	17	36	71	Intermediate	100%	CHOP	88%	5-y OS	90%	
Review	(localized 88%)					CMT	59%	(CMT group)		
Dubey (1997)[77]	45	52	53	Intermediate	96%	CMT	80%	5-y OS	68%	IPI predictive outcome
Review						XRT	11%	DSS	72%	
						chemoRX	9%			
Fairbanks (1994)[160]	44	55	54	Intermediate	94%	XRT	77%	5-y DFS		
Review 1970–1989						CMT	23%	-XRT	57%	Not randomized
								-CMT	90%	Univariable analysis
Heyning (1999)[161]	60	48	65	Intermediate	95%	XRT	8%	5-y		Heterogeneous treatment
Review 1943–1995	(localized 62%)					CMT	58%	PFS	46%	OS/PFS includes stage IV patients
						other	33%	OS	61%	

ChemoRx, chemotherapy, usually with anthracycline; CHOP, cyclophosphamide, doxorubicin, vincristine, prednisone; CMT, combined modality therapy; DSS, disease-specific survival; OS, overall survival; PFS, progression-free survival; OS, overall survival; WF, Working Formulation[103]; XRT, irradiation; y, years.

of developing thyroid lymphoma in patients with Hashimoto's thyroiditis is 40 to 80 times greater than that of the general population.[81]

The diagnosis of lymphoma of the thyroid is usually established by incisional biopsy or lobectomy, and does not require an extensive surgical resection. FNA is not sufficient for diagnosis, and frequently retrieves lymphocytes consistent only with a diagnosis of thyroiditis. A core biopsy is acceptable provided that the pathologist can unequivocally establish the diagnosis of malignancy as well as the particular subtype of lymphoma. At a minimum, this requires adequate tissue for light microscopy and immunohistochemistry. Molecular genetics and cytogenetic studies can refine the diagnosis in more challenging cases. It is important to obtain a representative sample of the lesion and correlate it with the clinical findings. For example, a diagnosis of an indolent lymphoma, such as a B-cell marginal zone lymphoma, is not compatible with a clinical picture of rapid growth and tissue infiltration, and should prompt additional biopsies.

Most thyroid lymphomas (about 80%) present with Stage I or II disease. When more extensive disease is present, it is usually part of a generalized process that sometimes includes other extranodal sites such as the GI tract.[78,82] Prior to the establishment of a malignant diagnosis, many patients will have had investigations including ultrasound and/or radioisotope scans. Ultrasound usually shows a solid mass in an enlarged gland, and can serve as a guide to the best region to biopsy. Most radioisotope scans show a cold nodule, although patchy background uptake can be seen. Although MRI can delineate soft tissue invasion better than CT, if combined modality treatment with chemotherapy is to be used, this superior resolution is not necessary.[83]

Over 80% of thyroid lymphomas are DLBCL, including its variants. Similar to the experience in general for DLBCL, the IPI can be applied to predict clinical outcome.[5] The second most common histology reported is the indolent B-cell marginal zone lymphoma, extranodal subtype, also known as MALToma (mucosa-associated lymphoid tissue lymphoma). MALTomas of the thyroid have a better prognosis than non-MALT lymphomas.[84] Several authors have reported an entity called "high-grade MALToma," which typically refers to an aggressive lymphoma resembling DLCL arising from background of MALToma. The demographics, histology, treatment, and outcomes for thyroid NHL from selected series in the literature are shown in Table 18–10.

There is an association between lymphoma of the thyroid and other extranodal sites of involvement.[82,85–87] In the setting of MALTomas, lymphocytes appear to "home" to certain tissues that include Waldeyer's ring, thyroid, and the GI tract. Although the predominant lymphoma of the thyroid gland is DLBCL, it is likely that some of these tumors arise from a background MALToma that has transformed to more aggressive disease.

The treatment of Stage I or II DLBCL of the thyroid is similar to that of nodal DLBCL of the same stage. Patients with localized disease should be given combined modality therapy, usually three cycles of CHOP plus rituximab followed by involved-region irradiation.[12,85] Prolonged chemotherapy for six to eight cycles is indicated for patients with more advanced disease including B symptoms, bulk of more than 10 cm, or Stage III or IV disease. For patients with localized MALT-type lymphomas of the thyroid, involved-field irradiation with doses from 35 to 45 Gy can achieve a 90% cause-specific survival at 5 years. This is the treatment of choice for radioencompassable indolent histology thyroid lymphomas. For more extensive or relapsed disease, treatment options include alkylators, such as chlorambucil or cyclophosphamide, fludarabine, or rituximab. It is important to anticipate that most patients treated with irradiation for lymphoma of the thyroid will become hypothyroid. Lifelong monitoring of the TSH level, and full replacement with thyroxin if the TSH becomes elevated, are necessary.

Lung

Primary B-cell pulmonary NHL is a heterogeneous entity including a spectrum of diseases ranging from indolent (marginal zone lymphoma, extranodal type, lymphoplasmacytic lymphoma, and small lymphocytic lymphoma) to aggressive disease (DLBCL). This section will only address the clinical scenario of lymphoma isolated to the lung, and not cases where the lung is involved as part of a widespread systemic process. Primary pulmonary lymphoma is uncommon. One Canadian series reported incidence of 1.1% of all extranodal presentations, which is slightly lower than the 4% that we have seen in British Columbia.[88]

The most common histologic type of primary pulmonary lymphoma is extranodal marginal zone B-cell lymphoma, which arises from bronchus-associated lymphoid tissue, a situation analogous to MALT in gastric tissue. There is currently no known infectious etiologic agent in this specific scenario, nor is there a definite correlation with an underlying autoimmune condition, although an association with Sjögren's syndrome and other autoimmune disorders has been reported.[38,89] It is likely that two previously occasionally diagnosed entities, pseudolymphoma and lymphocytic interstitial pneumonitis, were actually MALTomas. They are now only of historical interest. With refinement of pathologic techniques, including immunohistochemistry and molecular genetics, most cases thought to be one of these entities actually represent extranodal B-cell marginal zone lymphomas. The second most frequent NHL to involve the lung is DLBCL.

Many patients with primary pulmonary lymphoma are asymptomatic, and the disease is discovered incidentally on a chest radiograph done for other purposes. When patients have symptoms, they may include cough, dyspnea, hemoptysis, chest pain, or, rarely, wheezing due to diffuse submucosal infiltration causing airway narrowing. Constitutional symptoms are usually associated with more aggressive histology disease. The chest radiographs of patients with primary pulmonary lymphoma typically demonstrate a solitary frank consolidation nodule, mass, or infiltrate. In the minority of cases (<10%), multiple nodules or a diffuse alveolar or interstitial infiltrate is seen.[37,38,88,90,91] CT scan of the thorax can clarify the extent of the primary lesion and the presence of any extrapulmonary disease, such as involvement of chest wall, mediastinum, and nodes. Such extensive involvement is more common with DLBCL.[92,93] The diagnosis of primary pulmonary lymphoma requires an adequate biopsy specimen that is representative of the

Table 18–10. Overview of Recent Series in Literature Outlining Demographics, Histology, Therapy, and Outcome for Patients with Thyroid Non-Hodgkin's Lymphoma

Reference Study Type	Number	Median Age (y)	% Male	Histology		Treatment		Outcome		Comments
Ha (2001)[162] Retrospective review 1959–1994	51	59	35	WF intermediate or high grade	96%	Resection Resection + IRRT Biopsy and ChemoRx CMT	8% 35% 10% 47%	5-y OS FFS	 64% 76%	IPI predicted FFS and OS
Skacel (2000)[163] 18-year review	53 (90% localized)	66	28	DLBCL DLBCL + MALT MALT FL	51% 34% 6% 6%	IRRT ChemoRx CMT Surgery +CMT +IRRT +ChemoRx	21% 23% 24% 6% 4% 2%	5-y OS (a) DLBCL alone (b) DLBCL + MALT 5-y OS stage I	 75% 25% 100%	
Derringer (2000)[164] Review	108 (91% localized)	64	27	MALT DLBCL DLBCL + MALT FL	28% 38% 33% 1%	Surgery Excision + ChemoRx + IRRT + CMT	24% 15% 19% 42%	5-y DSS (a) Overall (b) MALT only	 79% 100%	Pre-existing lymphocytic thyroiditis in 94%. IPI predicts DSS
Pedersen (1996)[81] 1983–1991 population based	50 (76% localized)	73	20	DLBCL a) alone b) + MALT MALT	79% 36% 43% 17%	Not reported		5-y DSS OS	 46% 34%	Age > 66y Stage III confers poor prognosis
Matsuzuka (1993)[79] Retrospective review 1963–1990	119	60	28	WF intermediate or high grade	77%	IRRT CMT	26% 68%	8-y OS —In 16 pts given CHOP x 6 + IRRT —In 21 pts given CHOP x 2 + IRRT	100% 75%	68% Positive antimicrosomal antibodies
Tsang (1993)[85] Review 1978–1986	39	63	17	Diffuse (Histiocytic/mixed) Nodular	92% 8%	CMT ChemoRX IRRT	46% 8% 46%	5-y DSS OS	 73% 64%	
Logue (1992)[86] Retrospective review 1965–1983	70	67	11	Aggressive Indolent	95% 5%	IRRT	100%	5-y OS RFS	 49% 42%	Histologic Hashimoto's thyroiditis 66%

ChemoRx, chemotherapy, usually with anthracycline; CHOP, cyclophosphamide, doxorubicin, vincristine, prednisone; CMT, combined modality therapy; DSS, disease-specific survival; OS, overall survival; PFS, progression-free survival; OS, overall survival; WF, Working Formulation[103]; XRT, irradiation; y, years.

pathologic process. Although occasionally this can be achieved by bronchoscopy, bronchoalveolar lavage, and transbronchial biopsy, in most cases accurate diagnosis requires an open procedure. The staging work-up should include history and physical exam, blood tests, imaging studies, and bone marrow exam, as described in the introductory section. A common clinical finding in pulmonary MALT lymphoma is the presence of a monoclonal gammopathy in up to 40% of patients.[37,38]

An overview of recent series outlining the demographics, histology, therapy, and outcome for patients with primary pulmonary lymphoma is shown in Table 18–11.

Primary pulmonary NHL encompasses a number of different histologic subtypes, and the appropriate treatment depends primarily on the underlying histology. Other factors contributing to the treatment decision include the extent of the lymphomatous involvement, symptoms, and the patient's age and comorbid conditions. Indolent B-cell neoplasms account for the majority of cases in reported series of pulmonary lymphoma.[37,94,95] The majority are extranodal marginal zone lymphomas or MALTomas, but small lymphocytic, lymphoplasmacytic, and follicular lymphomas are also seen. Asymptomatic disease can be safely observed. If the disease is or becomes symptomatic, then systemic treatment with an alkylator such as chlorambucil or cyclophosphamide is a reasonable first choice. Options at further progression include a purine analogue such as fludarabine, rituximab or multiagent chemotherapy depending on clinical behavior and quality and duration of prior response to treatment. Although some investigators have reported very favorable outcomes with greater than 90% overall survival at 5 years,[37,96] others have recorded a 68% 5-year survival for this condition.[90] Because localized irradiation is seldom feasible for pulmonary lymphoma, the treatment of DLBCL of the lung should be the same as that used for advanced-stage DLBCL of any site: CHOP plus rituximab for six to eight cycles. With such treatment, the prognosis can be estimated by using the IPI.[5]

Salivary Glands and Parotid

Lymphomas of the salivary glands are rare tumors with a unique epidemiology. Typically, they are associated with an antecedent history of Sjögren's syndrome, the pathologic hallmark of which is lymphoid infiltration of the salivary gland or myoepithelial sialadenitis. It is postulated that chronic antigenic stimulation leads to development of a malignant B cell. Consistent with this hypothesis, the most common histology is extranodal marginal zone B-cell lymphoma or MALToma. Patients typically present with a painless salivary gland mass. In over 80% of cases, the parotid gland is the primary site of involvement.

Other histologies, including follicular lymphoma and DLBCL, can involve the salivary glands, but it is often difficult in these cases to determine whether the disease arose from a lymph node embedded within or adjacent to the gland that subsequently involved the salivary tissue or in the glandular tissue itself. This issue is academic, however, because the management of these tumors is not affected by this distinction. Those patients who present with limited-stage indolent B-cell lymphoma should be managed with involved-region irradiation. Those with symptomatic disease that is more extensive require systemic treatment appropriate for indolent disease. Patients with limited-stage DLBCL should receive combined modality therapy with brief chemotherapy, usually three cycles of CHOP plus rituximab and involved-region irradiation, while those with bulky or more extensive disease require a more prolonged course of systemic treatment.

Orbit

Primary malignant lymphomas of the orbital soft tissue account for about 10% of orbital tumors, and about 4% to 5% of all primary extranodal Stage I and II NHLs. Lymphomas of the extraocular orbital tissue are much more common than true intraocular lymphoma. The latter condition is an aggressive lymphoma often associated with primary CNS lymphoma, and is discussed further in Chapter 17C.

Orbital lymphomas typically arise from the conjunctiva, eyelids, lacrimal glands, or retro-orbital soft tissue. The usual conjunctival lesion appears as a salmon pink mass often associated with tearing, swelling, ptosis, or blurred vision. The retro-orbital soft tissue lesions can present with swelling, proptosis, and interference with extraocular movement causing diplopia. Only in cases where the optic nerve is involved is there visual impairment. Bilateral involvement, without other extranodal or nodal disease, is seen in at least 20% of cases. This pattern of spread implies a special relationship between the malignant B-lymphocytes and the microenvironment of the eye.

In the past, the majority of these localized orbital soft tissue lymphomas were classified as "pseudolymphoma," a term that reflected both the difficulty of making a definitive malignant diagnosis and the indolent nature of the condition. With the help of modern diagnostic tools, however, the vast majority of these malignancies are found to be indolent B-cell neoplasms. The histology most commonly diagnosed is mucosa-associated lymphoid tumor (MALT, now categorized as marginal zone lymphoma, extranodal type). Since chronic B-cell stimulation by infectious agents or autoimmune disorders is a common theme in the etiology of MALT lymphomas, it is not surprising that such stimuli may predispose to ocular lymphoma as well. Recently molecular evidence for an association between *Chlamydia psittaci* and ocular adnexal lymphoma has been demonstrated, but whether eradication of this organism can lead to regression of the lymphoma remains to be seen.[25,26] Other indolent NHLs such as small lymphocytic, lymphoplasmacytic, and follicular lymphomas, can present with exclusive orbital involvement. In about 10% of cases, the primary diagnosis is a more aggressive B-cell lymphoma such as DLBCL or mantle cell lymphoma.

Standard staging tests for lymphoma should be performed to rule out more disseminated disease, which is found approximately 15% to 20% of the time. In addition, detailed views of the periorbital structures should be obtained to document the local extent of disease and for radiation planning. CT and MRI scanning are equally capable of fully documenting the orbital disease for most patients. Occasionally, one or the other gives better delineation and that test should then be used for subsequent follow-up.

Table 18–11. Overview of Recent Series in Literature Outlining Demographics, Histology, Therapy, and Outcome for Patients with Primary Pulmonary Lymphoma

Reference Study Type	Number	Median Age (y)	% Male	Histology		Treatment		Outcome		Comments
Kurtin (2001)[38] Retrospective review 1979–1994	50	67	36	MALT DLBCL + MALT	82% 18%	Surgery alone ChemoRx Observation CMT	34% 24% 10% 8%	10-y LSS	72%	30% With associated autoimmune disorder
Cordier (1993)[37] Retrospective	70	58	50	Low grade High grade	87% 13%	Various including surgery, ChemoRX, CMT, XRT		5-y OS Low grade High grade	 94% 44%	
Ferraro (2000)[90] Retrospective	48	62	44	MALT Non-MALT	73% 27%	Complete resection Post-op ChemoRx XRT No adjuvant	40% 54% 4% 42%	5-y OS MALT Non MALT	 68% 65%	
Zinzani (2003)[91] 1992–2000	12 MALT only	61	60	MALT	100%	ChemoRx Resection CMT	67% 17% 16%	5-y OS RFS	 100% 75%	

ChemoRx, chemotherapy, usually with anthracycline; CMT, combined modality therapy; DLBCL, diffuse large B-cell lymphoma; LSS, lymphoma-specific survival; MALT, mucosa-associated lymphoid tissue; OS, overall survival; RFS, relapse-free survival; XRT, irradiation; y, years.

The treatment depends on the histology and extent of disease. For patients with indolent localized neoplasms irradiation is highly effective and potentially curative.[97–101] The dose can be kept in the 25-Gy to 30-Gy range to minimize the risks of cataract formation, xerophthalmia, and retinal damage.[102] Shielding of the lens also reduces the risk of cataract formation. After a complete response, the risk of locoregional relapse is very small. If the disease is more widespread at diagnosis or recurs after irradiation, or if the morbidity of irradiation is excessive, then treatment with systemic agents suitable for indolent B-cell lymphomas is indicated.[99]

The largest series of patients with periorbital lymphoma was reported by Bessell et al.[99] They described 115 patients seen between 1974 and 1980, of whom 89 had disease confined to the orbit. Five patients had bilateral disease. Ninety-one percent of patients had low-grade disease by the Working Formulation, and the remainder had intermediate- or high-grade lesions.[103] The median age of patients was 63 years and 53% were male. Ninety-five percent of patients were treated with orbital irradiation alone. The 5-year disease-free survival for patients with localized disease was 80% in the low-grade group, and 40% in those with more aggressive histology disease.

When the periorbital tissues are involved with diffuse large B-cell lymphoma, there is nothing unique about the natural history compared to presentation at other nodal or extranodal sites except when the orbital involvement is an extension of paranasal sinus presentation. Treatment should be based on the overall clinical picture, including the stage and bulk of disease, age, and overall condition of the patient. When the periorbital lymphoma also involves the paranasal sinuses, intrathecal chemotherapy to prevent CNS relapse should be added to the therapeutic regimen.

Extranodal B-Cell Lymphoma at Other Sites

Rarely, B-cell lymphomas can present at other sites than those mentioned above. Anecdotal case reports and small series have documented apparently localized lymphoma in such structures as the breast,[104–111] heart,[112–114] adrenal glands,[115–119] kidney,[120–122] ovary,[123–128] uterus,[129–131] prostate,[132–135] bladder,[136–141] pancreas,[142–144] and muscle.[145–151] As best can be determined from such limited experience localized lymphoma at any of these sites responds to treatment similarly to type- and stage-matched lymphomas presenting in nodal tissue. Indeed, the major challenge is diagnosis, not treatment. Once lymphoma is confirmed standard staging tests followed by stage- and type-directed treatments can be expected to cure the majority of patients with the same overall prognostic expectations as for localized lymphoma presenting in nodal tissue.

SUMMARY

The term "primary extranodal non-Hodgkin's lymphoma" encompasses a heterogeneous group of lymphomas, both indolent and aggressive, that may affect virtually any organ or tissue. It is relevant to consider these conditions unique from their nodal counterparts when special aspects of their etiology, pattern of spread, or pattern of relapse require a unique approach to their work-up, treatment, or follow-up. There are many special aspects of the natural history of extranodal lymphomas including a tendency toward bilateral involvement in paired organs or structures such the lungs, testicles, orbital soft tissue, and parotid glands; association with infectious agents as is seen with gastric and intestinal lymphoma; special patterns of recurrence such as spread to the CNS with paranasal sinus and testicular lymphomas; association with prior autoimmune disease as noted with thyroid and salivary gland lymphomas; and a wide spectrum of typical histologic types ranging from mostly MALT-type marginal zone lymphomas in lungs, stomach, periorbital, and pulmonary lymphomas to almost exclusively aggressive DLBCL in paranasal sinuses, bone, thyroid, and testicles. Careful consideration of these unique characteristics of extranodal lymphomas is necessary for their best management. With attention to these important differences from nodal lymphomas, most patients can be offered highly effective, often curative treatment.

REFERENCES

1. Zucca E, Roggero E, Bertoni F, et al. Primary extranodal non-Hodgkin's lymphomas. Part 2: Head and neck, central nervous system and other less common sites. Ann Oncol 1999;10:1023–33.
2. Zucca E, Roggero E, Bertoni F, et al. Primary extranodal non-Hodgkin's lymphomas. Part 1: Gastrointestinal, cutaneous and genitourinary lymphomas. Ann Oncol 1997;8:727–37.
3. Zucca E and Cavalli F. Extranodal lymphomas. Ann Oncol 2000;11(suppl 3):219–22.
4. Harris NL, Jaffe ES, Diebold J, et al. The World Health Organization classification of neoplastic diseases of the hematopoietic and lymphoid tissues. Report of the Clinical Advisory Committee meeting, Airlie House, Virginia, November, 1997. Ann Oncol 1999;10:1419–32.
5. The International Non-Hodgkin's Lymphoma Prognostic Factors Project. A predictive model for aggressive non-Hodgkin's lymphoma. 'sN Engl J Med 1993;329:987–94.
6. Zucca E, Conconi A, Mughal TI, et al. Patterns of outcome and prognostic factors in primary large-cell lymphoma of the testis in a survey by the International Extranodal Lymphoma Study Group. J Clin Oncol 2003;21:20–7.
7. Gurney KA, Cartwright RA, and Gilman EA. Descriptive epidemiology of gastrointestinal non-Hodgkin's lymphoma in a population-based registry. Br J Cancer 1999;79–:1929–34.
8. Doglioni C, Wotherspoon AC, and Moschini A. High incidence of primary gastric lymphoma in northeastern Italy. Lancet 1992;339:834–5.
9. Nakamura S, Matsumoto T, and Iida M. Primary gastrointestinal lymphoma in Japan: a clinicopathologic analysis of 455 patients with special reference to its time trends. Cancer 2003;97:2462–73.
10. Rohatiner A. Report on a workshop convened to discuss the pathological and staging classifications of gastrointestinal tract lymphoma. Ann Oncol 1994;5:397–400.
11. The Non-Hodgkin's Lymphoma Classification Project. A clinical evaluation of the International Lymphoma Study Group classification of non-Hodgkin's lymphoma. The Non-Hodgkin's Lymphoma Classification Project. Blood 1997;89:3909–18.
12. Miller TP, Dahlberg S, Cassady JR, et al. Chemotherapy alone compared with chemotherapy plus radiotherapy for localized intermediate- and high-grade non-Hodgkin's lymphoma. N Engl J Med 1998;339:21–6.

13. Chen MG, Prosnitz LR, and Gonzalez-Serva A. Results of radiotherapy in control of stage I and II non-Hodgkin's lymphoma. Cancer 1979;43:1245–54.
14. Hagberg H, Glimelius B, and Sundstrom C. Radiation therapy of non-Hodgkin's lymphoma stages I and II. Acta Radiol Oncol Radiat Ther Phys Biol 1982;21:145–50.
15. Kun LE, Cox JD, and Komaki R. Patterns of failure in treatment of stage I and II diffuse malignant lymphoid tumors. Radiology 1981;141:791–4.
16. Timothy AR, Lister TA, and Katz D. Localized non-Hodgkin's lymphoma. Eur J Cancer Clin Oncol 1980;16:799–807.
17. Lester JN, Fuller LM, Conrad FG, et al. The roles of staging laparotomy, chemotherapy, and radiotherapy in the management of localized diffuse large cell lymphoma: A study of 75 patients. Cancer 1982;49:1746–53.
18. Nissen NI, Ersboll J, Hansen HS, et al. A randomized study of radiotherapy versus radiotherapy plus chemotherapy in Stage I-II non-Hodgkin's lymphomas. Cancer 1983;52:1–7.
19. Sutcliffe SB, Gospodarowicz MK, Bush RS, et al. Role of radiation therapy in localized non-Hodgkin's lymphoma. Radiother Oncol 1985;4:211–23.
20. Shenkier TN, Voss N, Fairey R, et al. Brief chemotherapy and involved-region irradiation for limited-stage diffuse large-cell lymphoma: an 18-year experience from the British Columbia Cancer Agency. J Clin Oncol 2002;20:197–204.
21. Coiffier B, Lepage E, Briere J, et al. CHOP Chemotherapy plus rituximab compared with CHOP alone in elderly patients with diffuse large-B-cell lymphoma. N Engl J Med 2002;346:235–42.
22. Sehn L, Donaldson J, Chhanabhai M, et al. Introduction of combined CHOP-rituximab therapy dramatically improved outcome of diffuse large B-cell lymphoma (DLBCL) in British Columbia. J Clin Oncol 2005;23:5027–33.
23. Marcus KC, Imrie K, Belch A, et al. An international multicentre, randomized, open-lable, Phase III trial comparing Rituximab added to CVP chemotherapy to CVP chemotherapy alone in untreated stage III/IV follicular non-Hodgkin's lymphoma. Blood 2003;102[abstract]:902a-3a.
24. Lecuit M, Abachin E, Martin A, Poyart C, et al. Immunoproliferative Small Intestinal Disease Associated with Campylobacter jejuni. N Engl J Med 2004;350:239–48.
25. Ferreri AJ, Guidoboni M, Ponzoni M, et al. Evidence for association between chlamydia psitacci infection and ocular adnexal lymphoma (OAL). J Natl Cancer Inst 2004:96(8): 586–94.
26. Lietman T, Brooks D, and Moncada J. Chronic follicular conjunctivitis associated with Chlamydia psittaci or Chlamydia pneumoniae. Clin Infect Dis 1998;26:1335–40.
27. Cerroni L, Zochling N, and Putz B. Infection by Borrelia burgdorferi and cutaneous B-cell lymphoma. J Cutan Pathol 1997;24:457–61.
28. Li C, Inagaki H, and Kuo TT. Primary cutaneous marginal zone B-cell lymphoma: a molecular and clinicopathologic study of 24 Asian cases. Am J Surg Pathol 2003;27: 1061–9.
29. de la Fouchardiere A, Vandenesch F, and Berger F. Borrelia-associated primary cutaneous MALT lymphoma in a nonendemic region. Am J Surg Pathol 2003;27:702–3.
30. Roggero E, Zucca E, Mainetti C, et al. Eradication of Borrelia burgdorferi infection in primary marginal zone B-cell lymphoma of the skin. Hum Pathol 2000;31:263–8.
31. Conconi A, Martinelli G, Thieblemont C, et al. Clinical activity of rituximab in extranodal marginal zone B-cell lymphoma of MALT type. Blood 2003;102:2741–5.
32. Maloney DG, Grillo-Lopez AJ, White CA, et al. IDEC-C2B8 (Rituximab) anti-CD20 monoclonal antibody therapy in patients with relapsed low-grade non-Hodgkin's lymphoma. Blood 1997;90:2188–95.
33. Witzig TE, Gordon LI, Cabanillas F, et al. Randomized controlled trial of yttrium-90–labeled ibritumomab tiuxetan radioimmunotherapy versus rituximab immunotherapy for patients with relapsed or refractory low-grade, follicular, or transformed B-cell non-Hodgkin's lymphoma. J Clin Oncol 2002;20:2453–63.
34. Cheson BD, Horning SJ, Coiffier B, et al. Report of an international workshop to standardize response criteria for non-Hodgkin's lymphomas. J Clin Oncol 1999;17:1244.
35. Blade J and Kyle R. Monoclonal gammopathies of undetermined significance. In: Malpas JS, Kyle RA, Anderson KC, et al., eds. Myeloma Biology and Management, 2nd ed. New York: Oxford University Press, 1998:528–30.
36. Price SK. Immunoproliferative small intestinal disease: a study of 13 cases with alpha heavy-chain disease. Histopathology 1990;17:7–17.
37. Cordier J, Chailleux E, Lauque D, et al. Primary pulmonary lymphomas. A clinical study of 70 cases in nonimmunocompromised patients. Chest 1993;103:201–8.
38. Kurtin PJ, Myers JL, Adlakha H, et al. Pathologic and clinical features of primary pulmonary extranodal marginal zone B-cell lymphoma of MALT type. Am J Surg Pathol 2001; 25:997–1008.
39. Sackmann M, Morgner A, Rudolph B, Neubauer A, Thiede C, Schulz H, et al. Regression of gastric MALT lymphoma after eradication of Helicobacter pylori is predicted by endosonographic staging. MALT Lymphoma Study Group. Gastroenterology 1997;113(4):1087–90.
40. Thieblemont C, Berger F, Dumontet C, et al. Mucosa-associated lymphoid tissue lymphoma is a disseminated disease in one third of 158 patients analyzed. Blood 2000;95:802–6.
41. McGuigan JE. Helicobacter pylori: the versatile pathogen. Dig Dis 1996;14:289–303.
42. Bayerdorffer E, Neubauer A, Rudolph B, et al. Regression of primary gastric lymphoma of mucosa-associated lymphoid tissue type after cure of Helicobacter pylori infection. MALT Lymphoma Study Group. Lancet 1995;345:1591–4.
43. Isaacson PG and Spencer J. Gastric lymphoma and Helicobacter pylori. Important Adv Oncol 1996;111–21.
44. Roggero E, Zucca E, Pinotti G, et al. Eradication of Helicobacter pylori infection in primary low-grade gastric lymphoma of mucosa-associated lymphoid tissue. Ann Intern Med 1995;122:767–9.
45. Wotherspoon AC, Doglioni C, Diss TC, et al. Regression of primary low-grade B-cell gastric lymphoma of mucosa-associated lymphoid tissue type after eradication of Helicobacter pylori. Lancet 1993;342:575–7.
46. Nakamura S, Yao T, Aoyagi K, et al. Helicobacter pylori and primary gastric lymphoma. A histopathologic and immunohistochemical analysis of 237 patients. Cancer 1997;79:3–11.
47. Savio A, Franzin G, Wotherspoon AC, et al. Diagnosis and posttreatment follow-up of Helicobacter pylori-positive gastric lymphoma of mucosa-associated lymphoid tissue: histology, polymerase chain reaction, or both? Blood 1996;87:1255–60.
48. Isaacson PG. Primary gastric lymphoma. Br J Biomed Sci 1995;52:291–6.
49. Pinotti G, Zucca E, Roggero E, et al. Clinical features, treatment and outcome in a series of 93 patients with low-grade gastric MALT lymphoma. Leuk Lymphoma 1997;26:527–37.
50. Steinbach G, Ford R, Glober G, et al. Antibiotic treatment of gastric lymphoma of mucosa-associated lymphoid tissue. An uncontrolled trial. Ann Intern Med 1999;131:88–95.
51. Bertoni F, Conconi A, Capella C, et al. Molecular follow-up in gastric mucosa-associated lymphoid tissue lymphomas: early analysis of the LY03 cooperative trial. Blood 2002; 99:2541–4.

52. Neubauer A, Thiede C, Morgner A, et al. Cure of Helicobacter pylori infection and duration of remission of low-grade gastric mucosa-associated lymphoid tissue lymphoma. J Natl Cancer Inst 1997;89:1350–5.
53. Coiffier B and Salles G. Does surgery belong to medical history for gastric lymphomas? [comment]. Ann Oncol 1997;8:419–21.
54. Shchepotin IB, Evans SR, Shabahang M, et al. Primary non-Hodgkin's lymphoma of the stomach: three radical modalities of treatment in 75 patients. Ann Surg Oncol 1996; 3:277–84.
55. Rabbi C, Aitini E, Cavazzini G, et al. Stomach preservation in low- and high-grade primary gastric lymphomas: preliminary results. Haematologica 1996;81:15–9.
56. Ernst M, Stein H, Ludwig D, et al. Surgical therapy of gastrointestinal non-Hodgkin's lymphomas. Eur J Surg Oncol 1996;22:177–81.
57. Haim N, Leviov M, Ben-Arieh Y, et al. Intermediate and high-grade gastric non-Hodgkin's lymphoma: a prospective study of non-surgical treatment with primary chemotherapy, with or without radiotherapy. Leuk Lymphoma 1995;17–:321–6.
58. Tedeschi L, Romanelli A, Dallavalle G, et al. Stages I and II non-Hodgkin's lymphoma of the gastrointestinal tract. Retrospective analysis of 79 patients and review of the literature. J Clin Gastroenterol 1994;18:99–104.
59. Bozzetti F, Audisio RA, Giardini R, et al. Role of surgery in patients with primary non-Hodgkin's lymphoma of the stomach: an old problem revisited. Br J Surg 1993;80: 1101–6.
60. Thirlby RC. Gastrointestinal lymphoma: a surgical perspective. Oncology (Huntingt) 1993;7:29–32, 34;discussion 34, 37–8.
61. Taal BG, Burgers JM, van Heerde P, et al. The clinical spectrum and treatment of primary non-Hodgkin's lymphoma of the stomach [see comments]. Ann Oncol 1993;4:839–46.
62. Tondini C, Giardini R, Bozzetti F, et al. Combined modality treatment for primary gastrointestinal non-Hodgkin's lymphoma: the Milan Cancer Institute experience. Ann Oncol 1993;4:831–7.
63. Cortelazzo S, Rossi A, Roggero E, et al. Stage-modified international prognostic index effectively predicts clinical outcome of localized primary gastric diffuse large B-cell lymphoma. Ann Oncol 1999;10:1433–1440.
64. Domizio P, Owen RA, Shepherd NA, et al. Primary lymphoma of the small intestine. A clinicopathological study of 119 cases. Am J Surg Pathol 1993;17:429–42.
65. Radaszkiewicz T, Dragosics B, and Bauer P. Gastrointestinal malignant lymphomas of the mucosa-associated lymphoid tissue: factors relevant to prognosis. Gastroenterology 1992;102:1628–38.
66. Kohno S, Ohshima K, Yoneda S, et al. Clinicopathological analysis of 143 primary malignant lymphomas in the small and large intestines based on the new WHO classification. Histopathology 2003;43:135–43.
67. Daum S, Ullrich R, Heise W, et al. Intestinal non-Hodgkin's lymphoma: a multicenter prospective clinical study from the German Study Group on Intestinal non-Hodgkin's Lymphoma J Clin Oncol 2003;21:2740–6.
68. Ibrahim EM, Ezzat AA, El-Weshi AN, et al. Primary intestinal diffuse large B-cell non-Hodgkin's lymphoma clinical features, management, and prognosis of 66 patients. Ann Oncol 2001;12:53–58.
69. Johnson CD, Kent DM, Varjabedian GC, et al. Malignant lymphoma of the maxillary sinus. J Am Osteopath Assoc 1993;93:252, 255–8.
70. Juman S, Robinson P, Balkissoon A, et al. B-cell non-Hodgkin's lymphoma of the paranasal sinuses. J Laryngol Otol 1994;108:263–5.
71. Laskin J, Savage KJ, Gascoyne RD, et al. Primary paranasal sinus lymphoma: natural history and improved outcome with central nervous system chemoprophylaxis. Cancer 2005 (in press).
72. Connors JM. Problems in lymphoma management: special sites of presentation. Oncology (Huntingt) 1998;12: 185–91;discussion 192–5.
73. Saul SH and Kapadia SB. Primary lymphoma of Waldeyer's ring. Clinicopathologic study of 68 cases. Cancer 1985; 56:157–66.
74. Hoppe RT, Burke JS, Glatstein E, et al. Non-Hodgkin's lymphoma: involvement of Waldeyer's ring. Cancer 1978;42: 1096–104.
75. Aviles A, Delgado S, Ruiz H, et al. Treatment of non-Hodgkin's lymphoma of Waldeyer's ring: radiotherapy versus chemotherapy versus combined therapy. Eur J Cancer B Oral Oncol 1996;32B:19–23.
76. Bertoni F, Sanna P, Tinguely M, et al. Association of gastric and Waldeyer's ring lymphoma: a molecular study. Hematol Oncol 2000;18:15–9.
77. Dubey P, Ha CS, Besa PC, et al. Localized primary malignant lymphoma of bone. Int J Radiat Oncol Biol Phys 1997;37: 1087–1093.
78. Anscombe AM and Wright DH. Primary malignant lymphoma of the thyroid—a tumour of mucosa-associated lymphoid tissue: review of seventy-six cases. Histopathology 1985;9:81–97.
79. Matsuzuka F, Miyauchi A, Katayama S, et al. Clinical aspects of primary thyroid lymphoma: diagnosis and treatment based on our experience of 119 cases. Thyroid 1993;3:93–9.
80. Limanova Z, Neuwirtova R, and Smejkal V. Malignant lymphoma of the thyroid. Exp Clin Endocrinol 1987;90:113–9.
81. Pedersen RK and Pedersen NT. Primary non-Hodgkin's lymphoma of the thyroid gland: a population based study. Histopathology 1996;28:25–32.
82. McDermott EW, Cassidy N, and Heffernan SJ. Perforation through undiagnosed small bowel involvement in primary thyroid lymphoma during chemotherapy. Cancer 1992; 69:572–3.
83. Takashima S, Nomura N, Noguchi Y, et al. Primary thyroid lymphoma: evaluation with US, CT, and MRI. J Comput Assist Tomogr 1995;19:282–8.
84. Laing RW, Hoskin P, Hudson BV, et al. The significance of MALT histology in thyroid lymphoma: a review of patients from the BNLI and Royal Marsden Hospital. Clin Oncol (R Coll Radiol) 1994;6:300–4.
85. Tsang RW, Gospodarowicz MK, Sutcliffe SB, et al. Non-Hodgkin's lymphoma of the thyroid gland: prognostic factors and treatment outcome. Int J Radiat Oncol Biol Phys 1993;27:599–604.
86. Logue JP, Hale RJ, Stewart AL, et al. Primary malignant lymphoma of the thyroid: a clinicopathological analysis. Int J Radiat Oncol Biol Phys 1992;22:929–33.
87. Isaacson PG and Spencer J. Malignant lymphoma of mucosa-associated lymphoid tissue. Histopathology 1987;11:445–62.
88. Sutcliffe SB and Gospodarowicz MK. Localized extranodal lymphomas. In: Keating A, Burnett A, Newland A, eds. Haematological Oncology. Cambridge: Cambridge Medical Reviews, 1992:189–222.
89. Hansen LA, Prakash UB, and Colby TV. Pulmonary lymphoma in Sjögren's syndrome. Mayo Clin Proc 1989; 64:920–31.
90. Ferraro P, Trastek VF, Adlakha H, et al. Primary non-Hodgkin's lymphoma of the lung. Ann Thorac Surg 2000;69:993–7.
91. Zinzani PL, Tani M, Gabriele A, et al. Extranodal marginal zone B-cell lymphoma of MALT-type of the lung: single-center experience with 12 patients. Leuk Lymphoma 2003; 44:821–4.

92. Lewis ER, Caskey CI, and Fishman EK. Lymphoma of the lung: CT findings in 31 patients. Am J Roentgenol 1991; 156:711–4.
93. Khoury MB, Godwin JD, and Halvorson SJ. Role of chest CT in non-Hodgkin lymphoma. Radiology 1986;158:659–62.
94. Li G, Hansmann ML, Zwingers T, et al. Primary lymphomas of the lung: morphological, immunohistochemical and clinical features. Histopathology 1990;16:519–31.
95. Fiche M, Caprons F, Berger F, et al. Primary pulmonary non-Hodgkin's lymphomas. Histopathology 1995;26:529–37.
96. Zucca E, Conconi A, Pedrinis E, et al. Nongastric marginal zone B-cell lymphoma of mucosa-associated lymphoid tissue. Blood 2003;101:2489–95.
97. Smitt MC and Donaldson SS. Radiotherapy is successful treatment for orbital lymphoma. Int J Radiat Oncol Biol Phys 1993;26:59–66.
98. Esik O, Ikeda H, Mukai K, et al. A retrospective analysis of different modalities for treatment of primary orbital non-Hodgkin's lymphomas. Radiother Oncol 1996;38:13–8.
99. Bessell EM, Henk JM, Wright JE, et al. Orbital and conjunctival lymphoma treatment and prognosis. Radiother Oncol 1988;13:237–44.
100. Chao CK, Lin HS, Devineni VR, et al. Radiation therapy for primary orbital lymphoma. Int J Radiat Oncol Biol Phys 1995;31:929–34.
101. Minehan KJ, Martenson JA Jr, Garrity JA, et al. Local control and complications after radiation therapy for primary orbital lymphoma: a case for low-dose treatment. Int J Radiat Oncol Biol Phys 1991;20:791–6.
102. Bessell EM, Henk JM, Whitelocke RA, et al. Ocular morbidity after radiotherapy of orbital and conjunctival lymphoma. Eye 1987;1:90–6.
103. The Non-Hodgkin's Lymphoma Pathologic Classification Project. National Cancer Institute sponsored study of classifications of non-Hodgkin's lymphomas: summary and description of a working formulation for clinical usage. Cancer 1982;49:2112–35.
104. Park YH, Kim SH, Choi SJ, et al. Primary malignant lymphoma of the breast: clinicopathological study of nine cases. Leuk Lymphoma 2004;45:327–30.
105. Oksuzoglu B, Er O, Guler M, et al. Disseminated high-grade malignant lymphoma involving both breasts. Breast 2002;11:454–6.
106. Martinelli B, Giardina G, and Pinotti G. Primary breast lymphomas a review of the literature and report of four cases. Int J Med Biol Environ 2001;29:173–178.
107. Ribrag V, Bibeau F, El Weshi A, et al. Primary breast lymphoma: a report of 20 cases. Br J Haematol 2001;115:253–6.
108. Babovic N, Jelic S, and Jovanovic V. Primary non-Hodgkin lymphoma of the breast. Is it possible to avoid mastectomy? J Exp Clin Cancer Res 2000;19:149–154.
109. Arber DA, Simpson JF, Weiss LM, et al. Non-Hodgkin's lymphoma involving the breast. Am J Surg Pathol 1994;18:288–95.
110. Ho Jong J, Akagi T, Hoshida Y, et al. Primary non-Hodgkin malignant lymphoma of the breast: an immunohistochemical study of seven patients and literature review of 152 patients with breast lymphoma in Japan. Cancer 1992;70:2451–9.
111. Cohen PL and Brooks JJ. Lymphomas of the breast. A clinicopathologic and immunohistochemical study of primary and secondary cases. Cancer 1991;67:1359–69.
112. Chalabreysse L, Berger F, Loire R, et al. Primary cardiac lymphoma in immunocompetent patients: a report of three cases and review of the literature. Virchows Archiv 2002; 441:456–61.
113. Cohen Y, Daas N, Libster D, et al. Large B-cell lymphoma manifesting as an invasive cardiac mass: sustained local remission after combination of methotrexate and rituximab. Leuk Lymphoma 2002;43:1485–7.
114. Delmas-Marsalet B, Molinie V, Jary L, et al. Cardiac localization of non-Hodgkin's lymphoma: two case reports and review of the literature. Nouv Rev Franc Hematol 1995; 37:223–30.
115. Grigg AP and Connors JM. Primary adrenal lymphoma. Clin Lymphoma 2003;4:154–60.
116. Singh D, Kumar L, Sharma A, et al. Adrenal involvement in non-Hodgkin's lymphoma: four cases and review of the literature. Leuk Lymphoma 2004;45:789–94.
117. Xu A, Xiao X, Ye L, et al. Primary adrenal lymphoma. Leuk Lymphoma 2003;44:739–40.
118. Hahn JS, Choi HS, Suh CO, et al. A case of primary bilateral adrenal lymphoma (PAL) with central nervous system (CNS) involvement. Yonsei Med J 2002;43:385–90.
119. Al-Fiar FZ, Pantalony D, and Shepherd F. Primary bilateral adrenal lymphoma. Leuk Lymphoma 1997;27–:543–9.
120. Okuno SH, Hoyer JD, Ristow K, et al. Primary renal non-Hodgkin's lymphoma: an unusual extranodal site. Cancer 1995;75:2258–61.
121. Malbrain M, Lambrecht GLY, Daelemans R, et al. Acute renal failure due to bilateral lymphomatous infiltrates—primary extranodal non-Hodgkin's lymphoma (p-EN-NHL) of the kidneys: does it really exist? Clin Nephrol 1994;42:163–9.
122. Richards MA, Mootoosamy I, Reznek RH, et al. Renal involvement in patients with non-Hodgkin's lymphoma: clinical and pathological features in 23 cases. Hematol Oncol 1990;8:105–10.
123. Ambulkar I and Nair R. Primary ovarian lymphoma: report of cases and review of literature. Leuk Lymphoma 2003;44:825–7.
124. Abduljabbar H, Ghazzawi MB, and El-Hosseiny M. Primary ovarian lymphoma in pregnancy: a case report. Ann Saudi Med 1990;10:453–6.
125. Niitsu N, Nakamine H, Hayama M, et al. Ovarian follicular lymphoma: a case report and review of the literature. Ann Hematol 2002;81:654–8.
126. Mansouri H, Sifat H, Gaye M, et al. Primary malignant lymphoma of the ovary: an unusual presentation of a rare disease. Eur J Gynaecol Oncol 2000;21:616–8.
127. Dao AH. Malignant lymphoma of the ovary: report of a case successfully managed with surgery and chemotherapy. Gynecol Oncol 1998;70:137–40.
128. Skodras G, Fields V, and Kragel PJ. Ovarian lymphoma and serous carcinoma of low malignant potential arising in the same ovary: a case report with literature review of 14 primary ovarian lymphomas. Arch Pathol Lab Med 1994;118: 647–50.
129. Latteri MA, Cipolla C, Gebbia V, et al. Primary extranodal non-Hodgkin lymphomas of the uterus and the breast: report of three cases. Eur J Surg Oncol 1995;21:432–4.
130. Aozasa K, Saeki K, Ohsawa M, et al. Malignant lymphoma of the uterus: report of seven cases with immunohistochemical study. Cancer 1959;72:1959–64.
131. Matsuyama T, Tsukamoto N, Kaku T, et al. Primary malignant lymphoma of the uterine corpus and cervix. Report of a case with immunocytochemical analysis. Acta Cytol 1989;33:228–32.
132. Jhavar S, Agarwal JP, Naresh KN, et al. Primary extranodal mucosa associated lymphoid tissue (MALT) lymphoma of the prostate. Leuk Lymphoma 2001;41–:445–9.
133. Bostwick DG, Iczkowski KA, Amin MB, et al. Malignant lymphoma involving the prostate: report of 62 cases. Cancer 1998;83:732–8.
134. Bell CRW, Napier MP, Morgan RJ, et al. Primary non-Hodgkin's lymphoma of the prostate gland: case report and review of the literature. Clin Oncol 1995;7:409–10.

135. Patel DR, Gomez GA, Henderson ES, et al. Primary prostatic involvement in non-Hodgkin lymphoma. Urology 1988;32:96–8.
136. Coskun U, Gunel N, Eroglu A, et al. Primary high grade malignant lymphoma of bladder. Urol Oncol 2002;7:181–3.
137. Oscier D, Bramble J, Hodges E, et al. Regression of mucosa-associated lymphoid tissue lymphoma of the bladder after antibiotic therapy [5]. J Clin Oncol 2002;20.
138. Power RE, Kay EW, O'Connell F, et al. Primary lymphoma of the bladder: a report of three cases. Ir J Med Sci 2001;170: 196–7.
139. Al-Maghrabi J, Kamel-Reid S, Jewett M, et al. Primary low-grade B-cell lymphoma of mucosa-associated lymphoid tissue type arising in the urinary bladder: report of 4 cases with molecular genetic analysis. Arch Pathol Lab Med 2001;125:332–6.
140. Kempton CL, Kurtin PJ, Inwards DJ, et al. Malignant lymphoma of the bladder: evidence from 36 cases that low-grade lymphoma of the malt-type is the most common primary bladder lymphoma. Am J Surg Pathol 1997;21: 1324–33.
141. Ohsawa M, Aozasa K, Horiuchi K, et al. Malignant lymphoma of bladder: report of three cases and review of the literature. Cancer 1969;72:1969–74.
142. Arranz Arija F, Arizcun Sanchez-Morate AJ, Martin Serradilla JI, et al. Pancreas lymphoma. Report of a case [Spanish]. Oncologia 2003;26:49–52.
143. Soria MT, Gines A, Miquel R, et al. Follow-up of a large-B-cell pancreatic lymphoma by endoscopic ultrasonography. Endoscopy 2003;35:360–2.
144. Nishimura R, Takakuwa T, Hoshida Y, et al. Primary pancreatic lymphoma: clinicopathological analysis of 19 cases from Japan and review of the literature. Oncology 2001;60: 322–9.
145. Bertoni F, Sanna P, Zucca E, et al. Primary extranodal lymphoma of skeletal muscles: a report of four cases. Oncol Rep 1998;5:605–7.
146. Hatori Y, Sato H, and Adachi E. A case of MALT lymphoma originated from the medial rectus muscle [Japanese]. Neuro Ophthalmol Jpn 2003;20:191–6.
147. Chim CS, Choy C, and Liang R. Primary anaplastic large cell lymphoma of skeletal muscle presenting with compartment syndrome. Leuk Lymphoma 1999;33–:601–5.
148. Lee VS, Martinez S, and Coleman RE. Primary muscle lymphoma: clinical and imaging findings. Radiology 1997;203: 237–44.
149. Beggs I. Primary muscle lymphoma. Clin Radiol 1997;52: 203–12.
150. Keung YK and Liang R. Report of a case of primary skeletal muscle lymphoma and review of the literature. Acta Haematol 1996;96:184–6.
151. Eustace S, Winalski CS, McGowen A, et al. Skeletal muscle lymphoma: observations at MR imaging. Skeletal Radiol 1996;25:425–30.
152. Liang R, Todd D, Chan TK, et al. Prognostic factors for primary gastrointestinal lymphoma. Hematol Oncol 1995;13:153–63.
153. Ibrahim EM, Ezzat AA, Raja MA, et al. Primary gastric non-Hodgkin's lymphoma: clinical features, management, and prognosis of 185 patients with diffuse large B-cell lymphoma. Ann Oncol 1999;10:1441–9.
154. Nakamura S, Matsumoto T, Takeshita M, et al. A clinicopathologic study of primary small intestine lymphoma: prognostic significance of mucosa-associated lymphoid tissue-derived lymphoma. Cancer 2000;88:286–94.
155. Krol AD, Le Cessie S, Snijder S, et al. Waldeyer's ring lymphomas: a clinical study from the Comprehensive Cancer Center West population based NHL registry. Leuk Lymphoma 2001;42:1005–13.
156. Ezzat AA, Ibrahim EM, El Weshi AN, et al. Localized non-Hodgkin's lymphoma of Waldeyer's ring: clinical features, management, and prognosis of 130 adult patients. Head & Neck 2001;23:547–58.
157. Harabuchi Y, Tsubota H, Ohguro S, et al. Prognostic factors and treatment outcome in non-Hodgkin's lymphoma of Waldeyer's ring. Acta Oncol 1997;36:413–20.
158. Liang R, Chiu E, Todd D, et al. Combined chemotherapy and radiotherapy for lymphomas of Waldeyer's ring. Oncology 1991;48:362–4.
159. Baar J, Burkes RL, and Gospodarowicz M. Primary non-Hodgkin's lymphoma of bone. Semin Oncol 1999;26:270–5.
160. Fairbanks RK, Bonner JA, Inwards CY, et al. Treatment of stage IE primary lymphoma of bone. Int J Radiat Oncol Biol Phys 1994;28:363–72.
161. Heyning FH, Hogendoorn PCW, Kramer MHH, et al. Primary non-Hodgkin's lymphoma of bone: a clinicopathological investigation of 60 cases. Leukemia 1999;13:2094–8.
162. Ha CS, Shadle KM, Medeiros LJ, et al. Localized non-Hodgkin lymphoma involving the thyroid gland. Cancer 2001;91:629–35.
163. Skacel M, Ross CW, and Hsi ED. A reassessment of primary thyroid lymphoma: high-grade MALT-type lymphoma as a distinct subtype of diffuse large B-cell lymphoma. Histopathology 2000;37:10–8.
164. Derringer GA, Thompson LDR, Frommelt RA, et al. Malignant lymphoma of the thyroid gland: a clinicopathologic study of 108 cases. Am J Surg Pathol 2000;24:623–39.

19

Follicular Lymphoma

Ama Z. Rohatiner, M.D., F.R.C.P.
Andrew Davies, B.Sc., B.M., M.R.C.P.
Silvia Montoto, M.D.
T. Andrew Lister, M.D., F.R.C.P., F.R.C.Path.

Follicular lymphoma (FL) is the second most common B-cell lymphoma in the World Health Organization (WHO) classification and the most prevalent of the so-called "indolent" lymphomas, occurring with a frequency of approximately 2/100,000 in the Western world.[1] There is a notable variation in incidence, depending on geographical area, with the illness occurring less frequently in Asia and in developing countries than in Western Europe and the United States.[2] Moreover, the risk of developing FL has been reported to be lower in first-generation immigrants from Japan and China to the United States than for subsequent generations.[3]

The etiology of the illness is unknown, although much has recently been discovered about the molecular events culminating in its development, the nonrandom chromosomal translocation resulting in over expression of bcl-2 being critical. Interestingly, the frequency of the BLC2 translocation is lower in FLs occurring in Asian patients than that in Caucasians who develop FL in the West.[4] This may have relevance for the pathogenesis of the illness since the incidence of the BLC2 rearrangement has been reported to be the same among normal individuals from Asian countries as compared to those in the West.[4]

Therapeutic innovations, based in part on increased understanding of pathogenesis, have raised the possibility that it may shortly become curable as opposed to treatable: proof is awaited.

PATHOLOGY AND PATHOGENESIS

Morphology

Follicular lymphoma is a B-cell malignancy of follicle center cells, with at least a partial follicular growth pattern. Two principal cell types, present in normal follicle centers are involved. The centrocyte (small cleaved cell) is the predominant cell type, with centroblasts (large non-cleaved cells) present in variable numbers and typically in the minority. The neoplastic follicles are closely packed, effacing the nodal architecture, and are poorly defined. Lying between the follicles are areas of neoplastic cells with varying degrees of sclerosis. The WHO classification of FL[1] recommends histologic grading based on the cell counting method of Mann and Berard.[5] Diffuse areas of centrocytes and centroblasts may also be observed and the WHO has recommended that the degree of follicularity be described as follows: more than 75% follicular, 25% to 75% follicular, or less than 25% minimally follicular. Monocytoid B cells may also be present and may impact on prognosis,[6] and plasmacytoid differentiation may be seen with a dense meshwork of dendritic cells within the follicles. Grade 3 FL is heterogeneous and subclassified into 3a, where centrocytes are preserved among centroblasts, and 3b, where sheets of centroblasts are present. Differing antigen profiles and genomic changes suggest that such a distinction is biologically relevant, with 3a more akin to Grades 1 and 2 FL, and 3b similar to diffuse large B-cell (DLBC) lymphoma.[7]

This histologic pattern has been well documented to change with the passage of time and clinical progression. There may be an increase in the proportion of centroblasts, the follicular pattern being retained; there may be loss of the follicular pattern, the cellular morphology being unchanged, or there may be frank transformation to DLBC lymphoma (or much less frequently to lymphoblastic lymphoma).

Transformation, apparently successfully treated, may be followed by "reversion" to FL.[8] Both progression and transformation are associated with increasing cytogenetic and molecular abnormalities, without an absolutely consistent pattern (see below).

Two distinct variants of FL are described in the WHO classification[1]: primary cutaneous FL and diffuse FL. In the former, although a partially follicular pattern comprising both centrocytes and centroblasts is observed, these cells are typically BCL2-negative. The diffuse variant lacks recognizable follicular structures, and consists largely of centrocytes with some centroblasts in an entirely diffuse pattern. The neoplastic cells have the phenotypic features of FL cells.

Immunophenotype

The malignant cells express pan B-cell markers (CD19, CD20, CD22, and CD79a), and surface immunoglobulin (most commonly IgM).[1] CD10 is variably expressed, and appears to be less frequently expressed in those with higher histologic grade.[9] Conversely, *BLC6* is more frequently detected in the higher histologic Grade 3.[7] CD5 is negative, and CD43 only present in Grade 3.[10] *BLC2* is expressed in the majority of cases.[11,12] A meshwork of CD21 and CD23 positive follicular dendritic cells is also identified.[1]

Molecular and Cytogenetic Changes

The malignant cells have rearranged immunoglobulin genes, consistent with the postulated germinal center cell counterpart; this is readily detectable by polymerase chain reaction (PCR). Furthermore, consistent with their derivation from the germinal center, ongoing somatic hypermutation is observed in neoplastic cells with extensive diversity developing within some clones.[13,14] At the time of disease progression and transformation, longitudinal analysis of VDJ arrangement indicates a common origin for both follicular and transformed lymphoma.[15–18]

The t(14:18) Chromosomal Translocation

The t(14;18)(q32:q21) translocation is observed in 85% of cases of FL,[19,20] but is usually not the sole abnormality. Indeed the average number of cytogenetic abnormalities at presentation is six.[21] Common with other translocations in B-cell lymphomas, the Ig gene locus is juxtaposed with a proto-oncogene. Cloning of the translocation led to the identification of the BLC2 gene at 18q21.[22] The entire coding region of BLC2 is coupled to one of the IgH joining segments (J_H) on chromosome 14, the breakpoint lying either within the 3′ noncoding region of BLC2, the third exon, or 3′ to the gene. The result is transcription and ultimate translation of non-disrupted BLC2. The breakpoints on chromosome 18 are clustered in two main regions. The major breakpoint region (MBR) lies within a 150-bp region of the 2′ untranslated region,[23,24] and the minor cluster region (mcr) spans a region of some 500 pb to 20 Kb downstream of BLC2.[25,26] In keeping with the notion that the t(14:18) occurs as a result of erroneous VDJ recombination is the finding of breakpoints within the DH region.[27]

The consequence of the BLC2 gene coming under the control of the IgH enhancer is an increase in BLC2 transcript. In t(14;18)-bearing cells, there is a log increase in basal Bcl-2 expression,[28] with no modification in half-life of the IgH/bcl-2 fusion.[29] The Bcl-2 protein is the prototype of the Bcl-2 family of proteins that are important regulators of the apoptotic pathway. These proteins which largely reside within the mitochondrial membrane are able to homo- and hetero-dimerize to influence membrane permeability. Bcl-2 is an antiapoptic protein, reducing membrane permeability. The mitochondrial apoptotic pathway is mediated by changes in the electrical gradient across the mitochondrial membrane. Loss of this potential difference through increased permeability results in release of cytochrome-c, which is able to activate apoptosis-mediating caspases. By maintaining the mitochondrial membrane's integrity, Bcl-2 protein is thus able to inhibit cellular apoptosis in the face of numerous cytotoxic stimuli.[30]

The observed dysregulation of BLC2 expression in the presence of the IGH/BLC2 rearrangement suggests a clear oncogenic mechanism in the pathogenesis of FL. There are a number of lines of evidence however which indicate that further genomic "hits" are required for development of lymphoma. Using PCR, the IGH/BLC2 rearrangement has been identified in populations of healthy blood donors, typically at low levels,[31,32] at an increasing frequency in the older population. Furthermore, BLC2 transgenic mice develop polyclonal follicular hyperplasia and only after a latent period, go on to develop monoclonal immunoblastic lymphoma presumably on the acquisition of a second "hit."[33] The existence of FL lacking the t(14;18) additionally points to other oncogenic mechanisms in lymphomagenesis.

The ability to detect molecular evidence of disease at a very low level with PCR techniques has led to the concept of "molecular remission." This term was originally used to describe the absence of BLC2 rearrangement-containing cells at the molecular level. Thus, the presence (or absence) of such cells (in blood or bone marrow) has been used as a surrogate marker of disease activity. As such, it has been applied as a measure of efficacy following various treatment modalities, and in particular, high-dose therapy, fludarabine-containing regimens, and antibody treatment. Further refinement of the methodology (using quantitative or "real-time" PCR) has made it possible to quantify the "copy number" of BLC2 rearrangement–containing cells.

Other Oncogenic Events in Follicular Lymphoma

The majority of other cytogenetic changes in FL are either genomic gains or losses, although other translocations (including those involving 3q27) have been described. Such cytogenetic changes accumulate during disease progression and transformation.[21,34–38] Through the use of conventional comparative genomic hybridization (CGH) and more latterly, array-based CGH, documentation and localization of these regions of recurrent gain and loss have been refined. Large gains of chromosome 7 are frequently observed, as are gains at 1q, 2p, 12q, 18q, and X.[38] Speculation regarding candidate oncogenes (e.g., rel on 2p)[39] has been made for some of these regions, although in other cases, large regions of chromosomal involvement, without a definable minimal region of amplification are observed (e.g., on the X chromosome). Loss of 6q and 13q is also frequently reported, suggesting the presence of a number of candidate tumor suppressors within these regions.[38]

Loss of 17p, which includes the TP53 locus, is also frequently observed in FL.[40] This appears to be a late event with a detrimental effect on survival. The activated p53 protein acts on a number of effector pathways to inhibit cell cycle progression, allow DNA repair, or induce apoptosis in response to a number of cellular stresses. Mutations within the TP53 gene are infrequently documented in FL,[40] but at the time of transformation become more frequent and may be observed in between 30% to 70% of cases.[41,42] It appears that the acquisition of mutant TP53 results in selective growth advantage, but in itself may not be required for the transformation process. Rearrangement of the c-MYC oncogene may occur upon transformation,[43] although the frequency of this event is only 8%. Microarray studies however document much more frequent dysregulation of c-MYC expression and its numerous target genes.[44]

Translocation of the BLC6 transcriptional repressor to a number of partner genes is observed in FL, and may be of prognostic significance.[45] The accumulation of mutations in the 5' noncoding region of BLC6,[46,47] which might result in dysregulated expression has been reported, although it is likely that this phenomenon represents an unwanted effect of the somatic hypermutation machinery present in the germinal center reaction. The cell cycle regulators CDKN2A (p16) and CDKN2B (p15) (cyclin-dependent kinase inhibitors, which are tumor suppressor genes located at 9q21) are deleted in some FLs and may also be associated with transformation events.[48,49] Dysregulation of the RAS signaling and downstream MAP kinase pathways have also been implicated in the process of disease transformation by microarray studies,[50] yet mutations in the RAS gene are infrequently observed (3%) in both FL and transformed FL.[51]

Importantly, the critical role of the nonmalignant, cellular microenvironment in determining the behavior of the disease has been highlighted by recent microarray data.[52] The genes that determined survival were primarily derived from T cells, macrophages, and dendritic cells, highlighting the role of the immune response. Moreover, the fact that survival could be determined from the pattern of gene expression at presentation of FL, raises questions about how the apparent stochastic events described above that accumulated during disease progression interact with the microenvironment.

CLINICAL PERSPECTIVE

Presenting Features and Natural History

The earliest cases of what is now recognized as FL were identified early in the 20th century.[53,54] The first major series, published in an article entitled "Giant follicular lymphadenopathy with or without splenomegaly" by Symmers[55] outlined what came to be called "Brill–Symmers Disease." The description reflects most of the features of the disease seen today, even though the author was not absolutely convinced of its malignant nature, despite describing evolution into frank neoplasia. The majority of patients had extensive and often bulky lymphadenopathy and sometimes (massive) splenomegaly. In contrast to the situation today, a significant proportion of patients was quite young. The same spectrum of histologic presentation as now was reported, with some apparently presenting de novo with what today is called transformation. Spontaneous regression was seen and periods of quiescence were noted. Irradiation, the only treatment available at the time, resulted in reduction of lymphadenopathy and splenomegaly.

Gall, Morrison, and Scott in 1941 identified 63 cases of "the follicular type of malignant lymphoma" in biopsy or necropsy material from patients presenting to the Massachusetts General Hospital between 1917 and 1939.[56] The subsequent manuscript[57] incorporated "follicular lymphoma" into the first formal classification of malignant lymphoma. It accounted for 9%, Hodgkin 's disease excluded. Rappaport, Winter, and Hicks subsequently reviewed biopsy and necropsy material contributed to the Lymphatic Tumour Registry of the Armed Forces Institute of Pathology, describing 253 cases, and focused on the distinction between follicular hyperplasia and FL, and the different cellular composition of the follicles (in FL).[58] Rosenberg et al. found 162 cases of "giant follicle" lymphosarcoma in a series of 1296 patients (13%) with "lymphosarcoma" presenting between 1928 and 1958 to the Sloan Kettering Institute for Cancer Research and Cornell University Medical College.[59] The demographics of the patient populations (age and gender excepted for obvious reasons in the study from the Armed Forces Institute of Pathology) and the conclusions drawn from these sources about outcome are remarkably similar. The median age at diagnosis was about 50 years and the male:female ratio close to unity. The majority presented well, with painless lymphadenopathy which might have been present for several years before diagnosis. The median survival was about five years in all three series, responsiveness, often to irradiation, being the rule rather than the exception. Death was most commonly attributed to the disease itself. Changes in histology over time correlated with survival.

More recent data are entirely consistent with the above, taking into account the more rigorous investigation currently undertaken. The only interesting difference lies in the proportion of patients described as having FL being reported as 28% in 1982 and 22% in 1997, compared overall with about 10% previously. Currently, in most patients, the illness presents with generalized peripheral lymphadenopathy, which is characteristically painless. Further evaluation with CT scanning usually reveals intra-thoracic and intra-abdominal disease. Thus, the majority of patients present with advanced-stage disease, typically involving bone marrow. Beta 2 microglobulin levels may to some extent correlate with extent of disease.[60] The demographics of 4167 adults with FL, presenting between 1985 and 2002, who formed the basis of the data on which the Follicular Lymphoma International Prognostic Index was formulated (please Prognostic Factors)[61] may be considered representative (Table 19–1 and Table 19–2).

Table 19–1. Clinical Presenting Features

Feature	Proportion (%)
Gender (M:F)	51:49
Age <60 vs. ≧60 years	63:37
Stage I + II vs. III + IV	22:78
"B" symptoms absent vs present	81:19
Performance status (ECOG) 0–1 vs. >1	88:12
No. of nodal sites <4 vs. ≧4	65:35
Splenic involvement – vs. +	78:22
Bone marrow – vs. +	52:48
Histology: small cell vs. mixed pattern vs. large cell	50:41:9

From van Besien K, Sobocinski K, Rowlings P, et al. Allogenic bone marrow transplantation for low-grade lymphoma. Blood 1998; 92:1832–6.[265]

Table 19–2. Laboratory Presenting Features

Features		Proportion (%)
Hemoglobin	≧12 g/dL vs. <12 g/dL	82:18
Lymphocyte count × 10^9/L	≧1 vs. <1	80:20
Platelet count × 10^9/L	≧150 vs. <50	88:12
ESR	≦40 mm vs. >40 mm	89:11
Serum LDH	≦ULN vs. >ULN	79:21
Serum β-2 microglobulin	≦ULN vs. >ULN	59:41
Serum albumin (g/L)	≧3.5 vs. <3.5	90:10

ESR, erythrocyte sedimentation rate; LDH, lactate dehydrogenase; ULN, upper limit of normal.
From van Besien K, Sobocinski K, Rowlings P, et al. Allogenic bone marrow transplantation for low-grade lymphoma. Blood 1998; 92:1832–6.[265]

Follicular lymphoma occurs only rarely in childhood[62] representing about 1% of all pediatric lymphoma. There are suggestions that it may be a rather different disease than its adult counterpart. In the largest series comprising 21 cases from three institutions, the male:female ratio was 2.3:1 and the median age was 11 years.[62] More than 75% of patients had Stage I disease, and only one-third expressed bcl-2. Clinical outcome data are limited, and natural history is unknown, since all received therapy.

Further insight into the natural history of FL in adults comes from observation of patients electively managed expectantly during an era when both radiotherapy and chemotherapy have been available. Data from Stanford University Medical Center are particularly valuable. Eighty-three patients, 62 of whom had advanced-stage FL (the remainder having small lymphocytic lymphoma) were managed expectantly over a 20-year period for a variety of reasons including advanced age, and a history of waxing and waning lymphadenopathy antedating diagnosis.[63] Spontaneous regression, (usually partial), occurred in 16 of 62 patients with FL, over a range of 2 months to 10 years, with a median duration of regression of just over a year. Fifty-one of the original 83 patients had required treatment (at a median of 8 years for "follicular small cell'" lymphoma and about 2 years for "follicular mixed" lymphoma). In the majority, the indication was gradually increasing lymphadenopathy; in the remainder, there was rapid progression, systemic symptoms, or extranodal involvement.

A similar analysis has recently been conducted in patients with Stage I and II FL.[64] Forty-five (of 133) patients were identified who received no therapy for 3 months following diagnosis and continued to be managed expectantly. The remainder proceeded "conventionally." At a median follow-up of more than 6 years, more than half of the patients had not been treated. At the time of publication, 16 of 45 had been treated, 12 for significant progression and 4 because of transformation. The estimated median survival was 19 years. Another study, concerning 26 patients with Stage "O" disease (after surgery) with a median follow-up of 6 years, reported 13 progressions (6 local and 7 distant).[65]

Clinical Course

The clinical course of FL represents the influence of therapy on the natural history of the disease. Irrespective of where in the world patients have been treated, or the details of the specific therapy used, with conventional management in the late 20th century, the median survival is approximately 10 years.[66–69] It has, however, recently been suggested, on the basis of data for patients treated at M.D. Anderson Cancer Hospital in Houston,[70] those treated in Southwest Oncology Group trials,[71] and Cancer Registry (Surveillance Epidemiology and End Results [SEER]) data from the United States[72] that the median survival has increased (somewhat) in recent years, possibly as a result of new interventions. However, the overall pattern of the illness has not yet convincingly been shown to have been altered; repeated responses, usually incomplete, are almost always followed by recurrence (Fig. 19–1, Fig. 19–2, and Fig. 19–3).

Transformation to DLBC lymphoma at the time of recurrence usually has grave prognostic significance[73–80] as shown in Fig. 19–4, and may be the terminal event. This change in pathology may occur early in the course of the illness, after several recurrences many years after the diagnosis of FL, or never. The frequency with which it occurs is independent of whether treatment is started at the time of diagnosis or later. The change in pathology is generally associated with changes in the clinical behavior of the illness. Most patients develop rapidly progressive lymphadenopathy often associated with systemic symptoms; the serum lactate dehydrogenase may be raised.

The incidence of transformation to DLBC pathology has been variously reported as occurring in 10% to 70% of

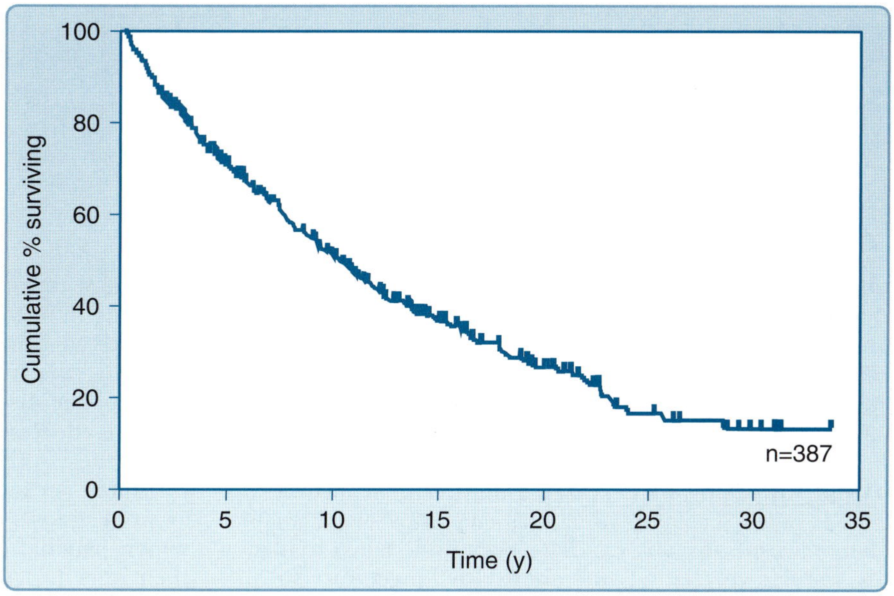

Figure 19–1. Overall survival in follicular lymphoma.

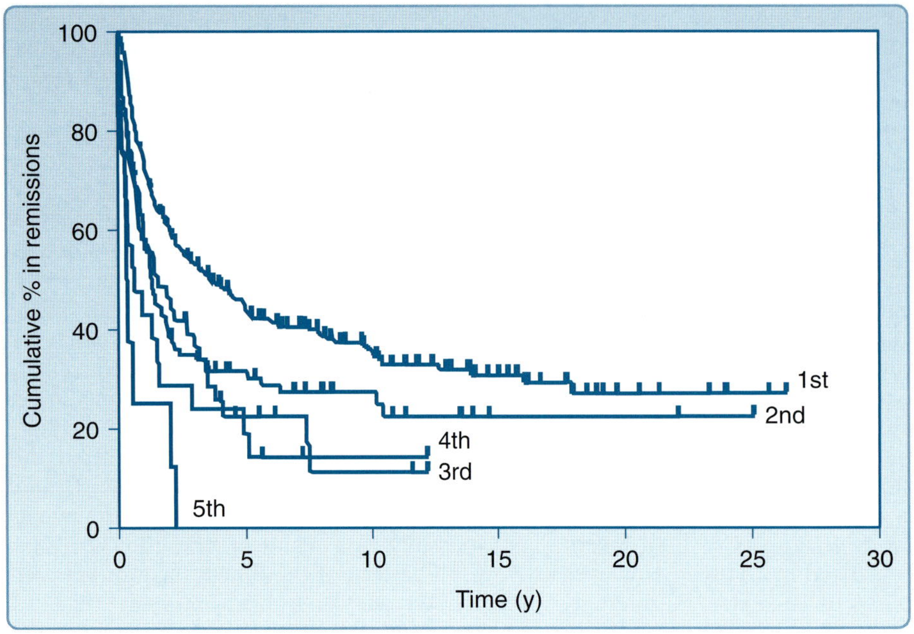

Figure 19–2. Duration of first to fifth remissions in follicular lymphoma.

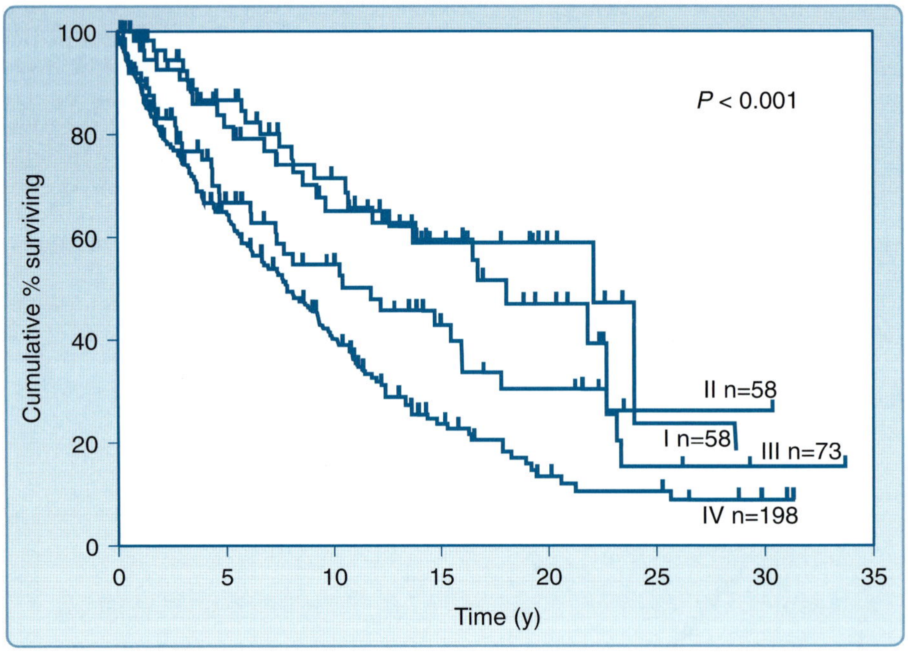

Figure 19–3. Overall survival according to stage in follicular lymphoma.

patients.[73–80] The reason for the variation relates to some extent to the rigor with which biopsies are performed at the time of recurrence. However, regardless of the pattern of evolution, most people who develop FL die as a consequence of the illness, or from complications of treatment for it.

PROGNOSTIC FACTORS

Many retrospective analyses have been undertaken to identify features correlating with shorter or longer survival in patients with FL, with the aim of determining which treatment might be most appropriate at a given time. All the data are derived from patients who received treatment, hence reflecting the impact of prognostic factors on the *clinical course* of the disease rather than the *natural history*. Almost all have addressed the prognosis from the time of the first treatment as opposed to later, in spite of the fact that the treatment decisions at first relapse are, at least, as difficult as at diagnosis and, hence, the importance of knowing which patients deserve a more aggressive approach given their poor prognosis. In the few series that have analyzed

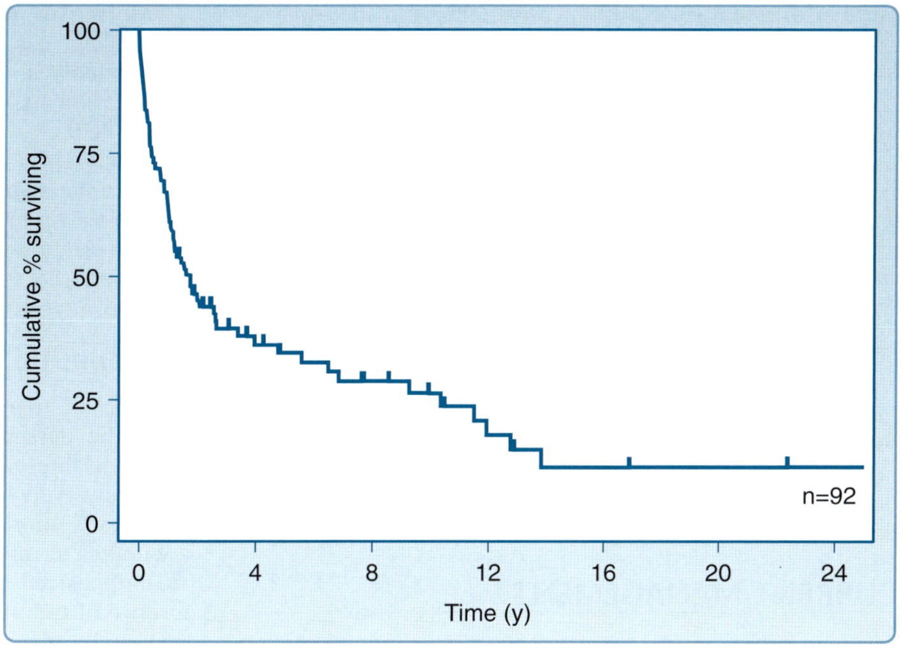

Figure 19–4. Survival from transformation at SBH in follicular lymphoma.

prognostic factors at first relapse, both features related to the response to initial therapy (i.e., the number of chemotherapy lines to achieve that response and the duration of first response) as well as factors related to clinical characteristics at relapse (including the Follicular Lymphoma International Prognostic Index [FLIPI]) have been demonstrated to influence outcome.[81]

Histology

There is strong evidence that overall survival is the same for Grades 1, 2 and 3a FL at the initial presentation, although there have been several reports showing that freedom from progression may be better for those (receiving combination chemotherapy) for Grades 2 and 3a than Grade 1.[82–84] Grade 3b is a small subset of FL that has in the past been considered as having a prognosis akin to that of diffuse large B-cell (DLBC) lymphoma. It is usually treated with combination chemotherapy (as for DLBC lymphoma).

As mentioned above, transformation to DLBC lymphoma (or less commonly Burkitt's lymphoma) later in the illness carries a particularly poor prognosis, but its significance as a "de novo" presentation is less clear. Even less satisfactory are the data about discordant pathology (usually "transformation" in a lymph node with paratrabecular involvement of the marrow with FL) and "composite histology" (when there is both follicular and DLBC lymphoma in the same lymph node).

Clinical Features

Advanced age,[85–92] male gender, advanced stage,[89–94] poor performance status,[89–93] elevated ESR, LDH,[89–93] and β-2-microglobulin,[60] reduced albumin, and reduced haemoglobin[69,91,94] have been variously demonstrated in univariate and multivariate analyses to confer a worse prognosis. Prognostic indices have been generated and applied locally,[91,92,95] but have found little general acceptance, certainly as a basis for determining therapy. Application of the IPI[96] has in the past been advocated since it has been shown to predict prognosis for three risk categories.[97] Its relevance, however, is severely limited by the fact that the "high-risk" group is very small.

A recent international collaboration retrospectively investigated the prognostic significance of 17 pretreatment variables in 4167 patients from Europe, North America, and China (66 cases) who had been treated according to generally accepted guidelines over the period 1985 to 2002, with a median follow-up of 10 years.[61] Four features that were highly significant on univariate analysis nonetheless had to be excluded from the final analysis for the following reasons: serum β-2 microglobulin and albumin (because of missing data), ESR (because data were only available in Europe), and performance status (due to discordance between European and North American patients and hence difficulty in interpretation).

On the basis of multivariate analysis, a five-variable prognostic index was constructed based on age, stage, number of nodal sites, and hemoglobin and LDH level. Grouping according to number of risk factors resulted in three risk categories (0–1, 2, and ≥3) containing approximately equal numbers of patients. The FLIPI, like the IPI, may be age adjusted, and has been validated in a separate retrospective series of almost 1000 patients not included in the initial analysis.

This is almost certainly the last attempt to create a prognostic index based on clinical factors. It remains to be seen whether it will find favor as a basis for therapeutic decisions. It deserves to be tested. It may, however, not be universally adopted for two reasons: accurate recording of the number of nodal sites is time consuming, and the integration of rituximab into first-line therapy *may* render the data obsolete.

Molecular Features

It has recently been shown that the prognosis of newly diagnosed patients with FL may correlate with the pattern of gene expression.[52] A collaborative group (Leukemia and Lymphoma Molecular Profiling Project), established through the National Cancer Institute (Bethesda, MD) has demonstrated that survival relates to specific "signatures" of gene expression reflecting proliferation and immune competence. If the signatures can be identified reproducibly (and cost-effectively), or if they can be validated at the protein expression level with immunohistochemistry, a major advance will have been made, not only in terms of determining prognosis and planning therapy, but also potentially in the identification of new therapeutic targets.

CURRENT MANAGEMENT

Diagnosis

The diagnosis should be made on the basis of excision biopsy, whenever possible. Core needle biopsy may be adequate,[98] but fine-needle aspiration is not. By choice, beyond making paraffin blocks for morphology and immunohistochemistry, fresh tissue should be frozen for molecular analyses with the potential for both prognostic and therapeutic relevance.

Under circumstances when peripheral node biopsy reveals Grade 1, 2 or 3a FL but there is another (often intra-abdominal) larger mass, second biopsy should be performed. The latter may confirm discordant pathology, with FL in the peripheral node but "transformation" in the abdominal mass. In the event of failure of therapy and at each recurrence or progression, repeat biopsy should be performed, once again to confirm or (rule out) transformation to DLBC pathology.

Further Investigation

As with other lymphomas, investigation begins with a full history and clinical examination. Full blood count and peripheral blood film, together with biochemical tests of renal and hepatic function, uric acid, and lactate dehydrogenase (some regard β_2 microglobulin as essential) are accompanied by unilateral bone marrow aspirate, and trephine biopsy and computed axial tomography. The relevance of positron emission tomography is currently not clear in FL.

These investigations are undertaken prior to starting treatment and are repeated at the time of outcome assessment. They should also be repeated if clinically relevant during surveillance; for example, if a patient is being managed expectantly in partial remission, it may be appropriate to repeat the CT scans 3 to 6 months after cessation of therapy. The same may apply to patients who have not yet had any treatment. In contrast, outside the demands of a clinical trial, there is no clinical evidence that aggressive investigation during surveillance is warranted, nor any evidence that it will influence survival.

"Molecular monitoring" is a research investigation. If undertaken, it should be performed against a background of knowledge about rearrangement of the BLC2 gene in the presentation tissue, and followed with quantitative ("real-time") PCR.

Investigation at the time of progression will depend on the circumstances. It may well be appropriate to allow some time to elapse to see if spontaneous regression occurs, and to assess the rate of progression. The patient's overall situation and the therapeutic options should determine the extent of investigation.

Therapeutic Strategy

The goal of treatment of FL (as that of any illness) is to make the person feel better, and if possible, to prolong (pleasant) life. Since the majority of patients with FL are physically well with "lumps," and since most treatments have some morbidity if not mortality, the first decision is whether to intervene or to manage expectantly. It should be emphasized that expectant management is *not* the absence of treatment. It involves the real practice of medicine, including an explanation to the patient of the justification for not intervening immediately in the face of malignancy.

If the patient has histologic evidence of transformation, constitutional "B" symptoms, "bulk," or vital organ impairment, systemic treatment should be instigated. In practice, most patients are treated for symptoms arising from progressive local, nodal disease, systemic symptoms, or concern about potential or actual compromise of organ function due to, for example, intra-abdominal disease. Other indications may be anemia, neutropenia, or thrombocytopenia due to bone marrow infiltration.

The rationale for intervention is based on the fact that most patients with this illness "respond to therapy" and that such response confers a survival advantage at least three times.[99] Furthermore, most treatments have "acceptable" toxicity at the time at which they are recommended.

The strategy following outcome of first treatment at St. Bartholomew's Hospital (London) has traditionally been as follows: Complete remission is managed expectantly. Partial remission is managed according to "how good" the partial remission is—either expectantly, or with further treatment given to improve outcome. Best response is then managed expectantly. Subsequent progression is managed according to the histology, other prognostic factors, and the persuasion of the patient and physician.

Changing the Criteria for Decision Making

During the past 10 years, beyond evaluation of response rate and complete response rate, progression-free survival has become a more popular endpoint of therapy than the traditional duration of remission and overall survival. This raises two important issues, namely: What is a sufficiently good response to justify stopping treatment, or is partial remission enough? (The corollary to this is: When is a response poor enough to mandate changing therapy?) The answers will be different in different patients.

The second issue is: Should decisions about selection of therapy be based on progression-free survival in a recurring/remitting disease? This assumes that the use of a new treatment (which is not curative) may never allow the demonstration of an overall survival advantage. If it is concluded that new treatments leading to improvement in progression-free survival should be incorporated into the algorithm of treatment overall, then the initial therapy of FL should incorporate rituximab. Hitherto, however, improvements in the freedom from recurrence pattern have rarely led to significant improvements in survival.

MANAGEMENT

Expectant Management (Observation Without Treatment)

Three randomized studies[100–102] initiated in the pre–high-dose therapy, pre-rituximab era strongly support the concept of not starting treatment until there is a specific indication to do so. The first, from the National Cancer Institute,[100] was designed to compare the use of intensive, combined modality therapy in newly diagnosed patients with FL, with observation alone. Patients initially randomized to observation received ProMACE-MOPP when therapy became indicated. At the last analysis, there was no difference in overall survival between patients randomized to be treated initially, and those who received treatment after a period of observation; 75% of patients in each group were alive at 5 years.

In the second study, from France,[101] patients deemed not "in need of" initial therapy (according to the criteria of the Groupe pour l'Etude de Lymphome Folliculaire [GELF]) were randomized to expectant management, or to receive interferon or prednimustine. No survival difference was noted among the three groups. However, despite well-established criteria to start treatment in the expectant management arm, one-third of the patients who commenced treatment did so without fulfilling the described criteria, reflecting the difficulty in managing patients without treatment and, thus, the difficulty in analyzing the results of this approach. A third study, published recently from the British National Lymphoma Investigation,[102] compared outcome for patients randomized to immediate treatment with chlorambucil, or to observation, treatment being delayed until disease progression. Local radiotherapy to symptomatic areas of lymphadenopathy was permissible in both arms. At the time of publication, with a median follow-up of 16 years, there was no significant difference in overall survival or cause-specific survival between the two patient groups.

The criteria for initiating treatment in the latter two studies were different (Table 19–3).

These results demand serious consideration and have formed the basis of contemporary management of newly diagnosed patients with FL worldwide. However, the evidence supporting an expectant approach is not a matter for congratulations, but rather a reflection of the current inability to eliminate the disease. It is to be hoped that the advances being made around the turn of the 21st century will make the foregoing redundant. In 2005, trials are in progress that may hold out more hope than ever before of curing FL (or treating it as effectively as today but with less toxicity).

Table 19–3. BNLI and GELF Criteria for Delaying Treatment

BNLI [Ardeshna et al. (2003)[102]]	Absence of all of the following: 1. Pruritus or B symptoms. 2. Rapid generalized disease progression. 3. "Life-endangering" organ involvement. 4. Marrow compromise (Hb ≤10.0g/L, WBC <3.0 or platelets <100). 5. Bone lesions. 6. Renal infiltration. 7. Macroscopic liver involvement.
GELF [Brice et al. (1997)[101]]	All of the following: 1. Maximum diameter of any site of disease <7 cm. 2. Fewer than 3 nodal sites with a diameter >3 cm 3. Absence of systemic symptoms. 4. No "substantial" splenic involvement (spleen <16 cm in length based on CT measurement). 5. No significant serious effusions clinically evident or on chest x-ray. 6. Absence of risk of local compressive symptoms (epidural, ureteral, etc.). 7. No circulating lymphoma cells or peripheral blood cytopenias (Hb >10g/dL, neutrophils >1.5 and platelets >100).

BNLI, British National Lymphoma Investigation; GELF, Groupe pour l'Etude de Lymphome Folliculaire.
Using these criteria, 36% of consecutive patients diagnosed with follicular lymphoma were considered to have a "low" tumor burden.

A study that is currently in progress in Europe compares an expectant approach with 4 weeks of treatment with the chimeric antibody, anti-CD20 (rituximab/mabthera), to determine whether the early use of antibody will result in deferral of the "need" for chemotherapy.

SPECIFIC THERAPEUTIC OPTIONS

Irradiation

Follicular lymphoma is extremely radiation sensitive (see Radioimmunotherapy). There is a dose-response relationship, "within field" recurrence being rare above 45Gy.[103] In most series, the dose is between 35 to 40 Gy.

Both involved-field (IFRT) and extended-field (EFRT) radiotherapy have been used extensively as the initial treatment of localized nodal disease.[104–111] The response rate is very high. Progression, if it occurs, is seen most frequently in the first 3 years, less often between 3 and 10 years, and rarely thereafter, the median overall survival comfortably exceeding 10 years.[104–111] It is also effective at the time of progression, although robust data are difficult to identify, and the impact on survival almost impossible to assess. At Stanford University, about half of a cohort of patients initially treated with irradiation received it again, on the basis of the "relapse stage." The median survival was 6 years (the same as for those managed expectantly).[112]

There is less experience with radiotherapy for more advanced nodal disease; however, some consider it curative for a proportion of patients.[113–115] In long follow-ups of 61 patients treated with total nodal irradiation or subtotal nodal irradiation (of which only a small number received additional chemotherapy), 40% were disease-free at 10 years.[115]

Superficial comparison of these results with those from studies in which irradiation was combined with chemotherapy, do not suggest much additional benefit from the chemotherapy.[116,117] A large randomized trial is in progress.

Low-dose total-body irradiation is also effective at inducing remission of clinically advanced FL, although the responses are not usually durable, and there is a risk of severe thrombocytopenia.[118–121] There has been a recent increase in interest in low-dose involved-field irradiation following the demonstration of its use in recurrent localized nodal disease. Almost 100 cases were treated with either 2 × 2 Gy or 1 × 4 Gy. The overall response rate was very high, and the median time to further progression was more than a year. This may be a highly relevant treatment for selected patients.[122]

Thus, irradiation is an effective tool in the treatment of FL. It is given with curative intent, and some anticipation of success for localized nodal disease, particularly Stage I at presentation, and may have an effective and relatively nontoxic role in the management of recurrent disease.

Radioimmunotherapy

Over a decade's experience has now been gained in the use of radioimmunoconjugates as treatment for B-cell lymphoma. By conjugating a radioisotope to a monoclonal antibody, systemic administration results in the delivery of radiation directly to the tumor. Such cytocidal activity will also result in the death of neighboring antibody-negative cells, the so-called "cross-fire" effect. Furthermore, antibody binding to antigen may also recruit a number of additional effector mechanisms including antibody-dependent cellular cytotoxicity, activation of complement, and induction of apoptosis. Although a number of cellular targets have been explored, the CD20 antigen has been the main focus of investigation. Two agents are now commercially available (at least in the United States), ^{131}I-labeled tositumomab (Bexxar), and ^{90}Y ibritumomomab tiuxetan (Zevalin).

^{131}I-Labeled Tositumomab (Bexxar)

Tositumomab (formerly anti-B1) is a murine IgG2a monoclonal antibody to which ^{131}I is covalently bound. ^{131}I is an attractive choice of isotope because its dual emission properties allow for detection ex vivo of γ emissions, while high-energy β emissions are locally lethal to the tumor. The isotope is administered in a standard, two-step schedule, in order to deliver a patient-specific, whole-body dose, dependent on individual patient pharmacokinetics. A dosimetric step is performed with administration of unlabeled Tositumomab to saturate antigen "sinks" and improve tumor targeting. An infusion of a small dose of radiolabeled antigen is then given (the "test" dose), with external gamma camera counts being obtained within 1 hour, and subsequently on two occasions within 7 days. Between 1 and 2 weeks after the test dose, the therapeutic dose (again preceded by unlabeled tositumomab) is given. The latter is calculated to deliver a total body dose of 75cGy (attenuated to 65cGy in patients with relative thrombocytopenia). In the United Kingdom, this treatment requires hospitalization for reasons of radiation protection to caregivers, while in the United States, changes in the Nuclear Regulatory Commission regulations allow outpatient administration in most states.

The efficacy of Bexxar has been documented in a number of clinical settings (Table 19–4). In a randomized study, radioiodination added significantly to the therapeutic activity of the parent monoclonal antibody.[123] In recurrent FL, the response rates have been high, and prolonged freedom from progression has been achieved in some cases, often in circumstances where expectation of success was limited.[124–129] In a Phase II trial, using a study design where the patient acted as his/her own control, 65% of 60 patients who had failed to respond to the last chemotherapy (or had progressed within 6 months) responded, with 23% entering a complete remission.[126] Fifty-three percent of patients had a longer duration of response to radioimmunotherapy than to their previous chemotherapeutic regimen. Bexxar also has efficacy in patients that have progressed after rituximab,[128] and following transformation of FL.[129]

When used alone in patients with newly diagnosed, advanced-stage FL, the overall response rate was 95%, with actuarial 5-year progression-free survival of 59%.[130] Given that concerns regarding hematologic toxicity have limited therapy to patients with less than 25% intertrabecular bone marrow involvement, and that radioimmunotherapy appears to perform best in nonbulky disease, sequential administration of Bexxar is currently being investigated after conventional chemotherapy.[131]

Although infusion-related reactions do occur, the principal short-term toxicity of conventional dose Bexxar is hematological. A single nadir is observed 4 to 6 weeks post-therapy, typically with complete recovery by week 9. The degree of cytopenias observed is similar to that observed with any moderately intensive chemotherapeutic regimen. Long-term concerns about the risk of therapy-related myelodysplasia (tMDS) and therapy-related acute myeloid leukemia (tAML) have been expressed. The incidence, however, appears consistent with that expected on the basis of conventional therapies,[132] and has not been described following the use of Bexxar as first-line therapy.[130] Further investigation is definitely warranted.

It has also been possible to incorporate targeted irradiation into myeloablative therapy, either alone,[133–135] or in combination with chemotherapy.[136,137] The results are excellent, although the complex logistics of such treatment may limit its use.

Table 19–4. Response Data from CD20-Directed Radioimmunotherapy

Reference		Patients (n)	Median Number of Prior Therapies (range)	ORR	CR/CR(u)	DR or PFS (months)	DR or PFS for Patients Achieving CR/CR(u) (months)
Yttrium 90 Ibritumomab (Zevalin)							
138	Phase I/II Relapsed refractory B cell	51 (FL 33 pts)	2 (1–7)	All 73% (FL 85%)	All 51% (FL 57%)	DR 11.7	DR 12.4
141	Relapsed/refractory Randomized study comparing yttrium 90 ibritumomab to rituximab	73 (FL 55 pts, Tx 9 pts) (Results for RIT arm only, total study population 143)	2 (1–6)	80	34	DR 14.2 (DR 18.5 FL pts)	
140	Mild thrombocytopenia (pl 100–149 × 10^9/L, dose reduction to 0.3 mCi/kg)	30 (FL 25, Tx 3)	2 (1–9)	83	44	DR 11.7	
139	Rituximab refractory FL	57 (54 FL)	4 (1–9)	FL 74%	FL 15%	DR 6.4	
Tositumomab and Iodine I 131 Tositumomab (Bexxar)							
124	Relapsed/refractory	47 (37 "low" grade, 10 Tx)	4 (1–8)	57 ("low" grade 57%)	32 ("low" grade 27%)	DR 9.9 (DR "low" grade 8.2)	DR 19.9 (DR "low" grade 25.5)
125	Phase I/II Relapsed/refractory Single center	59 ("low" grade 28 pts, transformed 14 pts)	4 (1–3)	71 ("low" grade 86%)	34 ("low" grade 46%)	PFS 12	PFS 20.3
126	Pivotal Phase III Chemotherapy refractory	60 ("low" grade 36 pts, Tx 23 pts)	4 (2–13)	65 ("low" grade 81%)	28%	DR 6.5	DR NR (>47)
127	First or second recurrence	41 (FL 29 pts, TX 7 pts)	1 (1–34)	76% (FL 79%)	49% (FL 59%	DR 15.6	DR 36
123	Relapsed/refractory Randomized study of tositumomab against iodine I 131 tositumomab	42 (low grade 36 pts Tx 6 pts) (results for RIT arm only, total study population 78)	2 (1–4)	55%	33%	DR 14.7	DR NR
128	Rituximab refractory	40 (FL 28 pts, Tx 10 pts)	4 (1–11)	65% (grade 1/2 FL 86%)	38% (grade 1/2 FL 57%)	PFS 10.4 (DR grade 1/2 FL NR)	PFS 24.5 (DR grade 1/2 FL NR)
130	Initial therapy for FL	76	0	95%	75%	PFS 73	PFS NR (77% at 5 years)

Note: "Low" grade refers to histology as given in the respective publications. (The majority of these patients will have had follicular lymphoma, although this is not stated by authors.)

CR, complete remission; CRu, complete response unconfirmed; DR, duration of response; FL, follicular lymphoma; Tx, transformed FL; ORR, overall response rate; PFS, progression-free survival; pl, platelets; RIT, radioimmunotherapy; NR, not reached.

^{90}Y Ibritumomab Tiuxetan (Zevalin)

^{90}Y ibritumomab tiuxetan (Zevalin) was, in fact, the first radioimmunoconjugate to receive U.S. Food and Drug Administration (FDA) approval. Unlike ^{131}I, ^{90}yttrium (^{90}Y) is a pure β emitter and cannot be used for imaging (although treatment may be performed on an outpatient basis). However, because of less interpatient variability in kinetics, dosing of Zevalin is based solely on weight, and an imaging phase using indium-labeled antibody is used only to confirm favorable biodistribution. The parent antibody is a murine kappa IgG1, and ^{90}Y is bound via the chelator tiuxetan. As with Bexxar, prior to administration of labeled antibody, a "cold" antibody infusion (in this case of the chimeric antibody rituximab) is given to improve tumor targeting. Therapy is given 1 week after administration of the imaging dose. Efficacy data suggest a similarity in response rates to those seen with Bexxar in the setting of recurrent disease[138–144] (Table 19–4).

At present, apart from local experience, there is little to guide physician choice between the two radioimmunoconjugates. An FDA-mandated trial directly comparing the two agents may help determine appropriate patient selection. Zevalin has, however, been tested directly against rituximab in a randomized Phase III study.[143] The overall response rate was 80% in the radioimmunotherapy arm, compared to 56% in the rituximab-treated group (CR 30% and 16%, respectively). Duration of response and time to progression, however, were not significantly different between the two arms. Short-term toxicity was again primarily hematological, with the nadir at 7 to 9 weeks post-therapy lasting between 1 and 4 weeks.[143] tMDS/tAML was reported in only 1% of the patient population. Importantly, it appears that subsequent chemotherapy regimens are well tolerated.[145]

Chemotherapy

The majority of those who develop FL will receive cytotoxic chemotherapy at some time because of the clinical course of the illness and its propensity to be disseminated. Many agents induce remissions when given alone: until quite recently, single-agent chemotherapy was the treatment of choice, repeatedly. Very high response rates (some "molecular") with combination chemotherapy, and more recently with chemoimmunotherapy, have made it generally much less popular. This is based largely on the view, as mentioned above, that progression-free survival rather than overall survival is the correct endpoint upon which to determine treatment choice.

Two groups of therapy, the alkylating agents and the purine analogues, are most widely perceived as the best single cytotoxic agents, and have been variously combined with corticosteroids, vinca alkaloids, and topoisomerase I inhibitors, all of which have been shown to induce remission alone (but with the exception of corticosteroids, are not used singly themselves).

Alkylating Agents

These remain the most widely used drugs in the treatment of FL. Chlorambucil alone induces regression of lymphadenopathy in at least 75% of patients.[69,99,146–148] This was first demonstrated almost a half-century ago by Galton,[146] and has been amply confirmed since. Relatively modest doses, given daily, result in clinical evidence of responsiveness, if it is to occur, within 6 weeks. Similar results may be achieved with cyclophosphamide.[149–151] The addition of prednisolone does not appear to confer any advantage.[152,153] There are many different regimens of schedule and dose in current use. At St. Bartholomew's Hospital, a daily dose of chlorambucil of 10 mg is given for 6 weeks, blood count permitting. A 2-week gap is followed by three 2-week pulses of 10 mg daily, with 2-week intervals. The response rate is more than 75% with relatively few complete remissions. As initial therapy, this results in a median freedom from recurrence of about 2 years, and no evidence of cure (Figure 19–3). Repeated cycles given at the time of progression result in repeated responsiveness.[69,99]

Purine Analogues

Purine analogues are the second most frequently used cytotoxic agents in the treatment of FL. As antimetabolites which mimic physiological nucleosides, they are incorporated into newly synthesized DNA, eventually causing cell death by apoptosis. By far the greatest experience has been gained with fludarabine,[154–160] the attraction of which has increased with its availability as an oral formulation with reasonably reproducible bioavailability.[161] The response rate lies between 30% and 70%,[154–160] being highest in newly diagnosed patients, with a complete remission rate of 38%.[162] The median duration of remission is somewhat in excess of a year.

Initial enthusiasm for this highly effective drug has been somewhat tempered by the risk of opportunistic infection, particularly with *Pneumocystis carinii*, as a consequence of T-cell dysfunction, which makes the use of prophylactic co-trimoxazole mandatory. There is also the potential for hemolytic anemia.

Alkylating Agent-Based Combination

CVP/COP

With the development of combination chemotherapy for other malignancies, a series of studies compared the use of chlorambucil (or in the United States, cyclophosphamide) with the combination CVP (cyclophosphamide, vincristine, and prednisolone).[148,163–165] CVP, in various doses and schedules, remains one of the most widely used combinations (at least in Europe), and is given a minimum of six times in responding patients. The regimen has been shown to result in a higher *complete* remission rate (although not overall response rate) than an alkylating agent alone when given as the first treatment for advanced disease. Although longer freedom from progression was observed, there was no survival advantage. It is difficult to understand why the combination is so popular (Table 19–5).

Topo-Isomerase I-Containing Regimens

The incorporation of doxorubicin into the CHOP combination (cyclophosphamide, daunorubicin, vincristine [Oncovin], and prednisone) also results in higher response rates and better freedom from progression, but again, in comparison with historical controls,[166] or in randomized clinical trials,[167–172] there is no evidence of a survival advantage, except possibly for patients with pathologies Grade 3a and 3b. Despite this, in the United States, CHOP is the most popular chemotherapy for FL, either early or late in the course of the disease. The combination CHVEP (cyclophosphamide, doxorubicin, vincristine, etoposide, and prednisolone) is very widely used in France, with good effect; it has not, however, been proven to improve survival.[173]

With regard to combining chemotherapy and radiotherapy for advanced-stage disease, only one study from the M.D. Anderson Cancer Center (in which CHOP with and without bleomycin was given with involved-field radiotherapy) resulted in an extremely high complete remission rate (81%) with a 75% 5-year survival rate and 52% recurrence-free survival rate[174] (Table 19–5).

Fludarabine-Based Combinations

The demonstration of an in vitro synergistic effect between fludarabine and other drugs[175,176] led to the development of clinical trials of fludarabine combinations, which showed better results overall than those achieved with fludarabine alone. Thus, the addition of cyclophosphamide with or

Table 19–5. Combination Chemotherapy as First-Line Therapy

Treatment		% CR	Median OS	References
CVP	Cy, VCR, PDN	37	NS	148; 163; 164; 165
CHOP	Cy, Dox, VCR, PDN	64	6.9 years	166; 167; 168; 169; 170; 171; 172
ProMACE-MOPP	PDN, MTX, Dox, CFM, VP-16, Mec,VCR, Proc	78	>60 months (75% at 5 years)	100
ATT	CHOD-Bleo/ESHAP/NOPP	87	>5.9 years (82% at 5 years)	181
CVP-R	Cy, VCR, PDN, Rituximab	41	89% at 30 months	263
CHOP-R	Cy, Dox, VCR, PDN, Rituximab	87	NS	255; 256

[a] Seventy-six percent first-line.
Cy, cyclophosphamide; VCR, vincristine; PDN, prednisolone; Dox, doxorubicin; Proc, procarbazine; MTX, methotrexate; VP-16, etoposide; Mec, mechlorethamine; CHOD, cyclophosphamide, doxorubicin, vincristine, dexamethasone; Bleo, bleomycin; ESHAP, etoposide, cytarabine, prednisolone, cisplatin; NOPP, mitoxantrone, vincristine, prednisone, procarbazine; DXM, dexamethasone; NS, not specified; CR, complete remission; OS, overall survival.

without mitoxantrone (FC[177], FCM[178,179]) or mitoxantrone and dexamethasone (FMD)[180,181] results in the achievement of CR in almost 80% of patients. Furthermore, even in heavily pretreated patients, achievement of a "molecular response" is possible in a considerable proportion of patients (Table 19–6).

Long-term toxicity in the form of bone marrow suppression is a matter of concern and the use of fludarabine or fludarabine combinations has been associated with difficulties in harvesting peripheral blood progenitor cells.[182,183] In addition, previous treatment with purine analogues can result in the development of myelodysplasia in patients subsequently receiving HDT followed by autologous stem cell rescue.[184]

Myeloablative Chemo/Chemo-Radiotherapy with Hematopoietic Stem Cell Rescue

Now considered to be the best standard of care for consolidation of second remission of "intermediate" and "high" grade non-Hodgkin's lymphoma, this therapeutic approach has had variable popularity in the treatment of FL. Its advocates have relied in the main on Phase II single center data, showing impressive freedom from progression and latterly, on two randomized trials which show a survival advantage. Its detractors point to the risk of myelodysplasia,[184–189] limited if any evidence of cure, and suggest that the advent of antibody therapy, and possibly vaccine therapy render it redundant. Any treatment with a potential long-term mortality of 20% can only be considered in light of the risk of the disease itself, highlighting the importance of prognostic factors.

The majority of data relate to the use of cyclophosphamide and total body irradiation or the combination of BEAM () or CBV given in second or subsequent remission, either in trials to test the curability of the therapy, or because the patient's circumstances were thought to warrant it. Both single center[190–201] and registry data[202] are valuable.

The risk of potentially reinfusing malignant cells in the stem cell harvest led first to the concept of "purging," either in vitro or in vivo. Early approaches concentrated on the in vitro manipulation of bone marrow with monoclonal antibodies and complement.[191–196] Currently, the potential benefit of pre-treating the patient with rituximab is being evaluated. The benefit of these procedures will ultimately be measured in terms of survival of the patient. Meanwhile, molecular monitoring has been used as a surrogate and is being correlated with survival and progression-free survival.[194,196,197,200,203] While different techniques may make comparison between different centers difficult, it does appear that the achievement of a persistent molecular remission is good for the patient.

Both single center and Registry data suggest that the freedom from recurrence is longer than would otherwise have been expected if myeloablative treatment is given in

Table 19–6. Fludarabine Combinations

Treatment	Disease Status	PR (%)	CR (%)	Molecular CR (%)	OS	FFS	References
FCM	Recurrence	7	50	21	NS	NS	179
FMD	Recurrence/newly diagnosed	48	20	23	10 months[a]	30 months[a]	180; 181
FC	Newly diagnosed	11	89	Not evaluated	66%[b]	53%[b]	177
FND	Newly diagnosed	18	79	66	84%[b]	39%[b]	284
FCM	Newly diagnosed	13	80	75	90%[c]	76%[c]	178

[a] Median.
[b] At 5 years.
[c] At 2 years.
CR, complete remission; FC, fludaribine and cyclophosphamide; FCM, fludaribine, cyclophosphamide, and mitoxantrone; FFS, failure-free survival; FND, fludaribine mitoxantrone (novantrone) and dexamethasone; NS, not specified; OS, overall survival; PR, partial remission.

second or subsequent remission.[194–201] Historical controls are difficult to find and generally distrusted.[194,204] Even with this caveat in mind, the combined data from St Bartholomew's Hospital and the Dana Farber Cancer Institute are encouraging. Analysis 12 years since Cy + TBI + ABMT, shows that only 50% of patients have developed recurrent lymphoma with freedom from recurrence at 5, 10, and 15 years being 55%, 48%, and 47% respectively. Forty-seven percent are still alive, overall survival at 5, 10, and 15 years being 70%, 54%, and 44%, respectively. These results are significantly better than those for the historical control, and there is a strong hint of a plateau on the curves.[205]

These results are supported by the outcome of the "CUP" trial, which compared conventional chemotherapy with high-dose therapy with purged and unpurged hematopoietic support showing an overall survival advantage to the patients receiving high-dose therapy either purged or unpurged.[206]

There is much less data about consolidation of first remission. Phase II trials were provocative[207–209] and, recently three Phase III studies have been reported.[210–212] The German Low-Grade Lymphoma Study Group[210] compared outcome of patients with FL, mantle cell lymphoma or lymphoplasmacytic lymphoma treated with cyclophosphamide +TBI in first remission to that of those receiving maintenance interferon. Patients in the high-dose arm had a longer progression-free survival than the remainder (64.7% vs. 33.3% at 5 years), although there was no difference in overall survival. A separate report comments on the significantly higher incidence of secondary myelodysplasia in the high-dose treatment arm (3.8% vs. 0.0% at 5 years).[213] Likewise, in the study recently published by the Groupe Ouest Est des Leucemies Aigues et des Maladies du Sang (GOELAMS)[211] patients were randomized to conventional chemotherapy followed by either: IFN maintenance or Cy +TBI. Again, an advantage in event-free survival was demonstrated for patients in the Cy +TBI arm, though no difference in overall survival was found. This was attributed to a higher risk of secondary malignancies after high-dose treatment.[211] In contrast, another French study comparing CHVP + IFN with CHOP + Cy + VP16 + TBI, reported longer survival for patients receiving high-dose treatment with no difference in event-free survival.[212]

Improvements in supportive care, coupled with potentially better methods of determining the future risk of myelodysplasia,[214] make this an important treatment to consider in patients at high-risk of early failure of "conventional therapy."

High-Dose Treatment Following Transformation to Diffuse Large B-Cell Pathology

The consensus is now that provided a complete or at least partial remission can be achieved (with treatment as for DLBC lymphoma), there is at least the possibility of cure following high-dose treatment in a proportion of patients. Several studies suggest that between 30% and 40% of patients may remain free of disease at 4-5 years.[215–217] A study from the European Bone Marrow Transplant Registry also showed progression-free survival of 30% for 50 patients at 5 years.[218] Importantly, in the latter studies as for DLBC lymphoma, there was a clear difference between patients with "responsive" disease, in whom a CR was achieved after high-dose treatment (overall survival of 69% at 5 years) compared with those who had resistant disease at the time of high-dose treatment, the latter all dying as a consequence of lymphoma. A further study from Toronto confirms this.[219]

Biological Therapies

Interferon-∝ (IFN-∝)

This treatment was first tested as treatment for lymphoma more than 25 years ago following preclinical studies of L1210 leukaemia[220] and AKR lymphoma[221] in mice. It induces remission of FL through mechanisms which remain unclear` in about 50% of patients, relatively slowly, at doses which most find "tolerable."[222–229] It has been tested in combination with chemotherapy, both as remission induction and maintenance, in randomized clinical trials.[230–238] A meta-analysis of all the Phase III trials, incorporating IFN-α as part of initial therapy revealed that, when combined with relatively intensive chemotherapy, it conferred an overall survival advantage.[239] Despite this, a rare achievement for any drug in the treatment of FL, it is not widely used. This may be a function of its toxicity, or possibly better newer therapy. It should not however be neglected for patients for whom other therapy has failed.

Rituximab

The identification of the B-1 antigen (CD20)[240] and the development of technology for producing monoclonal antibodies on a large scale paved the way for the introduction of rituximab/mabthera (anti-CD20) therapy for FL. As a result, almost as many patients with FL will now receive antibody therapy as chemotherapy at some time during the illness. This relatively non-toxic treatment is a major breakthrough: it remains yet to be shown how best it should be used.

Initial experience with rituximab alone in patients with recurrent FL revealed an overall response rate of about 50% following 4 injections of antibody at weekly intervals.[241–243] The first infusion, planned to last two hours was often prolonged because of fever and chills. Otherwise the treatment was very well tolerated. Most remissions were partial, and continued to occur for up to six months.[241–243] "Molecular remission" was observed, even in the presence of persistent adenopathy.[243] Patients with "bulky" disease respond[244] and re-treatment was effective.[245] Response has been shown to correlate with serum levels[246] and the concept of individualizing dosage has been proposed.[247]

The overall remission rate, and the complete remission rate are higher and freedom from progression is longer when rituximab is used as first line therapy, although there is no indication that it is curative.[248–250] Prolongation of treatment with rituximab alone, either as first line or as second line therapy has been investigated,[248,251] and in one study, compared with re-treatment with observation and rituximab alone at recurrence.[252] The complete remission rate and freedom from progression were both better for patients receiving prolonged therapy. Once again, however there was no suggestion of cure, or improvement on overall survival. Activity has been shown to be associated with polymorphisms in the IgG FL receptor,[253,254] and variations in gene expression.[255]

Thus, rituximab alone has been convincingly demonstrated to be a well-tolerated, safe, if rather expensive treatment for FL, with efficacy somewhat less than that of single agent chemotherapy. Its toxicity profile (or lack thereof) may make it the treatment of first choice in patients with considerable co-morbidity. The observation that "more is better" or "longer is better" must be treated with caution in the absence of a survival advantage, and be seen within the context of the results of combining rituximab with chemotherapy. (Its potential role in avoiding or postponing chemotherapy in newly diagnosed patients is being examined in a large European study.)

The theoretical advantages of enhancing recruitment of effector mechanisms have led to the construction of almost completely humanized, as opposed to chimeric, antibodies which are now in early clinical trial.[256] An alternative target, CD22 is also being exploited with epitruzimab.[257]

Antibody with Chemotherapy

Standard care of FL in the United States was altered by the results of a small Phase II trial testing the combination of rituximab with CHOP for patients with advanced disease, predominantly at presentation.[258] Almost all the patients responded and at the latest analysis, 70% were progression-free at 5 years.[259] Other Phase II data, particularly for combinations of fludarabine with rituximab are encouraging.[260,261]

Large Phase III trials comparing combination chemotherapy with or without Rituximab have been conducted both in the setting of recurrent disease and at presentation. The results are uniformly positive provided improvement in complete remission rate and progression-free survival, but not overall survival is the goal. Fludarabine, cyclophosphamide, and mitoxantrone + rituximab (FCM-R) had a highly significantly ($p = 0.001$) better complete remission rate than FCM at recurrence.[262] CVP-R was significantly better than CVP for newly diagnosed patients needing therapy, with the complete remission rate being 41% compared with 10% ($p = 0.0001$).[263] With a median follow-up of 2 years, the time to progression was doubled from 15 to 30 months. There was no hint however of a plateau on the curve, and it has been suggested that the CVP alone result is relatively poor. Similarly, CHOP-R yielded a higher response rate than CHOP alone. With a median follow-up of 3 years, the median time to treatment failure following CHOP-R has not been reached, while it is 2.6 years for CHOP alone.[264]

Do these results mean that all patients with "chemotherapy requiring" FL should receive "chemo-R," and if so, when? The question needs to be addressed if only from the viewpoint of health care economics.

On the positive side, the high complete remission rates are encouraging, as are the freedom from progression improvements. On the negative side, very few of the improvements in response rate and duration of remission achieved in the past with chemotherapy have converted into a survival advantage because none were curative and repeated responsiveness after treatment failure was observed. Paradoxically, as previously recorded, neither interferon nor high-dose therapy, both shown to improve overall survival, have been widely adopted.

A healthy approach is to view the results optimistically and conduct trials to demonstrate the best way to utilize an undoubted advance. The contribution of maintenance Rituximab following chemo-immunotherapy is being explored in a randomized trial for patients "needing therapy." Chemotherapy + rituximab followed by myeloablative therapy and rituximab maintenance is an appropriate strategy to treat with curative intent.

It is however clear that Rituximab is ineffective in some patients. As mentioned above, this relates to polymorphisms in the FC λIIIa receptor.[253,254] A satisfactory test might avoid the unnecessary prescription of the antibody.

Allogeneic Bone Marrow Transplantation

Small numbers of highly selected patients have received HLA-matched sibling allografts with myeloablative conditioning for FL.[265–272] The data derive from both the International Bone Marrow Transplant Registry and from single centers. In terms of Registry data,[266] for 113 patients with low-grade lymphoma, most of whom were treated in CR or PR at 3 years, only 16% of patients had developed recurrent disease, and the overall survival was 49% (Fig. 19–5). Furthermore, only 1 of 33 patients in whom at the time of publication follow-up exceeded 2 years had developed recurrent disease.

In an attempt to decrease the incidence and mortality of graft-versus-host disease, T-cell depletion has been evaluated with indeed a very low treatment-related mortality (at the DFCI) and a disease-free survival of 50%.[257] Results for patients treated in Vancouver (without T-cell depletion) show an equally low recurrence rate, although a higher initial mortality, largely as a result of graft-versus-host-disease (GVHD).[269] Thus, remarkably low recurrence rates have been demonstrated despite the treatment being given to a group of patients who often have resistant, late-stage disease and extensive bone marrow involvement, suggesting that there may be a "graft-versus-lymphoma" effect.

Several studies have retrospectively compared outcome following allogeneic marrow transplantation versus high-dose treatment in patients with indolent lymphoma[270–272] (Table 19–7). As would be expected, the treatment-related mortality following allografting was significantly higher; however, a lower recurrence rate resulted in no significant difference in overall survival despite the "poor risk" characteristics of the patients undergoing allogeneic transplantation. Disease-free survival (DFS) was significantly better in the allogeneic group in all three studies shown in Table 19–7 below.

Thus, the following can be concluded: complete responses have been achieved in a proportion of patients in whom no previous complete remission had been possible. There is a high treatment-related mortality, but for patients surviving the treatment, long-term disease-free survival has been observed with few recurrences after 2 years. A graft-versus-lymphoma effect has been postulated.

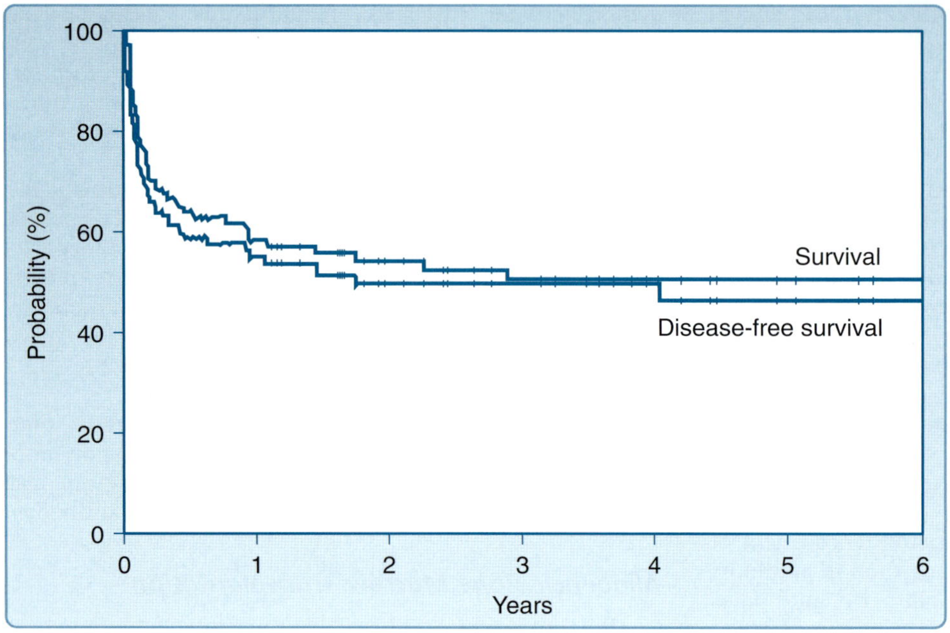

Figure 19–5. Disease-free survival and overall survival in a series of 113 patients treated with an allograft. (From Van Besien 1998, with permission.)

Nonmyeloablative (Reduced-Intensity) Stem Cell Transplantation

Hematopoietic engraftment following nonmyeloablative irradiation was originally demonstrated in the preclinical setting.[273] This was subsequently confirmed in patients with hematologic malignancy demonstrating that engraftment of allogeneic stem cells was feasible, with considerably less toxicity than that incurred with a standard allograft. Data for patients with FL are preliminary but interesting. Twenty patients with recurrent FL (18) or SLL (2) received nonmyeloablative conditioning with fludarabine and cyclophosphamide (with and without rituximab) followed by allogeneic stem transplantation from HLA identical siblings at M.D. Anderson Cancer Center in Houston.[274] The median age was 51; at the time of treatment, 12 were in CR, 6 in PR, and 2 had progressive disease. After treatment, all evaluable patients were in CR post-treatment; the 100-day mortality was 10%. With a median follow-up of 21 months at the time of publication, there had been no recurrences, but the number of deaths rose to three (15%). DFS at 2 years was 84%. The cumulative rate of chronic GVHD was, however, very high at 64% (Table 19–8).

The results for allogeneic stem cell transplantation using reduced-intensity conditioning comprising BEAM chemotherapy and alemtuzumab (Campath) have been reported for 65 patients with lymphoproliferative diseases, including 28 with low-grade NHL.[275] The overall survival at 2 years for this group was 74%, with a treatment-related mortality at 2 years of 16%. The recurrence risk at 2 years was 10%, with no relapses being seen after 1 year. The risk of developing GVHD was 17% for the 53 patients in the whole study group who were alive at 100 days.

Thus, there is no doubt that the mortality from the treatment is less than that following a "standard" allograft. However, it remains high at 10% to 25%, so is clearly not negligible. It remains to be seen whether this potential for cure will be realized. Trials with a "biological'" randomization comparing "mini-allografting" with myeloablative chemotherapy with autologous peripheral blood progenitor cell support are in progress.

Vaccination

The potential to derive meaningful clinical benefit from active immunotherapy directed at a tumor-associated antigen has been intensively investigated and holds much promise. The clonal immunoglobulin antigen receptor provides a unique tumor-associated antigen in FL.

The idiotype is the unique amino acid sequence derived from the variable regions of both the heavy and light

Table 19–7. Comparison of Allogeneic Bone Marrow Transplantation with HDT for Follicular Lymphoma

	Patients (n)	TRM (%)	Recurrence Rate	5-year DFS	5-year OS	Reference
HDT	18	0%	83%	16%	33%	272
Allogeneic	15	27%	0%	70%	70%	
HDT	728	8%–14%	43%–58%	31%–39%	55%–62%	271
Allogeneic	176	30%	21%	45%	51%	
HDT	68	6%	60%	34%	52%	270
Allogeneic	44	34%	19%	45%	49%	

DFS, disease-free survival; HDT, high-dose treatment; OS, overall survival; TRM, treatment-related mortality.

Table 19–8. Nonmyeloablative (Reduced-Intensity) Stem Cell Transplantation in Follicular Lymphoma

Reference	N[a]	Age	No. Previous Treatments	Conditioning Regimen	Post-Transplant IS	GVHD: Acute (II–IV)/Chronic	Graft Failure	Outcome
274	18/20	51	2	Cyclo-flu +/– Rit	Tacro + MTX	Acute: 20%, Chronic: 64%	0	20 CR, 2 died TRM, DFS: 84% 2 yrs
284	28/65	46	2	BEAM + alemtuzumab	CSA + MTX	Acute: 17%, Chronic: 17%, (38% post-DLI)	3	EFS: 69%, TRM: 8% 1 yr
285	29/88	48	3	Flu + mel + alemtuzumab	CSA	Acute: 15%, Chronic: 6.8%, (28% post-DLI)	4	PFS: 65% 3 yrs, TRM: 11% 3 yrs

Note: Data refer to whole series.
[a] Number of FL/total number of patients.
BEAM, BCNU, etoposide, ara-C, and melphalan; CSA, cyclosporine A; DLI, donor lymphocyte infusion; DFS, disease-free survival; EFS, event-free survival; GVHD, graft-versus-host disease; IS, immunosuppression; MTX, methotrexate; PFS, progression-free survival; TRM, treatment-related mortality.

immunoglobulin chains that identify tumor clonality and may be harnessed as an immunogenic antigen. Vaccination strategies have exploited this to generate a polyclonal antilymphoma response. Idiotype protein may be generated using the "classical'" approach of somatic cell hybridization between patient biopsy-derived lymphoma cells and a myeloma cell line. Protein is derived from the culture supernatant and conjugated to the immune "adjuvant," keyhole limpet hemocyanin. Kwak et al.[276,277] demonstrated that using this methodology, both a cellular and antibody-mediated immunologic response could be evoked in patients with B-cell lymphoma, and that mounting a specific response was associated with superior freedom from progression. In another study from the National Cancer Institute, co-administration of GM-CSF and protein idiotype vaccination enhanced the immune response, and was able to induce "molecular remission" in patients with FL at the time of first remission.[278] Despite the daunting nature of the logistics, this approach is currently being investigated in randomized Phase III studies.

The classical approach to idiotype protein production, however, remains challenging, and relies on the availability of viable tumor cells. In an alternative approach, the idiotype gene is cloned from patient material and inserted into a cell line–based expression system. Early data suggest promise, with a high percentage of patients mounting an immune response, and Phase III studies are in progress. Vaccination with autologous dendritic cells, pulsed with idiotype protein has also resulted in immune responses, and in some patients, tumor regressions.[279,280]

DNA vaccination strategies have focused on the cloning of idiotype genes (either those for immunoglobulin heavy and light chains[281] or represented as a single-chain antibody fragment [scFv]),[282] into DNA expression plasmid, which may be injected as "naked" DNA directly. Expression of in vivo transfected idiotype protein as scFV results from the plasmid's ability to exploit the patient's own intracellular protein production machinery. Additionally, the DNA itself may activate an immune response. To enhance immunogenicity, the idiotype gene is fused with a microbial protein gene, typically tetanus toxoid fragment C. These vaccines appear to be safe to administer, and have some advantage in the manufacturing process over their protein counterparts.[283] The results of ongoing trials are awaited.

Regardless of strategy, deficiencies in the immune responsiveness of patients with FL (whether as a consequence of the disease or treatment related) are a consideration. Some vaccination studies have therefore focused on patients early in the clinical course of the disease. Furthermore, in an attempt to offer the immune response the "best chance" of success, prior cytoreduction with chemotherapy is required. Most current studies therefore use the vaccine as a treatment given in first remission. Accrual to studies has been good; the outcomes are eagerly awaited.

What To Do, and When: The Doctor's Dilemma

Be as well informed as possible, both about the patient and about the treatment options. Both the histology and the other prognostic factors should be known at each decision time.

With our present state of knowledge, and the treatments available today, Grades 1, 2, and 3a should be treated the same. Grade 3b and FL that has transformed to DLBCL should be managed as DLBCL. Transformation to "Burkitt-like" or lymphoblastic leukemia should be treated as the circumstances dictate.

The Doctor's Dilemma, and the Authors' Persuasion

Both the strategic plan and the details of specific therapy should be based on the anticipated prognosis at the time of a therapeutic decision, and should take into account the general health of the patient and his or her philosophy. With the breadth of alternatives currently available, the benefit of which is obviously more proven for some than others, it is

Table 19–9. Open Trials for Follicular Lymphoma

Trial	Phase	Disease Status	Description
NCRI-Watch and Wait	Phase III	Diagnosis	Stages II–IV, asymptomatic, expectant management vs. rituximab
SWOG-S0016	Phase III	Diagnosis	Stages II bulky–IV, CHOP–rituximab vs. CHOP–Bexxar
EORTC-20971	Phase III	1st treatment	Stages I–II, Low-dose TBI
NCRI-MCD vs. FMD	Phase III	1st treatment	Stages III–IV, needing treatment, MCD vs. FMD
PRIMA	Phase III	1st treatment	Bulky disease, Rituximab–chemotherapy +/– rituximab maintenance
EORTC-20981	Phase III	1st/2nd relapse	No previous anthracyclines, CHOP vs. CHOP–rituximab
EBMT Lym1	Phase III	2nd or subsequent response	BEAM + PBPCR +/– prior rituximab +/– rituximab maintenance
CCBX001-053[a]	Phase III	3rd or subsequent relapse	Relapse after rituximab, Zevalin vs. Bexxar

[a] To be opened.

inappropriate to be over-proscriptive. With there being dramatic differences in the cost of different treatments, (national) guidelines may advocate what is best for the people but not necessarily for the individual. The patient should always be advised of potential clinical trials. Examples of these are shown in Table 19–9.

Sensible Approaches

At Initial Presentation

Expectant management, with reasonably close surveillance in the first instance is entirely appropriate for patients who are without a history of rapid progression, are well, and who have neither bulky disease nor evidence of vital organ compromise. The only exception is the patient with Stage I and possibly Stage II disease, for whom involved-field irradiation is almost universally regarded as the treatment of first choice. Even this may be debated in the light of the data shown above.

When Therapy Is First Indicated

When the patient presents with a history of rapid progression, is ill, has evidence of vital organ compromise or "bulky disease," or when progression occurs during initial surveillance (when repeat biopsy and complete restaging are indicated), it is customary to commence therapy.

It is at this point that the doctor's dilemma (or dilemmas) first surfaces, particularly for the younger patient. Should treatments for which there are great promise (but possibly much toxicity) be advocated (a) optimistically, and (b) because "we must help this younger person," despite little or no evidence base to indicate either curative potential or prolongation of life above that achieved hitherto? Or should the conservative approach be pursued: "Accept that the disease is incurable but very treatable and give what has been shown best so far"? For the most conservative, the initial therapy is still chlorambucil, since there are no data yet showing a major survival advantage for anything else.

For the majority of hemato-oncologists today, treatment with a chemotherapy-plus-rituximab combination to an arbitrary maximum of eight cycles, if response is obvious, has become the norm, expense not being spared. At present, superficial comparison of the alternatives suggests that CHOP-R and FCM-R or FMD-R may have a better progression-free survival than R-CVP. There is too little data about F-R (fluradibine and rituximab) to comment. Rituximab alone may be best for the patient with comorbidity. Total nodal irradiation with or without chemotherapy is an acceptable alternative for patients with Stage III disease, although rarely used today.

Most patients in complete remission or CR(u) should be managed expectantly until clinical evidence of progression. Those with lesser responses may also be observed, but should be considered for second-line therapy, and consolidation with high-dose therapy and stem cell rescue. Recent data showing a survival advantage for patients in first remission proceeding to cyclophosphamide and TBI make it worthy of consideration at this point for those predicted to be at high risk of progression according to the FLIPI.

At First Progression

This should be managed expectantly in the first instance, unless there is any evidence that transformation has occurred. The same criteria may be applied to deciding about re-treating as to treating in the first instance. There are some data suggesting that the prognosis from recurrence correlates with the survival pattern (not at St. Bartholomew's Hospital), suggesting that early and late progression should be treated differently. Histologic confirmation should always be obtained.

Once it is clear that intervention is indicated again, the choice of treatment is again heavily influenced by the age and general well-being of the patient. It is customary to attempt to re-induce remission. There is no evidence that one chemotherapy regimen is much better than another. Re-treating (certainly after a reasonably long remission) with the same chemotherapy that was "effective" the first time is entirely reasonable. The best published results are with FMD and FCM-R (in patients who had not received prior rituximab). It is not clear what the role of further rituximab is in this setting. Rituximab alone is reasonable. Low-dose involved-field irradiation should also be considered.

However, if consolidation of the second remission with HDT is being considered, this may influence the choice of the induction therapy, there having been many reports of difficulty obtaining sufficient numbers of CD34 positive cells after fludarabine-containing combinations. Patients at high risk of further recurrence in whom enough cells cannot be collected should be considered for allogeneic transplantation.

At the Time of Second and Subsequent Progressions

The art of the practice of medicine (*as opposed to quasi-science*) comes into play here more than earlier in the course of the illness. Once again, histologic confirmation and restaging are critical for the majority of patients. Once again, the age and general well-being of the patient are relevant, as is philosophy.

Expectant management may be appropriate. The second (and certainly the third) recurrence is probably the last opportunity for introducing an "aggressive" treatment that might confer a survival advantage. Remission induction should be attempted, and if successful, high-dose therapy should be considered, despite the fact that it is less effective in third and subsequent remissions than second. Regardless of whether a harvest can be obtained, reduced-intensity allogeneic transplantation, with its attendant greater risk, may be the treatment of choice.

As the illness progresses, particularly in older patients, high-risk treatments become progressively less relevant. Hence, the enormous importance of *relatively* nontoxic treatments such as single-agent chemotherapy and rituximab for the best delivery of care.

At the Time of Chemotherapy or Antibody Refractoriness

Local irradiation may be appropriate. Anecdotal evidence suggests that pulsed high-dose corticosteroids are beneficial. Phase I and II trials are very important.

THE BEST WAY FORWARD

Data have now been published (either as a full paper or as abstracts) indicating that at a single center (M.D. Anderson Cancer Center), in a cooperative group, Southwest Oncology Group and in several parts of the United States (Surveillance Epidemiology and End Results), the prognosis of FL improved as the result of treatments introduced late in the 20th century. From one source, it is suggested that the improvement is a function of better initial therapy, and from another that it is due to the increased number of treatments available to treat a repeatedly responsive disease.

The ability to quantify at very low levels the "molecular" evidence of disease, or the achievement and maintenance of molecular remission, presents the opportunity of testing the hypothesis that "molecular remission" may be a prerequisite to cure, and is a more desirable endpoint than "complete remission" alone. Regardless of the fact that the use of rituximab may, in the short term after its administration, obscure the meaning of molecular (plus clinical remission), now is the time to explore it.

Instead of designing Phase III trials to compare the outcome of treatment A versus treatment B, the alternative is to design trials to determine whether the goal of clinical or clinical plus molecular remission is more relevant to the patient. To prove the point, either from the time of presentation, first therapy, or second therapy, the perceived best algorithm of treatment, using the best treatments in sequence would be pursued in one arm until clinical remission, and on the other to molecular remission. Clearly such an approach would, in the first instance, only be relevant to the younger, fitter patient. But it might yield much. Otherwise, a best-bet algorithm should involve the concept of achieving the desired effect with the minimum of toxicity.

Acknowledgment

We are most grateful to Margaret Cresswell for her infinite patience in preparing and typing this manuscript, again and again.

References

1. Jaffe ES, Harris NL, Stein H, et al. World Health Organization Classification of Tumours. Pathology and Genetics of Tumours of Haematopoietic and Lymphoid Tissues. Lyon: IARC Press, 2001.
2. Groves F, Linet M, Travis L, et al. Cancer surveillance series: non-Hodgkin's lymphoma incidence by histologic subtype in the United States from 1978 through 1995. J Natl Cancer Inst 2000;92:1240–51.
3. Herrinton L, Goldoft M, Schwartz S, et al. The incidence of non-Hodgkin's lymphoma and its histologic subtypes in Asian migrants to the United States and their descendants. Cancer Causes Control 1996;7:224–30.
4. Biagi J, Seymour J. Insights into the molecular pathogenesis of follicular lymphoma arising from analysis of geographic variation. Blood 2002;99:4265–75.
5. Mann RB and Berard CW. Criteria for the cytologic subclassification of follicular lymphomas: a proposed alternative method. Hematol Oncol 1983;1:187–92.
6. Nathwani BN, Anderson JR, Armitage JO, et al. Clinical significance of follicular lymphoma with monocytoid B cells. Non-Hodgkin's Lymphoma Classification Project. Hum Pathol 1999;30:263–8.
7. Ott G, Katzenberger T, Lohr A, et al. Cytomorphologic, immunohistochemical, and cytogenetic profiles of follicular lymphoma: 2 types of follicular lymphoma grade 3. Blood 2002;99:3806–12.
8. Bastion Y, Brice P, Haioun C, et al. Intensive therapy with peripheral blood progenitor cell transplantation in 60 patients with poor-prognosis follicular lymphoma. Blood 1995;86:3257–62.
9. Eshoa C, Perkins S, Kampalath B, et al. Decreased CD10 expression in grade III and in interfollicular infiltrates of follicular lymphomas. Am J Clin Pathol 2001;115:862–7.
10. Lai R, Weiss LM, Chang KL, et al. Frequency of CD43 expression in non-Hodgkin lymphoma. A survey of 742 cases and further characterization of rare CD43+ follicular lymphomas. Am J Clin Pathol 1999;111:488–94.
11. Cattoretti G, Chang CC, Cechova K, et al. BCL-6 protein is expressed in germinal-center B cells. Blood 1995;86:45–53.
12. Nguyen PL, Zukerberg LR, Benedict WF, et al. Immunohistochemical detection of p53, bcl-2, and retinoblastoma proteins in follicular lymphoma. Am J Clin Pathol 1996;105: 538–43.
13. Cleary ML, Meeker TC, Levy S, et al. Clustering of extensive somatic mutations in the variable region of an immunoglobulin heavy chain gene from a human B cell lymphoma. Cell 1986;44:97–106.
14. Bahler DW, Campbell MJ, Hart S, et al. Ig VH gene expression among human follicular lymphomas. Blood 1991; 78:1561–8.
15. Aarts WM, Bende RJ, Bossenbroek JG, et al. Variable heavy-chain gene analysis of follicular lymphomas: subclone selec-

tion rather than clonal evolution over time. Blood 2001; 98:238–40.
16. Matolcsy A, Schattner EJ, Knowles DM, et al. Clonal evolution of B cells in transformation from low- to high-grade lymphoma. Eur J Immunol 1999;29:1253–64.
17. Ottensmeier CH, Thompsett AR, Zhu D, et al. Analysis of VH genes in follicular and diffuse lymphoma shows ongoing somatic mutation and multiple isotype transcripts in early disease with changes during disease progression. Blood 1998;91:4292–9.
18. Zelenetz AD, Chen TT, and Levy R. Histologic transformation of follicular lymphoma to diffuse lymphoma represents tumor progression by a single malignant B cell. J Exp Med 1991;173:197–207.
19. Yunis JJ, Frizzera G, Oken MM, et al. Multiple recurrent genomic defects in follicular lymphoma. A possible model for cancer. N Engl J Med 1987;316:79–84.
20. Tilly H, Rossi A, Stamatoullas A, et al. Prognostic value of chromosomal abnormalities in follicular lymphoma. Blood 1994;84:1043–9.
21. Horsman DE, Connors JM, Pantzar T, et al. Analysis of secondary chromosomal alterations in 165 cases of follicular lymphoma with t(14;18). Genes Chromosomes Cancer 2001;30:375–82.
22. Tsujimoto Y, Finger LR, Yunis J, et al. Cloning of the chromosome breakpoint of neoplastic B cells with the t(14;18) chromosome translocation. Science 1984;226:1097–9.
23. Tsujimoto Y, Gorham J, Cossman J, et al. The t(14;18) chromosome translocations involved in B-cell neoplasms result from mistakes in VDJ joining. Science 1985; 229:1390–3.
24. Cleary ML, Smith SD, and Sklar J. Cloning and structural analysis of cDNAs for bcl-2 and a hybrid bcl-2/immunoglobulin transcript resulting from the t(14;18) translocation. Cell 1986;47:19–28.
25. Buchonnet G, Lenain P, Ruminy P, et al. Characterisation of BCL2-JH rearrangements in follicular lymphoma: PCR detection of 3' BCL2 breakpoints and evidence of a new cluster. Leukemia 2000;14:1563–9.
26. Cleary ML, Galili N, and Sklar J. Detection of a second t(14;18) breakpoint cluster region in human follicular lymphomas. J Exp Med 1986;164:315–20.
27. Cotter F, Price C, Zucca E, et al. Direct sequence analysis of the 14q+ and 18q- chromosome junctions in follicular lymphoma. Blood 1990;76:131–5.
28. Graninger WB, Seto M, Boutain B, et al. Expression of Bcl-2 and Bcl-2-Ig fusion transcripts in normal and neoplastic cells. J Clin Invest 1987;80:1512–5.
29. Seto M, Jaeger U, Hockett RD, et al. Alternative promoters and exons, somatic mutation and deregulation of the Bcl-2-Ig fusion gene in lymphoma. EMBO J 1988;7: 123–31.
30. Zamzami N and Kroemer G. The mitochondrion in apoptosis: how Pandora's box opens. Nat Rev Mol Cell Biol 2001; 2:67–71.
31. Dolken G, Illerhaus G, Hirt C, et al. BCL-2/JH rearrangements in circulating B cells of healthy blood donors and patients with nonmalignant diseases. J Clin Oncol 1996; 14:1333–44.
32. Summers KE, Goff LK, Wilson AG, et al. Frequency of the Bcl-2/IgH rearrangement in normal individuals: implications for the monitoring of disease in patients with follicular lymphoma. J Clin Oncol 2001;19:420–4.
33. McDonnell TJ and Korsmeyer SJ. Progression from lymphoid hyperplasia to high-grade malignant lymphoma in mice transgenic for the t(14; 18). Nature 1991;349:254–6.
34. Whang-Peng J, Knutsen T, Jaffe ES, et al. Sequential analysis of 43 patients with non-Hodgkin's lymphoma: clinical correlations with cytogenetic, histologic, immunophenotyping, and molecular studies. Blood 1995;85:203–16.
35. Hoglund M, Sehn L, Connors JM, et al. Identification of cytogenetic subgroups and karyotypic pathways of clonal evolution in follicular lymphomas. Genes Chromosomes Cancer 2004;39:195–204.
36. Martinez-Climent JA, Alizadeh AA, Segraves R, et al. Transformation of follicular lymphoma to diffuse large cell lymphoma is associated with a heterogeneous set of DNA copy number and gene expression alterations. Blood 2003; 101:3109–17.
37. Hough RE, Goepel JR, Alcock HE, et al. Copy number gain at 12q12–14 may be important in the transformation from follicular lymphoma to diffuse large B cell lymphoma. Br J Cancer 2001;84:499–503.
38. Viardot A, Moller P, Hogel J, et al. Clinicopathologic correlations of genomic gains and losses in follicular lymphoma. J Clin Oncol 2002;20:4523–30.
39. Goff L, Neat M, Crawley C, et al. The use of real-time quantitative PCR and comparative genomic hybridisation to identify amplication of the REL gene in follicular lymphoma. Br J Haematol 2000;111:618–25.
40. Koduru PR, Raju K, Vadmal V, et al. Correlation between mutation in P53, p53 expression, cytogenetics, histologic type, and survival in patients with B-cell non-Hodgkin's lymphoma. Blood 1997;90:4078–91.
41. Lo Coco F, Gaidano G, Louie DC, et al. p53 mutations are associated with histologic transformation of follicular lymphoma. Blood 1993;82:2289–95.
42. Sander CA, Yano T, Clark HM, et al. p53 mutation is associated with progression in follicular lymphomas. Blood 1993;82:1994–2004.
43. Yano T, Jaffe ES, Longo DL, et al. MYC rearrangements in histologically progressed follicular lymphomas. Blood 1992;80:758–67.
44. Lossos IS, Alizadeh AA, Diehn M, et al. Transformation of follicular lymphoma to diffuse large-cell lymphoma: alternative patterns with increased or decreased expression of c-myc and its regulated genes. Proc Natl Acad Sci U S A 2002; 99:8886–91.
45. Akasaka T, Lossos IS, and Levy R. BCL6 gene translocation in follicular lymphoma: a harbinger of eventual transformation to diffuse aggressive lymphoma. Blood 2003;102:1443–8.
46. Szereday Z, Csernus B, Nagy M, et al. Somatic mutation of the 5' noncoding region of the BCL-6 gene is associated with intraclonal diversity and clonal selection in histological transformation of follicular lymphoma. Am J Pathol 2000; 156:1017–24.
47. Lossos IS and Levy R. Mutation analysis of the 5' noncoding regulatory region of the BCL-6 gene in non-Hodgkin lymphoma: evidence for recurrent mutations and intraclonal heterogeneity. Blood 2000;95:1400–5.
48. Elenitoba-Johnson KS, Gascoyne RD, Lim MS, et al. Homozygous deletions at chromosome 9p21 involving p16 and p15 are associated with histologic progression in follicle center lymphoma. Blood 1998;91:4677–85.
49. Pinyol M, Cobo F, Bea S, et al. p16(INK4a) gene inactivation by deletions, mutations, and hypermethylation is associated with transformed and aggressive variants of non-Hodgkin's lymphomas. Blood 1998;91:2977–84.
50. Elenitoba-Johnson KS, Jenson SD, Abbott RT, et al. Involvement of multiple signaling pathways in follicular lymphoma transformation: p38-mitogen-activated protein kinase as a target for therapy. Proc Natl Acad Sci U S A 2003; 100:7259–64.
51. Clark HM, Yano T, Sander C, et al. Mutation of the ras genes is a rare genetic event in the histologic transformation of follicular lymphoma. Leukemia 1996;10:844–7.

52. Dave SS, Wright G, Tan B, et al. Prediction of survival in follicular lymphoma based on molecular features of tumor-infiltrating immune cells. N Engl J Med 2004;351:2159–69.
53. Becker E. Ein beitrag zur lehre von den lymphomen. Deutsch Med Wchnschr 1917;27:726–8.
54. Brill NE, Baehr G, and Rosenthal N. Generalized giant lymph follicle hyperplasia of lymph nodes and spleen. A hitherto undescribed type. JAMA 1925;2:668–71.
55. Symmers D. Giant follicular lymphadenopathy with or without splenomegaly. Arch Pathol 1938;26:603–47.
56. Gall E, Morrison H, and Scott A. The follicular type of malignant lymphoma: a survey of 63 cases. Ann Intern Med 1941;14:2073.
57. Gall EA and Mallory TB. Malignant lymphoma: a clinicopathological survey of 618 cases. Am J Pathol 1942; 18:381–415.
58. Rappaport H, Winter H, and Hicks E. Follicular lymphoma: a re-evaluation of its place in the scheme of malignant lymphoma based on a survey of 253 cases. Cancer 1956;9:792.
59. Rosenberg SA, Diamond HD, and Craver LF. Lymphosarcoma: survival and the effects of therapy. Am J Roentgenol Radium Ther Nucl Med 1961;85:521–32.
60. Litam P, Swan F, Cabanillas F, et al. Prognostic value of serum b-2 microglobulin in low-grade lymphoma. Ann Intern Med 1991;114:855–60.
61. Solal-Celigny P, Roy P, Colombat P, et al. Follicular lymphoma international prognostic index. Blood 2004;104: 1258–65.
62. Pinto A, Hutchison R, Grant L, et al. Follicular lymphomas in paediatric patients. Mod Pathol 1990;3:308–13.
63. Horning S and Rosenberg S. The natural history of initially untreated low-grade non-Hodgkin's lymphoma. N Engl J Med 1984;311:1471–508.
64. Advani R, Rosenberg S, and Horning S. Stage I and II follicular non-Hodgkin's lymphoma: long-term follow-up of no initial therapy. J Clin Oncol 2004;22:1454–9.
65. Soubeyran P, Eghbali H, Torjani M, et al. Is there any place for a wait and see policy in Stage 0 follicular lymphoma? A study of 43 consectuve patients in a single centre. Ann Oncol 1996;7:713–8.
66. Jones S, Fuks Z, Bull M, et al. Non-Hodgkin's lymphoma: IV. Clinicopathologic correlation in 405 cases. Cancer 1973; 31:806–23.
67. Anderson T, De Vita V, Simon R, et al. Malignant lymphoma: II. Prognostic factors and response to treatment of 473 patients at the National Cancer Institute. Cancer 1982; 50:2708–21.
68. Brittinger G, Bartels H, Common H, et al. Clinical and prognostic relevance of the Kiel classification of non-Hodgkin's lymphomas: results of a prospective multicentre study of the Kiel lymphoma study group. Hematol Oncol 1984;2:269.
69. Gallagher CJ, Gregory WM, Jones AE, et al. Follicular lymphoma: prognostic factors for response and survival. J Clin Oncol 1986;4:1470–80.
70. Liu Q, Fayad L, Hagemeister F, et al. Stage IV indolent lymphoma: 25 years of treatment progress. Blood 2003;102: 1446a.
71. Fisher R, LeBlanc M, Press O, et al. New treatment options have changed the natural history of follicular lymphoma. Proc Am Soc Hematol 2004;104:168a.
72. Swenson W, Woodridge J, Lynch C, et al. Improved survival of follicular lymphoma patients in the United States. J Clin Oncol 2005; 23(22):4830–1.
73. Hubbard S, Chabner B, De Vita V, et al. Histologic progression in non-Hodgkin's lymphoma. Blood 1982;59:258–64.
74. Cullen M, Lister T, RL B, et al. Histologic transformation of non-Hodgkin's lymphoma: a prospective study. Cancer 1979;44:645–51.
75. Ostrow S, Digs C, Sutherland J, et al. Nodular poorly differentiated lymphocytic lymphoma: Changes in histology and survival. Cancer Treat Rep 1981;65:929–33.
76. Ersboll J, Schultz H, Pedersen-Bjergaard J, et al. Follicular low-grade non-Hodgkin's lymphoma: long-term outcome with or without tumor progression. Eur J Haematol 1989; 42:155 –63.
77. Armitage J, Dick F, and Corder M. Diffuse histiocytic lymphoma after histologic conversion: a poor prognostic variant. Cancer Treat Rep 1981;65:413–8.
78. Bastion Y, Sebban C, Berger F, et al. Incidence, predictive factors and outcome of lymphoma transformation in follicular lymphoma patients. J Clin Oncol 1997;15:1587–94.
79. Acker B, Hoppe R, Colby T, et al. Histologic conversion in the non-Hodgkin's lymphomas. J Clin Oncol 1983;1:11–6.
80. Yuen AR, Kamel OW, Halpern J, et al. Long-term survival after histologic transformation of low-grade follicular lymphoma. J Clin Oncol 1995;13:1726–33.
81. Montoto S, Lopez-Guillermo A, Ferrer A, et al. Survival after progression in patients with follicular lymphoma: analysis of prognostic factors. Ann Oncol 2002;13:523–30.
82. Longo D, Young R, Hubbard S, et al. Prolonged initial remission in patients with nodular mixed lymphomas. Ann Intern Med 1984;100:651–6.
83. Peterson B, Anderson J, Frizzera G, et al. Combination chemotherapy prolongs survival in follicular mixed lymphoma (FML) [abstract]. Proc Am Soc Clin Oncol 1990; 9:259.
84. Glick J, Barnes J, and Ezdinli E. Nodular mixed lymphoma: results of a randomized trial failing to confirm prolonged disease-free survival with COPP chemotherapy. Blood 1981; 58:920–5.
85. Horning S. Follicular lymphoma: have we made any progress? Ann Oncol 2000;11:23–7.
86. MacManus M and Seymour J. Management of localised low-grade follicular lymphomas. Australas Radiol 2001;45: 326–34.
87. Rudders R, Kaddis M, DeLellis R, et al. Nodular non-Hodgkin's lymphoma: factors influencing prognosis and indications for aggressive treatment. Cancer 1979;43: 1643–51.
88. Soubeyran P, Eghbali H, Bonichon F, et al. Low-grade follicular lymphomas: analysis of prognosis in a series of 281 patients. Eur J Cancer 1991;27:1606–13.
89. Gospodarowicz M, Bush R, Brown T, et al. Prognostic factors in nodular lymphomas: a multivariate analysis based on the Princess Margaret Hospital experience. Int J Radiat Oncol Biol Phys 1984;10:489–97.
90. Lepage E, Sebban D, Gisselbrecht C, et al. Treatment of low-grade non-Hodgkin's lymphomas: assessment of doxorubicin in a controlled trial. Hematol Oncol 1990;8:31–39.
91. Leonard R, Hayward R, Prescott R, et al. The identification of discrete prognostic groups in low grade non-Hodgkin's lymphoma. Ann Oncol 1991;2:655–62.
92. Romaguera J, McLaughlin P, North L, et al. Multivariate analysis of prognostic factors in stage IV follicular low-grade lymphoma: a risk model. J Clin Oncol 1991;9:762–9.
93. Steward W, Crowther D, McWilliam L, et al. Maintenance chlorambucil after CVP in the management of advanced stage, low-grade histologic type non-Hodgkin's lymphoma: a randomized prospective study with an assessment of prognostic factors. Cancer 1988;61:441–7.
94. Peterson B, Petroni G, Frizzera G, et al. Prolonged single-agent versus combination chemotherapy in indolent follicular lymphomas: a study of the cancer and leukemia group B. J Clin Oncol 2003;21:5–15.
95. Coiffier B, Gisselbrecht C, Vose J, et al. Prognostic factors in aggressive malignant lymphomas: description and validation

of a prognostic index that could identify patients requiring a more intensive chemotherapy. J Clin Oncol 1991;9:211–19.
96. Shipp M, Harrington D, Anderson J, et al. A predictive model for aggressive non-Hodgkin's lymphoma. The International Non-Hodgkin's Lymphoma Prognostic Factors Project. N Engl J Med 1993;329:987–94.
97. Coiffier B, Bastion Y, Berger F, et al, et al. Prognostic factors in follicular lymphomas. Semin Oncol 1993;20(suppl 5):89–95.
98. Pappa VI, Hussain HK, Reznek RH, et al. Role of image-guided core-needle biopsy in the management of patients with lymphoma. J Clin Oncol 1996;14:2427–30.
99. Johnson PW, Rohatiner AZ, Whelan JS, et al. Patterns of survival in patients with recurrent follicular lymphoma: a 20-year study from a single center. J Clin Oncol 1995;13:140–7.
100. Young R, Longo D, Glatstein E, et al. The treatment of indolent lymphomas: watchful waiting v aggressive combined modality treatment. Semin Hematol 1988;2(suppl 2):11–16.
101. Brice P, Bastion Y, Lepage E, et al. Comparison in low-tumor-burden follicular lymphomas between an initial no treatment policy, prednimustine or interferon-alpha: a randomized study from the Groupe d'Etude des Lymphomas Folliculaires. J Clin Oncol 1997;15:1110–17.
102. Ardeshna K, Smith P, Norton A, et al. Long-term effect of a watch and wait policy vs immediate systemic treatment for asymptomatic advanced stage non-Hodgkin's lymphoma: a randomised controlled trial. Lancet 2003;362:516–22.
103. Fuks Z and Kaplan H. Recurrence rates following radiation therapy of nodular and diffuse malignant lymphomas. Radiology 1973;108:675–84.
104. Chen M, Prosnitz L, Gonzales-Serva A, et al. Results of radiotherapy in control of Stage I and II non-Hodgin's lymphoma. Cancer 1979;43:1245–54.
105. Gomez G, Barlos M, Krishnamsetty R, et al. Treatment of early—stage I and I—nodular poorly differentiated lymphocytic lymphoma. Am J Clin Oncol 1986;9:40–4.
106. Gospodarowicz M, Bush R, Brown T, et al. Prognostic factors in nodular lymphomas: a multivariate analysis based on the Princess Margaret Hospital experience. Int J Radiat Oncol Biol Phy 1984;10:489–97.
107. Paryani S, Hoppe R, and Cox R. Analysis of non-Hodgkin's lymphomas with nodular and favorable histologies, stages I and II. Cancer 1983;52:2300–7.
108. Reddy S, Saxema V, Pellettiere E, et al. Stage I and II non-Hodgkin's lymphomas: Long-term results of radiation therapy. Int J Radiat Oncol Biol Phys 1989;16:687–92.
109. Mc Laughlin P, Fuller L, Velasquez W, et al. Stage I-II follicular lymphoma: treatment results of 76 patients. Cancer 1986;58:1596–602.
110. Richards M, Gregory W, Hall P, et al. Management of localized non-Hodgkin's lymphoma: the experience at St. Bartholomew's Hospital, 1972–1985. Hematol Oncol 1989; 7:1–18.
111. MacManus MP and Hoppe RT. Overview of treatment of localized low-grade lymphoma. Haematol Oncol Clin North Am 1997;11:901–8.
112. Murtha A, Rupnow B, Hansosn J, et al. Long-term follow-up of patients with Stage III follicular lymphoma treated with primary radiotherapy at Stanford University. Int J Radiat Oncol Biol Phy 2001;49:3–15.
113. Glatstein E, Fuks Z, Goffinet D, et al. Non-Hodgkin's lymphoma of stage III extent. Cancer 1976;37:2806–12.
114. Hoppe R, Kushlan P, Kaplan H, et al. The treatment of advanced stage favorable histology non-Hodgkin's lymphoma: a preliminary report of a randomized trial comparing single agent chemotherapy, combination chemotherapy and whole body irradiation. Blood 1981;58:592.
115. Jacobs JP, Murray KJ, Schultz CJ, et al. Central lymphatic irradiation for stage III nodular malignant lymphoma: long-term results. J Clin Oncol 1993;11:233–8.
116. Carde P, Burgers J, Van Glabbeke M, et al. Combined radiotherapy-chemotherapy for early stages in non-Hodgkin's lymphoma: the EORTC controlled lymphoma trial. Radiother Oncol 1984;2:301–12.
117. Monfardini S, Banfi A, Bonadonna G, et al. Improved five year survival after combined radiotherapy-chemotherapy for stage I and II non-Hodgkin's lymphoma. Int J Radiat Oncol Biol Phys 1980;6:125–34.
118. Mendenhall N, Noyes W, and Million R. Total body irradiation for stage II-IV non-Hodgkin's lymphoma: ten year follow-up. J Clin Oncol 1989;7:67–74.
119. Lybeert M, Meerwaldt J, Deneve W. Long-term results of low-dose total body irradiation for advanced non-Hodgkin's lymphoma. Int J Radiat Oncol Biol Phys 1987;13:1167–73.
120. Chaffey J, Hellman S, Rosenthal D, et al. Total body irradiation in the treatment of lymphocytic lymphoma. Cancer Treat Rep 1977;61:1149–52.
121. Choi C, Timothy A, Kaufman S, et al. Low-dose fractionated total body irradiation in the treatment of advanced non-Hodgkin's lymphoma. Cancer 1979;43:1636–42.
122. Haas R, Poortmans P, de Jong D, et al. High response rates and lasting remissions after low-dose involved field radiotherapy in indolent lymphomas. J Clin Oncol 2003;21: 2474–80.
123. Davis TA, Kaminski MS, Leonard JP, et al. The radioisotope contributes significantly to the activity of radioimmunotherapy. Clin Cancer Res 2004;10:7792–8.
124. Vose JM, Wahl RL, Saleh M, et al. Multicenter phase II study of iodine-131 tositumomab for chemotherapy-relapsed/refractory low-grade and transformed low-grade B-cell non-Hodgkin's lymphomas. J Clin Oncol 2000;18: 1316–23.
125. Kaminski MS, Estes J, Zasadny KR, et al. Radioimmunotherapy with iodine (131)I tositumomab for relapsed or refractory B-cell non-Hodgkin lymphoma: updated results and long-term follow-up of the University of Michigan experience. Blood 2000;96:1259–66.
126. Kaminski MS, Zelenetz AD, Press OW, et al. Pivotal study of iodine I 131 tositumomab for chemotherapy-refractory low-grade or transformed low-grade B-cell non-Hodgkin's lymphomas. J Clin Oncol 2001;19:3918–28.
127. Davies AJ, Rohatiner AZ, Howell S, et al. Tositumomab and iodine I 131 tositumomab for recurrent indolent and transformed B-cell non-Hodgkin's lymphoma. J Clin Oncol 2004; 22:1469–79.
128. Horning SJ, Younes A, Jain V, et al. Efficacy and safety of tositumomab and iodine-131 tositumomab (Bexxar) in B-cell lymphoma, progressive after rituximab. J Clin Oncol 2005; 23:712–9.
129. Zelenetz AD, Saleh M, Vose JM, et al. Patients with transformed low grade lymphoma attain durable responses following outpatient radioimmunotherapy with tositumomab and iodine I 131 tositumomab (Bexxar®) [abstract]. Blood 2002;100:357a.
130. Kaminski MS, Tuck M, Estes J, et al. 131I-tositumomab therapy as initial treatment for follicular lymphoma. N Engl J Med 2005;352:441–9.
131. Press OW, Unger JM, Braziel RM, et al. A phase 2 trial of CHOP chemotherapy followed by tositumomab/iodine I 131 tositumomab for previously untreated follicular non-Hodgkin lymphoma: Southwest Oncology Group Protocol S9911. Blood 2003;102:1606–12.
132. Bennett JM, Kaminski MS, Leonard JP, et al. Assessment of treatment-related myelodysplastic syndromes and acute myeloid leukemia in patients with non-Hodgkin's lymphoma

treated with Tositumomab and Iodine I 131 Tositumomab (BEXXAR(R)). Blood 2005;105(12): 4576–82.
133. Press OW, Eary JF, Appelbaum FR, et al. Radiolabeled-antibody therapy of B-cell lymphoma with autologous bone marrow support. N Engl J Med 1993;329:1219–24.
134. Press OW, Eary JF, Appelbaum FR, et al. Phase II trial of 131I-B1 (anti-CD20) antibody therapy with autologous stem cell transplantation for relapsed B cell lymphomas. Lancet 1995;346:336–40.
135. Gopal AK, Gooley TA, Maloney DG, et al. High-dose radioimmunotherapy versus conventional high-dose therapy and autologous hematopoietic stem cell transplantation for relapsed follicular non-Hodgkin lymphoma: a multivariable cohort analysis. Blood 2003;102:2351–7.
136. Vose JM, Bierman PJ, Enke C, et al. Phase I trial of iodine-131 tositumomab with high-dose chemotherapy and autologous stem-cell transplantation for relapsed non-Hodgkin's lymphoma. J Clin Oncol (prepublication release November 8, 2004 as 10.1200/JCO.2005.05.117, 2004).
137. Press OW, Eary JF, Gooley T, et al. A phase I/II trial of iodine-131-tositumomab (anti-CD20), etoposide, cyclophosphamide, and autologous stem cell transplantation for relapsed B-cell lymphomas. Blood 2000;96:2934–42.
138. Witzig TE, White CA, Wiseman GA, et al. Phase I/II trial of IDEC-Y2B8 radioimmunotherapy for treatment of relapsed or refractory CD20(+) B-cell non-Hodgkin's lymphoma. J Clin Oncol 1999;17:3793–803.
139. Witzig TE, Flinn IW, Gordon LI, et al. Treatment with ibritumomab tiuxetan radioimmunotherapy in patients with rituximab-refractory follicular non-Hodgkin's lymphoma. J Clin Oncol 2002;20:3262–9.
140. Wiseman GA, Gordon LI, Multani PS, et al. Ibritumomab tiuxetan radioimmunotherapy for patients with relapsed or refractory non-Hodgkin lymphoma and mild thrombocytopenia: a phase II multicenter trial. Blood 2002;99:4336–42.
141. Gordon LI, Molina A, Witzig T, et al. Durable responses after ibritumomab tiuxetan radioimmunotherapy for CD20+ B-cell lymphoma: long-term follow-up of a phase 1/2 study. Blood 2004;103:4429–31.
142. Knox SJ, Goris ML, Trisler K, et al. Yttrium-90–labeled anti-CD20 monoclonal antibody therapy of recurrent B-cell lymphoma. Clin Cancer Res 1996;2:457–70.
143. Witzig TE, Gordon LI, Cabanillas F, et al. Randomized controlled trial of yttrium-90–labeled ibritumomab tiuxetan radioimmunotherapy versus rituximab immunotherapy for patients with relapsed or refractory low-grade, follicular, or transformed B-cell non-Hodgkin's lymphoma. J Clin Oncol 2002;20:2453–63.
144. Witzig TE, White CA, Gordon LI, et al. Safety of yttrium-90 ibritumomab tiuxetan radioimmunotherapy for relapsed low-grade, follicular, or transformed non-Hodgkin's lymphoma. J Clin Oncol 2003;21:1263–70.
145. Ansell SM, Ristow KM, Habermann TM, et al. Subsequent chemotherapy regimens are well tolerated after radioimmunotherapy with yttrium-90 ibritumomab tiuxetan for non-Hodgkin's lymphoma. J Clin Oncol 2002;20:3885–90.
146. Galton D, Israels L, Nabarro J, et al. Clinical trial of p(dichloroethylamino) phenylbutyric acid (CB 1384) in malignant lymphoma. BMJ 1955;2:1172–6.
147. Israels L, Galton D, Till M, et al. Clinical evaluation of CB 1348 in malignant lymphoma and related diseases. Ann N Y Acad Sci 1958;68:915–25.
148. Lister A, Cullen M, Beard M, et al. Comparison of combined and single agent chemotherapy in non-Hodgkin's lymphoma of favourable histological subtype. BMJ 1978;1:533–41.
149. Jones S, Rosenberg S, Kaplan H, et al. Non-Hodgkin's lymphomas II. Single agent chemotherapy. Cancer 1972;30: 31–38.
150. Kennedy J, Bloomfield C, Kiang D, et al. Combination versus successive single agent chemotherapy in lymphocytic lymphoma. Cancer 1978;41:23–8.
151. Portlock C, Rosenberg S, Glatstein E, et al. Treatment of advanced non-Hodgkin's lymphomas with favorable histology: preliminary results of a prospective trial. Blood 1976; 47:747–56.
152. Cavallin-Stahl E and Moller T. With the Swedish Lymphoma Group. Predimustines: cyclophosphamide, vincristine, prednisolone in the treatment of non-Hodgkin's lymphoma with favorable histology: results of a national cancer care program in Sweden. Semin Oncol 1986;13:19–22.
153. Ezdinli E, Anderson J, Melvin F, et al. Moderate versus aggressive chemotherapy of nodular lymphocytic poorly differentiated lymphoma. J Clin Oncol 1985;3:769–75.
154. Hochster H and Cassileth P. Fludarabine phosphate therapy of non-Hodgkin's lymphoma. Semin Oncol 1990;17:63–5.
155. Leiby J, Snider K, Kraut E, et al. Phase II trial of 9-b-o-arabinofuranosyl-2-fluoroadenine 5'-monophosphate in non-Hodgkin's lymphoma: prospective comparison of response with deoxycytidine kinase activity. Cancer Res 1987;47:2719–22.
156. Whelan J, Davis C, Rule S, et al. Fludarabine phosphate for the treatment of low grade lymphoid malignancy. Br J Cancer 1991;64:120–3.
157. Redman J, Cabanillas F, Velasquez W, et al. Phase II trial of fludarabine phosphate in lymphoma: an effective new agent in low-grade lymphoma. J Clin Oncol 1992;10:790.
158. Hiddemann W, Unterhalt M, Pott C, et al. Fludarabine single agent therapy for relapsed low-grade non-Hodgkin's lymphomas—a phase II study of the German Low-Grade Non-Hodgkin's Lymphoma Study Group. Semin Oncol 1993; 20:28–31.
159. Zinzani P, Lauria F, Rondelli D, et al. Fludarabine—an active agent in the treatment of previously treated and untreated low-grade non-Hodgkin's lymphoma. Ann Oncol 1993;4: 575–8.
160. Pigaditou A, Rohatiner A, Whelan J, et al. Fludarabine in low-grade lymphoma. Semin Oncol 1993;20:24–7.
161. Foran J, Oscier D, Orchard J, et al. Pharmacokinetic study of single doses of oral fludarabine phosphate in patients with "low-grade" non-Hodgkin's Lymphoma and B-cell chronic lymphocytic leukemia. J Clin Oncol 1999;17:1574–9.
162. Solal-Celigny P, Brice P, Brousse N, et al. Phase II trial of fludarabine monophosphate as first line therapy in patients with advanced follicular lymphoma: a multicenter study by the Groupe d'Etude des Lymphomas de l'Adult. J Clin Oncol 1996;14:514–9.
163. Hoogstraten B, Owens A, Lenhard R, et al. Combination chemotherapy in lymphosarcoma and reticulum cell sarcoma. Blood 1969;33:370.
164. Luce J, Gamble J, Wilson H, et al. Combined cyclophosphamide, vincristine and prednisolone therapy of malignant lymphoma. Cancer 1971;28:306–17.
165. Bagley C, De Vita V, Berrard C, et al. Advanced lymphosarcoma: intensive cyclical combination chemotherapy with cyclophosphamide, vincristine and prednisolone. Ann Intern Med 1972;76:227–34.
166. Dana BW, Dahlberg S, Nathwani BN, et al. Long-term follow-up of patients with low-grade malignant lymphomas treated with doxorubicin-based chemotherapy or chemoimmunotherapy. J Clin Oncol 1993;11:644–51.
167. Rodriguez V, Cabanillas F, Burgess M, et al. Combination chemotherapy ("CHOP–bleo") in advanced non-Hodgkin's lymphoma. Blood 1977;49:325–33.
168. McKelvey E, Gottlieb J, Wilson H, et al. Hydroxydaunomycin (Adriamycin) in malignant lymphoma. Cancer 1976; 38:1484–93.

169. Jones S, Grozea P, Metz E, et al. Superiority of Adriamycin-containing combination chemotherapy in the treatment of diffuse lymphoma: a Southwest Oncology Group study. Cancer 1979;43:417–25.
170. Kalter S, Holmes L, and Cabanillas F. Long-term results of treatment of patients with follicular lymphomas. Hematol Oncol 1987;5:127–38.
171. Peterson B, Anderson J, Frizzera G, et al. Nodular mixed lymphoma: a comparative trial of cyclophosphamide and cyclophosphamide, adriamycin, vincristine, prednisolone and bleomycin [abstract]. Blood 1985;66:216a.
172. Anderson K, Skarin A, Rosenthal D, et al. Combination chemotherapy for advanced non-Hodgkin's lymphomas other than diffuse histiocytic or undifferentiated histologies. Can Treat Rep 1984;68:1343–50.
173. Carde P, Meerwaldt J, Van Glabbeke M, et al, et al. Superiority of second over first generation chemotherapy in a randomized trial for stage III-IV intermediate and high grade non-Hodgkin's lymphoma (NHL): the 1980–1985 EORTC trial. Ann Oncol 1991;2:431–5.
174. Sullivan M, Netman P, and Kadin M. Combined modality therapy of advanced non-Hodgkin's lymphoma: an analysis of remission duration and survival in 95 patients. Blood 1983;1:51–61.
175. Bellosillo B, Villamor N, Colomer D, et al. In vitro evaluation fludarabine in combination with cyclophosphamide and/or mitoxantrone in B-cell chronic lymphocytic leukemia. Blood 1999;94:2836–43.
176. Johnson S and Thomas W. Therapeutic potential of purine analogue combinations in the treatment of lymphoid malignancies. Hematol Oncol 2000;18:141–53.
177. Hochster H, Oken M, Winter J, et al. Phase I study of fludarabine plus cyclophosphamide in patients with previously untreated low-grade lymphoma: results and long-term follow-up: a report from the Eastern Co-operative Oncology Group. J Clin Oncol 2000;18:987–94.
178. Santini G, Chisesi T, Nati S, et al. Fludarabine, cyclophosphamide and mitoxantrone for untreated follicular lymphoma: a report from the Non-Hodgkin's Lymphoma Co-operative Study Group. Leuk Lymphoma 2004;45: 1141–7.
179. Bosch F, Perales M, Cobo F, et al. Fludarabine, cyclophosphamide and mitoxantrone (FCM) therapy in resistant or relapsed chronic lymphocytic leukemia (CLL) or follicular lymphoma (FL) [abstract]. Blood 1997;90:530a.
180. McLaughlin P, Hagemeister F, Romaguera J, et al. Fludarabine, mitoxantrone and dexamethasone: an effective new regimen for indolent lymphoma. J Clin Oncol 1996;14: 1262–72.
181. Crawley C, Foran J, Gupta R, et al. A Phase II study to evaluate the combination of fludarabine, mitoxantrone and dexamethsone (FMD) in patients with follicular lymphoma. Ann Oncol 2000;11:861–5.
182. Tournilhac O, Cazin B, Lepretre S, et al. Impact of frontline fludarabine and cyclophosphamide combined treatment on peripheral blood stem cell mobilsation in B-cell chronic lymphocytic leukemia. Blood 2004;103:363–5.
183. Micallef IN, Apostolidis J, Rohatiner AZ, et al. Factors which predict unsuccessful mobilisation of peripheral blood progenitor cells following G-CSF alone in patients with non-Hodgkin's lymphoma. Hematol J 2000;1:367–73.
184. Micallef IN, Lillington DM, Apostolidis J, et al. Therapy-related myelodysplasia and secondary acute myelogenous leukemia after high-dose therapy with autologous hematopoietic progenitor-cell support for lymphoid malignancies. J Clin Oncol 2000;18:947–55.
185. Miller J, Arthur D, Litz C, et al. Myelodysplastic syndrome after autologous bone marrow transplantation: an additional late complication of curative cancer therapy. Blood 1994;83: 3780–6.
186. Stone R, Neuberb D, Soiffer R, et al. Myelodysplastic syndrome as a late complication following autologous bone marrow transplantation for non-Hodgkin's lymphoma. J Clin Oncol 1994;12:2535–42.
187. Darrington D, Vose J, Anderson J, et al. Incidence and characterization of secondary myelodysplastic syndrome following high-dose chemotherapy and autologous stem cell transplantation for lympoid malignancies. J Clin Oncol 1994;12:2527–34.
188. Friedberg J, Neuberg D, Stone R, et al. Outcome in patients with myelodysplastic syndrome after autologous bone marrow transplantation for non-Hodgkin's lymphoma. J Clin Oncol 1999;17:3128–35.
189. Milligan DW, Ruiz De Elvira MC, Kolb HJ, et al. Secondary leukaemia and myelodysplasia after autografting for lymphoma: results from the EBMT. EBMT Lymphoma and Late Effects Working Parties. European Group for Blood and Marrow Transplantation. Br J Haematol 1999;106:1020–6.
190. Schouten H, Bierman P, Vaughan W, et al. Autologous bone marrow transplantation in follicular non-Hodgkin's lymphoma before and after histologic transformation. Blood 1989;74:2579–84.
191. Freedman A, Ritz J, Neuberg D, et al. Autologous bone marrow transplantation in 69 patients with a history of low-grade B cell non-Hodgkin's lymphoma. Blood 1991;77: 2524–9.
192. Rohatiner AZ, Johnson PW, Price CG, et al. Myeloablative therapy with autologous bone marrow transplantation as consolidation therapy for recurrent follicular lymphoma. J Clin Oncol 1994;12:1177–84.
193. Apostolidis J, Foran JM, Johnson PW, et al. Patterns of outcome following recurrence after myeloablative therapy with autologous bone marrow transplantation for follicular lymphoma. J Clin Oncol 1999;17:216–21.
194. Apostolidis J, Gupta RK, Grenzelias D, et al. High-dose therapy with autologous bone marrow support as consolidation of remission in follicular lymphoma: long-term clinical and molecular follow-up. J Clin Oncol 2000;18: 527–36.
195. Berglund A, Enblad G, Carlson K, et al. Long-term follow-up of autologous stem cell transplantation in follicular and transformed follicular lymphoma. Eur J Haematol 2000; 65:17–22.
196. Gonzales-Barca E, Fernandez de Sevilla A, Domingo-Claros A, et al. Autologous stem cell transplantation (ASCT) with immunologically purged progenitor cells in patients with advanced stage follicular lymphoma after early partial or complete remission: toxicity, follow-up of minimal residual disease and survival. Bone Marrow Transplant 2000;26: 1051–6.
197. Ladetto M, Corradini P, Vallet S, et al. High rate of clinical and molecular remissions in follicular lymphoma patients receiving high-dose sequential chemotherapy and autografting at diagnosis: multicenter, prospective study by the Gruppo Italiano Trapianto Midollo Osseo (GITMO). Blood 2002;100:1559–65.
198. Bierman PJ, Vose JM, Anderson JR, et al. High-dose therapy with autologous hematopoietic rescue for follicular low-grade non-Hodgkin's lymphoma. J Clin Oncol 1997;15: 445–50.
199. Corradini P, Ladetto M, Zallio F, et al. Long-term follow-up of indolent lymphoma patients treated with high-dose sequential chemotherapy and autografting evidence that durable molecular and clinical remission frequently can be attained only in follicular subtypes. J Clin Oncol 2004;22:1460–8.

200. Gopal A, Gooley T, Maloney D, et al. High-dose radioimmunotherapy versus conventional high-dose therapy and autologous hematopoietic stem cell transplantation for relapsed follicular non-Hodgkin's lymphoma: a multivariate cohort analysis. Blood 2003;102:2351–7.
201. Pettengell R. Autologous stem cell transplantation in follicular non-Hodgkin's lymphoma. Bone Marrow Transplant 2002;29:S1–4.
202. Freedman A, Neuberg D, Mauch P, et al. Long-term follow-up of autologous bone marrow transplantation in patients with relapsed follicular lymphoma. Blood 1999;94:3325–33.
203. Brice P, Simon D, Bouabdallah R, et al. High-dose therapy with autologous stem cell transplantation (ASCT) after first progression prolonged survival of follicular lymphoma patients included in the prospective GELF 86 protocol. Ann Oncol 2000;11:1585–90.
204. Rohatiner A, Davies A, Apostolidis J, et al. High dose therapy (HDT) with autologous haematopoietic progenitor cell support as consolidation of remission in patients with follicular lymphoma (FL); long follow-up of St Bartholomew's Hospital (SBH) and Dana-Farber Cancer Institute (DFCI) data [abstract]. Ann Oncol 2005;16(5):67.
205. Schouten H, Kvaloy S, Sydes M, et al. The CUP trial: a randomized study analysing the efficacy of high-dose therapy and purging in low-grade non-Hodgkin's lymphoma (NHL). Ann Oncol 2000;11:91–4.
206. Freedman A, Gribben J, Neuberg D, et al. High-dose therapy and autologous bone marrow transplantation in patients with follicular lymphoma during first remission. Blood 1996;88:2780–6.
207. Horning S, Negrin R, Hoppe R, et al. High-dose therapy and autologous bone marrow transplantation for follicular lymphoma in first complete or partial remission: results of a phase II clinical trial. Blood 2001;97:404–9.
208. Tarella C, Corradini P, Caracciolo D, et al. High-dose chemotherapy as upfront treatment in 35 patients with indolent lymphoma induces a high rate of durable clinical and molecular remission. Blood 1996;88:121–3.
209. Lenz G, Dreyling M, Schiegnitz E, et al. Myeloablative radiochemotherapy followed by autologous stem cell transplantation in first remission prolongs progression-free survival in follicular lymphoma—results of a prospective randomized trial of the German Low-Grade Lymphoma Study Group (GLSG). Blood 2004;104:2667–74.
210. Deconinck E, Foussard C, Milpied N, et al. High-dose therapy followed by autologous purged stem cell transplantation and doxorubicin-based chemotherapy in patients with advanced follicular lymphoma: a randomized mutlicentre study by GOELAMS. Blood 2005;105:3817–23.
211. Sebban C, Coiffier B, Belanger C, et al. A randomized trial in follicular lymphoma comparing a standard chemotherapy regimen with 4 courses of CHOP followed by autologous stem cell transplant with TBI: the GELF94 trial from GELA. Hematol J 2003;150.
212. Lenz G, Unterhalt M, Haferlach T, et al. Significant increase of secondary myelodysplasia and acute myeloid leukemia after myeloablative radiochemotherapy followed by autologous stem cell transplantation in indolent lymphoma patients: results of a prospective randomized study for the GLSG. Blood 2003;102:986.
213. Lillington DM, Micallef IN, Carpenter E, et al. Detection of chromosome abnormalities pre-high-dose treatment in patients developing therapy-related myelodysplasia and secondary acute myelogenous leukemia after treatment for non-Hodgkin's lymphoma. J Clin Oncol 2001;19:2472–81.
214. Foran JM, Apostolidis J, Papamichael D, et al. High-dose therapy with autologous haematopoietic support in patients with transformed follicular lymphoma: a study of 27 patients from a single centre. Ann Oncol 1998;9:865–9.
215. Friedberg J, Neuberg D, Gribben J, et al. Autologous bone marrow transplantation following histologic transformation of indolent B cell malignancies. Biol Blood Marrow Transplant 1999;5:262–8.
216. Gisselbrecht C, Lepage E, and Molina T. Shortened first line high dose chemotherapy for patients with poor prognosis aggressive lymphoma. J Clin Oncol 2002;20:2472–9.
217. Williams C, Harrison C, Lister T, et al. High dose therapy and autologous stem cell support for chemosensitive transformed low-grade follicular non-Hodgkin's lymphoma: a case-matched study from the European Bone Marrow Transplant Registry. J Clin Oncol 2001;19:727–35.
218. Chen C, Crump M, Tsang R, et al. Autotransplants for histologically transformed follicular non-Hodgkin's lymphoma. Br J Haematol 2001;113:202–8.
219. Gresser I, Maury C, and Tovey M. Interferon and murine leukaemia VII: therapeutic effect of interferon preparations after diagnosis of lymphoma in AKR mice. Int J Cancer 1976;17:647–51.
220. Gresser I, Brouty-Boye D, Thomas MT, et al. Interferon and cell division. I: Inhibition of the multiplication of mouse leukaemia L1210 cells in vitro by an interferon preparation. Proc Natl Acad Sci U S A 1970;66:1052–8.
221. Gutterman J, Blumenschein G, and Alexanian R. Leukocyte interferon-induced tumor regression in human metastatic breast cancer, multiple myeloma, and malignant lymphoma. Ann Intern Med 1980;93:399–406.
222. Horning S, Merigan T, and Krown S. Human interferon alpha in malignant lymphoma and Hodgkin's disease. Cancer 1985;56:1305–10.
223. Louie A, Gallagher J, Sikora K, et al. Follow-up observations on the effect of human leukocyte interferon in non-Hodgkin's lymphoma. Blood 1981;58:712–8.
224. Quesada J, Hawkins M, Horning S, et al. Collaborative phase I–II study of recombinant DNA-produced leukocyte interferon (clone A) in metastatic breast cancer, malignant lymphoma, and multiple myeloma. Am J Med 1984;77:427–32.
225. O'Connell M, Colgan J, Oken M, et al. Clinical trial of recombinant leukocyte A interferon as initial therapy for favorable histology non-Hodgkin's lymphomas and chronic lymphocytic leukaemia. J Clin Oncol 1986;4:128–36.
226. Wagstaff J, Loynds P, and Crowther D. A phase II study of human rDNA a-2 interferon in patients with low-grade non-Hodgkin's lymphoma. Can Chemo Pharmacol 1986;18:54.
227. Leavitt J, Ratanathathorn V, Ozer H, et al. Alfa-2b interferon in the treatment of Hodgkin's Disease and non-Hodgkin's lymphoma. Semin Oncol 1987;14:18–23.
228. Foon K, Roth M, and Bunn P. Interferon therapy of non-Hodgkin's lymphoma. Cancer 1987;59:601–4.
229. Arranz R, Garcia-Alfonso P, Sobrino P, et al. Role of interferon alfa-2b in the induction and maintenance treatment of low-grade non-Hodgkin's lymphoma: results from a prospective, multicentre trial with double randomisation. J Clin Oncol 1998;16:1538–46.
230. Aviles A, Duque G, Talavera A, et al. Interferon Alpha 2b as maintenance therapy in low grade malignant lymphoma improves duration of remission and survival. Leuk Lymphoma 1996;20:495–9.
231. Chisesi T, Congiu M, Confu A, et al. Randomized study of Chlorambucil (CB) compared to interferon (alfa-2b) combined with CB in low-grade non-Hodgkin's lymphoma: an interim report of a randomised study. Non-Hodgkin's Lymphoma Co-Operative Study Group. Eur J Cancer 1991; 27:S31–3.
232. Fisher R, Dana B, LeBlanc M, et al. Interferon alpha consolidation after intensive chemotherapy does not prolong the

progression-free survival of patients with low-grade non-Hodgkin's lymphoma: results of the Southwest Oncology Group randomized phase III study 8809. J Clin Oncol 2000;18:2010–16.
233. Hagenbeek A, Carde P, Meerwaldt J, et al. Maintenance of remission with human recombitant interferon alfa-2a in patients with stages III and IV low-grade malignant non-Hodgkin's lymphoma. European Organisation for Research and Treatment of Cancer, Lymphoma Co-Operative Group. J Clin Oncol 1998;16:41–7.
234. Peterson B, Petroni G, Oken M, et al. Cyclophosphamide vs cyclophosphamide plus interferon alfa-2b in follicular low-grade lymphomas: an intergroup phase III trial (CALGB 8691 and EST 7486) [abstract]. Proc Am Soc Clin Oncol 1997;16:14a.
235. Smalley R, Andersen J, Hawkins M, et al. Interferon alpha combined with cytotoxic chemotherapy for patients with non-Hodgkin's lymphoma. N Engl J Med 1992;327:1336–41.
236. Solal-Celigny P, Lepage E, Brousse N, et al. Recombinant interferon alfa-2b combined with a regimen containing doxorubicin in patients with advanced follicular lymphoma. N Engl J Med 1993;329:1608–14.
237. Unterhalt M, Hermann R, Koch P, et al. Long term interferon alpha maintenance prolongs remission duration in advanced low grade lymphomas and is related to the efficacy of initial cytoreductive chemotherapy [abstract]. Blood 1996;88: 1801a.
238. Rohatiner A, Gregory W, Peterson B, et al. Meta analysis to evaluate the role of Interferon in follicular lymphoma. J Clin Oncol 2005;23:2215–23.
239. Nadler LM, Stashenko P, Hardy R, et al. Serotherapy of a patient with a monoclonal antibody directed against a human lymphoma-associated antigen. Cancer Res 1980; 40:3147–54.
240. Maloney DG, Grillo-Lopez AJ, White CA, et al. IDEC-C2B8 (rituximab) anti-CD20 monoclonal antibody therapy in patients with relapsed low-grade non-Hodgkin's lymphoma. Blood 1997;90:2188–95.
241. McLaughlin P, Grillo-Lopez AJ, Link BK, et al. Rituximab chimeric anti-CD20 monoclonal antibody therapy for relapsed indolent lymphoma: half of patients respond to a four-dose treatment program. J Clin Oncol 1998;16: 2825–33.
242. Foran JM, Gupta RK, Cunningham D, et al. A UK multicentre phase II study of rituximab (chimaeric anti-CD20 monoclonal antibody) in patients with follicular lymphoma, with PCR monitoring of molecular response. Br J Haematol 2000;109:81–8.
243. Davis TA, White CA, Grillo-Lopez AJ, et al. Single-agent monoclonal antibody efficacy in bulky non-Hodgkin's lymphoma: results of a phase II trial of rituximab. J Clin Oncol 1999;17:1851–7.
244. Davis TA, Grillo-Lopez AJ, White CA, et al. Rituximab anti-CD20 monoclonal antibody therapy in non-Hodgkin's lymphoma: safety and efficacy of re-treatment. J Clin Oncol 2000;18:3135–43.
245. Berinstein NL, Grillo-Lopez AJ, White CA, et al. Association of serum Rituximab (IDEC-C2B8) concentration and anti-tumor response in the treatment of recurrent low-grade or follicular non-Hodgkin's lymphoma. Ann Oncol 1998;9: 995–1001.
246. Gordan LN, Grow WB, Pusateri A, et al. Phase II trial of individualized rituximab dosing for patients with CD20-positive lymphoproliferative disorders. J Clin Oncol 2005;23: 1096–102.
247. Hainsworth JD, Litchy S, Burris HA 3rd, et al. Rituximab as first-line and maintenance therapy for patients with indolent non-Hodgkin's lymphoma. J Clin Oncol 2002;20:4261–7.
248. Hainsworth JD, Burris HA 3rd, Morrissey LH, et al. Rituximab monoclonal antibody as initial systemic therapy for patients with low-grade non-Hodgkin lymphoma. Blood 2000;95:3052–6.
249. Witzig TE, Vukov AM, Habermann TM, et al. Rituximab therapy for patients with newly diagnosed, advanced-stage, follicular grade I non-Hodgkin's lymphoma: a phase II trial in the North Central Cancer Treatment Group. J Clin Oncol 2005;23:1103–8.
250. Ghielmini M, Schmitz SF, Cogliatti SB, et al. Prolonged treatment with rituximab in patients with follicular lymphoma significantly increases event-free survival and response duration compared with the standard weekly x 4 schedule. Blood 2004;103:4416–23.
251. Hainsworth JD, Litchy S, Shaffer DW, et al. Maximizing therapeutic benefit of rituximab: maintenance therapy versus re-treatment at progression in patients with indolent non-Hodgkin's lymphoma—a randomized phase II trial of the Minnie Pearl Cancer Research Network. J Clin Oncol 2005;23:1088–95.
252. Cartron G, Dacheux L, Salles G, et al. Therapeutic activity of humanized anti-CD20 monoclonal antibody and polymorphism in IgG Fc receptor FcgammaRIIIa gene. Blood 2002;99:754–8.
253. Weng WK and Levy R. Two immunoglobulin G fragment C receptor polymorphisms independently predict response to rituximab in patients with follicular lymphoma. J Clin Oncol 2003;21:3940–7.
254. Bohen SP, Troyanskaya OG, Alter O, et al. Variation in gene expression patterns in follicular lymphoma and the response to rituximab. Proc Natl Acad Sci U S A 2003;100:1926–30.
255. Stein R, Qu Z, Chen S, et al. Characterization of a new humanized anti-CD20 monoclonal antibody, IMMU–106, and its use in combination with the humanized anti-CD22 antibody, epratuzumab, for the therapy of non-Hodgkin's lymphoma. Clin Cancer Res 2004;10:2868–78.
256. Leonard JP, Coleman M, Ketas JC, et al. Phase I/II trial of epratuzumab (humanized anti-CD22 antibody) in indolent non-Hodgkin's lymphoma. J Clin Oncol 2003;21:3051–9.
257. Czuczman M. Immunochemotherapy in indolent non-Hodgkin's lymphoma. Semin Oncol 2002;29:11–17.
258. Czuczman M, Weaver R, Alkuzweny B, et al. Prolonged clinical and molecular remission in patients with low-grade or follicular non-Hodgkin's lymphoma treated with Rituximab plus CHOP chemotherapy: 9-year follow-up. J Clin Oncol 2004;22:4711–6.
259. Zinzani P, Pulsoni A, Perrotti A, et al. Fludarabine plus mitoxantrone with and without Rituximab versus CHOP with and without Rituximab as front line treatment for patients with follicular lymphoma. J Clin Oncol 2004;22: 2654–61.
260. Forstpointner R, Dreyling M, Repp R, et al. The addition of Rituximab to a combination of fludarabine, cyclophosphamide, mitoxantrone (FCM) significantly increases the response rate and prolongs survival as compared with FCM alone in patients with relapsed and refractory follicular and mantle cell lymphoma: results of a prospective randomized study of the German Low-Grade Lymphoma Study Group. Blood 2004;104:3064–71.
261. Hiddemann W, Dreyling M, Forstpointner R, et al. Combined immuno-chemotherapy (R-CHOP) significantly improves time to treatment failure in first line therapy of follicular lymphoma—results of a prospective randomized trial of the German Low Grade Lymphoma Study Group (GLSG) [abstract]. Blood 2003;11:104a.
262. Marcus R, Imrie K, Belch A, et al. CVP chemotherapy plus rituximab compared with CVP as first line treatment for advanced follicular lymphoma. Blood 2005;105:1417–23.

263. Dreyling M, Forstpointner R, Repp R, et al. Combined immuno-chemotherapy (R-FCM) results in superior remission and survival rates in recurrent follicular and mantle cell lymphoma—final results of a prospective randomized trial of the German Low Grade Lymphoma Study Group (GLSG) [abstract]. Blood 2003;102:103a.
264. van Besien KW, Mehra RC, Giralt SA, et al. Allogeneic bone marrow transplantation for poor-prognosis lymphoma: response, toxicity and survival depend on disease histology. Am J Med 1996;100:299–307.
265. van Besien K, Sobocinski K, Rowlings P, et al. Allogeneic bone marrow transplantation for low-grade lymphoma. Blood 1998;92:1832–6.
266. Yakoub-Agha I, Fawaz A, Foliot O, et al. Allogeneic bone marrow transplantation in patients with follicular lymphoma: a single center study. Bone Marrow Transplant 2002;30:229–34.
267. Forrest D, Thompson K, Nevill T, et al. Allogeneic hematopoietic stem cell transplantation for progressive follicular lymphoma. Bone Marrow Transplant 2002;29:973–8.
268. Toze C, Barnett M, Connors J, et al. Long-term disease-free survival of patients with advanced follicular lymphoma after allogeneic bone marrow transplantation. Br J Haematol 2004;127:311–21.
269. Hosing C, Saliba RM, McLaughlin P, et al. Long-term results favor allogeneic over autologous hematopoietic stem cell transplantation in patients with refractory or recurrent indolent non-Hodgkin's lymphoma. Ann Oncol 2003;14:737–44.
270. van Besien K, Loberiza F, Bajorunaite R, et al. Comparison of autologous and allogeneic hematopoietic stem cell transplantation for follicular lymphoma. Blood 2003;102:3521–9.
271. Verdonck L. Allogeneic versus autologous bone marrow transplantation for refractory and recurrent low-grade non-Hodgkin's lymphoma: updated results of the Utrecht experience. Leuk Lymphoma 1999;34:120–36.
272. Storb R, Yu C, Barnett T, et al. Stable mixed hematopoietic chimerism in DLA-identical littermate dogs given sublethal total body irradiation before and pharmacological immunosuppression after marrow transplantation. Blood 1997;89:3048–54.
273. Ho A, Devereux S, Mufti G, et al. Reduced-intensity rituximab-BEAM-CAMPATH allogeneic haematopoietic stem cell transplantation for follicular lymphoma is feasible and induces durable molecular remission. Bone Marrow Transplant 2003;31:551–7.
274. Khouri I, Saliba R, Giralt S, et al. Nonablative allogeneic hematopoietic transplantation as adoptive immunotherapy for indolent lymphoma: low incidence of toxicity, acute graft-versus-host disease, and treatment-related mortality. Blood 2001;98:3595–9.
275. Kwak LW, Campbell MJ, Czerwinski DK, et al. Induction of immune responses in patients with B-cell lymphoma against the surface-immunoglobulin idiotype expressed by their tumors. N Engl J Med 1992;327:1209–15.
276. Hsu FJ, Caspar CB, Czerwinski D, et al. Tumor-specific idiotype vaccines in the treatment of patients with B-cell lymphoma—long-term results of a clinical trial. Blood 1997; 89:3129–35.
277. Bendandi M, Gocke CD, Kobrin CB, et al. Complete molecular remissions induced by patient-specific vaccination plus granulocyte-monocyte colony-stimulating factor against lymphoma. Nat Med 1999;5:1171–7.
278. Timmerman JM, Czerwinski DK, Davis TA, et al. Idiotype-pulsed dendritic cell vaccination for B-cell lymphoma: clinical and immune responses in 35 patients. Blood 2002; 99:1517–26.
279. Hsu FJ, Benike C, Fagnoni F, et al. Vaccination of patients with B-cell lymphoma using autologous antigen-pulsed dendritic cells. 1996;Nat Med 2:52–8.
280. Stevenson FK, Ottensmeier CH, Johnson P, et al. DNA vaccines to attack cancer. Proc Natl Acad Sci U S A 2004; 101(suppl 2):14646–52.
281. Timmerman JM, Singh G, Hermanson G, et al. Immunogenicity of a plasmid DNA vaccine encoding chimeric idiotype in patients with B-cell lymphoma. Cancer Res 2002;62:5845–52.
282. Stevenson FK, Zhu D, King CA, et al. Idiotypic DNA vaccines against B-cell lymphoma. Immunol Rev 1995;145:211–28.
283. Tsimberidou A, McLaughlin P, Younes A, et al. Fludarabine, Mitoxantrone, Dexamethasone (FMD) compared with an alternating triple therapy (ATT) regimen in patients with Stage IV indolent lymphoma. Blood 2002;100:4351–7.
284. Morris E, Thomson K, Craddock C, et al. Outcome following Alemtuzumab (CAMPATH-IH)-containing reduced intensity allogeneic transplant regimen for relapsed and refractory non-Hodgkin's lymphoma (NHL). Blood 2004;104:3865–71.
285. Faulkner R, Craddock C, Byrne J, et al. Campath reduced intensity allogeneic stem cell transplantation for lymphoproliferative diseases: GVHD, toxicity and survival in 65 patients. Blood 2004;103:428–34.

20

Lymphoplasmacytic Lymphoma/ Waldenström's Macroglobulinemia

Magnus Björkholm M.D., Ph.D.

Lymphoplasmacytic lymphoma (LPL) has been recognized as a heterogeneous group of rare lymphomas, the diagnosis of which has shown a very low reproducibility.[1] In the present World Health Organization (WHO) classification, lymphoplasmacytic lymphoma/Waldenström's macroglobulinemia is defined as a neoplasm of small B lymphocytes, plasmacytoid lymphocytes, and plasma cells, usually involving bone marrow, lymph nodes, and spleen. Tumor cells usually lack CD5, and a serum monoclonal protein of IgM type is demonstrated in most cases. Plasmacytoid/cytic variants of other lymphomas are excluded.[2] Thus, this classification has introduced more strict criteria in the definition of this subtype of mature B-cell neoplasm which in the past were included in the following categories; Rappaport: well-differentiated lymphocytic, plasmacytoid; updated Kiel: immunocytoma, lymphoplasmacytic type; Lukes–Collins: plasmacytic-lymphocytic; Working Formulation: small lymphocytic, plasmacytoid, Waldenström's macroglobulinemia (WM). Although the pathologic basis for the LPL/WM diagnosis is provided in the REAL and also WHO classifications, WM is in these systems recognized as a clinical syndrome and not synonymous with lymphoplasmocytic lymphoma (LPL). Thus, also patients with IgM paraproteinemia and diseases other than LPL like splenic marginal zone lymphoma, B-cell chronic lymphocytic leukemia, and extranodal marginal zone lymphoma of the MALT type are included as WM. A recent international workshop on WM recommended that WM should be regarded as a distinct clinicopathologic entity rather than a clinical syndrome. In addition, a diagnosis of LPL/WM could be made irrespective of the magnitude of the monoclonal IgM concentration if other criteria are fulfilled.[3]

In a retrospective analysis of immunocytoma from St. Bartholomew's Hospital (London), 16 of 24 patients with lymphoplasmacytic immunocytoma (Kiel) had a monoclonal IgM component, with the remainder having IgG or IgA paraproteinemia.[4] The large majority of patients reported in earlier studies, lacking IgM paraproteinemia, would probably be classified as other "indolent" lymphomas with today's strict definition of LPL/WM (also excluding tumors that lack features of other lymphomas).[2,5] Also, within the defined LPL/WM subgroup, there is a variation in tumor cell and clinical characteristics.[6,7] Immunophenotypic, cytogenetic, and molecular studies will help to better define LPL/WM in the future.[8] In the following, LPL/WM will mainly be discussed as defined in the WHO classification with the modifications suggested above,[3] thus regarding WM as synonymous with LPL. However, apart from treatment of certain IgM-associated clinical manifestations, the principles of systemic lymphoma treatment of LPL/WM with IgM paraproteinemia or with no or other types of paraproteinemia are at present essentially the same.[4,9]

DIAGNOSIS

A diagnosis of LPL/WM can thus be made irrespective of the size of the monoclonal IgM component if other diagnostic criteria are fulfilled (see above). A trephine bone marrow biopsy should be regarded as mandatory, and lymph node biopsies are encouraged in patients with accessible nodes. In the few patients with nodal LPL/WM and no bone marrow involvement, the diagnosis is dependent upon an available lymph node section. Apart from other indolent lymphomas an important differential diagnosis is monoclonal IgM gammopathy of undetermined significance. These patients have by definition no symptoms attributable to IgM or morphologic evidence of bone marrow/tumor infiltration. Immunophenotypic studies are strongly recommended in routine clinical practice.

Variations in the immunophenotypic profile exist but the large majority of LPL/WM patients meet the newly proposed criteria: monoclonal sIg+ (5:1 κ:λ ratio), CD19+, CD20+, CD5–, CD10–, and CD23–.[3,6,10,11] This phenotype in combination with the presence of somatic mutations of V genes (IgM) without intraclonal diversity (but no evidence for isotype switch transcripts) strongly suggests that the malignant cells originate from cells at a late stage of differentiation.[12,13] Translocation t(9;14)(p13;q32) is reported in up to 50% of LPL patients, but apparently confined to patients with nodal based LPL, and no identifiable serum monoclonal spike.[14] This translocation leads to a rearrangement of the PAX5 gene encoding a protein involved in the regulation of B-cell proliferation and differentiation. In a more homogenous LPL/WM patient population, the only recurrent chromosome abnormality was del 6q21, appearing in 40% to 60% of patients, and also in other B-cell neoplasia,[7] a locus that may harbor a putative tumor-suppressor gene. Abnormal cytogenetic findings predict a poor prognosis in LPL/WM.[15] Diffuse large B-cell lymphoma, most likely as a result of histologic transformation, has been reported to occur in a subset (13%) of patients with LPL/WM.[16] These patients have an aggressive clinical course and a poor prognosis.

EPIDEMIOLOGY AND ETIOLOGY

Due to the rarity of LPL and the introduction of new lymphoma classifications, including the change of diagnostic criteria, no precise incidence data are available. However, accepting the diagnostic uncertainty, the overall incidence of WM has been estimated to be approximately 3/1 million/year (10% to 20% as common as multiple myeloma), constituting approximately 1% to 2% of hematologic malignancies,[17,18] with markedly higher rates for WM among Caucasians than African Americans.[19] The median age among large series of patients varies between 63 and 68 years, more than 50% to 70% being males.[20] LPL accounted for 1.5% of nodal lymphomas in another study.[21] The etiology of LPL/WM is virtually unknown. Recently, hepatitis C virus has been recognized as the etiologic agent of mixed cryoglobulinaemia, which can be considered as a benign lymphoproliferative disorder. Since mixed cryoglobulinaemia can frequently evolve into more aggressive hematologic disorders, an increased prevalence of hepatitis C virus infection in non-Hodgkin's lymphoma (NHL) has been found, especially in low-grade NHL including LPL/WM.[22] A genetic predisposition probably exists, as suggested by familial occurrences also in monozygotic twins.[23] Occupational exposure to leather, rubber, dyes, and paints has been suggested, but such association is not definitely confirmed.[20]

CLINICAL FEATURES

The clinical manifestations associated with LPL/WM can be related to those of direct organ tumor infiltration, IgM-related hyperviscosity, and deposition of IgM in various tissues. Some patients may have advanced lymphoma with pronounced organomegaly (lymphadenopathy dominating), severe constitutional symptoms, and anemia, even with a low or lacking M component. At the other end of the spectrum, many patients present with a high monoclonal IgM component, significant tumor infiltration of the bone marrow but with no constitutional symptoms, hepatosplenomegaly, lymphadenopathy, or significant anemia.[24] Manifestations related to the IgM paraproteinemia include hyperviscosity syndrome reported in 10% to 30% in some series.[20] IgM is a large pentameric molecule, and an increased concentration may result in increase of plasma viscosity and expansion of plasma volume. Symptoms usually appear when the relative (to water) serum viscosity is above 4 to 5 (normal values 1.4 to 1.8). In symptomatic patients, the corresponding serum IgM concentration is almost always above 30 to 40 g/L. The symptomatic threshold, however, varies quite broadly from patient to patient.[25] Clinical manifestations of hyperviscosity syndrome include mucosal hemorrhage, visual abnormalities, neurologic symptoms (headache, vertigo, somnolence, dizziness, and so on), and heart failure.

Cryoglobulins are detected in approximately 15% of patients with overt WM. Less than 5% of patients have symptoms or complications, including Raynaud's phenomenon, arthralgia, purpura, glomerulonephritis, peripheral neuropathy, liver function abnormalities, and renal failure.[20]

Cold agglutinin disease, caused by monoclonal IgM reactivity with specific red blood cell antigens at temperatures less than 37°, is manifested by usually mild and extravascular episodic or chronic hemolytic anemia in less than 10% of patients.

Peripheral neuropathy (sensory, motor or both) is a classical complication in 5% to 10% of patients with WM symptoms, including numbness, paresthesias, imbalance, and gait ataxia. These neuropathies may be subdivided into a demyelinating neuropathy with IgM anti-myelin–associated glycoprotein (MAG) antibodies, or with monoclonal IgM reacting with gangliosides (but not MAG). Other forms of neuropathy are caused by monoclonal IgM nonreactive with known peripheral nerve antigens, cryoglobulinemic neuropathy, and amyloid neuropathy.[20,26] Amyloidosis has developed in less than 5% of patients with WM. The clinical features are similar to those of patients with AL associated with IgG, IgA, or light-chain production. Cardiac, renal, hepatic, and pulmonary involvement predominated, and were the cause of death in more than 50% of patients.[27]

TREATMENT AND PROGNOSIS

Today there is no cure for patients with LPL/WM, although improvements have been made in controlling the disease with the introduction of new treatment modalities. While there has been no controlled comparison between initial and deferred treatment in LPL/WM, it is generally accepted that patients who do not have symptoms should be followed without any treatment until disease-related symptoms appear. Results from studies in other low-grade lymphoproliferative disorders support this notion.[25,28] Thus, because the LPL/WM patient population is quite heterogeneous,[24] the therapeutic approach must be individualized according to the nature of the clinical manifestations, patient's age, and performance status as far as possible. Common clinical features motivating treatment are symptoms of anemia, hyperviscosity syndrome, massive enlargement of lymphoid tissues, cryoglobulinemia, cold agglutinin disease, amyloidosis, peripheral neuropathy, and general symptoms including weight loss, night sweats, fever, and asthenia.

Comparisons of studies have been hampered by a rather broad variation in diagnostic criteria, indications for and choice of treatment. Criteria for response to treatment have also been rather poorly defined until recently.[29] Response criteria are a combination of those in patients with myeloma and low-grade malignant lymphoma:

- Complete response—Disappearance of monoclonal protein by immunofixation, resolution of lymphadenopathy and organomegaly, and no signs or symptoms attributable to LPL/MW and absence of malignant cells by bone marrow histologic evaluation.
- Partial response—A ≥50% reduction of serum monoclonal IgM and a ≥50% improvement in bulky adenopathy/organomegaly with no new signs, symptoms, or other evidence of disease.[29]

Overall, the median survival of patients with LPL/WM is approximately 5 years. However, at least 20%, and in certain series, more than 50% of patients survive for more than 10 years, and 10% to 20% die of unrelated causes.[24,25] Hemoglobin, β-2 microglobulin, and total number of cytopenias are important prognostic markers, influencing the timing of treatment and predicting survival. Age is also an independent predictor of response and survival.[5,25] Several prognostic models based on large patient series have recently been presented.[30–32]

TREATMENT OF IGM-ASSOCIATED CLINICAL MANIFESTATIONS

The IgM level per se should not influence the decision to start treatment. Eventually, most patients with manifestations related to the IgM component will require systemic therapy. However, in patients with clinical manifestations of hyperviscosity total plasma exchange plays a significant role, especially in newly diagnosed patients who need urgent therapy. Long-term maintenance plasmapheresis can also be considered in patients intolerant to or failing systemic treatment.[33] Funduscopic examination and serum viscosity determination (if available) are important tools for evaluation of hyperviscosity and patient monitoring. A 20% to 35% reduction in IgM can dramatically reduce viscosity (50% to 60%) with resolution of symptoms.[34,35] Intensive plasmapheresis has also been used successfully in patients with cryoglobulinemia and cold IgM antibody agglutinin disease,[35,36] and more rarely in patients with peripheral neuropathy.[37]

SYSTEMIC LYMPHOMA TREATMENT

Alkylating Agents

Chlorambucil was first used with response rates ranging from 31% to 72%, and is probably the most commonly used oral agent. Melphalan and cyclophosphamide were introduced later with a broadly clinical efficacy.[38] This has, however not been shown in prospective comparative trials. Daily and intermittent oral chlorambucil are equally effective.[39] The addition of corticosteroids appears not to increase response rates.[20,38] Combination chemotherapy protocols including the M2 protocol (melphalan, cyclophosphamide, carmustine, vincristine, and prednisone),[40] CMP (chlorambucil, melphalan, and prednisone),[41] COP (cyclophosphamide, vincristine, and prednisone),[42] and CHOP (cyclophosphamide, doxorubicin, vincristine, and prednisone)[43] have been used in previously untreated WM.

There are no prospective comparisons of these combination programs to single alkylating treatment, and no data to support their use in chemotherapy-naive WM patients.[44] The median survival of patients in these and other studies averages 5 to 6 years (range 4 to 10 years). Symptomatic patients who fail alkylating-based treatment have a worse prognosis than responders.[5,44] The existence of patients who do not require treatment for a long period of time should be borne in mind since alkylating agents may induce myelodysplasia and leukemia.[38,45,46]

Purine Nucleoside Analogues

The positive treatment results of nucleoside analogues in other low-grade lymphoma led to studies of these agents also in patients with primary refractory or relapsing disease. Fludarabine induced response rates between 30% and 45%,[30,47–54] and in most studies the treatment plan has been to give six cycles of fludarabine. In a randomized trial, patients with primary refractory disease or first-relapse patients received either fludarabine or CAP (cyclophosphamide, doxorubicin, and prednisone).[53] The response rate (30% vs. 11%) and duration of response (19 months vs. 3 months) were superior in fludarabine-treated patients, although no difference in median survival was observed (41 vs. 45 months). In general, patients who still are sensitive to their primary therapy have higher response rates and the highest response rates (≥80%) have been reported in previously untreated patients.[48,52] Complete remissions have been observed, but are mainly seen in previously untreated patients. Fludarabine has been combined with cyclophosphamide leading to an overall response rate of 55% in patients with progressive disease.[55] Response rates varying between 39% and 68% are reported with single-agent cladribine in WM patients, mainly receiving it as second line therapy.[56–62] Even higher response rates are seen in previously untreated patients, but the combination with prednisone, cyclophosphamide, or cyclophosphamide/rituximab has added no obvious clinical benefit.[62] In patients with disease resistance to fludarabine, cladribine has little activity,[63] and the reverse is probably true. Early responses are frequently seen with both cladribine and fludarabine, although late responses (after more than 6 months of treatment) were observed in 17% of a large series of patients.[30] Myelosuppression is the main side effect of fludarabine and cladribine, which in general seems modest and well tolerated. If high-dose treatment with autologous stem cell support (AutoSCT) is integrated in the treatment plan, the duration of exposure to nucleoside analogue (and alkylator) drugs should be considered due to potential stem cell damage.[44,64] These drugs are also well known to impair cell-mediated immunity due to reduction of CD4+ and CD8+ cell counts leading to an increased risk for various opportunistic infections.[65–67]

Rituximab

Rituximab has been used successfully in patients with CD-20 positive indolent and "aggressive" B-cell NHL.[68,69] Since LPL/WM tumor cells strongly express this antigen, CD20-directed therapy using standard-dose rituximab is a novel approach to treat this lymphoma subcategory. In an early study, three of seven chemotherapy refractory symptomatic patients showed a partial response,[70] and similar results have been reported in extended studies.[71,72] In a prospective Phase 2 study, a once-weekly standard dose of rituximab for four doses (nonprogressive patients at 3 months after completion received repeat 4-week courses) induced a partial response in 44% of 27 patients (40% and 50% of previously untreated and pretreated patients, respectively).[73] The median time to response was 3.3 months and the median time to progression was 16 months. Nine of 12 responding patients remained free of progression at follow-up. With a more extended rituximab treatment, a response rate of 35% and a median time to progression of 17 months were documented in 17 previously untreated symptomatic WM patients.[74] Patients with progressive neuropathy may also respond.[75] Nucleoside analogues in combination with rituximab are being evaluated in clinical trials. However, the experience with such treatment combinations is today too limited, also regarding alkylator agents, in order to make any treatment recommendations.[62,76]

In summary, there are obviously no data from prospective randomized studies to guide the choice among alkylating agents, nucleoside analogues, and rituximab for first-line therapy of LPL/WM. Important aspects to consider are patient's age and performance status, treatment-related side effects, the overriding treatment strategy, and costs of therapy.

Thalidomide

The growing interest in tumor angiogenesis as a novel therapeutic target has led to a number of studies using thalidomide with its known antiangiogenic properties, particularly in multiple myeloma (MM). In MM, overall response rates of 25% to 45% are reported in patients with relapsed/refractory disease.[77] Accumulating data have revealed that thalidomide has complex effects and the exact mechanism of action is not known and may not be related to its antiangiogenic properties. In LPL/WM, only 30% of patients had increased angiogenesis as compared to 64% of patients with MM.[78,79] Notwithstanding this, in a prospective Phase 2 study, 5 of 20 patients (25%) achieved a partial response on thalidomide.[80] The time to response was short, and treatment was associated with several side effects including constipation, somnolence/fatigue, and depression, which were more common among older patients. In two subsequent studies, low-dose thalidomide was combined with clarithromycin (due to its immunomodulatory effects) and dexamethasone, given the high response rate observed with this combination in MM.[81] At least a partial response was seen in 83%[81] and 25%[82] of patients, respectively. Again, many patients had to be taken off the study due to side effects, including neurotoxicity in particular, as well as thrombosis, skin rash, and hyperglycemia. However, the combination may be considered as a useful salvage regimen for some heavily pretreated patients with cytopenia.

High-Dose Therapy with Stem Cell Support

In MM, AutoSCT performed early in the course of disease improves response rates, relapse-free and overall survival in patients less than 65 years,[82] and has become the treatment of choice for MM patients in many centers.[83] The role of AutoSCT in indolent lymphoma is much less clear,[84] and particularly for LPL/WM, where the published experience is limited to small rather heterogeneous patient series including a total of 48 patients.[64,85–91] Almost all patients responded to treatment, and the toxic mortality in the largest series was 6%. Thus, responses were also observed in a rather heavily pretreated patient population, chemosensitivity being an important predictor of response. The rather limited follow-up time also hampers the possibility of drawing conclusions about this therapeutic approach. However, although most patients are likely to relapse, approximately 50% of patients in the three series including eight or more patients had prolonged responses.[64,85,91] A broad range of preparative regimens has been used. In elderly patients, high-dose melphalan may be recommended because of the age-dependent toxicity associated with TBI, BEAM, and some other regimens. Previous exposure to nucleoside analogue (and alkylator) drugs may complicate stem cell harvesting.[64,91]

The experience with allogeneic stem cell transplantation (AlloSCT) is even more limited, being restricted to 16 patients, and associated with a high treatment-related mortality rate (35% to 40%). In the largest series AlloSCT was performed in 10 patients with a median age of 46 years (range 38 to 56 years), and most patients had received three or more previous treatments.[91] Six patients were alive and free from progression at more than 3 to more than 76 months, one patient eventually achieving a complete remission. Interestingly, one patient with progressive disease responded to donor lymphocyte infusion supporting the existence of a graft-versus-WM effect described in other indolent lymphoproliferative disorders.[92]

In summary, additional studies will hopefully define the role for AutoSCT and AlloSCT in LPL/WM but such an approach may for some patients result in prolonged remissions and even long-term disease control.

Corticosteroids, Splenectomy, Radiotherapy, and Interferon-Alpha

Responses to high-dose dexamethasone have been reported in patients with severe pancytopenia who were not candidates for other therapy.[93] Patients with bony lesions may benefit from local palliative radiotherapy.[94] Splenectomy is rarely indicated but may be a therapeutic option in patients with hypersplenism, painful splenomegaly, and/or disease predominantly involving this organ.[95–97] In the elderly patient, splenic irradiation may be a noninvasive alternative. In some reports on the benefit of splenectomy, a splenic marginal-zone lymphoma may have been misdiagnosed as LPL/WM, contributing to the relatively high reported success rate.[98] Interferon-alpha was found to be effective in one controlled trial of patients with peripheral neuropathy.[99] In a few Phase 2 trials, responses to low-dose interferon-alpha treatment have been reported in patients with progressive disease, and this may be a therapeutic option in this clinical setting if side effects are manageable.[100,101]

Potential New Therapeutics

Alemtuzumab (CAMPATH-1H) had a significant but limited activity in patients with advanced, heavily pretreated indolent NHL.[102] In a small study, promising effects have been seen in refractory WM patients.[103] CD22, which is expressed by more than 50% of tumor cells from the large majority (88%) of LPL/WM patients, is another potential target of passive immunotherapy in this disease.[104] Radioimmunotherapy targeting CD20 is a promising novel treatment for NHL, but myelosuppression, which increases with the degree of bone marrow tumor involvement, may limit its use in LPL/WM.[105] Thalidomide derivatives (lenalidomide [revlimid, CC-5013] and actimid [CC-4047]) are also explored in LPL/WM,[106,107] like the proteasome inhibitor bortezomib (Velcade).[107,108] Another experimental strategy is to boost WM-specific immunity with the use of autologous tumor cell–loaded dendritic cells. However, no clinical data are available.[109]

References

1. Harris NL. Mature B-cell neoplasms: introduction. In: Jaffe ES, Lee Harris N, Stein H, et al., eds., World Health Organization Classification of Tumours. Lyon: IARC Press, 2001:121–26.

2. Berger F, Isaacson PG, Piris MA, et al. Lymphoplasmacytic lymphoma/Waldenström macroblobulinemia. In Jaffe ES, Lee Harris N, Stein H, et al., eds., World Health Organization Classification of Tumours. Lyon: IARC Press, 2001:132–37.
3. Owen RG, Treon SP, Al-Katib A, et al. Clinicopathological definition of Waldenstrom's macroglobulinemia: consensus panel recommendations from the Second International Workshop on Waldenstrom's macroglobulinemia. Semin Oncol 2003;30:110–15.
4. Papamichael D, Norton AJ, Foran JM, et al. Immunocytoma: A retrospective analysis from St Bartholomew's Hospital—1972 to 1996. J Clin Oncol 1999;17:2847–53.
5. Rohatiner A, Lister TA: "Diffuse" low-grade B-cell lymphomas. In: Canellos GP, Lister TA, Sklar JL, eds., The Lymphomas. Philadelphia: WB Saunders, 1998:389–98.
6. San Miguel JF, Vidriales MB, Ocio E, et al. Immunophenotypic analysis of Waldenstrom's macroglobuliniemia. Semin Oncol 2003;30:187–95.
7. Schop RFJ and Fonseca R. Genetics and cytogenetics of Waldenstrom's macroglobulinemia. Semin Oncol 2003;30:142–5.
8. Kraus MD. Lymphoplasmacytic lymphoma/Waldenström macroglobulinemia. One disease or three? Am J Clin Pathol 2001;116:799–801.
9. Clavio M, Quintino S, Venturino C, et al. Lymphoplasmacytic lymphoma/immunocytoma: towards a disease-targeted treatment? J Exp Clin Cancer Res 2001;20:351–8.
10. Owen RG. Developing diagnostic criteria in Waldenstrom's macroglobulinemia. Semin Oncol 2003;30:196–200.
11. Remstein ED, Hanson CA, Kyle RA, et al. Despite apparent morphologic and immunophenotypic heterogeneity, Waldenstrom's macroglobulinemia is consistently composed of cells along a morphologic continuum of small lymphocytes, plasmacytoid lymphocytes, and plasma cells. Semin Oncol 2003;30:182–6.
12. Wagner SD, Martinelli V, and Luzzatto L. Similar patterns of V kappa gene usage but different degrees of somatic mutation in hairy cell leukemia, prolymphocytic leukemia, Waldenstrom's macroglobulinemia, and myeloma. Blood 1994;83:3647–53.
13. Sahota SS, Forconi F, Ottensmeier CH, et al. Origins of the malignant clone in typical Waldenstrom's macroglobulinemia. Semin Oncol 2003;30:136–41.
14. Iida S, Rao PH, Ueda R, et al. Chromosomal rearrangement of the PAX-5 locus in lymphoplasmacytic lymphoma with t(9;14)(p13;q32). Leuk Lymphoma 1999;34:25–33.
15. Mansoor A, Jeffrey Medeiros L, Weber DM, et al. Cytogenetic findings in lymphoplasmacytic lymphoma/Waldenström macroglobulinemia chromosomal abnormalities are associated with the polymorphous subtype and an aggressive clinical course. Am J Clin Pathol 2001;116:543–9.
16. Lin P, Mansoor A, Bueso-Ramos C, et al. Diffuse large B-cell lymphoma occurring in patients with lymphoplasmacytic lymphoma/Waldenström macroglobulinemia. Am J Clin Pathol 2003;120:246–53.
17. Herrinton LJ and Weiss NS. Incidence of Waldenstrom's macroglobulinemia. Blood 1993;82:3148–50.
18. Groves FD, Travis LB, Devesa SS, et al. Waldenstrom's macroglobulinemia: incidence patterns in the United States, 1988–1994. Cancer 1998;82:1078–81.
19. Benjamin M, Reddy S, and Brawley OW. Myeloma and race: a review of the literature. Cancer Metastasis Rev 2003; 22:87–93.
20. Dimopoulos MA, Panayiotidis P, Moulopoulos LA, et al. Waldenstrom's macroglobulinemia: clinical features, complications, and management. J Clin Oncol 2000;18:214–26.
21. A clinical evaluation of the International Lymphoma Study Group classification of non-Hodgkin's lymphoma. The Non-Hodgkin's Lymphoma Classification Project. Blood 1997;89: 3909–18.
22. Mazzaro C, Efremov DG, Burrone O, et al. Hepatitis C virus, mixed cryoglobulinaemia and non-Hodgkin's lymphoma. Ital J Gastroenterol Hepatol 1998;30:428–34.
23. McMaster M.: Familial Waldenstrom's macroglobulinemia. Semin Oncol 2003;30:146–52.
24. Björkholm M, Johansson E, Papamichael D, et al. Patterns of clinical presentation, treatment and outcome in patients with Waldenstrom's macroglobulinemia: a two-institution study. Semin Oncol 2003;30:226–30.
25. Kyle RA, Treon SP, Alexanian R, et al. Prognostic markers and criteria to initiate therapy in Waldenstrom's macroglobulineamia: consensus panel recommendations from the Second International Workshop on Waldenstrom's macroglobulinemia. Semin Oncol 2003;30:116–20.
26 Kyle RA. Monoclonal proteins in neuropathy. Neurol Clin 1992;10:713–34.
27. Gertz MA and Kyle RA. Amyloidosis with IgM monoclonal gammapathies. Semin Oncol 2003;30:325–8.
28. Solal-Celigny P. Increasing treatment options in indolent non-Hodgkin's lymphoma. Semin Oncol 2002;29:2–6.
29. Weber D, Treon SP, Emmanouilides C, et al. Uniform response criteria in Waldenstrom's macroglobulinemia: consensus panel recommendations from the Second International Workshop on Waldenstrom's Macroglobulinemia. Semin Oncol 2003;30:127–31.
30. Dhodapkar MV, Jacobson JL, Gertz MA, et al. Prognostic factors and response to fludarabine therapy in patients with Waldenstrom macroglobulinemia: results of United States intergroup trial (Southwest Oncology Group S9003). Blood 2001;98:41–8.
31. Gobbi PG, Bettini R, Montecucco C, et al. Study of prognosis in Waldenstrom's macroglobulinemia: a proposal for a simple binary classification with clinical and investigational utility. Blood 1994;83:2939–45.
32. Morel P, Monconduit M, Jacomy D, et al. Prognostic factors in Waldenström macroglobulinemia: a report on 232 patients with the description of a new scoring system and its validation on 253 other patients. Blood 2000; 6:852–8.
33. Buskard NA, Galton DA, Goldman JM, et al. Plasma exchange in the long-term management of Waldenstrom's macroglobulinemia. CAMJ 1977;117:135–7.
34. Reinhart WH, Lutolf O, Nydegger UR, et al. Plasmapheresis for hyperviscosity syndrome in macroglobulinemia Waldenstrom and multiple myeloma: influence on blood rheology and the microcirculation. J Lab Clin Med 1992;119:69–76.
35. Drew MJ. Plasmapheresis in the dysproteinemias. Ther Apher 2002;6:45–52.
36. Siami GA and Siami FS. Plasmapheresis and paraproteinemia: cryoprotein-induced diseases, monoclonal gammopathy, Waldenstrom's macroglobulinemia, hyperviscosity syndrome, multiple myeloma, light chain disease, and amyloidosis. Ther Apher 1999;3:8–19.
37. Meier T and Meyer M. Peripheral neuropathy with monoclonal gammopathy. Schweiz Med Wochenschr 1990;120: 417–25.
38. Waldenström JG. Macroglobulinemia—a review. Haematologica 1986;71:437–40.
39. Kyle RA, Greipp PR, Gertz MA, et al. Waldenstrom's macroglobulinaemia: a prospective study comparing daily with intermittent oral chlorambucil. Br J Haematol 2000; 108:737–42.
40. Case DC Jr, Ervin TJ, Boyd MA, et al. Waldenstrom's macroglobulinemia: long-term results with the M-2 protocol. Cancer Invest 1991;9:1–7.

41. Petrucci MT, Avvisati G, Tribalto M, et al. Waldenstrom's macroglobulinaemia: results of a combined oral treatment in 34 newly diagnosed patients. J Intern Med 1989;226:443–7.
42. Garcia-Sanz R, Montoto S, Torrequebrada A, et al. Waldenstrom macroglobulinaemia: presenting features and outcome in a series with 217 cases. Br J Haematol 2001;115:575–82.
43. Dimopoulos MA and Alexanian R. Waldenstrom's macroglobulinemia. Blood 1994;83:1452–9.
44. Gertz MA, Anagnostopoulos A, Anderson K, et al. Treatment recommendations in Waldenstrom's macroglobulinemia: consensus panel recommendations from the Second International Workshop on Waldenstrom's Macroglobulinemia. Semin Oncol 2003;30:121–6.
45. Waldenström J: To treat or not to treat, this is the real question. Leuk Res 1991;15:407–8.
46. Rodriguez JN, Fernandez-Jurado A, Martino ML, et al. Waldenstrom's macroglobulinemia complicated with acute myeloid leukemia. Report of a case and review of the literature. Haematologica 1998;83:91–2.
47. Kantarjian HM, Alexanian R, Koller CA, et al. Fludarabine therapy in macroglobulinemic lymphoma. Blood 1990;75: 1928–31.
48. Dimopoulos MA, O'Brien S, Kantarjian HM, et al. Fludarabine therapy in Waldenström's macroglobulinemia. Am J Med 1993;95:49–52.
49. Zinzani PL, Gherlinzoni F, Bendandi M, et al. Fludarabine treatment in resistant Waldenstrom's macroglobulinemia. Eur J Haematol 1995;54:120–3.
50. Thalhammer-Scherrer R, Geissler K, Schwarzinger I, et al. Fludarabine therapy in Waldenstrom's macroglobulinemia. Ann Hematol 2000;79:556–9.
51. Leblond V, Ben-Othman T, Deconinck E, et al. Activity of fludarabine in previously treated Waldenstrom's macroglobulinemia: a report of 71 cases. Groupe Cooperatif Macroglobulinemie. J Clin Oncol 1998;16:2060–4.
52. Foran JM, Rohatiner AZ, Coiffier B, et al. Multicenter phase II study of fludarabine phosphate for patients with newly diagnosed lymphoplasmacytoid lymphoma, Waldenstrom's macroglobulinemia, and mantle-cell lymphoma. J Clin Oncol 1999;17:546–53.
53. Leblond V, Levy V, Maloisel F, et al. Multicenter, randomized comparative trial of fludarabine and the combination of cyclophosphamide-doxorubicin-prednisone in 92 patients with Waldenstrom macroglobulinemia in first relapse or with primary refractory disease. Blood 2001;98:2640–4.
54. Björkholm M: Treatment options in Waldenstrom's macroglobulinemia. Clin Lymphoma 2005 (in press).
55. Dimopoulos MA, Hamilos G, Efstathiou E, et al. Treatment of Waldenstrom's macroglobulinemia with the combination of fludarabine and cyclophosphamide. Leuk Lymphoma 2003;44:993–6.
56. Dimopoulos MA, Kantarjian H, Estey E, et al. Treatment of Waldenstrom macroglobulinemia with 2-chlorodeoxyadenosine. Ann Intern Med 1993;118:195–8.
57. Delannoy A, Ferrant A, Martiat P, et al. 2-Chlorodeoxyadenosine therapy in Waldenstrom's macroglobulinaemia. Nouv Rev Fr Hematol 1994;36:317–20.
58. Dimopoulos MA, Kantarjian H, Weber D, et al. Primary therapy of Waldenstrom's macroglobulinemia with 2-chlorodeoxyadenosine. J Clin Oncol 1994;12:2694–8.
59. Betticher DC, Hsu Schmitz SF, Ratschiller D, et al. Cladribine (2-CDA) given as subcutaneous bolus injections is active in pretreated Waldenstrom's macroglobulinaemia. Swiss Group for Clinical Cancer Research (SAKK). Br J Haematol 1997;99:358–63.
60. Liu ES, Burian C, Miller WE, et al. Bolus administration of cladribine in the treatment of Waldenstrom macroglobulinaemia. Br J Haematol 1998;103:690–5.
61. Hellmann A, Lewandowski K, Zaucha JM, et al. Effect of a 2-hour infusion of 2-chlorodeoxyadenosine in the treatment of refractory or previously untreated Waldenstrom's macroglobulinemia. Eur J Haematol 1999;63:35–41.
62. Weber DM, Dimopoulos MA, Delasalle K, et al. 2-Chlorodeoxyadenosine alone and in combination for previously untreated Waldenstrom's macroglobulinemia. Semin Oncol 2003;30:243–7.
63. Dimopoulos MA, Weber D, Kantarjian H, et al. 2Chlorodeoxyadenosine therapy of patients with Waldenström macroglobulinemia previously treated with fludarabine. Ann Oncol 1994;5:288–9.
64. Munshi NC and Barlogie B. Role for high-dose therapy with autologous hematopoietic stem cell support in Waldenstrom's macroglobulinemia. Semin Oncol 2003;30:282–5.
65. Cheson BD. Infectious and immunosuppressive complications of purine analog therapy. J Clin Oncol 1995;13: 2431–48.
66. Björkholm M, Celsing F, Runarsson G, et al. Successful intravenous immunoglobulin therapy for severe and persistent astrovirus gastroenteritis after fludarabine treatment in a patient with Waldenstrom's macroglobulinemia. Int J Hematol 1995;62:117–20.
67. Costa P, Luzzati R, Nicolato A, et al. Cryptococcal meningitis and intracranial tuberculoma in a patient with Waldenstrom's macroglobulinemia treated with fludarabine. Leuk Lymphoma 1998;28:617–20.
68. Petryk M and Grossbard ML. Rituximab therapy of B-cell neoplasms. Clin Lymphoma 2000;1:186–94;discussion 195–6.
69. Boye J, Elter T, and Engert A. An overview of the current clinical use of the anti-CD20 monoclonal antibody rituximab. Ann Oncol 2003;14:520–35.
70. Byrd JC, White CA, Link B, et al. Rituximab therapy in Waldenstrom's macroglobulinemia: preliminary evidence of clinical activity. Ann Oncol 1999;10:1525–7.
71. Foran JM, Rohatiner AZS, Cunningham D, et al. European phase II study of Rituximab (chimeric anti-CD20 monoclonal antibody) for patients with newly diagnosed mantle-cell lymphoma and previous treated mantle-cell lymphoma, immunocytoma, and small B-cell lymphocytic lymphoma. J Clin Oncol 2000;18:317–24.
72. Treon SP, Agus DB, Link B, et al. CD20-directed antibody-mediated immunotherapy induces responses and facilitates hematologic recovery in patients with Waldenstrom's macroglobulinemia. J Immunother 2001;24:272–9.
73. Dimopoulos MA, Zervas C, Zomas A, et al. Treatment of Waldenstrom's macroglobulinemia with rituximab. J Clin Oncol 2002;20:2327–33.
74. Dimopoulos MA, Zervas C, Zomas A, et al. Extended rituximab therapy for previously untreated patients with Waldenstrom's macroglobulinemia. Clin Lymphoma 2002;3:163–6.
75. Weide R, Heymanns J, and Koppler H. The polyneuropathy associated with Waldenstrom's macroglobulinaemia can be treated effectively with chemotherapy and the anti-CD20 monoclonal antibody rituximab. Br J Haematol 2000; 109:838–41.
76. Mohammad RM, Aboukameel A, Nabha S, et al. Rituximab, cyclophosphamide, dexamethasone (RCD) regimen induces cure in WSU-WM xenograft model and a partial remission in previously treated Waldenstrom's macroglobulinemia patient. J Drug Target 2002;10:405–10.
77. Singhal S, Mehta J, Desikan R, et al. Antitumor activity of thalidomide in refractory multiple myeloma. N Engl J Med 1999;341:1565–71.
78. Rajkumar SV, Leong T, Roche PC, et al. Prognostic value of bone marrow angiogenesis in multiple myeloma. Clin Cancer Res 2000;6:3111–16.

79. Rajkumar SV, Hayman S, and Greipp PR. Angiogenesis in Waldenstrom's macroglobulinemia. Semin Oncol 2003; 30:262–4.
80. Dimopoulos MA, Zomas A, Viniou NA, et al. Treatment of Waldenstrom's macroglobulinemia with thalidomide. J Clin Oncol 2001;19:3596–601.
81. Coleman M, Leonard J, Lyons L, et al. Treatment of Waldenstrom's macroglobulinemia with clarithromycin, low-dose thalidomide, and dexamethasone. Semin Oncol 2003;30:270–4.
82. Attal M, Harousseau JL, Stoppa AM, et al. A prospective, randomized trial of autologous bone marrow transplantation and chemotherapy in multiple myeloma. Intergroupe Francais du Myelome. N Engl J Med 1996;335:91–7.
83. Harousseau JL and Attal M. The role of stem cell transplantation in multiple myeloma. Blood Rev 2002;16:245–53.
84. Gribben JG. Autologous hematopoietic transplantation for low-grade lymphomas. Cytotherapy 2002;4:205–15.
85. Dreger P, Seyfarth B, Sonnen R, et al. Follow-up of autologous stem cell transplantation (SCT) for treatment of Waldenstrom's macroglobulinemia. Poster Session, 8th Annual Congress of the European Hematology Association, Lyon, France 2003, 107.
86. Mustafa M, Powles R, and Treleaven Jea. Total therapy with VAMP/CVAMP + high dose melphalan and autograft for IgM lymphoplasmacytoid disease. Blood 1998;92:281b.
87. Mazza P, Palazzo G, Amurri B, et al. Analysis of feasibility of myeloablative therapy and autologous peripheral stem cell (PBSC) transplantation in the elderly: an interim report. Bone Marrow Transplant 1999;23:1273–8.
88. Yang L, Wen B, Li H, et al. Autologous peripheral blood stem cell transplantation for Waldenstrom's macroglobulinemia. Bone Marrow Transplant 1999;24:929–30.
89. Anagnostopoulos A, Dimopoulos MA, Aleman A, et al. High-dose chemotherapy followed by stem cell transplantation in patients with resistant Waldenstrom's macroglobulinemia. Bone Marrow Transplant 2001;27:1027–9.
90. Desikan R, Dhodapkar M, Siegel D, et al. High-dose therapy with autologous haemopoietic stem cell support for Waldenstrom's macroglobulinaemia. Br J Haematol 1999;105: 993–6.
91. Tournilhac O, Leblond V, Tabrizi R, et al. Transplantation in Waldenstrom's macroglobulinemia—the French experience. Semin Oncol 2003;30:291–6.
92. Khouri IF, Keating M, Korbling M, et al. Transplant-lite: induction of graft-versus-malignancy using fludarabine-based nonablative chemotherapy and allogeneic blood progenitor-cell transplantation as treatment for lymphoid malignancies. J Clin Oncol 1998;16:2817–24.
93. Jane SM and Salem HH. Treatment of resistant Waldenstrom's macroglobulinemia with high dose glucocorticosteroids. Aust N Z J Med 1988;18:77–8.
94. Shehata WM. Report of a case of Waldenstrom macroglobulinemia treated and controlled by radiotherapy. Blood 1977;49:1023–4.
95. Nagai M, Ikeda K, Nakamura H, et al. Splenectomy for a case with Waldenstrom macroglobulinemia with giant splenomegaly. Am J Hematol 1991;37:140.
96. Humphrey JS and Conley CL. Durable complete remission of macroglobulinemia after splenectomy: a report of two cases and review of the literature. Am J Hematol 1995;48: 262–6.
97. Gertz MA. Waldenstrom's macroglobulinemia: a review of therapy. Leuk Lymphoma 2002;43:1517–26.
98. Thieblemont C, Felman P, Callet-Bauchu E, et al. Splenic marginal-zone lymphoma: a distinct clinical and pathological entity. Lancet Oncol 2003;4:95–103.
99. Mariette X, Chastang C, Clavelou P, et al. A randomised clinical trial comparing interferon-alpha and intravenous immunoglobulin in polyneuropathy associated with monoclonal IgM. The IgM-Associated Polyneuropathy Study Group. J Neurol Neurosurg Psychiatry 1997;63:28–34.
100. Rotoli B, De Renzo A, Frigeri F, et al. A phase II trial on alpha-interferon (alpha IFN) effect in patients with monoclonal IgM gammopathy. Leuk Lymphoma 1994;13:463–9.
101. Legouffe E, Rossi JF, Laporte JP, et al. Treatment of Waldenstrom's macroglobulinemia with very low doses of alpha interferon. Leuk Lymphoma 1995;19:337–42
102. Lundin J, Osterborg A, Brittinger G, et al. CAMPATH-1H monoclonal antibody in therapy for previously treated low-grade non-Hodgkin's lymphomas: a phase II multicenter study. European Study Group of CAMPATH-1H Treatment in Low-Grade Non-Hodgkin's Lymphoma. J Clin Oncol 1998; 16:3257–63.
103. Owen R, Rawstron, A, Österborg A, Lundin J, Nilsson G, Hillmen P. Activity of alemtuzumab in relapsed/refractory Waldenstrom's Macroglobulinemia. Blood 2003;102(11): 645a.
104. Cesano A and Gayko U. CD22 as a target of passive immunotherapy. Semin Oncol 2003;30:253–7.
105. Emmanouilides C. Radioimmunotherapy for Waldenstrom's macroglobulinemia. Semin Oncol 2003;30:258–61.
106. Richardson PG, Schlossman RL, Weller E, et al. Immunomodulatory drug CC-5013 overcomes drug resistance and is well tolerated in patients with relapsed multiple myeloma. Blood 2002;100:3063–7.
107. Mitsiades CS, Mitsiades N, Richardson PG, et al. Novel biologically based therapies for Waldenstrom's macroglobulinemia. Semin Oncol 2003;30:309–12.
108. Richardson PG, Barlogie B, Berenson J, et al. A phase 2 study of bortezomib in relapsed, refractory myeloma. N Engl J Med 2003;348:2609–17.
109. Dhodapkar MV. Dendritic cell-mediated immunization in macroglobulinemia. Semin Oncol 2003;30:305–8.

21

Marginal Zone B-Cell Lymphomas

Emanuele Zucca, M.D.
Francesco Bertoni, M.D.
Franco Cavalli, M.D., F.R.C.P.

In the early 1990s, the term "marginal zone lymphoma" (MZL) was proposed in the REAL classification[1] to encompass two apparently closely related lymphoma subtypes, namely the "low-grade B-cell lymphoma of MALT type," currently named MALT lymphoma, and the "nodal marginal zone B-cell lymphoma," also known as "monocytoid lymphoma." A third MZL subtype, with similar immunophenotype, but distinct clinical and morphologic features was also provisionally included in the REAL classification, that is, the "primary splenic MZL with or without villous lymphocytes." At that time, no recurrent balanced translocation had yet been reported in MZL, and the available cytogenetic data seemed to suggest that all these three lymphomas share similar cytogenetic alterations, including whole or partial trisomy 3, trisomy 18, and structural rearrangements of chromosome 1.[2,3] In following years, several important cytogenetic/molecular genetic observations have shed light on the distinctiveness of these lymphoid neoplasms, and each is now considered a unique lymphoma subtype in the World Health Organization (WHO) classification.[4–6] While extranodal marginal zone lymphoma of MALT type is relatively common, the nodal and splenic marginal-zone lymphomas appear to be quite rare. Each entity will be addressed separately in this chapter.

EXTRANODAL MARGINAL ZONE LYMPHOMA OF MALT TYPE (MALT LYMPHOMA)

Although MALT lymphomas occur in many different anatomic sites, this discussion will focus primarily on gastric MALT lymphomas as the most common and best-known site of involvement.

In a survey of more than 1400 non-Hodgkin's lymphomas from nine institutions in the United States, Canada, United Kingdom, Switzerland, France, Germany, South Africa, and Hong Kong, marginal zone B-cell MALT lymphomas represented 7.6% of the total number of cases, including both the most common gastrointestinal (GI) and the less usual non-GI localizations.[7] Some additional information is available regarding primary MALT lymphomas of the stomach: the highest prevalence has been reported in northeastern Italy (13.2:100,000/year, which is 13 times higher than in corresponding U.K. communities), suggesting the existence of important geographic variations.[8] The incidence in the United States has been estimated to be between 1:30,000 and 1:80,000 among the *Helicobacter pylori*–infected populations.[9]

Pathology

The term MZL means that extranodal MZL, nodal MZL, and splenic MZL are believed to derive from B cells normally present in the marginal zone. The latter is the outer part of the mantle zone of B-cell follicles, and it is more developed in the lymphoid organs, which have to face high influx of antigens, such as the spleen, Peyer's patches, and mesenteric lymph nodes. In the spleen, the marginal zone is a compartment localized at the outer limit of the white pulp, bordered by a sinus and outermost by the red pulp.[10–13] The sinus surrounds B-cell follicles and T-cell areas. The most common B cells resident in the marginal zone are naive B cells, with a restricted immunoglobulin (Ig) repertoire and with B-cell receptors properties that are involved in the T-cell–independent early immune response. Post-germinal center memory B cells necessary for T-cell–dependent immune response are also localized in the marginal zone, as well as plasma cells, macrophages, T cells, and granulocytes.

Histologic Features of Extranodal Lymphomas of MALT Type

The histologic features of extranodal B-cell lymphomas of MALT type are largely similar regardless of the site of origin.[4,14–17] The main morphologic and histologic features recall the structure of the MALT tissue, the highly specialized lymphoid and epithelial tissue that can be found in most mucosal sites and that represents the mucosal immune system.

The morphology of MALT lymphoma cells is heterogeneous. Marginal zone cells are the predominant component, and are small- to medium-sized cells with small- to medium-sized, irregularly shaped nuclei, resembling those of centrocytes, and with moderately abundant cytoplasm (centrocyte-like cells). Other cell types comprise monocytoid cells (abundant pale cytoplasm, well-defined cell borders, bean-shaped nuclei), and small B lymphocytes, sometimes with lymphoplasmacytic differentiation (as in the immunocytoma of the Kiel classification). A range of plasma cell differentiation is often present. Any of these cytologic aspects can predominate, or they can coexist to various degrees within the same case. Scattered large basophilic blast cells (immunoblast and centroblast-like) can also be found. An abundance of T cells is sometimes associated with the neoplastic B cells as well.

The most striking feature of MALT lymphoma is the presence of a variable number of lymphoepithelial lesions defined by evident invasion and partial destruction of mucosal glands by the tumor cells. Lymphoepithelial lesions are typically seen in MALT lymphomas of the stomach, thyroid, salivary glands, and lungs. They can be less numerous or not well developed in other extranodal sites, such as the lachrymal glands or the skin. Despite being almost exclusive to MALT lymphoma, lymphoepithelial lesions can be sometimes detected also in the context of florid chronic gastritis and in extranodal localizations of other lymphoma subtypes, such as mantle cell lymphomas and follicular lymphomas.[18,19]

MALT lymphoma growth first involves the marginal zone areas around the reactive follicles. Later, the lymphoma cells can extend into the follicles ("follicular colonization") as well, and infiltrate the surrounding lamina propria and muscularis mucosae. In case of follicular colonization, neoplastic cells frequently show a more evident plasma cell differentiation. The pattern of infiltration is similar in lymph node involvement, with a conservation of the general lymph node architecture. An initial interfollicular spreading of centrocyte-like or monocytoid neoplastic determining an expansion of the marginal zones is followed by the replacement of normal lymphoid follicles and of the whole lymph node.

High-Grade Lesions

As mentioned above, there are almost always some scattered blast cells among the small- to medium-sized neoplastic cells. Their prognostic significance is not fully understood. De Jong and colleagues found a prognostic relevance of the presence of a minor large-cell component in MALT lymphoma patients treated with local radiotherapy (plus chemotherapy in cases of advanced or bulky disease).[20] However, a general agreement has never been achieved. When the blast cells form solid or sheet-like proliferations, the diagnosis of a diffuse, large B-cell lymphoma (DLBCL) has to be formulated. The term "high-grade" MALT lymphomas must not be used anymore, but the presence or absence of a "low-grade" MALT lymphoma component should be included in the report.[4]

Immunophenotype

The immunophenotypic features of MZLs are summarized in Table 21–1. There is no antigen specific for MALT lymphoma. The B cells of MALT lymphoma show the immunophenotype of the normal marginal zone B cells present in spleen, Peyer's patches, and lymph nodes. Therefore, the tumor B cells have positivity for surface immunoglobulins and pan-B antigens (CD19, CD20, and CD79a), express the marginal zone–associated antigens CD35 and CD21, and have a lack of CD5, CD10, CD23, and cyclin D1 expression.

The T-cell component can be identified and characterized by staining with CD3, CD4, CD8, and CD45RO. MALT lymphoma often presents a rich CD4+ T-cell fraction. The T cells are likely to sustain the initial lymphoma growth, and they are not evident in the DLBCL lesions. Lymphoepithelial lesions can be highlighted using anti-CD20 and anti-pan-cytokeratin KL1. Staining with antibodies for follicular dendritic cells (CD23, CDCD35, KiM4p) can help in identifying the reactive follicles.

Table 21–1. Immunophenotype of Marginal Zone B-Cell Lymphomas

	Extranodal MZL	Nodal MZL	Splenic MZL
CD20	+	+	+
CD79a	+	+	+
CD21	+		+/–
CD35	+		+/–
CD43	+/–	–/+	–
CD38	–/+[a]		–
CD45RA		+	+
CD11c	+/– (Weak)	+	–
CD5	–	–	–
CD23	–	–	–
CD10	–	–	–
CD25	–	–	–
CCND1	–	–	–
BCL6	–	–	–
BCL2	+	+	+
TRAP[b]	–	–	–
Ki67+ fraction	Low		Low
sIgM	+	+	+
sIgA	–/+	–	–
sIgG	–/+	–/+	–
sIgD	–	–/+	–/+
cIgM	–/+[a]	+/–	–
IgH mutations	Yes	Yes/No	Yes/No

[a] In case of plasma cell differentiation.
[b] Tartrate-resistant acid phosphatase, positive in hairy cell leukemia.

While the expression of sIgA or sIgG is not common on MALT lymphoma neoplastic cells, it is normal for the reactive plasma cells present within the lymphoma tissue.

Differential Diagnosis

The main conditions that must be taken in consideration are the benign lymphoid hyperplasia that can arise in the different extranodal sites: *H. pylori*–associated chronic gastritis, myoepithelial sialoadenitis (MESA)/Sjögren syndrome, allergic follicular conjunctivitis, and Hashimoto thyroiditis. From a morphologic viewpoint, the most important criteria for a diagnosis of extranodal MZL are the monomorphism of lymphoid infiltrate, cellular atypia, and distortion of the normal architectural pattern. In addition, the presence of Dutcher bodies in plasma cells, and especially of lymphoepithelial lesions, also suggests the diagnosis of lymphoma, more than a benign condition, even if lymphoepithelial lesions are not exclusively specific of a neoplastic nature. Besides the morphologic features, the demonstration of B-cell monoclonality, either by immunoglobulin light-chain restriction at immunohistochemistry or by a polymerase chain reaction (PCR) assay for rearranged immunoglobulin heavy-chain genes, can also help in the differential diagnosis process. Since lymphoma represents a clonal outgrowth of cells that have acquired certain genetic alterations, finding a monoclonal B-cell population might provide support for a diagnosis, but the significance of, especially PCR-detected, monoclonality in

Table 21–2. Wotherspoon and GELA Scoring/Grading System for Gastric MALT Lymphoma

A: The Wotherspoon histological score for diagnosis and post-treatment evaluation of gastric MALT lymphoma

Score	Description	Histological Features
0	Normal	Scattered plasma cells in LP
1	Chronic active gastritis	Small clusters of lymphocytes in LP; no lymphoid follicles; no LELs
2	Chronic active gastritis with lymphoid follicles	Prominent lymphoid follicles with surrounding mantle zone and plasma cells; no LELs
3	Suspicious lymphoid infiltrate, probably reactive	Lymphoid follicles surrounded by small lymphocytes that infiltrate diffusely in LP and occasionally into epithelium
4	Suspicious lymphoid infiltrate, probably lymphoma	Lymphoid follicles surrounded by CCL cells that infiltrate diffusely in LP and into epithelium in small groups
5	Low-grade MALT lymphoma	Dense diffuse infiltrate of CCL cells in LP with prominent LELs

B: The GELA histological grading system for post-treatment evaluation of gastric MALT lymphoma

Score	Description	Histological Features
CR	Complete histological remission	Normal or empty LP and/or fibrosis with absent or scattered plasma cells and lymphoid cells in LP; no LELs
pMRD	Probable minimal residual disease	Empty LP and/or fibrosis with aggregates of lymphoid cells or lymphoid nodules in the LP/MM and/or SM; no LELs
rRD	Responding residual disease	Focal empty LP and/or fibrosis; dense, diffuse, or nodular lymphoid infiltrate, extending around glands in the LP; focal LELs or absent
NC	No change	Dense, diffuse, or nodular lymphoid infiltrate with LELs (LELs "may be absent")

CCL, centrocyte-like; LP, lamina propria; MM, muscularis mucosa; SM, submucosa; LEL, lymphoepithelial lesion.
Modified from Wotherspoon AC, Doglioni C, Diss TC, et al. Regression of primary low-grade B-cell gastric lymphoma of mucosa-associated lymphoid tissue type after eradication of Helicobacter pylori. Lancet 1993;342:575–7,[21]; and Copie-Bergman C, Gaulard P, Lavergne-Slove A, et al. Proposal for a new histological grading system for post-treatment evaluation of gastric MALT lymphoma. Gut 2003;52:1656,[98] with permission.

absence of histologic evidence of lymphoma is still uncertain. The interpretation of the molecular results must always be done in the context of the histologic findings (see below). The histologic score proposed by Wotherspoon and colleagues can be helpful to differentiate gastric MALT lymphoma from chronic gastritis[21] (Table 21–2).

Because of the different natural history and clinical management, it is important to differentiate extranodal MZL from the other small B-cell lymphomas that may arise or disseminate at extranodal sites.

Follicular lymphoma (FL) can be difficult to distinguish from extranodal MZL with follicular colonization. MALT lymphoma cells within follicles may closely resemble centroblasts, but typically are CD10 and BCL6 (nuclear) negative in contrast to FL cells, which usually express both antigens.

The cytologic features of mantle cell lymphoma (MCL) can closely simulate those of extranodal MZL. The expression of CD5, IgD, and cyclin D1 together with the absence of transformed blasts, helps to identify MCL.

Small lymphocytic lymphoma/chronic lymphocytic leukemia (SLL/CLL) is characterized by small round lymphocytes, with, in CLL, peripheral blood lymphocytosis. Expression of CD5, CD23, and IgD without nuclear cyclin D1 serves to distinguish from extranodal MZL.

Pattern of Immunoglobulin Gene Rearrangements: Cell of Origin, an Antigen-Driven Process

The sequence analysis of the immunoglobulin genes expressed by the gastric MALT lymphoma B cells shows a pattern of somatic hypermutation and rearrangement suggesting that the tumor cell has undergone antigen selection in germinal centers and they continue to be at least partially driven by direct antigen stimulation.[22–25] The cell of origin appears to be a post-germinal center marginal zone B cell. Interestingly, among the three lymphomas believed to derive from marginal zone B cells, extranodal MZL of MALT type is the only one to consistently present a unique pattern with somatically mutated IgH genes. As shown later on, both splenic MZL and nodal MZL can be subdivided in two subsets based on IgH status.

Helicobacter pylori and Other Infectious Agents

Histologic features, such as scattered transformed blasts, plasma cell differentiation, presence of reactive T cells, and follicular colonization, suggest that MALT lymphoma cells may be participating in an immunologic process. Extranodal MZL usually arises in mucosal sites where lymphocytes are not normally present, and where a MALT is acquired in response to either chronic infectious conditions or autoimmune processes: *H. pylori* gastritis, Hashimoto's thyroiditis, and Sjögren syndrome.[26]

A whole series of evidence supports the hypothesis that the *H. pylori* may provide the antigenic stimulus for sustaining the growth of the lymphoma in the stomach to gastric lymphoma.[27–29] Epidemiologic studies confirm the link between *H. pylori* infection and gastric lymphomas of either low-grade or high-grade histology.[30] In vitro experiments have demonstrated that the neoplastic cells of low-grade gastric MALT lymphoma proliferate in a strain-specific response to *H. pylori*, and that this response is dependent on T-cell activation by the microorganism.[31] The presence of the B-cell clone that will become predominant in the transformation to MALT lymphoma has been demonstrated in the chronic *H. pylori* gastritis that preceded the lymphoma.[32] A regression of gastric MALT lymphoma after antibiotic eradication of *H. pylori* has been reported in more than half of the treated patients.[21,33,34]

Besides *H. pylori*, other infectious agents are being associated to particular extranodal MZL. *Borrelia burgdorferi*, the spirochete responsible for Lyme disease, may be implicated in the pathogenesis of at least a subset of cutaneous marginal zone B-cell lymphomas. We and others[35–37] have shown that the microorganism can be cultured or its DNA amplified from skin MZL, and a lymphoma complete remission can be achieved with antibiotics therapy aimed at the spirochete.

Ferreri et al.[38] demonstrated the presence of *Chlamydia psittaci* in up to 80% of ocular adnexal lymphomas: in 21 of 24 extranodal MZLs, in 3 of 5 diffuse large B-cell lymphomas, and 8 of 11 other lymphoma subtypes. Seven patients underwent eradication therapy with doxycycline, and one of the four patients with lymphoma at the time of antibiotic treatment obtained complete remission of at least 18 months.

Campylobacter jejuni has been associated with the immunoproliferative small intestine disease (IPSID, also known as alpha chain disease).[39] IPSID is now considered an extranodal MZL, more frequent in the Middle East, especially in the Mediterranean area.[17] It was already known that cases of IPSID could respond to antibiotic treatment,[40] but Lecuit et al.[39] have now demonstrated the presence of *C. jejuni* in five of seven patients, linking this extranodal MZL to a specific pathogen.

All these data strongly associate the origin of extranodal MZLs with chronic inflammations, often related to infectious conditions and/or autoimmune conditions. Together with the IgH data (see below), it seems that an antigen (bacterial, self-antigen, or cross-reactive?) could directly stimulate the lymphoma growth in its early stages. The long-term antigenic stimulation might give the B-cell clones with increased affinity a growth advantage over those that cannot respond or that respond less efficiently to the antigen. Hence, due to antigenic selection and clonal expansion, such a B-cell clone could become predominant by a Darwinian mechanism. Because of the persistent antigenic stimulation, the clone may become more susceptible to genetic alterations that can result in neoplastic transformation and tumor progression. It remains to be defined why different conditions would determine very specific chromosomal translocations such as the t(11;18) or the t(14;18).

Genetic Abnormalities

About 30% to 50% of MALT lymphomas show the presence of the t(11;18)(q21;q21), often as the sole abnormality.[41–50] The translocation appears to be specifically associated with MALT lymphoma; it is not detected in nodal MZL, splenic MZL, and in *H. pylori*–associated gastritis.[50] The data concerning its presence in extranodal DLBCL are still controversial.[42–44,46,51–53]

The frequency of the t(11;18) in MALT lymphoma is site related.[54] The translocation is more frequent in lesions of the GI tract (stomach, 24%; small intestine, 62%; large intestine, 20%) and the lung (38%). It is less common in conjunctiva (18%) and orbit (14%), and absent or almost absent in salivary glands (1%), thyroid (0%), liver (0%), and skin (0%).[54]

The t(11;18) translocation causes reciprocal fusion of API2--MALT1 on derivative chromosome 11 and MALT1-API2 (or the downstream gene in the presence of 3' API2 deletion) on derivative chromosome 18.[55–57] API2 (cIAP2, HIAP1, MIHC, BIRC3) belongs to the inhibitor of apoptosis proteins (IAP) family, which includes XIAP, cIAP1, NAIP, Survivin, and Apollon, all characterized by the presence of one to three baculovirus IAP repeat (BIR) domains.[58] The API2 gene contains three N-terminal baculovirus IAP repeats (BIR), a middle caspase recruitment domain (CARD), and a C-terminal zinc binding RING finger domain.[59] The MALT1 (MLT) gene codes for a paracaspase, comprising an N-terminal death domain (DD), followed by two Ig-like C2 domains and a caspase-like domain.[60] All the breakpoints in the API2 gene occur downstream of the third BIR domain, but upstream of the C-terminal RING, with more than 90% of them just before the CARD.[43,45,46,48–50,61] In contrast, the breakpoints in the MALT1 gene are more variable, occurring in four different introns, but always upstream of the caspase-like domain.[43,46,48–51,61] The resulting API2–MALT1 fusion transcripts always comprise the N-terminal region of API2 with three intact BIR domains and the C-terminal MALT1 region containing an intact caspase-like domain. Replacement of the C-terminal of API2 with the C-terminal of MALT1 by the fusion product would give origin to a new antiapoptotic molecule.

The MALT1 gene is also involved in another chromosomal translocation, the t(14;18)(q32;q21).[62,63] It has to be noted that the MALT lymphoma associated-t(14;18) is cytogenetically indistinguishable from the one occurring in FL and DLBCL, which determines the over-expression of BCL2 due to its juxtaposition with IgH. The MALT1/IgH has been found in extranodal MZL of the liver (100%, 4 of 4), ocular adnexa (38%, 3 of 8), skin (27%, 3 of 11), and salivary gland (18%, 2 of 11), but not in lesions of the gastrointestinal tract, lung, and thyroid.[63] Interestingly, the t(14;18) is present in those sites that rarely show the presence of the t(11;18), and vice versa. Moreover, the genomic region containing MALT1 can be amplified in up to 30% of the cases on MALT lymphomas,[62,64] also possibly leading to MALT1 over-expression. It has to be noted that rearrangement involving MALT1 occurs also in DLBCL.[62,65]

Other uncommon but recurrent MALT lymphoma–specific translocations are the t(1;14)(p22;q32)[66,67] and the t(1;2)(p22;p12),[68] which juxtapose BCL10 (hE10, CIPER) to the immunoglobulin heavy-chain (IgH) and Ig light-kappa-chain genes, respectively. BCL10 contains a CARD in its N-terminal, and is rich in serine and threonine residues in its C-terminal.[66,67,69–72] BCL10 may promote growth and is a positive regulator of antigen receptor–mediated NFκB activation.[73,74] BCL10 protein is expressed primarily in the cytoplasm of normal B cells including those from the marginal zone of B-cell follicles, the normal cell counterpart of MALT lymphoma.[75] In contrast, BCL10 is highly expressed predominantly in the nuclei of MALT lymphoma cells with the t(1;14),[75] and, again predominantly in the nucleus but at a moderate level, also in 50% of MALT lymphomas without the translocation.[75] BCL10 nuclear expression correlates also significantly with the presence of the t(11;18),[50,54] but the reason is not yet clear. Liu et al. have shown that the t(11;18) was present in only 10% of tumors confined to the gastric wall but in 78% of those disseminated beyond the stomach.[50] Similarly, the proportion of cases expressing nuclear BCL10 is significantly higher in tumors disseminated to local lymph nodes or to distal sites (more than 90%) than in those confined to the stomach (less than half of cases).[50,75]

All the recurrent and mutually exclusive translocations t(11;18), t(14;18), and t(1;14) act via NFκB activation.[60,76,77] In normal unstimulated cells, NFκB, a transcription factor member of the rel family, is localized in the cytoplasm due to the binding with IκB. After a variety of stimuli, IκB is degraded after phosphorylation by IK kinases, activated by the interaction between BCL10 and MALT1; NFκB is released and moves to the nucleus to activate a variety of genes involved in immunity and inflammation, as well as apoptosis. In MALT lymphomas, the fusion protein API2-MALT1 can replace the BCL10-MALT1 interaction to activate NFκB in the absence of external stimuli. The t(1;14), the t(14;18), and genomic amplifications lead to the overexpression of BCL10 and MALT1, which can interact with their normal partners and trigger NFκB activation, also in the absence of external stimuli.

Clinical Features

The presenting symptoms of MALT lymphomas are nonspecific and mainly related to the primary location.[27,78,79] Few patients present with elevated lactate dehydrogenase (LDH) or beta-2 microglobulin levels. Constitutional B symptoms are exceedingly uncommon. MALT lymphoma usually remains localized for a prolonged period within the tissue of origin, but involvement of multiple mucosal sites is not uncommon, being reported in up to one-fourth of cases. It has been postulated that this dissemination may be due to specific expression of special homing receptors or adhesion molecules on the surface of most MALT lymphoma cells and normal B cells of MALT.[80–82] Bone marrow involvement is reported in up to 20% of cases.[14] A gastroduodenal endoscopy with multiple biopsies may lead to detecting a concomitant GI and non-GI involvement in approximately 10% of cases.

Within the stomach, low-grade MALT lymphoma is often multifocal, and this may explain the report of relapses in the gastric stump after surgical excision. Gastric MALT lymphoma can often disseminate to the splenic marginal zone where it is usually undetectable by conventional histopathology. The incidental discovery of secondary small intestinal MALT lymphoma during gastrectomy for MALT lymphoma has been reported as well.

Disseminated disease appears to be more common in non-GI MALT lymphomas, in which about one-fourth of cases have been reported to present with involvement of multiple mucosal sites or nonmucosal sites such as bone marrow.[79,83,84]

The stomach is the most common and best-studied organ involved with extranodal MZL, and it will be helpful to discuss the clinical aspects of diagnosis, staging, and treatment of gastric MALT lymphoma separately from all other sites.

Diagnosis and Staging of Gastric MALT Lymphoma

The most common presenting symptoms of gastric MALT lymphoma are nonspecific dyspepsia, epigastric pain, nausea, and chronic manifestations of GI bleeding such as anemia. The upper GI complaints often lead to an endoscopy that usually reveals nonspecific gastritis or peptic ulcer with mass lesions being unusual.[27,79]

The best staging system is still controversial.[79,85] We use the modification of the Blackledge staging system recommended at an international workshop.[86]

The initial staging should include a gastroduodenal endoscopy with multiple biopsies from each region of the stomach, duodenum, gastroesophageal junction, and from any abnormal appearing site. Fresh biopsy and washings material should be available for cytogenetic studies in addition to routine histology and immunohistochemistry. A molecular genetic or a FISH analysis for detection of t(11;18) is recommended for identifying disease that is unlikely to respond to antibiotic therapy. The presence of active *H. pylori* infection must be determined by histochemistry (Genta stain or Warthin-Starry stain) and breath test; serology studies are recommended when the results of histology are negative. Endoscopic ultrasound is recommended in the initial follow-up for evaluation of depth of infiltration and presence of perigastric lymph nodes. A deep infiltration of the gastric wall is associated with a higher risk of lymph node involvement, and a lower response rate with antibiotic therapy alone.[87–90] Presentation with multiple MALT localizations is more frequent in patients with non-GI lymphoma. Regardless of the presentation site, work-up studies should include complete blood counts, basic biochemical studies (including LDH and beta-2 microglobulin), computed tomography (CT) of the chest, abdomen, and pelvis, and a bone marrow biopsy. Although the disease remains usually localized in the stomach, systemic dissemination and bone marrow involvement should be excluded at presentation since prognosis is worse with advanced-stage disease or with an unfavorable International Prognostic Index (IPI) score.[27]

Treatment

The Role of H. pylori *Eradication in Gastric MALT Lymphoma*

It is generally accepted that eradication of *H. pylori* with antibiotics should be employed as the sole initial treatment of localized (i.e., confined to the gastric wall) MALT lymphoma. Actually, this is at present the best-studied therapeutic approach with more than 20 reported studies.[91–93]

The regression of gastric MALT lymphoma after antibiotic eradication of *H. pylori* was first reported in 1993 by Wotherspoon and colleagues, who described the efficacy of antibiotic therapy in six patients with superficially invasive gastric MALT lymphoma.[21] Post-treatment biopsies were performed to evaluate the histologic changes of lymphomas, the persistence of *H. pylori* infection, and the molecular evidence of a monoclonal B-cell population. In all cases, *H. pylori* was successfully eradicated, and in five of the six patients, a histologic remission of the lymphoma was achieved. A long-term follow-up report of these six patients, published in 1999, confirmed the achievement of prolonged lymphoma remissions, and revealed that transient histologic and molecular relapses have occurred, suggesting that the neoplastic clone can re-expand, but without the growth stimulus from *H. pylori*, this may remain a self-limiting event.[94]

Several groups thereafter confirmed the efficacy of antibiotics in inducing apparently durable lymphoma remissions in 60% to 100% of patients with localized *H. pylori*–positive gastric MALT lymphoma.[78,87,88,90,95–97] The histologic remission can usually be documented within 6 months from the *H. pylori* eradication, but sometimes the period required is more prolonged and the therapeutic response may be delayed up to more than 1 year.[27]

Histologic Evaluation of Lymphoma Response to Antibiotic Therapy

The interpretation of residual lymphoid infiltrate in post-treatment gastric biopsies can be very difficult, and there are no uniform criteria in the literature for the definition of histologic remission. The Wotherspoon score reported in Table 21–2, part A[21] was initially proposed to express the degree of confidence in the diagnosis of MALT lymphoma on small gastric biopsies. It has been used to evaluate the response to therapy in some trials, but many investigators found it difficult to apply in this setting, and other criteria have been proposed.[95] The lack of standardized and easily reproducible criteria can affect comparison of the results of the different clinical trials. A novel histologic grading system has been proposed by Copie-Bergman and colleagues[98] with the aim of providing clinically relevant information to the clinician. This system, which is summarized in Table 21–2, part B, appears to be highly reproducible and classifies the histologic features in post-treatment gastric biopsies as "complete histologic remission," "probable minimal residual disease," "responding residual disease," and "no change." Assessing treatment response is of great clinical relevance, and this scheme may become a useful tool if its reproducibility will be confirmed by further testing on larger series.

Predictors of Lymphoma Response to Antibiotic Therapy

Endoscopic ultrasound can be useful to predict the lymphoma response to *H. pylori* eradication. Several studies showed that there is a significant difference between the response rates of lymphomas restricted to the gastric mucosa and those with less superficial lesions. The response rate is highest for the mucosa-confined lymphomas (approximately 70% to 90%), and then decreases markedly and progressively for the tumors infiltrating the submucosa, the muscularis propria, and the serosa. In cases with documented nodal involvement, the response is very unlikely.[88,90]

Presence of the t(11;18) translocation can predict the therapeutic response of gastric MALT lymphoma to *H. pylori* eradication.[50,61,99] The translocation is absent in gastric MALT lymphomas showing complete regression,[100] but present in 77% of nonresponsive tumors, including 68% of those with the disease confined to the gastric wall.[61] These data indicate that at least the t(11;18) is a molecular marker for the gastric MALT lymphomas that will be nonresponsive to *H. pylori* eradication, and its detection is valuable in choosing the best therapeutic approach.

Clinical and Molecular Follow-up

Several studies of postantibiotic molecular follow-up showed that histologic and endoscopic remission does not necessarily mean a cure. The long-term persistence of monoclonal B cells after histologic regression of the lymphoma has been reported in about half of the cases, suggesting that *H. pylori* eradication suppresses but does not eradicate the lymphoma clones.[97,101,102] The clinical significance of the detection of monoclonal B cells by molecular methods remains unclear, and histologic evaluation of repeated biopsies remains a fundamental follow-up procedure, despite the reproducibility problems discussed above. Some cases of lymphoma recurrence following *H. pylori* reinfection have been reported, suggesting that residual dormant tumor cells can be present despite clinical and histologic remission.[95] Relapses have also been documented in the absence of *H. pylori* reinfection, indicating the presence of B-cell lymphoma clones that have escaped the antigenic drive.[95] On the other hand, in the long-term follow-up of some cases with minimal residual disease who refused further treatment, neither lymphoma progression nor histologic transformation was documented despite persistent clonality, suggesting that a watch-and-wait policy could be feasible and safe.[103] Nevertheless, histologic transformation into DLBCL has also been described in some cases.[78,104] A strict follow-up is strongly advisable. We perform a breath test 2 months after treatment to document *H. pylori* eradication, and repeat post-treatment endoscopies with multiple biopsies every 6 months for 2 years, and then yearly to monitor the histologic regression of the lymphoma.

Management of H. pylori*–Negative or Antibiotic-Resistant Cases*

No definite guidelines exist for the management of the subset of *H. pylori-negative* cases and for the patients who fail antibiotic therapy. A choice can be made between conventional oncologic modalities, but there are no published randomized studies to help the decision. In two retrospective series of patients with gastric low-grade MALT lymphoma, no statistically significant difference was apparent in survival between patients who received different initial treatments (including chemotherapy alone, surgery alone, surgery with additional chemotherapy or radiation therapy, or antibiotics against *H. pylori*).[78,105]

Excellent disease control using radiation therapy has been reported by several institutions supporting the approach that modest-dose involved-field radiotherapy (30 Gy given in 4 weeks radiation to the stomach and perigastric nodes) is the treatment of choice for patients with Stage I–II MALT lymphoma of the stomach without evidence of *H. pylori* infection or with persistent lymphoma after antibiotics.[106–108] Surgery has been widely and successfully used in the past, but the precise role for surgical resection should nowadays be redefined in view of the promising results of the conservative approach.[27]

Patients with systemic disease should be considered for systemic treatment (i.e., chemotherapy and/or immunotherapy with anti-CD20 monoclonal antibodies).[109] In the presence of disseminated or advanced disease, chemotherapy is an obvious choice, but only a few compounds and regimens have been tested specifically in MALT lymphomas. Oral alkylating agents (either cyclophosphamide or chlorambucil, with median treatment duration of 1 year) can result in a high rate of disease control.[110,111] More recent Phase II studies demonstrated some antitumor activity of the purine analogues fludarabine[112] and cladribine (2-CDA),[113] which might, however, be associated with an increased risk of secondary myelodysplastic syndrome,[114] and of a combination regimen of chlorambucil/mitoxantrone/prednisone.[115] The activity of the anti-CD20 monoclonal antibody rituximab has also been shown in a Phase II study (with a response rate of about 70%), and may represent an additional option for the treatment of systemic disease.[109,116]

*Anti–*H. pylori *Therapy in Diffuse Large B-Cell Lymphoma of the Stomach*

The use of antibiotics in the treatment for DLBCL of the stomach is highly controversial. Because a subset of cases may have been derived from an extranodal MZL, eradication of *H. pylori* may be of benefit. Antibiotics may eliminate a residual or relapsed low-grade component that can be responsible for tumor recurrence following antigen stimulation. Cases of regression of high-grade lesions after anti–*H. pylori* therapy, have been reported suggesting that high-grade transformation is not necessarily associated with the loss of *H. pylori* dependence.[117] At present, however, the sole antibiotic therapy for gastric DLBCL cannot be advised. Therefore, these tumors, even if restricted to the mucosa, must be considered aggressive and need aggressive chemotherapy.

Management of Nongastric Localizations

The stomach is the most common and best-studied site of involvement, but MALT lymphomas have also been described in various non-GI sites, such as salivary gland, thyroid, skin, conjunctiva, orbit, larynx, lung, breast, kidney, liver, prostate, and even in the intracranial dura.[83,84,118,119] Nongastric MALT lymphomas have been difficult to characterize because these tumors, numerous when considered together, are distributed so widely throughout the body that it is difficult to assemble adequate series of any given site. One-fourth of non-GI MALT lymphomas have been reported to present with involvement of multiple mucosal sites or nonmucosal sites such as bone marrow.[83,84] Non-GI MALT lymphomas, despite presenting more often with Stage IV disease than the gastric variant, usually have a quite indolent course regardless of treatment type (5-year survival of 90%). The rate of histologic transformation seems much lower than in follicular lymphomas. Patients at high risk according to the IPI and those with lymph node involvement at presentation, but not those with involvement of multiple MALT sites, have a worse outcome. Localization may have prognostic relevance. In a radiotherapy study from Toronto, gastric and thyroid MALT lymphomas had the best outcome, whereas distant failures were more common for other sites. However, despite frequent relapses, the disease most often maintained an indolent course.[106]

In a multicentric retrospective survey of 180 nongastric cases observed over a long period of time, patients were treated according to the current policy of each institution at the time of diagnosis, and the presence of organ-specific problems presumably had a role in the choice of treatment. This study showed no evidence of a clear advantage for any type of therapy, and, despite the high proportion of cases with disseminated disease, which should require a systemic approach, no clear advantage was associated with a chemotherapy program.[83]

In general, the consideration previously done regarding the treatment of *H. pylori*–negative cases can be applied to nongastric MALT lymphoma. Radiation therapy is the best-studied approach, and is the treatment of choice for localized lesions.[108,120] The optimal management of disseminated MALT lymphomas is less clearly defined. The treatment choice should be "patient tailored," taking into account the site, stage, and clinical characteristics of the individual patient. The anti-CD20 antibody rituximab has shown clinical activity, and the efficacy of its combination with chemotherapy is being explored in a randomized study of the International Extranodal Study Group (IELSG). The finding that *C. psittaci* is associated with MALT lymphoma of the ocular adnexa may provide the rationale for the antibiotic treatment of localized lesions, and preliminary encouraging results have been reported, but this approach remains investigational and will need to be confirmed by larger clinical studies.

SPLENIC MARGINAL ZONE LYMPHOMA

Pathology

Splenic MZL is a very rare disorder, comprising less than 1% of lymphomas.[7] The disease is characterized by a lymphoid infiltrate in the splenic white pulp that grows in a nodular pattern replacing pre-existing follicles.[16,121–124] A variable degree of red pulp infiltration is also often present. The neoplastic cells present a biphasic morphology. Small lymphocytes (resembling the mantle zone cells) are predominant in central areas, while medium-sized lymphocytic cells with slightly irregular nuclei and a moderate amount of pale cytoplasm (resembling splenic, marginal zone lymphocytes) are present in the periphery. Plasmacytic differentiation as well, and rarely, clusters of plasma cells, can be present.

Up to two-thirds of patients with splenic MZL present circulating villous lymphocytes with characteristic fine, short, cytoplasmic polar projections. When these comprise more than 20% of the lymphocyte count, the term "splenic lymphoma with villous lymphocytes" is commonly used.[125]

Bone marrow is usually involved, even in cases with no circulating neoplastic cells. The pattern of infiltration is typically nonparatrabecular, intrasinusoidal only. This pattern of bone marrow involvement is not exclusive of splenic MZL, and it can also be found in other small cell lymphomas.[126–128]

When biopsied, the liver is usually involved with a nodular infiltration of portal tracts; hilar splenic lymph node involvement is common as well. According to the WHO classification, peripheral lymph node involvement is typically absent.[121] Transformation to DLBCL occurs in about 15% of cases.[129]

Immunophenotype and Differential Diagnosis

The neoplastic cells show typical positivity for surface (and sometimes cytoplasmic) monotypic immunoglobulins and pan-B antigens (CD19, CD20, and CD22), and usually coexpress the monocytic/histiocytic antigen CD11c, and they lack CD5, CD10, and CD23 expression.

Distinction from non-neoplastic monocytoid reactions is based on the greater degree of polymorphism in the lymphomatous lesions, but a search for monotypic surface immunoglobulins may be necessary in order to distinguish between reactive lymphoid infiltrate (e.g., toxoplasmosis lymphadenitis) and monocytoid B lymphoma in cases where the morphologic pattern is equivocal. Some confusion in the differential diagnosis can arise with hairy cell leukemia, since morphology and phenotype are similar (pan-B and CD11c coexpression); however, in contrast to hairy cell leukemia, marginal zone lymphomas are usually CD25−, PCA-1−, and tartrate-resistant acid phosphatase (TRAP)-negative.

Splenic MZL has to be differentiated from other small B-cell lymphomas. MCL can be identified by immunohistochemistry (CD5+, CCND1+) and its morphology is usually more homogenous without any blast cells. A process morphologically resembling an MZL is the monocytoid B-cell differentiation that can be seen in other primary low-grade nodal lymphomas, mainly in FL, where a monocytoid component appears to occupy the marginal zone. The immunophenotypic and genotypic features of the neoplastic cells are those of FL. FL are CD10+ and have no reactive germinal centers left. Hairy cell leukemia, which has similar clinical features, is easily differentiated on histologic and immunohistochemistry. In hairy cell leukemia, the pattern of both bone marrow and spleen involvement is different, and the neoplastic cells are TRAP, CD25, and CD103-positive. CLL cells are CD5 and CD23+, and there are prolymphocytes and paraimmunoblasts that are absent in splenic MZL. The differential diagnosis with lymphoplasmacytic lymphoma (immunocytoma) is difficult, since splenic MZL can have a serum M component and also plasmacytic differentiation. Indeed, lymphoplasmacytic lymphoma is a diagnosis of exclusion, done after having ruled out other B-cell lymphomas. Lymphoplasmacytic lymphoma is very rare, and concerning the differential diagnosis with splenic MZL, it can be diagnosed only in the complete absence of marginal or monocytoid cells.

In patients coming from Africa, especially in regions endemic for malaria infection, splenic MZL has to be differentiated from hyper-reactive malarial splenomegaly.[130] The demonstration of monoclonal B-cell population, an age at diagnosis below 40 years, lymphocyte count of less than 10×10^9/L, and IgM concentration of less than 3.4 g/L are useful in the differential diagnosis.

Pattern of Immunoglobulin Gene Rearrangements: Cell of Origin

The sequence analysis of the immunoglobulin genes expressed by splenic MZL cells shows that approximately half of the cases bear unmutated IgH and half-mutated IgH genes,[131,132] suggesting the possibility that this lymphoma subtype derives from different B-cell subsets that are normally present in the marginal zone. Cases with unmutated IgH genes have a poorer prognosis, and are more commonly associated with the presence of chromosome 7q loss.[131] Splenic MZL show a biased usage of VH1-2 gene, occurring in almost half of the cases, indicating a very selected B-cell subset as origin for part of splenic MZL.[131] All nine cases of "tropical splenic lymphoma" that have been molecularly analyzed have revealed unmutated immunoglobulin genes.[133]

Role of Infectious Agents

Despite relevant geographic variations, hepatitis C virus (HCV) seems to be involved in lymphomagenesis, especially regarding splenic MZL and nodal MZL.[12,28,134–139] Very interesting is the observation that seven out of nine patients with splenic lymphoma with villous lymphocytes and HCV infection obtained a complete remission after treatment with interferon alpha with or without concomitant ribavirin, and two had a partial remission.[140] These data, confirmed also by other groups,[139] suggest a strict relationship between HCV and splenic marginal zone lymphoma, indicating the necessity to search for HCV infection in patients affected by this lymphoma subtype.

An association with malaria and with EBV infection, both of which may act as strong polyclonal B-cell activators, and with the hyper-reactive malarial splenomegaly, has been shown in tropical Africa, especially in Ghana.[130,141,142] Tropical splenic lymphoma appears as a form of splenic MZL, characterized by a high percentage of circulating villous lymphocytes, unmutated immunoglobulin genes, and a predilection for middle-aged women more frequently than elderly men.

Genetic Abnormalities

Rearrangements and deletions affecting chromosome 7q are common in splenic MZL. An apparently heterogeneous pattern of 7q deletions (7q31-q33) can be shown in up to 50% of splenic MZL.[131,143–147] No gene has been identified as the target of the deletion, which is a relatively common chromosomal abnormality among hematologic malignancies. Conversely, the gene coding for CDK6, on 7q21-22 is affected by 7q chromosomal translocations, such as the t(7;21)(q21-22;q22) and the t(2;7)(p12;q21-22).[148] In particular, the latter juxtaposes CDK6 to the kappa IgL locus on 2p12, determining a deregulated gene expression. Another recurrent translocation is the t(9;14)(p13;q32), which juxtaposes the IgH locus to the PAX5 gene.[149,150] The latter codes for a transcriptional factor, called BSAP, which is expressed starting at the very early B-cell stages until its expression is down-regulated during the plasma cell differentiation. The translocation, described especially in cases of lymphoplasmacytoid lymphoma and splenic MZL with plasmacytoid differentiation, would maintain the gene switched on. However, its frequency is controversial.[151]

Genomic regions that appear to be amplified in splenic MZL comprise 3q23-q25, 4q25-q28, 5q13-q15, 9q31, 12q15-q21, and 20q.[145] Similarly, with extranodal MZL and nodal MZL, a gain of chromosome 3 (3q13-q29) appears as the most common abnormality.[2,64,143,144,152]

Using the cDNA microarray technique, Thieblemont et al. compared the gene expression profile of splenic MZL, MCL, and SLL.[153] The gene coding for AKT1 was the most representative among the genes cluster specific for splenic MZL. AKT1, mapped at 14q32, is a serine threonine kinase, and participates in the PI3-kinase/AKT cell survival pathway. Thieblemont et al.[153] also confirmed some previous reports that suggested the presence of cases of splenic MZL bearing the chromosomal translocation t(11;14)(q13;32), which juxtaposes the gene coding for the cyclin D1 to the IgH locus, and is believed to be specific for MCL and, despite difference in where the breakpoints occur, for multiple myeloma. The association of splenic MZL with the t(11;14) has still to be studied in detail, it seems likely that the translocation breakpoints in MZL are not the same of MCL and this translocation does not appear to cause a more aggressive course in splenic MZL[153].

Clinical Features

Most patients are over 50 with a similar incidence in males and females.[121] The disease usually presents with massive splenomegaly, which produces abdominal discomfort and pain. Diagnosis is often made at a splenectomy performed to establish the cause of unexplained spleen enlargement. B symptoms are present in 25% to 60% of cases; anemia, trombocytopenia, or leukocytosis is reported in approximately 25% of cases. Autoimmune hemolitical anemia is not uncommon, being found in up to 15% of patients. The splenic hilar lymph nodes appear involved in about one-fourth of cases, and approximately one-third of cases have liver involvement.[154–158]

According to the WHO classification, the peripheral lymph node involvement is typically absent,[121] but some reports refer to splenic MZL, even with some evidence of peripheral nodal or extranodal involvement.[157] Patients with disseminated marginal zone lymphomas can be observed in advanced stages of splenic MZL, nodal MZL, or extranodal MZL,[124] and a precise diagnosis can be very difficult in cases presenting with concomitant splenic, extranodal, and nodal involvement. In a retrospective French series of 124 patients with non–MALT-type MZL from Lyon,[156] four clinical subtypes were observed: splenic (48% of cases), nodal (30%), disseminated (splenic and nodal, 16%), and leukemic (not splenic or nodal, 6%). These lymphomas were usually CD5–, CD10–, CD23–, and CD43–, but the detection of one or, rarely, two of these antigens may be observed. Bone marrow and blood infiltrations were frequent, except in the nodal subtype. Even when the disease is restricted to the cases presenting with splenomegaly, nearly all patients have bone marrow involvement, often accompanied by involvement of peripheral blood (defined as the presence of absolute lymphocytosis of more than 5%).[157] Because of the high frequency of bone marrow or liver involvement, about 95% of cases are classified as Ann Arbor Stage IV. Serum paraproteinemia is observed in about 10% to 25% of cases, and is most frequently of the IgM type, which poses the problem of the differential diagnosis with lymphoplasmacytic lymphoma/Walderström macroglobulinemia.[155–157,159] The two diseases often present with similar clinical features (splenomegaly, bone marrow lymphoplasmacytic infiltration, anemia), but marked hyperviscosity and hypergammaglobulinemia are uncommon in splenic MZL,[156,160] and splenic involvement by lymphoplasmacytic lymphoma is usually recognizable, affecting both white and red pulp, with periarteriolar lymphoid aggregates and no marginal zone differentiation.[122]

Treatment

The clinical course is most usually indolent, with 5-year overall survival ranging from 65% to 80%. In the above-mentioned study from Lyon,[156] the subgroup of patients with splenic lymphoma had the more favorable outcome, with a median survival of more than 9 years. The reported largest series[155,157,158] show that a significant group of patients can be managed with an initial wait-and-see policy, and they did not seem to have a worse outcome than those initially treated.[124,154,156]

When treatment is needed, this is usually because of large symptomatic splenomegaly or cytopenias. Splenectomy appears to be the treatment of choice; it allows a reduction/disappearance of circulating tumor lymphocytes and recovery from the lymphoma-associated cytopenia.[124,154,155,158,161] The benefit of splenectomy often persists for several years, and time to next treatment can be longer than 5 years in cases where lymphocytosis persists and/or progresses after splenectomy.[124] Adjuvant chemotherapy after splenectomy may result in a higher rate of complete responses; however, there is no evidence of a survival benefit.[124]

Chemotherapy alone may be considered for patients who require treatment, but have a contraindication to splenectomy, and also for patients with clinical progression after spleen removal. Alkylating agents (chlorambucil or cyclophosphamide) have been reported to be active, and can be used as a single agent or in combination (as in the CVP and CHOP regimens). Among the purine analogues, fludarabine has been shown to be effective,[162,163] and, curiously, cladribine seems not to be active.[164] The anti–B-cell monoclonal antibody rituximab, alone or in combination with chemotherapy, is capable—according to a few case reports—of inducing good responses in cases refractory to standard chemotherapy.[124,165,166] The reported association with HCV infection led Hermine and colleagues[140] to treat this infection in a series of nine patients with splenic lymphoma with villous lymphocyte and HCV infection. Treatment consisted of interferon alpha alone or in combination with ribavirine. Of the nine treated patients who received interferon alpha, seven had a complete remission of the lymphoma after the loss of detectable HCV RNA. Another two patients had a partial and complete remission after the addition of ribavirine and the loss of detectable HCV RNA. One patient relapsed when HCV RNA became detectable again in blood. No HCV-negative patient had a lymphoma response to interferon therapy.[140] Analogous to the *H. pylori* infection in the gastric MZL, it appears that HCV may be responsible for an antigen-driven stimulation of the lymphoma clone. This report suggests that all cases should be tested for HCV infection, and antiviral therapy should be considered in the positive cases before any decision about more aggressive therapeutic approaches. Prospective studies are warranted to confirm this interesting finding.

NODAL MARGINAL ZONE LYMPHOMA (MONOCYTOID LYMPHOMA)

Pathology

In contrast with mucosa-based extranodal MALT lymphoma, nodal MZL lymphoma is typically lymph node based. The tumor cell morphology is heterogeneous, and resembles the lymph node involvement of extranodal and splenic MZL. Sometimes the tumor cells are usually small-to-medium-sized lymphocytes with oval or reniform nuclei, abundant pale cytoplasm, and well-defined cell borders, resembling monocytes. The marginal zone and interfollicular areas are infiltrated by marginal zone B cells, monocytoid B cells, or small B lymphocytes. Plasma cell differentiation can be present, as well as variable content of medium to large cells (centroblast- or immunoblast-like cells), which sometimes can be higher than 20%.[5,16,167–169]

Immunophenotype and Differential Diagnosis

Most cases have an immunophenotype profile similar to extranodal MZL. However, some cases have been reported to be IgD+ (Table 21–1). Follicular hyperplasia with monocytoid B-cell reaction, FL with marginal zone differentiation, MCL, extranodal MZL, splenic MZL, SLL, and lymphoplasmacytic lymphoma (immunocytoma) are the conditions to be excluded. Immunohistochemistry, demonstration of Ig light-chain restriction, and bcl-2 positivity help in distinguishing nodal MZL from follicular hyperplasia with monocytoid B-cell reaction that is associated with toxoplasmosis, AIDS, and infectious mononucleosis. The absence of a t(14;18)(q32;q21), the FL-related translocation, can often be the only way to differentiate nodal MZL from FL with marginal zone differentiation. The presence of monoclonal plasma cells or blast cells and the negativity for cyclin D1 allow the diagnosis of nodal MZL versus MCL. CLL cells are CD5 and CD23+, and there are prolymphocytes and paraimmunoblasts that are absent in splenic MZL. Similar to splenic MZL, the distinction between nodal MZL and the lymphoplasmacytic lymphoma can be vague. Extranodal MZL and SMLZ are to be excluded on the basis of the clinical features. Involvement of extranodal sites and of the spleen has to be ruled out before making the diagnosis of nodal MZL. Some authors reported nodal MZL in association with dissemination of extranodal MZL to lymph nodes or spleen; in these cases, the recognition of a primary extranodal disease can be difficult, since the distant spread of extranodal MZL may occur many years after initial diagnosis. The histologic pattern of lymph node involvement by extranodal MZL is often indistinguishable from that of primary nodal MZL.

Pattern of Immunoglobulin Gene Rearrangements: Cell of Origin

Analysis of the IgH genes suggests a prevalence of cases with mutated IgH genes, but, similar to splenic MZL, unmutated cases do exist.[170–172] These data are in accordance with the various normal B-cell populations resident within the marginal zone that comprise both naive and postgerminal center B cells.[11] Of interest, HCV-positive nodal MZL have a biased usage of the VH1-69, while HCV-negative MSL might preferentially use the VH4-34 gene.[170]

Role of Infectious Agents

As mentioned previously, both nodal MZL and splenic MZL have been associated with HCV infection.[12,28,134–136,138,139]

Genetic Abnormalities

No specific genomic alteration is known to occur in nodal MZL. The most common alterations, such as gain of 3q, are also present in extranodal MZL and splenic MZL.

Clinical Features

The clinical data are sparse and have been largely drawn from pathologic series rather than clinical centers.[173,174] Nodal MZL is a disease of older people, with the median age at presentation in the 6th decade, and affects both genders, with an unusual (albeit slight) female predominance. The most common presenting feature is a localized adenopathy, most often in the neck around the parotid gland. Concurrent extranodal involvement, most often of the salivary gland, is not rare, and many patients have a history of Sjögren's syndrome or other autoimmune diseases, suggesting a possible overlap with extranodal MALT lymphomas.[175,176] Bone marrow is involved at presentation in less than half of the cases. Transformation to high-grade lymphoma has been described in some cases.

Treatment and Outcome

There is at present no consensus about the best treatment, individual cases being managed differently according to site and stage. Indeed, there are very few studies comparing nodal MZL with the other low-grade B-cell lymphomas. The most important study was recently published by the Southwest Oncology Group (SWOG), comparing various low-grade lymphomas presenting with advanced disease (Stage III–IV). This study reviewed the pathology and clinical course of 376 patients previously classified within the Working Formulation categories A, B, C, D, or E, and uniformly treated with the standard combination-chemotherapy CHOP regimen. Twenty-one patients with nodal MZL (monocytoid B-cell lymphoma), and 19 patients with extranodal MZL (MALT lymphoma) were identified. Advanced-stage MALT lymphoma appeared to carry a worse prognosis than nodal MZL (10-year actuarial survivals of 21% versus 53%, respectively).[177] All nodal MZL patients were given full-dose CHOP, and showed a survival pattern superimposable on that of advanced FL, but how they would behave with other treatment strategies frequently employed in low-grade lymphomas (such as watchful waiting, single alkylating agents, new purine analogues, rituximab) is still to be ascertained.

The previously mentioned international collaborative survey for the validation of the REAL classification, which included patients of any stage treated with heterogeneous modalities, showed 5-year survivals of 57% for MZBCL and 74% for MALT lymphomas. Comparisons of patients with IPI scores of 0 to 3 showed that those with nodal MZL had lower 5-year overall survival (52% vs. 88%, p = 0.025) and failure-free survival (30% vs. 75%, p = 0.007) rates than those with extranodal MZL. This discrepancy with the SWOG study might be at least partially due to the higher incidence of advanced disease in the nodal MZBCL group (82%, versus 44% in the extranodal MALT-type group).[173,178] In a French series of non-MALT–type MZL from Lyon,[156] four clinical subtypes were identified: splenic, nodal, disseminated (splenic and nodal), and leukemic (not splenic or nodal). The nodal cases comprised 30% of patients and showed a more aggressive behavior. Nodal and disseminated subtypes had shorter median time to progression (about 1 year) in comparison with the splenic and leukemic subtypes (median time to progression longer than 5 years). The cases with disseminated disease more often presented with poor prognosis parameters (high LDH and beta-2 microglobulin, poor performance status, bulky disease), and might represent the end stage of the other subtypes.[124,156] However, in all subsets, even if the median time to progression was short, prolonged survival was observed (splenic, 9 years; nodal, 5.5 years; disseminated, 15 years; and leukemic, 7 years). About half of the nodal and one-fourth of the disseminated cases presented with more than 50% of large cells or sheets of large B cells. These patients' cases may be considered as having a "transformed" lymphoma at diagnosis, or a composite lymphoma with MZL aspect and features of DLBCL. Large-cell–rich cases were definitely less common in the splenic subsets. This finding may at least partially explain the observed differences in the outcome of different subsets.

The retrospective nature of this study precludes any conclusion on the therapeutic aspects, but conservative treatments seem recommended for leukemic and splenic subtypes, while in nodal and disseminated subtypes frontline chemotherapy may be considered. Treatment options may include single-agent chlorambucil or fludarabine or combination chemotherapy regimens (such as the CVP or CHOP).[156] Rituximab may also have some efficacy.[179] Autologous transplantation has been used in younger patients with adverse prognostic factors and a high number of large cells. However, no prospective studies have been conducted so far and treatment decision should be based on the histologic and clinical features of the individual patient.[12,167]

References

1. Harris NL, Jaffe ES, Stein H, et al. A revised European–American classification of lymphoid neoplasms: a proposal from the International Lymphoma Study Group. Blood 1994;84:1361–92.
2. Dierlamm J, Pittaluga S, Wlodarska I, et al. Marginal zone B-cell lymphomas of different sites share similar cytogenetic and morphologic features. Blood 1996;87:299–307.
3. De Wolf-Peeters C, Pittaluga S, Dierlamm J, et al. Marginal zone B-cell lymphomas including mucosa-associated lymphoid tissue type lymphoma (MALT), monocytoid B-cell lymphoma and splenic marginal zone cell lymphoma and their relation to the reactive marginal zone. Leuk Lymphoma 1997;26:467–78.
4. Isaacson PG, Muller-Hermelink HK, Piris MA, et al. Extranodal marginal zone B-cell lymphoma of mucosa-associated lymphoid tissue (MALT lymphoma). In: Jaffe ES, Harris NL, Stein H, et al., eds. World Health Organization Classification of Tumours. Pathology and Genetics of Tumours of Haematopoietic and Lymphoid Tissues. Lyon: IARC Press, 2001:157–60.
5. Isaacson PG, Nathwani BN, Piris MA, et al. Nodal marginal zone B-cell lymphoma. In: Jaffe ES, Harris NL, Stein H, et al., eds. World Health Organization Classification of Tumours. Pathology and Genetics of Tumours of Haematopoietic and Lymphoid Tissues. Lyon: IARC Press, 2001:161.
6. Isaacson PI, Piris MA, Catovsky D, et al. Splenic marginal zone lymphoma. In: Jaffe ES, Harris NL, Stein H, et al., eds. World Health Organization Classification of Tumours. Pathology and Genetics of Tumours of Haematopoietic and Lymphoid Tissues. Lyon: IARC Press, 2001:135–7.
7. The Non-Hodgkin's Lymphoma Classification Project. A clinical evaluation of the International Lymphoma Study Group classification of non-Hodgkin's lymphoma. Blood 1997;89:3909–18.
8. Doglioni C, Wotherspoon AC, Moschini A, et al. High incidence of primary gastric lymphoma in northeastern Italy. Lancet 1992;339:834–5.
9. Zaki M and Schubert ML. Helicobacter pylori and gastric lymphoma. Gastroenterology 1995;108:610–12.
10. Lopes-Carvalho T and Kearney JF. Development and selection of marginal zone B cells. Immunol Rev 2004;197: 192–205.
11. Martin F and Kearney JF. Marginal-zone B cells. Nat Rev Immunol 2002;2:323–35.
12. Arcaini L, Paulli M, Boveri E, et al. Marginal zone-related neoplasms of splenic and nodal origin. Haematologica 2003; 88:80–93.
13. Sagaert X and De Wolf-Peeters C. Classification of B-cells according to their differentiation status, their micro-anatomical localisation and their developmental lineage. Immunol Lett 2003;90:179–86.
14. Cavalli F, Isaacson PG, Gascoyne RD, et al. MALT Lymphomas. Hematology (Am Soc Hematol Educ Program) 2001:241–58.
15. Yahalom J, Isaacson PG, and Zucca E. Extranodal marginal zone B-cell lymphoma of mucosa-associated lymphoid tissue. In: Mauch PM, Armitage J, Coiffier B, et al, eds. Non-Hodgkin's Lymphomas. Philadelphia: Lippincott Williams & Wilkins, 2004:345–60.
16. Feller AC and Diebold J. Histopathology of nodal and extranodal non-Hodgkin's lymphomas, 3rd ed. Berlin: Springer Verlag, 2004.
17. Pozzi B, Cerati M, and Capella C. MALT lymphoma: pathology. In: Bertoni F and Zucca E, eds. MALT Lymphomas. Georgetown, TX: Landes Bioscience/Eurekah.com and New York, NY: Kluwer Academic/Plenum Publishers, 2004:17–45.
18. Lavergne A, Brouland JP, Launay E, et al. Multiple lymphomatous polyposis of the gastrointestinal tract. An extensive histopathologic and immunohistochemical study of 12 cases. Cancer 1994;74:3042–50.
19. Chan JK. Gastrointestinal lymphomas: an overview with emphasis on new findings and diagnostic problems. Semin Diagn Pathol 1996;13:260–96.

20. de Jong D, Boot H, van Heerde P, et al. Histological grading in gastric lymphoma: pretreatment criteria and clinical relevance. Gastroenterology 1997;112:1466–74.
21. Wotherspoon AC, Doglioni C, Diss TC, et al. Regression of primary low-grade B-cell gastric lymphoma of mucosa-associated lymphoid tissue type after eradication of Helicobacter pylori. Lancet 1993;342:575–7.
22. Qin Y, Greiner A, Trunk MJ, et al. Somatic hypermutation in low-grade mucosa-associated lymphoid tissue-type B-cell lymphoma. Blood 1995;86:3528–34.
23. Du M, Diss TC, Xu C, et al. Ongoing mutation in MALT lymphoma immunoglobulin gene suggests that antigen stimulation plays a role in the clonal expansion. Leukemia 1996;10:1190–7.
24. Bertoni F, Cazzaniga G, Bosshard G, et al. Immunoglobulin heavy chain diversity genes rearrangement pattern indicates that MALT-type gastric lymphoma B cells have undergone an antigen selection process. Br J Haematol 1997;97:830–6.
25. Zucca E, Bertoni F, Roggero E, et al. Autoreactive B cell clones in marginal-zone B cell lymphoma (MALT lymphoma) of the stomach. Leukemia 1998;12:247–9.
26. Isaacson P and Wright DH. Extranodal malignant lymphoma arising from mucosa-associated lymphoid tissue. Cancer 1984;53:2515–24.
27. Zucca E, Bertoni F, Roggero E, et al. The gastric marginal zone B-cell lymphoma of MALT type. Blood 2000;96:410–9.
28. Luppi M and Negrini R. MALT lymphoma: epidemiology ad infectious agents. In: Bertoni F and Zucca E, eds. MALT Lymphomas. Georgetown, TX: Landes Bioscience/Eurekah.com and New York, NY: Kluwer Academic/Plenum Publishers, 2004:17–45.
29. Du MQ and Isaacson PG. Gastric MALT lymphoma: from aetiology to treatment. Lancet Oncol 2002;3:97–104.
30. Parsonnet J, Hansen S, Rodriguez L, et al. Helicobacter pylori infection and gastric lymphoma. N Engl J Med 1994; 330:1267–71.
31. Hussell T, Isaacson PG, Crabtree JE, et al. Helicobacter pylori-specific tumour-infiltrating T cells provide contact dependent help for the growth of malignant B cells in low-grade gastric lymphoma of mucosa-associated lymphoid tissue. J Pathol 1996;178:122–7.
32. Zucca E, Bertoni F, Roggero E, et al. Molecular analysis of the progression from Helicobacter pylori–associated chronic gastritis to mucosa-associated lymphoid-tissue lymphoma of the stomach. N Engl J Med 1998;338:804–10.
33. Roggero E, Zucca E, Pinotti G, et al. Eradication of Helicobacter pylori infection in primary low-grade gastric lymphoma of mucosa-associated lymphoid tissue. Ann Intern Med 1995;122:767–9.
34. Bayerdorffer E, Neubauer A, Rudolph B, et al. Regression of primary gastric lymphoma of mucosa-associated lymphoid tissue type after cure of Helicobacter pylori infection. MALT Lymphoma Study Group. Lancet 1995;345:1591–4.
35. Garbe C, Stein H, Dienemann D, et al. Borrelia burgdorferi–associated cutaneous B cell lymphoma: clinical and immunohistologic characterization of four cases. J Am Acad Dermatol 1991;24:584–90.
36. Kutting B, Bonsmann G, Metze D, et al. Borrelia burgdorferi-associated primary cutaneous B cell lymphoma: complete clearing of skin lesions after antibiotic pulse therapy or intralesional injection of interferon alfa-2a. J Am Acad Dermatol 1997;36:311–14.
37. Roggero E, Zucca E, Mainetti C, et al. Eradication of Borrelia burgdorferi infection in primary marginal zone B-cell lymphoma of the skin. Hum Pathol 2000;31:263–8.
38. Ferreri AJ, Guidoboni M, Ponzoni M, et al. Evidence for an association between Chlamydia psittaci and ocular adnexal lymphomas. J Natl Cancer Inst 2004;96:586–94.
39. Lecuit M, Abachin E, Martin A, et al. Immunoproliferative small intestinal disease associated with Campylobacter jejuni. N Engl J Med 2004;350:239–48.
40. Zucca E, Roggero E, Bertoni F, et al. Primary extranodal non-Hodgkin's lymphomas. Part 1: Gastrointestinal, cutaneous and genitourinary lymphomas. Ann Oncol 1997;8:727–37.
41. Auer IA, Gascoyne RD, Connors JM, et al. t(11;18)(q21;q21) is the most common translocation in MALT lymphomas. Ann Oncol 1997;8:979–85.
42. Ott G, Katzenberger T, Greiner A, et al. The t(11;18)(q21;q21) chromosome translocation is a frequent and specific aberration in low-grade but not high-grade malignant non-Hodgkin's lymphomas of the mucosa-associated lymphoid tissue (MALT-) type. Cancer Res 1997; 57:3944–8.
43. Dierlamm J, Baens M, Stefanova-Ouzounova M, et al. Detection of t(11;18)(q21;q21) by interphase fluorescence in situ hybridization using API2 and MLT specific probes. Blood 2000;96:2215–8.
44. Rosenwald A, Ott G, Stilgenbauer S, et al. Exclusive detection of the t(11;18)(q21;q21) in extranodal marginal zone B cell lymphomas (MZBL) of MALT type in contrast to other MZBL and extranodal large B cell lymphomas. Am J Pathol 1999;155:1817–21.
45. Remstein ED, James CD, and Kurtin PJ. Incidence and subtype specificity of API2-MALT1 fusion translocations in extranodal, nodal, and splenic marginal zone lymphomas. Am J Pathol 2000;156:1183–8.
46. Baens M, Maes B, Steyls A, et al. The product of the t(11;18), an API2-MLT fusion, marks nearly half of gastric MALT type lymphomas without large cell proliferation. Am J Pathol 2000;156:1433–9.
47. Maes B, Baens M, Marynen P, et al. The product of the t(11;18), an API2-MLT fusion, is an almost exclusive finding in marginal zone cell lymphoma of extranodal MALT-type. Ann Oncol 2000;11:521–6.
48. Motegi M, Yonezumi M, Suzuki H, et al. API2-MALT1 chimeric transcripts involved in mucosa-associated lymphoid tissue type lymphoma predict heterogeneous products. Am J Pathol 2000;156:807–12.
49. Nakamura T, Nakamura S, Yonezumi M, et al. Helicobacter pylori and the t(11;18)(q21;q21) translocation in gastric low-grade B-cell lymphoma of mucosa-associated lymphoid tissue type. Jpn J Cancer Res 2000;91:301–9.
50. Liu H, Ye H, Dogan A, et al. T(11;18)(q21;q21) is associated with advanced mucosa-associated lymphoid tissue lymphoma that expresses nuclear BCL10. Blood 2001;98: 1182–7.
51. Kalla J, Stilgenbauer S, Schaffner C, et al. Heterogeneity of the API2-MALT1 gene rearrangement in MALT-type lymphoma. Leukemia 2000;14:1967–74.
52. Inagaki H, Okabe M, Seto M, et al. API2-MALT1 fusion transcripts involved in mucosa-associated lymphoid tissue lymphoma: multiplex RT-PCR detection using formalin-fixed paraffin-embedded specimens. Am J Pathol 2001;158: 699–706.
53. Takada S, Yoshino T, Taniwaki M, et al. Involvement of the chromosomal translocation t(11;18) in some mucosa-associated lymphoid tissue lymphomas and diffuse large B-cell lymphomas of the ocular adnexa: evidence from multiplex reverse transcriptase-polymerase chain reaction and fluorescence in situ hybridization on using formalin-fixed, paraffin-embedded specimens. Mod Pathol 2003;16:445–52.
54. Ye H, Liu H, Attygalle A, et al. Variable frequencies of t(11;18)(q21;q21) in MALT lymphomas of different sites: significant association with CagA strains of H. pylori in gastric MALT lymphoma. Blood 2003;102:1012–8.

55. Morgan JA, Yin Y, Borowsky AD, et al. Breakpoints of the t(11;18)(q21;q21) in mucosa-associated lymphoid tissue (MALT) lymphoma lie within or near the previously undescribed gene MALT1 in chromosome 18. Cancer Res 1999;59:6205–13.
56. Dierlamm J, Baens M, Wlodarska I, et al. The apoptosis inhibitor gene API2 and a novel 18q gene, MLT, are recurrently rearranged in the t(11;18)(q21;q21) associated with mucosa-associated lymphoid tissue lymphomas. Blood 1999;93:3601–9.
57. Akagi T, Motegi M, Tamura A, et al. A novel gene, MALT1 at 18q21, is involved in t(11;18) (q21;q21) found in low-grade B-cell lymphoma of mucosa-associated lymphoid tissue. Oncogene 1999;18:5785–94.
58. Reed JC. Mechanisms of apoptosis. Am J Pathol 2000;157:1415–30.
59. Deveraux QL, Reed JC. IAP family proteins—suppressors of apoptosis. Genes Dev 1999;13:239–52.
60. Uren GA, O'Rourke K, Aravind L, et al. Identification of paracaspases and metacaspases: two ancient families of caspase-like proteins, one of which plays a key role in MALT lymphoma. Mol Cell 2000;6:961–7.
61. Liu H, Ruskon-Fourmestraux A, Lavergne-Slove A, et al. Resistance of t(11;18) positive gastric mucosa-associated lymphoid tissue lymphoma to Helicobacter pylori eradication therapy. Lancet 2001;357:39–40.
62. Sanchez-Izquierdo D, Buchonet G, Siebert R, et al. MALT1 is deregulated by both chromosomal translocation and amplification in B-cell non-Hodgkin lymphoma. Blood 2003;101:4539–46.
63. Streubel B, Lamprecht A, Dierlamm J, et al. T(14;18) (q32;q21) involving IGH and MALT1 is a frequent chromosomal aberration in MALT lymphoma. Blood 2003;101: 2335–9.
64. Dierlamm J, Rosenberg C, Stul M, et al. Characteristic pattern of chromosomal gains and losses in marginal zone B cell lymphoma detected by comparative genomic hybridization. Leukemia 1997;11:747–58.
65. Cook JR, Sherer M, Craig FE, et al. T(14;18)(q32;q21) involving MALT1 and IGH genes in an extranodal diffuse large B-cell lymphoma. Hum Pathol 2003;34:1212–15.
66. Zhang Q, Siebert R, Yan M, et al. Inactivating mutations and overexpression of BCL10, a caspase recruitment domain-containing gene, in MALT lymphoma with t(1;14)(p22;q32). Nat Genet 1999;22:63–8.
67. Willis TG, Jadayel DM, Du MQ, et al. Bcl10 is involved in t(1;14)(p22;q32) of MALT B cell lymphoma and mutated in multiple tumor types. Cell 1999;96:35–45.
68. Achuthan R, Bell SM, Leek JP, et al. Novel translocation of the BCL10 gene in a case of mucosa associated lymphoid tissue lymphoma. Genes Chromosomes Cancer 2000;29: 347–9.
69. Costanzo A, Guiet C, and Vito P. c-E10 is a caspase-recruiting domain-containing protein that interacts with components of death receptors signaling pathway and activates nuclear factor-kappaB. J Biol Chem 1999;274: 20127–32.
70. Yan M, Lee J, Schilbach S, et al. mE10, a novel caspase recruitment domain-containing proapoptotic molecule. J Biol Chem 1999;274:10287–92.
71. Srinivasula SM, Ahmad M, Lin JH, et al. CLAP, a novel caspase recruitment domain-containing protein in the tumor necrosis factor receptor pathway, regulates NF-kappaB activation and apoptosis. J Biol Chem 1999;274:17946–54.
72. Koseki T, Inohara N, Chen S, et al. CIPER, a novel NF kappaB-activating protein containing a caspase recruitment domain with homology to herpesvirus-2 protein E10. J Biol Chem 1999;274:9955–61.
73. Zhang Q, Cui X, Sangster MY, et al. Selective hyperexpansion of marginal zone (MZ) B-cells in Em-BCL10 mice. Blood 2000;96:822a.
74. Ruland J, Duncan GS, Elia A, et al. Bcl10 is a positive regulator of antigen receptor-induced activation of NF-kappaB and neural tube closure. Cell 2001;104:33–42.
75. Ye H, Dogan A, Karran L, et al. BCL10 expression in normal and neoplastic lymphoid tissue: nuclear localization in MALT lymphoma. Am J Pathol 2000;157:1147–54.
76. Lucas PC, Yonezumi M, Inohara N, et al. Bcl10 and MALT1, independent targets of chromosomal translocation in MALT lymphoma, cooperate in a novel NF-kappa B signaling pathway. J Biol Chem 2001;276:19012–19.
77. McAllister-Lucas LM, Inohara N, Lucas PC, et al. Bimp1, a MAGUK family member linking PKC activation to Bcl10-mediated NF-kB induction. J Biol Chem 2001;276: 30589–97.
78. Pinotti G, Zucca E, Roggero E, et al. Clinical features, treatment and outcome in a series of 93 patients with low-grade gastric MALT lymphoma. Leuk Lymphoma 1997;26:527–37.
79. Thieblemont C, Coiffier B. MALT lymphoma: Sites of presentations, clinical features and staging procedures. In: Bertoni F, Zucca E, eds. MALT lymphomas. Georgetown TX: Landes Bioscience/Eurekah.com and New York, NY: Kluwer Academic/Plenum Publishers, 2004:60–80.
80. Dogan A, Du M, Koulis A, et al. Expression of lymphocyte homing receptors and vascular addressins in low-grade gastric B-cell lymphomas of mucosa-associated lymphoid tissue. Am J Pathol 1997;151:1361–9.
81. Drillenburg P, van der Voort R, Koopman G, et al. Preferential expression of the mucosal homing receptor integrin alpha 4 beta 7 in gastrointestinal non-Hodgkin's lymphomas. Am J Pathol 1997;150:919–27.
82. Drillenburg P and Pals ST. Cell adhesion receptors in lymphoma dissemination. Blood 2000;95:1900–10.
83. Zucca E, Conconi A, Pedrinis E, et al. Nongastric marginal zone B-cell lymphoma of mucosa-associated lymphoid tissue. Blood 2003;101:2489–95.
84. Thieblemont C, Berger F, Dumontet C, et al. Mucosa-associated lymphoid tissue lymphoma is a disseminated disease in one third of 158 patients analyzed. Blood 2000;95:802–806.
85. de Jong D, Aleman BM, Taal BG, et al. Controversies and consensus in the diagnosis, work-up and treatment of gastric lymphoma: an international survey. Ann Oncol 1999;10: 275–80.
86. Rohatiner A, d'Amore F, Coiffier B, et al. Report on a workshop convened to discuss the pathological and staging classifications of gastrointestinal tract lymphoma. Ann Oncol 1994;5:397–400.
87. Sackmann M, Morgner A, Rudolph B, et al. Regression of gastric MALT lymphoma after eradication of Helicobacter pylori is predicted by endosonographic staging. MALT Lymphoma Study Group. Gastroenterology 1997;113:1087–90.
88. Ruskone-Fourmestraux A, Lavergne A, Aegerter PH, et al. Predictive factors for regression of gastric MALT lymphoma after anti–Helicobacter pylori treatment. Gut 2001;48: 297–303.
89. Eidt S, Stolte M, and Fischer R. Factors influencing lymph node infiltration in primary gastric malignant lymphoma of the mucosa-associated lymphoid tissue. Pathol Res Pract 1994;190:1077–81.
90. Steinbach G, Ford R, Glober G, et al. Antibiotic treatment of gastric lymphoma of mucosa-associated lymphoid tissue. An uncontrolled trial. Ann Intern Med 1999;131:88–95.
91. Stolte M, Bayerdorffer E, Morgner A, et al. Helicobacter and gastric MALT lymphoma. Gut 2002;50(Suppl 3): III19–24.

92. Ahmad A, Govil Y, and Frank BB. Gastric mucosa-associated lymphoid tissue lymphoma. Am J Gastroenterol 2003; 98:975–86.
93. Conconi A, Cavalli F, Zucca E. Gastric MALT lymphomas: The role of antibiotics. In: Bertoni F, Zucca E, eds. MALT lymphomas. Georgetown TX: Landes Bioscience/ Eurekah.com and New York, NY: Kluwer Academic/Plenum Publishers, 2004:81–90.
94. Isaacson PG, Diss TC, Wotherspoon AC, et al. Long-term follow-up of gastric MALT lymphoma treated by eradication of H. pylori with antibodies. Gastroenterology 1999;117: 750–1.
95. Neubauer A, Thiede C, Morgner A, et al. Cure of Helicobacter pylori infection and duration of remission of low-grade gastric mucosa-associated lymphoid tissue lymphoma. J Natl Cancer Inst 1997;89:1350–5.
96. Nakamura S, Matsumoto T, Suekane H, et al. Predictive value of endoscopic ultrasonography for regression of gastric low grade and high grade MALT lymphomas after eradication of Helicobacter pylori. Gut 2001;48:454–60.
97. Bertoni F, Conconi A, Capella C, et al. Molecular follow-up in gastric mucosa-associated lymphoid tissue lymphomas: early analysis of the LY03 cooperative trial. Blood 2002;99: 2541–4.
98. Copie-Bergman C, Gaulard P, Lavergne-Slove A, et al. Proposal for a new histological grading system for post-treatment evaluation of gastric MALT lymphoma. Gut 2003; 52:1656.
99. Liu H, Ye H, Ruskone-Fourmestraux A, et al. T(11;18) is a marker for all stage gastric MALT lymphomas that will not respond to H. pylori eradication. Gastroenterology 2002;122: 1286–94.
100. Alpen B, Neubauer A, Dierlamm J, et al. Translocation t(11;18) absent in early gastric marginal zone B-cell lymphoma of MALT type responding to eradication of Helicobacter pylori infection. Blood 2000;95:4014–15.
101. Thiede C, Wundisch T, Alpen B, et al. Persistence of monoclonal B cells after cure of Helicobacter pylori infection and complete histologic remission in gastric mucosa-associated lymphoid tissue B-cell lymphoma. J Clin Oncol 2001;19: 1600–9.
102. Wotherspoon AC, Savio A. Molecular follow-up in gastric MALT lymhomas. In: Bertoni F, Zucca E, eds. MALT lymphomas. Georgetown TX: Landes Bioscience/Eurekah.com and New York, NY: Kluwer Academic/Plenum Publishers, 2004:91–98.
103. Fischbach W, Goebeler-Kolve M, Starostik P, et al. Minimal residual low-grade gastric MALT-type lymphoma after eradication of Helicobacter pylori. Lancet 2002;360: 547–8.
104. Montalban C, Manzanal A, Castrillo JM, et al. Low grade gastric B-cell MALT lymphoma progressing into high grade lymphoma. Clonal identity of the two stages of the tumour, unusual bone involvement and leukemic dissemination. Histopathology 1995;27:89–91.
105. Thieblemont C, Dumontet C, Bouafia F, et al. Outcome in relation to treatment modalities in 48 patients with localized gastric MALT lymphoma: a retrospective study of patients treated during 1976–2001. Leuk Lymphoma 2003;44: 257–62.
106. Tsang RW, Gospodarowicz MK, Pintilie M, et al. Localized mucosa-associated lymphoid tissue lymphoma treated with radiation therapy has excellent clinical outcome. J Clin Oncol 2003;21:4157–64.
107. Schechter NR, Portlock CS, and Yahalom J. Treatment of mucosa-associated lymphoid tissue lymphoma of the stomach with radiation alone. J Clin Oncol 1998;16: 1916–21.
108. Gospodarowicz M, Tsang R. Radiation therapy of mucosa-associated lymphoid tissue (MALT) lymphomas. In: Bertoni F, Zucca E, eds. MALT lymphomas. Georgetown TX: Landes Bioscience/Eurekah.com and New York, NY: Kluwer Academic/Plenum Publishers, 2004:104–29.
109. Conconi A, Cavalli F, Zucca E. MALT lymphomas: The role of chemotherapy. In: Bertoni F, Zucca E, eds. MALT lymphomas. Georgetown TX: Landes Bioscience/Eurekah.com and New York, NY: Kluwer Academic/Plenum Publishers, 2004:93–103.
110. Hammel P, Haioun C, Chaumette MT, et al. Efficacy of single-agent chemotherapy in low-grade B-cell mucosa-associated lymphoid tissue lymphoma with prominent gastric expression. J Clin Oncol 1995;13:2524–9.
111. Levy M, Copie-Bergman C, Traulle C, et al. Conservative treatment of primary gastric low-grade B-cell lymphoma of mucosa-associated lymphoid tissue: predictive factors of response and outcome. Am J Gastroenterol 2002;97:292–7.
112. Zinzani PL, Stefoni V, Musuraca G, et al. Fludarabine-containing chemotherapy as frontline treatment of nongastrointestinal mucosa-associated lymphoid tissue lymphoma. Cancer 2004;100:2190–4.
113. Jager G, Neumeister P, Brezinschek R, et al. Treatment of extranodal marginal zone B-cell lymphoma of mucosa-associated lymphoid tissue type with cladribine: a Phase II study. J Clin Oncol 2002;20:3872–7.
114. Jager G, Hofler G, Linkesch W, et al. Occurence of a myelodysplastic syndrome (MDS) during first-line 2-chloro-deoxyadenosine (2-CDA) treatment of a low-grade gastrointestinal MALT lymphoma. Case report and review of the literature. Haematologica 2004;89:ECR01.
115. Wohrer S, Drach J, Hejna M, et al. Treatment of extranodal marginal zone B-cell lymphoma of mucosa-associated lymphoid tissue (MALT lymphoma) with mitoxantrone, chlorambucil and prednisone (MCP). Ann Oncol 2003;14: 1758–61.
116. Conconi A, Martinelli G, Thieblemont C, et al. Clinical activity of rituximab in extranodal marginal zone B-cell lymphoma of MALT type. Blood 2003;102:2741–5.
117. Chen LT, Lin JT, Shyu RY, et al. Prospective study of Helicobacter pylori eradication therapy in Stage I(E) high-grade mucosa-associated lymphoid tissue lymphoma of the stomach. J Clin Oncol 2001;19:4245–51.
118. Thieblemont C, Bastion Y, Berger F, et al. Mucosa-associated lymphoid tissue gastrointestinal and nongastrointestinal lymphoma behavior: analysis of 108 patients. J Clin Oncol 1997;15:1624–30.
119. Zinzani PL, Martelli M, Magagnoli M, et al. Treatment and clinical management of primary mediastinal large B-cell lymphoma with sclerosis: MACOP-B regimen and mediastinal radiotherapy monitored by (67)gallium scan in 50 patients. Blood 1999;94:3289–93.
120. Schechter NR and Yahalom J. Low-grade MALT lymphoma of the stomach: a review of treatment options. Int J Radiat Oncol Biol Phys 2000;46:1093–103.
121. Isaacson PG. Splenic marginal zone B cell lymphoma. In: Mason DY and Harris NL, eds. Human Lymphoma: Clinical Implications of the REAL Classification. London: Springer-Verlag, 1999:7.1–7.6.
122. Piris MA, Mollejo M, Chacon I, et al. Splenic marginal zone B-cell lymphoma. In: Mauch PM, Armitage J, Coiffier B, et al., eds. Non-Hodgkin's Lymphomas. Philadelphia: Lippincott Williams & Wilkins, 2004:275–82.
123. Franco V, Florena AM, and Iannitto E. Splenic marginal zone lymphoma. Blood 2003;101:2464–72.
124. Thieblemont C, Felman P, Callet-Bauchu E, et al. Splenic marginal-zone lymphoma: a distinct clinical and pathological entity. Lancet Oncol 2003;4:95–103.

125. Isaacson PG, Matutes E, Burke M, et al. The histopathology of splenic lymphoma with villous lymphocytes. Blood 1994;84:3828–34.
126. Schenka AA, Gascoyne RD, Duchayne E, et al. Prominent intrasinusoidal infiltration of the bone marrow by mantle cell lymphoma. Hum Pathol 2003;34:789–91.
127. Kent SA, Variakojis D, and Peterson LC. Comparative study of marginal zone lymphoma involving bone marrow. Am J Clin Pathol 2002;117:698–708.
128. Audouin J, Le Tourneau A, Molina T, et al. Patterns of bone marrow involvement in 58 patients presenting primary splenic marginal zone lymphoma with or without circulating villous lymphocytes. Br J Haematol 2003;122: 404–12.
129. Camacho FI, Mollejo M, Mateo MS, et al. Progression to large B-cell lymphoma in splenic marginal zone lymphoma: a description of a series of 12 cases. Am J Surg Pathol 2001; 25:1268–76.
130. Bedu-Addo G and Bates I. Causes of massive tropical splenomegaly in Ghana. Lancet 2002;360:449–54.
131. Algara P, Mateo MS, Sanchez-Beato M, et al. Analysis of the IgV(H) somatic mutations in splenic marginal zone lymphoma defines a group of unmutated cases with frequent 7q deletion and adverse clinical course. Blood 2002;99: 1299–304.
132. Tierens A, Delabie J, Malecka A, et al. Splenic marginal zone lymphoma with villous lymphocytes shows on-going immunoglobulin gene mutations. Am J Pathol 2003;162: 681–9.
133. Zhu D, Thompsett AR, Bedu-Addo G, et al. VH gene sequences from a novel tropical splenic lymphoma reveal a naive B cell as the cell of origin. Br J Haematol 1999; 107:114–20.
134. Gisbert JP, Garcia-Buey L, Pajares JM, et al. Prevalence of hepatitis C virus infection in B-cell non-Hodgkin's lymphoma: systematic review and meta-analysis. Gastroenterology 2003;125:1723–32.
135. Chan CH, Hadlock KG, Foung SK, et al. V(H)1-69 gene is preferentially used by hepatitis C virus-associated B cell lymphomas and by normal B cells responding to the E2 viral antigen. Blood 2001;97:1023–6.
136. Karavattathayyil SJ, Kalkeri G, Liu HJ, et al. Detection of hepatitis C virus RNA sequences in B-cell non-Hodgkin lymphoma. Am J Clin Pathol 2000;113:391–8.
137. Zucca E, Roggero E, Maggi-Solca N, et al. Prevalence of Helicobacter pylori and hepatitis C virus infections among non-Hodgkin's lymphoma patients in Southern Switzerland. Haematologica 2000;85:147–53.
138. Thalen DJ, Raemaekers J, Galama J, et al. Absence of hepatitis C virus infection in non-Hodgkin's lymphoma. Br J Haematol 1997;96:880–1.
139. Arcaini L, Paulli M, Boveri E, et al. Splenic and nodal marginal zone lymphomas are indolent disorders at high hepatitis C virus seroprevalence with distinct presenting features but similar morphologic and phenotypic profiles. Cancer 2004;100:107–15.
140. Hermine O, Lefrere F, Bronowicki JP, et al. Regression of splenic lymphoma with villous lymphocytes after treatment of hepatitis C virus infection. N Engl J Med 2002;347: 89–94.
141. Bates I, Bedu-Addo G, Rutherford T, et al. Splenic lymphoma with villous lymphocytes in tropical West Africa. Lancet 1992;340:575–7.
142. Bates I, Bedu-Addo G, Jarrett RF, et al. B-lymphotropic viruses in a novel tropical splenic lymphoma. Br J Haematol 2001;112:161–6.
143. Boonstra R, Bosga-Bouwer A, van Imhoff GW, et al. Splenic marginal zone lymphomas presenting with splenomegaly and typical immunophenotype are characterized by allelic loss in 7q31-32. Mod Pathol 2003;16:1210–17.
144. Sole F, Salido M, Espinet B, et al. Splenic marginal zone B-cell lymphomas: two cytogenetic subtypes, one with gain of 3q and the other with loss of 7q. Haematologica 2001; 86:71–7.
145. Hernandez JM, Garcia JL, Gutierrez NC, et al. Novel genomic imbalances in B-cell splenic marginal zone lymphomas revealed by comparative genomic hybridization and cytogenetics. Am J Pathol 2001;158:1843–50.
146. Gruszka-Westwood AM, Hamoudi R, Osborne L, et al. Deletion mapping on the long arm of chromosome 7 in splenic lymphoma with villous lymphocytes. Genes Chromosomes Cancer 2003;36:57–69.
147. Andersen CL, Gruszka-Westwood A, M OS, et al. A narrow deletion of 7q is common to HCL, and SMZL, but not CLL. Eur J Haematol 2004;72:390–402.
148. Brito-Babapulle V, Gruszka-Westwood AM, Platt G, et al. Translocation t(2;7)(p12;q21-22) with dysregulation of the CDK6 gene mapping to 7q21-22 in a non-Hodgkin's lymphoma with leukemia. Haematologica 2002;87: 357–62.
149. Iida S, Rao PH, Nallasivam P, et al. The t(9;14)(p13;q32) chromosomal translocation associated with lymphoplasmacytoid lymphoma involves the PAX-5 gene. Blood 1996; 88:4110–7.
150. Ohno H, Ueda C, Akasaka T. The t(9;14)(p13;q32) translocation in B-cell non-Hodgkin's lymphoma. Leuk Lymphoma 2000;36:435–45.
151. Cook JR, Aguilera NI, Reshmi-Skarja S, et al. Lack of PAX5 rearrangements in lymphoplasmacytic lymphomas: reassessing the reported association with t(9;14). Hum Pathol 2004;35:447–54.
152. Gazzo S, Baseggio L, Coignet L, et al. Cytogenetic and molecular delineation of a region of chromosome 3q commonly gained in marginal zone B-cell lymphoma. Haematologica 2003;88:31–8.
153. Thieblemont C, Nasser V, Felman P, et al. Small lymphocytic lymphoma, marginal zone B-cell lymphoma, and mantle cell lymphoma exhibit distinct gene-expression profiles allowing molecular diagnosis. Blood 2004;103:2727–37.
154. Catovsky D and Matutes E. Splenic lymphoma with circulating villous lymphocytes/splenic marginal-zone lymphoma. Semin Haematol 1999;36:148–54.
155. Troussard X, Valensi F, Duchayne E, et al. Splenic lymphoma with villous lymphocytes: clinical presentation, biology and prognostic factors in a series of 100 patients. Groupe Francais d'Hematologie Cellulaire (GFHC). Br J Haematol 1996; 93:731–6.
156. Berger F, Felman P, Thieblemont C, et al. Non-MALT marginal zone B-cell lymphomas: a description of clinical presentation and outcome in 124 patients. Blood 2000;95: 1950–6.
157. Chacon JI, Mollejo M, Munoz E, et al. Splenic marginal zone lymphoma: clinical characteristics and prognostic factors in a series of 60 patients. Blood 2002;100:1648–54.
158. Thieblemont C, Felman P, Berger F, et al. Treatment of splenic marginal zone B-cell lymphoma: an analysis of 81 patients. Clin Lymphoma 2002;3:41–7.
159. Berger F, Isaacson PG, Piris MA, et al. Lymphoplasmacytic lymphoma/Waldenstroem macroglobulinemia. In: Jaffe ES, Harris NL, Stein H, et al., eds. World Health Organization Classification of Tumours. Pathology and Genetics of Tumours of Haematopoietic and Lymphoid Tissues. Lyon: IARC Press, 2001:135–7.
160. Mollejo M, Menarguez J, Lloret E, et al. Splenic marginal zone lymphoma: a distinctive type of low-grade B-cell lymphoma. A clinicopathological study of 13 cases. Am J Surg Pathol 1995;19:1146–57.

161. Mulligan SP, Matutes E, Dearden C, et al. Splenic lymphoma with villous lymphocytes: natural history and response to therapy in 50 cases. Br J Haematol 1991;78:206–9.
162. Lefrere F, Hermine O, Belanger C, et al. Fludarabine: an effective treatment in patients with splenic lymphoma with villous lymphocytes. Leukemia 2000;14:573–5.
163. Bolam S, Orchard J, and Oscier D. Fludarabine is effective in the treatment of splenic lymphoma with villous lymphocytes. Br J Haematol 1997;99:158–61.
164. Lefrere F, Hermine O, Francois S, et al. Lack of efficacy of 2-chlorodeoxyadenoside in the treatment of splenic lymphoma with villous lymphocytes. Leuk Lymphoma 2000;40:113–7.
165. Arcaini L, Orlandi E, Scotti M, et al. Combination of rituximab, cyclophosphamide, and vincristine induces complete hematologic remission of splenic marginal zone lymphoma. Clin Lymphoma 2004;4:250–2.
166. Paydas S, Yavuz S, Disel U, et al. Successful rituximab therapy for hemolytic anemia associated with relapsed splenic marginal zone lymphoma with leukemic phase. Leuk Lymphoma 2003;44:2165–6.
167. Berger F, Traverse-Glehen A, and Salles G. Nodal marginal zone B-cell lymphoma. In: Mauch PM, Armitage J, Coiffier B, et al., eds. Non-Hodgkin's Lymphomas. Philadelphia: Lippincott Williams & Wilkins, 2004:361–5.
168. Armitage JO, Cavalli F, Zucca E, and Longo DL. Nodal and splenic marginal zone B-cell lymphomas. In: Armitage JO, Cavalli F, Zucca E and Longo DL eds. Text atlas of lymphomas, Revised edition. London: Martin Dunitz; 2002:123–131.
169. Grogan TM. Does nodal marginal zone lymphoma exist? In: Mason DY and Harris NL, eds. Human Lymphoma: Clinical Implications of the REAL Classification. London: Springer-Verlag, 1999:18.11–18.15.
170. Marasca R, Vaccari P, Luppi M, et al. Immunoglobulin gene mutations and frequent use of VH1-69 and VH4-34 segments in hepatitis C virus–positive and hepatitis C virus–negative nodal marginal zone B-cell lymphoma. Am J Pathol 2001;159:253–61.
171. Conconi A, Bertoni F, Pedrinis E, et al. Nodal marginal zone B-cell lymphomas may arise from different subsets of marginal zone B lymphocytes. Blood 2001;98:781–6.
172. Camacho FI, Algara P, Mollejo M, et al. Nodal marginal zone lymphoma: a heterogeneous tumor: a comprehensive analysis of a series of 27 cases. Am J Surg Pathol 2003;27: 762–71.
173. Nathwani BN, Anderson JR, Armitage JO, et al. Marginal zone B-cell lymphoma: a clinical comparison of nodal and mucosa-associated lymphoid tissue types. Non-Hodgkin's Lymphoma Classification Project. J Clin Oncol 1999;17: 2486–92.
174. Sheibani K, Burke JS, Swartz WG, et al. Monocytoid B-cell lymphoma. Clinicopathologic study of 21 cases of a unique type of low-grade lymphoma. Cancer 1988;62:1531–8.
175. Royer B, Cazals-Hatem D, Sibilia J, et al. Lymphomas in patients with Sjogren's syndrome are marginal zone B-cell neoplasms, arise in diverse extranodal and nodal sites, and are not associated with viruses. Blood 1997;90:766–75.
176. Shin SS, Sheibani K, Fishleder A, et al. Monocytoid B-cell lymphoma in patients with Sjogren's syndrome: a clinicopathologic study of 13 patients. Hum Pathol 1991;22: 422–30.
177. Fisher RI, Dahlberg S, Nathwani BN, et al. A clinical analysis of two indolent lymphoma entities: mantle cell lymphoma and marginal zone lymphoma (including the mucosa-associated lymphoid tissue and monocytoid B-cell subcategories): a Southwest Oncology Group study. Blood 1995;85:1075–82.
178. Nathwani BN, Drachenberg MR, Hernandez AM, et al. Nodal monocytoid B-cell lymphoma (nodal marginal-zone B-cell lymphoma). Semin Haematol 1999;36:128–38.
179. Koh LP, Lim LC, and Thng CH. Retreatment with chimeric CD 20 monoclonal antibody in a patient with nodal marginal zone B-cell lymphoma. Med Oncol 2000;17:225–8.

Mantle Cell Lymphoma

Georg Lenz, M.D.
Martin Dreyling, M.D., Ph.D.
Wolfgang Hiddemann, M.D., Ph.D.

DEFINITION

Several years ago mantle cell lymphoma (MCL) was finally accepted as a distinct entity of malignant lymphoma by the World Health Organization lymphoma classification.[1] Thirty years ago it was already described as centrocytic lymphoma in the Kiel classification,[2] whereas in the International Working Formulation, MCL was grouped into different subtypes (mainly diffuse, small cleaved-cell lymphoma, small lymphocytic lymphoma, follicular small cleaved-cell lymphoma, and diffuse, mixed small- and large-cell lymphoma).[3]

EPIDEMIOLOGY AND ETIOLOGY

With a median age of 65 years at first presentation, and a male-to-female ratio of 3 to 4:1, MCL primarily represents a disorder of the elderly male. The incidence of MCL is approximately 2 to 3/100,000/year,[4,5] representing 5% to 10% of all lymphoma cases in North America and Europe.[6,7] MCL is characterized by an aggressive clinical course and poor prognosis with virtually no long-term survivors[8] (Fig. 22–1). Similar to other lymphoma subentities, etiology and epidemiologic risk factors are largely unknown.

BIOLOGY

Histology and Immunophenotype

MCL is derived from a subset of naive pre-germinal center cells, localized in primary follicles or in the mantle region of secondary follicles. Accordingly, the majority of cases display an unmutated immunoglobulin heavy chain locus. Some cases with mutated Ig locus have recently been described.[9] MCL is characterized by atypical small- to medium-sized cells. Nodular or diffuse and less frequently mantle zone growth pattern may be observed.[7,10] Cytologically, two subsets can be distinguished: classical MCL and the blastoid or pleomorphic variants (approximately 20% of cases[5]). Classical MCL is characterized by a population of atypical small lymphoid cells with irregular and indented nuclei, moderately coarse chromatin, inconspicuous nucleoli, and scant cytoplasm. In the blastoid variant, the neoplastic cells are larger and have a more finely dispersed nuclear chromatin and small nucleoli.[11–13]

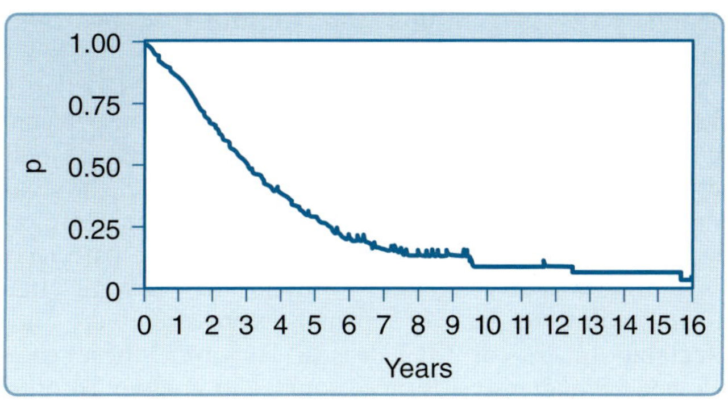

Figure 22–1. Overall survival of patients with mantle cell lymphoma.

The characteristic immunophenotype of mantle cells includes the co-expression of a variety of pan–B-cell antigens (CD19, CD20, CD22, and CD79a) and the pan–T-cell antigen CD5. The neoplastic cells may also bear the T-cell–associated antigens CD43 and Leu8, but fail to stain for other pan–T-cell antigens. In contrast to chronic lymphocytic leukemia (CLL), the cells are usually negative for CD23, although a weak expression may be detected in some cases. They almost always bear surface IgM and often IgD, whereas surface IgG is expressed in only about 20% of cases.[5]

Cytogenetics

Genetically, MCL is characterized by the chromosomal translocation t(11; 14) (q13; q32), which is detectable in 60% to 70% of cases.[14] This genomic rearrangement results in a juxtaposition of the *bcl-1* gene locus to the Ig heavy-chain promoter, and subsequently to constitutive overexpression of the cell cycle regulator protein cyclin D1. Cyclin D1 plays an important role in the cell cycle regulation by propelling cells from the G1 into the S phase as the complex of cyclin D1/cyclin-dependent kinase (CDK) inactivates the tumor suppressor retinoblastoma protein (pRb).[5] However, cyclin D1 overexpression alone is not sufficient for lymphoma development.[15,16] Accordingly, in more than 80% of MCL cases, secondary alterations are detectable.[17–19] These alterations include the loss of chromosomes 13 and Y, deletions of chromosomes 1p, 6q, 11q22–23, 13q14, and 17p, and gains at chromosome 3q26–29, as well as trisomy 12.[20,21]

CLINICAL FEATURES OF PRESENTATION

With a median age of 65 years at diagnosis and a male-to-female ratio of 3 to 4:1, MCL primarily represents a disorder of the male elderly. The majority of cases is diagnosed at

Table 22–1. Clinical Characteristics of Mantle Cell Lymphoma

Author	n	Median Age (years)	Stage IV	Sex (m/f)	Bone Marrow	Leukemic Expression	GI Tract
Zucca et al. (1995)[8]	65	64	72%	2/1	58%	20%	15%
Norton et al. (1995)[38]	66	62	82%	3.7/1	80%	N.A.	12%
Fisher et al. (1995)[95]	36	55	N.A.	4/1	53%	N.A.	19%
Hiddemann et al. (1996)[22]	573	63	75%	2.5/1	69%	N.A.	N.A.
Majlis et al. (1997)[37]	46	54	82% (III + IV)	1.7/1	69%	N.A.	24%
Bosch et al. (1998)[24]	59	63	95% (III + IV)	3/1	81%	58%	17%
Andersen et al. (2002)[30]	105	66	80%	3/1	72%	N.A.	12%

n, number of patients; m, male; f, female; N.A., not available.

advanced Ann Arbor Stages III or IV. Extranodal involvement is found in approximately 90% of cases, including bone marrow, liver, and gastrointestinal tract[22–26] (Table 22–1). A characteristic extranodal presentation of MCL is multiple lymphomatous polyposis of the intestine. However, this feature is frequently not diagnosed due to incomplete staging procedures.[27] Less common extranodal sites are skin, lung, breast, or soft tissues. Central nervous system involvement is found in up to 20% of relapsed MCL cases.[28] B symptoms are described in less than 50% of cases (Table 22–1).

PROGNOSTIC FACTORS

Clinical Prognostic Factors

Important clinical prognostic factors that are correlated with an adverse outcome include poor performance status, splenomegaly, anemia, and age.[24,29,30] Contradictory reports on the value of the International Prognostic Index (IPI),[31] which considers age (≤60 years vs. >60 years), performance status (ECOG 0–1 vs. 2–4), Ann Arbor stage (I–II vs. III–IV), extranodal involvement (less than two vs. two or more involved sites), and serum LDH level (normal vs. elevated), have been published. Weissenburger et al.[32] reported a high prognostic value of high risk IPI, predictive for short survival. Similarly, Bosch et al.[24] claimed that patients with high-risk IPI had lower response rates to chemotherapy. This observation was supported by a retrospective study of Zucca et al.,[8] which demonstrated a benefit of anthracycline-containing chemotherapeutic regimens in patients with a favorable IPI. In contrast, the studies of Andersen et al.[30] and Samaha et al.[23] suggested that the IPI has no impact on the patients' survival. In the largest retrospective series published, the IPI identified different risk groups of patients, but a significant overlap of the survival curves was observed.[22] Thus, the IPI is of limited impact in predicting clinical outcome of MCL patients.

A recent study by Pott et al. investigated the value of molecular remission as a prognostic factor in MCL patients following high-dose radiochemotherapy and autologous stem cell transplantation.[33] Similar to follicular lymphoma, molecular remission was a strong prognostic factor predicting progression-free survival (PFS). In contrast, in the study by Howard et al., patients who achieved a molecular remission after a combined immuno-chemotherapy had a similar PFS as patients without molecular remission.[34] Thus, future studies have to further evaluate the prognostic value of the molecular remission status.

Biological Prognostic Factors

Various studies investigated the value of biological parameters to predict outcome in MCL. The correlation between cytologic forms of MCL and prognosis has intensively been studied. In the study of Bernard et al.,[35] median overall survival (OS) for the blastoid variant was only 14.5 months as compared to 53 months for patients with the common form of MCL. These data were confirmed by Bosch et al.[24] However, in the largest series published so far, cytology showed only a borderline significance.[36]

Similarly, the published data on the prognostic value of the growth pattern are contradictory. Weisenburger et al. reported a poor prognosis of patients showing the diffuse growth pattern compared to those with nodular tumor architecture[32] (16 months median survival vs. 50 months). This finding was confirmed by the study of Majlis et al., which demonstrated poor treatment response and short OS in patients with diffuse or nodular growth pattern.[37] In contrast, Norton et al. showed that growth pattern had no impact on the prognosis.[38]

Various studies confirmed the poor outcome of patients with *p53* gene mutations. *p53* aberrations have been detected especially in high-grade lymphomas and secondary transformed follicular lymphoma. The study of Greiner et al. detected *p53* gene mutations in 15% (8 out of 53) of investigated MCL cases.[39] These cases were characterized by a short median survival of only 1.3 years, as compared to a median survival of 5.1 years in cases with germline *p53*. These results were confirmed by two other studies.[40,41]

p16 is a cyclin-dependent kinase inhibitor (CKI) that is involved in the cell cycle control. Alterations of the *p16* gene are detectable in various B-cell malignancies.[42] These neoplasias, irrespective of their histologic grade, show an increased clinical aggressivity and more frequent treatment resistance. The influence of the *p16* gene on the pathogenesis of MCL was investigated by Pinyol et al.[43] Genetic alterations leading to loss of normal expression were only detectable in 5% of MCL cases. However, these cases followed an aggressive clinical course. In analogy to other lymphoid malignancies, Pinyol et al. concluded that *p16*

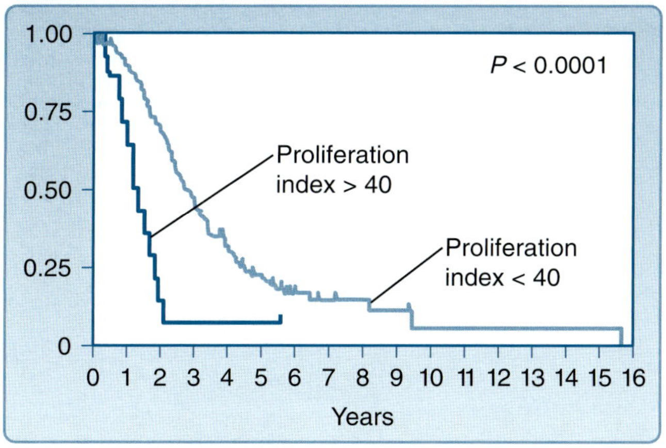

Figure 22–2. Patients with low proliferation rate experience significantly longer overall survival in comparison to patients with high proliferation.

genetic alterations are relatively infrequent in MCL but are associated with a poor clinical outcome. In contrast, in another study, genomic alterations of the *p16* region were more frequently detected and closely related to cell proliferation.[44]

The most important biological prognostic factor in multiple series was the proliferation rate determined by the number of mitoses or the Ki-67 staining index. In a study by Bosch et al. patients with more than 2.5 mitoses/high power field (HPF) had a median survival of only 24 months, whereas those with ≤2.5 mitoses/HPF had a survival of 50 months.[24] Similarly, in a large retrospective study of 350 patients with a confirmed diagnosis of MCL, various proliferation indices represented the most powerful prognostic marker clearly superior to cytomorphology and clinical parameters[29] (Fig. 22–2). These results have just recently been confirmed by a microarray study of Rosenwald et al.[45]

THERAPY

Radiation in Early Stages

The small number of patients with limited Ann Arbor Stage I–II may potentially be cured by modified extended or involved field radiation. In addition, a recent study suggested an advantage of sequential radiochemotherapy.[46] In contrast, in advanced-stage III–IV, the benefit of radiation therapy in addition to chemotherapy is not proven, and is not recommended outside of controlled clinical trials.

Conventional Chemotherapy

MCL has the poorest long-term survival of all lymphoma subtypes. Consequently, a wait-and-watch strategy is not justified, although in advanced stages conventional chemotherapy is a noncurative approach. Various chemotherapeutic regimens achieve overall response rates of approximately 70% with complete remissions in up to 20% to 30% of cases.[8,47]

The use of anthracycline-containing regimens was evaluated in various studies. In the only randomized trial, no advantage of the CHOP regimen (cyclophosphamide, doxorubicin, vincristine and prednisone) in comparison to a nonanthracycline combination (COP: cyclophosphamide, vincristine, and prednisone) was detectable.[48] The overall response rate was 84% after COP, as compared to 89% after CHOP, with a median OS of 32 months and 37 months, respectively (Table 22–2). In contrast, in a retrospective study, Zucca and colleagues claimed a superiority of anthracycline-containing regimens in the low and low-intermediate risk group of MCL patients[8] (Table 22–2). Thus, although clinical trials did not clearly prove a superiority of anthracycline-containing combinations, CHOP-like regimens may represent the most established chemotherapeutic approach.

Table 22–2. Anthracyclines in the Therapy of Mantle Cell Lymphoma

Author	n	Regimen	CR/OR
Meusers et al. (1989)[48]	37	COP: Cyclophosphamide 400 mg/m²/d × 5 Vincristine 1.4 mg/m²/d × 1 Prednisone 100 mg/m²/d × 5	41%/84%
	26	CHOP: Cyclophosphamide 750 mg/m²/d × 1 Doxorubicin 50 mg/m²/d × 1 Vincristine 1.4 mg/m² × 1 (maximum 2 mg) Prednisone 100 mg/m²/d × 5	58%/89%
Hiddemann et al. (1996)[96]	20	COP: Cyclophosphamide 400 mg/m²/d × 5 Vincristine 1.4 mg/m²/d × 1 Prednisone 100 mg/m²/d × 5	5%/80%
	19	PmM: Prednimustine 100 mg/m²/d × 5 Mitoxantrone 8 mg/m²/d × 2	27%/80%
Zinzani et al. (2000)[97]	18	Fludarabine 25 mg/m²/d × 3 Idarubicin 12 mg/m²/d × 1	33%/61%
	11	Fludarabine 25 mg/m²/d × 5	27%/73%

n, number of patients; OR, overall response, CR, complete remission.

Table 22–3. Efficacy of Fludarabine in Mantle Cell Lymphoma Therapy

Author	n	Regimen	Disease Status	CR/OR
Decaudin et al. (1998)[50]	15	Fludarabine 25 mg/m^2/d × 5	Untreated and relapsed	0%/33%
Foran et al. (1999)[49]	17	Fludarabine 25 mg/m^2/d × 5	Untreated	29%/41%
Flinn et al. (2000)[51]	10	Fludarabine 20 mg/m^2/d × 5 Cyclophosphamide 600 mg/m^2/d × 1	Untreated	40%/80%
Cohen et al. (2001)[52]	30	Fludarabine 20–25 mg/m^2/d × 3 Cyclophosphamide 600 mg/m^2/d × 1	Untreated and relapsed	30%/63%
Seymour et al. (2002)[98]	8	Fludarabine 30 mg/m^2/d × 2 Cisplatin 25 mg/m^2/d × 4 Cytarabine 500 mg/m^2/d × 2	Relapsed	N.A./88%
Hiddemann et al. (2003)[64]	24	Fludarabine 25 mg/m^2/d × 3 Cyclophosphamide 200 mg/m^2/d × 3 Mitoxantrone 8 mg/m^2/d × 1	Relapsed	0%/46%

n, number of patients; CR, complete remission; OR, overall response; N.A., not available.

The efficacy of purine analogs (fludarabine or cladribine) has been investigated.[23,49,50] Single-agent fludarabine, which has significant activity in follicular lymphoma, showed only moderate activity with response rates of 30% to 40% (Table 22–3). In contrast, combinations with either alkylating agents (e.g., cyclophosphamide) or anthracyclines (e.g., mitoxantrone, idarubicin) were able to achieve significantly higher remission rates (Table 22–3). In a study by Flinn et al., the combination of fludarabine and cyclophosphamide achieved an overall response rate of 80%.[51] Similarly, in the study of Cohen and colleagues, fludarabine and cyclophosphamide was highly effective in newly diagnosed and relapsed or refractory disease.[52] Previously untreated patients had a remarkable overall response rate of 100% (70% complete and 30% partial remissions) with a PFS of 28.1 months (Table 22–3).

Encouraging results were also achieved in various Phase II studies implementing high-dose cytarabine (Ara-C). Lefrere et al. showed that after a sequential CHOP-DHAP regimen (dexamethasone, high-dose cytarabine, and cisplatin), over 80% of the treated patients obtained a complete remission.[53] Similarly, high response rates of more than 90% could be demonstrated by a dose-intensified approach of the M.D. Anderson Cancer Center, applying an alternating regimen of Hyper-CVAD (fractionated cyclophosphamide, vincristine, doxorubicin, and dexamethasone) with high-dose cytarabine and methotrexate in elderly patients not suitable for stem cell transplantation.[54] Because these data suggest a high efficacy of high-dose cytarabine in MCL, this concept is currently being tested in various Phase III trials.

Interferon-α

Two Phase III studies investigated the efficacy of interferon-α maintenance (IFNα) following induction therapy.[55,56] Both trials showed a tendency towards a prolonged PFS with IFNα. However, the number of investigated patients was too small to definitely answer the question as to what extent IFNα may be of benefit.

Monoclonal Antibodies

Another encouraging approach is the application of the anti-CD20 antibody rituximab. Rituximab is a chimeric murine/human monoclonal antibody that binds the B-cell specific antigen CD20. In vitro studies demonstrated that rituximab lyses CD20+ cells by complement activation or antibody-dependent, cell-mediated cytotoxicity.[57,58] In the past few years, various studies investigated the efficacy of rituximab in MCL. Rituximab as a single agent showed only a moderate activity with partial response rates of approximately 20% to 40%[59–62] (Table 22–4). In contrast, based on a proposed in vitro synergism, a combined immunochemotherapy of rituximab and CHOP (R-CHOP) achieved remarkably high overall and complete remission rates in a recent Phase II study[34] (Table 22–5). Nevertheless, the higher response rates did not translate into a prolonged PFS. These results were confirmed by a recent randomized trial of the German Low Grade Lymphoma Study Group that evaluated the efficacy of R-CHOP in comparison to CHOP alone in previously untreated patients with MCL.[63] In patients receiving CHOP alone, an overall response rate of 75% with only 7% complete remissions was detectable. In contrast, in the R-CHOP study arm, 94% of patients achieved a complete or partial remission (34% complete response, 60% partial response; $p = 0.00024$). Although the time to treatment failure was significantly prolonged in the immunochemotherapy arm, no

Table 22–4. Rituximab as Single Agent in Mantle Cell Lymphoma Therapy

Author	n	Disease Status	OR
Coiffier et al. (1998)[99]	12	Resistant/ relapsed	4 (33%)
Nguyen et al. (1999)[100]	10	Resistant/ relapsed	2 (20%)
Foran et al. (2000)[60]	34 40	Untreated Relapsed	13 (38%) 15 (37%)
Ghielmini et al. (2000)[61]	39	Relapsed	9 (23%)
Tobinai et al. (2002)[62]	13	Relapsed	6 (46%)

n, number of patients; OR, overall response.

Table 22–5. Combined Immunochemotherapy in Mantle Cell Lymphoma

Author	n	Regimen	CR/OR
Howard et al. (2002)[34]	40	R-CHOP	48%/96%
Hiddemann et al. (2003)[64]	24	R-FCM	33%/62%[a]
Lenz et al. (2003)[63]	62	R-CHOP	34%/94%[a]

[a] Significant improvement in comparison to chemotherapy alone.
n, number of patients; CR, complete remission, OR, overall response.

plateau in the OS was observed indicating the absence of durable remissions (Table 22–5). Thus, R-CHOP may become the standard therapeutic approach in the first-line therapy of MCL but multimodal consolidation concepts are warranted to translate this high response rate into long-term remissions.

More encouraging results were recently published by Hiddemann et al.[64] In a randomized trial, the combination of FCM chemotherapy (fludarabine, cyclophosphamide, and mitoxantrone) and rituximab was compared to chemotherapy alone in refractory and relapsed MCL. The addition of rituximab resulted in significantly improved complete remission rates (33% vs. 0%; $p = 0.003$), clearly indicating the superiority of a combined immunochemotherapy in MCL (Table 22–5). However, more importantly after a median follow-up of 19 months, a significantly improved OS was detectable in the R-FCM study arm ($p = 0.004$) (Fig. 22–3). Future study concepts will focus on the role of rituximab maintenance and in vivo purging prior to autologous stem cell transplantation.

Another innovative approach is the application of radio (^{131}iodine or ^{90}yttrium) labeled anti-CD20 antibodies in a conventional or myeloablative dosage. Some studies have achieved remarkably high and long-lasting remissions in relapsed or refractory MCL patients.[65,66] Gopal and colleagues investigated the efficacy of the ^{131}iodine labeled anti-CD20 antibody tositumomab in 16 heavily pretreated patients with MCL in combination with high-dose chemotherapy followed by autologous stem cell transplantation.[65] High overall response rates of 100% with 91% complete remissions were reported, and the estimated 3-year OS of 93% was remarkable. Thus, the concept of a radioimmunotherapy in combination with various effective chemotherapy regimens is currently being investigated in Phase II studies.

Autologous Stem Cell Transplantation

Recently the potentially curative concept of high-dose therapy followed by autologous stem cell transplantation was introduced to eliminate residual lymphoma cells after conventional induction chemotherapy. In several Phase II studies, promising results were achieved.[67–75] In order to assess the role of myeloablative radiochemotherapy followed by ASCT as consolidation in first remission, the European MCL Network embarked on a randomized comparison of this approach versus IFNα maintenance in patients up to 65 years of age after a CHOP-like induction.[76]

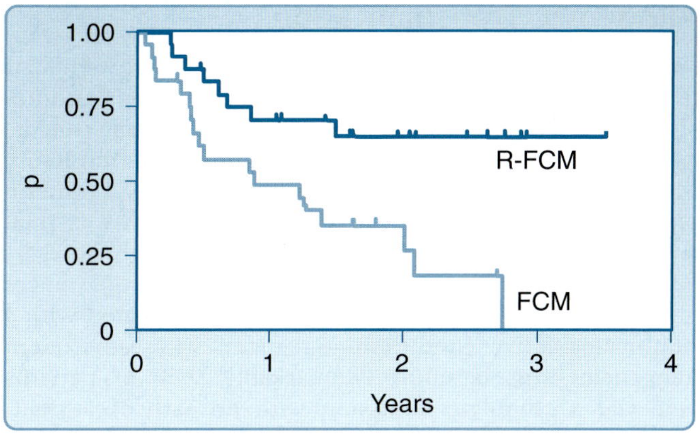

Figure 22–3. Randomized comparison of overall survival following R-FCM and FCM, respectively. Patients assigned to R-FCM experience significantly longer overall survival.

Patients receiving high-dose therapy achieved a significantly longer PFS (Fig. 22–4). Thus, high-dose consolidation in first remission represents a promising therapeutic approach in MCL patients up to 65 years of age. However, the concept of autologous stem cell transplantation is potentially hampered by the risk of secondary myelodysplastic syndromes (MDS) and acute leukemias as various studies claimed an increased risk of secondary hematological neoplasias.[77–79]

However, even after a dose-intensified approach the majority of patients will finally relapse, in part possibly due to a contamination of the harvested stem cells with lymphoma cells. Different approaches are currently being applied to eliminate these contaminations. They comprise either conventional purging procedures[80] or "in vivo" purging with monoclonal anti-CD20 antibodies as rituximab.[81–84] In particular, antibody-based purging seems to be very efficient in killing residual lymphoma cells, as encouraging data on the OS have been reported in various Phase II studies.

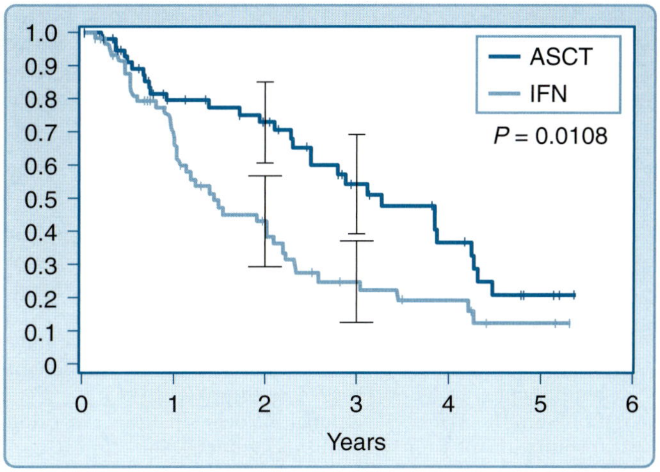

Figure 22–4. Progression-free survival after high-dose radiochemotherapy followed by autologous stem cell transplantation and interferon-α maintenance in mantle cell lymphoma. Patients assigned to stem cell transplantation experience significantly longer progression-free survival.

Allogeneic Transplantation

In advanced-stage MCL, the only curative therapy thus far is allogeneic stem cell transplantation. Various studies showed that long-lasting complete remissions can be achieved even in patients with relapsed or refractory MCL.[85–89] However, infectious complications are common and transplantation-related toxicity, and mortality is relatively high. Promising results were recently published by Khouri et al.[88] In a study by the M.D Anderson Cancer Center, 18 patients with relapsed MCL were treated with a nonmyeloablative conditioning regimen with subsequent allogeneic transplantation. Remarkably, 94% of patients achieved a complete remission with no early treatment-related (day 100) mortality. The estimated event-free survival was 82% at 3 years. Thus, the application of nonmyeloablative conditioning regimens in MCL is currently being investigated in multicenter trials.

New Therapeutic Strategies

A new molecular targeting agent in the treatment of MCL is the cyclin-dependent kinase inhibitor flavopiridol. Kouroukis et al.[90] investigated the efficacy of flavopiridol given three times per week, every 3 weeks, in a recent Phase II study. However, neither this regimen (no complete remissions and only 11% partial responses) nor a 72-hour continuous infusion showed significant efficacy in relapsed or refractory MCL.[91] However, as cell culture experiments suggest a chemosensitizing effect, flavopiridol might be more effective in combination with chemotherapy.

Encouraging results were obtained in a small Phase II study applying the combination of rituximab and thalidomide.[92] In patients with relapsed or refractory MCL, an overall response in over 90% of cases was observed indicating the antilymphoma activity of this regimen. Thus, this concept should be further investigated in additional trials.

The proteasome inhibitor bortezomib (Velcade, formerly PS-341) represents another molecular-targeted approach in the treatment of MCL. Bortezomib is highly effective in MCL-derived cell lines and SCID mouse models by sensitizing lymphoma cells to apoptosis.[93] In addition, bortezomib showed its efficacy in a recent Phase II study of the M.D. Anderson Cancer Center[94]; 53% previously heavily pretreated MCL patients responded to a bortezomib therapy at a dose of 1.5 mg/m^2.

References

1. Jaffe ES, Harris NL, Stein H, et al. World Health Organization Classification of Tumours. Pathology and Genetics of Tumours of Haematopoietic and Lymphoid Tissues. Lyon: IARC Press, 2001.
2. Lennert K, Stein H, and Kaiserling E. Cytological and functional criteria for the classification of malignant lymphomata. Br J Cancer 1975;31(suppl 2):29–43.
3. Robb-Smith AH. US National Cancer Institute working formulation of non-Hodgkin's lymphomas for clinical use. Lancet 1982;2:432–4.
4. Hiddemann W, Dreyling MH, Tiemann M, et al. Mantle cell lymphomas. Haematologica 1999;84:93–5.
5. Campo E, Raffeld M, and Jaffe ES. Mantle-cell lymphoma. Semin Hematol 1999;36:115–27.
6. Meusers P, Hense J, and Brittinger G. Mantle cell lymphoma: diagnostic criteria, clinical aspects and therapeutic problems. Leukemia 1997;11(Suppl 2):S60–4.
7. Weisenburger DD and Armitage JO. Mantle cell lymphoma—an entity comes of age. Blood 1996;87:4483–94.
8. Zucca E, Roggero E, Pinotti G, et al. Patterns of survival in mantle cell lymphoma. Ann Oncol 1995;6:257–62.
9. Walsh SH, Thorselius M, Johnson A, et al. Mutated VH genes and preferential VH3–21 use define new subsets of mantle cell lymphoma. Blood 2003;101:4047–54.
10. Banks PM, Chan J, Cleary ML, et al. Mantle cell lymphoma. A proposal for unification of morphologic, immunologic, and molecular data. Am J Surg Pathol 1992;16:637–40.
11. Swerdlow SH, Zukerberg LR, Yang WI, et al. The morphologic spectrum of non-Hodgkin's lymphomas with BCL1/cyclin D1 gene rearrangements. Am J Surg Pathol 1996;20:627–40.
12. Ott G, Kalla J, Hanke A, et al. The cytomorphological spectrum of mantle cell lymphoma is reflected by distinct biological features. Leuk Lymphoma 1998;32:55–63.
13. Lai R and Medeiros LJ. Pathologic diagnosis of mantle cell lymphoma. Clin Lymphoma 2000;1:197–206; discussion 207–8.
14. Swerdlow SH and Williams ME. From centrocytic to mantle cell lymphoma: a clinicopathologic and molecular review of 3 decades. Hum Pathol 2002;33:7–20.
15. Bodrug SE, Warner BJ, Bath ML, et al. Cyclin D1 transgene impedes lymphocyte maturation and collaborates in lymphomagenesis with the myc gene. EMBO J 1994;13:2124–30.
16. Lovec H, Grzeschiczek A, Kowalski MB, et al. Cyclin D1/bcl-1 cooperates with myc genes in the generation of B-cell lymphoma in transgenic mice. EMBO J 1994;13:3487–95.
17. Cuneo A, Bigoni R, Rigolin GM, et al. Cytogenetic profile of lymphoma of follicle mantle lineage: correlation with clinicobiologic features. Blood 1999;93:1372–80.
18. Scheubner M, Huebler K, Ott G, et al. Genotyping of mantle cell lymphoma identifies a new tumor suppressor gene on 17p13.3. Ann Oncol 2002;13:8[abstract].
19. Wlodarska I, Pittaluga S, Hagemeijer A, et al. Secondary chromosome changes in mantle cell lymphoma. Haematologica 1999;84:594–9.
20. Cuneo A, Bigoni R, Rigolin GM, et al. 13q14 deletion in non-Hodgkin's lymphoma: correlation with clinicopathologic features. Haematologica 1999;84:589–93.
21. Bentz M, Plesch A, Bullinger L, et al. t(11;14)-positive mantle cell lymphomas exhibit complex karyotypes and share similarities with B-cell chronic lymphocytic leukemia. Genes Chromosomes Cancer 2000;27:285–94.
22. Hiddemann W, Brittinger G, Tiemann M, et al. Presentation features and clinical course of Mantle Cell Lymphomas—Results a European survey. Ann Oncol 1996;7:22[abstract].
23. Samaha H, Dumontet C, Ketterer N, et al. Mantle cell lymphoma: a retrospective study of 121 cases. Leukemia 1998;12:1281–7.
24. Bosch F, Lopez-Guillermo A, Campo E, et al. Mantle cell lymphoma: presenting features, response to therapy, and prognostic factors. Cancer 1998;82:567–75.
25. Pittaluga S, Wlodarska I, Stul MS, et al. Mantle cell lymphoma: a clinicopathological study of 55 cases. Histopathology 1995;26:17–24.
26. Velders GA, Kluin-Nelemans JC, De Boer CJ, et al. Mantle-cell lymphoma: a population-based clinical study. J Clin Oncol 1996;14:1269–74.
27. Kadayifci A, Benekli M, Savas MC, et al. Multiple lymphomatous polyposis. J Surg Oncol 1997;64:336–40.
28. Oinonen R, Franssila K, and Elonen E. Central nervous system involvement in patients with mantle cell lymphoma. Ann Hematol 1999;78:145–9.

29. Dreyling M. The increasing role of prognostic factotors in the choice of treatment—Mantle Cell Lymphoma Ann Oncol 2002;13[abstract].
30. Andersen NS, Jensen MK, de Nully Brown P, et al. A Danish population-based analysis of 105 mantle cell lymphoma patients. incidences, clinical features, response, survival and prognostic factors. Eur J Cancer 2002;38:401–8.
31. The International Non-Hodgkin's Lymphoma Prognostic Factors Project. A predictive model for aggressive non-Hodgkin's lymphoma. N Engl J Med 1993;329:987–94.
32. Weisenburger DD, Vose JM, Greiner TC, et al. Mantle cell lymphoma. A clinicopathologic study of 68 cases from the Nebraska Lymphoma Study Group. Am J Hematol 2000;64:190–6.
33. Pott C, Schrader C, Dermer N, et al. Molecular remission predicts progression-free survival in mantle cell lymphoma after peripheral blood stem cell transplantation. Ann Oncol 2002;69[abstract].
34. Howard OM, Gribben JG, Neuberg DS, et al. Rituximab and CHOP induction therapy for newly diagnosed mantle-cell lymphoma: molecular complete responses are not predictive of progression-free survival. J Clin Oncol 2002;20:1288–94.
35. Bernard M, Gressin R, Lefrere F, et al. Blastic variant of mantle cell lymphoma: a rare but highly aggressive subtype. Leukemia 2001;15:1785–91.
36. Tiemann M and Dreyling MH. Pathology, proliferation indices and survival in 304 patients. Ann Oncol 1999;10[abstract].
37. Majlis A, Pugh WC, Rodriguez MA, et al. Mantle cell lymphoma: correlation of clinical outcome and biologic features with three histologic variants. J Clin Oncol 1997;15: 1664–71.
38. Norton AJ, Matthews J, Pappa V, et al. Mantle cell lymphoma: natural history defined in a serially biopsied population over a 20-year period. Ann Oncol 1995;6:249–56.
39. Greiner TC, Moynihan MJ, Chan WC, et al. p53 mutations in mantle cell lymphoma are associated with variant cytology and predict a poor prognosis. Blood 1996;87: 4302–10.
40. Hernandez L, Fest T, Cazorla M, et al. p53 gene mutations and protein overexpression are associated with aggressive variants of mantle cell lymphomas. Blood 1996;87:3351–9.
41. Zoldan MC, Inghirami G, Masuda Y, et al. Large-cell variants of mantle cell lymphoma: cytologic characteristics and p53 anomalies may predict poor outcome. Br J Haematol 1996;93:475–86.
42. Sanchez-Beato M, Sanchez-Aguilera A, et al. Cell cycle deregulation in B-cell lymphomas. Blood 2003;101:1220–35.
43. Pinyol M, Cobo F, Bea S, et al. p16(INK4a) gene inactivation by deletions, mutations, and hypermethylation is associated with transformed and aggressive variants of non-Hodgkin's lymphomas. Blood 1998;91:2977–84.
44. Dreyling MH, Bullinger L, Ott G, et al. Alterations of the cyclin D1/p16-pRB pathway in mantle cell lymphoma. Cancer Res 1997;57:4608–14.
45. Rosenwald A, Wright G, Wiestner A, et al. The proliferation gene expression signature is a quantitative integrator of oncogenic events that predicts survival in mantle cell lymphoma. Cancer Cell 2003;3:185–97.
46. Leitch HA, Gascoyne RD, Chhanabhai M, et al. Limited-stage mantle-cell lymphoma. Ann Oncol 2003;14:1555–61.
47. Vandenberghe E, De Wolf-Peeters C, Vaughan Hudson G, et al. The clinical outcome of 65 cases of mantle cell lymphoma initially treated with non-intensive therapy by the British National Lymphoma Investigation Group. Br J Haematol 1997;99:842–7.
48. Meusers P, Engelhard M, Bartels H, et al. Multicentre randomized therapeutic trial for advanced centrocytic lymphoma: anthracycline does not improve the prognosis. Hematol Oncol 1989;7:365–80.
49. Foran JM, Rohatiner AZ, Coiffier B, et al. Multicenter Phase II study of fludarabine phosphate for patients with newly diagnosed lymphoplasmacytoid lymphoma, Waldenstrom's macroglobulinemia, and mantle-cell lymphoma. J Clin Oncol 1999;17:546–53.
50. Decaudin D, Bosq J, Tertian G, et al. Phase II trial of fludarabine monophosphate in patients with mantle-cell lymphomas. J Clin Oncol 1998;16:579–83.
51. Flinn IW, Byrd JC, Morrison C, et al. Fludarabine and cyclophosphamide with filgrastim support in patients with previously untreated indolent lymphoid malignancies. Blood 2000;96:71–5.
52. Cohen BJ, Moskowitz C, Straus D, et al. Cyclophosphamide/fludarabine (CF) is active in the treatment of mantle cell lymphoma. Leuk Lymphoma 2001;42:1015–22.
53. Lefrere F, Delmer A, Suzan F, et al. Sequential chemotherapy by CHOP and DHAP regimens followed by high-dose therapy with stem cell transplantation induces a high rate of complete response and improves event-free survival in mantle cell lymphoma: a prospective study. Leukemia 2002;16:587–93.
54. Romaguera JE, Khouri IF, Kantarjian HM, et al. Untreated aggressive mantle cell lymphoma: results with intensive chemotherapy without stem cell transplant in elderly patients. Leuk Lymphoma 2000;39:77–85.
55. Hiddemann W, Unterhalt M, Herrmann R, et al. Mantle-cell lymphomas have more widespread disease and a slower response to chemotherapy compared with follicle-center lymphomas: results of a prospective comparative analysis of the German Low-Grade Lymphoma Study Group. J Clin Oncol 1998;16:1922–30.
56. Teodorovic I, Pittaluga S, Kluin-Nelemans JC, et al. Efficacy of four different regimens in 64 mantle-cell lymphoma cases: clinicopathologic comparison with 498 other non-Hodgkin's lymphoma subtypes. European Organization for the Research and Treatment of Cancer Lymphoma Cooperative Group. J Clin Oncol 1995;13:2819–26.
57. Manches O, Lui G, Chaperot L, et al. In vitro mechanisms of action of rituximab on primary non-Hodgkin lymphomas. Blood 2003;101:949–54.
58. Smith MR. Rituximab (monoclonal anti-CD20 antibody): mechanisms of action and resistance. Oncogene 2003;22: 7359–68.
59. Foran JM, Rohatiner AZ, Cunningham D, et al. European Phase II study of rituximab (chimeric anti-CD20 monoclonal antibody) for patients with newly diagnosed mantle-cell lymphoma and previously treated mantle-cell lymphoma, immunocytoma, and small B-cell lymphocytic lymphoma. J Clin Oncol 2000;18:317–24.
60. Foran JM, Cunningham D, Coiffier B, et al. Treatment of mantle-cell lymphoma with Rituximab (chimeric monoclonal anti-CD20 antibody): analysis of factors associated with response. Ann Oncol 2000;11:117–21.
61. Ghielmini M, Schmitz SF, Burki K, et al. The effect of rituximab on patients with follicular and mantle-cell lymphoma. Swiss Group for Clinical Cancer Research (SAKK). Ann Oncol 2000;11:123–6.
62. Tobinai K. Monoclonal antibody therapy for B-cell lymphoma: clinical trials of an anti-CD20 monoclonal antibody for B-cell lymphoma in Japan. Int J Hematol 2002;76:411–9.
63. Hiddemann W, Dreyling MH, Forstpointner R, et al. Combined immuno-chemotherapy (R-CHOP) significantly improves time to treatment failure in first-line therapy of follicular lymphoma—results of a prospective randomized trial of the German Low-Grade lymphoma Study Group (GLSG). Blood 2003;102:352[abstract].

64. Dreyling MH, Forstpointner R, Repp R, et al. Combined immuno-chemotherapy (R-FCM) results in superior remission and survival rates in recurrent follicular and mantle cell lymphoma—final results of a prospective randomized trial of the GLSG. Hematol J 2003;4:484[abstract].
65. Gopal AK, Rajendran JG, Petersdorf SH, et al. High-dose chemo-radioimmunotherapy with autologous stem cell support for relapsed mantle cell lymphoma. Blood 99:3158–62, 2002.
66. Younes A, Pro B, Delpassand E, et al. A Phase II study of 90yttrium-ibritumomab (Zevalin) for the treatment of patients with relapsed and refractory mantle cell lymphoma (MCL). Blood 2003;102:1476[abstract].
67. Stewart DA, Vose JM, Weisenburger DD, et al. The role of high-dose therapy and autologous hematopoietic stem cell transplantation for mantle cell lymphoma. Ann Oncol 1995;6:263–6.
68. Haas R, Brittinger G, Meusers P, et al. W Myeloablative therapy with blood stem cell transplantation is effective in mantle cell lymphoma. Leukemia 1996;10:1975–9.
69. Ketterer N, Salles G, Espinouse D, et al. Intensive therapy with peripheral stem cell transplantation in 16 patients with mantle cell lymphoma. Ann Oncol 1997;8:701–4.
70. Freedman AS, Neuberg D, Gribben JG, et al. High-dose chemoradiotherapy and anti-B-cell monoclonal antibody-purged autologous bone marrow transplantation in mantle-cell lymphoma: no evidence for long-term remission. J Clin Oncol 1998;16:13–8.
71. Decaudin D, Brousse N, Brice P, et al. Efficacy of autologous stem cell transplantation in mantle cell lymphoma: a 3-year follow-up study. Bone Marrow Transplant 2000;25:251–6.
72. Vose JM, Bierman PJ, Weisenburger DD, et al. Autologous hematopoietic stem cell transplantation for mantle cell lymphoma. Biol Blood Marrow Transplant 2000;6:640–5.
73. Vandenberghe E, Ruiz de Elvira C, Loberiza FR, et al. Outcome of autologous transplantation for mantle cell lymphoma: a study by the European Blood and Bone Marrow Transplant and Autologous Blood and Marrow Transplant Registries. Br J Haematol 2003;120:793–800.
74. Andersen NS, Pedersen L, Elonen E, et al. Primary treatment with autologous stem cell transplantation in mantle cell lymphoma: outcome related to remission pretransplant. Eur J Haematol 2003;71:73–80.
75. Dreger P, Martin S, Kuse R, et al. The impact of autologous stem cell transplantation on the prognosis of mantle cell lymphoma: a joint analysis of two prospective studies with 46 patients. Hematol J 2000;1:87–94.
76. Hiddemann W, Dreyling MH, Pfreundschuh M, et al. Myeloablative Radiochemotherapy followed by autologous Blood stem cell transplantation leads to a significant prolongation of the event-free survival in patients with mantle cell lymphoma (MCL)—results of a prospective randomized European Intergroup study. Blood 2001;98:861 [abstract].
77. Lenz G, Unterhalt M, Haferlach T, et al. Significant increase of secondary myelodysplasia and acute myeloid leukemia after myeloablative radiochemotherapy followed by autologous stem cell transplantation in indolent lymphoma patients—results of a prospective randomized study for the GLSG. Blood 2003;102:986[abstract].
78. Micallef IN, Lillington DM, Apostolidis J, et al. Therapy-related myelodysplasia and secondary acute myelogenous leukemia after high-dose therapy with autologous hematopoietic progenitor-cell support for lymphoid malignancies. J Clin Oncol 2000;18:947–55.
79. Howe R, Micallef IN, Inwards DJ, et al. Secondary myelodysplastic syndrome and acute myelogenous leukemia are significant complications following autologous stem cell transplantation for lymphoma. Bone Marrow Transplant. 2003;32:317–24.
80. Van Besien K, Loberiza FR, Bajorunaite R, et al. Comparison of autologous and allogeneic hematopoietic stem cell transplantation for follicular lymphoma. Blood 2003;102: 3521–9.
81. Gianni AM, Magni M, Martelli M, et al. Long-term remission in mantle cell lymphoma following high-dose sequential chemotherapy and in vivo rituximab-purged stem cell autografting (R-HDS regimen). Blood 2003;102:749–55.
82. Magni M, Di Nicola M, Devizzi L, et al. Successful in vivo purging of CD34-containing peripheral blood harvests in mantle cell and indolent lymphoma: evidence for a role of both chemotherapy and rituximab infusion. Blood 2000; 96:864–9.
83. Hess G, Flohr T, and Derigs HG. Rituximab as in vivo purging agent in autologous stem cell transplantation for relapsed B-NHL Ann Hematol 2002;81(Suppl 2):S54–5.
84. Tothova E, Kafkova A, Guman T, et al. Efficiency of in vivo purging with autologous stem cell transplantation and monoclonal antibody in B-cell lymphomas. Neoplasma 2003;50:22–5.
85. Adkins D, Brown R, Goodnough LT, et al. Treatment of resistant mantle cell lymphoma with allogeneic bone marrow transplantation. Bone Marrow Transplant 1998;21: 97–9.
86. Kroger N, Hoffknecht M, Kruger W, et al. Allogeneic bone marrow transplantation for refractory mantle cell lymphoma. Ann Hematol 2000;79:578–80.
87. Martinez C, Carreras E, Rovira M, et al. Patients with mantle-cell lymphoma relapsing after autologous stem cell transplantation may be rescued by allogeneic transplantation. Bone Marrow Transplant 2000;26:677–9.
88. Khouri IF, Lee MS, Saliba RM, et al. Nonablative allogeneic stem-cell transplantation for advanced/recurrent mantle-cell lymphoma. J Clin Oncol 2003;21:4407–12.
89. Khouri IF, Lee MS, Romaguera J, et al. Allogeneic hematopoietic transplantation for mantle-cell lymphoma: molecular remissions and evidence of graft-versus-malignancy. Ann Oncol 1999;10:1293–9.
90. Kouroukis CT, Belch A, Crump M, et al. Flavopiridol in untreated or relapsed mantle-cell lymphoma: results of a Phase II study of the National Cancer Institute of Canada Clinical Trials Group. J Clin Oncol 2003;21: 1740–5.
91. Lin TS, Howard OM, Neuberg DS, et al. Seventy-two hour continuous infusion flavopiridol in relapsed and refractory mantle cell lymphoma. Leuk Lymphoma 2002;43: 793–7.
92. Drach J, Kaufmann H, Puespoek A, et al. Marked anti-tumor activity of rituximab plus thalidomide in patients with relapsed/resistant mantle cell lymphoma. Blood 2002; 100:606[abstract].
93. Pham L, Tamayo A, Lo P, et al. Anti-tumor activity of the proteasome inhibitor PS-341 in mantle cell lymphoma B cells. Blood 2001;98:465b[abstract].
94. Goy A, Hart S, Pro B, et al. Report of a Phase II study of proteasome inhibitor Bortezombin (Velcade) in patients with relapsed or refractory indolent or aggressive Lymphomas. Blood 2003;102:627[abstract].
95. Fisher RI, Dahlberg S, Nathwani BN, et al. A clinical analysis of two indolent lymphoma entities: mantle cell lymphoma and marginal zone lymphoma (including the mucosa-associated lymphoid tissue and monocytoid B-cell subcategories): a Southwest Oncology Group study. Blood 1995;85:1075–82.
96. Unterhalt M, Herrmann R, Tiemann M, et al. Prednimustine, mitoxantrone (PmM) vs cyclophosphamide, vincristine,

prednisone (COP) for the treatment of advanced low-grade non-Hodgkin's lymphoma. German Low-Grade Lymphoma Study Group. Leukemia 1996;10:836–43.

97. Zinzani PL, Magagnoli M, Moretti L, et al. Randomized trial of fludarabine versus fludarabine and idarubicin as frontline treatment in patients with indolent or mantle-cell lymphoma. J Clin Oncol 2000;18:773–9.
98. Seymour JF, Grigg AP, Szer J, et al. Cisplatin, fludarabine, and cytarabine: a novel, pharmacologically designed salvage therapy for patients with refractory, histologically aggressive or mantle cell non-Hodgkin's lymphoma. Cancer 2002;94:585–93.
99. Coiffier B, Haioun C, Ketterer N, et al. Rituximab (anti-CD20 monoclonal antibody) for the treatment of patients with relapsing or refractory aggressive lymphoma: a multicenter Phase II study. Blood 1998;92:1927–32.
100. Nguyen DT, Amess JA, Doughty H, et al. IDEC-C2B8 anti-CD20 (rituximab) immunotherapy in patients with low-grade non-Hodgkin's lymphoma and lymphoproliferative disorders: evaluation of response on 48 patients. Eur J Haematol 1999;62:76–82.
101. Ghielmini M, Hsu Schmitz SF, Cogliatti SB, et al. Prolonged treatment with rituximab in patients with follicular lymphoma significantly increases event-free survival and response duration compared with the standard weekly × 4 schedule. Blood 2004;103:4416–23.

23

Small Lymphocytic Lymphoma/ Chronic Lymphocytic Leukemia

Emili Montserrat, M.D., Ph.D.

Elias Campo, M.D., Ph.D.

Small lymphocytic lymphoma/chronic lymphocytic leukemia (SLL/CLL) is a lymphoproliferative disorder resulting from the proliferation of lymphoid cells arrested at a mature stage of their differentiation pathway. This disease has its origin in mature (peripheral) CD5+ lymphoid cells of B-cell origin. Formerly envisaged as two separate entities, SLL and CLL are now considered to be the same disease.

DISEASE DEFINITION

The first name that SLL received was "diffuse, well-differentiated lymphocytic lymphoma," a term that actually included a variety of neoplasias that are now recognized as separate entities, such as SLL/CLL, marginal zone lymphoma, lymphoplasmacytic lymphoma, and mantle cell lymphoma.

In the World Health Organization classification, CLL/SLL is defined as a neoplasm of monomorphic, small, round B lymphocytes, admixed with prolymphocytes and paraimmunoblasts, usually expressing CD5 and CD23.[1] The term SLL is restricted to cases with the tissue morphology and immunophenotype of CLL, but which are non-leukemic. However, with the use of immunophenotyping as a diagnostic tool, it has become clear that, in virtually all SLL cases, it is possible to demonstrate cells with the typical immunophenotype of CLL in peripheral blood. Therefore, SLL and CLL can be considered as the two ends of a continuous spectrum in which either lymphadenopathy or peripheral blood involvement are the most prominent features (Fig. 23–1).

EPIDEMIOLOGY

The median age of patients at diagnosis is about 70 years.[2–4] SLL/CLL is rare in people under the age of 40. The incidence of SLL/CLL varies according to the series and to whether this is evaluated in lymphoma series or in leukemia series. In the study from the Non-Hodgkin's Lymphoma Classification Project, SLL accounts for 6% of all non-Hodgkin's lymphomas (2). When considering CLL, its overall incidence is about 5 cases per 100,000 people per year, increasing with age.[5] SLL/CLL, in its typical leukemic presentation, is the most frequent form of leukemia in Western countries, where it accounts for 30% of all leukemias. In contrast, SLL/CLL constitutes only 10% of all leukemias in Asian populations.[6] In most series, SLL/CLL is more frequent in males than in females.

ETIOLOGY

The etiology of SLL/CLL is unknown. SLL/CLL is not associated with exposure to radiation or other cytotoxic agents.[6] Familial cases of SLL/CLL support the existence of a genetic basis for this disease.[7] In about 5% of first-degree relatives of patients with CLL, it is possible to demonstrate in peripheral blood a population immunophenotypically identical to that of SLL/CLL; the clinical significance of this observation is still unclear.[7,8] An interesting observation is the so-called "anticipation phenomenon," whereby in younger members of the affected family, CLL presents, on average, 20 years earlier than in the older members.[9]

BIOLOGY

The CD5+ B cells from which SLL/CLL arise constitute a small subpopulation of B lymphocytes with a characteristic immunophenotype resembling that of lymphocytes normally present in the mantle zone of lymphoid follicles; these cells may also been found in the peripheral blood of a small proportion (2% to 3%) of normal subjects, a finding of uncertain clinical significance.[10] SLL/CLL results from the neoplastic transformation and accumulation of such B lymphocytes. The majority of these cells are arrested in the G_0 phase of the cell cycle. They also express large amounts of antiapoptotic Bcl-2 proteins, whereas the pro-apoptotic Bcl-X proteins are decreased. This, together with the interaction of neoplastic and stromal cells through a number of chemokines, leads to the accumulation of leukemic cells.[4]

Immunophenotypically, the neoplastic lymphocytes from SLL/CLL express surface membrane immunoglobulin (SmIg), usually of IgM or IgM and IgD types, in small amounts ("weak" SmIg expression), and a single Ig light chain (κ or λ). They also express CD5, HLA-DR, and B-cell antigens (e.g., CD19, CD20); in most cases they are CD23+, whereas CD22, CD79a, and CD79b are infrequently or weakly expressed.[4]

From the cytogenetic standpoint, in approximately 90% of the patients with CLL, it is possible to demonstrate chromosomal abnormalities by FISH.[11–14] The most frequent abnormalities are del(13q), del (11q), trisomy 12, and del(6q). Karyotypic evolution is observed in around 20% of the patients, usually in relation to disease progression.[15,16]

No genes have been consistently associated with SLL/CLL. Putative oncogenes have been identified in the

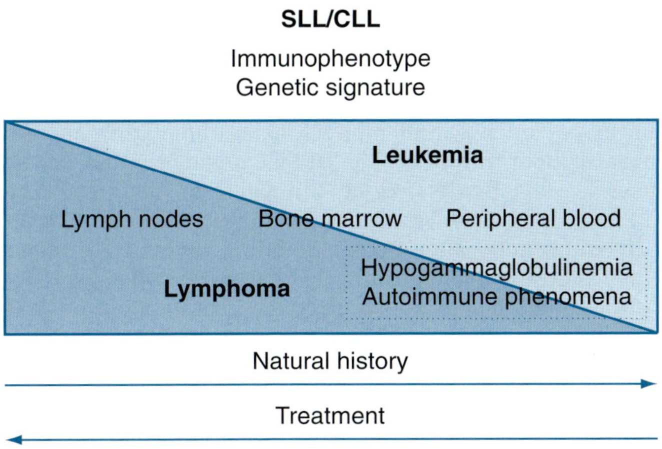

Figure 23–1. SLL and CLL can be regarded as two ends of the same disease: SLL (when lymphadenopathy is the major clinical finding), CLL (when the leukemic component predominates). In the natural history of SLL/CLL, there are cases with lymph node involvement only at diagnosis that eventually present leukemic involvement. On the other hand, treatment may reverse the clinical picture, with cases in which, after effective treatment of the leukemic component, residual lymphadenopathy remains. No consistent differences in immunophenotype or genetic signature have been identified between these two forms of the disease. Certain adhesion molecules might facilitate the predominant "lymphoma" or "leukemia" expression of the disease.

band 13q14.[17,18] In cases of disease progression, del(11q), over-expression of the c-myc oncogene, deletions of the *Rb1* gene, and mutations of the p53 tumor-suppressor gene have been reported.[15,16]

SLL/CLL has long been considered a homogeneous disease of naive CD5+ B cells, pre-germinal cells not exposed to antigenic stimulation. However, it is now clear that in some SLL/CLL cases IgV_H genes are mutated, which indicates interaction of the neoplastic cells with antigens in the germinal center of lymph nodes.[19,20] As discussed later, the unmutated and mutated forms have different clinical behavior. These two forms, however, share the same genetic signature as determined by microarrays, and, accordingly, SLL/CLL is considered a single disease with two variants (i.e., mutated, unmutated).[21] ZAP-70 can be detected by either cytofluorometry or PCR in peripheral blood cells or immunohistochemistry in lymph nodes and correlates with the IgV_H status: cases with unmutated IgV_H highly express ZAP-70.[22–24]

CLINICAL FEATURES

About 70% of SLL/CLL patients are diagnosed in asymptomatic phase on a routine medical examination. In symptomatic patients, the most frequent finding is lymphadenopathy. General symptoms such as fever, night sweats, or weight loss are not frequent in this variety of lymphoma. Sometimes the patient refers a history of repeated infections or autoimmune hemolytic anemia in the preceding months. The majority of the patients (80%) have advanced disease (Ann Arbor Stage III or IV) upon careful staging. Flow cytometry can demonstrate peripheral blood involvement in cases in which this is not detectable by routine methods.

The infiltration of extralymphatic tissues (e.g., pleura, lung, skin, and the central nervous system) is extremely rare. In addition, vasculitis, hypercalcemia and nephrotic syndrome have occasionally been described. In rare cases (<1% of patients), spontaneous remissions may be observed at some time during the course of the disease.[3]

Some cytogenetics abnormalities correlate with particular clinical features. Thus, del(11q) is particularly frequent in young males with bulky disease; trisomy 12 is commonly associated with atypical morphology of the lymphocytes in peripheral blood; del(6q) may be more common in cases with lymphoplasmacytoid cells in blood; and finally, del (17p) with mutations of p53 are observed in transforming disease and convey refractoriness to treatment.[11–14]

LABORATORY FEATURES

Patients with CLL present with absolute lymphocytosis in peripheral blood. A lymphocyte count greater than 5000/mL is usually employed as threshold to separate SLL from CLL. Usually, the more advanced the disease, the higher the WBC count. About 20% of patients present with anemia or thrombocytopenia. Autoimmune phenomena are frequent. A positive direct antiglobulin test may be found in less than 2% to up to 35% of patients with CLL.[25–27] Autoimmune hemolytic anemia occurs in 10% to 25% of patients, and may be triggered by treatment. Immune thrombocytopenia is observed in only 2% of cases. Pure red-cell aplasia and immune neutropenia are even less frequent, and, as it occurs with immune thrombocytopenia, can be difficult to document. Hypogammaglobulinemia, may be observed in about 60% of patients, particularly in the advanced phases of the disease.[28]

HISTOPATHOLOGY

The lymph nodes involved by SLL/CLL usually show a total effacement of the architecture by a diffuse proliferation of small lymphocytes. In addition, the tumor contains a variable number of intermediate-sized cells with central nucleoli, which resemble prolymphocytes. These cells are usually associated with the so-called paraimmunoblasts. In some cases, the prolymphocytes and paraimmunoblasts tend to accumulate in vaguely nodular aggregates. These nodules have been denominated *pseudofollicles* because they are poorly circumscribed and lack a well-developed meshwork of follicular dendritic cells (FDC), or *proliferation growth centers* because most of the tumor-proliferative cells accumulate in these nodules. These pesudofollicles contain also a high number of CD4+ cells.

In some cases, the nodal involvement is characterized by an interfollicular pattern preserving reactive follicles. Interestingly, these interfollicular patterns are frequently associated with an absence of malignant cells in peripheral blood, although bone marrow infiltration is common. In addition, cases with a perifollicular growth pattern tend to be associated with hypermutations of the IgV_H genes.[30]

SLL/CLL may involve any organ and tissue. Bone marrow is infiltrated in virtually all cases with different patterns, the more advanced the disease, the heavier the infiltration. Paratrabecular infiltration, a characteristic feature of follicular lymphoma, is not found in SLL/CLL. Splenic involvement is usually associated with splenomegaly. Histologically the tumor cells expand the white pulp with presence of multiple small nodules in the red pulp. These nodules tend to coalesce creating some areas with diffuse appearance. Red pulp infiltration is common, including sinuses and cords.

A few cases of CLL/SLL associated with a second malignant lymphoma (follicular lymphoma, mantle cell lymphoma) in the same topographic site (*composite* lymphoma) have been reported. Molecular studies have identified unrelated clonal rearrangement in these tumors, suggesting distinct clonal origins.[31] Mycosis fungoides and peripheral T-cell lymphomas, mainly of cytotoxic phenotype have been also described in association with CLL.[32]

Although the histologic aspect of SLL/CLL is relatively characteristic, immunophenotypic analysis may be helpful in cases in which the differential diagnosis with other small B-cell lymphomas is entertained (Table 23–1). SLL/CLL is positive for B-cell markers, but CD20 tends to be weaker and even negative in the smaller cell component whereas CD79a staining is more homogenously positive. The tumor cells coexpress the T-cell–associated antigens CD5 and CD43, and are also commonly positive for CD23. The cyclin D1 negativity and strong p27 expression in SLL/CLL are helpful findings in the differential diagnosis with mantle cell lymphoma.[33] Follicular dendritic cells may be recognized in the proliferative growth centers. Contrary to follicular lymphomas or MCL, the FDC in SLL/CLL form small groups without a well-developed meshwork. The germinal center–associated marker CD10 is negative. ZAP-70 expression may be examined in tissue by immunohistochemistry and correlates with ZAP-70 detected by flow cytometry in peripheral blood cells, IgV_H mutational status, and prognosis.[34,35]

DISEASE TRANSFORMATION

In about 10% of patients the disease undergoes transformation into a more aggressive tumor, most commonly diffuse large B-cell lymphoma (DLBCL), also known as Richter's syndrome.[36,37] In such cases, fever, weight loss, night sweats, enlarged lymphadenopathy, increased lactate dehydrogenase (LDH) serum levels, anemia, hypercalcemia, thrombocytopenia, and monoclonal gammopathy are the most frequent features.[37] The DLBCL arising in this context may be clonally related or unrelated to the preceding SLL/CLL.[38,39] SLL/CLL transformation is associated with different genetic alterations, including increased number of chromosomal alterations, losses of 8p, 9p, and 17p, homozygous deletions of p16, and mutations of p53 gene.[39–41] The prognosis in cases of transformation into DLBCL is poor, with a median survival of less than 6 months.[37] DLBCL associated with the presence of EBV in the transformed tumor cells has been observed in some patients.[42] Usually, these tumors are not clonally related to the previous SLL/CLL. SLL/CLL can also transform into Hodgkin's lymphoma. This transformation is usually also associated with EBV, and may be clonally related or unrelated to the preceding SLL/CLL.[43,44] Transformation of CLL into prolymphocytic leukemia can also be observed.[45]

INFECTIONS

Infections are frequent. Common bacteria such as *Streptococcus pneumoniae*, *Staphylococcus*, and *Haemophilus influenzae* cause most of the infections. Herpes zoster is also common. The use of new treatment agents with a highly immunosuppressive effect has led to the observation of infections due to *Legionella pneumophila*, *Pneumocystis carinii*, *Listeria monocytogenes*, and cytomegalovirus (CMV). *Candida* and *Aspergillus* species are also of concern.[46,47]

SECOND MALIGNANCIES

Patients with SLL/CLL have an increased risk of suffering second cancers.[48,49] In a study based on data from population-based cancer registries, the observed/expected ratio was 1.20, with an increased risk for Kaposi sarcoma, malig-

Table 23–1. SLL/CLL Versus Other Chronic B-Cell Malignancies: Immunophenotype, Cytogenetic, and Molecular Features

Disease	SmIg	CD5	CD43	CD22	CD23	CD25	FMC7	CD103	CD11c	CD10	CD79b	Other Features
CLL	−/+	+	+	−/+	+	+/−	−/+	−	−/+	−	−	del(13q), trisomy 12, del(6q), del
LP/WM	++	−	+/−	+	−	−/+	+	−	−/+	−	+/−	(11q), del(17p)
PL	++	−/+	+	+	−/+	−	+	−	−	−/+	+	CIg+, CD38+, CD71+, trisomy 12
HCL	++	−	+	+	−	+	+	+	+	−	−/+	del(13q)
SLVL	++	−/+	−/+	+	+/−	−/+	+	−/+	+/−	−/+	+	t(11;14), 14q+
MCL	++	+	+	+/−	−	−	+/−	−	−	−/+	+	HC2+, trisomy 5
FL	++	−	−	+/−	−/+	−	+	−	−	+/−	+	del(7q)
												t(11;14), Cyclin-D1
												t(14;18), bcl-2

Note: All express pan-B cell markers (e.g., CD19, CD20) and HLA-DR Class II antigens.
CLL, chronic lymphocytic leukemia; LP/WM, lymphoplasmacytic lymphoma/Waldenström's macroglobulinemia; PL, prolymphocytic leukemia; HCL, hairy cell leukemia; SLVL, splenic lymphoma with villous lymphocytes; MCL, mantle cell lymphoma; FL, follicular lymphoma; CIg, cytoplasmic immunoglobulin.

nant melanoma, larynx cancers, lung cancer, and also bladder and gastric cancer in men. No relationship was found between the characteristics of the disease and its treatment and the incidence of second cancers.[49]

DIAGNOSIS

In those cases in which SLL/CLL presents with lymphadenopathy and no apparent analytical abnormalities, the disease is usually diagnosed through a lymph node biopsy. Currently, however, the majority of patients with SLL/CLL are diagnosed on the occasion of a blood analysis performed because of trivial reasons or as part of the work-up to study fatigue, anemia, or other symptoms.

The histopathologic features of SLL/CLL have been described above (see Histopathology section). In cases in which the diagnosis is based on the histopathologic findings of an enlarged lymph node, peripheral blood should be screened to rule out the presence of leukemic cells.

With regard to the leukemic form, CLL, a number of diagnostic criteria have been proposed,[50,51] including an absolute increase (e.g., >5000 to 10,000/mL) of mature-looking lymphocytes in peripheral blood, with a characteristic immunophenotype (SmIg+/– CD5+, CD19++, CD20+, CD23++, FMC 7–), and bone marrow infiltration. The differential diagnosis with other B-cell chronic malignancies may require the integration of immunophenotypic, cytogenetic, and molecular data (Fig. 23–1).

In practice, CLL can be diagnosed whenever there is an absolute increase in the number of lymphocytes in blood that are morphologically and immunophenotypically consistent with the diagnosis. Although bone marrow examination should no longer be considered necessary to diagnose SLL/CLL, it may be useful in cases without obvious peripheral blood involvement, as staging procedure, and also to provide a clue on the origin of cytopenias (central vs. peripheral).

PROGNOSIS

The prognosis of patients with SLL/CLL is extremely variable. The overall median survival is about 10 years, but aside from patients whose disease has an indolent course and have a survival that is not different from that of the general population, there are others who have a rapidly evolving and fatal course.

Clinical stages have been the most useful prognostic parameters in CLL (Table 23–2).[52,53] However, they have some limitations. For example, indolent and progressive forms of the disease are not identified. Moreover, the mechanisms accounting for cytopenias are not taken into consideration. However, patients with cytopenias of immune origin may have a better outcome than those in whom the cytopenia is caused by a massive infiltration of the bone marrow by neoplastic cells.[62] For all these reasons, many other prognostic factors have been proposed to complement clinical stages[54–61] (Table 23–3).

The correlation of the mutational status of IgV_H genes with the clinical outcome has signified an important progress in the understanding of the natural history of SLL/CLL.[19,20] The mutational status of IgV_H genes separates SLL/CLL into two forms with distinct presenting features and outcome. Thus, patients with unmutated forms have a more malignant disease than those with mutated IgV_H. Unfortunately, studying IgV_H mutations is difficult on a routine basis. CD38 expression correlates, although not absolutely, with IgV_H mutations; moreover, CD38 expression may vary over time.[63] Recently, it has been demonstrated that ZAP-70 expression, as evaluated by

Table 23–2. Staging Systems for CLL

Staging System	Stage	Clinical Features	Median Survival (years)
Rai			
Low-risk	0	Lymphocytosis alone	14.5
Intermediate-risk	I	Lymphocytosis Lymphadenopathy	7.5
	II	Lymphocytosis Spleen or liver enlargement	
High-risk	III	Lymphocytosis Hemoglobin <11 g/dL	2.5
	IV	Lymphocytosis Platelets <100,000/mL	
Binet			
Low-risk	A	No anemia, no thrombocytopenia <3 Lymphoid areas[a] enlarged	15.5
Intermediate-risk	B	No anemia, no thrombocytopenia >3 Lymphoid areas enlarged	5.5
High-risk	C	Hemoglobin <10 g/dL or Platelets <100,000/mL	3

[a]The Binet staging system takes into consideration the following lymphoid areas: lymph nodes (whether unilateral or bilateral) in the head and neck, axillae, and groin; spleen, and liver. Results shown are based on the series by the authors at the Hospital Clinic of Barcelona (n = 465).

Table 23–3. Parameters with Prognostic Significance in CLL

Parameter	Low-Risk	High-Risk
Clinical stage		
Binet	A	B, C
Rai	0	I, II, III, IV
Bone marrow infiltration		
Biopsy	Nondiffuse pattern	Diffuse pattern
Aspirate	≤80% Lymphocytes	>80% Lymphocytes
WBC count (× 10^9/L)[a]	≤50	>50
Prolymphocytes in peripheral blood (%)[a]	≤10	>10
Lymphocyte doubling time[a]	≤12 months	>12 months
Serum markers[b]	Normal	Increased
Cytogenetics	Normal del (13q) isolated	del(11q) del(17p)
C38 expression	≤30%	>30%
IgV_H genes	Mutated	Unmutated
ZAP-70[c]	Low (<20%)	High (≥20%)

[a] Continuous variables.
[b] LDH, 2 microglobulin, thymidin-kinase, CD23, and others.
[c] As detected by cytofluorometry.

cytofluorometry, immunohistochemistry, or PCR, strongly correlates with IgV_H mutations and has important prognostic significance.[22–24]

TREATMENT

Therapy is considered justified when any of the following features is present:

- General symptoms (i.e., weight loss, extreme fatigue, night sweats, or fever without evidence of infection)
- Increasing anemia or thrombocytopenia due to bone marrow failure
- Bulky or progressive lymphadenopathy
- Massive or progressive splenomegaly
- Autoimmune cytopenias not responsive to corticosteroids
- Rapidly increasing lymphocyte counts in peripheral blood

A marked hypogammaglobulinemia or increased white blood cell (WBC) counts, in the absence of any of the above criteria, are not sufficient to initiate treatment.[51]

Treatment Approaches

The current evidence regarding the optimal therapy for patients with SLL/CLL has been obtained in clinical trials performed in patients with the leukemic form of the disease.

Treatment of patients in early stage (Binet A, Rai 0) has resulted in a delay in the rate of disease progression but no survival benefit.[64,65]

A proportion of patients in intermediate stage (Rai I and II, Binet B) have indolent disease; these patients may be followed with no therapy, like those in the early stage. However, the majority of patients with intermediate stage and virtually all patients with advanced stage (Rai III and IV, Binet C) due to bone marrow infiltration require therapy.

Over the last 20 years, chlorambucil has been the treatment of choice. The number of complete responses obtained with chlorambucil is low (10%) and, besides symptoms palliation, it is doubtful that it has any impact on the natural history of the disease. Because of this, chorambucil is usually given to patients not likely to tolerate more intensive therapies. Likewise, radiation therapy has a limited role in the treatment of SLL/CLL, although it may be useful to treat bulky lymphadenopathy or splenomegaly causing compressive problems in patients not suitable for chemotherapy, and also patients in whom the disease is confined to localized lymph nodes (<10%).

Purine analogues, particularly fludarabine, are the most effective agents to treat SLL/CLL. Treatment with fludarabine results in a much higher complete response (CR) rate than chlorambucil or alkylating based chemotherapies (20% to 40% vs. 10%) and a longer disease-free interval, although survival is not prolonged.[66–68] The efficacy of fludarabine may be improved by combining it with other agents (e.g., cyclophosphamide, mitoxantrone, rituximab).[69–72] There are already data indicating that the combination of fludarabine plus cyclophosphamide not only results in a superior response rate than fludarabine alone, but also longer freedom from progression and, perhaps, longer survival.[71,72]

The most important side effects of purine analogues are myelosuppression and infections, including opportunistic ones. This seems to be more frequent in patients receiving corticosteroids, and, particularly, in those who have been heavily pretreated.[73] Therefore, antibiotic and antiviral prophylaxis (e.g., cotrimoxazole, acyclovir) is recommended in patients receiving purine analogues.

Another side effect of concern is autoimmune hemolytic anemia (AIHA), which in some cases can be fatal.[74] Because of this, purine analogues should be avoided in patients with AIHA or a positive Coombs' test.

In patients treated with purine analogues, anecdotal cases of pulmonary toxicity,[75,76] tumor lysis syndrome,[77] and acute myelofibrosis have been reported.[78,79] In addition, several cases of transfusional acute graft-versus-host disease have been described.[80,81] Regarding long-term complications, several cases of myelodysplasia have been reported.[82,83]

Treatment of Complications

Patients with *autoimmune hemolytic anemia* (AIHA) should initially be treated with corticosteroids, with cytotoxic agents added only in the case of no response after 2 to 4 weeks of treatment. In patients with AIHA not responding to or difficult to control with corticosteroids plus cytotoxic agents, high-dose immunoglobulin, cyclosporin, or rituximab may be tried. A proportion of these patients, however, will eventually require splenectomy.[84] *Pure red-cell aplasia* (PRCA) may occasionally be associated with SLL/CLL; the treatment of choice is cyclosporine, and rituximab can also be effective.[4,85]

Hypogammaglobulinemia is the major cause of infections, which are the major cause of death and a significant cause of morbidity. Although high and intermediate doses of immunoglobulin have been found to be of some value in preventing infections,[86] cost–benefit considerations make the routine use of immunoglobulin questionable.[87] Hematopoietic growth factors (i.e., G-CSF) may overcome treatment-related *neutropenia*.[88] Finally, erythropoietin may be useful to treat *anemia unresponsive to other measures*.[89]

The prognosis of patients who suffer *disease transformation* is very poor (median survival <6 months), but patients responding to aggressive lymphoma-type chemotherapy may have longer survival.[37]

Patients *refractory to treatment*, or those who progress soon after therapy, have a very poor prognosis. Treatment options in these patients, particularly those who have received fludarabine, are limited to new or experimental treatment approaches or stem cell transplants.

New Treatment Approaches

Alemtuzumab (Campath 1H) is a humanized anti-CD52 monoclonal antibody that results in 40% to 89% responses, including 2% to 50% CR. Responses are better in patients without prior therapy. Toxicity includes rigors, chills, fever, immunosuppression, and lymphocytopenia. Opportunistic infections can be observed. CMV reactivation is a problem that deserves monitorization and pre-emptive therapy.[90–95]

Responses to alemtuzumab vary in different disease sites, being higher in peripheral blood and bone marrow than in lymph nodes. Interestingly, alemtuzumab may induce responses in patients refractory to fludarabine, this indicating that well-known mechanisms of resistance to the drug (e.g., p53 mutations) either do not apply to, or can be overcome, by the monoclonal antibody. Current studies with alemtuzumab include its subcutaneous administration and in combination with other agents (e.g., fludarabine, rituximab).

Rituximab is an anti-CD20 antibody. In SLL/CLL the amount of CD20 on the surface of neoplastic cells is moderate, this being a possible reason for the low response rate to rituximab when given alone.[94,95] However, rituximab acts synergistically with fludarabine and cyclophosphamide, with impressive preliminary treatment results having been reported. Patients with high WBC counts (i.e., >50,000/mL) may develop the so-called *cytokine-release syndrome* characterised by fever, rigors, skin rash, nausea, vomiting, hypotension, and dyspnea, upon rituximab administration.

A number of new monoclonal antibodies are under investigation in PhaseI/II trials. These include IDEC-152 (anti-CD23), Apolizumab (Hu1D10, Remitogen), and BL-22 (anti-CD22(Fv)-PE38), among others.[95]

Although there are many results showing cross-resistance between the different purine analogues, there is some renewed interest to investigate purine analogues other than fludarabine (i.e., cladribine, pentostatin) along with other cytotoxic agents or monoclonal antibodies (e.g, pentosatin + cyclophosphamide + rituximab) in patients failing under fludarabine treatment. High-dose methylprednisolone may be useful in flurarabine-resistant cases.

Other agents which are being studied include denileukin diftitox fusion protein (Ontak) and bcl-2 antisense (Genasense).[95]

An increasing number of subjects with SLL/CLL are being offered stem cell transplants.[96–101] The necessary condition for the success of an autologous transplant is to achieve CR prior to the procedure, which is extremely unlikely in patients refractory to the newer chemotherapy or chemoimmunotherapy regimens. Moreover, unfavorable prognostic factors for response to conventional chemotherapy (e.g., del(17p), del(11q), unmutated VH genes) also predict poor results with autologous transplants. Autologous transplants do not cure CLL but may prolong survival in selected patients (i.e., sensititive to chemotherapy, without unfavorable prognostic factors, and transplanted early in the course of the disease). In contrast, allogeneic transplants can cure about 40% of the patients, but at the cost of high toxicity and mortality. Because of this and the advanced age of most patients with CLL, the role of allotransplants with reduced-intensity conditioning regimens is being intensively investigated; preliminary results are encouraging. The possibility of performing an allogeneic transplant should be seriously considered in any patient with refractory CLL, an acceptable clinical condition, and willing to accept the risk of the procedure. Stem cell transplants, however, should not be performed outside clinical trials.

References

1. Müller-Hermelink HK, Catovsky D, et al. Chronic lymphocytic leukaemia/small lymphocytic lymphoma. In: Jaffe ES, Harris NL, Stein H, et al., eds. "World Health Organization Classification of Tumours. Pathology and Genetics of Tumours of Haematopoietic and Lymphoid Tissues. " Lyon: IARC Press, 2001:127–30.
2. Armitage JO and Weisenburger DD's. New approach to classifying non-Hodgkin's lymphomas: clinical features of the major histologic subtypes. J Clin Oncol 1998; 16:2780–95.
3. Rozman C and Montserrat E. Chronic lymphocytic leukemia. N Engl J Med 1995;333:1052–7.
4. Keating MJ, Chiorazzi N, Messmer B, et al. Biology and treatment of chronic lymphocytic leukemia. Hematology (Am Soc Hematol Educ Program) 2003:153–75.
5. Ries LAG, Eismer MP, Kosary CL, et al., eds. SEER Cancer Statistics Review, 1993–1997. Bethesda MD: National Cancer Institute, 2000.
6. Finch SC and Linet MS. Chronic leukaemias. Baillière's Clin Haematol 1992;5:27–56.
7. Cuttner J. Increased incidence of hematologic malignancies in first-degree relatives of patients with chronic lymphocytic leukemia. Cancer Invest 1992;10:103–9.
8. Rawstron C, Yuille R, Fuller R, et al. Inherited predisposition to CLL is detectable as sub-clinical monoclonal B-lymphocyte expansion. Blood 2002;100:2289–90.
9. Goldin LR, Sgambati M, Marti GE, et al. Anticipation in familial chronic lymphocytic leukemia. Am J Hum Genet 1999 65:265–9.
10. Rawstron AC, Green MJ, Kuzmicki A, et al. Monoclonal B lymphocytes with the characteristics of "indolent" chronic lymphocytic leukemia are present in 3.5% of adults with normal blood counts. Blood 2002;100:635–9.
11. Döhner H, Stilgenbauer S, Benner A, et al. Genomic aberrations and survival in chronic lymphocytic leukemia. N Engl J Med 2000;343:1910–16.
12. Döhner H, Stilgenbauer S, Döhner K, et al. Chromosome aberrations in B-cell chronic lymphocytic leukemia: reassessment based on molecular cytogenetic analysis. J Mol Med 1999;77:266–81.
13. Döhner H, Stilgenbauer S, Fischer K, et al. Cytogenetic and molecular cytogenetic analysis of B cell chronic

lymphocytic leukemia: specific chromosome aberrations identify prognostic subgroups of patients and point to loci for candidate genes. Leukemia 1997;11(suppl 2): S19–24.
14. Stilgenbauer S, Bullinger L, Benner A, et al. Incidence and clinical significance of 6q deletions in B cell chronic lymphocytic leukemia. Leukemia 1999:13:1331–4.
15. Oscier O, Fitchett M, Herbert T, et al. Karyotypic evolution in B-cell chronic lymphicytic leukemia. Gene Chromosomes Cancer 1991;3:16–20.
16. Fegan C, Robinson H, Thompson P, et al. Karyotypic evolution in CLL: identification of a new subgroup of patients with deletions of llq and advanced or progressive disease. Leukemia 1995;9:2003–8.
17. Migliazza A, Bosch F, Komatsu H, et al. Nucleotide sequence, transcription map, and mutation analysis of the 13q14 chromosomal region deleted in B-cell chronic lymphocytic leukemia. Blood 2001;97:2098–104.
18. Bullrich F, Fujii H, Calin G, et al. Characterization of the 13q14 tumor suppressor locus in CLL: identification of ALT1, an alternative splice variant of the LEU2 gene. Cancer Res 2001;61:6640–8.
19. Hamblin TJ, Davis Z, Gardiner A, et al. Unmutated Ig V(H) genes are associated with a more aggressive form of chronic lymphocytic leukemia. Blood 1999;94:1848–54.
20. Damle RN, Wasil T, Fais F, et al. Ig V gene mutation status and CD38 expression as novel prognostic indicators in chronic lymphocytic leukemia. Blood 1999;94:1840–7.
21. Rosenwald A, Alizadeh AA, Widhopf G, et al. Relation of gene expression phenotype to immunoglobulin mutation genotype in B cell chronic lymphocytic leukaemia. J Exp Med 2001;194:1639–47.
22. Crespo M, Bosch F, Villamor N, et al. ZAP-70 expression as a surrogate for immunoglobulin-variable-region mutations in chronic lymphocytic leukemia. N Engl J Med 2003;348:1764–75.
23. Wiestner A, Rosenwald A, Barry TS, et al. ZAP-70 expression identifies a chronic lymphocytic leukemia subtype with unmutated immunoglobulin genes, inferior clinical outcome, and distinct gene expression profile. Blood 2003;101:4944–51.
24. Orchad JA, Ibbotson RW, Davis Z, et al. ZAP-70 expression and prognosis in chronic lymphocytic leukemia. Lancet 2004;363:105–11.
25. Kipps TJ and Carson DA. Autoantibodies in chronic lymphocytic leukemia and related systemic autoimmune diseases. Blood 1993;81:2475–87.
26. Hamblin TJ, Oscier DG, and Young BJ. Autoimmunity in chronic lymphocytic leukemia. J Clin Pathol 1986;39: 713–16.
27. Ward JH. Autoimmunity in chronic lymphocytic leukemia. Curr Treat Options Oncol 2001;2:253–7.
28. Rozman C, Montserrat E, and Viñolas N. Serum immunoglobulins in B-chronic lymphocytic leukaemia. Natural history and prognostic significance. Cancer 1988;61:279–83.
29. Pangalis GA, Moutsdopoulos HM, Papadopoulos NM, et al. Monoclonal and oligoclonal immunoglobulins in the serum of patients with B-chronic lymphocytic leukemia. Acta Haematol 1988;80:23–7.
30. Bahler DW, Aguilera NS, Chen CC, et al. Histological and immunoglobulin VH gene analysis of interfollicular small lymphocytic lymphoma provides evidence for two types. Am J Pathol 2000;157:1063–70.
31. Fend F, Quintanilla-Martinez L, Kumar S, et al. Composite low grade B-cell lymphomas with two immunophenotypically distinct cell populations are true biclonal lymphomas. A molecular analysis using laser capture microdissection. Am J Pathol 1999;154:1857–66.
32. Martinez A, Pittaluga S, Villamor N, et al. Clonal T-cell populations and increased risk for cytotoxic T-cell lymphomas in B-CLL patients: clinicopathologic observations and molecular analysis. Am J Surg Pathol 2004;28:849–58.
33. Quintanilla-Martinez L, Thieblemont C, Fend F, et al. Mantle cell lymphomas lack expression of p27Kip1, a cyclin dependent kinase inhibitor. Am J Pathol 1998;153:175–82.
34. Admirand JH, Rassidakis GZ, Abruzzo LV, et al. Immunohistochemical detection of ZAP-70 in 341 cases of non-Hodgkin and Hodgkin lymphoma. Mod Pathol 2004;17: 954–61.
35. Villamor N, Carreras J, Colomo L, et al. ZAP-70 expression in B-cell lymphoid neoplasms. An immunohistochemical study. J Pathol 2005;205:507–13.
36. Richter MN. Generalized reticular cell sarcoma of lymph nodes associated with lymphatic leukaemia. Am J Pathol 1928;4:285–92.
37. Robertson LE, Pugh W, O'Brien S, et al. Richter's syndrome: a report on 39 patients. J Clin Oncol 1993;11:1985–9.
38. Matolcsy A, Inghirami G, and Knowles DM. Molecular genetic demonstration of the diverse evolution of Richter's syndrome (chronic lymphocytic leukemia and subsequent large cell lymphoma). Blood 1994;83:1363–72.
39. Bea S, Lopez-Guillermo A, Ribas M, et al. Genetic imbalances in progressed B-cell chronic lymphocytic leucemia and transformed large-cell lymphoma (Richter's syndrome). Am J Pathol 2002;161:957–68.
40. Gaidano G, Ballerini P, Gong JZ, et al. p53 mutations in human lymphoid malignancies: association with Burkitt lymphoma and chronic lymphocytic leukemia. Proc Natl Acad Sci U S A 1991;88:5413–17.
41. Cobo F, Martinez A, Pinyol M, et al. Multiple cell cycle regulator alterations in Richter's transformation of chronic lymphocytic leukemia. Leukemia 2002;16:1028–34.
42. Abruzzo LV, Rosales CM, Medeiros LJ, et al. Epstein–Barr virus-positive B-cell lymphoproliferative disorders arising in immunodeficient patients previously treated with fludarabine for low-grade B-cell neoplasms. Am J Surg Pathol 2002;26:630–6.
43. Momose H, Jaffe ES, Shin SS, et al. Chronic lymphocytic leukemia/small lymphocytic lymphoma with Reed-Sternberg–like cells and possible transformation to Hodgkin's disease. Mediation by Epstein–Barr virus. Am J Surg Pathol 1992;16:859–67.
44. Kanzler H, Kuppers R, Helmes S, et al. Hodgkin and Reed-Sternberg-like cells in B- cell chronic lymphocytic leukemia represent the outgrowth of single germinal-center B-cell-derived clones: potential precursors of Hodgkin and Reed-Sternberg cells in Hodgkin's disease. Blood 2000;95: 1023–31.
45. Enno A, Catovsky D, O'Brien M, et al. "Prolymphocytoid" transformation of chronic lymphocytic leukemia. Br J Haematol 1979;41:9–18.
46. Molica S. Infections in chronic lymphocytic leukemia: risk factors and impact on survival, and treatment. Leuk Lymphoma 1994;13:203–14.
47. Morrison VA. The infectious complications of chronic lymphocytic leukemia. Semin Oncol 1998;25:98–106.
48. Greene MH, Hoover RN, and Fraumeni JF. Subsequent cancer in patients with chronic lymphocytic leukemia. A possible immunologic mechanism. J Natl Cancer Inst 1978;61:337–40.
49. Hisada M, Biggar RJ, Greene MH, et al. Solid tumors after chronic lymphocytic leukemia. Blood 2001;98:1979–81.
50. International Workshop on Chronic Lymphocytic Leukemia. Chronic lymphocytic leukemia: recommendations for diagnosis, staging, and response criteria. Ann Intern Med 1989;110:236–8.

51. Cheson BD, Bennett JM, Grever M, et al. National Cancer Institute-sponsored working group guidelines for chronic lymphocytic leukemia: revised guidelines for diagnosis and treatment. Blood 1996;87:4990–7.
52. Rai KR, Sawitsky A, Cronkite EP, et al. Clinical staging of chronic lymphocytic leukemia. Blood 1975;46:219–34.
53. Binet JL, Auquier A, Dighiero G, et al. A new prognostic classification of chronic lymphocytic leukemia derived from a multivariate survival analysis. Cancer 1981;48:198–206.
54. Montserrat E Classical and new prognostic factors in chronic lymphocytic leukemia: where to now? Hematol J 2002;3:7–9.
55. Montserrat E, Viñolas N, Reverter JC, et al. Natural history of chronic lymphocyhic leukemia: on the progression and prognosis of early clinical stages. Nouv Rev Franc 1988; 30:359–61.
56. Hallek M, Langenmayer I, Nerl C, et al. Elevated serum thymidin kinase levels identify a subgroup at high risk of disease progression in early, nonsmoldering chronic lymphocytic leukemia. Blood;1999;93:1732–7.
57. Reinisch W, Wiliheim M, Hilgarth M, et al. Soluble CD23 reliably reflects disease actlvity in B-cell chronic lymphocytic leukemia. J Clin Oncol 1994;12:2146–52.
58. Lavabre-Bertrand T, Exbrayat C, Bourquard P, et al. CD23 antigen density is related to gamma globulin level, bone marrow reticulin pattern, and treatment in B chronic lymphocytic leukemia. Leuk Lymphoma 1994;13: 89–94.
59. Manshouri T, Do KA, Wang X, et al. Circulating CD20 is detectable in the plasma of patients with chronic lymphocytic leukaemia and is of prognostic significance. Blood 2003;101:2507–13.
60. El Rouby S, Thomas A, Costin D, et al. p53 gene mutation in B-cell chronic lymphocytic leukemia is associated with drug resistance and is independent of MDR1 /MDR3 gene expression. Blood 1993;82:3452–9.
61. Catovsky D, Fooks I, Richards S. Prognostic factors in chronic lymphocytic leukaemia: the importance of age, sex, and response to treatment in survival. Br J Haematol 1989;72:141–9.
62. Mauro FR, Foa R, Cerretti R, et al. Autoimmune hemolytic anemia in chronic lymphocytic leukemia: clincial, therapeutic, and prognostic features. Blood 2000;95:2788–92.
63. Hamblin TJ, Orchad JA, Ibbotson RE, et al. CD38 expression and immunoglobulin variable region mutations are independent prognostic variables in chronic lymphocytic leukemia, but CD38 expression may vary during the course of the disease. Blood 2002;99:1023–9.
64. Dighiero G, Maloum K, Desablens B, et al. Chlorambucil in indolent chronic lymphocytic leukemia. N Engl J Med 1998;338:1506–11.
65. Chemotherapeutic options in chronic lymphocytic leukemia: a meta-analysis of the randomized trials. CLL Trialists' Collaborative Group. J Natl Cancer Inst 1999;91: 861–8.
66. The French Cooperative Group on CLL, Johnson S, Smith AG, et al. Multicentre prospective randomized trial of fludarabine versus cyclophosphamide, doxorubicin, and prednisone (CAP) for treatment of advanced-stage chronic lymphocytic leukemia. Lancet 1996;347:1432–8.
67. Rai KR, Peterson BL, Appelbaum FR, et al. Fludarabine compared with chlorambucil as primary therapy for chronic lymphocytic leukemia. N Engl J Med 2000;343: 1750–7.
68. Leporrier M, Chevret S, Cazin B, et al. Randomized comparison of fludarabine, CAP, and ChOP in 938 previously untreated stage B and C chronic lymphocytic leukemia patients. Blood 2001;98:2319–25.
69. Bosch F, Ferrer A, Lopez-Guillermo A, et al. Fludarabine, cyclophosphamide, and mitoxantrone in the treatment of resistant or relapsed chronic lymphocytic leukaemia. Br J Haematol 2002;119:976–84.
70. Eichorst BF, Busch R, Hopfinger G, et al. Fludarabine plus cyclophosphamide (FC) induces higher remission rates and longer progression free survival than fludarabine (F) alone in first-line therapy of advanced chronic lymphocytic leukemia (CLL): results of a Phase III study (CLL4 protocol) of the German Study Group (GCLLSG). Blood 2003;102 [abstract 243].
71. Wierda W, O'Brien S, Faderi S, et al. Improved survival in patients with relapsed—refractory chronic lymphocytic leukemia (CLL) treated with fludarabine, cyclophosphamide, and rituximab (FCR) combination. Blood 2003; 102[abstract 373].
72. Byrd JC, Peterson BL, Morrison VA, et al. Randomized phase 2 study of fludarabine with concurrent versus sequential treatment with rituximab in symptomatic, untreated patients with B-cell chronic lymphocytic leukemia: results from Cancer and Leukemia Group B 9712 (CALGB 9712). Blood 2003;101:6–14.
73. Cheson BD. Infectious and immunosuppresive complications of purine analog therapy. J Clin Oncol 1995;13: 2431–48.
74. Di Raimondo F, Giustolisi R, Cacciola E, et al. Autoimmune hemolytic anemia in chronic lymphocytic leukemia patients treated with fludarabine. Leuk Lymphoma 1993;11:63–8.
75. Hurst PG, Habib MP, Garewall H, et al. Pulmonary toxicity associated with fludarabine monophosphate. Invest New Drugs 1987;5:207–10.
76. Cervantes F, Salgado C, Montserrat E, et al. Fludarabine for prolymphocytic leukaemia and risk of interstitial pneumonitis. Lancet 1990;2:1130.
77. Frame JN, Dahut WL, and Crowley S. Fludarabine and acute tumor lysis in chronic lymphocytic leukemia. N Engl J Med 1992;327:1396.
78. Palomera L, Azaceta G, Varo MJ, et al. Fatal myelofibrosis following fludarabine administration in a patient with indolent lymphoma. Haematologica 1998;83:1045–6.
79. Paydas S, Disel U, Yavuz S, et al. Fludarabine as the possible cause of acute myelofibrosis. Hematol J 2004;5:283–4.
80. Maung ZT, Wood AC, Jackson GH, et al. Transfusion-associated graft-versus-host disease in fludarabine-treated B-chronic lymphocytic leukaemia. Br J Haematol 1994;88: 649–52.
81. Briz M, Cabrera R, Sanjuan I, et al. Diagnosis of transfusion-associated graft versus-host disease by polymerase chain reaction in fludarabine treated B-chronic lymphocytic leukaemia. Br J Haematol 1995;91:409–11.
82. Morrison VA, Rai KR, Peterson BL, et al. Therapy-related leukemias are observed in patients with chronic lymphocytic leukemia after treatment with fludarabine and chlorambucil: results of an intergroup study of the Cancer and Leukemia Group B 9011. J Clin Oncol 2002;20:3878–84.
83. Orchad JA, Bolam S, and Oscier DG. Association of myelodysplastic syndromes with purine analogues. Br J Haematol 1998;100:677–9.
84. Majumdar C and Singh AK. Role of splenectomy in chronic lymphocytic leukaemia with massive splenomegaly and cytopenia. Leuk Lymphoma 1992;7:131–4.
85. Chikkappa G, Pasquale D, Zarrabi MH, et al. Cyclosporine and prednisone therapy for pure red cell aplasia in patients with chronic lymphocytic leukemia. Am J Hematol 1992;41: 5–12.
86. Cooperative Group for the Study of Immunoglobulin in Chronic Lymphocytic Leukemia. Intravenous immunoglobulin for the prevention of infection in chronic lymphocytic

leukemia. A randomized, controlled clinical trial. N Engl J Med 1988;319:902–7.
87. Weeks JC, Tiemey MR, and Weinstein MC. Cost effectiveness of prophylactic intravenous immune globulin in chronic lymphocytic leukemia. N Engl J Med 1991;325: 81–6.
88. Hollander AAMJ, Kluin-Nelemans HC, Haak HR, et al. Correction of neutropenia associated with chronic lymphocytic leukemia following treatment with granulocyte-macrophage colony stimulating factor. Ann Hematol 1991;62:32–4.
89. Straus DJ. Epoetin alfa therapy for patients with hematologic malignancies and mild anemia. Clin Lymphoma 2003; (suppl 1):S13–7.
90. Tallman MS. Monoclonal antiboidy therapies in leukemias. Semin Hematol 2002;39(suppl 3):12–9.
91. Osterborg A, Dyer MJ, Bunjes D, et al. Phase II multicenter study of human CD52 antibody in previously treated chronic lymphocytic leukemia. European Study Group of CAMPATH-1H Treatment in Chronic Lymphocytic Leukemia J Clin Oncol 1997;4:1567–74.
92. Osterborg A, Fassas AS, Anagnostopoulos A, et al. Humanized CD52 monoclonal antibody Campath-1H as first line treatment in chronic lymphocytic leukemia. Br J Haematol 1996;93:151–3.
93. Dyer MJ, Kelsey SM, Mackay HJ, et al. In vivo "purging" of residual disease in CLL with Campath-1H Br J Haematol 1997;97:669–72.
94. Huhn D, von Schilling C, Wilhelm M, et al. Rituximab therapy of patients with B-cell chronic lymphocytic leukemia. Blood 2001;98:1326–1331.
95. Mavromaties BH and Cheson BD. Novel therapies for chronic lymphocytic leukemia. Blood Rev 2004;18:137–48.
96. Esteve J, Villamor N, Colomer D, et al. Stem cell transplantation for chronic lymphocytic leukemia: different outcome after autologous and allogeneic transplantation and correlation with minimal residual disease status. Leukemia 2001; 15:445–51.
97. Dreger P and Montserrat E. Autologous and allogeneic stem cell transplantation for chronic lymphocytic leukemia. Leukemia 2002;16:985–92.
98. Schetelig J, Thiede C, Bornhäuser M, et al. Evidence of a graft-versus-leukemia effect in chronic lymphocytic leukemia after reduced-intensity conditioning and allogeneic stem-cell transplantation: the Cooperative German Transplant Study Group. J Clin Oncol 2003;21:2747–53.
99. Dreger P, Brand R, Hansz J, et al. Treatment-related mortality and graft-versus-leukemia activity after allogeneic stem cell transplantation for chronic lymphocytic leukemia using intensity-reduced conditioning. Leukemia 2003;17:841–8.
100. Ritgen M, Lange A, Stilgenbauer S, et al. Unmutated immunoglobulin variable heavy-chain gene status remains an adverse prognostic factor after autologous stem cell transplantation for chronic lymphocytic leukemia. Blood 2003;101:2049–53.
101. Dreger P, Stilgenbauer S, Benner A, et al. The prognostic impact of autologous stem cell transplantation in patients with chronic lymphocytic leukemia: a risk-matched analysis based on the V_H gene mutational status. Blood 2004;103: 2850–8.

24

Cutaneous B-Cell Lymphoma

Rein Willemze, M.D.

The term "cutaneous B-cell lymphoma" (CBCL) refers to a heterogeneous group of B-cell lymphomas that present in the skin without evidence of extracutaneous disease at the time of diagnosis.[1] These CBCL have to be differentiated from B-cell lymphomas involving the skin secondarily. The existence of this group of CBCL has been recognized only recently. Until the 1980s, malignant lymphomas other than mycosis fungoides were considered invariably as manifestations of systemic disease. In retrospective studies, distinction between benign and malignant cutaneous lymphoproliferative disorders was generally based on clinical criteria, in particular the outcome of the disease.[2] Thus, patients developing extracutaneous disease or patients who died of lymphoma within 5 years after diagnosis were considered to have malignant lymphoma, whereas patients with an uneventful follow-up were considered to have a benign condition. Given their excellent prognosis many primary CBCL would have been considered as a benign condition using this criterion.

The introduction of immunohistochemistry in the late 1970s had a major impact on the diagnosis and classification of B-cell proliferations in the skin. Accepting the presence of monotypic immunoglobulin light-chain expression on frozen or paraffin sections as golden standard for the diagnosis of a malignant B-cell lymphoma did not only facilitate differentiation between malignant B-cell lymphomas and reactive B-cell proliferations, but also led to the recognition that malignant B-cell lymphomas can present in the skin without concurrent extracutaneous disease being detectable. The simple distinction between primary and secondary CBCL proved extremely important. Studies on well-defined groups of patients showed that the different types of primary CBCL have a highly distinctive clinical presentation, often have a completely different clinical behaviour compared to systemic B-cell lymphomas with or without secondary skin involvement and therefore require a different therapeutic approach. These studies resulted in the delineation of distinct types of CBCL, which were included in recent classification systems for cutaneous lymphomas.

EPIDEMIOLOGY

Primary CBCL are much less frequent than primary cutaneous T-cell lymphomas (CTCL). Several European studies indicate that CBCL constitute about 20% to 25% of all primary cutaneous lymphomas.[1,3] In contrast, the percentages of CBCL newly registered between 1995 and 1998 in three institutions in the United States varied between 3.2% and 7.7% of all primary cutaneous lymphomas.[4] Whether these differences in the incidence of CBCL relate to differences in diagnostic procedures or classification systems, or represent true regional differences, is as yet unknown.

ETIOLOGY AND PATHOGENESIS

In contrast to T lymphocytes, B lymphocytes are not found in normal human skin and skin-specific homing receptors used by benign or malignant B-cells to accumulate preferentially in the skin have not been identified. However, several antigenic stimuli are known to result in a reactive B-cell response. These reactions are designated variously as cutaneous lymphoid hyperplasia, pseudo–B-cell lymphoma, or lymphadenosis benigna cutis, and may be caused by insect bites, in particular tick bites transmitting a *Borrelia burgdorferi* infection, acupuncture, antigen injections, and tattoo pigments.[5] *B. burgdorferi* infection[6–10] and tattoo pigments[11–12] have also been implicated in the development of CBCL, and particularly marginal zone B-cell lymphomas. Interestingly, *B. burgdorferi*–specific DNA sequences have been demonstrated in a significant minority of CBCL from European regions with endemic *Borrelia* infections,[6,7] but could not be detected in 38 CBCL from several geographical areas in the United States,[13] nor in 24 Asian cases.[14]

There is accumulating evidence to suggest that these low-grade malignant CBCL and cutaneous lymphoid hyperplasia represent a spectrum of cutaneous B-cell lymphoproliferative disorders with a stepwise progression from a reactive to a neoplastic state.[5,12,15,16] This also explains why it can be so difficult to differentiate early stages of these low-grade CBCL from cutaneous lymphoid hyperplasias. Apart from clinical and histological similarities, and the shared association with *B. burgdorferi* infection and tattoo pigments, clonal Ig gene rearrangements have been demonstrated not only in primary CBCL, but also in a proportion of pseudo-B-cell lymphomas, as defined by immunohistochemical criteria.[12,17,18]

The *B. burgdorferi*–associated CBCL resemble in many ways gastric MALT lymphomas that develop in association with *Helicobacter pylori* infection, including resolution of the skin lymphoma after antibiotic therapy in some cases.[8,9] However, the various translocations associated with the subsequent steps of evolution of gastric MALT lymphomas are rarely found in these primary cutaneous marginal zone B-cell lymphomas.[14,19–22]

Recent studies have started to evaluate the genetic mechanisms involved in the development and progression of these lymphomas. However, in contrast to many types of nodal B-cell lymphomas, specific cytogenetic abnormalities have not been identified yet in the different types of CBCL.

CLASSIFICATION

In recent years, primary cutaneous lymphomas were classified either by the European Organization for Research and Treatment of Cancer (EORTC) classification[1] or by the World Health Organization (WHO) classification.[23]

Whereas there was consensus between the EORTC and WHO classification schemes regarding the categorization of most types of CTCL, differences in the definition and terminology of the various types of CBCL have evoked much debate and confusion. However, during recent consensus meetings, representatives of both classification systems proved successful in resolving the existing controversies and a new classification was developed.[24] In this chapter, this new WHO-EORTC classification for cutaneous lymphomas will be used. In this classification, three main types of primary CBCL are recognized: *primary cutaneous marginal zone B-cell lymphoma* (PCMZL), *primary cutaneous follicle center lymphoma* (PCFCL), and *primary cutaneous large B-cell lymphoma, leg type* (PCLBCL, leg type). The term PCFCL is used for cutaneous lymphomas composed of neoplastic follicle center cells, usually a mixture of centrocytes (small and large cleaved follicle center cells) and centroblasts (large non-cleaved follicle center cells with prominent nucleoli), which may show a follicular, a follicular and diffuse, or a diffuse growth pattern. Clinically, most patients present with localized skin lesions on the head or trunk and, irrespective of the growth pattern or number of blast cells, are highly responsive to radiotherapy and have an excellent prognosis.[25–28] In the WHO classification, these lymphomas were categorized in a different way. Cases with a (partly) follicular growth pattern were included as a variant of follicular lymphoma, and designated cutaneous follicle center lymphoma, while the much more common cases with a diffuse growth pattern were classified as diffuse large B-cell lymphoma, which could easily lead to overtreatment with multiagent chemotherapy rather than radiotherapy. The PCFCL in the WHO-EORTC classification differ from the group of primary cutaneous follicle center-cell lymphomas in the EORTC classification by the fact that uncommon cases with confluent sheets of centroblasts and immunoblasts not localized on the leg are classified as PCLBCL. This is in line with the results of a recent multicenter study showing that cases with a predominance of round cells have a more unfavorable prognosis than cases with a predominance of large cleaved cells.[29] There was agreement that PCLBCL, leg, as defined in the EORTC classification is a distinct entity with a characteristic clinical presentation (tumors on the [lower] legs, particularly in elderly patients), morphology (predominance or confluent sheets of centroblasts and immunoblasts) and immunophenotype (strong expression of bcl-2 and Mum-1/IRF4), and an intermediate prognosis.[29,30] It was, however, also recognized that cases with a similar morphology, immunopehnotype, and prognosis may sometimes arise at sites other than the legs.[29] In the WHO-EORTC classification, the term PCLBCL, leg type, is used for both the typical lesions on the legs and similar lesions at other sites. Rare cases of PCLBCL that do not belong to the group of PCLBCL, leg type, or the group of PCFCL are designated as PCLBCL, other.

PRIMARY CUTANEOUS MARGINAL ZONE B-CELL LYMPHOMA

Primary cutaneous marginal zone B-cell lymphoma is an indolent lymphoma composed of small B cells including marginal zone (centrocyte-like) cells, lymphoplasmacytoid cells, and plasma cells. They include cases previously designated as primary cutaneous immunocytoma,[31] and cases of cutaneous follicular lymphoid hyperplasia with monotypic plasma cells.[32] Rare cases of primary cutaneous plasmacytoma (extramedullary plasmacytoma of the skin) show considerable overlap with PCMZL, both clinically and histologically, and are therefore included in this category.[33]

Clinical Features

In most cases, PCMZL presents with red to violaceous papules, plaques, or nodules localized preferentially on the trunk or extremities. In contrast to PCFCL, presentation with multifocal skin lesions is frequently observed (Fig. 24–1). Ulceration is uncommon. PCMZL have a tendency to recur in the skin, but dissemination to extracutaneous sites is exceedingly rare.[14,31,34–36] In some cases, spontaneous resolution of the skin lesions may be observed. These lymphomas can develop in areas of acrodermatitis chronica atrophicans, indicative of an association with *B. burgdorferi* infection.[34] This association has been reported in a significant minority of European cases of PCMZL, but not in Asian cases or cases from the United States.[6,7,13,14] Associated autoimmune diseases are uncommon in PCMZL, but rather suggest secondary cutaneous involvement of a systemic lymphoma.[31] Unlike MZL occurring at other sites, PCMZL rarely show transformation into a diffuse large B-cell lymphoma. The prognosis of these primary cutaneous MZL is excellent with a 5-year survival close to 100%.[14,31–16]

Histopathology

Histologically these lymphomas show nodular to diffuse infiltrates with sparing of the epidermis (Fig. 24–2A). The infiltrates are composed of small lymphocytes, marginal zone B-cells (centrocyte-like cells), lymphoplasmacytoid cells, and plasma cells, admixed with small numbers of centroblast- or immunoblast-like cells and many reactive T cells. Reactive follicle centers are frequently observed. They may be surrounded by a population of small- to medium-sized cells with irregular nuclei, inconspicuous nucleoli, and abundant pale cytoplasm (marginal zone B cells). Monotypic plasma cells are often located at the periphery

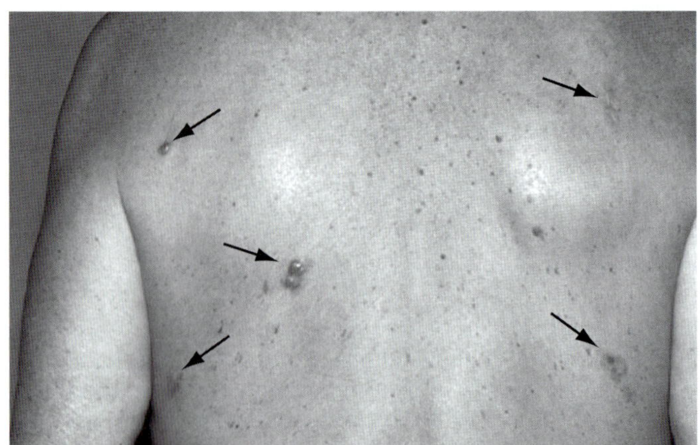

Figure 24–1. Primary cutaneous marginal zone B-cell lymphoma. Typical clinical presentation with multiple nodules on the back. (See color insert.)

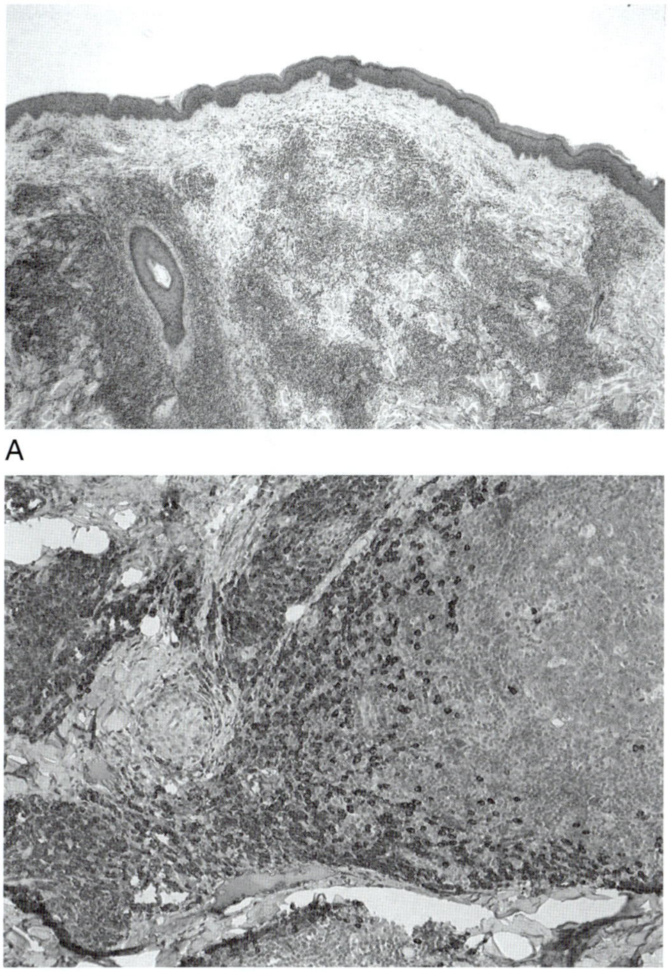

A

B

Figure 24–2. Primary cutaneous marginal zone B-cell lymphoma. **A:** Patchy infiltrates throughout the dermis. (See color insert.) **B:** Detail of dermal infiltrate with reactive follicle center and monotypic IgA, kappa-positive, plasma cells at the periphery of the infiltrate (IgA staining).

of the infiltrates and in the superficial dermis beneath the epidermis[31,32,34,35] (Fig. 24–2B). PAS-positive intranuclear or intracytoplasmic inclusions may be present. Lymphoepithelial lesions are extremely rare in PCMZL, and if present are highly suggestive of secondary cutaneous involvement. Exceptional cases showing a predominance of monotypic plasma cells and no or few admixed small lymphocytes classified previously as primary cutaneous plasmacytoma[33] are now included in this group of PCMZL.

Immunophenotype

The marginal zone B-cells express CD20, CD79a and bcl-2, but are negative for CD5, CD10, and bcl-6, which may serve as an useful adjunct to differentiate these PCMZL from PCFCL.[37,38] Reactive germinal centers are typically bcl-6+, CD10+, and bcl–2–. Plasma cells express CD38 and CD79a positive, but generally not CD20, and show monotypic cytoplasmic immunoglobulin light-chain expression on paraffin sections.

Genetic Features

Immunoglobulin heavy-chain (IgH) genes are clonally rearranged. Whether skin lesions showing a clonal IgH gene rearrangement, but no monotypic Ig light-chain expression, should be labeled CBCL or still considered as a benign condition (clonal cutaneous lymphoid hyperplasia) is a matter of debate.[12,18]

Several translocations including the t(14;18)(q32;q21) involving the IGH gene on chromosome 14 and the MLT gene on chromosome 18, and the t(3;14)(p14.1;q32) involving IGH and FOXP1 genes, have been reported in a proportion of PCMZL.[19,39] However, other translocations observed in gastric MALT lymphomas, such as t(11;18)(q21;q21) and t(1;14)(p22;q32) have not been found in primary cutaneous MZL.[20–22,40]

Therapy

Patients with a solitary lesion or a few lesions can be treated with radiotherapy or surgical excision.[36] In patients with associated *B. burgdorferi* infection, systemic antibiotics should be tried first, before more aggressive therapies are employed.[41] For patients presenting with multifocal skin lesions, intralesional or subcutaneous administration of interferon alpha may produce complete responses in approximately 50% of patients.[8] Similar results can be obtained with chlorambucil.[36] Skin relapses are common, in particular in patients with multifocal skin disease. In many patients, a wait-and-see strategy can be followed, similar to that used in indolent B-cell lymphomas and leukemias at extracutaneous sites. Alternatively, one may consider treating small and superficial lesions with topical or intralesional steroids, while only the most infiltrated lesions are treated with radiotherapy.

PRIMARY CUTANEOUS FOLLICLE CENTER LYMPHOMA

Primary cutaneous follicle center lymphoma (PCFCL) is defined as a tumor of neoplastic follicle center cells, usually a mixture of centrocytes (small and large cleaved follicle center cells) and variable numbers of centroblasts (large non-cleaved follicle center cells with prominent nucleoli). It includes cases with a follicular, a follicular and diffuse, or a diffuse growth pattern, and generally presents on the head or trunk. In the WHO-EORTC classification, lymphomas with a diffuse growth pattern and a monotonous proliferation or confluent sheets of centroblasts and immunoblasts are, irrespective of site, classified as PCLBCL.

Clinical Features

PCFCL show a characteristic clinical presentation with solitary or grouped plaques and tumors, preferentially located on the scalp or forehead or on the trunk[25–28] (Fig. 24–3). In particular, on the trunk these tumors may be surrounded by papules and slightly indurated plaques, which may precede the development of tumorous lesions for months or even many years. In the past, PCFCL with such a typical presentation on the back were referred to as "reticulohistiocytoma of the dorsum" or "Crosti's lymphoma."[26] Presentation with multifocal skin lesions is observed in a small

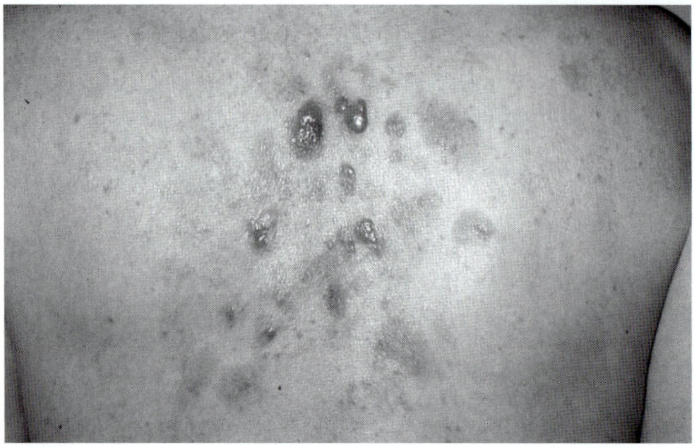

A

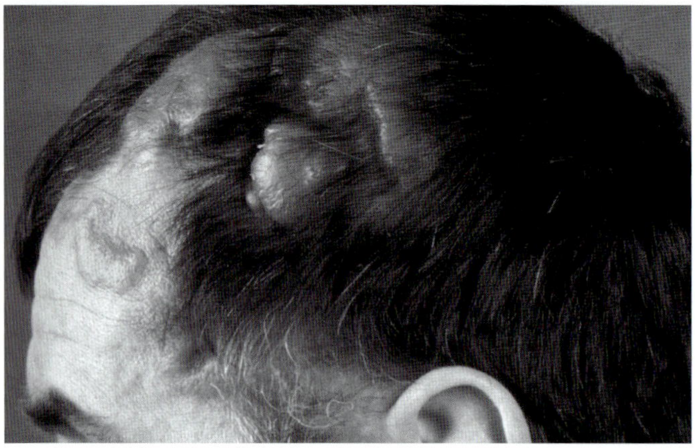

B

Figure 24–3. Primary cutaneous follicle center lymphoma. Characteristic clinical presentation with localized skin lesions (**A**) on the back (Crosti's lymphoma) and (**B**) on the scalp. (See color insert.)

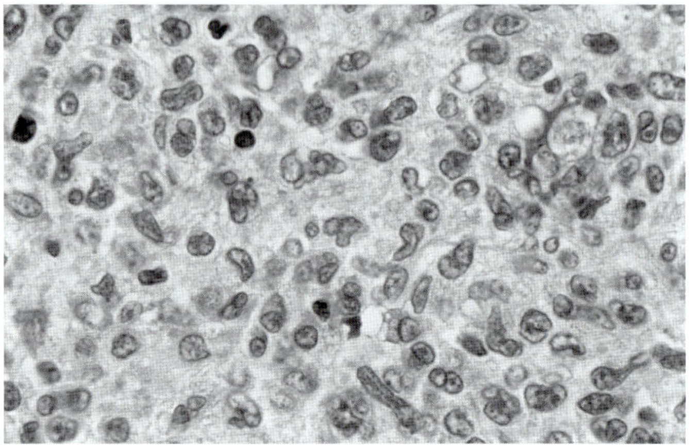

A

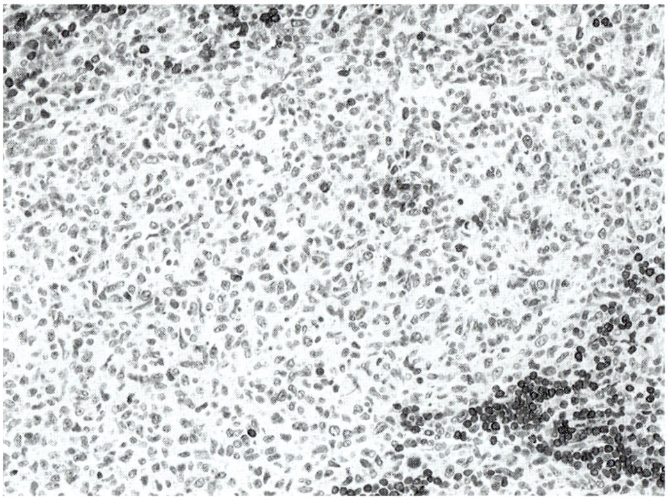

B

Figure 24–4. Primary cutaneous follicle center lymphoma. **A:** Histology of a skin tumor showing a diffuse infiltrate of large centrocytes (large cleaved cells) including many cells with multilobated nuclei. (See color insert.) **B:** Bcl-2 staining showing positive reactive T-cells, whereas the tumor cells are bcl-2 negative.

minority of patients, but is not associated with a more unfavorable prognosis.[29,42] If left untreated, the skin lesions gradually increase in size over the years, but dissemination to extracutaneous sites is uncommon. Irrespective of the growth pattern (follicular or diffuse) or the number of blast cells, these PCFCL have an excellent prognosis with a 5-year survival over 95%.[1,25–28,42–44]

Histopathology

PCFCL show nodular to diffuse infiltrates with almost constant sparing of the epidermis. The histologic picture is variable, which relates primarily to the age and the growth rate of the biopsied skin lesion.[1,27] Small and early lesions contain a mixture of centrocytes, relatively few centroblasts and many reactive T cells. In such lesions, a clear-cut follicular growth pattern or remnants of a follicular growth pattern may be observed. If present, the abnormal follicles show malignant bcl6+ follicle center cells enmeshed in a network of CD21+ or CD35+ follicular dendritic cells, are ill-defined, lack tangible body macrophages, and generally have a reduced or absent mantle zone.[43,44] With progression to tumorous lesions, the neoplastic B cells increase both in number and size, whereas the number of reactive T cells steadily decreases. Follicular structures, if present before, are no longer visible except for occasional scattered CD21+ or CD35+ follicular dendritic cells. Rapidly growing tumors generally show a monotonous population of large follicle center cells, generally large centrocytes, including multilobated cells, and in rare cases, spindle-shaped cells, with a variable admixture of centroblasts and immunoblasts[26,27,29,45,46] (Fig. 24–4A).

Immunophenotype

The neoplastic follicle center cells express B-cell–associated antigens CD20 and CD79a, and may show monotypic staining for surface immunoglobulins (sIg). However, absence of detectable sIg is common in tumorous lesions showing a diffuse population of large follicle center cells. PCFCL consistently express bcl-6.[37,38,44] CD10 expression is particularly observed in cases with a follicular growth pattern, but is uncommon in PCFCL with a diffuse growth pattern.[38] Staining for CD5 and CD43 is negative. Unlike nodal and secondary cutaneous follicular lymphomas, most PCFCL do not express bcl-2 protein or show faint bcl-2 staining in a minority of neoplastic B-cells[43,47,48] (Fig. 24–4B). Staining for Mum-1/IRF4 is negative.[49]

Genetics

Clonally rearranged immunoglobulin genes are present, and several studies demonstrated somatic hypermutation of variable heavy- and light-chain genes, which further supports the follicle center cell origin of these lymphomas.[50,51] In most studies, PCFCL, including cases with a follicular growth pattern, do not show the t(14;18), which is characteristically found in systemic follicular lymphomas and a considerable proportion of systemic diffuse large B-cell lymphomas.[44,48,52] In contrast, recent studies report the presence of t(14;18), as well as bcl-2 expression in a significant minority of PCFCL with a follicular growth pattern.[53,54] The reasons for this discrepancy are as yet unexplained.

These PCFCL have the gene expression profile of germinal center-like large B-cell lymphomas.[49] Array-based comparative genomic hybridization (CGH) studies in combination with interphase fluorescence in situ hybridization (FISH) analysis revealed high-level DNA amplifications of a small region of chromosome 2p16.1 containing both the C-REL and BCL11A genes in 63%, and loss of chromosome 14q32.33 containing the IGH chain locus in 68% of PCFCL, as compared to 17% and 25% of PCLBCL, leg type, respectively.[55] Inactivation of p15 and p16 tumor suppressor genes by promotor hypermethylation is rarely found in these PCFCL.[55] In studies using interphase FISH, no evidence for translocations involving IGH, Myc, or bcl-6 loci were found.[40]

Therapy

In patients with localized or few scattered skin lesions, radiotherapy is the preferred mode of treatment, also in cases with a diffuse large-cell infiltrate.[28,42,56–58] Cutaneous relapses, observed in approximately 20% of patients, do not indicate progressive disease, and can be treated with radiotherapy as well. Only in patients with very extensive cutaneous disease and patients developing extracutaneous disease, is anthracycline-based chemotherapy required.[29,42] Recent studies report beneficial effects of systemic or intralesional administration of anti-CD20 antibody (rituximab) therapy in small series of PCFCL, but the long-term effects of this approach have yet to be determined.[59–61]

PRIMARY CUTANEOUS LARGE B-CELL LYMPHOMA, LEG TYPE

Primary cutaneous large B-cell lymphomas (PCLBCL), leg type, are diffuse large-cell B-cell lymphomas with a predominance or confluent sheets of centroblasts and immunoblasts. Characteristically, they present with tumorous skin lesions on the (lower) legs, but uncommonly can arise at other sites as well.

Clinical Features

PCLBCL, leg type, predominantly affect elderly patients. Females are more often affected than males.[29,30,62] Patients present with red or bluish-red tumors on one or both (lower) legs (Fig. 24–5). In contrast to the group of PCFCL, these lymphomas are not preceded by papular skin lesions or annular erythemas with or without a follicular growth pattern, but develop de novo. In addition, these PCLBCL,

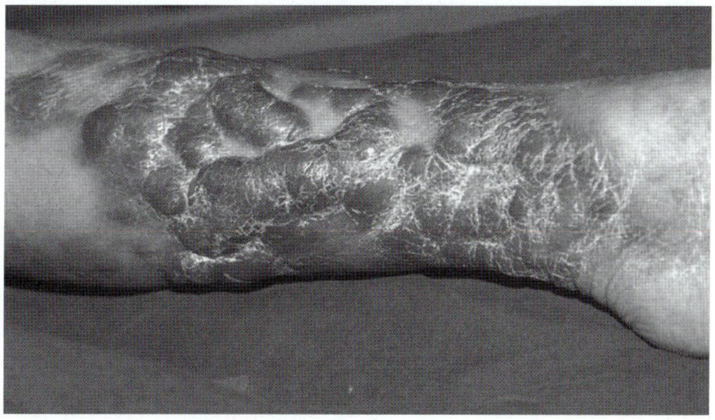

Figure 24–5. Primary cutaneous large B-cell lymphoma, leg type. (See color insert.)

leg type, more often disseminate to extracutaneous sites, and have a more unfavorable prognosis with a 5-year survival of approximately 50%.[29,30] Unlike PCFCL, the presence of multiple skin lesions at diagnosis is a significant adverse risk factor in this group. In a recent study, patients presenting with a single skin tumor on one leg had a disease-related 5-year-survival of 100%, whereas patients presenting with multiple skin lesions on one or both legs had a disease-related 5-year-survival of 45% and 36%, respectively.[29] Reports on PCLBCL, leg type, arising at other sites than the legs are few. In a European multicenter study, which included 17 such cases, 16 of 17 patients presented with solitary or localized skin lesions either on the trunk or head, 7 of 17 patients developed extracutaneous disease, and the 5-year disease-related 5-year survival was 72%.[29]

Histopathology

These lymphomas show diffuse nonepidermotropic infiltrates, which often extend into the subcutaneous tissue. These infiltrates generally show a monotonous population or confluent sheets of centroblasts and immunoblasts[29,30] (Fig. 24–6A). Mitotic figures are frequently observed. Small B cells are lacking, and reactive T cells are relatively few and often confined to perivascular areas.

Immunophenotype

The neoplastic B cells express monotypic sIg and/or cIg and B-cell–associated antigens CD20 and CD79a. In contrast to the group of PCFCL, these PCLBCL, leg type, consistently show strong bcl-2 and Mum-1/IRF4 expression[38,48,49,62–64] (Fig. 24–6B). Bcl-6 is expressed by most cases, whereas CD10 staining is generally absent.[38]

Genetics

Recent studies suggest that these PCLBCL, leg type, have an activated B-cell gene expression profile.[49] The t(14;18) is not found in these lymphomas, although they consistently show strong bcl-2 expression.[48,62] In a number of cases, bcl-2 over-expression may result from chromosomal amplification of the bcl-2 gene.[55,65] Using classical CGH, chromosomal imbalances have been identified in up to 85% of PCLBCL, with gains in 18q and 7p and loss of 6q as most common findings.[65,66] Using array-based CGH and FISH analyses, high-level DNA amplifications of

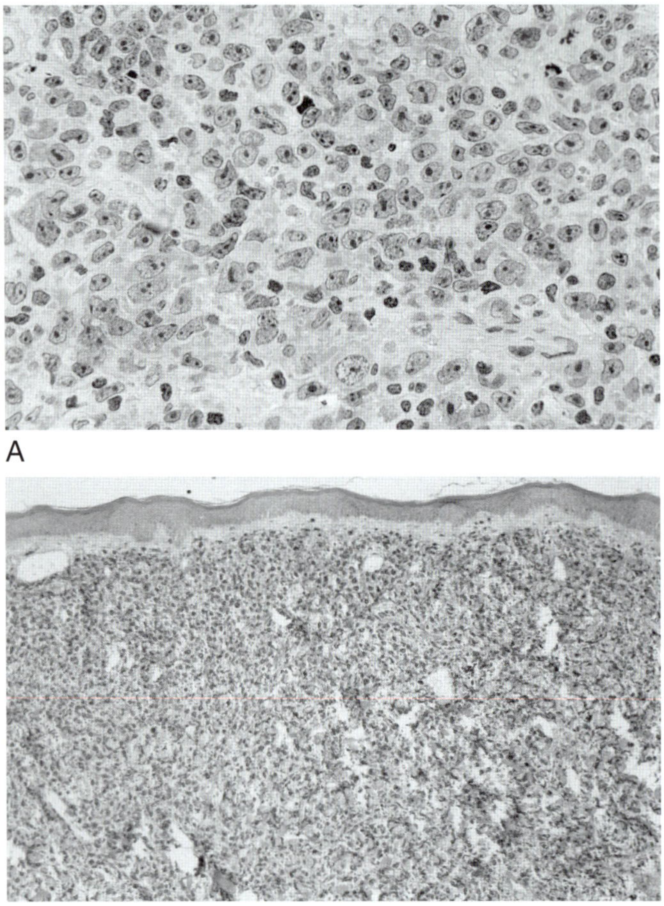

Figure 24–6. Primary cutaneous large B-cell lymphoma, leg type. A: diffuse proliferation of centroblasts and immunoblasts. B: Tumor cells show strong reactivity for bcl-2. (See color insert.)

18q21.31–q21.31, including the BCL2 and MALT1 genes, were detected in 67% of PCLBCL, leg type, but in only 11% of PCFCL.[55] Deletion of a small region on chromosome 9p21.3 containing the CDKN2a and CDKN2B gene loci was detected in 67% of PCLBCL, leg type, but not in the group of PCFCL.[55] More importantly, inactivation of CDKN2A either by deletion or promoter hypermethylation was found to be an important prognostic parameter in this group.[55] Interphase FISH analysis demonstrated translocations involving myc, bcl-6, and IgH genes in 11 of 14 PCLBCL-leg, but not in patients with a PCFCL.[40] Taken together, these findings suggest that these PCLBCL are similar to diffuse large B-cell lymphomas arising at other sites, whereas PCFCL including cases with a diffuse large-cell morphology clearly represent a separate group.

Therapy

PCLBCL should be treated as systemic diffuse large B-cell lymphomas with anthracycline-based chemotherapy.[29,30] Only in some patients presenting with a single skin tumor radiotherapy may be considered.[29] Systemic administration of anti-CD20 antibody (rituximab) has proved effective in some patients, but long-term follow-up data are not available, and the place of rituximab, either as single-agent therapy or in combination with systemic chemotherapy in the treatment of PCLBCL remains to be established.[59,67]

PRIMARY CUTANEOUS INTRAVASCULAR B-CELL LYMPHOMA, OTHER

In the WHO-EORTC classification, the term "PCLBCL, other" is used for rare cases of PCLBCL that do not belong to the group of PCLBCL, leg type, or the group of PCFCL. These include morphologic variants of diffuse large B-cell lymphoma, such as rare cases of anaplastic or plasmablastic lymphoma, rare primary cutaneous T-cell/histiocyte-rich B-cell lymphomas, and primary cutaneous, intravascular large B-cell lymphomas.

Primary Cutaneous T-Cell/Histiocyte-Rich B-Cell Lymphoma

T-cell/histiocyte-rich B-cell lymphomas are characterized by the presence of large scattered B cells in a background of numerous reactive T cells. Cutaneous involvement is considered extremely uncommon. Nevertheless, rare cases of primary cutaneous T-cell/histiocyte-rich B-cell lymphoma have been reported.[68,69] Clinically, they show similarities with the groups of PCFCL and PCMZL. These lymphomas commonly present with skin lesions on the head, trunk, or extremities, and, unlike their nodal counterpart, appear to have an excellent prognosis.[68,69] Whether all published cases are genuine T-cell/histiocyte-rich B-cell lymphomas, or in fact represent an exaggerated T-cell infiltrate in other types of CBCL, such as PCFCL or PCMZL, is questionable.

Primary Cutaneous Intravascular Large B-Cell Lymphoma

Intravascular large B-cell lymphomas are characterized by an accumulation of large neoplastic B-cells within blood vessels. These lymphomas preferentially affect the central nervous system, lungs, and skin, and are generally associated with a poor prognosis. Intravascular lymphomas presenting with only skin lesions may occur.[70,71]

Intravascular CBCL present with violaceous indurated patches and plaques or telangiectatic skin lesions usually on the (lower) legs or the trunk (Fig. 24–7A). Patients presenting with only skin lesions appear to have a significantly better survival than patients with other clinical presentations (3-year overall survival 56% vs. 22%, respectively).[71]

Histologically, dilated blood vessels in the dermis and subcutis are filled and often extended by a proliferation of large neoplastic B cells (Fig. 24–7B). These cells may cause vascular occlusion of venules, capillaries, and arterioles. In some cases, small numbers of tumor cells can also be observed around blood vessels.

Multiagent chemotherapy is the preferred mode of treatment, also in patients presenting with skin-limited disease.[71]

B-LYMPHOBLASTIC LYMPHOMA

B-lymphoblastic lymphoma is a malignant proliferation of precursor B lymphocytes. Although skin lesions are usually

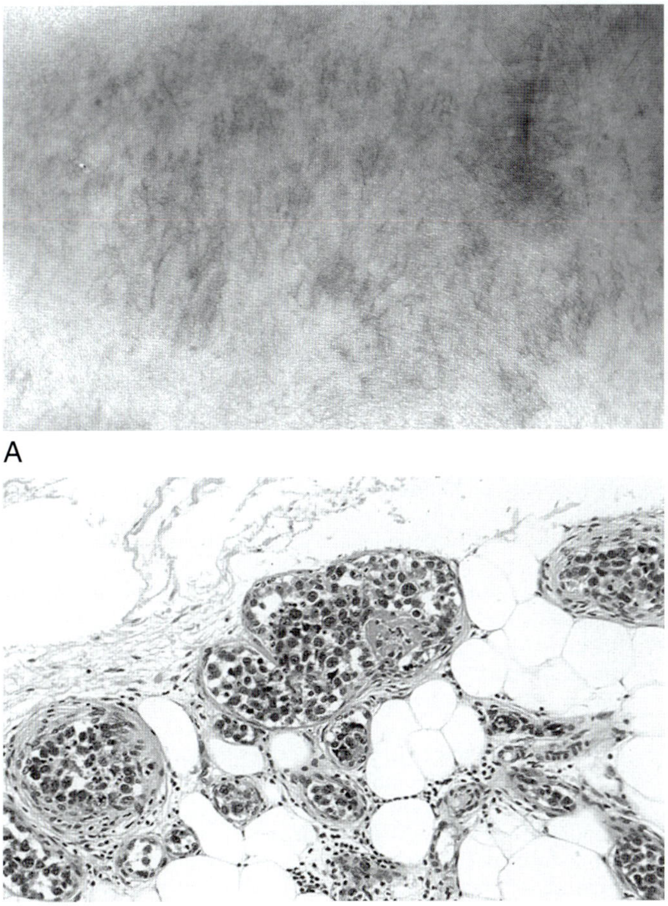

A

B

Figure 24–7. Primary cutaneous intravascular large B-cell lymphoma. **A:** Erythematous skin lesions on the chest. **B:** Intravascular population of large neoplastic B cells. (See color insert.)

a manifestation of acute lymphoblastic leukemia with bone marrow and peripheral blood involvement, B-lymphoblastic lymphomas may also present with localized disease involving extracutaneous sites, and in particular, the skin, soft tissue, and bone. The disease usually affects children and young adults.[72] Large erythematous skin tumors in the head and neck region are a characteristic clinical presentation.[73] Histologically, these lymphomas are characterized by the presence of a monotonous proliferation of medium-sized cells with round or convoluted nuclei showing fine chromatin and inconspicuous nucleoli and scanty cytoplasm. The tumor cells show expression of CD79, CD20, CD10, and TdT. Aggressive systemic chemotherapy, similar to that designed for patients with B-ALL, is the treatment of choice, also in patients presenting with only skin lesions.[72]

CONCLUSION

It is now well established that malignant B-cell lymphomas may arise primarily in the skin, and that these primary CBCL differ clinically and biologically from their nodal counterparts. It is therefore extremely important that every patient with or suspected to have a CBCL is adequately staged, which should always include bone marrow examination and appropriate imaging. PCMZL, PCFCL, and PCLBCL, leg type are the most common types of CBCL, each of them with a characteristic clinical presentation and clinical behavior in terms of relapse rate, tendency to involve extracutaneous sites, and prognosis. The WHO-EORTC classification is a major step forward, and is expected to contribute to a more uniform diagnosis, and hence more uniform treatment of patients with a CBCL. Recently, studies have started to investigate gene and protein expression profiles in the various types of CBCL. It is expected that these studies will not only contribute to a better understanding of the molecular pathways involved in the development and progression of these lymphomas, but will also provide new diagnostic and prognostic criteria as well as molecular targets for therapeutic intervention.

REFERENCES

1. Willemze R, Kerl H, Sterry W, et al. EORTC classification for primary cutaneous lymphoma: a proposal from the Cutaneous Lymphoma Study Group of the European Organization for Research and Treatment of Cancer. Blood 1997;90:354–71.
2. Evans H, Winkelmann R, and Banks P. Differential diagnosis of malignant and benign cutaneous infiltrates. Cancer 1979; 44:699–717.
3. Pink-Fuches R, Zenahlik P, Bäck B, et al. Primary cutaneous lymphomas: applicability of current classification schemes (EORTC, WHO) based on clinicopathologic features observed in a large group of patients. Blood 2002;99:800–5.
4. Zackheim HS, Vonderheid EC, Ramsay DL, et al. Relative frequency of various forms of primary cutaneous lymphomas. J Am Acad Dermatol 2000:43:793–6.
5. Rijlaarsdam JU and Willemze R. Cutaneous pseudolymphomas: classification and differential diagnosis. Semin Dermatol 1994;13:187–96.
6. Cerroni L, Zöchling N, Pütz B, et al. Infection by Borrelia burgdorferi and cutaneous B-cell lymphoma. J Cutan Pathol 1997;24:457–61.
7. Goodlad JR, Davidson MM, Hollowood K, et al. Primary cutaneous B-cell lymphoma and Borrelia burgdorferi infection in patients from the Highlands of Scotland. Am J Surg Pathol 2000;24:1279–85.
8. Kütting B, Bonsmann G, Metze D, et al. Borrelia burgdorferi-associated primary cutaneous B-cell lymphoma: complete clearing of skin lesions after antibiotic pulse therapy or intralesional injection of interferon alfa-2a. J Am Acad Dermatol 1997;36:311–4.
9. Roggero E, Zucca E, Mainetti C, et al. Eradication of Borrelia burgdorferi infection in primary marginal zone B-cell lymphoma of the skin. Hum Pathol 2000;31:263–8.
10. Garbe C, Stein H, Dienemann D, et al. Borrelia burgdorferi associated cutaneous B cell lymphoma: clinical and immunohistochemical characterization of four cases. J Am Acad Dermatol 1991;24:584–90.
11. Sangueza OP, Yadav S, White CR, et al. Evolution of B-cell lymphoma from pseudolymphoma. Am J Dermatopathol 1992;14:408–13.
12. Gilliam AC and Wood GS. Cutaneous lymphoid hyperplasias. Semin Cutan Med Surg 2000;19:133–41.
13. Wood GS,Kamath NV, Guitart J, et al. Absence of Borrelia burgdorferi DNA in cutaneous B-cell lymphomas from the United States. J Cutan Pathol 2001;28:502–7.
14. Li C, Inagaki H, Kuo T, et al. Primary cutaneous marginal zone B-cell lymphoma. A molecular and clinicopathologic study of 24 Asian cases. Am J Surg Pathol 2003;27:1061–9.
15. Slater DN. MALT and SALT: the clue to cutaneous B-cell lymphoproliferative disease. Br J Dermatol 1994;131:557–61.

16. Goodlad JR and Hollowood K. Primary cutaneous B-cell lymphoma. Curr Diag Pathol 2001;7:33–44.
17. Rijlaarsdam, JU, Bakels V, van Oostveen JW, et al. Demonstration of clonal immunoglobulin gene rearrangements in cutaneous B-cell lymphomas and pseudo-B-cell lymphomas: differential diagnostic and pathogenetic aspects. J Invest Dermatol 1992;99:749–54.
18. Nihal M, Mikkola D, Horvath N, et al. Cutaneous lymphoid hyperplasia. A lymphoproliferative continuum with lymphomatous potential. Hum Pathol 2003;34:617–22.
19. Streubel B, Lamprecht A, Dierlamm J, et al. T(14;18)(q32;q21) involving IGH and MALT1 is a frequent chromosomal aberration in MALT lymphoma. Blood 2003; 101:2335–9.
20. Ye H, Liu H, Attygalle A, et al. Variable frequencies of t(11;18)(q21;q21) in MALT lymphomas of different sites: significant association with CagA strains of H pylori in gastric MALT lymphoma. Blood 2003;102:1012–8.
21. Gronbaek K, Ralfkiaer E, Kalla J, et al. Infrequent somatic Fas mutations but no evidence of Bcl-10 mutations or t(11;18) in primary cutaneous MALT-type lymphoma. J Pathol 2003;201: 134–40.
22. Schreuder MI, Hoefnagel JJ, Jansen PM, et al. FISH analysis of MALT lymphoma-specific translocations and aneuploidy in primary cutaneous marginal zone lymphoma. J Pathol 2005;205:302–10.
23. Jaffe ES, Harris NL, Stein H, et al. World Health Organization Classification of Tumours. Pathology and Genetics of Tumours of Haematopoietic and Lymphoid Tissues. Lyon: IARC Press, 2001.
24. Willemze R, Jaffe ES, Burg G, et al. WHO-EORTC classification for cutaneous lymphomas. Blood 2005;105: 68–85.
25. Willemze R, Meijer CJLM, Sentis HJ, et al. Primary cutaneous large cell lymphomas of follicular center cell origin. J Am Acad Dermatol 1987;16:518–26.
26. Berti E, Alessi E, Caputo R, et al. Reticulohistiocytoma of the dorsum. J Am Acad Dermatol 1988;19:259–72.
27. Santucci M, Pimpinelli N, and Arganini L. Primary cutaneous B-cell lymphoma: A unique type of low-grade lymphoma. Cancer 1991;67:2311–26.
28. Rijlaarsdam JU, Toonstra J, Meijer CJLM, et al. Treatment of primary cutaneous B-cell lymphomas of follicular center cell origin. A clinical follow-up study of 55 patients treated with radiotherapy or polychemotherapy. J Clin Oncol 1996;14:549–55.
29. Grange F, Bekkenk MW, Wechsler J, et al. Prognostic factors in primary cutaneous large B-cell lymphomas: A European multicenter study. J Clin Oncol 2001;19:3602–10.
30. Vermeer MH, Geelen FAMJ, van Haselen CW, et al. Primary cutaneous large B-cell lymphomas of the legs. A distinct type of cutaneous B-cell lymphoma with an intermediate prognosis. Arch Dermatol 1996;132:1304–8.
31. Rijlaarsdam JU, van der Putte SCJ, Berti E, et al. Cutaneous immunocytomas: a clinicopathologic study of 26 cases. Histopathology 1993;23:119–25.
32. Schmid U, Eckert F, Griesser H, et al. Cutaneous follicular lymphoid hyperplasia with monotypic plasma cells. A clinicopathologic study of 18 patients. Am J Surg Pathol 1995;19:12–20.
33. Torne R, Su WPD, Smolle J, et al. Clinicopathologic study of cutaneous plasmacytoma. Int J Dermatol 1990;29:562–6.
34. Cerroni L, Signoretti S, Höfler G, et al. Primary cutaneous marginal zone B-cell lymphoma: a recently described entity of low-grade malignant cutaneous B-cell lymphoma. Am J Surg Pathol 1997;21:1307–15.
35. Bailey EM, Ferry JA, Harris NL, et al. Marginal zone lymphoma (low-grade B-cell lymphoma of mucosa-associated lymphoid tissue type) of skin and subcutaneous tissue: a study of 15 patients. Am J Surg Pathol 1996;20:1011–23.
36. Hoefnagel JJ, Vermeer MH, Jansen PM, et al. Primary cutaneous marginal zone B-cell lymphoma: clinical and therapeutic features of 50 patients. Arch Dermatol 2005 (in press).
37. de Leval L, Harris NL, Longtine J, et al. Cutaneous B-cell lymphomas of follicular and marginal zone types. Use of Bcl-6, CD10, Bcl-2, and CD21 in differential diagnosis and classification. Am J Surg Pathol 2001;25:732–741.
38. Hoefnagel JJ, Vermeer MH, Janssen PM, et al. Bcl-2, Bcl-6 and CD10 expression in cutaneous B-cell lymphoma: further support for a follicle centre cell origin and differential diagnostic significance. Br J Dermatol 2003;149:1183–1191.
39. Streubel B, Vinatzer U, Lamprecht A, et al. T(3;14)(p14.1;q32) involving IGH and FOXP1 is a novel recurrent chromosomal aberration in MALT lymphoma. Leukemia 2005;19: 652–8
40. Hallermann C, Kaune KM, Gesk S, et al. Molecular cytogenetic analysis of chromosomal breakpoints in the IGH, MYC, BCL6 and MALT1 gene loci in primary cutaneous B-cell lymphomas. J Invest Dermatol 2004:123:213–9.
41. Zenahlik P, Pink-Fuches R, Kapp KS, et al. Therapy of primary cutaneous B-cell lymphomas. Hautarzt 2000;51:19–24.
42. Bekkenk M, Vermeer MH, Geerts ML, et al. Treatment of multifocal primary cutaneous B-cell lymphoma: guidelines of the Dutch Cutaneous Lymphoma Group. J Clin Oncol 1999;17: 2471–8.
43. Cerroni L, Arzberger E, Pütz B, et al. Primary cutaneous follicular center cell lymphoma with follicular growth pattern. Blood 2000;95:3922–8.
44. Goodlad JR, Krajewski AS, Batstone PJ, et al. Primary cutaneous follicular lymphoma. A clinicopathologic and molecular study of 16 cases in support of a distinct entity. Am J Surg Pathol 2002;26:733–41.
45. Willemze R, Meijer CJLM, and Scheffer E. Diffuse large cell lymphomas of follicle center cell origin presenting in the skin. A clinicopathologic and immunologic study of 16 patients. Am J Pathol 1987;126:325–33.
46. Cerroni L, El-Shabrawi-Caelen L, Pink-Fuches R, et al. Cutaneous spindle-cell lymphoma: a morphologic variant of cutaneous large B-cell lymphoma. Am J Dermatopathol 2000;22:299–309.
47. Cerroni L, Volkenandt M, Rieger E, et al. Bcl-2 protein expression and correlation with the interchromosomal (14;18) translocation in cutaneous lymphomas and pseudolymphomas. J Invest Dermatol 1994;102:231–5.
48. Geelen FAMJ, Vermeer MH, Meijer CJLM, et al. Bcl-2 expression in primary cutaneous large B-cell lymphoma is site-related. J Clin Oncol 1998;16:2080–5.
49. Hoefnagel JJ, Dijkman R, Basso K, et al. Distinct types of primary cutaneous large B-cell lymphoma identified by gene expression profiling. Blood 2005;105:3671–9.
50. Aarts WM, Willemze R, Bende RJ, et al. VH gene analysis of primary cutaneous B-cell lymphomas: evidence for ongoing somatic hypermutation and isotype switching. Blood 1998; 92:3857–64.
51. Gellrich S, Rutz S, Golembowski S, et al. Primary cutaneous follicle center cell lymphomas and large B-cell lymphomas of the leg descend from germinal center cells. A single cell polymerase chain reaction analysis. J Invest Dermatol 2001;117:1512–20.
52. Child FJ, Russell-Jones R, Woolford AJ, et al. Absence of the t(14,18) chromosomal translocation in primary cutaneous B-cell lymphoma. Br J Dermatol 2001;144:735–44.
53. Aguilera NS, Tomaszewski MM, Moad JC, et al. Cutaneous follicle center lymphoma: a clinicopathologic study of 19 cases. Mod Pathol 2001;14:828–35.

54. Mirza I, Macpherson S, Paproski S, et al. Primary cutaneous follicular lymphoma: an assessment of clinical, histopathologic, immunophenotypic, and molecular features. J Clin Oncol 2002;20:647–55.
55. Dijkman R, Tensen CP, Jordanova ES, et al. Array-based CGH analysis reveals recurrent chromosomal alterations and prognostic parameters in primary cutaneous large B-cell lymphoma. J Clin Oncol 2005 (in press).
56. Pimpinelli N and Vallecchi C. Local orthovolt radiotherapy in primary cutaneous B-cell lymphomas. Results in a series of 115 patients. Skin Cancer 1999;14:219–24.
57. Piccino R, Caccialanza M, and Berti E. Dermatologic radiotherapy of primary cutaneous follicle center cell lymphoma. Eur J Dermatol 2003;13:49–52.
58. Smith BD, Glusac EJ, McNiff JM, et al. Primary cutaneous B-cell lymphoma treated with radiotherapy: acomparison of the European Organization for Research and Treatment of Cancer and the WHO classification systems. J Clin Oncol 2004;22:634–9.
59. Heinzerling LM, Urbanek M, Funk JO, et al. Reduction of tumor burden and stabilization of disease by systemic therapy with anti-CD20 antibody (rituximab) in patients with primary cutaneous B-cell lymphoma. Cancer 2000;89:1835–44.
60. Gellrich S, Muche JM, Pelzer K, et al. Anti-CD20 antibodies in primary cutaneous B-cell lymphoma. Initial results in dermatologic patients. Hautarzt 2001;52:205–10.
61. Paul T, Radny P, Krober SM, et al. Intralesional rituximab for cutaneous B-cell lymphoma. Br J Dermatol 2001;144: 1239–43.
62. Goodlad JR, Krajewski AS, Batstone PJ, et al. Primary cutaneous diffuse large B-cell lymphoma. Prognostic significance and clinicopathologic subtypes. Am J Surg Pathol 2003;27:1538–45.
63. Grange F, Petrella T, Beylot-Barry M, et al. Bcl-2 protein expression is the strongest independent prognostic factor of survival in primary cutaneous large B-cell lymphomas. Blood 2004;103:3662–8.
64. Paulli M, Viglio A, Vivenza D, et al. Primary cutaneous large B-cell lymphoma of the leg: histogenetic analysis of a controversial clinicopathologic entity. Hum Pathol 2002;33: 937–43.
65. Mao X, Lillington D, Child FJ, et al. Comparative genomic hybridization analysis of primary cutaneous B-cell lymphomas: identification of common genomic alterations in disease pathogenesis. Genes Chromosomes Cancer 2002;35:144–55.
66. Hallerman C, Kaune K, Siebert R, et al. Cytogenetic aberration patterns differ in subtypes of primary cutaneous B-cell lymphomas. J Invest Dermatol 2004;122:1495–502.
67. Brogan BL, Zic JA, Kinney MC, et al. Large B-cell lymphoma of the leg: clinical and pathologic characteristics in a North American series. J Am Acad Dermatol 2003;49:223–8.
68. Sander CA, Medeiros LJ, Abruzzo LV, et al. Lymphoblastic lymphoma presenting in cutaneous sites. A clinicopathologic analysis of six cases. J Am Acad Dermatol 1991;25:1023–31.
69. Sander CA, Kaudewitz P, Kutzner H, et al. T-cell rich B-cell lymphoma presenting in the skin. A clinicopathologic analysis of six cases. J Cutan Pathol 1996;23:101–8.
70. Perniciaro C, Winkelmann RK, Daoud MS, et al. Malignant angioendotheliomatosis is an angiotropic intravascular lymphoma. Immunohistochemical, ultrastructural and molecular genetic studies. Am J Dermatopathol 1995;17:242–48.
71. Ferreri AJM, Campo E, Seymour JF, et al. Intravascular lymphoma: clinical presentation, natural history, management and prognostic factors in a series of 38 cases with special emphasis on the "cutaneous variant." Br J Haematol 2004; 127:173–83.
72. Lin P, Jones D, Dorfman DM, et al. Precursor B-cell lymphoblastic lymphoma. A predominantly extranodal tumor with low propensity for leukemic involvement. Am J Surg Pathol 2000;24:1480–90.
73. Li S, Griffin CA, Mann RB, et al. Primary cutaneous T-cell rich B-cell lymphoma: clinically distinct from its nodal counterpart? Mod Pathol 2001;14:10–3.

25

Primary Cutaneous Lymphomas

Richard T. Hoppe, M.D.
Youn Y. Kim, M.D.
Ranjana Advani, M.D.

Primary cutaneous lymphomas involve only the skin and affect other sites only secondarily. They include mycosis fungoides (MF) and Sézary syndrome (SS), as well as other T-cell, B-cell, and miscellaneous non-Hodgkin's lymphomas.

MYCOSIS FUNGOIDES AND SÉZARY SYNDROME

Mycosis fungoides is a cutaneous lymphoma of mature, predominately CD4+ T cells. It is the most common type of cutaneous T-cell lymphoma. The Sézary syndrome is an erythrodermic, leukemic variant of MF.[1] Other cutaneous T-cell lymphomas include some anaplastic large-cell lymphomas and peripheral T-cell lymphoma.

Epidemiology

Mycosis fungoides accounts for only 2% to 3% of cases of non-Hodgkin's lymphoma. The estimated annual incidence rate in the United States is 0.29 per 100,000, which is nearly twice that reported in Western Europe.[2] There are 500 to 600 new cases and 100 to 200 deaths attributable to MF in the United States annually. It commonly affects older adults (median age 55 to 60 years), and the male-to-female ratio is 2:1.

Etiology

The etiology of MF/SS is unknown. Some retrospective studies have suggested a role for chemical exposure as a source of either chronic antigenic stimulation or toxic exposure. However, recent case–control studies refute this hypothesis.[3,4] Although a viral etiology for MF was once proposed, based on the isolation of human T-cell leukemia/lymphoma virus 1 (HTLV-1) from the peripheral blood lymphocytes of a patient with a cutaneous lymphoma that resembled MF, HTLV-1–associated T-cell lymphoma is now recognized as an independent entity.

Pathology

The essential criteria for a diagnosis of MF vary among pathologists, and there may be inter- and intraobserver disagreement.[5] The characteristic histopathology of MF includes mild epidermal hyperplasia, a perivascular or band-like infiltrate of atypical lymphocytes, and an intraepidermal infiltrate of mononuclear cells that may be present in clusters, called "Pautrier's microabscesses." Although these clusters are not essential, abnormal cells must be present in the epidermis ("epidermotropism") to make a firm diagnosis. An upper dermal infiltrate includes similar cells, in addition to histiocytes, eosinophils, and plasma cells. Under oil immersion light microscopy, the nuclei of the neoplastic mononuclear cells have a hyperconvoluted surface. Electron microscopic studies demonstrate marked infolding of the nuclear membrane, which produces a cerebriform appearance.[6] As lesions evolve clinically from patches to plaques, the density of neoplastic cells within the dermis may increase. In tumorous lesions, the dermal infiltrate may involve the full thickness of the dermis. However, the infiltrate density and extent of involvement of the epidermis may be minimal in patients with the SS or erythrodermic variant of MF.

Functional studies and monoclonal antibody staining demonstrate that most cases of MF are associated with the helper T-cell phenotype (CD4+).[7] However, there may be a loss of other mature T-cell antigens such as CD-7, and this may help in the differential diagnosis of MF.[8] Most cases of conventional MF are CD2+, CD3+, CD4+, CD8–, CD5+, CD7–, CD25–/+, and CD30–. Rare cases have a CD8+ (cytotoxic/suppressor) T-cell phenotype.

Lymph nodes involved with MF show a range of histologic features. Often, they only demonstrate the changes of dermatopathic lymphadenitis with a small number of atypical lymphocytes with cerebriform nuclei. The potential prognostic relevance of various degrees of infiltration by these abnormal cells led to the development of a lymph node classification system.

Lymph nodes are classified as LN-0 to LN-4 corresponding to lymph node involvement ranging from "no atypical lymphocytes" (LN-0) to "partial or complete replacement of nodal architecture by atypical lymphocytes or frankly neoplastic cells" (LN-4). This descriptive system for grading lymph node involvement has been shown to have prognostic relevance.[9]

Southern blot analysis has demonstrated monoclonal rearrangements of the T-cell receptors in the skin, lymph nodes, and peripheral blood of patients with MF. These rearrangements are concordant about 80% of the time in multiple lesions from a single patient.[10,11] Genotyping, the evaluation of skin biopsies to detect T-cell receptor gene rearrangements, is sometimes helpful in the differential diagnosis of early lesions of MF.

Natural History

Mycosis fungoides often has a long natural history. A "premycotic" phase is characterized by nonspecific, slightly scaling skin lesions and nondiagnostic biopsies. These lesions may wax and wane over a period of years, and during this phase, patients may respond to treatment with topical corticosteroids. Some experience an evolution of the disease and develop more typical patches or infiltrated plaques with diagnostic biopsy changes.

The typical patches of MF are erythematous and slightly scaling. The disease is often present in the "bathing trunk" distribution, although any part of the body may be involved. Sometimes the sites of disease are curiously symmetric. The palms or soles may be heavily involved, or they may be spared. Scalp involvement may cause alopecia. Pruritus is common.

More infiltrated lesions are present as palpable plaques that are erythematous, slightly scaling, and have variable shape and well-defined borders. Infiltrated plaques may evolve into nodules, or ulcerated or exophytic tumors. These may become infected, and sepsis secondary to infection may ensue. Generalized dermal thickening from infiltrative disease may cause the classic but highly unusual "leonine facies" of MF.

Some patients may demonstrate only the patch phase throughout the course of their disease. However, others demonstrate progression from patches to plaques and finally to tumorous involvement. The rapidity of this progression is unpredictable. The development of extracutaneous disease may be accompanied by cytologic transformation, with the appearance of large cells comprising greater than 25% of the dermal infiltrate, similar to those seen in large-cell lymphoma. The large cells may express lymphocyte activation markers such as CD30 and CD25, and there may be an increase in Ki-67 positivity.[12,13]

Another manifestation of skin involvement in MF is generalized erythroderma. The skin may be either atrophic or lichenified. The erythroderma is accompanied by cold intolerance and intense pruritus. These patients may also have lymphadenopathy and circulating abnormal cells in the peripheral blood, known as the Sézary syndrome.[14] Although patients with erythroderma usually present in that phase of skin involvement, patients occasionally develop erythroderma superimposed over preexisting plaque or tumorous disease.

In individual patients, MF may have systemic manifestations from the outset, but progressive skin disease usually precedes lymph node and visceral involvement. The likelihood of developing clinical evidence of extracutaneous disease during a patient's lifetime ranges from 2% for limited plaque disease to 40% for tumorous involvement.[15] The first manifestation of extracutaneous disease is often in peripheral nodes draining the sites of the most extensive skin involvement. Lymph node involvement tends to be peripheral, with central nodal areas such as the mediastinum and para-aortic nodes involved only late in the course of disease. Visceral disease may follow documented lymph node involvement. The involved visceral sites most commonly identified include the lungs, upper aerodigestive tract, central nervous system, spleen, and liver, but virtually any organ may be involved at autopsy.[16]

Staging

The most useful staging classification system for MF is the Tumor, Node, Metastasis, Blood (TNMB) system first proposed at the Workshop on Mycosis Fungoides held at the National Cancer Institute (NCI) in 1978.[17] Tables 25–1 and 25–2 summarize the TNMB categories and staging classification.

Table 25–1. TNMB Classification for Mycosis Fungoides

T (Skin)	
T1	Limited patch/plaque (<10% of total skin surface)
T2	Generalized patch/plaque (≧10% of total skin surface)
T3	Tumors
T4	Generalized erythroderma
N (Nodes)	
N0	Lymph nodes clinically uninvolved
N1	Lymph nodes enlarged, histologically uninvolved (includes "reactive" and "dermatopathic" nodes)
N2	Lymph nodes clinically uninvolved, histologically involved
N3	Lymph nodes enlarged and histologically involved
M (Viscera)	
M0	No visceral involvement
M1	Visceral involvement
B (Blood)	
B0	No circulating atypical (Sézary) cells (<5% of lymphocytes)
B1	Circulating atypical (Sézary) cells (≧5% of lymphocytes)

The T stage represents the extent of skin involvement, and it correlates closely with survival.[18] The N stage indicates the presence or absence of lymph node involvement. A biopsy specimen of enlarged lymph nodes should always be obtained, since palpable enlargement may be associated only with dermatopathic lymphadenitis, which has only minor prognostic significance.[9,19] It is only when frank lymph node involvement is detected (LN-3 or LN-4) that the prognosis is substantially worse.

The M category defines visceral disease. Suspected sites of visceral involvement should be confirmed by biopsy. Other neoplasms, as well as benign diseases, may be confused with MF if a diagnosis is based solely on imaging studies. This is important, since the presence of visceral disease has important prognostic implications.[20] Treatment

Table 25–2. Clinical Staging System for Mycosis Fungoides

Clinical Stages	Tumor, Node, Metastasis Classification[a]		
IA	T1	N0	M0
IB	T2	N0	M0
IIA	T1-2	N1	M0
IIB	T3	N0-1	M0
IIIA	T4	N0	M0
IIIB	T4	N1	M0
IVA	T1-4	N2-3	M0
IVB	T1-4	N0-3	M1

[a]The "B" classification does not alter clinical stage.

programs for visceral disease should be considered only if definite proof of extracutaneous disease exists.

The B category signifies the absence or presence of a significant proportion of abnormal cells in the peripheral blood. For a definitive diagnosis, they should number at least 1000/mm^3. Alternatively, there may be an increased ratio of CD4:CD8 T lymphocytes that is greater than 10:1, or molecular evidence of a T-cell receptor gene rearrangement within either the peripheral blood or skin.[21] The presence of blood involvement is not an independent prognostic factor and does not alter the stage classification, but it is closely linked with the extent of skin involvement and presence of extracutaneous disease.[9]

All patients with MF should undergo at least a limited staging evaluation, including a careful examination of the skin and lymph nodes, complete blood count, Sézary count, screening chemistries, including lactose dehydrogenase (LDH) and a chest radiograph. Additional imaging studies for patients with T1 or T2 skin involvement are not recommended unless the patient has lymphadenopathy. However, patients with T3 or T4 disease are at increased risk for extracutaneous involvement, and further imaging such as a chest/abdomen/pelvis CT scan is reasonable. The utility of nuclear medicine scans such as PET has not been established, but is being studied. Lymph node biopsies should be obtained if lymphadenopathy is present. Suspected sites of visceral involvement should be confirmed by appropriate biopsy. Bone marrow involvement may often be detected in patients who meet the clinical criteria for Sézary syndrome,[22] but is extremely uncommon in classic MF. Therefore, a bone marrow biopsy is not routinely used as part of the initial staging.

Therapy

The treatment intent for MF/SS is usually palliative. Although some patients with minimal manifestations of disease may have prolonged disease-free intervals following limited therapy, this is the exception. The majority of patients will experience intermittent, albeit often nonthreatening, manifestations of disease, throughout their lifetimes.

For the treatment of minor manifestations of MF, topical corticosteroids may achieve good responses and provide short-term palliation for pruritus and xerosis. However, complete responses are uncommon, and this treatment does not alter the long-term course of the disease. Additional symptomatic measures include aggressive emolliation and oral antipruritics.

More definitive treatment of MF is often challenging, but the response rates to standard topical therapies such as phototherapy, topical chemotherapy, or irradiation are gratifying. Many patients are symptomatic at the time of diagnosis, warranting the prompt initiation of treatment.

Phototherapy

Phototherapy includes ultraviolet (UV) radiation in the form of UVA or UVB wavelengths, used alone, together, or with psoralen, a photosensitizing agent, as psoralen plus UVA or PUVA. Long-wave UVA has the advantage over UVB in its greater depth of penetration. For early patch disease, UVB alone or home UV phototherapy (UVA + UVB) has been shown to be effective.[23,24]

Psoralen plus ultraviolet A (PUVA) therapy consists of treatment with 8-methoxypsoralen, an oral photosensitizing drug, followed by controlled exposure to long-wave ultraviolet light (UVA) in a specially designed box. Psoralen intercalates with DNA in the presence of UVA in the 320- to 400-nm range, forming monofunctional and bifunctional adducts with DNA base pairs, which inhibit DNA synthesis. The effective depth of penetration of the UVA includes the epidermis and upper dermis, making it ideally suited for the treatment of MF, especially patches or minimally infiltrated plaques.

During the induction (clearing) phase, which may require as long as 6 months, patients are treated two or three times weekly with a dose (in joules) that varies with the patient's skin type, severity of skin reaction, and degree of response. After the clearing phase has been completed, patients continue on a less frequent maintenance program. If the disease begins to recur during the maintenance phase, then the frequency of treatment is increased to achieve better control.

The most common acute complications of PUVA therapy include erythema and blistering. These risks are highest among patients with erythroderma, who must be treated with very low exposures to UVA. Patients shield their skin from sunlight with sunscreens and protective clothing for at least 24 hours following psoralen ingestion. Cataract formation and secondary cutaneous malignancies are the most important potential long-term complications of PUVA. To reduce the risk of cataracts, patients wear specially designed ultraviolet glasses while outdoors.

The results of PUVA therapy have been reported from several centers. The clearance rate is 50% to 90% and varies with the initial extent of skin involvement. Studies using PUVA alone for erythrodermic (Stage III) patients have reported complete response rates of 33% to 70%.[25–27] The response of infiltrated plaques or tumors may be accelerated by the addition of localized irradiation.

Indications for PUVA treatment include the primary therapy of patients with T1 or T2 disease or as a secondary therapy following the failure of other topical modalities. Patients with erythroderma may also be suitable candidates for PUVA, provided that very low daily exposures are used to avoid phototoxic reactions.[25] PUVA, combined with systemic biologic therapy such as interferon or bexarotene, or chemotherapy such as chlorambucil, is one approach to the management of patients with SS.

Home phototherapy is another form of phototherapy.[24] Home phototherapy units with light sources that emit ultraviolet light in the UVA and UVB range (280 to 350 nm) are available for general use. Patients expose themselves to the ultraviolet treatment without using psoralen. Exposures are timed carefully to minimize adverse skin reactions. This treatment approach is most useful in patients who are fair skinned and have minimally infiltrative disease. Some of these patients may remain disease-free, even after discontinuation of therapy.

Topical Chemotherapy

Topical nitrogen mustard (mechlorethamine, HN2) is an effective topical therapy for MF.[28–30] The mechanism of action when HN2 is applied topically is not clear, and may not be related simply to its alkylating agent properties. Its activity may be mediated by immune mechanisms or by interaction with the epidermal cell/Langerhans cell/T-cell axis. There is no detectable systemic absorption of topical HN2; hematologic monitoring during therapy is unnecessary.[31]

Nitrogen mustard may be mixed in water or in an ointment base (Aquaphor), generally in a concentration of 10 to 20 mg/dL. It is applied at least once daily during the clearing phase. The HN2 may be applied locally or to the entire skin. New areas of disease activity may become evident secondary to the inflammatory reaction provoked by the HN2. After a period of several weeks, treatment may then be limited to the affected region. Alternatively, if the disease is initially limited in distribution, the HN2 may be applied only to the affected anatomical region(s), with careful follow-up to detect any new areas of involvement. The concentration of the drug and frequency of application may be changed, depending on tolerance and response. The average time to skin clearance is 6 to 8 months. Maintenance treatment is continued for 1 to 3 months following documentation of response.

The most common complication of topical HN2 is a cutaneous hypersensitivity reaction, which occurs in as many as 30% of patients treated with the aqueous solution, and about 5% of patients treated with the ointment base.[32] Hypersensitivity reactions may be overcome by a variety of topical or systemic desensitization programs.[28] The primary long-term hazard of long-term HN2 use is the potential development of secondary squamous and basal cell cancers.[28,30] This risk is the greatest among patients who have had long-term sequential therapy with HN2, PUVA, and irradiation, and is only a minor risk after treatment with HN2 alone.[33]

Nearly all patients treated with topical HN2 respond to treatment. The complete response rate for limited patch/plaque (T1) disease is 70% to 80%. When treatment is discontinued, more than half of patients will relapse in the skin, but most will respond to a resumption of therapy. The proportion of patients treated with topical HN2 who have a durable complete response (more than 10 years) is 20% to 25%. In patients with a discrete number of refractory lesions, treatment may be supplemented with local irradiation.

Topical Retinoids

Bexarotene (Targretin) 1% gel is the most commonly used topical retinoid for treating MF. The reported overall response rate is 63%, and the complete response rate is 21%.[34] Bexarotene gel is applied with a thin application to the patches or plaques only, and is most effective when used twice daily. Due to its irritant effect, it is only feasible to use bexarotene when there is a discrete number of patches or plaques. It is not intended for generalized application. The most common toxicity of bexarotene is irritation at the sites of application, which occurs in the majority of patients, but with variable intensity. Because of the erythema from the irritant reaction, it may be necessary to withhold therapy for a few weeks to assess for residual active disease.

Radiation Therapy

Mycosis fungoides is an exquisitely radiosensitive neoplasm, and ionizing irradiation is the most effective agent for its treatment. Irradiation may be exploited in multiple ways.[35] Individual plaques or tumors may be treated with small-field irradiation for palliation. Complete response of individual lesions is generally achieved with doses greater than 20 Gy, although higher doses may be necessary to ensure long-term local control. Since the response to treatment is prompt, the total dose may be titrated to response. Small daily doses (1.25 to 1.5 Gy) may be used, especially in areas such as the eyelids and face, to minimize normal tissue reactions.

Radiation may be an effective palliative treatment for patients with extracutaneous MF, especially involving lymph nodes. Extensive or symptomatic nodal involvement may be treated with total doses similar to those used for cutaneous disease (~30 Gy). Other extracutaneous sites that may be palliated effectively with irradiation include the brain, upper aerodigestive, and gastrointestinal tracts.

In the late 1950s, techniques were developed to permit the treatment of large skin surfaces by means of electrons.[36,37] Commercially available linear accelerators may be modified to treat patients in the standing position at an extended distance to achieve the large field size. By standing in multiple positions (or on a rotational platform), the entire skin surface may be irradiated. The total skin electron beam therapy (TSEBT) technique employed at Stanford University Medical Center (and adopted at many other specialized centers) uses a six-field technique (anterior, posterior, and four opposed oblique fields). Treatment is administered four times per week, 4 Gy per week, to a total dose of 30 to 36 Gy. An electron energy of 9 MeV provides an 80% depth dose at 0.8 cm.[38] Only the eyes are shielded routinely.

The acute complications of TSEBT include acute erythema, desquamation, and temporary epilation. Patients experience temporary loss of their fingernails and toenails (usually after the completion of therapy), as well as an inability to sweat for 6 to 12 months. In most patients, a few scattered telangiectasia and tendency to dry skin are the only long-term effects of treatment when the technique was administered properly. There may be an increased risk of secondary squamous and basal cell cancers of the skin in long-term follow-up, but this is most evident in patients who have received protracted therapy with a variety of topical agents, including PUVA and topical HN2.[33]

A number of centers have developed expertise in the use of TSEBT.[37,39,40,41] Nearly all patients respond to treatment, with response rates dependent on the extent of skin involvement. At Stanford, the reported complete response rates are 98%, 64%, 34%, and 36% for patients with T1, T2, T3, and T4 disease, respectively. Topical treatment with HN2 is often employed as an adjuvant after completion of TSEBT to prolong the response duration.[42] Maintenance PUVA treatment may be used in a similar fashion.

Just over one half of patients with limited plaque disease (T1) and about 20% of patients with generalized plaque disease (T2) remain free of disease more than 5 years after completion of a single course of TSEBT.[37,41] Although the curative potential of this treatment is questioned, it definitely provides an important palliative benefit, especially for patients with extensive disease. In addition, when disease recurs after TSEBT, it is often in a limited distribution and may be controlled readily with local topical therapy.

Occasionally, patients who have had an initial good response to TSEBT and later develop progressive disease may be candidates for a repeat course of treatment. In addition to an initial good response, these patients should have exhausted other topical therapies and have generalized progressive or refractory disease. Ideally, they should also have had a good duration of initial response. Second courses of treatment to total doses of 20 to 35 Gy with standard fractionation are tolerated well.[43]

Chemotherapy

The efficacy of systemic chemotherapy in the management of MF has been disappointing.[44,45] Although only a minority of patients with MF (10% to 20%) require chemotherapy for systemic disease, it may be an important component of palliative treatment for patients with SS or refractory cutaneous disease.[14,44] There are many chemotherapeutic agents that are active in the treatment of lymphomas, including alkylating agents, antimetabolites, antitumor antibiotics, vinca alkaloids, topoisomerase II inhibitors, corticosteroids, and others. Virtually all of these drugs that are effective as single agents or in combination therapy in the treatment of patients with other lymphomas have been tested in MF.[45]

SINGLE AGENT CHEMOTHERAPY

A review by Bunn et al.[46] summarized the experience from several single-agent trials. Among 526 patients reported in these trials, the complete remission (CR) rate was 32%, and the median duration of response ranged from 3 to 22 months. Based on this review, the authors suggested that no particular single agent is preferred to another.

No large randomized studies comparing different single agents have been reported. Most of the existing data pertain to methotrexate, which is active in many doses and schedules.[47–49] It is not clear that high-dose methotrexate with leucovorin rescue is superior to lower-dose methotrexate therapy without leucovorin rescue.[48–50] Recently, Zackheim and Epstein[50] updated their experience with low-dose methotrexate. The overall response rate (ORR) was 33% and the time-to-treatment failure (TTTF) was 15 months in T2 disease. In an earlier report, the same group had reported an overall response rate of 58% and TTTF of 31 months in 29 patients with erythrodermic MF. A possible reason for the inferior outcome in the more current series of patients with T2 disease was attributed to the fact that the erythrodermic patients in the prior study were less heavily pretreated. However, it may also simply be that patients with erythroderma are simply more responsive to systemic therapy than patients with more classic, infiltrative disease.

Another commonly used chemotherapy is chlorambucil[51] administered daily in 2-mg doses, titrating the dose according to hematologic toxicity. Prednisone may also be given in combination with chlorambucil, generally at a dose of 20 mg/day, with a taper as palliation is achieved.

Some newer drugs have shown encouraging single activity and are summarized in Table 25–3. The purine analogues are drugs that have demonstrated activity in MF and a variety of other lymphomas. T cells have a high level of adenosine deaminase (ADA), a key enzyme in the purine degradation pathway. The purine analogues pentostatin (deoxycofromycin), fludarabine, and cladribine (2 CDA) are a group of structurally similar agents that were developed to target ADA. They have different interactions with ADA, but all result in DNA damage. The most experience has been with pentostatin.[52] In these small studies, the response rates vary from 14% to 70%.[52–54] 2-CDA[55,56] and fludarabine[57,58] have also been used, with response rates reported to be 20% to 40%. It is not clear whether one agent is superior to another. Hematologic toxicities and infection are the most common toxicities associated with this class of drugs. A decrease in the CD4 count is consistently seen, leading to long-term immunosuppression that may increase

Table 25–3. Systemic Chemotherapy in the Management of Mycosis Fungoides

Study	Therapy	Patients	ORR n (%)	CR n (%)	Median Duration of Response (months)
Single-Agent Therapy					
Bunn (1994)[46]	Single-agent chemotherapy	528	329 (62)	91 (33)	3–32
Zackheim (1989)[50]	Low-dose methotrexate	69	20 (33)	13 (22)	15
Winkleman (1984)[101]	Chlorambucil + prednisone	21	11 (57)	3 (14)	Not reported
Dearden (2000)[52]	Pentostatin	13	7 (54)	1 (7)	Not reported
Tsimberidon (2004)[53]	Pentostatin	32	13 (54.8)	6 (14)	4.3
Saven (1992)[55]	2 CDA	15	7 (47)	3 (20)	5
Kuzel (1996)[56]	2 CDA	21	6 (28)	3 (14)	2–16
Zinzani (2000)[61]	Gemcitabine	30	21 (70)	5 (11)	6–22
Wollina (2000)[62]	Liposomal doxorubicin	6	5 (83)	4/6	Not reported
Combination Therapy					
Bunn (1994)[46]	Combination	331	(81)	(38)	5–41
Kaye (1989)[90]	CAVE	52	47 (90)	20 (38)	Not reported
Fierro (1997)[68]	VICOB-P	25	(80)	(36)	7–8

CR, complete remission; ORR, overall response rate.

the risk for opportunistic infections. Prophylactic antibiotics against *Pneumocystis carinii* and antivirals to prevent herpes virus infection are routinely administered.

Combinations of purine analogues with interferon have also been utilized in small studies and show an increased response rate compared with historic data for these agents alone.[59]

Gemcitabine (2'2'-difluorodeoxycytidine, Gemzar™) is a novel deoxycytidine analogue with excellent antitumor activity against a number of solid tumors and lymphoproliferative disorders.[60] Gemcitabine needs to be activated by deoxycytidine kinase and other kinases to its triphosphate, gemcitabine triphosphate, which can be incorporated into RNA and DNA.[60] The latter effect is considered to be responsible for its antitumor effect, and causes masked chain termination and inhibition of DNA repair. This agent inhibits DNA synthesis through chain termination and ribonucleotide reductase inhibition. Overall response rates are reported to be as high as 70%,[61] but the complete response rate has been low.

Pegylated liposomes are stable, long-circulating carriers useful for delivering doxorubicin to tumor sites, and have less toxicity than free doxorubicin, used in several treatment protocols for non-Hodgkin's lymphoma. In a study of patients who had refractory or relapsed MF, Doxil was given in a dose of 20 mg/m^2 every month until a complete response had been achieved or a total dose of 400 mg had been administered.[62] An overall response rate of 80% and response duration of 15 months were reported. The responders showed a decrease of lymphocytic infiltrates and activated T-cells in skin biopsy specimens. Temporary Grade 0 to 3 side effects were reported. The most frequent side effects were mild anemia and lymphopenia, not requiring intervention.

An exciting new cytotoxic agent is temozolamide, which showed encouraging activity in MF in Phase I studies and requires further study.[63] Its mechanism of action is similar to other alkylating agents; it induces DNA damage by cross-linking. Resistance to alkylating agents in general, and temozolamide in particular, has been associated with high levels in tumor cells of the scavenger protein 06-alkylguanine DNA alkyltransferase (AGT). The neoplastic T lymphocytes in patients with MF have been shown to have only low levels of AGT.[64] Levels of AGT were also studied and correlated with response to temozolamide in patients with MF/SS. Response to treatment and development of resistance correlated with AGT levels.[65]

Combination Chemotherapy

Bunn et al. have also reviewed and summarized the role of combination therapy in MF and the SS (Table 25–3).[46] In a review of the literature that included 331 patients, the objective response rate was 81%, the complete response rate was 38%, and the response duration ranged from 5 to 41 months. The authors concluded that although these figures were slightly higher than for single-agent therapy, the differences were not striking.

There are no randomized trials comparing combination chemotherapy with single-agent regimens. For combination therapy, the greatest experience is with combinations that include cyclophosphamide, vincristine, and prednisone with or without doxorubicin.[66,67] Complete response rates are only about 25% (range 11% to 57%), and response duration is 3 to 20 months.[44,45]

Most of the patients who have been treated with combination chemotherapy had advanced disease (IIB to IV) and treatment was not curative. A few patients with early-stage disease (1A to IIA) have had complete responses, and were disease-free at the time of the reports.[46] However, the follow-up durations were too short to determine whether any of them were long-term, disease-free survivors.

An intensive third-generation regimen as front-line therapy has also been reported using VICOB-P (etoposide, idarubicin, cyclophosphamide, vincristine, prednisone, and bleomycin).[68] This intensive regimen was administered weekly for 12 weeks with a reported response rate of 80% (CR 36%). The median duration of response was 8 to 17 months, similar to that reported for CHOP chemotherapy. No response was seen in patients with SS.

One randomized study by the NCI compared combination chemotherapy (cyclophosphanide, doxorubin, vincristine, and etoposide) plus total skin electron beam irradiation with conservative therapy and topical nitrogen mustard.[69] The objective response rates (90% vs. 65%) and complete response rates (38% vs. 18%) were higher with the combined therapy approach. However, there was no difference in overall survival and considerably greater toxicity compared to conservative therapy.

There are several reports of cytotoxic chemotherapy with biological modalities such as targeted toxins and immunomodulating agents that appear encouraging and need to be confirmed in larger studies.[70]

High-Dose Therapy with Hematopoietic Cell Support

Recently, investigators have shown interest in using very high-dose chemotherapy followed by hematopoietic cell support (autologous or allogeneic) based on experience in patients with relapsed chemosensitive lymphomas. Given the small number of patients treated thus far, there are no appropriate prognostic factors to identify the patients for whom this therapy is beneficial. Some recent studies are summarized in Table 25–4.

Bigler et al. reported complete responses in five of six patients treated with an autologous approach.[71] However, three of the responses lasted less than 100 days and only two patients were disease-free at 1 year. In another study from the United Kingdom,[72] eight of nine patients achieved a complete response, but this was only 2 months in four of those patients. In both of the above studies, all patients relapsed, suggesting that this autologous approach is not a curative one.

Autologous transplant with T-cell depletion has also been reported. In a pilot study,[73] nine patients had the apheresis product treated with immunomagnetic methods for T-cell depletion. Eight of nine patients engrafted, and seven achieved a complete response. All patients relapsed, with a median time to relapse of 7 months. However, at the time of relapse, these patients appeared to have more indolent disease that responded to conventional therapy.

The use of allogeneic hematopoietic cell transplantation is provocative, since in the absence of a complete response,

Table 25–4. Autologous Transplant

Study	Stage	N	Complete Remission (n)	Relapse
Bigler (1991)[71]	IIB-IV B	5	4	4 patients <1 year, 1 patient >1 year
Russell-Jones (2001)[72]	IIB-IV B	9	8	4 patients <3 months, 3 patients 11 months
Olavarria	IIB-IV B	9	7	All in 1 year
Allogeneic Transplant				
Soligo (2003)[76]	IV	3	3	16 months, 12 months
Guitart (2002)[72]	IIB-IV A	3	3	10 months, >26 months, >67 months

an allogeneic graft-versus-tumor effect may provide an immune mechanism to control the malignant T-cell process, and thereby alter the natural history of the disease. In a report by Guitart et al. three patients received allografts from HLA-matched siblings.[74] Complete and sustained clinical and histologic remission was achieved in two patients, with durations of more than 15 months and more than 4.5 years. One additional patient was in complete response for 9 months, followed by a limited cutaneous recurrence.

In another series using allogeneic support, Molina and associates reported complete response in all six patients treated for refractory disease.[75] Five patients remained in complete response at a median follow-up of 17 months (range 3 to 65 months). Mild acute and chronic GVHD developed in all patients.

A nonmyeloablative approach has also been reported.[76] All three patients achieved a durable complete response, but there was a high incidence of infection.

Thus, it appears that in contrast to autologous grafts, allogeneic hematopoeitic cell transplants may result in durable long-term remissions. With better understanding of the disease biology and with newer molecular characteristics it may be possible to identify patients and develop prognostic factors so that these aggressive approaches can be offered to suitable patients. Larger studies will be required to identify the best conditioning regimen, efficacy, safety, and impact on quality of life.

Interferon

There is substantial experience in the use of interferon for MF. The interferons have antiproliferative, cytotoxic, and immunoregulatory functions. IFN-α is indicated primarily for the palliative management of refractory or advanced disease. It may be used alone or more often combined with topical or other systemic therapies. Treatment with IFN-α is usually initiated at 3 million to 5 million units daily or three times per week, and the dose is gradually increased, depending on the clinical response and the severity of adverse effects. The likelihood of response correlates with stage of disease, intensity of prior therapy, and dose of interferon. The greatest likelihood of response is in limited disease, little prior therapy, and interferon doses as high as 5 million to 10 million U/day, three times per week. Reported overall response rates when used alone are 50% to 75%, with complete response rates of 20% to 35%, and a median duration of 6 months.[77,78] The primary complications include mild to moderate systemic reactions, such as fatigue, anorexia, decreased performance status, and leukopenia.

Photopheresis

Extracorporeal photopheresis (ECPP or systemic photochemotherapy) is a method of delivering PUVA systemically by utilizing an extracorporeal technique.[79] The patient's white blood cells are collected (leukapheresis), exposed to a photoactivating drug, and then irradiated with UVA. The irradiated cells then are returned to the patient. The mechanism of action of ECPP remains unclear. It is hypothesized that there may be a direct cytotoxic or antiproliferative effect on the neoplastic cells and an immune-enhancing effect on the competent lymphocytes against the neoplastic cells. Photopheresis is usually administered every 4 weeks, but in patients with severe disease, the frequency can be as often as every 2 or 3 weeks. Once complete clearance is achieved, the frequency can be gradually reduced and then discontinued. Patients with erythroderma, especially those with low CD4+ : CD8+ ratios in the peripheral blood, are the most likely to respond. Responses are less likely in patients who present with a large number of circulating Sézary cells. The overall response rate to ECPP is 80%, with half of those patients demonstrating at least a 50% improvement. Unfortunately, this treatment approach has little usefulness among patients with more classic infiltrative disease.

Compared with other systemic therapies, ECPP has minimal adverse effects.[79] Some patients may experience nausea, mostly due to the ingested psoralen, and some have a transient low-grade fever or slight malaise after treatment. There are no reports of organ injury or bone marrow or immune suppression.

Systemic Retinoids

Systemic therapy with retinoids, most commonly bexarotene, may be effective for MF and Sézary syndrome. The reported response rate to bexarotene approximates 45%, with a 20% complete response rate. Systemic retinoids are indicated for palliative therapy for refractory or advanced disease, often in combination with other topical or systemic therapies, including PUVA, IFN-α, or TSEBT.[80–84]

Bexarotene is administered orally. The initial dose is 300 mg/m^2/day, which can be adjusted according to clinical response and the severity of adverse effects. The most common adverse effects include photosensitivity, xerosis, myalgia, arthralgia, headaches, and impaired night vision. Because of their known teratogenic effects, retinoids are often avoided for young female patients. Because of their potential hepatotoxic and hyperlipidemic effects, liver function and serum lipid levels must be monitored. In addition, central hypothyroidism is often induced. Patients are routinely started on levothyroxin (Synthroid) and a cholesterol-lowering agent immediately before or simultaneously with bexarotene.

Recombinant Fusion Proteins

Recombinant fusion proteins, such as the IL-2-diphtheria toxin fusion protein (Ontak, denileukin diftitox), incorporate growth factor-diphtheria toxin fusion proteins designed specifically to kill defined neoplastic cell populations. Denileukin diftitox has undergone a multicenter Phase III trial in patients with IL-2 receptor (CD25+)–expressing MF.[85] Patients with intermediate or advanced stages of disease were included in the Phase III trial. The overall response rate was 30%, with complete response and partial response rates of 10% and 20%, respectively. The main complication related to a "capillary leak" syndrome may be ameliorated by pretreatment with corticosteroids.

Combined Modality Therapy

Combined modality therapy plays an important role in the management of patients with MF. This may take the form of sequential topical therapies or combined topical and systemic treatment with either chemotherapy or biologic agents.[81,83,86] For example, following TSEBT, response may be prolonged by use of a topical adjuvant, such as HN2 or PUVA.[87–89] Combined topical therapies may be helpful in the palliative management of patients with persistent skin disease. Treatment with topical HN2 may be supplemented by the judicious use of irradiation to tumors or symptomatic plaques, and PUVA or photopheresis may be combined with interferon-alfa,[86] bexarotene, or topical HN2. The main risk to consider in these cases is the potential for developing squamoproliferative lesions of the skin after prolonged topical therapy.[33]

A routine, combined modality approach as initial therapy for patients with MF was evaluated in a prospective, randomized clinical trial reported from the NCI.[90] Patients were randomized to an aggressive treatment program that included electron beam therapy and chemotherapy with cyclophosphamide, doxorubicin, VP-16, and vincristine, or a conservative treatment program with sequential topical and then systemic therapies. There were no differences in outcome (survival) for conservative versus aggressive therapy for patients with either limited or advanced disease.

Novel Therapies

Anti–T-cell monoclonal antibodies have also been used for the management of patients with MF. There have been trials with a pan–T-cell murine monoclonal antibody (anti–Leu-1), an ^{131}I radiolabeled version of a similar antibody (T101), and a pan–T-cell anti-CD5 antibody linked to ricin.[91–93] Responses to antibody therapy are generally brief, and the duration of treatment is commonly limited by the development of human antimouse antibodies (HAMAs). In a more recent trial, a chimeric antihelper T-cell (anti-CD4) antibody has been used to minimize the development of HAMA and provide a more specific treatment against the subset of T cells.[94] The responses to this antibody were also modest and short-lived. Despite the minimal responses to antibody therapy that have been observed thus far, further studies are appropriate with different antibodies or with radiolabeled versions of existing antibodies. It is possible that antibody therapy will have a role to play in the management of minimal disease, perhaps as an adjuvant after TSEBT.

Therapeutic Approaches and Prognosis

The median survival of patients with MF is nearly 10 years.[15] The long-term disease-specific survival of a cohort of more than 500 patients with all stages of MF seen at Stanford since 1960 is displayed in Fig. 25–1. Treatment selection and prognosis are both linked closely to the extent of skin involvement and the presence of extracutaneous disease. Among patients who have disease apparently limited to the skin, the prognosis is linked closely to the extent of skin involvement. Patients who present with extracutaneous disease have a median survival just slightly longer than 1 year.

Limited Plaque Disease

Patients with limited plaque (T1) disease are usually treated effectively with topical therapies such as HN2, bexarotene, local radiation therapy or phototherapy (UVB or PUVA). The prognosis of these patients is quite good. In the experience at Stanford, less than 10% of patients treated in the limited plaque phase later progress to a more advanced stage of disease.[95] Nearly all deaths are due to causes other than MF, including cardiopulmonary disease and other cancers, and the long-term life expectancy is similar to an age-, gender-, and race/ethnicity-matched control population.

Generalized Plaque Disease

Patients with generalized plaque disease (T2) may be treated with HN2, PUVA, or TSEBT. Irradiation should be considered for patients with very thickened plaques (since its depth of penetration is better than that of either HN2 or PUVA) and for patients with a recent history of rapid progression of disease (because of its more prompt effect). Patients treated with either HN2 or PUVA should be followed closely, and treatment with electron beam therapy should be initiated if disease progresses despite treatment intensification. Generally, following completion of TSEBT, adjuvant treatment with topical HN2, PUVA, other topical agents, or a systemic biologic is appropriate and may be continued for as long as 6 months. In patients treated with PUVA, the complete response rate ranges from 50% to 80%.[25,27,96] Complete response rates using topical HN2 are 50% to 70%,[30,97,98] whereas the complete response rate for total skin electron beam therapy is 80% to 90%.[97,99] However, patients treated with TSEBT do not have an improved long-term survival compared to those who received topical HN2 as initial therapy, despite the superior complete response rate. Combination topical or topical plus biologic therapies may also be used as initial therapy for patients with T2 disease. This may provide for better long-term control of disease, but the ultimate outcome is not usually affected.[87,89,100] Patients with limited or generalized

MYCOSIS FUNGOIDES, DISEASE-SPECIFIC SURVIVAL

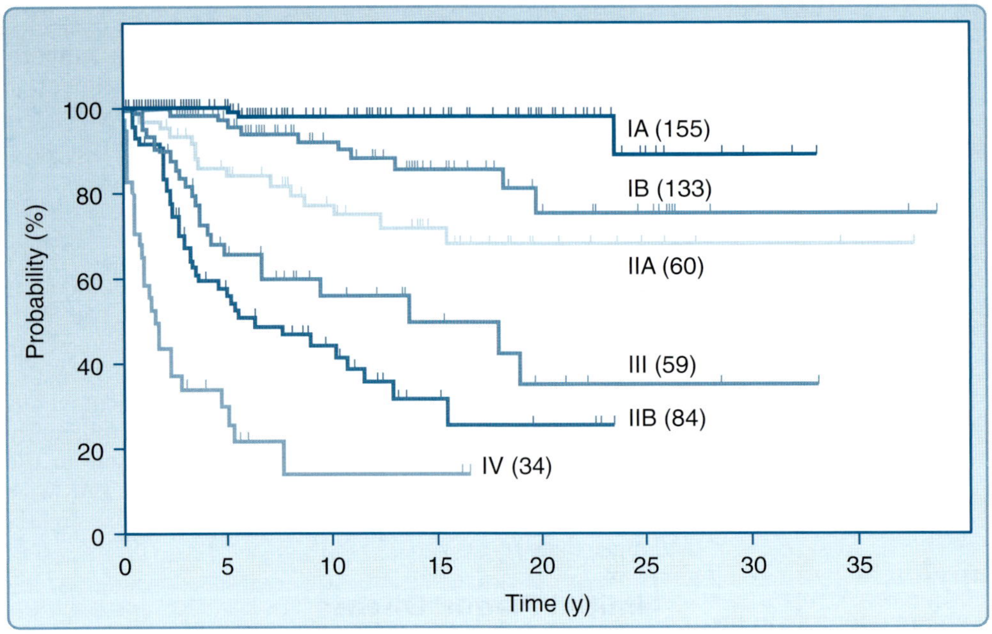

Figure 25–1. Disease-specific survival of 525 patients with a confirmed diagnosis of MF or SS seen and treated at Stanford University Medical Center. Patients are categorized according to disease stage at presentation (see Table 25–2 for stage classification).

plaque disease who fail to respond to one therapy, or who begin to progress after an initial response, may be treated with an alternative topical therapy. There is no evidence that development of resistance to one modality affects subsequent response to an alternative topical therapy.[95,97]

Patients with generalized disease (T2) at diagnosis are at greater risk for disease progression (30%) than patients with limited plaque. About one-quarter of deaths among patients with T2 disease are from causes related to MF, such as infection.

Tumorous Disease

Most patients with tumorous involvement (T3) have generalized cutaneous disease, and the greatest likelihood of a response is with TSEBT, generally followed by adjuvant topical HN2.[89] Others may be treated with combinations of PUVA and IFN-α or PUVA plus oral bexarotene. Some patients, with a discrete number of tumors, may be treated with either topical HN2 or PUVA, combined with localized irradiation to individual tumors. These patients have a median survival of 3.2 years, and the majority die of MF. There is no evidence that treatment has any curative potential in this stage, but it does have tremendous palliative benefit.

Erythroderma

Patients with erythroderma (T4) are challenging to manage. Common treatments for these patients include extracorporeal photopheresis, PUVA, oral bexarotene, IFN-α, and single-agent methotrexate. If there is no peripheral blood involvement, treatment may be initiated cautiously with low-dose PUVA. Photopheresis may also be effective treatment for these patients. If SS is present, systemic management such as chemotherapy or biologicals may have an important palliative role.[101] If there is a systemic response, but cutaneous symptoms persist, topical therapy such as low-potency corticosteroids, low-dose PUVA, or low concentrations of HN2 may be added. Patients who are young and have no peripheral blood involvement or extracutaneous disease may live quite long with palliative therapy only (median survival of 10 years).[102] However, once a patient develops SS, with circulating peripheral cells, the median survival is only about 3 years.

Extracutaneous Disease

Patients with extracutaneous disease may be treated with systemic chemotherapy or biologic therapies. Irradiation may be used for palliation, especially for disease involving lymph nodes. Because of the inadequacy of standard therapy, all patients with extracutaneous disease should be considered candidates for investigational therapies. Patients with extracutaneous disease and any extent of skin involvement have a median survival of only 1 year, and nearly all die of causes directly related to MF.[15,20]

OTHER CUTANEOUS LYMPHOMAS

The other primary cutaneous lymphomas represent only 5% to 7% of extranodal non-Hodgkin's lymphoma (see also Chapter 24). These are predominantly B-cell lymphomas and a minority are T-cell lymphomas. They may be further categorized according to the World Health Organization classification,[103] and include follicular lymphoma, marginal zone lymphoma, diffuse large B-cell lymphoma, peripheral T-cell lymphoma, NK/T-cell lymphoma, and CD-30 lymphoproliferative disease, including anaplastic large-cell lymphoma.

The cutaneous lymphomas other than MF are generally nonepidermatropic. That is, the neoplastic cells are usually absent from the epidermis and involve primarily the dermis and subcutaneous tissues. The region between the dermis and epidermis (the Grenz zone) is spared; however, relatively advanced lesions may ulcerate secondarily into the epidermis.

There is some site predilection for the subtypes of cutaneous lymphoma; follicular lymphoma more commonly arises on the scalp, marginal zone lymphoma on the trunk or upper extremities, and aggressive large B-cell lymphoma usually arises on the lower leg. Nevertheless, all types of cutaneous lymphoma can occur at any site, such that the site of presentation is not particularly useful when approaching the diagnosis in an individual patient.

The philosophy for staging patients with cutaneous lymphoma is to exclude extracutaneous disease. Therefore, one generally includes those studies employed for evaluating patients with non-Hodgkin's lymphomas in other sites. These include a thorough physical examination with detailed examination of the skin, complete blood counts, screening chemistries including LDH, chest radiograph, CT scan of the chest abdomen, and pelvis and bone marrow biopsy.

Primary Cutaneous T-Cell Lymphomas Other than Mycosis Fungoides

The non-MF primary cutaneous T-cell lymphomas have a variable presentation, and their behavior is less predictable than MF or the B-cell lymphomas. Management often includes both chemotherapy and radiation with or without biological agents, even for patients with isolated lesions.

Anaplastic Large-Cell Lymphoma

A distinct subtype of lymphoma, anaplastic large cell lymphoma (ALCL) of the skin, has been described.[104] These lymphomas are generally CD30+ and are part of the spectrum of cutaneous CD30+ lymphoproliferative disease (CLPD). They may arise de novo (primary) or develop in the face of preexisting cutaneous T-cell lymphoproliferative diseases such as MF and lymphomatoid papulosis (LyP) (secondary).[105]

The presentation of CD30+ CLPD may pose a difficult diagnostic dilemma. Histologically, LyP and ALCL may be difficult to distinguish, especially in cases of LyP where numerous CD30+ large atypical cells are present. Clinicopathologic correlation is necessary to establish a diagnosis. Misdiagnosis has led to patients occasionally receiving inappropriate and excessive therapy. Local excision and radiation is appropriate for patients with limited disease. Sequential biological agents (e.g., interferon-alpha and bexarotene) as well as combination chemotherapy may be used for patients with generalized disease. The survival of patients with ALCL is excellent, 75% to 80% at 10 years, with a disease-specific survival of 80% to 90%.[104,106]

Primary Cutaneous NK/T-Cell Lymphoma

NK/T-cell lymphoma is a CD56+ lymphoma. In its systemic form, it follows an aggressive course. Reports on patients with primary cutaneous NK/T-cell lymphoma are few in number.[107] Disease usually presents as plaques or tumors on the trunk or extremities. The outcome of therapy is worse than for patients with other forms of primary cutaneous lymphoma, with a median survival of less than 4 years.

Primary Peripheral T-Cell Lymphoma

Other T-cell lymphomas of the skin are CD-30-negative. Their prognosis is variable, and may reflect histologic variables such as tumor cell size, extent of disease, and immunophenotype.[108] The limited reports that have appeared in the literature do not permit definition of specific treatment guidelines.

References

1. Hoppe RT, Wood GS, Abel EA. Mycosis fungoides and the Sezary syndrome: pathology, staging, and treatment. Curr Prob Cancer 1990;14:293–371.
2. Weinstock M. Mycosis fungoides in the United States—increasing incidence and descriptive epidemiology. J Clin Oncol 1988;260:42–60.
3. Whittemore A, Holly E, Lee I, et al. Mycosis fungoides in relation to environmental exposures and immune response: a case-control study. J Natl Cancer Inst 1989;81:1560–7.
4. Tuyp E, Burgoyne A, Aitchison T, et al. A case-control study of possible causative factors in mycosis fungoides. Arch Dermatol 1987;123:196–200.
5. Olerud JE, Kulin PA, Chew DE, et al. Cutaneous T-cell lymphoma: evaluation of pretreatment skin biopsy specimens by a panel of pathologists. Arch Dermatol 1992;128:501–7.
6. Lutzner MA, Edelson RL, Schein P, et al. Cutaneous T cell lymphomas: the Sezary syndrome, mycosis fungoides, and related disorders. Ann Intern Med 1975;83:534–52.
7. Wood G, Weiss LM, Warnke R, et al. The immunopathology of cutaneous lymphomas: Immunophenotypcic and immunogenotypic characteristics. Semin Dermatol 1986;5:334.
8. Michie SA, Abel EA, Hoppe RT, et al. Expression of T-cell receptor antigens in mycosis fungoides and inflammatory skin lesions. J Invest Dermatol 1989;93:116–20.
9. Sausville EA, Eddy JL, Makuch RW, et al. Histopathologic staging at initial diagnosis of mycosis fungoides and the Sezary syndrome. Definition of three distinctive prognostic groups. Ann Intern Med 1988;109:372–82.
10. Weiss LM, Wood GS, Hu E, et al. Detection of clonal T-cell receptor gene rearrangements in the peripheral blood of patients with mycosis fungoides/Sezary syndrome. J Invest Dermatol 1989;92:601–4.
11. Bignon YJ, Souteyrand P, Roger H, et al. Clonotypic heterogeneity in cutaneous T-cell lymphomas. Cancer Res 1990;50:6620–5.
12. Dmitrovsky E, Matthews M, Bunn PA, et al. Cytologic transformation in cutaneous T cell lymphoma: a clinicopathologic entity associated with poor prognosis. J Clin Oncol 1987;5:208–15.
13. Cerroni L, Rieger E, Hodl S, et al. Clinicopathologic and immunologic features associated with transformation of mycosis fungoides to large-cell lymphoma. Am J Surg Pathol 1992;16:543–52.
14. Wieselthier JS, Koh HK. Sezary syndrome: diagnosis, prognosis, and critical review of treatment options. J Am Acad Dermatol 1990;22:381–401.
15. Kim YH, Liu HL, Mraz-Gernhard S, et al. Longterm outcome of 525 patients with mycosis fungoides and Sezary syndrome at Stanford: clinical porgnostic factors and risks of disease progression and second cancer. Arch Dermatol 2003;139:857–66.

16. Epstein EH Jr, Levin DL, Croft JD Jr, et al. Mycosis fungoides. Survival, prognostic features, response to therapy, and autopsy findings. Medicine (Baltimore) 1972;51:61–72.
17. Bunn PA, Lamberg SI. Report of the Committee on Staging and Classification of Cutaneous T-Cell Lymphomas. Cancer Treat Rep 1979;63:725–8.
18. Fuks Z, Bagshaw MA, Farber EM. Prognostic signs in the management of the mycosis fungoides. Cancer 1973; 32:1385–95.
19. Hoppe RT, Cox RS, Fuks Z, et al. Electron-beam therapy for mycosis fungoides: the Stanford University experience. Cancer Treat Rep 1979;63:691–700.
20. de Coninck EC, Kim YH, Varghese A, et al. Clinical characteristics and outcome of patients with extracutaneous mycosis fungoides. J Clin Oncol 2001;19:779–84.
21. Kim YH, Hoppe RT. Mycosis fungoides and the Sezary syndrome. Semin Oncol 1999;26:276–89.
22. Salhany KE, Greer JP, Cousar JB, et al. Marrow involvement in cutaneous T-cell lymphoma. A clinicopathologic study of 60 cases. Am J Clin Pathol 1989;92:747–54.
23. Ramsay DL, Lish KM, Yalowitz CB, et al. Ultraviolet-B phototherapy for early-stage cutaneous T-cell lymphoma. Arch Dermatol 1992;128:931–3.
24. Resnik KS, Vonderheid EC. Home UV phototherapy of early mycosis fungoides: long-term follow-up observations in thirty-one patients. J Am Acad Dermatol 1993; 29:73–7.
25. Abel EA, Sendagorta E, Hoppe RT, et al. PUVA treatment of erythrodermic and plaque-type mycosis fungoides. Ten-year follow-up study. Arch Dermatol 1987;123:897–901.
26. Rosenbaum MM, Roenigk HH Jr, Caro WA, et al. Photochemotherapy in cutaneous T-call lymphoma and parapsoriasis en plaques: long-term follow-up in forty-three patients. J Am Acad Dermatol 1985;13:613–22.
27. Herrmann JJ, Roenigk HH Jr, Hurria A, et al. Treatment of mycosis fungoides with photochemotherapy (PUVA): long-term follow-up. J Am Acad Dermatol 1995;33:234–42.
28. Kim YH, Martinez G, Varghese A, et al. Management with topical nitrogen mustard in mycosis fungoides: update of the Stanford experience. Arch Dermatol 2003;139:165–73.
29. Ramsey D, Halperin P, Zeleniuch-Jacquotte A. Topical mechlorethamine therapy for early stage mycosis fungoides. J Am Acad Dermatol 1988;19:684–91.
30. Vonderheid EC, Tan ET, Kantor AF, et al. Long-term efficacy, curative potential, and carcinogenicity of topical mechlorethamine chemotherapy in cutaneous T cell lymphoma. J Am Acad Dermatol 1989;20:416–28.
31. Studstrup L, Beck HI, Bjerring P, et al. No detectable increase in sister chromatid exchanges in lymphocytes from mycosis fungoides patients after topical treatment with nitrogen mustard. Br J Dermatol 1988;119:711–5.
32. Hoppe RT, Abel EA, Deneau DG, et al. Mycosis fungoides: management with topical nitrogen mustard. J Clin Oncol 1987;5:1796–803.
33. Abel EA, Sendagorta E, Hoppe RT. Cutaneous malignancies and metastatic squamous cell carcinoma following topical therapies for mycosis fungoides. J Am Acad Dermatol 1986;14:1029–38.
34. Breneman D, Duvic M, Kuzel T, et al. Phase 1 and 2 trial of bexarotene gel for skin-directed treatment of patients with cutaneous T-cell lymphoma. Arch Dermatol 2002;138: 325–32.
35. Hoppe R. Mycosis fungoides: radiation therapy. Dermatol Ther 2003;16:347–54.
36. Hoppe RT, Fuks Z, Bagshaw MA. Radiation therapy in the management of cutaneous T-cell lymphomas. Cancer Treat Rep 1979;63:625–32.
37. Hoppe RT. Total skin electron beam therapy in the management of mycosis fungoides. Front Radiat Ther Oncol 1991; 25:80–9.
38. Cox RS, Heck RJ, Fessenden P, et al. Development of total skin electron therapy at two energies. Int J Radiat Oncol Biol Phys 1990;18:659–69.
39. Lo TCM, Salzman FA, Moschella SL, et al. Whole-body surface electron irradiation in the treatment of mycosis fungoides: an evaluation of 200 patients. Radiology 1979; 130:453–7.
40. Nisce LZ, Safai B, Kim JH. Effectiveness of once weekly total skin electron beam therapy in mycosis fungoides and Sezary syndrome. Cancer 1981;47:870–6.
41. Jones GW, Tadros A, Hodson DI, et al. Prognosis with newly diagnosed mycosis fungoides after total skin electron radiation of 30 or 35 GY. Int J Radiat Oncol Biol Phys 1994; 28:839–45.
42. Price NM, Hoppe RT, Constantine VS, et al. The treatment of mycosis fungoides: adjuvant topical mechlorethamine after electron beam therapy. Cancer 1977;40:2851–3.
43. Becker M, Hoppe RT, Knox SJ. Multiple courses of high-dose total skin electron beam therapy in the management of mycosis fungoides. Int J Radiat Oncol Biol Phys 1995; 32:1445–9.
44. Abel EA, Wood GS, Hoppe RT. Mycosis fungoides: clinical and histologic features, staging, evaluation, and approach to treatment. CA Cancer J Clin 1993;43:93–115.
45. Kemme DJ, Bunn PA Jr. State of the art therapy of mycoses fungoides and sezary syndrome. Oncology 1992;6: 31–42.
46. Bunn PA Jr, Hoffman SJ, Norris D, et al. Systemic therapy of cutaneous T-cell lymphomas (mycosis fungoides and the Sezary syndrome). Ann Intern Med 1994;121:592–602.
47. Bunn PA Jr, Fuks Z. Cutaneous and acute T call lymphomas. In: DeVita V, Hellman SA, Rosenberg S, eds. Principles and Practice of Oncology, 3rd ed, vol. 2. Philadelphia: JB Lippincott, 1988:1799–808.
48. McDonald C, Bertino JR. Treatment of mycosis fungoides lymphoma: effectiveness of infusions of methotrexate followed by oral citrovorum factor. Cancer Treat Rep 1978; 62:1009–14.
49. Schappell DL, Alper JC, McDonald C. Treatment of advanced mycosis fungoides and Sezary syndrome with continuous infusions of methotrexate followed by fluorouracil and leucovorin rescue. Arch Dermatol 1995;131: 307–13.
50. Zackheim HS, Epstein EH Jr. Low-dose methotrexate for the Sezary syndrome. J Am Acad Dermatol 1989;21:757–62.
51. Holmes RC, McGibbon DH, Black MM. Mycosis fungoides: progression towards Sezary syndrome reversed with chlorambucil. Clin Exp Dermatol 1983;8:429–35.
52. Dearden C, Matutes E, Catovsky D, et al. Pentostatin treatment of cutaneous T-cell lymphoma. Oncology 2000;14: 37–40.
53. Tsimberidon AM, Giles F, Duvic M, et al. Phase II study of pentostatin in advanced T-cell lymphoid malignancies: update of an M.D. Anderson Cancer Center series. Cancer 2004;100:342–9.
54. Greiner D, Olsen EA, Petroni G. Pentostatin (2'-deoxycoformycin) in the treatment of cutaneous T-cell lymphoma. J Am Acad Dermatol 1997;36:950–5.
55. Saven A, Carrera CJ, Carson DA, et al. 2-chlorodeoxyadenosine: an active agent in the treatment of cutaneous T-cell lymphoma. Blood 1992;80:587–92.
56. Kuzel T, Hurria A, Samuelson E, et al. Rose Phase II trial of 2-chlorodeoxyadenosine for the treatment of cutaneous T-cell lymphoma. Blood 1996;87:906–11.
57. Quaglino P, Fierro MT, Rossotto GL, et al. Treatment of advanced mycosis fungoides/Sezary syndrome with fludara-

bine and potential adjunctive benefit to subsequent extracorporeal photochemotherapy. Br J Dermatol 2004;150:327–36.
58. Von Hoff D, Dahlberg S, Hartsock R, et al. Activity of fludarabine monophosphate in patients with advanced mycosis fungoides: a Southwest Oncology Group study. J Natl Cancer Inst 1990;82:1353–5.
59. Foss F, Waldmann TA. Interluekin-2 receptor–directed therapies for cutaneous lymphomas. Oncol Clin North Am 2003;17:1449–58.
60. Fossa A, Santoro A, Hiddemann W, et al. Gemcitabine as a single agent in the treatment of relapsed or refractory aggressive non-Hodgkin's lymphoma. J Clin Oncol 1999;17:3786–92.
61. Zinzani PL, Baliva G, Magagnoli M, et al. Gemcitabine treatment in pretreated cutaneous T-cell lymphoma: experience in 44 patients. J Clin Oncol 2000;18:2603–6.
62. Wollina U, Graefe T, Karte K. Treatment of relapsing or recalcitrant cutaneous T-cell lymphoma with pegylated liposomal doxorubicin. J Am Acad Dermatol 2000;42(1 Pt 1):40–6.
63. Newlands ES, Blackledge G, Slack JA, et al. Phase I trial of temozolomide (CCRG 81045: M&B 38931:NSC 362856. Br J Cancer 1992;65:287–91.
64. Dolan ME, McRae BL, Ferries-Rowe E, et al. 06-alkylguanine-DNA alkyltransferase in cutaneous T-cell lymphoma: implications for treatment with alkylating agents. Clin Cancer Res 1999;5:2059–64.
65. Kuzel TM, et al. Phase II trial of temozolamide for treatment of mycosis fungoides/Sezary syndrome. Proc Am Soc Clin Oncol 2002;21:286a [abstract].
66. Molin L, Thomsen K, Volden G, et al. Combination chemotherapy in the tumour stage of mycosis fungoides with cyclophosphamide, vincristine, vp-16, adriamycin and prednisone (COP, CHOP, CAVOP): a report from the Scandinavian Mycosis Fungoides Study Group. Acta Derm Venereol 1980;60:542–4.
67. Tirelli U, Carbone A, Zagonel V, et al. Staging and treatment with cyclophosphamide, vincristine and prednisone (CVP) in advanced cutaneous T-cell lymphomas. Hematol Oncol 1986;4:83–90.
68. Fierro MT, Doveil GC, Quaglino P, et al. Combination of etoposide, idarubicin, cyclophosphamide, vincristine, prednisone and bleomycin (VICOP-B) in the treatment of advanced cutaneous T-cell lymphoma. Dermatology 1997;194:268–72.
69. Kaplan HS. The radical radiotherapy of regionally localized Hodgkin's disease. Radiology 1962;78:553–61.
70. Duvic M, Apisarnthanarax M, Cohen DS, et al. Analysis of longterm outcomes of combined modality therapy for cutaneous T-cell lymphoma. J Am Acad Dermatol 2003;49:35–49.
71. Bigler RD, Crilley P, Micaily B, et al. Autologous bone marrow transplantation for advanced stage mycosis fungoides. Bone Marrow Transplant 1991;7:133–7.
72. Russell-Jones R, Child F, Olavarria E, et al. Autologous peripheral blood stem cell transplantation in tumor-stage mycosis fungoides: predictors of disease-free survival. Ann N Y Acad Sci 2001;941:147–54.
73. O'Brien PC, Parnis FX. Salvage radiotherapy following chemotherapy failure in Hodgkin's disease—what is its role? Acta Oncol 1995;34:99–104.
74. Guitart J, Wickless SC, Oyama Y, et al. Longterm remission after allogeneic hematopoietic stem cell transplantation for refactory cutaneous T-cell lymphoma. Arch Dermatol 2002;138:1359–65.
75. Molina A, Aber D, Collins JL, et al. Clinical, cytogenetic and molecular remission after allogenic hematopoietic stem cell transplantation for refractory Sezary syndrome and tumor stage mycoses fungoides. Blood 2001;98(Suppl):409a [abstract].
76. Soligo D, Ibatici A, Berti E, et al. Treatment of advanced mycosis fungoides by allogeneic stem-cell transplantation with a nonmyeloablative regimen. Bone Marrow Transplant 2003;31:663–6.
77. Olsen EA, Rosen ST, Vollmer RT, et al. Interferon alfa-2a in the treatment of cutaneous T cell lymphoma. J Am Acad Dermatol 1989;20:395–407.
78. Vagna M, Papa G, Defazio D, et al. Interferon alpha-2a in cutaneous T-cell lymphoma. Eur J Haematol 1990;52:32–5.
79. Edelson RL, Heald P, Perez M, et al. Photopheresis update. Prog Dermatol 1991;25:1–6.
80. Kessler JF, Jones SE, Levine N, et al. Isotretinoin and cutaneous helper T-cell lymphoma (mycosis fungoides). Arch Dermatol 1987;123:201–4.
81. Duvic M, Lemak NA, Redman JR, et al. Combined modality therapy for cutaneous T-cell lymphoma. J Am Acad Dermatol 1996;34:1022–9.
82. Knobler RM, Trautinger F, Radaszkiewicz T, et al. Treatment of cutaneous T cell lymphoma with a combination of low-dose interferon alfa-2b and retinoids. J Am Acad Dermatol 1991;24:247–52.
83. Thomsen K, Hammar H, Molin L, et al. Retinoids plus PUVA (RePUVA) in mycosis fungoides, plaque stage. A report from the Scandinavian Mycosis Fungoides Group. Acta Dermatol Venereol (Stockh) 1989;69:217–22.
84. Jones G, McLean J, Rosenthal D, et al. Combined treatment with oral etretinate and electron beam therapy in patients with cutaneous T-cell lymphoma (mycosis fungoides and Sezary syndrome). J Am Acad Dermatol 1992;26:960–7.
85. Olsen EA, Duvic M, Martin A, et al. Pivotal phase III trial of two dose levels of DAB389IL-2 (Ontak) for the treatment of cutaneous T-cell lymphoma (CTCL). J Invest Dermatol 1998;110:678.
86. Kuzel TM, Roenigk HH Jr, Samuelson E, et al. Effectiveness of interferon alfa-2a combined with phototherapy for mycosis fungoides and the Sezary syndrome. J Clin Oncol 1995;13:257–63.
87. Quiros PA, Jones GW, Kacinski BM, et al. Total skin electron beam therapy followed by adjuvant psoralen/ultraviolet-A light in the management of patients with T1 and T2 cutaneous T-cell lymphoma (mycosis fungoides). Int J Radiat Oncol Biol Phys 1997;38:1027–35.
88. Wilson LD, Licata A, Braverman IM, et al. Systemic chemotherapy and extracorporeal photochemotherapy to T3 and T4 cutaneous T-cell lymphoma patients who have achieved a complete response to total skin electron beam therapy. Int J Radiat Oncol Biol Phys 1995;32:987–95.
89. Chinn DM, Chow S, Kim YH, et al. Total skin electron beam therapy with or without adjuvant topical nitrogen mustard or nitrogen mustard alone as initial treatment of T2 and T3 mycosis fungoides. Int J Radiat Oncol Biol Phys 2000.
90. Kaye FJ, Bunn PA Jr, Steinberg SM, et al. A randomized trial comparing combination electron-beam radiation and chemotherapy with topical therapy in the initial treatment of mycosis fungoides. N Engl J Med 1989;321:1784–90.
91. Miller RA, Oseroff A, Stratte PT, et al. Monoclonal antibody therapeutic trials in seven patients with T-cell lymphoma. Blood 1983;62:988–95.
92. Dillman RO, Beauregard J, Shawler DL, et al. Continuous infusion of T101 monoclonal antibody in chronic lymphocytic leukemia and cutaneous T-cell lymphoma. J Biol Resp Mod 1986;5:394–410.
93. LeMaistre CF, Rosen S, Frankel A, et al. Phase I trial of H65-RTA immunoconjugate in patients with cutaneous T-cell lymphoma. Blood 1991;78:1173–82.

94. Knox S, Levy R, Hodgkinson S, et al. Observations on the effect of chimeric–anti-CD4 monoclonal antibody in patients with mycosis fungoides. Blood 1991;77:20–30.
95. Kim YH, Jensen RA, Watanabe GL, et al. Clinical stage IA (limited patch and plaque) mycosis fungoides. A long-term outcome analysis. Arch Dermatol 1996;132:1309–13.
96. Honigsmann H, Brenner W, Rauschmeier W, et al. Photochemotherapy for cutaneous T cell lymphoma. A follow-up study. J Am Acad Dermatol 1984;10:238–45.
97. Kim YH, Chow S, Varghese A, et al. Clinical characteristics and long-term outcome of patients with generalized patch and/or plaque (T2) mycosis fungoides. Arch Dermatol 1999;135:26–32.
98. Ramsay DL, Zackheim HS. Topical treatment of early cutaneous T-cell lymphoma. Hematol Oncol Clin North Am 1995;9:1031–56.
99. Jones GW, Hoppe RT, Glatstein E. Electron beam treatment for cutaneous T-cell lymphoma. Hematol Oncol Clin North Am 1995;9:1057–76.
100. Roenigk HJ, Kuzel TM, Skoutelis A, et al. Photochemotherapy alone or combined with interferon alpha-2a in the treatment of cutaneous T-cell lymphoma. J Invest Dermatol 1990;95:198S–205S.
101. Winkelmann RK, Diaz-Perez JL, Buechner SA, et al. The treatment of Sezary syndrome. J Am Acad Dermatol 1984; 10:1000–4.
102. Kim YH, Bishop K, Varghese A, et al. Prognostic factors in erythrodermic mycosis fungoides and the Sezary syndrome. Arch Dermatol 1995;131:1003–8 [see comments].
103. Jaffe ES, Harris NL, Stein H, et al. World Health Organization Classification of Tumours. Pathology and Genetics of Tumours of Haematopoietic and Lymphoid Tissues. Lyon: IARC Press, 2001.
104. Kaudewitz P, Stein H, Dallenback F, et al. Primary and secondary Ki-1+ (CD30+) anaplastic large cell lymphomas: morphologic, immunohistologic, and clinical characteristics. Am J Pathol 1989;135:359–67.
105. Willemze R, Beljaard R. Spectrum of primary cutaneous CD30 (Ki-1) positive lymphoproliferative disorders. J Am Acad Dermatol 1993;28:973–80.
106. Liu HL, Hoppe R, Kohler S, et al. CD30+ cutaneous lymphoproliferative disorders: the Stanford experience in lymphomatoid papulosis and primary cutaneous anaplastic large cell lymphomas. J Am Acad Dermatol 2003;1049–58.
107. Mraz-Gernhard S, Natkunam Y, Hoppe RT, et al. Natural killer/natural killer–like T-cell lymphoma, CD56+, presenting in the skin: an increasingly recognized entity with an aggressive course. J Clin Oncol 2001;19:2179–88.
108. Bekkenk MW, Vermeer MH, Jansen PM, et al. Peripheral T-cell lymphomas unspecified presenting in the skin: analysis of prognostic factors in a group of 82 paients. Blood 2003; 102:2213–9.

26

Peripheral T-Cell Lymphoma

James O. Armitage, M.D.

T-cell lymphomas have been less studied and are less well understood than their B-cell counterparts. This is, undoubtedly, due in large part to the relative infrequency of these lymphomas. In most of the industrialized world, T-cell lymphomas represent approximately 10% of all non-Hodgkin's lymphomas. In most clinical trials, they have been lumped together with aggressive B-cell lymphomas such as diffuse large B-cell lymphoma. T-cell lymphomas have made up a small number of the patients in any particular study. Thus, the treatments that we have today have been largely derived for their effectiveness in aggressive B-cell lymphomas. It is perhaps not surprising that they are considerably less effective in the treatment of T-cell lymphomas.

The phrase "peripheral T-cell lymphoma" has undoubtedly added to confusion about these disorders. The name has nothing to do with the site of involvement by lymphoma. Rather, it refers to lymphomas of a mature, rather than immature, T-cell immunophenotype. Thus, the distinction is between immature, central, or thymic lymphomas (e.g., lymphoblastic lymphoma) and those T-cell lymphomas with a more mature immunophenotype. Peripheral T-cell lymphomas as a group make up the great majority of T-cell non-Hodgkin's lymphomas found in adults.

The worldwide acceptance of the World Health Organization (WHO) classification of non-Hodgkin's lymphomas has helped focus more attention on those disorders characterized as peripheral T-cell lymphoma (Table 26–1).[1] Several distinctive, albeit rare, clinical pathologic syndromes are now recognized. These include angioimmunoblastic T-cell lymphomas, enteropathy-associated T-cell lymphomas, natural killer (NK)/T-nasal T-cell lymphomas, adult T-cell lymphoma/leukemia, hepatosplenoic gamma/delta T-cell lymphomas, subcutaneous paniculitis-like T-cell lymphoma, mycosis fungoides/Sézary syndrome, blastic NK cell lymphoma, and anaplastic large T/null-cell lymphoma. Lymphomas that do not fit into one of these syndromes are lumped together under the term "peripheral T-cell lymphoma-not otherwise specified" (NOS). Unfortunately, for our understanding of these disorders, the peripheral T-cell lymphoma/NOS is the largest subgroup (Table 26–2).[2–4]

Several of these lymphomas are dealt with in other sections of this text. These include NK/T nasal lymphomas, cutaneous T-cell lymphomas, and adult T-cell lymphoma/leukemia (i.e., the disorder associated with infection by HTLV-1). The remainder of the T-cell lymphomas are the subject of this chapter.

FREQUENCY/EPIDEMIOLOGY

T-cell lymphomas are one of the subtypes of non-Hodgkin's lymphoma that vary in incidence geographically. In a study of consecutive series of patients with non-Hodgkin's lymphoma from eight countries, the difference in frequency of peripheral T-cell lymphomas was striking (Table 26–3).[5] Adult T-cell lymphoma/leukemia that is associated with infection with HTLV1 is predominantly seen in southern Japan and the Caribbean. NK/T nasal lymphomas occur most frequently in Southeast Asia and certain areas in Latin America. However, for most of the peripheral T-cell lymphomas, and particularly those considered in this chapter, there does not appear to be an equally striking geographic variation in frequency. The one exception to this is enteropathy-associated peripheral T-cell lymphoma that is highly associated with untreated celiac disease. Thus, areas such as parts of the United Kingdom where celiac disease is more common seem to have a higher incidence of this fairly rare subtype of lymphoma.[6,7]

In one international study, the relative frequency of the subtypes of peripheral T-cell lymphoma versus B-cell non-Hodgkin's lymphomas was studied (Table 26–2).[2–4] Overall, peripheral T-cell lymphomas represented about 9% of non-Hodgkin's lymphomas. Two percent were anaplastic large T/null cell lymphoma. The most common subgroup was peripheral T-cell lymphoma not otherwise specified, which represented 55% of the remaining peripheral T-cell lymphomas. Angiocentric nasal lymphoma represented 20% and angioimmunoblastic lymphoma 18%. Enteropathy-associated T-cell lymphomas represented 5%, and the other types were rare. Angioimmunoblastic T-cell lymphomas represent approximately 15% to 20% of all peripheral T-cell lymphomas in Europe and North America.

EPSTEIN–BARR VIRUS AND PERIPHERAL T-CELL LYMPHOMA

Epstein–Barr virus has been associated with a number of malignancies, including Burkitt's lymphoma, nasopharyngeal carcinoma, Hodgkin's disease, post-transplant immunoproliferative disease and lymphoma, and peripheral T-cell lymphoma. The association of this virus with peripheral T-cell lymphoma has fairly recently been recognized.

Although Epstein–Barr virus is widely known to infect B cells, it is also capable of infecting certain T lymphocytes.[8] Three patients who developed an illness characterized by fever, pneumonia, abnormal immunoglobulins, hemato-

Table 26–1. World Health Organization Classification of—Peripheral T-Cell Lymphomas

Extranodal	Nodal
Mycosis fungoides	Angioimmunoblastic
Cutaneous anaplastic large cell	Peripheral T-cell lymphoma, unspecified
Extranodal NK/T cell	Anaplastic large T/null cell
Enteropathy type	**Uncertain**
Hepatosplenic	Blastic NK cell
Subcutaneous panniculitis-like	

logic abnormalities, and extraordinarily high titers of antibody to components of the Epstein–Barr virus were described in 1988.[8] Each of these patients was identified as having peripheral T-cell lymphoma of the helper T-cell phenotype. The Epstein–Barr virus genome was found by in situ hybridization in the tumors of each patient. The tumor in each patient had an aggressive course and led to the patient's death.

Subsequent reports have confirmed the association of Epstein–Barr virus infection and peripheral T-cell lymphoma.[9–17] Peripheral T-cell lymphomas that have been demonstrated to have evidence of tumor cell infection by Epstein–Barr virus include those with the angioimmunoblastic lymphadenopathy and dysproteinemia type,[11] lethal midline granuloma with angiocentric lesions,[12,15] pleomorphic cell type,[14] and a tumor presenting like malignant histiocytosis with the hemophagocytic syndrome that was shown to be peripheral T-cell lymphoma.[17] The peripheral T-cell lymphomas have been shown to be both of helper and suppressor phenotypes.

The chances that a peripheral T-cell lymphoma might be associated with infection of the tumor cells by the Epstein–Barr virus seems to vary according to the lymphoma site of origin. One study from Holland demonstrated that peripheral T-cell lymphomas originating in the nose or nasal sinuses (100%) and lung (33%) were more likely to be associated with Epstein–Barr virus than lymphomas of the skin (0%) or gastrointestinal tract (8%).[18] The association of infection seemed to be by site of origin of the lymphoma rather than by the presence or absence of an angiocentric tumor growth pattern.

Table 26–2. Relative Frequency of Aggressive PTCLs

Types	% of All Non-Hodgkin's Lymphomas	% of PTCLs
PTCL-NOS	3.7%	39%
Anaplastic large T/null cell	2.4%	25%
Nasal NK/T-cell lymphoma	1.4%	15%
AILD	1.2%	13%
Others	<1%	—

AILD, angioimmunoblastic lymphadenopathy; NK, natural killer; NOS, not otherwise specified; PTCL, peripheral T-cell lymphoma.

Table 26–3. Geographical Distribution of Relative Frequency of PTCL (Excluding Anaplastic Large Cell) Versus B-Cell Lymphoma in Eight Countries

Country (City)	PTCL/All NHL	% PTCL
United States (Omaha)	6/200	3.0
Canada (Vancouver)	3/200	1.5
South Africa (Cape Town)	16/18	8.5
United Kingdom (London)	11/119	9.2
Switzerland (Locarno)	5/79	6.3
France (Lyon)	10/192	5.2
Germany (Wurzburg)	9/203	4.4
China (Hong Kong)	36/197	18.3

NHL, non-Hodgkin's lymphoma; PTCL, peripheral T-cell lymphoma.
From Rudiger T, Weisenburger DD, Anderson JR, et al. Peripheral T-cell lymphoma (excluding anaplastic large-cell lymphoma): results from the Non-Hodgkin's Lymphoma Classification Project. Ann Oncol 2002;13:140–9,[27] with permission.

Infection by Epstein–Barr virus is frequently associated with lymphomas that occur in immunosuppressed patients. The occurrence of such high-grade B-cell lymphomas has been a major problem in patients after organ transplantation. T-cell lymphomas have been rarely reported in this setting. However, post-transplant peripheral T-cell lymphomas have been reported.[13] In at least 5 of 22 reported cases, there was an association with Epstein–Barr virus in the tumor cells.[13]

IMMUNOLOGY/GENETICS

Peripheral T-cell lymphomas usually, but not always, express CD4 or CD8, with CD4 being the most common.[1] Most peripheral T-cell lymphomas express the alpha-beta T-cell receptor, but a minority of tumors expressed the more immature gamma-delta T-cell receptor.[1] Most likely to express the gamma-delta T-cell receptor are hepatosplenic lymphomas and subcutaneous panniculitis-like T-cell lymphomas.[1] There is no simple way to demonstrate clonality in T-cell lymphomas analogous to documenting clonality in B-cell lymphomas by restriction to either kappa or lambda light-chain expression using immunophenotyping. Clonality in T-cell lymphomas is best documented by demonstrating the unique T-cell receptor using the polymerase chain reaction. In some cases of angioimmunoblastic T-cell lymphomas, clonality has been difficult to demonstrate.[19]

In addition to aiding in an accurate diagnosis of T-cell lymphoma as opposed to B-cell lymphoma, immunophenotyping can help in identifying certain subtypes of peripheral T-cell lymphoma. CD30 positivity is a hallmark of anaplastic large T/null-cell lymphoma. While occasionally seen in other lymphomas and regularly seen in Hodgkin's disease, it is characteristic of anaplastic large T/null-cell lymphoma and its absence would put the diagnosis in doubt. Staining for CD56 is characteristic of nasal NK/T-cell lymphomas and can aid in this diagnosis.

In contrast to B-cell lymphomas, characteristic cytogenetic abnormalities in the peripheral T-cell lymphomas have been few. The one exception is the t(2;5)(p23;q35), which involves the anaplastic lymphoma kinase (alk) gene and the nucleophosmin (npm) gene.[20] Over-expression of the fusion protein produced by this translocation is associated with a good prognosis. Hepatosplenic T-cell lymphoma has been associated with i(7q) and trisomy 8.[21] Gains at chromosome 9q have been associated with enteropathy-type T-cell lymphomas.[22] Unfortunately, there has been no characteristic genetic abnormality associated with the largest subgroup of peripheral T-cell lymphoma-NOS. Identifying those genes and associated proteins involved in the pathogenesis of these lymphomas is an important goal. In this regard, gene expression profiling has great potential but has not yet been extensively studied. An early report suggested that gene expression profiling might be able to distinguish peripheral T-cell lymphomas from lymphoblastic lymphoma.[23] As might be expected, genes associated with tumor proliferation and cell death appear to be those most likely to be expressed abnormally in these lymphomas.

HISTOPATHOLOGY

The World Health Organization classification of non-Hodgkin's lymphomas is an important advance in understanding and diagnosing peripheral T-cell lymphomas. The WHO classification for mature T-cell and natural killing–cell neoplasms is listed in Table 24–1.[1] While there are leukemic subtypes classified as peripheral T-cell lymphomas, they are not considered in this chapter. There are separate chapters on extranodal NK/T-cell lymphoma of nasal type, mycosis fungoides/Sézary syndrome, and adult T-cell lymphoma/leukemia.

The most frequent subtype of peripheral T-cell lymphoma is peripheral T-cell lymphoma-NOS. The tumor cells in this subtype of lymphoma can be predominantly large, predominantly small, or most commonly, a mixture of atypical large and small lymphocytes. Typically, the tumor cells show a preference for involvement of the pericortical regions of lymph nodes, but this is not always the case. Frequently, these lymphomas are recognized as peripheral T-cell lymphomas only after immunophenotyping. In an international study of non-Hodgkin's lymphomas, expert hematopathologists were able to accurately diagnosis peripheral T-cell lymphomas only 41% to 46% of the time without the availability of immunophenotyping (Table 26–4).[2]

The angioimmunoblastic T-cell lymphoma has a histologic appearance that often can be confused with the entity formally called "angioimmunoblastic lymphadenopathy and dysproteinemia."[24,25] The typical morphologic appearance of angioimmunoblastic lymphadenopathy and dysproteinemia was a proliferation of small arborizing vessels and a pleomorphic cellular infiltrate. In angioimmunoblastic T-cell lymphoma, the same appearance combined with absence of or "burned-out" germinal centers is typical. Tumor cells in this disorder are sometimes positive for the Epstein–Barr virus. On occasion, this type of lymphoma can be confused with Hodgkin's disease because of large atypical cells.

Table 26–4. Reproducibility of Diagnosis of Peripheral T-Cell Lymphoma

Type	Based on Histology Alone	Based on Histology plus Immunophenotype
Anaplastic large T/null cell	46%	85%
Peripheral T-cell-NOS	41%	86%
Diffuse large B-cell	73%	97%
Follicular	93%	94%

NOS, not otherwise specified.

A variety of rare, extranodal peripheral T-cell lymphomas can cause difficulties in diagnosis. The hepatosplenic T-cell lymphoma often has a gamma-delta immunophenotype rather than the alpha-beta immunophenotype of more mature T-cell lymphomas. This type of T-cell lymphoma frequently does not express CD4 or CD8. The tumor cells infiltrate the sinusoids of involved organs and the diagnosis can be difficult. Sometimes only the identification of a T-cell receptor gene rearrangement allows accurate diagnosis. The enteropathy-type T-cell lymphoma most often occurs in patients with untreated celiac disease. The small bowel frequently shows villous atrophy, and the tumor usually presents as an ulcerating mass. These lymphomas are usually Epstein–Barr virus negative. Subcutaneous panniculitis-like T-cell lymphoma is an extremely unusual disease that is often misdiagnosed as benign panniculitis. The tumors often contain a mixture of small and large atypical lymphoid cells with clear cytoplasm. They usually have the alpha-beta immunophenotype, but in a minority of cases a gamma-delta immunophenotype can be seen. Tumor cells are generally confined to the subcutaneous tissue. Diagnosis might require recognition of a T-cell receptor gene rearrangement and is usually only made by experienced hematopathologists.

CLINICAL MANIFESTATIONS

Patients with peripheral T-cell lymphoma can present with an extraordinarily wide variety of clinical syndromes. When encountering an unusual condition such as the hemophagocytic syndrome or necrotic nasal/facial lesions, the possibility that the underlying condition might be a peripheral T-cell lymphoma should be considered. However, most patients with peripheral T-cell lymphomas present with nodal or extranodal masses in a manner analogous to that of patients with B-cell lymphomas.

A series of 134 patients with peripheral T-cell lymphoma was collected from Tennessee, Southern California, and Nebraska.[26] The clinical characteristics of these patients are summarized in Table 26–5. The median age was 57 years, with an age range of 4 to 97 years. Fifty-nine percent of the patients were male. Twenty-seven percent of the patients had previously been diagnosed as having some other disorder of the immune system. Eleven percent had had another lymphoproliferative disorder (e.g., angioimmunoblastic

Table 26–5. Peripheral T-Cell Lymphoma Series: Patient Characteristicsa[a]

Characteristic	Patients n (%)
Total number of patients	134
Male/female	79/55
Preceding immune systemdisorder	36 (27)
Other lymphoproliferative disorders	15 (11)
Angioimmunoblastic lymphadenopathy	6
Atypical dermatitis	4
Mononucleosis	2
Lymphomatoid papulosis	2
Lymphomatoid granulomatosis	1
Different lymphoma	11 (8)
"Autoimmune" arthritis	6 (4)
Preceding nonhematologic malignancy	4 (3)
Stage	
I	10 (7)
II	28 (21)
III	29 (22)
IV	67 (50)
Symptom status	
A	58 (43)
B	76 (57)
Histologic group	
Large cell	58 (43)
Mixed	53 (40)
Small cell	23 (17)
Hypercalcemia (Ca2+ measured in 122 patients)	3 (2)
HTLV-I positive (measured in 24 patients)	1 (4)
Elevated LDH level (measured in 113 patients)	98 (87)
Bone marrow involvement	41 (35)
Large cell	12 (24)
Mixed	16 (33)
Small cell	13 (68)

[a]Median age is 57 years (range of 4 to 97 years).
Includes only patients who had bone marrow biopsy.
HTLV-I, human T-cell lymphoma lymphotrophic virus, type I; LDH, lactate dehydrogenase.
From Armitage JO, Greer JP, Levine AM, et al. Peripheral T-cell lymphoma. Cancer 1989;63:158–63,[26] with permission.

lymphadenopathy), which might have represented an early phase of the lymphoma. Some patients had previously been diagnosed as having B-cell lymphoma or Hodgkin's disease. Four percent of the patients had been diagnosed as having an autoimmune arthritis before the appearance of the lymphoma. The occurrence of a peripheral T-cell lymphoma as a complication of other immune disorders is a real phenomenon that occurs at a higher-than-expected incidence.

Patients with peripheral T-cell lymphoma not associated with HTLV-I infection are not likely to present with hypercalcemia.[26] However, a number of adverse factors are frequent in these patients. For example, in an international study of 96 patients with peripheral T-cell lymphoma, excluding those with the anaplastic large-cell subtype, the median age was 61 years and 53% of the patients had an International Prognostic Index (IPI) score of 3 or greater. Sixty-one patients were Stage IV at presentation, and 40% presented with B symptoms. An elevated serum lactic dehydrogenase level was found in 61% of the patients, and 29% were nonambulatory at diagnosis. Thirteen percent of the patients had circulating tumor cells identified. More than half of the patients had both nodal and extranodal sites of involvement at diagnosis. However, as can be seen in Table 26–6, the various subtypes of peripheral T-cell lymphoma have different characteristics.[27]

Whether skin involvement occurs more frequently in patients with peripheral T-cell lymphomas than in those with B-cell lymphomas is unclear. Because it has been widely believed that patients with peripheral T-cell lymphomas are more likely to have cutaneous involvement, it may be that the frequent incidence of skin involvement in some reports relates to more patients with skin involvement having tumors immunotyped.

Peripheral T-cell lymphomas seem to share the same characteristics as B-cell lymphomas in the frequency of bone marrow involvement.[26] However, one report has suggested a very high incidence of marrow involvement when immunohistochemical studies were performed.[28,29] Patients with predominantly large cells are less likely to have bone marrow involvement (24% in one series) than those with mixed small and large cells (33%) or those with small cells

Table 26–6. Characteristics of Patients with Peripheral T-Cell Lymphoma from an International Study Involving Eight Countries

	Peripheral T-Cell Lymphoma-NOS	Angioimmunoblastic T-Cell Lymphoma	Anaplastic Large T/Null Cell
Median age	59	65	34
Male	44%	53%	69%
Stage IV	60%	83%	39%
B symptoms	41%	65%	51%
Elevated serum LDH	65%	60%	45%
Tumor diameter >10 cm	9%	17%	17%
Nonambulatory performance status	28%	38%	26%
Presentation			
Nodal only	22%	12%	39%
Extranodal only	16%	6%	12%

LDH, lactate dehydrogenase; NOS, not otherwise specified.
From Rudiger T, Weisenburger DD, Anderson JR, et al. Peripheral T-cell lymphoma (excluding anaplastic large-cell lymphoma): results from the Non-Hodgkin's Lymphoma Classification Project. Ann Oncol 2002;13:140–9,[27] with permission.

(68%). However, unlike patients with B-cell lymphomas, the patients with large-cell peripheral T-cell lymphoma did not have a worse prognosis than those with predominately small cells.

The ability to perform immunophenotyping on paraffin-embedded specimens has led to the recognition that a significant number of patients with extranodal anaplastic lesions that were believed to represent undifferentiated carcinomas in fact had anaplastic large-cell lymphoma. It was subsequently demonstrated that most of these patients had T-cell lymphomas that were Ki-1, or CD30, positive.[30] Ki-1 is an antigen that was originally recognized on Hodgkin's disease tumor cells.[31] It can be found occasionally on all types of non-Hodgkin's lymphomas, but is especially likely to be present on anaplastic large-cell lymphomas.[32–34]

It has become apparent that patients with Ki-1–positive anaplastic large-cell lymphoma represent many cases that were formerly called "malignant histiocytosis."[35] A characteristic chromosomal abnormality, t(2;5), and overexpression of the anaplastic lymphoma kinase (ALK) protein, are frequently associated with this subtype of lymphoma.[36] Although sometimes presenting in an extranodal site, this subtype usually presents in lymph nodes.[4]

Peripheral T-cell lymphomas are sometimes associated with a clinical syndrome manifested by fever, hepatosplenomegaly, liver function abnormalities, thrombocytopenia, and erythrophagocytosis seen on bone marrow biopsy and, occasionally, biopsy of other organs. The association is sufficiently strong that some have suggested that any patient presenting with the hemophagocytic syndrome should undergo an evaluation aimed at finding a peripheral T-cell lymphoma.[37,38]

Peripheral T-cell lymphomas have been reported in patients with a variety of immunologic abnormalities. As described earlier, peripheral T-cell lymphoma can occur in patients who are immunosuppressed after solid organ transplantation.[39] Peripheral T-cell lymphomas have been reported with unusual extranodal localizations in patients infected by human immunodeficiency virus.[40] There are also reports of peripheral T-cell lymphoma developing in patients with hypogammaglobulinemia[41] and Chediak–Higashi syndrome.[42]

Patients can present with a clinical syndrome of systemic illness, liver dysfunction, and unusual organ infiltration by post-thymic T cells. Documentation of the clonal origin of the T cells and their atypical characteristics can lead to the diagnosis of peripheral T-cell lymphoma. This usually leads to the diagnosis of hepatosplenic gamma/delta T-cell lymphoma.

Patients with adult celiac disease are at increased risk for developing intestinal peripheral T-cell lymphoma.[43] Peripheral T-cell lymphoma has been reported presenting with profound eosinophilia.[44] This syndrome has been found in patients who present with what appears to be systemic vasculitis.[45] Peripheral T-cell lymphomas have been diagnosed in patients who initially appeared to have dysmyelopoietic syndrome.[46] Peripheral T-cell lymphomas have been reported masquerading as hairy cell leukemia.[47] Other unusual presentations include peripheral neuropathy, granulomatous liver disease, and angioedema with diffuse pulmonary infiltrates.[48,49] Peripheral T-cell lymphomas have been reported to involve essentially all organs, including the central nervous system.[50]

THE PROGNOSIS OF T-CELL VERSUS B-CELL LYMPHOMAS

There has been a disagreement in the literature on the prognostic significance of a particular lymphoma having a B-cell or a T-cell immunophenotype. Some authors have found that peripheral T-cell lymphomas have a worse outlook than corresponding B-cell lymphomas, whereas others have found no difference. These results are summarized in Table 26–7. At least nine studies have contrasted the results between patients with B-cell lymphomas and those with peripheral T-cell lymphomas.[29,51–58] Seven studies found T-cell lymphomas to have a worse prognosis, whereas two studies found no difference.[29,57] No studies have found B-cell lymphoma to have a poorer prognosis than T-cell lymphoma.

One large study from Japan compared 449 patients with B-cell lymphoma to 92 patients with peripheral T-cell lymphoma; cases of adult T-cell leukemia/lymphoma were excluded.[59] The authors found that B-cell lymphomas were more likely to present with low and intermediate histologic grades, whereas patients with peripheral T-cell lymphoma were more likely to have a higher histologic grade, B symptoms, and poor performance status. The

Table 26–7. Comparative Prognosis for Patients with T-Cell and B-Cell Lymphoma

Reference	Patients with T-Cell Lymphoma (n)	Factors Favoring Patients with B-Cell NHL	Factors Favoring Patients with T-Cell NHL
Schimoyama (1993)[51]	552	Survival	—
Coiffier (1990)[52]	361	Freedom from relapse	—
Armitage (1989)[53]	110	Survival and progression-free survival	—
Lippman (1988)[54]	103	Disease-free survival	—
Kwak (1991)[29]	98	—	—
NHL Classification Project (1997)[55]	96	Survival, failure-free survival	—
Shimizu (1989)[56]	48	Complete remission rate survival	—
Cheng (1989)[57]	70	—	—
Brown (1989)[58]	51	Survival	—

NHL, non-Hodgkin's lymphoma.

overall survival of the patients with the B-cell lymphoma was superior.

A study from France reported 361 patients with aggressive non-Hodgkin's lymphoma who were immunophenotyped and received treatment with the LNH-84 regimen.[52] More than 90% of the patients had diffuse mixed cell, diffuse large-cell, or immunoblastic lymphoma using the Working Formulation classification. Seventy percent of the patients had a B-cell immunophenotype, and 30% a T-cell immunophenotype. Patients with peripheral T-cell lymphoma were more likely to present with an advanced stage ($p = 0.0002$) and to have B symptoms ($p \geq 0.01$). Although there was no difference in response rate to the chemotherapy regimen, patients with peripheral T-cell lymphoma were more likely to relapse from remission (43% vs. 29%, $p < 0.001$). Patients with peripheral T-cell lymphoma had a shorter overall survival (42 vs. 50 months, $p < 0.05$). A multivariate analysis showed that the T-cell immunophenotype was a significant adverse prognostic factor, independent of other adverse risk factors.

A total of 110 patients treated by physicians participating in the Nebraska Lymphoma Study Group had a diffuse mixed, diffuse large-cell, or immunoblastic lymphoma, and all patients were prospectively immunophenotyped.[53] All patients received the same six-drug chemotherapy regimen. Patients with peripheral T-cell lymphoma had significantly worse survival and progression-free survival rates. However, this poorer outlook was a result of the especially poor outcome seen in patients with Stage IV disease. Patients with less extensive lymphomas did equally well whether they had a B-cell or T-cell immunophenotype.

An Arizona study of 103 consecutively accrued patients with diffuse large-cell lymphoma found 83 to have a B-cell immunophenotype and 20 a T-cell immunophenotype.[60] Patients with B-cell lymphoma were more likely to have bulky disease, and patients with T-cell lymphoma were more likely to have skin involvement. Eight-three percent of the patients with each immunophenotype received a doxorubicin-containing combination chemotherapy regimen. Disease-free survival was significantly shorter in the patients with T-cell lymphoma (median 11 months vs. 43 months, $p = 0.01$). In fact, no patient with peripheral T-cell lymphoma remained disease-free for longer than 2 years, in contrast with 55% of the patients with B-cell lymphoma. However, the actuarial overall survival did not vary significantly between the two groups ($p = 0.23$).

An international study of patients from eight countries and four continents included 422 patients with diffuse large B-cell lymphoma, and 129 patients with aggressive peripheral T-cell lymphoma. Thirty-three patients had anaplastic large T/null-cell lymphomas and 96 patients other peripheral T-cell lymphomas.[2] The patients with anaplastic large T/null-cell lymphomas were younger with a median age of 33 years and 69% were male, while the patients with other peripheral T-cell lymphomas had a median age of 61 years and 56% were male. Patients with diffuse large B-cell lymphoma had a median age of 64 years and 55% were male. The patients were consecutive patients from their institutions were included regardless of therapy received. Patients with anaplastic large T/null-cell lymphoma had significantly better survival than patients with diffuse large B-cell lymphoma (i.e., 77% vs. 46%), while those with other types of aggressive peripheral T-cell lymphoma had a significantly poorer survival (i.e., 25% vs. 46%) (Fig. 26–1).[61]

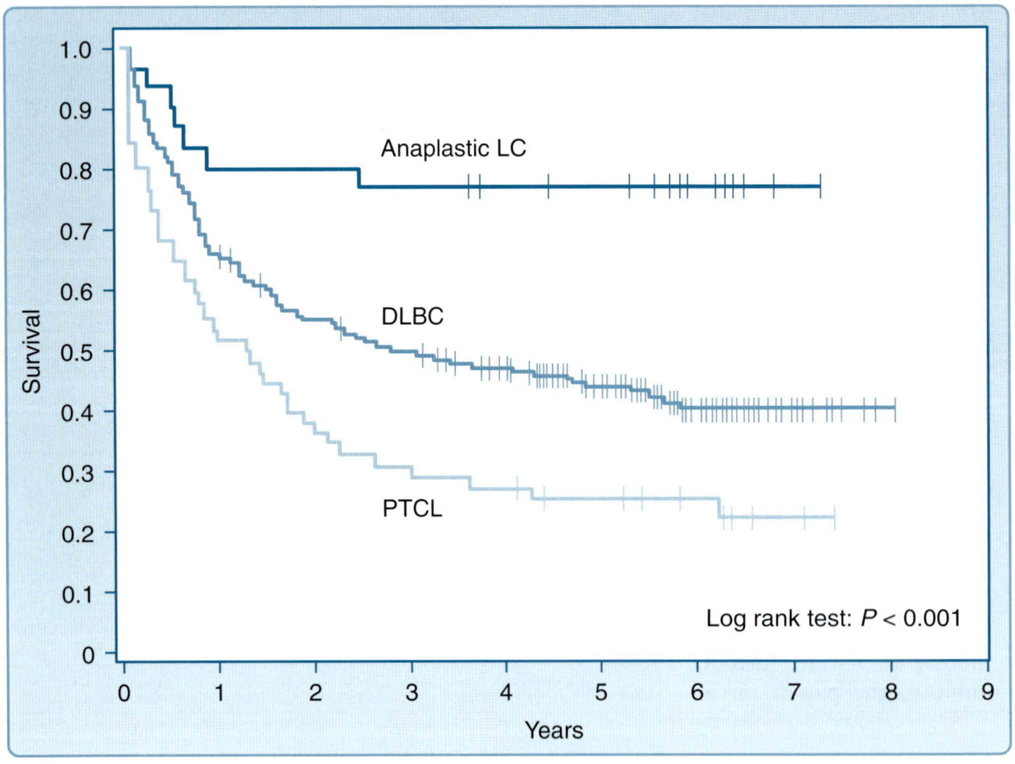

Figure 26–1. Survival of patients with anaplastic large T/null-cell lymphoma and other peripheral T-cell lymphomas compared to patients with diffuse large B-cell lymphoma. (From The Non-Hodgkin's Lymphoma Classification Project. A clinical evaluation of the International Lymphoma Study Group classification of non-Hodgkin's lymphoma. Blood 1997;89:3909–18,[2] with permission.)

The prognostic significance of having a peripheral T-cell lymphoma rather than a B-cell lymphoma remains somewhat controversial. However, most studies have shown poorer progression-free survival in patients with peripheral T-cell lymphoma, and several have shown worse overall survival.

AN APPROACH TO PATIENTS WITH POSSIBLE PERIPHERAL T-CELL LYMPHOMA

One of the problems in caring for these patients is determining when a patient with an atypical T-cell proliferative process actually has lymphoma. With B-cell proliferations, this process is somewhat easier. B-cell proliferations can be more easily identified as being clonal (i.e., κλ light-chain restricted), and B-cell lymphoma seems more likely to grow as a tumorous mass or to infiltrate the bone marrow and peripheral blood. There are several T-cell proliferations that can be difficult to classify. For example, the entity often referred to as "angioimmunoblastic lymphadenopathy with dysproteinemia" has been a source of controversy.[62,63] Although this has often been referred to as a "benign" proliferation of a mixture of cell types, it is now clear using T-cell gene rearrangement studies that these processes often have a clonal T-cell proliferation, and they certainly often have a rapidly fatal course.[5] A number of angiocentric T-cell proliferations have also caused confusion. Processes that in the past might have been called "lethal midline granuloma" now are frequently recognized as representing peripheral T-cell lymphomas.[64] Once again, this is based on a proliferation of atypical T-cells, demonstration of a monoclonal T-cell population using T-cell receptor gene rearrangement studies, and a rapidly fatal natural history that can be modified with chemotherapy. Finally, there are patients who present with a systemic illness and organ infiltration by atypical T lymphocytes.[65] With the same criteria, some of these patients can be identified as having peripheral T-cell lymphoma. The broader spectrum of illness seen with peripheral T-cell lymphomas than with the more common B-cell lymphomas has made these malignancies frequently challenging clinical problems for clinicians.

A useful way to consider the spectrum of peripheral T-cell lymphoma is to recognize the numerous clinical "syndromes" with which they can present. The most common presentation of both peripheral T-cell lymphoma and B-cell lymphoma is as a nodal or extranodal tumor. With peripheral T-cell lymphomas, biopsy reveals the tumor to represent a proliferation of atypical lymphoid cells that have a T-cell immunophenotype. The only distinction between B-cell and T-cell lymphomas with this presentation is documentation of the immunophenotype or finding characteristic gene rearrangements.

However, there are a number of more unusual presentations that are highly associated with the peripheral T-cell lymphomas. Peripheral T-cell lymphomas can present with a wide spectrum of clinical and histopathologic features. Because available treatments can modify the natural history of these disorders in a way favorable to the patient, it is important to recognize this variety of appearances so that a diagnosis can be reached quickly.

STAGING/PROGNOSIS (PREDICTING OUTCOME)

A number of studies have identified factors that predict treatment outcome in patients treated for peripheral T-cell lymphoma.[26,27,52,65–72] These have included histopathologic, immunologic, and clinical characteristics. Immunologic characteristics (e.g., helper vs. suppressor immunophenotype) have generally, but not always,[70] failed to predict treatment outcome. However, tumors that overexpress CD30 and the ALK protein have a better prognosis.[73–75] These findings go with the anaplastic large T/null-cell lymphoma, which has a better survival than other types of peripheral T-cell lymphoma.

The clinical characteristics of patients with peripheral T-cell lymphomas, like those in patients with B-cell lymphomas, are predictive of treatment outcome. Localized versus disseminated disease, poor performance status, elevated serum LDH level, older age, bone marrow involvement, and tumor mass size have all been found to be important predictors of treatment outcome.[26,27,52,65–72] Some authors have found a high tumor proliferative rate to be an adverse prognostic factor.[76,77]

The IPI is useful in predicting treatment outcome in patients with peripheral T-cell lymphoma[2,78–80] (Fig. 26–2). A recent study suggested a new prognostic model for predicting outcome in patients with peripheral T-cell lymphoma. The major factors in this analysis were age, performance status, serum LDH level, and bone marrow involvement. With this system, patients with no adverse prognostic factors had a 5-year survival rate of 62% in contrast to patients with three or four adverse risk factors who had a 5-year survival rate of only 18%.[81]

MANAGEMENT OF SPECIFIC SUBTYPES

Peripheral T-Cell Lymphoma-NOS

The most common subgroup of peripheral T-cell lymphomas are those that would be confused with diffuse large B-cell lymphoma if immunophenotyping were not carried out. These patients are somewhat more likely than those with diffuse large B-cell lymphoma to be at the advanced

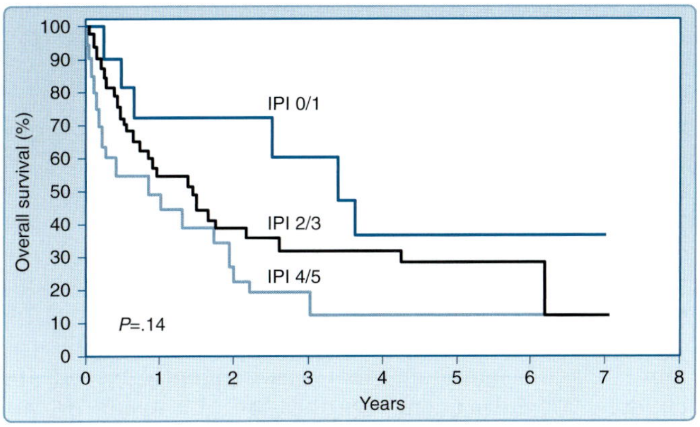

Figure 26–2. Overall survival by International Prognostic Index score for patients with peripheral T-cell lymphoma.

stage. However, there are no absolutely characteristic clinical findings to predict the T-cell immunophenotype, and the staging evaluation is the same.

The treatment for patients with peripheral T-cell lymphoma-NOS has generally been the same regimens used for diffuse large B-cell lymphoma. However, as noted in a previous section, the results tend to be poorer. Clinical trials have some times lumped together patients with different subtypes of peripheral T-cell lymphomas, although the majority of patients were those with peripheral T-cell lymphoma-NOS. Complete remission rates have varied from 24% to 77%, with failure-free survivals varying from 12% to 45%.[26,27,69,70,82–85]

Because the results for patients treated with anthracycline-contained regimens typically used for diffuse large B-cell lymphoma have been disappointing, several centers are now trying alternative approaches. These include the primary use of platinum-containing chemotherapy regimens, and very intensive regimens such as HyperCVAD. However, for documentation of the superiority of one of these approaches, clinical trials will have to be carried out. Because of the relative rarity of this disease, this will require cooperation among different institutions and perhaps among different countries.

Salvage therapy in patients with peripheral T-cell lymphoma-NOS has been reported using a wide variety of treatment approaches. Autologous bone marrow transplantation can certainly be curative.[83,84,86] For chemotherapy-sensitive relapsed patients, results appear to be similar to what has been seen for relapsed, diffuse large B-cell lymphoma. Because of this treatment outcome, some clinicians favor offering autologous bone marrow transplantation to patients achieving an initial complete remission with high-stage peripheral T-cell lymphoma. Other salvage therapies have been utilized including purine analogs, gemcitabine, retinoids, denileukin diftitox, interferon, and platinum-based chemotherapy.[87–94] Good results have been reported with several of these regimens, and utilized in combination they need to be studied as part of the initial therapy of patients with this disorder.

Anaplastic Large T/Null Lymphoma

The disorder now classified as anaplastic large T/null lymphoma has only been known for approximately 15 years. These highly anaplastic-appearing tumors were once usually diagnosed as anaplastic carcinoma or melanoma, undifferentiated malignant neoplasm, and more recently as malignant histiocytosis. In fact, the t(2;5)(p23;q35) was initially described as a characteristic chromosomal abnormality of malignant histiocytosis.[95] The identification of a monoclonal antibody to a protein typically seen on Reed–Sternberg cells accomplished by German scientists in the mid-1980s was an important step in identifying this disease.[64,65] The antigen recognized by the monoclonal antibody was originally designated Ki-1 and more recently CD30. By 1989, reports were appearing that associated this antigen and the t(2:5) with a particular subtype of large-cell non-Hodgkin's lymphoma that was frequently seen in the children.[96–99] Subsequent identification of a fusion protein involving the alk and npm genes that was characteristic of this lymphoma, and could be identified by immunophenotyping, solidified the recognition of anaplastic large T/null lymphoma as a specific entity.[100–102]

Patients with anaplastic large T/null-cell lymphoma have strikingly different clinical characteristics from those with other peripheral T-cell lymphomas (Table 26–6). Patients with anaplastic large T/null-cell lymphoma are much more likely to be young and male, but less likely to have Stage IV disease and elevated serum LDH level. Lymphomas with an anaplastic appearance frequently present with skin involvement, but when the disease is confined to the skin, it frequently follows a much more benign course. In the WHO classification of lymphoid malignancies, purely cutaneous, anaplastic large T/null-cell lymphoma, and a related entity, lymphomatoid papulosis, are recognized as separate disorders.[1] If the lymphomas over-express the ALK protein, they are probably part of a systemic disease. Patients with ALK-negative, cutaneous-only disease have a much more indolent process than the patients discussed in this section, and should be managed conservatively.

Patients with systemic anaplastic, large T/null-cell lymphoma do not all over-express the ALK protein. Over-expression of the ALK protein is more likely in young patients,[103] and associated with a much better prognosis.[104–107]

Patients with anaplastic large T/null-cell lymphoma have generally been treated with the same regimens as patients with other types of aggressive non-Hodgkin's lymphoma. Young patients, and those who overexpress the ALK protein, have had an excellent response to therapy.[103,108–110] In adults, using anthracycline containing chemotherapy regimens has produced complete remission rates from 49% to 95%,[111–117] and 5-year survival from 35% to 76% (Table 26–6). In studies that analyze patients by over-expression of the ALK protein, the survival for ALK-positive patients varied from 71% to 79%, while that for ALK-negative patients varied from 15% to 46%. The IPI and the status of the expression of the ALK protein are the major prognostic factors. At present in the United States, most adult patients with this lymphoma are treated with CHOP.

Relapses have been treated with a variety of salvage chemotherapy regimens, but the most effective treatment appears to be autologous bone marrow transplantation with results comparable to those seen in aggressive B-cell lymphomas.[118] Allogeneic bone marrow transplantation can also be effective, but because of its high treatment-related mortality, it might be most useful in young patients.[119]

Angioimmunoblastic Peripheral T-Cell Lymphoma

First reported by Flandrin in 1972 and Frizzera in 1974,[62,63] angioimmunoblastic lymphadenopathy with dysprotinemia was characterized by generalized lymphadenopathy, hepatosplenomegaly, hypergammaglobulinemia, fever, and immune abnormalities sometimes including a positive Coombs test. Shimoyama et al. in 1979 described immunoblastic lymphadenopathy–like T-cell lymphoma.[120] Brice et al. in 1987 described the same entity.[121]

Today it is clear that most patients formerly diagnosed with angioimmunoblastic lymphadenopathy with dysprotinemia had peripheral T-cell lymphoma. The rapidly fatal course in most patients originally diagnosed as angioimmunoblastic lymphadenopathy with dysprotinemia is consistent with this outcome. However, an occasional patient diagnosed with angioimmunoblastic lymphadenopathy with dysprotinemia had a durable response to prednisone causing concern in some physicians about immediately initiating therapy for lymphoma. This is particularly true since patients diagnosed with angioimmunoblastic T-cell lymphoma do not always have an abnormal T-cell clone identified on studies of T-cell receptor genes.[19] However, one study that compared initial treatment with prednisone to that using an anthracycline-containing combination chemotherapy regimen found far better survival in the patients initially treated with chemotherapy.[122] When therapy is required because of symptoms, unless strong evidence can be generated to the contrary, patients are probably best treated as having T-cell lymphoma.

Patients with angioimmunoblastic T-cell lymphoma usually present with systemic symptoms such as fever and weight loss, generalized lymphadenopathy, skin rashes, and frequently splenomegaly on physical exam, and have polyclonal hyperglobulinemia and an elevated serum LDH.[123] Patients often have a history of repeated infections and other immunologic abnormalities. Patients with angioimmunoblastic T-cell lymphoma are older, more frequently Stage IV, and more frequently present with systemic symptoms than peripheral T-cell lymphoma-NOS (Table 26–6).

As is true for most types of peripheral T-cell lymphoma, the optimal treatment for patients with angioimmunoblastic T-cell lymphoma is not known. Even when these patients are treated with an anthracycline-containing chemotherapy regimen, some studies suggest a poorer outcome than with peripheral T-cell lymphoma-NOS.[108,123,124] Autologous bone marrow transplantation has been reported to be effective in angioimmunoblastic peripheral T-cell lymphoma.[108] Salvage therapies have included alternate chemotherapy regimens such as those including platinum derivatives, lodes oral methotrexate, interferon, and cyclosporine.[103,108,125,126]

Enteropathy-Type Peripheral T-Cell Lymphoma

Enteropathy-type intestinal T-cell lymphoma frequently occurs in patients with celiac disease. The patients may have a long history of celiac disease and have become unresponsive to a gluten-free diet, or the two diagnoses may be made simultaneously. A characteristic HLA genotype has been associated with both celiac disease and enteropathy-type T-cell lymphoma.[96] In one study from the British National Lymphoma Investigation, 9% of lymphomas involving the intestine were enteropathy-type intestinal T-cell lymphoma.[127] In patients known to have celiac disease, this should be the first consideration when a patient develops a gastrointestinal lymphoma. While 5% or more of patients with adult-onset celiac disease have been reported to develop lymphoma,[128,129] not all patients who develop enteropathy-type T-cell lymphoma have celiac disease.[130]

The disease is usually confined to the jejunum or ileum. However, involvement of the colon, duodenum, and stomach occur rarely. Disease is metastatic to regional lymph nodes approximately one-third of the time.[130] In a large series of patients from the United Kingdom, the median age at diagnosis was 55 years and there was a striking male predominance.[130] The presenting symptoms were most commonly abdominal pain, weight loss, and, less frequently, diarrhea and vomiting. Unfortunately, perforation or bowel obstruction is seen in almost half the patients. Spread to distant sites is unusual, accounting for only approximately 20% of the patients in the United Kingdom.

When possible, resection is the best initial management. However, without subsequent therapy, relapse almost always occurs. Combination chemotherapy should be administered even to patients who have achieved complete remission after surgery. Unfortunately, these patients tolerate chemotherapy poorly, partly because of the frequency of untreated or poorly treated celiac disease and malnutrition. In addition, many of the patients, present with perforation or bowel obstruction. In one series of patients from the United Kingdom, the 1-year and 5-year survival rates were only 39% and 20%, with all but 3% of the patients either relapsing or dying from treatment-related complications.[130] In a study from Ireland, 9 of 23 patients were alive and disease-free at a median of 74 months.[131] A German group reported a 28% 2-year survival rate in patients with intestinal T-cell lymphoma.[132]

Enteropathy-associated intestinal T-cell lymphoma has a less than optimal response to combination chemotherapy regimens such as CHOP and poor survival rates. While the best approach to managing this disease is prevention by optimal management of celiac disease, new approaches to management of patients who develop this lymphoma are needed.

Hepatosplenic Gamma/Delta Peripheral T-Cell Lymphoma

This lymphoma typically presents in young men with systemic symptoms, hepatosplenomegaly, cytopenias, and bone marrow infiltration.[101,133] The disease often presents difficulties in diagnosis because of the absence of tumorous masses and the sinusoidal infiltration of the lymphoma cells in the spleen, liver, and bone marrow. Identification of rearranged T-cell receptor genes is sometimes necessary for the diagnosis. It will often be missed unless the tissue is reviewed by an experienced hematopathologist.

In a series of 21 patients reported from France, 15 patients were males and the median age was 34 years.[134] All 21 had splenomegaly, 15 had hepatomegaly, and thrombocytopenia was found in 20 patients at diagnosis. Marrow involvement was sometimes difficult to see by typical light microscopy, but involvement was documented in all patients by immunophenotyping. Lymphoma cells were CD3-positive, CD5-negative, and expressed a gamma/delta T-cell receptors. Fifteen of 18 lymphomas that were typed expressed CD56. Eighteen of 20 were negative for Epstein–Barr virus. Nine of thirteen patients who were studied showed an isochromosome 7q. Eight patients had a history of immune disease including kidney transplantation, systemic lupus, Hodgkin's disease, or malaria.

Patients were treated with multiagent chemotherapy regimens including, in 19 patients, an anthracycline.[134] Three patients died in the initial 2 months of treatment and four others failed to respond. Fourteen of the 21 patients responded to induction therapy and nine patients achieved a complete remission. Five relapsed between 10 and 44 months. Six patients received autologous bone marrow transplantation in first complete remission and two remain in remission at 42 and 42 months at the time of the report. The other 19 patients died of lymphoma or treatment-related toxicity.

This lymphoma often presents a diagnostic challenge. It should be considered, particularly in young patients, who present with a systemic illness manifested by fever, hepatosplenomegaly, and cytopenias. Unfortunately, making the diagnosis does not lead to a good treatment outcome in most patients. New treatment approaches are badly needed.

Subcutaneous Panniculitis-Like Peripheral T-Cell Lymphoma

This unusual and extremely rare disorder typically presents with subcutaneous nodules primarily involving the extremities.[135–138] The lesions range in size from less than 1 cm to several centimeters and at times can be necrotic. Frequently these are originally thought to represent panniculitis. To complicate matters, a diagnosis of benign panniculitis is usual at first biopsy, particularly when made by a pathologist not acquainted with this rare disease.

Typically, biopsies demonstrate a mixture of atypical small and large lymphoid cells mixed with reactive histiocytes.[139] The tumor cells can display either alpha-beta (more frequently) or gamma-delta T-cell receptors. In at least one series, patients who expressed the gamma-delta T-cell receptors were older, more likely to be male, more likely to have presented with systemic symptoms, more likely to have the hemophagocytic syndrome, and had a shorter survival.[140]

The clinical syndrome typically consists of progressive subcutaneous nodules, often accompanied by systemic symptoms such as fever. The hemaphagocytic syndrome has been frequently reported in patients with subcutaneous panniculitis-like T-cell lymphoma. Interestingly, there is one case of subcutaneous panniculitis-like T-cell lymphoma being transmitted to the recipient of an allogeneic bone marrow transplantation.[141]

Therapy for patients with this lymphoma has generally been unsuccessful.[135,138,142–145] In our experience involved-field radiotherapy consistently causes regression of the individual tumors, but is followed by relapse in new sites. Patients who have indolent disease can be followed with minimal treatment or involved-field radiotherapy to control symptomatic sites. However, patients with more aggressive illness have not had durable remissions, and sometimes are initially resistant to traditional antilymphoma regimens such as CHOP. Multiple alternative treatment regimens have been utilized including platinum-based regimens, cis-retinoic acid, interferon, immunosuppressive drugs such as cyclosporine, and denileukin diftitox.[3,138,143,146] No treatment has been consistently effective, although good responses have been described.

CONCLUSION

Our knowledge of peripheral T-cell lymphomas continues to evolve. Unfortunately, for most patients the outcome of therapy is still poor. New insights into the biology of these disorders might provide new targets for therapy. Clinical trials aimed specifically at finding the best treatments for T-cell lymphomas, rather than mixing T-cell and B-cell lymphomas together, will almost certainly improve our ability to benefit these patients. Hopefully, the years ahead will change the previous dismal prognosis for most patients with these disorders.

References

1. Jaffe E, Harris N, Stein H, et al., eds. World Health Organization Classification of Tumours. Pathology and Genetics of Tumours of Haematopoietic and Lymphoid Tissues. Lyon: IARC Press, 2001.
2. The Non-Hodgkin's Lymphoma Classification Project. A clinical evaluation of the International Lymphoma Study Group classification of non-Hodgkin's lymphoma. Blood 1997;89:3909–18.
3. Salhany KE, Macon WR, Choi JK, et al. Subcutaneous panniculitis-like T-cell lymphoma: clinicopathologic, immunophenotypic, and genotypic analysis of alpha/beta and gamma/delta subtypes. Am J Surg Pathol 1998; 22:881–93.
4. Weisenburger DD, Anderson JR, Diebold J, et al. Systemic anaplastic large-cell lymphoma: results from the non-Hodgkin's lymphoma classification project. Am J Hematol 2001;67:172–8.
5. Anderson JR, Armitage JO, Weisenburger DD. Epidemiology of the non-Hodgkin's lymphomas: distributions of the major subtypes differ by geographic locations. Non-Hodgkin's Lymphoma Classification Project. Ann Oncol 1998;9:717–20.
6. Isaacson P, Wright DH. Intestinal lymphoma associated with malabsorption. Lancet 1978;1:67–70.
7. Gough K, Read A, Naish J. Intestinal reticulosis as a complication of idiopathic steatorrhoea. Gut 1962;3:232–9.
8. Jones JF, Shurin S, Abramowsky C, et al. T-cell lymphomas containing Epstein–Barr viral DNA in patients with chronic Epstein–Barr virus infections. N Engl J Med 1988; 318:733–41.
9. Quintanilla-Martinez L, Fend F, Moguel LR, et al. Peripheral T-cell lymphoma with Reed–Sternberg-like cells of B-cell phenotype and genotype associated with Epstein–Barr virus infection. Am J Surg Pathol 1999;23:1233–40.
10. Richel DJ, Lepoutre JM, Kapsenberg JG, et al. Epstein–Barr virus in a CD8-positive T-cell lymphoma. Am J Pathol 1990;136:1093–9.
11. Anagnostopoulos I, Hummel M, Finn T, et al. Heterogeneous Epstein–Barr virus infection patterns in peripheral T- cell lymphoma of angioimmunoblastic lymphadenopathy type. Blood 1992;80:1804–12.
12. Harabuchi Y, Yamanaka N, Kataura A, et al. Epstein–Barr virus in nasal T-cell lymphomas in patients with lethal midline granuloma. Lancet 1990;335:128–30.
13. van Gorp J, Doornewaard H, Verdonck LF, et al. Posttransplant T-cell lymphoma. Report of three cases and a review of the literature. Cancer 1994;73:3064–72.
14. Korbjuhn P, Anagnostopoulos I, Hummel M, et al. Frequent latent Epstein–Barr virus infection of neoplastic T cells and bystander B cells in human immunodeficiency virus-negative European peripheral pleomorphic T-cell lymphomas. Blood 1993;82:217–23.

15. Mishima K, Horiuchi K, Kojya S, et al. Epstein–Barr virus in patients with polymorphic reticulosis (lethal midline granuloma) from China and Japan. Cancer 1994;73:3041–6.
16. Cheng AL, Su IJ, Chen YC, et al. Characteristic clinicopathologic features of Epstein–Barr virus-associated peripheral T-cell lymphoma. Cancer 1993;72:909–16.
17. Su IJ, Hsu YH, Lin MT, et al. Epstein–Barr virus-containing T-cell lymphoma presents with hemophagocytic syndrome mimicking malignant histiocytosis. Cancer 1993;72: 2019–27.
18. de Bruin PC, Jiwa M, Oudejans JJ, et al. Presence of Epstein–Barr virus in extranodal T-cell lymphomas: differences in relation to site. Blood 1994;83:1612–18.
19. Jaffe ES. Angioimmunoblastic T-cell lymphoma: new insights, but the clinical challenge remains. Ann Oncol 1995;6:631–2.
20. Ott G, Katzenberger T, Siebert R, DeCoteau JF, et al. Chromosomal abnormalities in nodal and extranodal CD30+ anaplastic large cell lymphomas: infrequent detection of the t(2;5) in extranodal lymphomas. Genes Chromosomes Cancer 1998;22:114–21.
21. Weidmann E. Hepatosplenic T cell lymphoma. A review on 45 cases since the first report describing the disease as a distinct lymphoma entity in 1990. Leukemia 2000;14: 991–7.
22. Zettl A, Ott G, Makulik A, et al. Chromosomal gains at 9q characterize enteropathy-type T-cell lymphoma. Am J Pathol 2002;161:1635–45.
23. Martinez-Delgado B, Melendez B, et al. Expression profiling of T-cell lymphomas differentiates peripheral and lymphoblastic lymphomas and defines survival related genes. Clin Cancer Res 2004;10:4971–82.
24. Medeiros LJ, Harris NL. Lymphoid infiltrates of the orbit and conjunctiva. A morphologic and immunophenotypic study of 99 cases. Am J Surg Pathol 1989;13:459–71.
25. Wotherspoon AC, Doglioni C, Diss TC, et al. Regression of primary low-grade B-cell gastric lymphoma of mucosa-associated lymphoid tissue type after eradication of Helicobacter pylori. Lancet 1993;342:575–7 [see comments].
26. Armitage JO, Greer JP, Levine AM, et al. Peripheral T-cell lymphoma. Cancer 1989;63:158–63.
27. Rudiger T, Weisenburger DD, Anderson JR, et al. Peripheral T-cell lymphoma (excluding anaplastic large-cell lymphoma): results from the Non-Hodgkin's Lymphoma Classification Project. Ann Oncol 2002;13:140–9.
28. Gaulard P, Kanavaros P, Farcet JP, et al. Bone marrow histologic and immunohistochemical findings in peripheral. T-cell lymphoma: a study of 38 cases. Hum Pathol 1991; 22:331–8.
29. Kwak LW, Wilson M, Weiss LM, et al. Similar outcome of treatment of B-cell and T-cell diffuse large-cell lymphomas: the Stanford experience. J Clin Oncol 1991;9:1426–31.
30. Stein H, Mason DY, Gerdes J, et al. The expression of the Hodgkin's disease associated antigen Ki-1 in reactive and neoplastic lymphoid tissue: evidence that Reed–Sternberg cells and histiocytic malignancies are derived from activated lymphoid cells. Blood 1985;66:848–58.
31. Schwab U, Stein H, Gerdes J, et al. Production of a monoclonal antibody specific for Hodgkin and Sternberg-Reed cells of Hodgkin's disease and a subset of normal lymphoid cells. Nature 1982;299:65–7.
32. Sandlund JT, Pui CH, Santana VM, et al. Clinical features and treatment outcome for children with CD30+ large- cell non-Hodgkin's lymphoma. J Clin Oncol 1994;12:895–8.
33. Penny RJ, Blaustein JC, Longtine JA, et al. Ki-1–positive large cell lymphomas, a heterogenous group of neoplasms. Morphologic, immunophenotypic, genotypic, and clinical features of 24 cases. Cancer 1991;68:362–73.
34. Piris M, Brown DC, Gatter KC, et al. CD30 expression in non-Hodgkin's lymphoma. Histopathology 1990;17:211–8.
35. Delsol G, Al Saati T, Gatter KC, et al. Coexpression of epithelial membrane antigen (EMA), Ki-1, and interleukin-2 receptor by anaplastic large cell lymphomas. Diagnostic value in so-called malignant histiocytosis. Am J Pathol 1988;130: 59–70.
36. Bitter MA, Franklin WA, Larson RA, et al. Morphology in Ki-1(CD30)-positive non-Hodgkin's lymphoma is correlated with clinical features and the presence of a unique chromosomal abnormality, t(2;5)(p23;q35). Am J Surg Pathol 1990;14:305–16.
37. Chan EY, Pi D, Chan GT, et al. Peripheral T-cell lymphoma presenting as hemophagocytic syndrome. Hematol Oncol 1989;7:275–85.
38. Falini B, Pileri S, De Solas I, et al. Peripheral T-cell lymphoma associated with hemophagocytic syndrome. Blood 1990;75:434–44 [see comments].
39. Garvin AJ, Self S, Sahovic EA, et al. The occurrence of a peripheral T-cell lymphoma in a chronically immunosuppressed renal transplant patient. Am J Surg Pathol 1988; 12:64–70.
40. Lum GH, Cosgriff TM, Byrne R, et al. Primary T-cell lymphoma of muscle in a patient infected with human immunodeficiency virus. Am J Med 1993;95:545–6.
41. Durham JC, Stephens DS, Rimland D, et al. Common variable hypogammaglobulinemia complicated by an unusual T-suppressor/cytotoxic cell lymphoma. Cancer 1987;59:271–6.
42. Argyle JC, Kjeldsberg CR, Marty J, et al. T-cell lymphoma and the Chediak-Higashi syndrome. Blood 1982;60:672–6.
43. Hamada S, Nishimura T, Hayashida K, et al.. Intracardiac malignant lymphoma detected by gallium-67 citrate and thallium-201 chloride. J Nucl Med 1988;29:1868–70.
44. O'Shea JJ, Jaffe ES, Lane HC, et al. Peripheral T cell lymphoma presenting as hypereosinophilia with vasculitis. Clinical, pathologic, and immunologic features. Am J Med 1987;82:539–45.
45. Foley JF, Linder J, Koh J, et al. Cutaneous necrotizing granulomatous vasculitis with evolution to T cell lymphoma. Am J Med 1987;82:839–44.
46. Auger MJ, Nash JR, Mackie MJ. Marrow involvement with T cell lymphoma initially presenting as abnormal myelopoiesis. J Clin Pathol 1986;39:134–7.
47. Greenberg BR, Grogan TM, Takasugi BJ, et al. A unique malignant T-cell lymphoproliferative disorder with neutropenia simulating hairy cell leukemia. Cancer 1985; 56:2823–30.
48. Gherardi R, Gaulard P, Prost C, et al. T-cell lymphoma revealed by a peripheral neuropathy. A report of two cases with an immunohistologic study on lymph node and nerve biopsies. Cancer 1986;58:2710–6.
49. Saito K, Nakanuma Y, Ogawa S, et al. Extensive hepatic granulomas associated with peripheral T-cell lymphoma. Am J Gastroenterol 1991;86:1243–6.
50. Morgello S, Maiese K, Petito CK. T-cell lymphoma in the CNS: clinical and pathologic features. Neurology 1989; 39:1190–6.
51. Shimoyama M, Oyama A, Tajima K, et al. Differences in clinicopathological characteristics and major prognostic factors between B-lymphoma and peripheral T-lymphoma excluding adult T-cell leukemia/lymphoma. Leuk Lymphoma 1993; 10:335–42.
52. Coiffier B, Brousse N, Peuchmaur M, et al. Peripheral T-cell lymphomas have a worse prognosis than B-cell lymphomas: a prospective study of 361 immunophenotyped patients treated with the LNH-84 regimen. The GELA (Groupe d'Etude des Lymphomes Agressives). Ann Oncol 1990; 1:45–50.

53. Armitage JO, Vose JM, Linder J, et al. Clinical significance of immunophenotype in diffuse aggressive non-Hodgkin's lymphoma. J Clin Oncol 1989;7:1783–90.
54. Lippman SM, Miller TP, Spier CM, et al. The prognostic significance of the immunotype in diffuse large-cell lymphoma: a comparative study of the T-cell and B-cell phenotype. Blood 1988;72:436–41.
55. The Non-Hodgkin's Lymphoma Classification Project. A clinical evaluation of the International Lymphoma Study Group classification of non-Hodgkin's lymphoma. Blood 1997;89:3909–18.
56. Shimizu K, Hamajima N, Ohnishi K, et al. T-cell phenotype is associated with decreased survival in non-Hodgkin's lymphoma. Jpn J Cancer Res 1989;80:720–6.
57. Cheng AL, Chen YC, Wang CH, et al. Direct comparisons of peripheral T-cell lymphoma with diffuse B-cell lymphoma of comparable histological grades—should peripheral T-cell lymphoma be considered separately? J Clin Oncol 1989; 7:725–31.
58. Brown DC, Heryet A, Gatter KC, et al. The prognostic significance of immunophenotype in high-grade non-Hodgkin's lymphoma. Histopathology 1989;14:621–7.
59. Pittaluga S, Bijnens L, Teodorovic I, et al. Clinical analysis of 670 cases in two trials of the European Organization for the Research and Treatment of Cancer Lymphoma Cooperative Group subtyped according to the Revised European-American Classification of Lymphoid Neoplasms: a comparison with the Working Formulation. Blood 1996;87:4358–67.
60. Melo JV, Hegde U, Parreira A, et al. Splenic B cell lymphoma with circulating villous lymphocytes: differential diagnosis of B cell leukaemias with large spleens. J Clin Pathol 1987;40:642–51.
61. van Krieken JH, von Schilling C, Kluin PM, et al. Splenic marginal zone lymphocytes and related cells in the lymph node: a morphologic and immunohistochemical study [see comments]. Hum Pathol 1989;20:320–5.
62. Frizzera G, Moran EM, Rappaport H. Angio-immunoblastic lymphadenopathy with dysproteinaemia. Lancet 1974;1: 1070–3.
63. Flandrin G, Daniel M, Yafi G, et al. Sarcomatoses ganglionnaires diffuses a differenciation plasmocytaire avec anemie hemolytique auto-immune. In: Actualites Hematologiques. Paris: Masson, 1972.
64. Lennert K and Feller A. Histopathology of non-Hodgkin's lymphomas. New York: Springer-Verlag, 1992.
65. Ascani S, Zinzani PL, Gherlinzoni F, et al. Peripheral T-cell lymphomas. Clinico-pathologic study of 168 cases diagnosed according to the R.E.A.L. Classification. Ann Oncol 1997;8:583–92.
66. Lopez-Guillermo A, Cid J, Salar A, et al. Peripheral T-cell lymphomas: initial features, natural history, and prognostic factors in a series of 174 patients diagnosed according to the R.E.A.L. Classification. Ann Oncol 1998;9:849–55.
67. Liang R, Todd D, Ho FC. Aggressive non-Hodgkin's lymphoma: T-cell versus B-cell. Hematol Oncol 1996;14:1–6.
68. Gisselbrecht C, Gaulard P, Lepage E, et al. Prognostic significance of T-cell phenotype in aggressive non-Hodgkin's lymphomas. Groupe d'Etudes des Lymphomes de l'Adulte (GELA). Blood 1998;92:76–82.
69. Liang R, Todd D, Chan TK, et al. Peripheral T cell lymphoma. J Clin Oncol 1987;5:750–5.
70. Coiffier B, Berger F, Bryon PA, et al. T-cell lymphomas: immunologic, histologic, clinical, and therapeutic analysis of 63 cases. J Clin Oncol 1988;6:1584–9.
71. Liang R, Loke SL, Chan AC. The prognostic factors for peripheral T-cell lymphomas. Hematol Oncol 1992;10: 135–40.
72. Haioun C, Gaulard P, Bourquelot P, et al. Clinical and biological analysis of peripheral T-cell lymphomas: a single institution study. Leuk Lymphoma 1992;7:449–55.
73. Fiorani C, Vinci G, Sacchi S, et al. Primary systemic anaplastic large-cell lymphoma (CD30+): advances in biology and current therapeutic approaches. Clin Lymphoma 2001;2: 29–37;discussion 38–9.
74. Gascoyne RD, Aoun P, Wu D, et al. Prognostic significance of anaplastic lymphoma kinase (ALK) protein expression in adults with anaplastic large cell lymphoma. Blood 1999;93: 3913–21.
75. Falini B, Pileri S, Zinzani PL, et al. ALK+ lymphoma: clinico-pathological findings and outcome. Blood 1999;93: 2697–706.
76. Chott A, Augustin I, Wrba F, et al. Peripheral T-cell lymphomas: a clinicopathologic study of 75 cases. Hum Pathol 1990;21:1117–25.
77. Grierson HL, Wooldridge TN, Purtilo DT, et al. Low proliferative activity is associated with a favorable prognosis in peripheral T-cell lymphoma. Cancer Res 1990;50:4845–8.
78. Greiner TC, Raffeld M, Lutz C, et al. Analysis of T cell receptor-gamma gene rearrangements by denaturing gradient gel electrophoresis of GC-clamped polymerase chain reaction products. Correlation with tumor-specific sequences. Am J Pathol 1995;146:46–55.
79. Ansell SM, Habermann TM, Kurtin PJ, et al. Predictive capacity of the International Prognostic Factor Index in patients with peripheral T-cell lymphoma. J Clin Oncol 1997;15:2296–301.
80. Armitage JO, Weisenburger DD. New approach to classifying non-Hodgkin's lymphomas: clinical features of the major histologic subtypes. Non-Hodgkin's Lymphoma Classification Project. J Clin Oncol 1998;16:2780–95.
81. Gallamini A, Stelitano C, Calvi R, et al. Peripheral T-cell lymphoma unspecified (PTCL-U): a new prognostic model from a retrospective multicentric clinical study. Blood 2004;103:2474–9.
82. Greer JP, York JC, Cousar JB, et al. Peripheral T-cell lymphoma: a clinicopathologic study of 42 cases. J Clin Oncol 1984;2:788–98.
83. Vose JM, Peterson C, Bierman PJ, et al. Comparison of high-dose therapy and autologous bone marrow transplantation for T-cell and B-cell non-Hodgkin's lymphomas. Blood 1990;76:424–31.
84. Rodriguez J, Munsell M, Yazji S, et al. Impact of high-dose chemotherapy on peripheral T-cell lymphomas. J Clin Oncol 2001;19:3766–70.
85. Blystad AK, Enblad G, Kvaloy S, et al. High-dose therapy with autologous stem cell transplantation in patients with peripheral T cell lymphomas. Bone Marrow Transplant 2001;27:711–16.
86. Rodriguez J, Caballero MD, Gutierrez A, et al. High-dose chemotherapy and autologous stem cell transplantation in peripheral T-cell lymphoma: the GEL-TAMO experience. Ann Oncol 2003;14:1768–75.
87. Cooper DL, Braverman IM, Sarris AH, et al. Cyclosporine treatment of refractory T-cell lymphomas. Cancer 1993; 71:2335–41.
88. Mercieca J, Matutes E, Dearden C, et al. The role of pentostatin in the treatment of T-cell malignancies: analysis of response rate in 145 patients according to disease subtype. J Clin Oncol 1994;12:2588–93.
89. Saven A, Carrera CJ, Carson DA, et al. 2-Chlorodeoxyadenosine: an active agent in the treatment of cutaneous T-cell lymphoma. Blood 1992;80:587–92.
90. Zinzani PL, Baliva G, Magagnoli M, et al. Gemcitabine treatment in pretreated cutaneous T-cell lymphoma: experience in 44 patients. J Clin Oncol 2000;18:2603–6.

91. Cheng AL, Su IJ, Chen CC, et al. Use of retinoic acids in the treatment of peripheral T-cell lymphoma: a pilot study. J Clin Oncol 1994;12:1185–92.
92. Dang N, Hagemeister F, Fayad L, et al. Phase II study of delineuki diftitox (ONTAK) for relapsed/refractory B and T-cell non-Hodkgin's lymphoma. Blood 2002;100:154 [abstract 1405].
93. Mehta A, Hutchison R, Himpler B, et al. Treatment of T-cell anaplastic large cell lymphoma (ALCL) relapsing after autologous stem cell transplant (ASCT) with denileukin difitox (Ontak). Blood 2002;100:160–1 (abstract 4772).
94. Armitage JO, Coiffier B. Activity of interferon-alpha in relapsed patients with diffuse large B-cell and peripheral T-cell non-Hodgkin's lymphoma. Ann Oncol 2000;11: 1–3.
95. Jaffe ES, Chan JK, Su IJ, et al. Report of the Workshop on Nasal and Related Extranodal Angiocentric T/Natural Killer Cell Lymphomas. Definitions, differential diagnosis, and epidemiology. Am J Surg Pathol 1996;20:103–11.
96. Howell WM, Leung ST, Jones DB, et al. HLA-DRB, -DQA, and -DQB polymorphism in celiac disease and enteropathy-associated T-cell lymphoma. Common features and additional risk factors for malignancy. Hum Immunol 1995;43:29–37.
97. Egan LJ, Stevens FM, McCarthy CF. Celiac disease and T-cell lymphoma. N Engl J Med 1996;335:1611–12 [letter, comment].
98. Spits H, Blom B, Jaleco AC, et al. Early stages in the development of human T, natural killer and thymic dendritic cells. Immunol Rev 1998;165:75–86.
99. Delves PJ, Roitt IM. The immune system. First of two parts. N Engl J Med 2000;343:37–49.
100. Arnulf B, Copie-Bergman C, Delfau-Larue MH, et al. Non-hepatosplenic gamma delta T-cell lymphoma: a subset of cytotoxic lymphomas with mucosal or skin localization. Blood 1998;91:1723–31.
101. Cooke CB, Krenacs L, Stetler-Stevenson M, et al. Hepatosplenic T-cell lymphoma: a distinct clinicopathologic entity of cytotoxic gamma delta T-cell origin. Blood 1996;88:4265–74 [see comments].
102. Toro JR, Beaty M, Sorbara L, et al. gamma delta T-cell lymphoma of the skin: a clinical, microscopic, and molecular study. Arch Dermatol 2000;136:1024–32.
103. Quintini G, Iannitto E, Barbera V, et al. Response to low-dose oral methotrexate and prednisone in two patients with angio-immunoblastic lymphadenopathy-type T-cell lymphoma. Hematol J 2001;2:393–5.
104. Smith JL, Hodges E, Quin CT, et al. Frequent T and B cell oligoclones in histologically and immunophenotypically characterized angioimmunoblastic lymphadenopathy. Am J Pathol 2000;156:661–9.
105. Crouzier R, Martin T, Pasquali JL. Monoclonal IgM rheumatoid factor secreted by CD5-negative B cells during mixed cryoglobulinemia. Evidence for somatic mutations and intraclonal diversity of the expressed VH region gene. J Immunol 1995;154:413–21.
106. Attygalle A, Al-Jehani R, Diss TC, et al. Neoplastic T cells in angioimmunoblastic T-cell lymphoma express CD10. Blood 2002;99:627–33.
107. Lipford EH, Smith HR, Pittaluga S, et al. Clonality of angioimmunoblastic lymphadenopathy and implications for its evolution to malignant lymphoma. J Clin Invest 1987; 79:637–42.
108. Pautier P, Devidas A, Delmer A, et al. Angioimmunoblastic-like T-cell non Hodgkin's lymphoma: outcome after chemotherapy in 33 patients and review of the literature. Leuk Lymphoma 1999;32:545–52.
109. Liang R, Loke SL, Ho FC, et al. Histologic subtypes and survival of Chinese patients with non-Hodgkin's lymphomas. Cancer 1990;66:1850–5.
110. Chan JK, Ng CS, Ngan KC, et al. Angiocentric T-cell lymphoma of the skin. An aggressive lymphoma distinct from mycosis fungoides. Am J Surg Pathol 1988;12:861–76.
111. Frizzera G, Moran EM, Rappaport H. Angio-immunoblastic lymphadenopathy. Diagnosis and clinical course. Am J Med 1975;59:803–18.
112. Ng CS, Lo ST, Chan JK, et al. CD56+ putative natural killer cell lymphomas: production of cytolytic effectors and related proteins mediating tumor cell apoptosis? Hum Pathol 1997;28:1276–82.
113. Tsang WY, Chan JK, Yip TT, et al. In situ localization of Epstein–Barr virus encoded RNA in non- nasal/nasopharyngeal CD56-positive and CD56-negative T-cell lymphomas. Hum Pathol 1994;25:758–65.
114. Wong N, Wong KF, Chan JK, et al. Chromosomal translocations are common in natural killer-cell lymphoma/leukemia as shown by spectral karyotyping. Hum Pathol 2000; 31:771–4.
115. Ho FC, Srivastava G, Loke SL, et al. Presence of Epstein–Barr virus DNA in nasal lymphomas of B and 'T' cell type. Hematol Oncol 1990;8:271–81.
116. Wong KF, Zhang YM, Chan JK. Cytogenetic abnormalities in natural killer cell lymphoma/leukaemia—is there a consistent pattern? Leuk Lymphoma 1999;34:241–50.
117. Siu LL, Wong KF, Chan JK, et al. Comparative genomic hybridization analysis of natural killer cell lymphoma/leukemia. Recognition of consistent patterns of genetic alterations. Am J Pathol 1999;155:1419–25.
118. Medeiros LJ, Peiper SC, Elwood L, et al. Angiocentric immunoproliferative lesions: a molecular analysis of eight cases. Hum Pathol 1991;22:1150–7.
119. Ng CS, Lo ST, Chan JK. Peripheral T and putative natural killer cell lymphomas commonly coexpress CD95 and CD95 ligand. Hum Pathol 1999;30:48–53.
120. Shimoyama M, Minato K, Saito H, et al. Immunoblastic lymphadenopathy (IBL)–like T-cell lymphoma. Jpn J Clin Oncol 1979;9:347.
121. Brice P, Calvo F, d'Agay MF, et al. Peripheral T cell lymphoma following angioimmunoblastic lymphadenopathy. Nouv Rev Fr Hematol 1987;29:371–7.
122. Siegert W, Agthe A, Griesser H, et al. Treatment of angioimmunoblastic lymphadenopathy (AILD)-type T-cell lymphoma using prednisone with or without the COPBLAM/IMVP-16 regimen. A multicenter study. Kiel Lymphoma Study Group. Ann Intern Med 1992;117:364–70.
123. Siegert W, Nerl C, Agthe A, et al. Angioimmunoblastic lymphadenopathy (AILD)–type T-cell lymphoma: prognostic impact of clinical observations and laboratory findings at presentation. The Kiel Lymphoma Study Group. Ann Oncol 1995;6:659–64.
124. Miller CB, Rowlings PA, Zhang MJ, et al. The effect of graft purging with 4-hydroperoxycyclophosphamide in autologous bone marrow transplantation for acute myelogenous leukemia. Exp Hematol 2001;29:1336–46.
125. Advani R, Warnke R, Sikic BI, et al. Treatment of angioimmunoblastic T-cell lymphoma with cyclosporine. Ann Oncol 1997;8:601–3.
126. Takemori N, Kodaira J, Toyoshima N, et al. Successful treatment of immunoblastic lymphadenopathy-like T-cell lymphoma with cyclosporin A. Leuk Lymphoma 1999;35: 389–95.
127. Morton JE, Leyland MJ, Vaughan Hudson G, et al. Primary gastrointestinal non-Hodgkin's lymphoma: a review of 175 British National Lymphoma Investigation cases. Br J Cancer 1993;67:776–82.

128. Cooper BT, Holmes GK, Cooke WT. Lymphoma risk in coeliac disease of later life. Digestion 1982;23:89–92.
129. Holmes GK, Stokes PL, McWalter R, et al. Proceedings: coeliac disease, malignancy, and gluten-free diet. Gut 1974;15:339.
130. Gale J, Simmonds PD, Mead GM, et al. Enteropathy-type intestinal T-cell lymphoma: clinical features and treatment of 31 patients in a single center. J Clin Oncol 2000;18:795–803.
131. Egan LJ, Walsh SV, Stevens FM, et al. Celiac-associated lymphoma. A single institution experience of 30 cases in the combination chemotherapy era. J Clin Gastroenterol 1995;21:123–9.
132. Daum S, Ullrich R, Heise W, et al. Intestinal non-Hodgkin's lymphoma: a multicenter prospective clinical study from the German Study Group on Intestinal Non-Hodgkin's Lymphoma. J Clin Oncol 2003;21:2740–6.
133. Farcet JP, Gaulard P, Marolleau JP, et al. Hepatosplenic T-cell lymphoma: sinusal/sinusoidal localization of malignant cells expressing the T-cell receptor gamma delta. Blood 1990;75:2213–19.
134. Belhadj K, Reyes F, Farcet JP, et al. Hepatosplenic gammadelta T-cell lymphoma is a rare clinicopathologic entity with poor outcome: report on a series of 21 patients. Blood 2003;102: 4261–9.
135. Gonzalez CL, Medeiros LJ, Braziel RM, et al. T-cell lymphoma involving subcutaneous tissue. A clinicopathologic entity commonly associated with hemophagocytic syndrome. Am J Surg Pathol 1991;15:17–27.
136. Ashworth J, Coady AT, Guy R, et al. Brawny cutaneous induration and granulomatous panniculitis in large cell non-Hodgkin's (T suppressor/cytotoxic cell) lymphoma. Br J Dermatol 1989;120:563–9.
137. Tanaka K, Hagari Y, Sano Y, et al. A case of T-cell lymphoma associated with panniculitis, progressive pancytopenia and hyperbilirubinaemia. Br J Dermatol 1990;123: 649–52.
138. Wang CY, Su WP, Kurtin PJ. Subcutaneous panniculitic T-cell lymphoma. Int J Dermatol 1996;35:1–8.
139. Kundrat H. Lymphosarcomatosis. Klin Wochenschr (Wien) 1893;6:211.
140. Wang H, Medeiros LJ, Jones D. Subcutaneous penniculitis-like T-cell lymphoma. Clin Lymphoma 2002;3:181–3.
141. Berg KD, Brinster NK, Huhn KM, et al. Transmission of a T-cell lymphoma by allogeneic bone marrow transplantation. N Engl J Med 2001;345:1458–63.
142. Perniciaro C, Zalla MJ, White JW Jr, et al. Subcutaneous T-cell lymphoma. Report of two additional cases and further observations. Arch Dermatol 1993;129:1171–6.
143. Matsue K, Itoh M, Tsukuda K, et al. Successful treatment of cytophagic histiocytic panniculitis with modified CHOP-E. Cyclophosphamide, adriamycin, vincristine, predonisone, and etoposide. Am J Clin Oncol 1994;17:470–4.
144. Weenig RH, Ng CS, Perniciaro C. Subcutaneous panniculitis–like T-cell lymphoma: an elusive case presenting as lipomembranous panniculitis and a review of 72 cases in the literature. Am J Dermatopathol 2001;23:206–15.
145. Santucci M, Pimpinelli N, Massi D, et al. Cytotoxic/natural killer cell cutaneous lymphomas. Report of EORTC Cutaneous Lymphoma Task Force Workshop. Cancer 2003;97:610–27.
146. Papenfuss JS, Aoun P, Bierman PJ, et al. Subcutaneous panniculitis-like T-cell lymphoma: presentation of 2 cases and observations. Clin Lymphoma 2002;3:175–80.

27

Nasal T/NK-Cell Lymphoma

Raymond Liang, M.D., F.R.C.P., F.R.A.C.P.

Most lymphomas are of B-cell origin. T-cell or NK-cell tumors are uncommon.[1,2] The new WHO classification has for the first time separately classified NK-cell neoplasms together with the T-cell tumors (Table 27–1). Extranodal NK/T-cell lymphoma, nasal type, is now considered to be a distinctive pathologic entity, and it typically affects the midline nasal region. With better understanding of its pathology, terms such as polymorphic reticulosis, lethal midline granuloma, and midline malignant reticulosis, which have previously been used to describe this destructive tumor of the midline facial structure, can now be abandoned.[3,4] Nasal T/NK-cell lymphoma should also be distinguished from lymphomas of the Waldeyer's ring and the nasal sinuses, which usually have the histology of diffuse large B-cell lymphoma and run a different clinical course.[5,6]

Nasal T/NK-cell lymphoma has a most peculiar epidemiologic pattern, and is seen predominantly in China, Japan, Korea, Malaysia, and other Asian countries, as well as in some parts of Central and South America, including Mexico and Peru.[7–11] Sporadic cases are only occasionally observed in other parts of the world. Isolated cases have also been reported in severely immunocompromised patients, such as those receiving immunosuppressive drugs following organ transplantation or those with HIV infection.[12,13] Primary nasal T/NK-cell lymphoma remains a rare tumor. Even in places where it is regularly seen, such as Hong Kong, it accounts for only about 5% of all lymphomas diagnosed.[8]

Nasal T/NK-cell lymphoma typically affects middle-aged adults with a median age of around 50 years. There is also a slight male predominance.[14] Patients often present with a nasal mass with symptoms of obstruction and bleeding.[14] Symptoms related to local invasion to the upper aerodigestive tract, including the nasal cavity, nasopharynx, palate, and larynx, are common (Fig. 27–1). The orbit and the cranial nerves are also sometimes involved.[15] A small proportion of patients may present with more disseminated disease. Common metastatic sites include skin, soft tissue, gastrointestinal tract, and genital organs. The tumor may also present as a primary lesion in one of these sites without clinically obvious nasal involvement.[15–22] Bone marrow involvement is uncommon at presentation. The presence of pancytopenia may alert clinicians to the possible presence of hemophagocytosis. Some patients may also have marked systemic symptoms in the form of high swinging fever and marked weight loss.[22,23]

A high index of suspicion is essential for prompt clinical diagnosis. Differential diagnoses include infections and nasopharygeal cancer.[24] A CT or an MRI scan may show up the tumor mass and demonstrate the extent of its local involvement[25–27] (Fig. 27–2). The tumor is frequently locally destructive with obliteration of the nasal passages and maxillary sinuses. Involvement of the adjacent alveolar bone, hard palate, orbits, and nasopharynx is found in more than 50% of cases, and is associated with extensive soft tissue masses. Presence of bone erosion is highly characteristic of this tumor. However, precise diagnosis can only be established by carefully performed nasal endoscopy and biopsy.[28–31] Because the biopsy specimens are often small in size and necrotic in nature, repeated examinations may be necessary before an adequate sample is available to obtain an accurate diagnosis. An experienced pathologist is most helpful, as interpretation may be quite difficult.[28–31] A delay in diagnosis can be catastrophic, as the clinical course may be very aggressive, requiring prompt therapy. In places where this tumor is not commonly seen, it is not unusual that the diagnosis can only be established postmortem.

Histologically, nasal T/NK-cell lymphoma has a very broad morphologic spectrum.[28–31] There is often a highly pleomorphic cellular infiltrate with a highly variable cytology.[32] The presence of angioinvasion and angiodestruction is highly characteristic, and is typical of this tumor[2] (Fig. 27–3). Vascular occlusion and marked tissue ischemia are often present, resulting in marked tissue necrosis. There may also be a significant amount of reactive inflammatory cells. Rarely, dysplastic changes in the overlying epithelium, mimicking nasopharygeal cancer, have been reported.[2]

Immunophenotyping is most helpful in confirming diagnosis.[2] The NK-cell marker CD56 is usually positive (Fig. 27–4). A negative surface CD3 staining on fresh tissue, but positive cytoplasmic CD3 epsilon on paraffin, supports the NK-cell origin of the tumor. This may further be confirmed by the germline configuration of T-cell receptor gene (TCR). However, it has been recognized that less than 10% of cases may express surface CD3 antigen, and also show clonal TCR gene rearrangement, suggesting a T-cell rather than NK-cell origin of the tumor.[33]

A very strong association of the nasal T/NK-cell lymphoma with Epstein–Barr virus (EBV) infection is well recognized.[34–37] The presence of the virus can be demonstrated by Southern analysis, polymerase chain reaction, or in situ hybridization (EBER) (Fig. 27–5). Clonal EBV proliferation has also been demonstrated with the assistance of the Dhet marker.[34] Abnormal cytogenetic and molecular genetic findings are present in about 80% of cases. They are often complex and nonspecific. Deletions of chromosome 6 at around q21-23 are most commonly found.[38–42] Fluorescence in situ hybridization studies have also confirmed the frequent presence of deletions at 6q22–23 in the CD3–/CD56+ tumor cells. Other cytogenetic abnormalities include +X, i(1q), i(7q), +8, del(13q), del(17p), i(17q), and 11aq23 rearrangement. Other genetic abnormalities include the include methylation of the p73 gene and genetic alterations

Table 27–1. World Health Organization Histologic Classification of Mature T-Cell and NK-Cell Neoplasms

Leukemic/Disseminated
T-cell prolymphocytic leukemia
T-cell large granular lymphocytic leukemia
Aggressive NK-cell leukemia
Adult T-cell leukemia/lymphoma
Cutaneous
Mycosis fungoides
Sézary syndrome
Primary cutaneous anaplastic large-cell lymphoma
Lymphomatoid papulosis
Other Extranodal
Extranodal NK/T-cell lymphoma, nasal type
Enteropathy-type T-cell lymphoma
Hepatosplenic T-cell lymphoma
Subcutaneous panniculitis-like T-cell lymphoma
Nodal
Angioimmunoblastic T-cell lymphoma
Peripheral T-cell lymphoma, unclassified
Anaplastic large-cell lymphoma
Neoplasm of Uncertain Lineage and Stage of Differentiation
Blastic NK-cell lymphoma

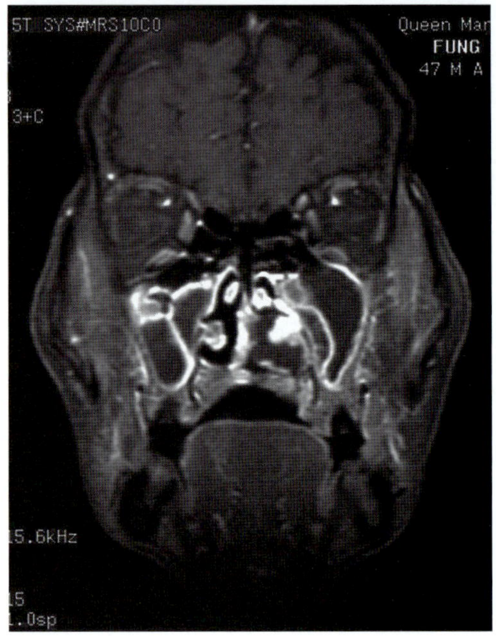

Figure 27–2. MRI image of nasal NK-cell lymphoma involving left nasal cavity.

of the Fas, Fas legend, and p53 genes. These genetic changes may significantly contribute to the clinical behaviors of the tumor.[10,43–47]

The clinical course of this lymphoma is often very aggressive, and the disease carries a poor prognosis. With the use of aggressive chemotherapy and local radiotherapy, prolonged remission is possible in less than half of cases of clinically localized tumors; the disseminated form of the disease is almost invariably fatal.[48–50] While a cure may be assumed in the minority of patients with prolonged remission, late relapses up to more than 10 years from the time of initial diagnosis have been observed.

The optimal therapeutic strategy remains uncertain, and large clinical trials are not available because of the rarity of this tumor.[51–54] A combination of intensive chemotherapy and local radiotherapy is often given. The CHOP chemotherapy regimen is commonly used, and it remains unconfirmed whether the more complicated regimens, such as ProMACE-cytaBOM, may be superior. Radiotherapy has been shown to be a key element in management. Local radiotherapy is very effective in achieving local control, and should be given to all patients.[48] It is important that vigilant follow-up should be part of the treatment plan. Frequent reassessment by nasal endoscopy and biopsy is essential for every patient treated.[7] Multiple biopsies should be performed even if the nasal mucosa is grossly normal, as residual tumor cells may still be demonstrable in this situation. Interpretation of the follow-up biopsy specimens can be very difficult, but can be assisted by the use of EBV staining by in situ hybridization. The molecular genetic abnor-

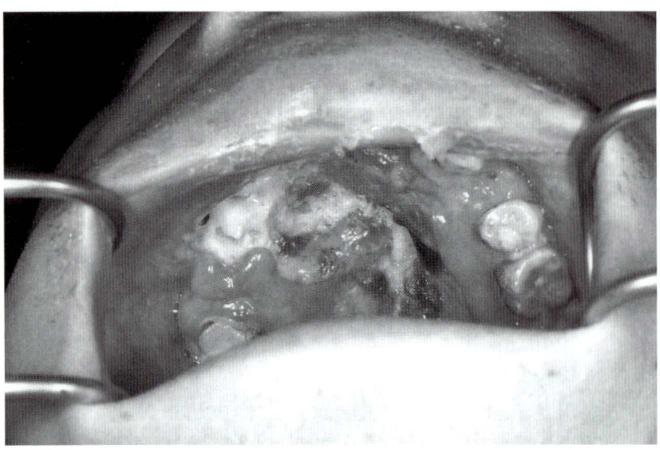

Figure 27–1. Primary nasal NK-cell lymphoma infiltrating hard palate. (See color insert.)

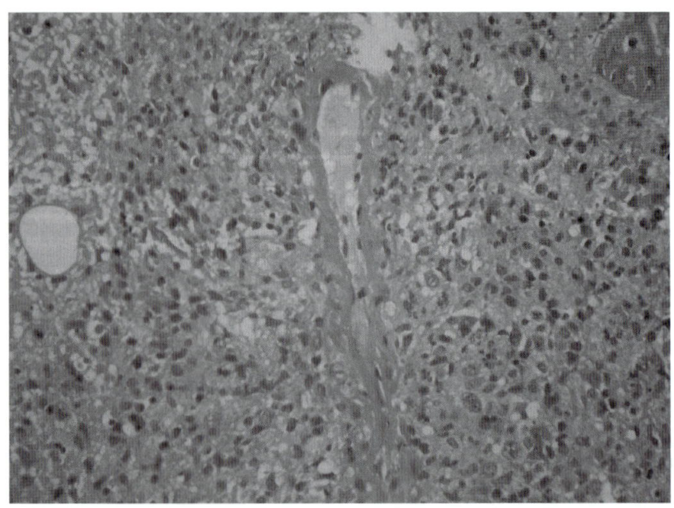

Figure 27–3. Nasal NK-cell lymphoma showing angiocentricity. (See color insert.)

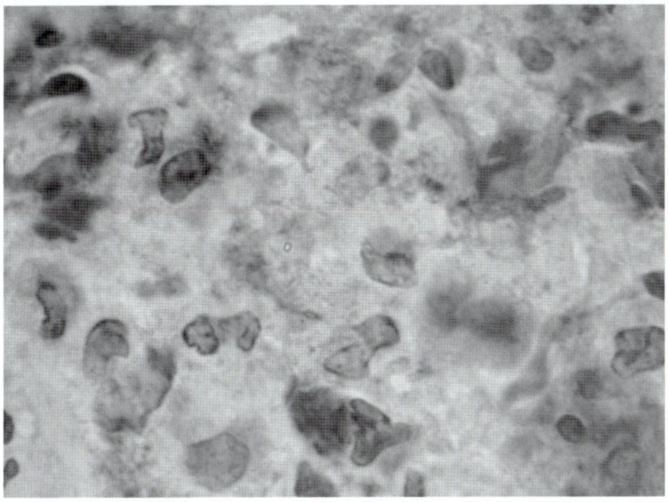

Figure 27–4. Nasal NK-cell lymphoma showing positive CD56 immunostaining. (See color insert.)

malities, such as gene methyalation, may potentially be useful as a marker of residual disease.[43] Also, studies have shown that the detection of plasma EBV DNA by quantitative PCR may have good correlation with tumor response and may again potentially be used as an adjunct for monitoring disease progress.[55]

For patients failing primary therapy, the prognosis is usually very poor. Local radiotherapy should be used early if it has not been given already. Response to second-line chemotherapy is often unsatisfactory. Isolated studies have demonstrated the effectiveness of L-asparaginase, and the usefulness of this agent should be further explored.[56–58]

High-dose chemotherapy with autologous peripheral blood stem cell rescue has been used for this tumor. Some benefit has been observed when it is used early for patients who are in first remission.[59–63] For those with refractory or disseminated disease, the treatment results remain disappointing. Further studies are ongoing to investigate the usefulness of allogeneic transplant, including the use of nonmyeloablative transplants, for nasal T/NK-cell lymphoma.[64]

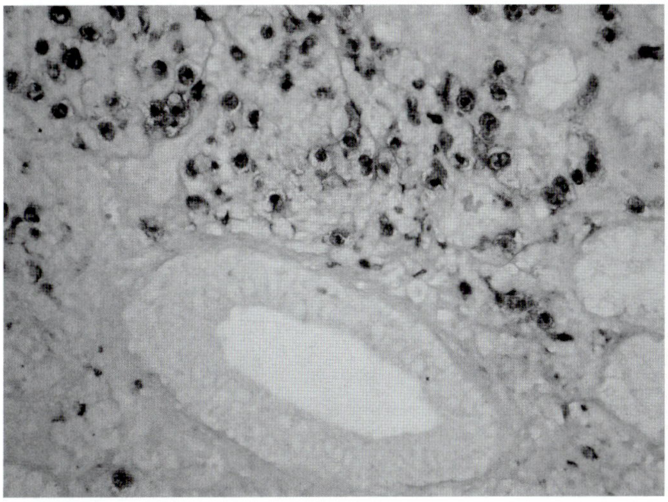

Figure 27–5. Nasal NK-cell lymphoma showing positive EBER staining on in situ hybridization. (See color insert.)

In summary, nasal NK/T-cell is a highly aggressive tumor, with unique epidemiology and pathology. Its strong association with EBV infection suggests that the virus may play an important role in the pathogenesis. The diagnosis can sometimes be problematic because of the difficulty in getting optimal biopsy specimens. Aggressive treatment with chemotherapy and radiotherapy results in favorable outcome in only a minority of patients. Locally advanced or disseminated disease predicts poor clinical outcome. The clinical usefulness of autologous or allogeneic haematopoietic stem cell transplant remains to be further defined.

References

1. Kwong YL, Chan ACL, Liang R. Natural killer cell lymphoma/leukemia: pathology and treatment. Hematol Oncol 1977;15:71–9.
2. Chan JKC, Jaffe ES, Ralfkiaer E. Extranodal NK/Tcell lymphoma, nasal type. In: Jaffe ES, Harris NL, Stein H, et al., eds. World Health Organization Classification of Tumours. Pathology and Genetics of Tumours of Haematopoietic and Lymphoid Tissues. Lyon: IARC Press, 2001:204–7.
3. Ho FCS, Choy D, Loke SL, et al. Polymorphic reticulosis and conventional lymphomas of the nose and upper aerodigestive tract. Hum Pathol 1990;21:1041–50.
4. Chim CS, Ooi GC, Shek TW, et al. Lethal midline granuloma revisited: nasal T/Natural-killer cell lymphoma. J Clin Oncol 1999;17:1322–5.
5. Vidal RW, Devaney K, Ferlito A, et al. Sino-nasal malignant lymphomas: a distinct clinico-pathological category. Ann Otol Rhinol Laryngol 1999;108:411–19.
6. Liang R, Ng RP, Todd D, et al. Management of stage I and II diffuse aggressive non-Hodgkin's lymphoma of the Waldeyer's ring: combined modality therapy versus radiotherapy alone. Hematol Oncol 1987;5:223–30.
7. Jaffe ES, Krenacs L, Kumar S, et al. Extranodal peripheral T-cell and NK-cell neoplasms. Am J Clin Pathol 1999;111(Suppl 1):S46–55.
8. Non-Hodgkin's Lymphoma Classification Project. A clinical evaluation of the international lymphoma study group classification of non-Hodgkin's lymphoma. Blood 1997;89:3909–18.
9. Liang R, Loke SL, Ho FCS, et al. The histology and survival of 840 Chinese patients with non-Hodgkin's lymphomas. Cancer 1990;66:1850–6.
10. Quintanilla-Martinez L, Franklin JL, Guerrero I, et al. Histological and immunophenotypic profile of nasal NK/T cell lymphoma from Peru: high prevalence of p53 overexpression. Hum Pathol 1999;30:849–55.
11. Peh SC, Quen QW. Nasal and nasal-type natural killer (NK)/T-cell lymphoma: immunophenotype and Epstein–Barr virus (EBV) association. Med J Malaysia 2003;58:196–204.
12. Kunisada M, Adachi A, Matsumoto S, et al. Nasal-type natural killer cell lymphoma preceded by benign panniculitis arising in an asymptomatic HTLV–1 carrier. Int J Dermatol 2003;42:710–14.
13. Tsao L, Draoua HY, Mansukhani M, et al. EBV-associated, extranodal NK-cell lymphoma, nasal type of the breast, after heart transplantation. Mod Pathol 2004;17:125–30.
14. Liang R, Todd D, Chan TK, et al. Nasal lymphoma: a retrospective analysis of 60 cases. Cancer 1990;66:2205–8.
15. Yeh KH, Lien HC, Hsu SM, et al. Quiescent nasal T-/NK-cell lymphoma manifested as primary central nervous system lymphoma. Am J Hematol 1999;60:161–3.

16. Chim CS, Choy C, Liang R, et al. Isolated uterine relapse of nasal T/NK cell lymphoma. Leuk Lymphoma 1999;34: 629–32.
17. Kato N, Yasukawa K, Onozuka T, et al. Nasal and nasal-type T/NK cell lymphoma with cutaneous involvement. J Am Acad Dermatol 1999;40:850–6.
18. Au WY, Chan ACL, Kwong YL. Scrotal skin ulcer in a patient with a previous tonsillectomy because of natural killer cell lymphoma. Am J Dermatopathol 1998;20:582–5.
19. Au WY, Liang R. Peripheral T-cell lymphoma. Curr Oncol Rep 1002;4:434–42.
20. Liang R. Diagnosis and management of primary nasal lymphoma of T-cell or NK-cell origin. Clin Lymphoma 2000;1:33–7.
21. Liang R, Todd D, Chan TK, et al. Treatment outcome and prognostic factors for primary nasal lymphoma. J Clin Oncol 1995;13:666–70.
22. Chan JKC, Sin VC, Wong KF, et al. Non-nasal lymphoma expressing the natural killer cell marker CD56: a clinicopathologic study of 49 cases of an uncommon aggressive neoplasm. Blood 1997;89:4501–13.
23. Han JY, Seo EJ, Kwon HJ, et al. Nasal angiocentric lymphoma with hemophagocytic syndrome. Korean J Intern Med 1999; 14:41–6.
24. Chen SH, Wu CS, Chan KH, et al. Primary sinonasal non-Hodgkin's lymphoma masquerading as chronic rhinosinusitis: an issue of routine histopathological examination. J Laryngol Otol 2003;117:404–7.
25. Chim CS, Ooi GC, Shek TWH, et al. Lethal midline granuloma revisited. J Clin Oncol 1999;17:728–9.
26. Ooi GC, Chim CS, Liang R, et al. Nasal T/NK cell lymphoma: CT and MR imaging features of a new clinico-pathological entity. Am J Roentgen 2000;174:1141–5.
27. King AD, Lei KI, Richards PS, et al. Non-Hodgkin's lymphoma of the nasopharynx: CT and MR imaging. Clin Radiol 2003;58:621–5.
28. Chan JKC. Peripheral T-cell and NK-cell neoplasms: an integrated approach to diagnosis. Mod Pathol 1999;12:177–99.
29. Jaffe ES, Chan JK, Su IJ, et al. Report of the Workshop on nasal and related extranodal angiocentric T/natural killer cell lymphomas. Definitions, differential diagnosis and epidemiology. Am J Surg Pathol 1996;20:103–11.
30. Chan JKC. Natural killer cell neoplasms. Anat Pathol 1998;3:77–145.
31. Ohsawa M, Nakatsuka S, Kanno H, et al. Immunopheotypic and genotypic characterization of nasal lymphoma with polymorphic reticulosis morphology. Int J Cancer 1999:81: 865–70.
32. Chan AB, Chan WY, Chow JH. Cytologic features of NK/T-cell lymphoma. Acta Cytol 2003;47:595–601.
33. Yoon TY, Lee HT, Chang SH. Nasal-type T/NK-cell angiocentric lymphoma, EBV associated, and showing T-cell receptor gamma gene rearrangement. Br J Dermatol 1999;140: 505–8.
34. Ho FCS, Srivastava G, Loke SL, et al. Presence of Clonal Epstein–Barr virus DNA in nasal lymphomas of B and T cell type. Hematol Oncol 19991;8:271–8.
35. Chiang AK, Wong KY, Liang AC, et al. Comparative analysis of Epstein–Barr virus gene polymorphisms in nasal T/NK cell and normal nasal tissues: implications on virus strain selection in malignancy. Int J Cancer 1999;80:356–64.
36. Chiang AK, Chan AC, Srivastava G, et al. Nasal T/NK-cell lymphomas are derived from Epstein–Barr virus infected cytotoxic lymphocytes of both NK- and T-cell lineage. Int J Cancer 1997;73:332–8.
37. Zhang Y, Nagata H, Ikeuchi T, et al. Common cytological and cytogenetic features of Epstein–Barr virus (EBV)–positive natural killer (NK) cells and cell lines derived from patients with nasal T/NK-cell lymphomas, chronic active EBV infection and hydroa vacciniforme-like eruptions. Br J Haematol 2003;121:805–14.
38. Wong KF, Zhang YM, Chan JKC. Cytogenetic abnormalities in natural killer cell lymphoma and leukaemia-is there a consistent pattern? Leuk Lymphoma 1999;34:241–50.
39. Wong KF, Chan JKC, Kwong YL. Identification of del (q21q25) as a recurrent chromosomal abnormality in putative NK cell lymphoma/leukaemia. Br J Haematol 1997;98:922–6.
40. Siu LL, Wong KF, Chan JKC, et al. Comparative genomic hybridization analysis of natural killer cell leukemia/ leukemia. Recognition of consistent patterns of genetic alterations. Am J Path 1999;155:1419–25.
41. Siu LL, Chan V, Chan JKC, et al. Consistent patterns of allelic loss in natural killer cell lymphoma. Am J Pathol 2000;157: 1803–9.
42. Sun HS, Su IJ, Lin YC, et al. A 2.6 Mb interval on chromosome 6q25.2-q25.3 is commonly deleted in human nasal natural killer/T-cell lymphoma. Br J Haematol 2003;122: 590–9.
43. Siu LL, Chan JKC, Wong KF, et al. Specific patterns of gene methylation in natural killer cell lymphomas: p73 is consistently involved. Am J Pathol 2002;160:59–66.
44. Shen L, Liang AC, Au WY, et al. BCL10 mutations are irrelevant to its aberrant nucler localization in nasal NK/T cell lymphoma. Leukemia 203;17:2240–2.
45. Shen L, Liang AC, Lu L, et al. Aberrant BCL10 nuclear expression in nasal NK/T cell lymphoma. Blood 2003;102:1553–4.
46. Shen L, Liang AC, Lu L, et al. Frequent deletion of Fas gene sequences encoding death and transmembrane domains in nasal natural killer/T-cell lymphoma. Am J Pathol 2002;161: 2123–31.
47. Shen L, Chiang AK, Liu WP, et al. Expression of HLA class I, beta-microglobulin, TAP1 and IL-10 in Epstein–Barr virus–associated nasal NK/T-cell lymphoma: Implications for tumor immune escape mechanism. Int J Cancer 2001;92:692–6.
48. Chim CS, Ma SY, Au WY, et al. Primary nasal natural killer cell lymphoma: long-term treatment outcome and relationship with the International Prognostic Index. Blood 2004; 103:216–21.
49. Strickler JG, Meneses MF, Habermann TM, et al. Polymorphic reticulosis: a reappraisal. Hum Pathol 1994;25;659–65.
50. Kwong YL, Chan AC, Liang R, et al. CD56+ NK lymphomas: clinicopathological features and prognosis. Br J Haematol 1997;97:821–9.
51. Kim BS, Kim TY, Kim CW, et al. Therapeutic outcome of extranodal NK/T-cell lymphoma initially treated with chemotherapy-result of chemotherapy in NK/T-cell lymphoma. Acta Oncol 2003;42:779–83.
52. Kim GE, Cho JH, Yang WI, et al. Angiocentric lymphoma of the head and neck: pattern of systemic failure after radiation treatment. J Clin Oncol 2000;18:54–63.
53. Cheung MM, Chan JK, Lau WH, et al. Primary non-Hodgkin's lymphoma of the nose and nasopharynx, clinical features, tumor immunophenotype and treatment outcome in 113 patients. J Clin Oncol 1998;16:70–7.
54. Lei KI, Suen JJ, Hui P, et al. Primary nasal and nasopharyngeal lymphomas: a comparative study of clinical presentation and treatment outcome. Clin Oncol (R Coll Radiol) 1999;11:379–87.
55. Lei KI, Chan LY, Chan WY, et al. Diagnostic and prognostic implications of circulating cell-free Epstein–Barr virus DNA in natural killer/T-cell lymphoma. Clin Cancer Res 2002;8: 29–34.
56. Obama K, Tara M, Niina K. L-asparaginase–based induction therapy for advanced extranodal NK/T-cell lymphoma. Int J Hematol 2003;78:248–50.

57. Yong W, Zheng W, Zhang Y, et al. L-asparaginase-based regimen in the treatment of refractory midline nasal/nasal-type T/NK-cell lymphoma. Int J Hematol 2003;78:163–7.
58. Matsumoto Y, Nomura K, Kanda-Akano Y, et al. Successful treatment with Erwinia L-asparaginase for recurrent natural killer/T cell lymphoma. Leuk Lymphoma 2003;44: 879–82.
59. Liang R, Chen F, Lee CK, et al. Autologous bone marrow transplantation for primary nasal T/NK-cell lymphoma. Bone Marrow Transplant 1997;19:91–3.
60. Y Nawa, Takenaka K, Shinagawa K, et al. Successful treatment of advanced natural killer cell lymphoma with high-dose chemotherapy and syngeneic peripheral blood stem cell transplantation. Bone Marrow Transplant 1999;23:1321–2.
61. Mukai HY, Kojima H, Suzukawa K, et al. High dose chemotherapy with peripheral blood stem cell rescue in blastoid natural killer cell lymphoma. Leuk Lymphoma 1999;32:583–8.
62. Au WY, Lie AK, Liang R, et al. Autologous stem cell transplantation for nasal NK/T-cell lymphoma: a progress report on its value. Ann Oncol 2003;14:1673–6.
63. Cheung MM, Chan JK, Wong KF. Natural killer cell neoplasms: a distinctive group of highly aggressive lymphomas/leukemias. Semin Hematol 2003;40:221–32.
64. Yagi T, Fujino H, Hirai M, et al. Esophageal actinomycosis after allogeneic peripheral blood stem cell transplantation for extranodal natural killer /T cell lymphoma, nasal type. Bone Marrow Transplant 2003;32:451–3.

28

Precursor T-Cell Lymphoblastic Lymphoma

John W. Sweetenham, M.D.

Precursor T-cell lymphoblastic leukemia/lymphoma is a neoplasm of T lymphoblasts. Until recently, the designation of lymphoblastic lymphoma was used to describe precursor B- and T-cell tumors with predominant lymph node involvement. Since the clinical distinction between lymphoblastic lymphoma and leukemia is arbitrary, and since these entities are identical at the morphologic, immunophenotypic, and molecular level, the World Health Organization classification has unified these entities as precursor B- or T-cell lymphoblastic leukemia/lymphoma. Lymphoblastic lymphoma is a clinically aggressive disease, frequently presenting with bulky mediastinal disease, and with a predilection for central nervous system (CNS) and bone marrow involvement. With the use of dose-intensive multiagent chemotherapy regimens, with CNS prophylaxis, with or without stem cell transplantation, long-term disease-free survival is achieved in 50% to 60% of adult patients with this disease.

FREQUENCY

Lymphoblastic lymphoma accounts for about 2% of all non-Hodgkin's lymphomas.[1] About 85% to 90% of adult cases are of T-cell phenotype, and occur most frequently in adolescent and young adult males.[2–5] The median age at diagnosis is around 20 years, with most series reporting male predominance. There have been no recent reports suggesting a change in the incidence of this disease.

DIAGNOSIS

Most cases of lymphoblastic lymphoma are diagnosed based on cellular morphology and flow cytometry or immunophenotyping. Lymphoblastic lymphoma is composed of medium-sized cells with finely dispersed chromatin and little cytoplasm[3] with inconspicuous nucleoli. High mitotic activity with frequent apoptotic bodies that often results in a "starry sky" pattern is characteristic.

Differential diagnosis includes lymphocyte-rich thymoma, which may be problematic since the lymphoid cells in both tumors have a thymic T-cell phenotype. However, the cytology of the cells is generally different, and the characteristic epithelial distribution of thymoma is not seen in lymphoblastic lymphoma.

Most lymphoblastic lymphomas are tumors of precursor T lymphocytes,[6,7] and express CD7, CD5, and CD2. CD3 is often present in the cytoplasm, but surface expression of CD3 is rare.[8] By immunocytochemistry, most cases are CD3-positive, while the sCD3-negative, cCD3+ phenotype is best demonstrated by flow cytometry. CD4 and CD8 can be expressed in any combination. Expression of non–lineage-specific immature markers such as TdT or CD99, or in some cases CD34,[9,10] is the most reliable way of distinguishing lymphoblastic lymphoma from peripheral T-cell lymphomas. If present, CD1a is relatively specific.

Most T-lymphoblastic lymphomas have clonal T-cell receptor gene rearrangements, most commonly TCRδ. However, gene rearrangement studies have a limited role in the diagnosis of this disease. Many precursor T-cell lymphoblastic lymphomas have translocations involving the T-cell receptor gene.

About one-third of patients with T-lymphoblastic lymphoma have translocations involving the alpha and delta T-cell receptor loci at 14q11.2, the beta locus at 7q35, and the gamma locus at 7p14-5,[11] resulting in juxtaposition of promoter and enhancer elements producing high levels of T-cell receptor gene expression, with transcription factor genes such as *HOX11/TLX1, TAL1/SCL, TAL 2*, and *LYL 1*.[12–14]

Gene expression profiles have identified molecular subtypes of precursor T-cell lymphoblastic disease that characterize different stages in thymocyte maturation, and which may identify prognostic subgroups.[15] For example, patients with *HOX11* expression show a pattern of gene expression corresponding to the early cortical thymocyte. This subgroup appears to have a more favorable clinical outcome, possibly related to the lower frequency of expression of the antiapoptotic *bcl-2* gene. These cells are apparently developmentally arrested at a stage in which they are particularly sensitive to drug-induced apoptosis.

In contrast, those samples with gene expression profiles associated with *TAL1* or *LYL1* expression resemble late cortical and early pro-T thymocytes, respectively, and show more drug resistance and correspondingly higher levels of *bcl-2*.

CLINICAL FEATURES

Typical clinical features of T-lymphoblastic lymphoma include peak incidence in the second and third decades, male predominance, mediastinal involvement in 60% to 70% of patients, and pleural and pericardial effusions, the latter occasionally producing cardiac tamponade. Superior vena caval obstruction may also be a presenting feature.

Peripheral lymph node involvement is present in 60% to 80% of patients at diagnosis, most commonly in cervical, supraclavicular, and axillary regions.

Bone marrow and CNS involvement are frequent. In a recent study, 21% of adult patients with lymphoblastic lymphoma had bone marrow involvement at presentation,[16] although it is important to emphasize that the reported incidence of marrow involvement is obscured by inconsistencies in distinction between lymphoblastic lymphoma and acute lymphoblastic leukemia.

CNS involvement occurs in 5% to 10% of patients at presentation. Several reports suggest that it is more common in patients with bone marrow involvement. Typical manifestations of CNS involvement include meningeal involvement with a pleocytosis in the cerebrospinal fluid, or cranial nerve involvement, which characteristically involves ophthalmic or facial nerves. Other less common sites of involvement include the liver, spleen, and subdiaphragmatic lymph nodes, as well as bone, skin, and testes. The CNS is a frequent site of relapse in the absence of adequate prophylaxis, when it may occur in up to 30% of patients.[17]

PROGNOSTIC AND PREDICTIVE FACTORS

"Biologic" Predictive Factors

Although genetic abnormalities have been described in around 30% of cases of T-cell lymphoblastic disease, particularly involving alpha and delta T-cell receptor loci, or deletion of 9p, none of these has prognostic significance.[18] In adult patients with acute lymphoblastic leukemia, expression of T-cell antigens including CD1, CD2, CD4, and CD5 has been associated with a more favorable prognosis. In the Cancer and Leukemia Group B 8364 study, overall and disease-free survival rates correlated with the number of T-cell antigens expressed.[19] Similar studies have not been performed in patients with lymphoblastic lymphoma. As mentioned above, there is emerging evidence that certain gene expression patterns may have predictive value.

Clinical Predictive Factors

Several small retrospective series of patients with lymphoblastic lymphoma identified adverse clinical prognostic factors for overall and disease-free survival.[20–22] These have varied among series, reflecting small patient numbers and variable criteria for categorizing acute lymphoblastic leukemia and lymphoblastic lymphoma. Few of these have been consistent across different retrospective series.

Until description of the IPI, the most widely accepted prognostic factors were those described by Coleman et al.[17] Patients with Ann Arbor Stage 1 to 3, or Ann Arbor Stage IV but without bone marrow or CNS involvement, with a serum lactate dehydrogenase (LDH) level of less than 300 IU/L (normal is 200 IU/L) were considered good risk, with a 5-year freedom-from-relapse rate of 94%. All other patients were considered poor risk, with a 5-year freedom from relapse of only 19%.

The applicability of the IPI for aggressive non-Hodgkin's lymphomas has now been investigated in three studies. A retrospective analysis of a small sample of 26 patients with a median age of 28 years with lymphoblastic lymphoma was reported by the Non-Hodgkin's Lymphoma Classification Project.[23] The 5-year overall and failure-free survival rates were approximately 20%. The number of IPI risk factors was not predictive of overall or failure-free survival in this series. A retrospective series of 62 patients from France also concluded that the IPI did not have prognostic significance in adults with lymphoblastic lymphoma.[24]

The predictive value of the IPI was also explored in the context of a European randomized trial in adults with lymphoblastic lymphoma.[16] Sixty patients had complete data. This represents the only prospectively collected data set in a relatively unselected population of adult patients with lymphoblastic lymphoma. This study showed a statistically significant trend for lower overall survival with an increasing number of adverse factors according to the age-adjusted IPI ($p = 0.016$). However, although survival in patients with three adverse factors was clearly inferior, there was little distinction between those with zero to two factors, and the value of the IPI as a prognostic model remains unclear.

Larger patient samples will be needed to determine whether the IPI will prove to be a suitable staging and prognostic system for lymphoblastic lymphoma, although since all of these patients require intensive multiagent chemotherapy, its relevance in terms of risk stratification for treatment or clinical trials is doubtful.

TREATMENT

Early trials in lymphoblastic lymphoma used chemotherapy regimens initially developed for the treatment of other, less aggressive types of non-Hodgkin's lymphoma.[3,4,25–27] Results with these regimens were poor. Nathwani et al. reported results in 95 adult and pediatric patients with lymphoblastic lymphoma treated on a variety of collaborative group protocols, none of which included CNS prophylaxis.[3] This series included some patients with leukemic involvement. The complete response rate was only 24%, and the median survival was 17 months, with less than 10% of patients alive and disease-free at 5 years. Similar results were reported for other low-intensity chemotherapy regimens.

The introduction of intensive chemotherapy and radiation therapy protocols in childhood lymphoblastic lymphoma produced marked improvements in outcome. Protocols such as the LSA_2L_2 regimen combined intensive chemotherapy, comparable to that used in childhood acute lymphoblastic leukemia, with CNS irradiation.[28] Long-term disease-free survival rates between 60% and 80% were reported for children treated with this and similar regimens. A subsequent randomized trial, comparing the LSA_2L_2 regimen with COMP (cyclophosphamide, vincristine, methotrexate, prednisone) demonstrated a 2-year actuarial, failure-free survival of 76% for children with lymphoblastic lymphoma receiving LSA_2L_2 compared with only 26% for those receiving COMP ($p = 0.0002$).[29] Subsequently, chemo/radiotherapy regimens similar in design to LSA_2L_2, adapted from those in adult acute lymphoblastic leukemia, have been applied to adult patients with lymphoblastic lymphoma.[17,20,21,30–33] Most of these regimens are characterized by intensive remission induction chemotherapy, CNS prophylaxis, a phase of consolidation chemotherapy, and a prolonged maintenance phase, often lasting for 12 to 18 months. Results from some of these regimens are summarized in Table 28–1. Most of these studies report long-term disease-free survival rates between 40% and 60%. Since all of these patient series are relatively small, the apparent minor differences in reported outcomes according to treat-

Table 28–1. Results of Intensive Combination Chemotherapy Regimens in Adults with Lymphoblastic Lymphoma

Reference	Regimen	Number of Patients	Response Rate	Failure-Free Survival/ Relapse-Free Survival	Overall Survival
Coleman (1986)[17]	ALL-type protocols, intensified CNS prophylaxis in second	44	100% (95% CR, 5% PR)	3-year FFS = 56%	3-year = 56%
Slater (1986)[20]	Various ALL protocols	51	80% CR for "nonleukemic" 77% CR for leukemic	N/A	5-year actuarial OS = 45%
Bernasconi (1990)[21]	Various ALL protocols	31	77%	3-year RFS = 45%	3-year = 59%
Morel (1992)[22]	CHOP plus various ALL protocols	80	82% CR	46% at 30 months	51% at 30 months
Levine (1983)[30]	Modified LSA_2L_2	15	73% CR 27% PR	5-year actuarial FFS = 35%	5-year actuarial OS = 40%
Weinstein (1983)[31]	APO	21	95% CR	3-year actuarial FFS = 58%	5-year actuarial OS = 69%
Hoelzer (2002)[32]	2 ALL-type protocols, including CNS and mediastinal irradiation	45	93% CR	7-year actuarial DFS = 62%	7-year actuarial OS = 51%

ALL, acute lymphoblastic leukemia; CNS, central nervous system; CR, complete response; DFS, disease-free survival; FFS, failure-free survival; N/A, not available; OS, overall survival; PR, partial response; RFS, relapse-free survival.

ment regimens are unlikely to be significant. Results from the unselected patient series reported by the Non-Hodgkin's Lymphoma Classification Project are inferior to this, with a reported 5-year actuarial overall survival of only approximately 20%.[23] This may reflect selection bias in the clinical series.

RADIATION THERAPY

In addition to the use of cranial radiation for prophylaxis of CNS disease, some protocols have also included mediastinal radiation for patients who present with isolated or bulky mediastinal disease. The benefit of mediastinal radiation in adults with lymphoblastic lymphoma is unclear, and has not been systematically studied.

A retrospective report from M.D. Anderson Cancer Center describes 47 patients who received mediastinal radiation as a component of their initial induction therapy over an 18-year period.[34] They report that the use of mediastinal irradiation reduced the incidence of mediastinal relapse, but had no effect on failure-free or overall survival. The 5-year overall and progression-free survival rates of 66% and 64%, respectively, reported in this series are comparable to many other regimens that do not include mediastinal radiation. Although no conclusive evidence exists, there is no clear role of mediastinal radiation.

AUTOLOGOUS STEM CELL TRANSPLANTATION IN FIRST REMISSION

Despite the high remission rates reported for first-line therapy in lymphoblastic lymphoma, relapse rates are also relatively high. As a result, several groups have investigated of the role of high-dose therapy with autologous or allogeneic stem cell transplantation in first remission, in an attempt to reduce the incidence of relapse after induction therapy.[24,33,35,36] In retrospective single-institution and registry studies, the results of this approach have appeared superior to those achieved with conventional dose consolidation and maintenance chemotherapy, and these are summarized in Table 28–2. Long-term disease-free survival in most of these series has been between 60% and 80%, although many of these series are not analyzed according to intention to treat. The study reported by Jost et al. includes a true intent-to-treat analysis, with follow-up on all patients from diagnosis. The 3-year actuarial overall and event-free survival rates were 48% and 31%, respectively.[35] These results do not appear to be superior to those reported for conventional dose first-line therapy.

A single, small, randomized trial has compared the use of high-dose therapy and autologous stem cell transplantation with conventional dose consolidation and maintenance therapy in adult patients with lymphoblastic lymphoma.[16] This study included 119 adult patients who were treated with intensive, acute lymphoblastic leukemia-type induction chemotherapy, of whom 111 were assessable for response to induction therapy. The overall response rate to induction chemotherapy was comparable to other series at 82%. However, of 98 patients eligible for randomization, only 65 were actually randomized. Reasons for failure to randomize included elective allogeneic transplantation in patients with HLA-matched sibling donors, early disease progression prior to transplantation, and patient refusal. The 3-year, actuarial relapse-free survival rate was 24% for patients receiving conventional consolidation and mainte-

Table 28–2. Results of First-Remission Stem Cell Transplantation in Adults with Lymphoblastic Lymphoma

Reference	Induction Therapy/ High-Dose Regimen/ Stem Cell Source	Number of Patients	Event-Free Survival/ Progression-Free Survival	Overall Survival
Bouabdallah (1998)[24]	Various ALL type induction regimens/high-dose cyclophosphamide and TBI/allogeneic and autologous BMT	62 (30 received bone marrow transplant in first CR)	5-year EFS = 58%	5-year OS = 60%
Verdonck (1992)[33]	CHOP or ALL-like induction/high-dose cyclophosphamide and TBI/autologous BMT	9	6/9 in long-term remission	6/9 long-term survivors
Jost (1995)[35]	MACOP-B or VACOP-B induction/high-dose cyclophosphamide and TBI or CBV/ autologous BMT	20	3-year EFS = 31%	3-year OS = 48%
Sweetenham (1994)[36]	Multiple induction and high-dose regimens/autologous BMT	105	6-year PFS = 63%	6-year OS = 64

BMT, bone marrow transplant; EFS, event-free survival; PFS, progression-free survival; OS, overall survival; TBI, total body irradiation.

nance therapy, compared with 55% for those receiving high-dose therapy and autologous stem cell transplantation (p = 0.065). The corresponding values for overall survival were 45% and 56% (p = 0.71) (Fig. 28–1). The fact that there was a nonsignificant trend for improved relapse-free survival in the transplant arm, but no difference in overall survival, may be due to the fact that some patients who relapsed after conventional dose consolidation therapy were "rescued" by high-dose therapy in second remission. On the basis of the above data, many centers now use high-dose therapy and autologous stem cell transplantation in first remission as the standard therapy for adults with lymphoblastic lymphoma.

AUTOLOGOUS STEM CELL TRANSPLANTATION FOR RELAPSED OR REFRACTORY DISEASE

Results of salvage therapy for adult patients with lymphoblastic lymphoma are very poor. The use of second-line conventional dose regimens in this situation produces response rates of less than 10%, and median overall survival in these series is only around 9 months.[17,20–22]

Very few published studies have addressed the role of autologous stem cell transplantation in this situation. In a retrospective study from Morel et al. of 37 patients with adult lymphoblastic lymphoma who required salvage therapy, 14 achieved a second complete remission with conventional dose reinduction.[22] Seven of these patients underwent consolidation with autologous stem cell transplantation, of whom three achieved long-term disease-free survival.

In a retrospective study from the European Group for Blood and Marrow Transplantation, 41 patients underwent high-dose therapy and autologous stem cell transplantation in second complete remission.[36] The 3-year actuarial progression-free survival and overall survival for this group were 30% and 31%, respectively (Fig. 28–2). As with other types of non-Hodgkin's lymphoma, the responsiveness of the disease to conventional dose therapy given prior to the transplant was predictive of outcome. The 5-year actuarial overall survival for those with chemosensitive relapse was 31% compared with 18% for those with chemorefractory disease (Fig. 28–3).

Since patients in chemosensitive relapse have a superior outcome to those with chemorefractory relapse, all relapsing patients should receive conventional dose salvage therapy in an attempt to induce a second remission prior to high-dose therapy. However, even in those patients with refractory disease, the reported long-term disease-free survival of 18% is superior to that achieved with conventional dose salvage, and these patients should also be offered high-dose therapy.

ALLOGENEIC STEM CELL TRANSPLANTATION

In view of the relatively young age of adult patients with lymphoblastic lymphoma, it is anticipated that their regimen-related mortality after allogeneic transplantation is likely to be relatively low. If a graft-versus-lymphoma effect exists in this disease, then the low relapse rate observed in patients who survive allogeneic transplantation might result in improved overall survival compared with

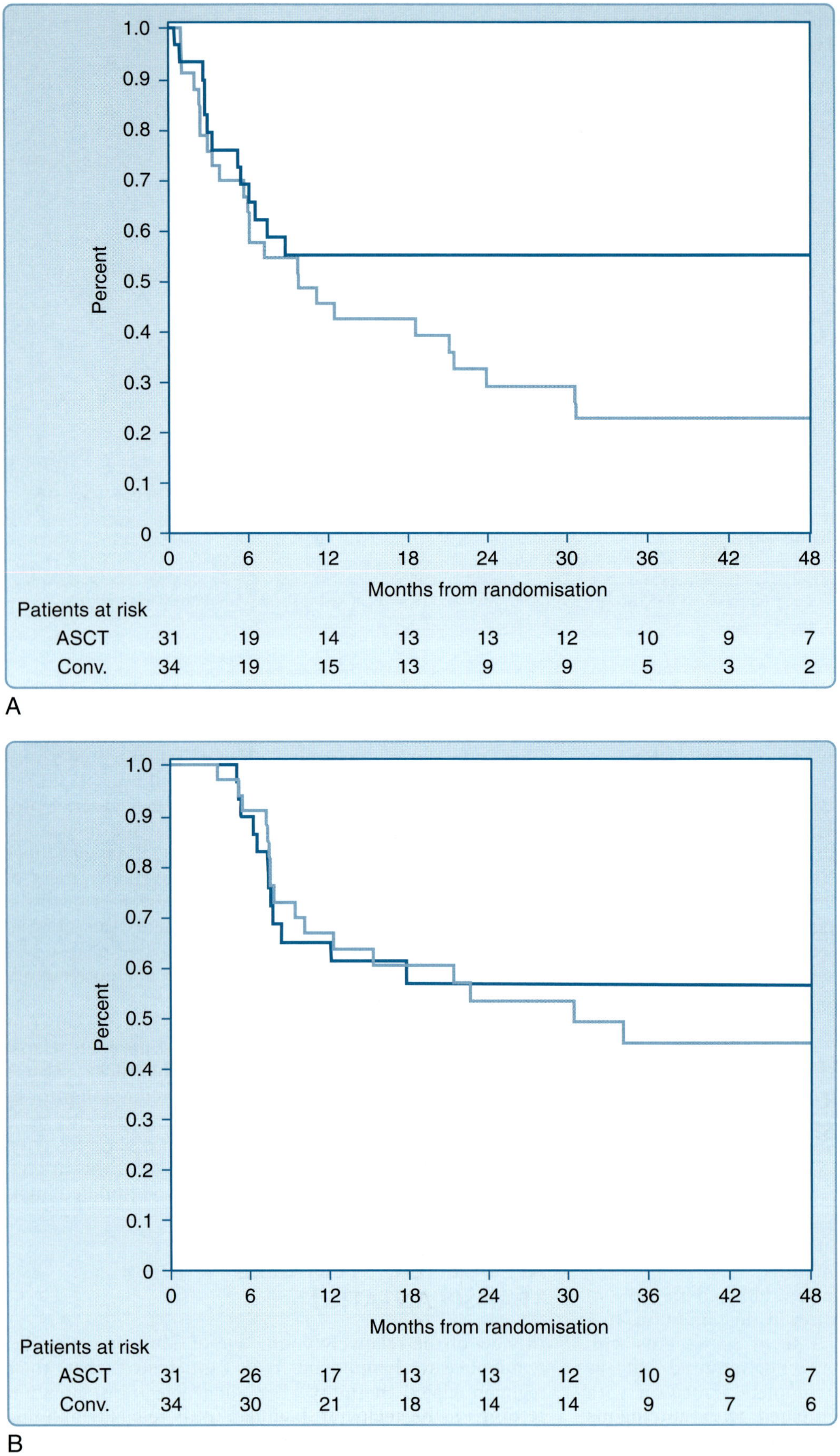

Figure 28–1. Results from the UKLG/EBMT randomized trial of high-dose therapy and stem cell transplantation versus conventional consolidation therapy in adult lymphoblastic lymphoma. Results shown are for relapse-free survival (**A**) and overall survival (**B**). (From Sweetenham JW, Santini G, Qian W, et al. High-dose therapy and autologous stem-cell transplantation versus conventional dose consolidation/maintenance therapy as post-remission therapy for adult patients with lymphoblastic lymphoma: results of a randomized trial of the European Group for Blood and Marrow Transplantation and the United Kingdom Lymphoma Group. J Clin Oncol 2001;19:2927–36,[16] with permission.)

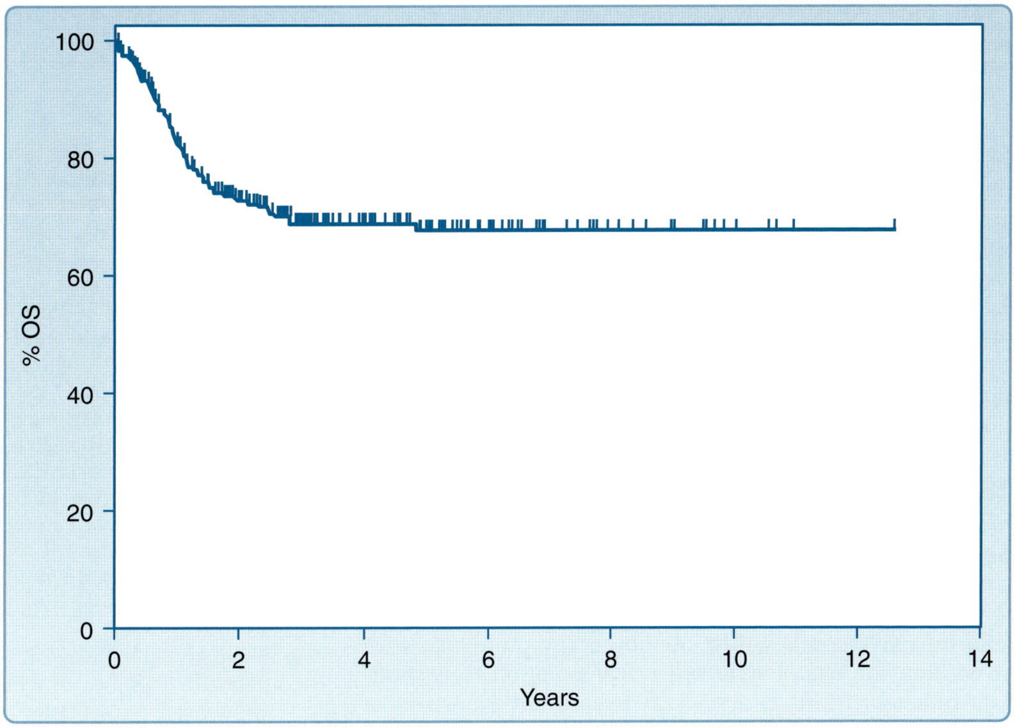

Figure 28–2. Results of high-dose therapy and autologous stem cell transplantation in adult patients with lymphoblastic lymphoma who received transplant in second complete remission. (From Jost LM, Jacky E, Dommann-Scherrer C, et al. Short-term weekly chemotherapy followed by high dose therapy with autologous bone marrow transplantation for lymphoblastic and Burkitt's lymphomas in adult patients. Ann Oncol 1995;6: 445–51,[35] with permission.)

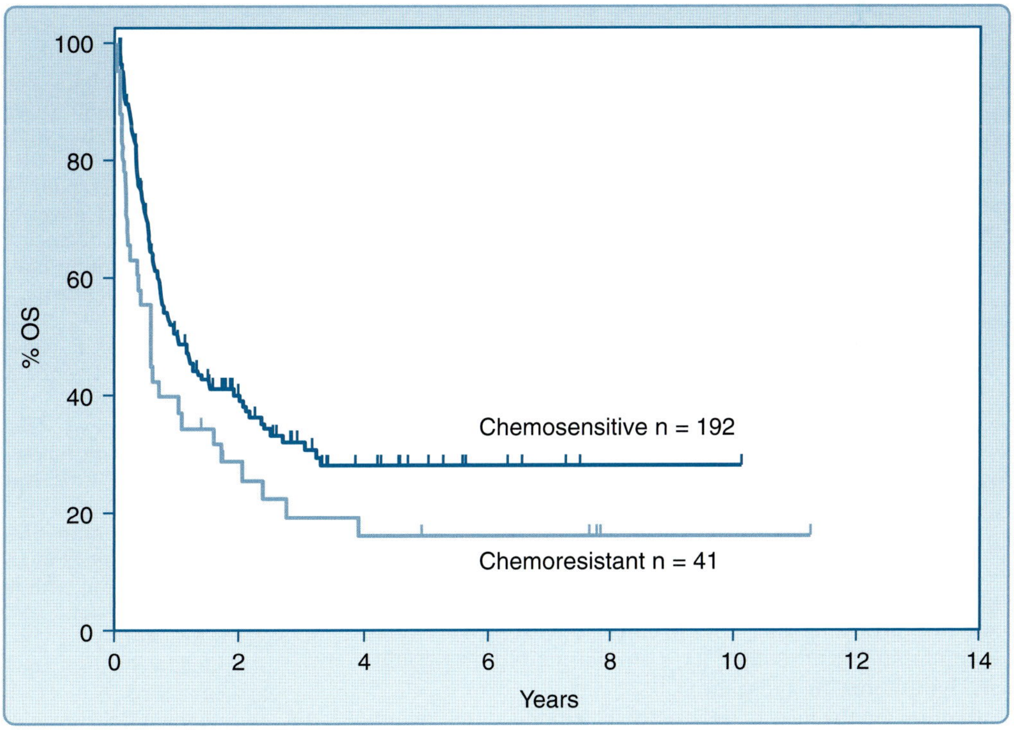

Figure 28–3. Results of high-dose therapy and autologous stem cell transplantation in adult patients with lymphoblastic lymphoma who received transplant in chemosensitive or chemoresistant relapse. (From Jost LM, Jacky E, Dommann-Scherrer C, et al. Short-term weekly chemotherapy followed by high dose therapy with autologous bone marrow transplantation for lymphoblastic and Burkitt's lymphomas in adult patients. Ann Oncol 1995;6: 445–51,[35] with permission.)

autologous transplantation. A retrospective, case-controlled analysis from the European Group for Blood and Marrow Transplantation comparing autologous with allogeneic stem cell transplantation reported a lower relapse rate for patients receiving allogeneic compared with autologous stem cell transplantation (2% vs. 48%, respectively, $p = 0.035$).[37] However, progression-free survival for both groups was equivalent because of the higher procedure-related mortality in the allogeneic group. Although one other series has reported a superior outcome for patients receiving HLA-matched allogeneic transplants, this was also a small retrospective series.[24] Patients proceeding to allogeneic transplant are likely to be favorable in terms of age, performance status, and time in remission prior to transplant—all factors that might bias for improved survival.

The only prospectively collected data on the role of allogeneic transplantation were reported in the context of the European randomized trial.[16] In this study, a small series of 12 patients with HLA-identical sibling donors were treated with allogeneic transplantation in first remission. The 3-year actuarial overall survival of 58% for this group is comparable to results in patients receiving autologous transplants. A recent study from the International Bone Marrow Transplant registry compared outcomes for autologous and allogeneic stem cell transplantation in adult patients with lymphoblastic lymphoma. No difference in survival was observed.[38]

There are currently no convincing data to suggest that allogeneic stem cells are a better stem cell source, or that a clinically significant graft versus lymphoma effect is active in this disease. Autologous stem cells should still be regarded as the preferred source of hematopoietic rescue.

PROGNOSIS AND MEDIAN SURVIVAL

Most published series that include adult patients treated with intensive combination chemotherapy protocols, with or without the use of stem cell transplantation to consolidate first remission report 5-year overall survival rates of 50% to 65%, respectively, with no obvious benefit from stem cell transplantation. Although the IPI may have predictive value, there are inadequate data to support the use of a risk-stratified approach to treatment.

Following relapse after first-line chemotherapy, subsequent prognosis is poor, with typical reported median survival rates of 6 to 9 months when conventional chemotherapy is used, although for relapsed, and primary refractory patients, long-term survival rates of approximately 30% and 20%, respectively, are reported after stem cell transplantation.

FUTURE DIRECTIONS

Dose-intensive multiagent induction chemotherapy, similar to that used in acute lymphoblastic leukemia has increased response rates and overall survival for adult patients with lymphoblastic lymphoma compared with standard non-Hodgkin's lymphoma–type regimens. Whether further enhancement of dose intensity will improve response rates further is unclear. The use of very intensive induction therapy, such as HyperCVAD, has been reported to produce high overall response rates in acute lymphoblastic leukemia, and some subtypes of non-Hodgkin's lymphoma. Regimens such as this may have similar activity in patients with lymphoblastic lymphoma.[39]

Reports of the use of relatively T-cell "specific" agents such as 506U78 suggest that such agents may have useful activity in this disease.[40]

Stem cell transplant strategies also require further evaluation. In particular, nonmyeloablative stem cell transplantation offers an opportunity to exploit the reported graft versus tumor effect in this disease, with lower risk of regimen-related mortality. The early experience with Hyper-CVAD for lymphoblastic lymphoma demonstrated a 91% complete remission rate with 66% progression-free survival at 3 years. The program included intrathecal prophylaxis, radiation therapy, if mediastinal mass was present, and maintenance therapy.[41]

References

1. The Non-Hodgkin's Lymphoma Classification Project. A clinical evaluation of the International Lymphoma Study Group classification of non-Hodgkin's lymphomas. Blood 1997;89:3909–18.
2. Rosen PJ, Feinstein DI, Pattengale PK, et al. Convoluted lymphocytic lymphoma in adults: a clinicopathological entity. Ann Intern Med 1978;89:319–24.
3. Nathwani BN, Diamond LW, Winberg CD, et al. Lymphoblastic lymphoma: a clinicopathologic study of 95 patients. Cancer 1978;48:2347–57.
4. Murphy SB. Management of childhood non-Hodgkin's lymphoma. Cancer Treat Rep 1977;61:1161–73.
5. Warnke RA, Weiss LM, Chan JKC, et al. Tumors of the lymph nodes and spleen. In: Atlas of Tumor Pathology. : Armed Forces Institute of Pathology, 1995: Washington, D.C.
6. Griffith RC, Kelly DR, Nathwani BN, et al. A morphologic study of childhood lymphoma of the lymphoblastic type: the Pediatric Oncology Group experience. Cancer 1987;59(6): 1126–31.
7. Sheibani K, Nathwani BN, Winberg CD, et al. Antigenically defined subgroups of lymphoblastic lymphoma: relationship to clinical presentation and biological behavior. Cancer 1987;60:183–90.
8. Link MP, Stewart SJ, Warnke RA, et al. Discordance between surface and cytoplasmic expression of the Leu-4(T3) antigen I thymocytes and in blast cells from childhood T lymphoblastic malignancies. J Clin Invest 1985;76:248–53.
9. Chilosi M, Pizzolog G. Review of terminal deoxynucleotidyl transferase: biological aspects, methods of detection, and selected diagnostic applications. Appl Immunohistochem 1995;3:209–21.
10. Borowitz MJ, Ferrando AA, Neuberg D, et al. Gene expression signatures define novel oncogenic pathways in T cell acute lymphoblastic leukemia. Cancer Cell 2002;1:75–87.
11. Borowitz MJ. Immunologic markers in childhood acute lymphoblastic leukemia. Hematol Oncol Clin North Am 1990;4:743–65.
12. Okuda T, Fisher R, Downing JR. Molecular diagnostics in pediatric acute lymphoblastic leukemia. Mol Diagn 1996; 1:139–51.
13. Finger LR, Kagan J, Christopher G, et al. Involvement of the TCL5 gene on human chromosome 1 in T-cell leukemia and melanoma. Proc Natl Acad Sci U S A 1989;86:5039–43.
14. Mellentin JD, Smith SD, Cleary ML. Lyl-1, A novel gene altered by chromosomal translocation in T-cell leukemia, codes for a protein with helix-loop-helix DNA binding motif. Cell 1989;58:77–83.
15. Xia Y, Brown L, Yang CY, et al. TAL2, a helix-loop-helix gene activated by the t(7;9)(q34;q32) translocation in human T-cell leukemia. Proc Natl Acad Sci U S A 1989;88:11416–20.
16. Sweetenham JW, Santini G, Qian W, et al. High-dose therapy and autologous stem-cell transplantation versus conventional dose consolidation/maintenance therapy as post-remission therapy for adult patients with lymphoblastic lymphoma: results of a randomized trial of the European Group for Blood and Marrow Transplantation and the United Kingdom Lymphoma Group. J Clin Oncol 2001;19:2927–36.
17. Coleman NC, Picozzi VJ, Cox RS, et al. Treatment of lymphoblastic lymphoma in adults. J Clin Oncol 1986;4:1626–37.
18. Okuda T, Fisher R, and Downing JR. Molecular diagnostics in pediatric acute lymphoblastic leukemia. Mol Diag 1996; 1:139–51.

19. Czuczman MS, Dodge RK, Stewart CC, et al. Value of imunophenotype in intensively treated adult acute lymphoblastic leukemia: Cancer and Leukemia Group B study 8364. Blood 1999;93:3931–9.
20. Slater DE, Mertelsmann R, Koriner B, et al. Lymphoblastic lymphoma in adults. J Clin Oncol 1986;4:57–67.
21. Bernasconi C, Brusamolino E, Lazzarino M, et al. Lymphoblastic lymphoma in adult patients;clnicopathological features and response to intensive multi-agent chemotherapy analogous to that used in acute lymphoblastic leukemia. Ann Oncol 1990;1:141–60.
22. Morel P, Lepage E, Brice P, et al. Prognosis and treatment of lymphoblastic lymphoma in adults: a report on 80 patients. J Clin Oncol 1992;10:1078–85.
23. Armitage JO, Weisenberger DD. New approach to classifying non-Hodgkin's lymphomas: clinical features of the major histologic subtypes. J Clin Oncol 1998;16:2780–95.
24. Bouabdallah R, Xerri L, Bardou V-J, et al. Role of induction chemotherapy and bone marrow transplantation in adult lymphoblastic lymphoma: a report on 62 patients from a single center. Ann Oncol 1998;9:619–25.
25. Voakes JB, Jones SE, McKelvey EM. The chemotherapy of lymphoblastic lymphoma. Blood 1981;57:186–8.
26. Colgan JP, Anderson J, Habermann TM, et al. Long-term follow-up of a CHOP-based regimen with maintenance chemotherapy and central nervous system prophylaxis in lymphoblastic non-Hodgkin's lymphoma. Leuk Lymphoma 1994;15:291–6.
27. Kaiser U, Uebelacker I, Havemann K. Non-Hodgkin's lymphoma protocols in the treatment of patients with Burkitt's lymphoma and lymphoblastic lymphoma: a report on 58 patients. Leuk Lymphoma 1999;36:101–8.
28. Woolner N, Burchenal JH, Liberman PH, et al. Non-Hodgkin's lymphoma in children. A progress report on the original patient treated with the LSA_2L_2 protocol. Cancer 1979; 44:1990–9.
29. Anderson JR, Wilson JF, Jenkin RDT, et al. Childhood non-Hodgkin's lymphoma. The results of a randomized therapeutic trial comparing a 4-drug regimen (COMP) with a 10-drug regimen (LSA_2L_2). N Engl J Med 1983;308;559–65.
30. Levine AM, Forman SJ, Meyer PR, et al. Successful therapy of convoluted T-lymphoblastic lymphoma in the adult. Blood 1983;61:92–9.
31. Weinstein HJ, Cassady JR, Levey R. Long-term results of the APO protocol (vincristine, doxorubicin [adriamycin] and prednisone) for the treatment of mediastinal lymphoblastic lymphoma. J Clin Oncol 1983;1:537–41.
32. Hoelzer D, Gokbuget N, Digel W, et al. Outcome of adult patients with T-lymphoblastic lymphoma treated according to protocols for acute lymphoblastic leukemia. Blood 2002;99:4379–85.
33. Verdonck LF, Dekker AW, deGast GC, et al. Autologous bone marrow transplantation for adult poor risk lymphoblastic lymphoma in first remission. J Clin Oncol 1992;4:644–6.
34. Dabaja BS, Ha CS, Thomas DA, et al. The role of local radiation therapy for mediastinal disease in adults with T-cell lymphoblastic lymphoma. Cancer 2002;94:2738–44.
35. Jost LM, Jacky E, Dommann-Scherrer C, et al. Short-term weekly chemotherapy followed by high dose therapy with autologous bone marrow transplantation for lymphoblastic and Burkitt's lymphomas in adult patients. Ann Oncol 1995;6:445–51.
36. Sweetenham JW, Santini G, Pearce R, et al. High-dose therapy and autologous bone marrow transplantation for adult patients with lymphoblastic lymphoma: results from the European Group for Bone Marrow Transplantation. J Clin Oncol 1994;12:1358–65.
37. Chopra R, Goldstone AH, Pearce R, et al. Autologous versus allogeneic bone marrow transplantation for non-Hodgkin's lymphoma: a case controlled analysis of the European Bone Marrow Transplant Group registry data. J Clin Oncol 1992;10:1690–5.
38. Levine JE, Harris RE, Loberiza FR, et al. A comparison of allogeneic and autologous bone marrow transplantation for lymphoblastic lymphoma. Blood 2003;101:2476–82.
39. Kantarjian HM, O'Brien S, Smith TL, et al. Results of treatment with HyperCVAD, a dose-intensive regimen, in adult acute lymphocytic leukemia. J Clin Oncol 2000;18: 547–61.
40. Kurtzberg J, Keating M, Moore JO, et al. 2-amino-9-B-D-arabinosyl-6-methoxy-9H-guanine (GW506U;compound 506U) is highly active in patients with T-cell malignancies: results of a phase I trial in pediatric and adult patients with refractory hematological malignancies. Blood 1996;88: 2666a.
41. Thomas DA, O'Brien S, Cortes J, et al. Outcome with the hyper-CVAD regimens in lymphoblastic lymphoma. Blood 2004;104:1624–30.

29

Human T-Cell Leukemia Virus Type I

Masao Matsuoka, M.D., Ph.D.

Human T-cell leukemia virus type I (HTLV-I) is the first human retrovirus shown to be linked with human disease. In 1977, adult T-cell leukemia/lymphoma (ATL) was proposed as a distinct clinical entity from its unique geographic distribution and clinical features.[1] Then, its causative retrovirus, HTLV-I, was identified in the human T-cell line,[2] which finally clarified that HTLV-I was the causative virus of ATL.[3] The discovery of HTLV-I leads to further characterization of ATL and HTLV-I infection, and discloses the virologic mechanism of transformation.

VIROLOGY OF HTLV-I

HTLV-I belongs to the delta-type retroviruses, which also include bovine leukemia virus (BLV), human T-cell leukemia virus type II (HTLV-II), and simian T-cell leukemia virus (STLV).[4] BLV and STLV have also been associated with neoplastic diseases as well as HTLV-I. The structure of HTLV-I provirus is similar to other retroviruses that contain *gag*, *pol*, and *env* genes flanked by long terminal repeat (LTR) sequences at both ends.[5] A unique structure was found between *env* and the 3'-LTR, denoted the pX region, which encodes the regulatory proteins, $p40^{tax}$ (Tax), $p27^{rex}$ (Rex), p12, p13, p30, p21, and HBZ (Fig. 29–1). The presence of accessory genes is the characteristics of delta-type retroviruses as well as foamy virus and lentivirus including human immunodeficiency virus type 1 (HIV-1).

Function of Tax

Among these accessory proteins encoded by HTLV-I, Tax protein plays a central role in the proliferation of infected cells and the leukemogenesis because of its pleiotropic actions (Fig. 29–2).[6] Tax potently increases the expression of viral genes through the viral LTR and stimulates the transcription of cellular genes through cellular signaling pathways of NF-κB, CREB, SRF, and AP-1. Tax does not bind to promoter or enhancer sequences by itself, but it interacts with cellular proteins that are transcriptional factors or modulators of cellular functions.

Transcriptional Activation

Tax can activate the NF-κB pathway by interacting with IKKγ. IKKα, β, and γ form a 700-kDa complex in which IKKγ functionally adapts Tax into this large complex.[7] The activated complex phosphorylates IκB, which detach NF-κB, result in activation of NF-κB. Among the various functions of the Tax protein, activation of NF-κB has been shown to be essential to transformation by HTLV-I.[8] Activation of the NF-κB pathway induces transcription of various cytokines and their receptor genes as well as numerous genes associated with apoptosis and the cell cycle. For example, Tax can activate the transcription of interleukin (IL)-2Rα and IL-2 genes through the NF-κB pathway. In addition, the transcription of IL-6, IL-15, and GM-CSF genes can be activated by the Tax protein via NF-κB. Such activation of genes associated with cell proliferation seems to be involved in the growth of HTLV-I–infected cells both in vitro and in vivo. Tax can also induce expression of Bcl-xL via activation of NF-κB, which renders ATL cells apoptosis-resistant.[9] As well as HTLV-I–transformed cell lines, increased expression of Bcl-xL was observed in fresh ATL cells,[10] which may account for the resistance of ATL cells to chemotherapy.

For activation of the viral LTR, Tax requires at least two 21-bp enhancers containing an imperfect cAMP-responsive element bound to a cyclicAMP response element binding protein (CREB).[11] Tax can bind to both CREB- and CREB-binding protein (CBP), the latter of which is a transcriptional co-activator.[12] Under physiologic conditions, only phosphorylated CREB induced by stimulation can bind to CBP. Tax shunts this pathway, resulting in stimulation-independent activation of the CREB pathway. CBP acetylates histone and opens the nucleosome structure around the transcriptional site.

Transcriptional Repression

Conversely, Tax can trans-repress transcription of certain genes, such as DNA polymerase β, *lck*, *p18*, and *p53* genes. For trans-repression of *p18* gene transcription, the E-box, which binds to transcriptional factor E47, is critical. Tax protein itself could not bind to E-box or E47, but interferes with binding of E47 to the transcriptional co-activator, p300, resulting in repression of transcription.[13] p53-dependent transcription is also repressed by Tax protein. Similar to trans-repression of p18, Tax does not bind to the p53- or p53-binding site, but rather inhibits the recruitment of CBP to p53 on the p53-binding sites.[13] This mechanism of trans-repression contrasts with that of trans-activation of the CREB pathway by Tax protein. Although both mechanisms depend on binding the Tax protein to the transcriptional activator, CBP/p300, their effect on transcription is quite different.[6]

Functional Inhibition

Apart from transcriptional regulation, Tax can influence the function of cellular factors. Tax protein can interact with a negative inhibitor of cyclin-dependent kinase (CDK) 4, $p16^{INK4a}$, via its ankyrin motif, and impair its function.[14] Since $p16^{INK4a}$ is an inhibitor of CDK4, its functional inactivation leads to activation of CDK4/6, phosphorylation of Rb, and finally G1/S transition.

Transforming growth factor β (TGF-β) is an inhibitory cytokine that plays important roles in development, the

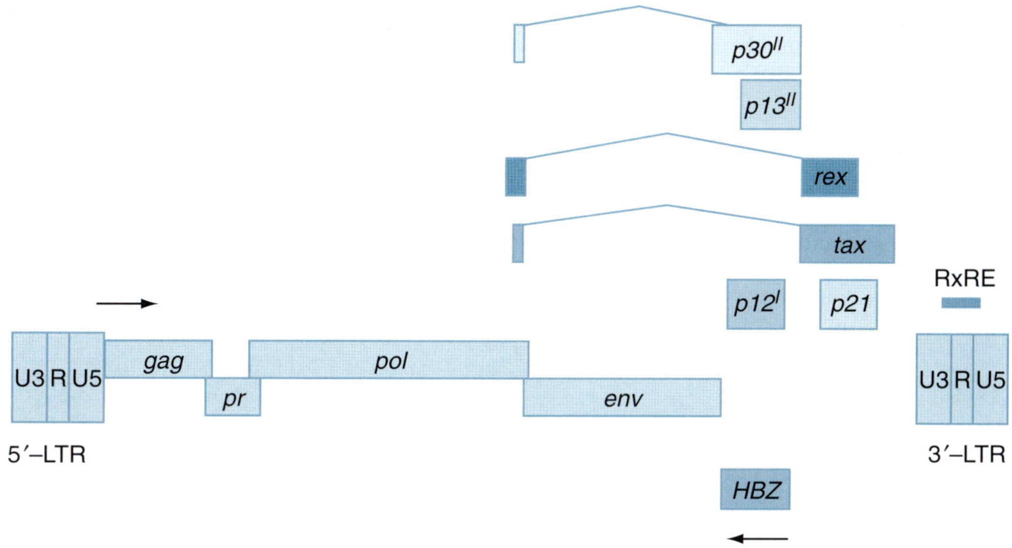

Figure 29–1. Structure of HTLV-I provirus and its encoding genes. The structure of HTLV-I provirus genome, and its encoded accessory gene have been shown. *Arrows* indicate orientation of viral gene transcription. Pr, protease.

immune system, and oncogenesis. Since TGF-β generally suppresses the growth of tumor cells, most tumor cells acquire escape mechanisms to inhibit signaling from TGF-β, which include mutation of its receptor and mutation of Smad molecules that transduce the signal from the receptor. Tax is also reported to inhibit the signal of TGF-β by its binding to Smad2, 3, and 4, or CBP/p300.[15,16] Inhibition of TGF-β signaling enables HTLV-I–infected cells to escape TGF-β–mediated growth inhibition.

ATL cells are well known to show remarkable chromosomal abnormalities, which are thought to reflect chromosomal instability. Tax has been reported to interact with the checkpoint protein, MAD1, which forms a complex with MAD2 and controls the mitotic checkpoint. The functional hindrance of MAD1 by Tax protein causes chromosomal instability, suggesting the involvement of this mechanism in oncogenesis.[17]

Rex

Rex acts at the post-transcriptional level to regulate viral gene expression, which enhances the expression of the unspliced *gag/pol* and singly spliced *env* transcripts, and decreases *tax/rex* mRNAs.[6] Therefore, Rex is a negative regulator for viral transcription by inhibiting the expression of the *tax* gene. Rex binds to the Rex-responsive elements (RxRE), which is located in the 3'-LTR (R/U3 region) (Fig. 29–1), which mediates the nuclear transport of unspliced viral mRNA, and also regulates RNA processing.

p30

p30 interacts with the transcriptional co-activator, CBP/p300, which competes with Tax at 5'-LTR, resulting in reduced viral gene expression. In addition, p30 specifically binds to *tax/rex* mRMA, and retains it in the nucleus. Thus,

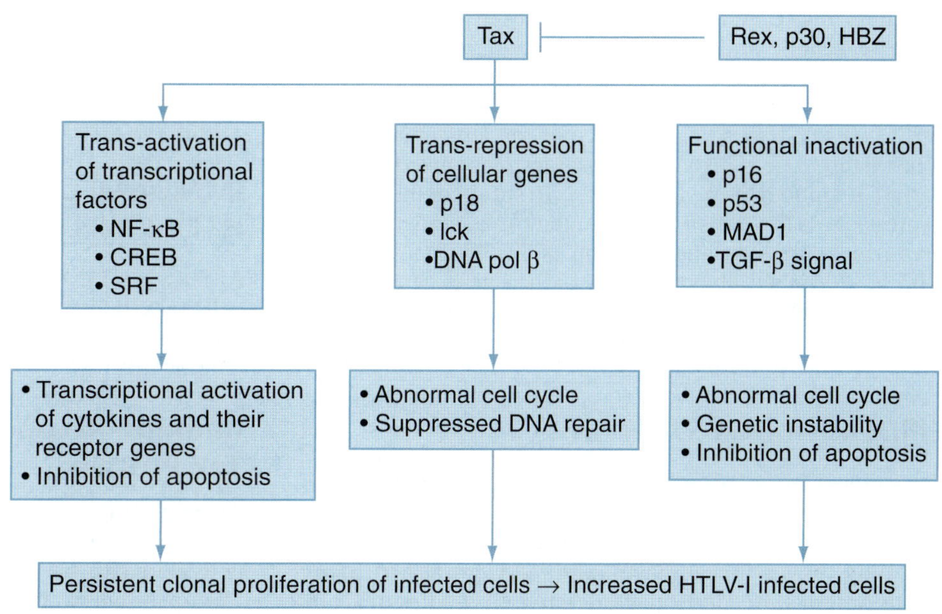

Figure 29–2. Pleiotropic actions of Tax. Pleiotropic actions of Tax proteins are summarized. Expression of Tax is also down-regulated by Rex, p30, and HBZ.

p30 reduces the production of Tax protein by a post-transcriptional mechanism, leading to suppression of viral gene transcription.[18]

HBZ

HBZ, which is encoded by the complementary strand of HTLV-I (Fig. 29–1), binds to c-Jun and JunB, and decreases the DNA-binding activity of these transcriptional factors,[19] which in turn reduces the viral transcription from LTR. This finding shows that HBZ is another negative regulator for virus gene expression.

p12

Open reading frame (ORF) 1 of the pX region encodes p12 (Fig. 29–1), which is present in the endoplastimic reticulum and Golgi apparatus. p12 has been shown to play an important role in establishment of HTLV-I infection and optimal viral infectivity in vivo and quiescent primary lymphocytes.[20,21] As a mechanism, p12 has been shown to interact with calreticulin and calnexin, and increase cytoplasmic calcium, leading to NFAT activation in T lymphocytes.[22] With this action, p12 facilitates host cell activation and establishment of persistent infection. Although the expression of p12 protein in vivo has remained obscure, cytotoxic T lymphocytes (CTLs) against p12 have been demonstrated in individuals infected with HTLV-I, indicating that p12 protein is expressed in vivo.[23]

p13

p13 is gene product encoded by ORFII of pX region, and selectively targeted to mitochondria, which is inserted in the inner mitochondrial membrane.[24] The presence of cytotoxic T cells against p13 in the carriers shows its expression in vivo.[23] Expression of p13 suppresses the growth of tumor cells and also increases the sensitivity to Ca2+-mediated stimuli.[25] The function of p13 in viral replication and cell proliferation needs further study.

Thus, HTLV-I has redundant strategies to increase infected cells through its encoded proteins, Tax and p12, which promote cell proliferation, inhibit apoptosis, and increase genetic and chromosomal instability (Fig. 29–2). With these strategies, HTLV-I increases its copies in vivo by promoting the proliferation and survival of infected cells, and causes ATL as a consequence of the strategies. On the other hand, Tax is also a major target recognized by cytotoxic T lymphocytes (CTL) in vivo. To suppress the *tax* gene expression, HTLV-I also has redundant mechanisms to suppress the expression and function of Tax by Rex, p30, and HBZ as described above, which reduce viral gene expression and virus production. Such mechanism enables HTLV-I–infected cells to suppress viral gene expression and escape from the host immune system.

EPIDEMIOLOGY OF HTLV-I

On a global basis, 10 million to 20 million people are estimated to be infected with HTLV-I. HTLV-I is endemic in southwest Japan, the Caribbean Islands, countries surrounding the Caribbean Basin, parts of Central Africa, and South America. In addition, epidemiologic studies of HTLV-I revealed high seroprevalence rates in Melanesia, Papua New Guinea, and the Solomon Islands, and among Australian aborigines.[26] In Japan, approximately 1.2 million individuals were estimated to be infected by HTLV-I, and more than 800 cases of ATL are diagnosed each year.[27] The cumulative risk of ATL among HTLV-I carriers in Japan was estimated at about 6.6% for men and 2.1% for women, indicating that most of HTLV-I carriers are asymptomatic throughout their lives.[28]

TRANSMISSION OF HTLV-I

HTLV-I is transmitted by three routes: (1) mother to infant (via breast milk); (2) horizontal (sexual); and (3) parenteral (blood transfusion or intravenous drug use). Infected cells are essential for transmission of HTLV-I via any of these routes, which has been demonstrated by the absence of seroconvertors among recipients of fresh frozen plasma transfusions.[29] The transmission efficiency of free virion is estimated to be 1 in 10^5 to 10^6 virion, whereas cell-to-cell transmission is much more efficient.[30] Thus, transmission of HTLV-I requires cell-to-cell contact. Such contact induces polarizations of the cytoskeleton of an infected cell to the cell-to-cell junction (virologic synapse), and then Gag protein complexes containing the virus genome accumulate at this junction, finally leading to the transfer of these complexes to uninfected cells.[31] This mechanism can explain why cell-to-cell contact is essential to transmission of HTLV-I.

HTLV-I can infect various cell types, including B lymphocytes, dendritic cells, fibroblast, rat cells, and mouse cells, indicating that its receptor is ubiquitously expressed on cell surfaces. Glucose transporter, GLUT-1, has been identified as a receptor of HTLV-I,[32] which also proved that the receptor for HTLV-I is ubiquitously expressed. However, after transmission in vivo, HTLV-I provirus was predominantly found in the CD4-positive T lymphocytes.[33] This suggests that HTLV-I could increase the number of infected CD4-positive T lymphocytes in vivo after infection, coinciding with the finding that HTLV-I can transform only T lymphocytes in vitro, most of which were CD4-positive. Even a retrovirus vector expressing only Tax could transform CD4-positive T lymphocytes in vitro.[34] Taken together, these findings suggest that Tax promotes proliferation, and inhibits apoptosis, of HTLV-I–infected CD4-positive T lymphocytes in vivo.

IMMUNOLOGICAL CONTROLS OF HTLV-I INFECTION

Although HTLV-I can promote the proliferation of infected cells by viral gene products such as Tax, it also induces the immune response to HTLD-1 to eliminate the infected cells (Fig. 29–3).

Immune Response Against Tax Protein

Among viral proteins, Tax has been shown to be a major target of CTLs in vivo.[35] Therefore, Tax-expressing cells are considered to be eliminated in vivo. Indeed, depletion of CD8-positive T lymphocytes from the peripheral blood

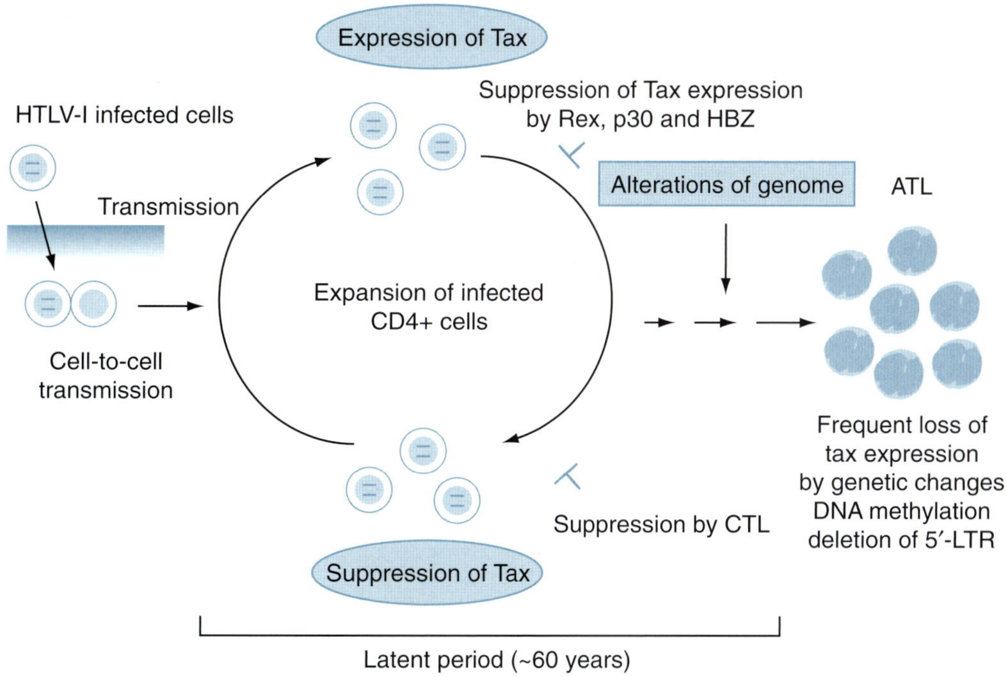

Figure 29–3. Natural course from the infection of HTLV-I to onset of ATL. HTLV-I is transmitted via three routes, and infected cells are necessary in all three. After infection, HTLV-I promotes clonal proliferation of infected cells by pleiotropic actions of Tax. Proliferation of HTLV-I–infected cells is controlled by cytotoxic T cells in vivo. After a long latent period, ATL develops in about 5% of asymptomatic carriers. The expression of Tax is inactivated by several mechanisms, suggesting that Tax is not necessary in this stage. Alternatively, alternations in the host genome accumulate during the latent period, finally leading to onset of ATL.

mononuclear cells of HTLV-I–infected individuals in vitro promoted Tax expression in the CD4-positive subpopulation, indicating that CD8-positive CTLs suppressed Tax expression in vivo.[36] Thus, the survival of HTLV-I–infected cells depends on the balance of proliferative actions of Tax and the host immune system. These findings suggest that in asymptomatic carriers, CTLs against HTLV-I can control the growth of cells carrying the HTLV-I provirus, resulting in preventing the development of ATL.

Immunodeficiency and Development of ATL

Opportunistic infections such as fungal, protozoal, and viral infections are common in patients with ATL due to the inevitable impairment of T-cell function. To a lesser extent, impaired cell-mediated immunity has also been demonstrated in HTLV-I carriers. Such immunodeficiency in the carrier state might be associated with leukemogenesis of ATL by allowing proliferation of HTLV-I–infected cells. A prospective study of HTLV-I–infected individuals identified carriers who later developed ATL and showed that the anti-Tax antibody level was low in all ATL cases for up to 10 years preceding their diagnosis. This finding indicates that HTLV-I carriers with a higher anti–HTLV-I titer, which is roughly correlated with HTLV-I provirus load, and a lower anti-Tax reactivity may be at greatest risk of ATL.[37] The levels of anti–HTLV-I antibody and soluble IL-2 receptor (sIL-2R) have been shown to be correlated with HTLV-I provirus load,[38] and high antibody titers, and high sIL-2R were risk factors for developing ATL among carriers.[39] Taken together, these findings suggest that a higher proliferation of HTLV-I–infected cells, and a low immune response against Tax, might be associated with the onset of ATL. Given this finding, potentiation of CTLs against Tax by a vaccine strategy might be useful in preventing the onset of ATL.[40]

EBV-associated lymphomas frequently develop in individuals with an immunodeficient state associated with transplantation or AIDS. Does such an immunodeficient state, which abrogates the immune function suppressing HTLV-I–infected cells, affect the onset of ATL? Among 24 patients with post-transplantation lymphoproliferative disorders (PT-LPD) after renal transplantation in Japan, five cases of ATL have been reported. Considering that most of PT-LPD is of B-cell origin in Western countries, this frequency of ATL was quite high. Although high seroprevalence of HTLV-I is due to blood transfusion during hemodialysis, the immunodeficient state during renal transplantation apparently promotes the onset of ATL.[41]

Impaired cell-mediated immunity, such as suppressed T-cell response to EBV, and seronegativity against purified protein derivative, has been reported in HTLV-I carriers, also indicating relationship to immunodeficiency. One mechanism of immunodeficiency is that HTLV-I infects CD8-positive T lymphocytes, which might impair the function of CD8-positive T lymphocytes.[33] Indeed, the immune response against Tax, via HTLV-I–infected CD8-positive T cells, renders these cells susceptible to fratricide mediated by autologous HTLV-I–specific CD8-positive T lymphocytes.[42] Fratricide among virus-specific CTLs could impair the immune control of HTLV-I. Another mechanism of immunodeficiency is based on the observation that the number of naive T cells decreased in individuals infected with HTLV-I via decreased thymopoiesis.[33]

HTLV-I–INFECTED CELLS IN VIVO

HTLV-I provirus load, which is correlated with the number of HTLV-I–infected cells, varied by more than 100-fold among HTLV-I carriers. When the sequential DNA samples from peripheral blood mononuclear cells of the same HTLV-I carriers who were followed in a cohort study were analyzed, provirus loads fluctuated only 2- to 4-fold in most carriers, showing that provirus loads were relatively constant over time for up to 7 years in individual carriers.[38] Analyses of HTLV-I provirus load in seroconverters showed that the same virus sequences were identified in the married couples (infected persons transmitted virus to partners); however, their provirus loads were quite different, suggesting that provirus load was determined not by HTLV-I itself, but rather by host factors.[43] One of the candidates for such host factors is the immune response, especially CTLs against HTLV-I, which control the number of HTLV-I–infected cells (Fig. 29–3).[44]

Clonal Expansion of HTLV-I–Infected Cells

Since HTLV-I provirus is randomly integrated in the host genome,[45] the integration site is specific to each HTLV-I–infected cell. When integration sites of HTLV-I provirus were identified in infected cells by inverse PCR, HTLV-I–infected cells clonally proliferated in carriers, some clones were shown to persist for a long time in the same individuals.[46,47] Most of these persistent clones were CD4-positive lymphocytes, which is consistent with the finding that HTLV-I predominantly immortalizes CD4-positive T lymphocytes in vitro.

The HTLV-I provirus is genetically stable, especially compared with the other major human retrovirus, human immunodeficiency virus (HIV). It has been postulated that increased HTLV-I load is achieved not by virus replication, but by clonal proliferation of infected cells. Since reverse transcriptase is an error-prone DNA polymerase, a higher replication rate generates the vast diversity in the virus genome. In HIV, a higher rate of mutation generated in the viral replication results in acquisition of drug resistance, and escape from the host immune system. On the other hand, HTLV-I increases its copies mainly by proliferation of HTLV-I–infected cells. In such situation, HTLV-I provirus in the host cells is replicated by cellular DNA polymerase with proofreading activity. Therefore, HTLV-I provirus is genetically stable in striking contrast to HIV-I. Such clonal expansion of HTLV-I–infected cells is directly associated with the onset of ATL (Fig. 29–3).

However, the reverse transcriptase (RT) inhibitor inhibits the replication of HTLV-I in vitro,[48] and in addition, in vivo administration of RT inhibitor also suppresses the provirus load.[49] This finding shows the possibility that HTLV-I replicates in vivo, although it remains unknown how much such replication can account for provirus load in vivo.

GENETIC FACTORS AFFECTING PROVIRUS LOAD AND SUSCEPTIBILITY TO HTLV-I–ASSOCIATED DISEASES

Cellular immunity, including MHC molecules, influences the provirus load in HTLV-I–infected individuals. In addition, other polymorphisms of genes might influence the provirus load. For example, although the higher provirus load is associated with the risk of HAM/TSP, polymorphism of the TNF gene (*TNF-863A*) increases susceptibility to the disease, whereas SDF-1 (*SDF-1 +801A* 3'UTR), and IL-15 (*IL-15 191C*) gene polymorphism are protective at onset.[50] Among these polymorphisms, *IL-15 191C* has been implicated in reducing the provirus load. Familial clustering of ATL patients has been reported, suggesting predisposing genetic factors. Polymorphism of tumor necrosis factor α (TNF-α) has been shown to be associated with ATL in comparison with asymptomatic carriers, suggesting that genetic polymorphism, which increases the production of TNF-α, is associated with susceptibility to ATL.[51] Such genetic analysis utilizing rapidly accumulating knowledge and developing technology will clarify the genetic basis of the familial clustering of ATL patients.

ADULT T-CELL LEUKEMIA/LYMPHOMA

Clinical Features of ATL

The onset of ATL is slightly more common in males (male-to-female ratio is 1.16:1). However, since female carriers are predominant in HTLV-I infection, the risk for developing ATL is three times higher for males. Average age at the onset of ATL is 60 years in Japan. On the other hand, the average age of Caribbean and African ATL patients is about 43 years, suggesting that the onset is influenced by genetic or environmental factors.[52]

The findings at onset are abdominal pain, diarrhea, pleural effusion, ascites, cough, sputum, and an abnormal shadow on chest x-ray films. Predominant physical findings are peripheral lymph node enlargement (72%), hepatomegaly (47%), splenomegaly (25%), and skin lesions (53%).[52] ATL cells tend to infiltrate into various organs/tissues, including skin, liver, lung, gastrointestinal tract, central nervous system, and bone. Various skin lesions, such as papules, erythema, and nodules are frequently observed in ATL patients (Fig. 29–4). In the skin, ATL cells densely infiltrate the dermis and epidermis, forming Pautrier's microabscesses in the epidermis (Fig. 29–5). In the bone, infiltration of ATL cells causes punched-out lesions (Fig. 29–6). Pulmonary complication is also frequently observed in patients with ATL, which includes leukemic infiltration (Fig. 29–7) and pulmonary infections. The high frequency of hypercalcemia is the most striking feature of ATL; about 70% of ATL patients have high serum Ca2+ levels during the clinical course of the disease, particularly during the aggressive stage of ATL. In the bone of ATL patients with hypercalcemia, the number of activated osteoclasts increase (Fig. 29–8).

White blood cell (WBC) count ranges from normal to 500×10^9/L. Blood involvement is frequently observed in patients with ATL, and leukemic cells in peripheral blood resemble Sézary cells, having indented or lobulated nuclei (Fig. 29–9). Since infiltration of ATL cells into bone marrow is usually not so dense, anemia and thrombocytopenia are rare. Eosinophilia is frequently observed in ATL patients, as well as other T-cell malignancies.

Serum lactate dehydrogenase (LDH) is elevated in most ATL patients, and higher LDH levels indicate an advanced or aggressive disease state. Thus, serum calcium and LDH levels reflect the extent of disease, and are useful for monitoring the remaining tumor or disease activity. Hyper-

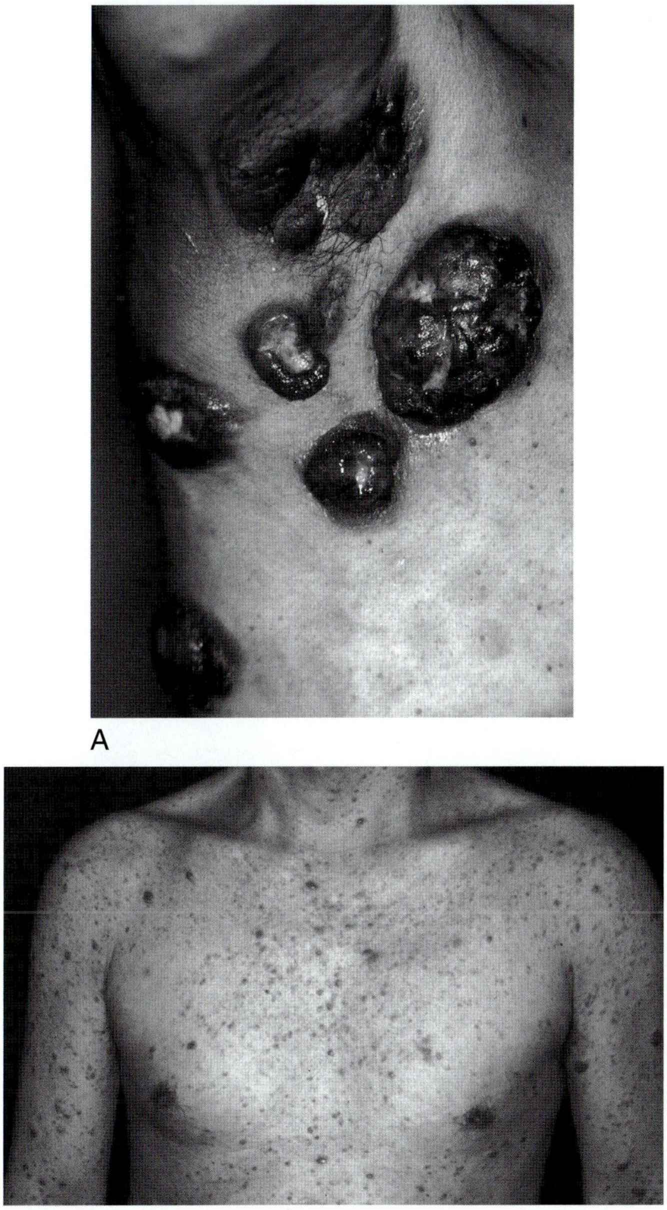

Figure 29–4. Skin lesions in ATL patients. Skin lesions observed in ATL patients are variable. Tumor formation is common among skin involvement in ATL patients (**A**). Papule is also observed in a patient with acute ATL (**B**). (See color insert.)

bilirubinemia, observed when ATL cells infiltrate the liver, indicates a poor prognosis. Hypergammaglobulinemia is very rare in ATL, which is consistent with the fact that ATL cells have suppressor-inducer activity to immunoglobulin synthesis in vitro. ATL cells are known to express interleukin 2 (IL-2) receptor alpha chain on their surfaces, and also secrete its soluble forms. Therefore, levels of SIL-2R are elevated in the sera of patients with ATL, the levels of SIL-2R being correlated with the tumor mass and clinical course.

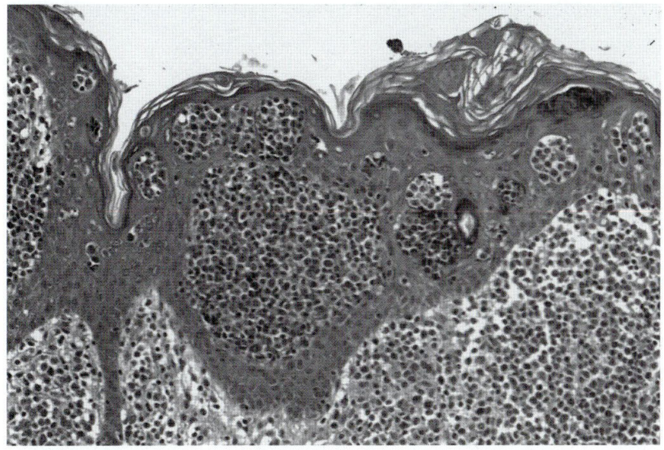

Figure 29–5. Skin involvement of ATL. ATL cells infiltrate into epidermis and form Pautrier's microabscesses. (See color insert.)

Pathogenesis of ATL

ATL is a neoplasm of activated helper T lymphocytes, which elaborate various cytokines, and express the immunoregulatory molecules on the surface. Such cytokines produced by ATL cells influence the pathophysiology of ATL. Eosinophilia is frequently observed in patients with ATL, which is caused by elevated IL-5. In addition, elaborated parathyroid hormone–related protein (PTH-rP) from ATL cells activates osteoclasts and promotes bone resorption, which is implicated in hypercalcemia. ATL cells produce

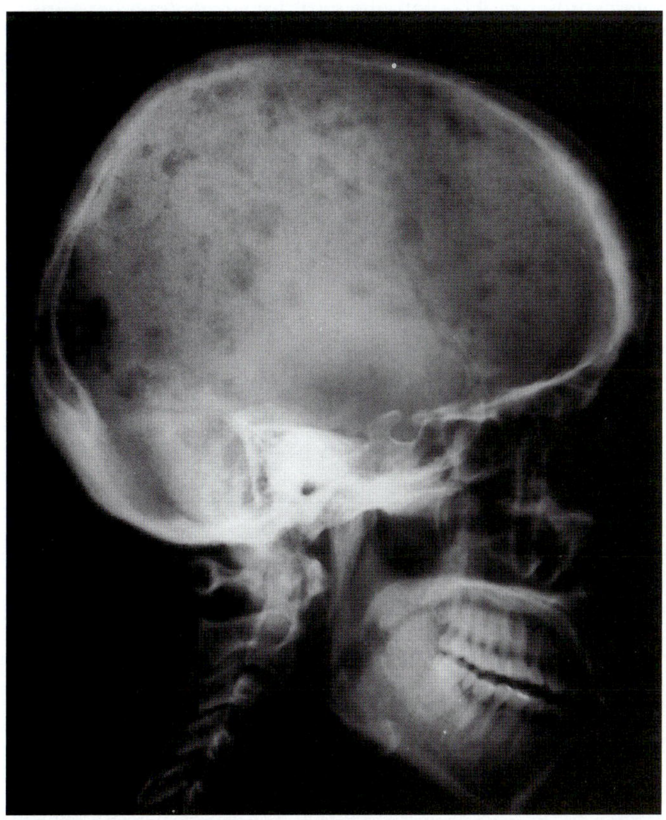

Figure 29–6. Punched-out lesions in the skull of an acute ATL patient.

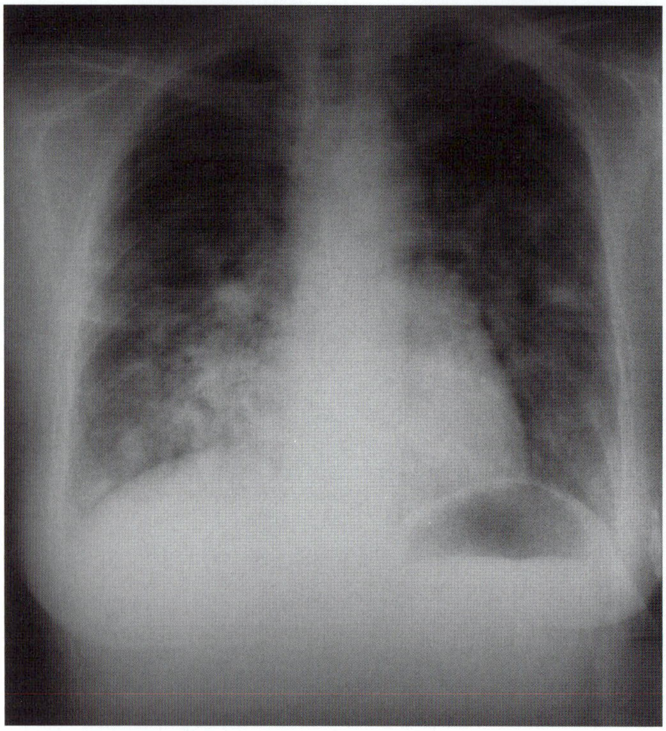

Figure 29–7. Pulmonary infiltration of ATL cells.

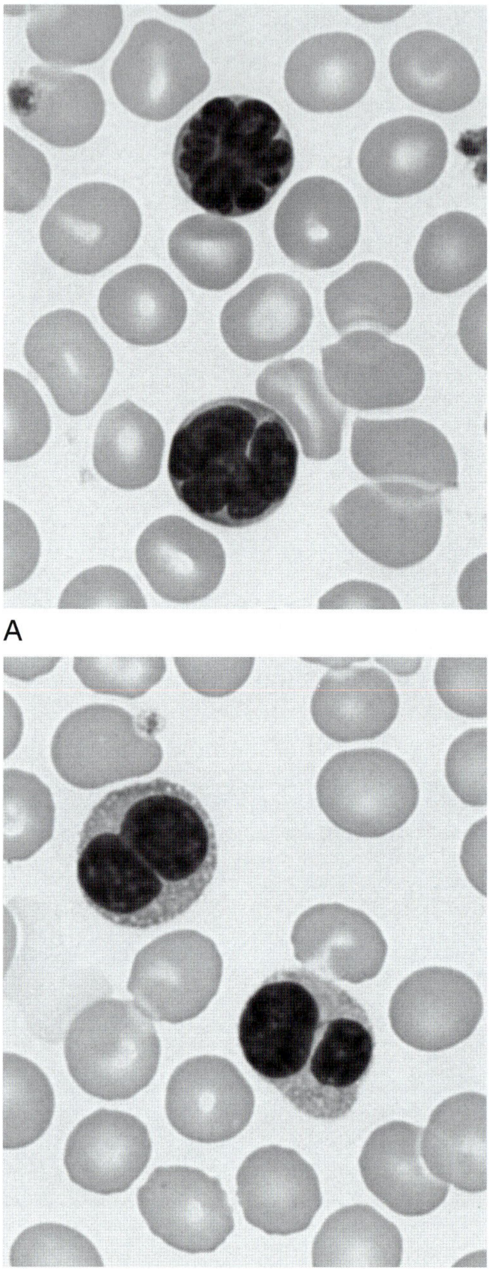

A

B

Figure 29–9. Cell morphology of ATL cells. ATL cells from an acute ATL (**A**) and a chronic ATL (**B**) are shown. (See color insert.)

other cytokines, including TGF-β, IL-10, IL-8, and M-CSF, which modify the pathogenesis of ATL.

Hypercalcemia is more severe in patients with ATL than those with other hematologic malignancies. Several pathologic studies of ATL patients with hypercalcemia have indicated that high serum Ca2+ levels are due to an increased number of osteoclasts and accelerated bone resorption (Fig. 29–8). Bone is constitutively remodeled by osteoblasts (matrix synthesis) and osteoclasts (bone resorption). Osteoclasts are derived from hematopoietic precursor cells and belong to the monocyte macrophage lineage. During differentiation of osteoclasts, precursor cells sequentially express c-Fms (receptor of M-CSF) followed by receptor activator nuclear factor κB (RANK).[53] M-CSF and RANK ligand (RANKL) have been shown to be critical factors for the differentiation of osteoclasts, which are physiologically produced by stromal cells and osteoblasts. ATL cells from patients with hypercalcemia, which highly expressed the transcripts of the RANKL gene, induced the differentiation of hematopoietic precursor cells into osteoclasts in vitro in the presence of M-CSF.[54] It showed that RANKL expressed on ATL cells induced the differentiation into osteoclasts, resulting in increased number of osteoclasts and hypercalcemia in cooperation with PTH-rP. Thus, the immunoregulatory molecules on the ATL cells modify the pathogenesis.

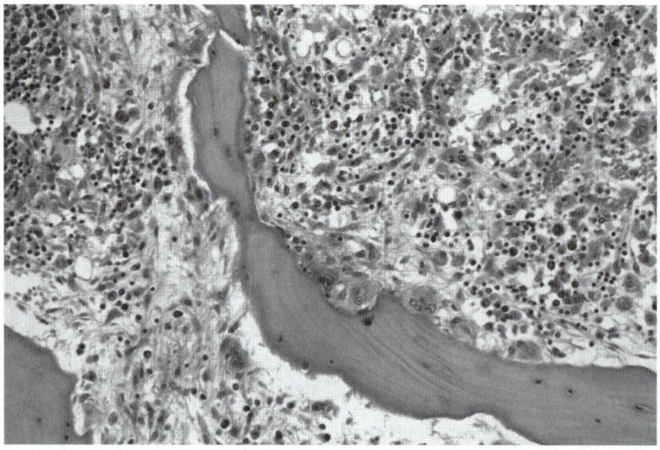

Figure 29–8. Increased osteoclasts in a hypercalcemic ATL patient. In a hypercalcemic patient, the number of osteoclast increased in the bone, which accelerated bone resorption. (See color insert.)

Chemokines and their receptors have been implicated in the migration and tissue localization of lymphocytes. ATL cells are well known to infiltrate into various organs or tissues, frequently invading skin or lymphoid tissues, which suggests that the differential expression of chemokine receptors might determine the migration of ATL cells. Analysis of chemokine receptor expression revealed that CCR4 was frequently expressed on HTLV-I–transformed cell lines and fresh ATL cells.[55] CCR4-positive T lymphocytes contain skin-seeking memory T cells, suggesting that expression of CCR4 accounts for frequent infiltration of ATL cells into skin. On the other hand, expression of CCR7 was reported to be associated with involvement of lymphoid tissues and lymph node enlargement.[56]

Diagnosis of ATL

The diagnostic criteria for ATL have been defined as follows: (1) histologically and/or cytologically proven lymphoid malignancy with T-cell surface antigens; and (2) abnormal T lymphocytes present in the peripheral blood except for the lymphoma-type. These abnormal T lymphocytes include not only typical ATL cells, the so-called flower cells, but also the small and mature T lymphocytes with incised or lobulated nuclei that are characteristic of the chronic or smoldering type. Additional criteria follow: (3) antibody to HTLV-I present in the sera at diagnosis; and (4) demonstration of monoclonal integration of HTLV-I provirus by the Southern blot method.

Morphology of ATL Cells

Most ATL cells characteristically exhibit lobular division of their nuclei; most are bi- or multi-foliate, and are separated by deep indentations. Cells with such a nuclear configuration are designated as "flower cells" (Fig. 29–9A). Cells from chronic ATL are relatively uniform in size and nuclear configuration, and smaller than those seen in either acute or smoldering ATL (Fig. 29–9B). Cells in this type also exhibit lobular division of their nuclei. However, most of the lobulated nuclei are bi- or tri-foliate. Cells from the smoldering type are relatively large and lack cytoplasmic granules or vacuoles. The nuclear chromatin is in coarse strands and is deeply stained.

Serology of HTLV-I

Anti-HTLV-I antibodies are positive in almost all patients with ATL, although seronegative ATL cases have been rarely reported.[52] The presence of serum antibodies against HTLV-I can be demonstrated by enzyme-linked immunosorbence, gelatin particle hemagglutination, indirect immunofluorescence, and the Western blot method.

Immunologic Characterization of ATL Cells

Surface phenotype of typical ATL cells is positive for CD2, 3, 4, 25, and HLA-DR, and is negative for CD7 and 8, indicating that ATL cells are derived from activated helper T lymphocytes. A characteristic feature of ATL cells is the decreased expression of T-cell receptor (TCR)/CD3 complex on their surfaces. There are several reports of ATL cases with different leukemic cell phenotypes, such as CD4+ and CD8+, CD4– and CD8–, and CD4– and CD8+.[29] Most of these variant forms are observed in patients with acute ATL and indicate poor prognosis. CD95 (Fas/APO-1) antigen is highly expressed on the leukemic cells in most patients with ATL, and such ATL cells are highly susceptible to antibody against Fas antigen. On the other hand, Fas-negative ATL cases were also reported and underlying mutations of the Fas gene were identified.[52]

HTLV-I Provirus Genome in Leukemic Cells of ATL

Definitive diagnosis of ATL requires detection of monoclonal integration of HTLV-I provirus in genomic DNA from tumor cells, especially in endemic areas. Monoclonal integration of HTLV-I provirus can be detected by the Southern blot method.

Tax plays a critical role in the proliferation of HTLV-I–infected cells and leukemogenesis. However, it is a major target of cytotoxic T cells. Thus, the presence of Tax in HTLV-I–infected cells provides advantages and disadvantages for survival of HTLV-I–infected cells. Since Tax expression is not frequently detected in ATL cells,[58] they presumably acquire the ability to proliferate independent of Tax function during the leukemogenesis. ATL cells frequently lose Tax expression by several mechanisms. Although the 5′-LTR is a viral promoter for transcription of viral genes, it was reported that 5′-LTR of HTLV-I provirus was deleted in 39% of cases examined, indicating that the viral gene transcription was impaired in ATL cells with such a provirus.[59] The second mechanism is the nonsense or missense mutation of the *tax* gene in fresh ATL cells. It is noteworthy that ATL cells in some cases had mutations in the Class I MHC recognition site of the Tax protein, resulting in escape from immune recognition.[60] The third mechanism is epigenetic change of the 5′-LTR: the 5′-LTR was selectively methylated, which silenced the transcription of viral genes.[58,61] With these mechanisms, ATL cells lost Tax expression, and could escape from the host immune surveillance system. It is speculated that Tax plays an important role in persistent proliferation of HTLV-I–infected cells during the carrier state, and then genetic and epigenetic changes accumulate in the host genome mediated by mutator phenotype of Tax,[62] which finally leads to Tax-independent proliferation and escape from the host immune system by inactivation of the *tax* gene.[4]

Chromosomal Abnormalities of ATL Cells

Karyotype analyses of 107 patients with ATL revealed several chromosomal abnormalities[63]: trisomies of chromosome 3 (21%), 7 (10%), and 21 (9%); monosomy of the X chromosome (38%) in females; loss of a Y chromosome (17%) in males; structural abnormalities, including translocations involving 14q32 (28%) or 14q11 (14%), and deletion of 6q (23%). Although there is no specific chromosomal abnormality for ATL, chromosomal abnormalities accumulate during disease progression. Comparative genomic hybridization (CGH) analyses of ATL revealed gains at chromosome 14q, 7q, and 3p. Genomic alterations increase in aggressive ATL compared with indolent forms (chronic and smoldering), which indicate the marked chromosomal instability in ATL cells.[64]

Classification of ATL

Clinical features of ATL vary among patients. Therefore, ATL patients can be classified into four clinical subtypes according to the clinical features: acute, chronic, smoldering, and lymphoma type. The Lymphoma Study Group (1984–1987) in Japan proposed the following diagnostic criteria for classifying ATL into the following four subtypes[65]:

1. *Smoldering type.* Five percent or more abnormal lymphocytes of T-cell nature in peripheral blood (PB); normal lymphocyte level (<4×10⁹/L); no hypercalcemia; LDH value of up to 1.5 times the normal upper limit; no lymphadenopathy; no involvement of liver, spleen, central nervous system (CNS), bone, or gastrointestinal tract; and neither ascites nor pleural effusion. Skin and pulmonary lesion(s) may be present. In patients with less than 5% abnormal T lymphocytes in PB, at least one histologically proven skin or pulmonary lesion should be present.
2. *Chronic type.* Absolute lymphocytosis of more than 3.5×10⁹/L; LDH value up to twice the normal upper limit; no hypercalcemia; no involvement of CNS, bone, or gastrointestinal tract; and neither ascites nor pleural effusion. There may be histologically proven lymphadenopathy with or without extranodal lesions, and there may be involvement of liver, spleen, skin, and lung, and 5% or more abnormal lymphocytes.
3. *Lymphoma type.* No lymphocytosis, 1% or less abnormal lymphocytes; histologically proven lymphadenopathy with or without extranodal lesions.
4. *Acute type.* The most common subtype, highly aggressive malignancy that shows lymphadenopathy, hepatosplenomegaly, and skin lesions, but does not meet the criteria of the other types.

Treatment and Prevention of ATL

Aggressive forms of ATL (acute and lymphoma-type) are generally treated with combination chemotherapy, although long-term success has been very limited. The acute form, with hypercalcemia, high LDH levels, and an elevated white blood cell count, carries a particularly poor prognosis. Sequential trials in Japan have resulted in the complete remission rate being increased from 16% with a four-drug combination to 43% with eight drugs.[66] In the recent study by Lymphoma Study Group in Japan, the improved survival of ATL patients has been reported by a granulocyte colony–stimulating factor–supported multiagent chemotherapy protocol. Although the median survival remains 13 months in this study, the estimated 2-year survival was 31.3%.[67] In contrast, smoldering ATL, or some cases of chronic ATL, may have a more protracted natural course, which may be compromised by aggressive chemotherapy. Alternative strategies for both acute and chronic forms are clearly needed.

The major obstacles in the treatment of patients with ATL include drug resistance and development of opportunistic infections caused by various organisms, such as *Pneumocystis jiroveci*, cytomegalovirus, *Strongyloidiasis*, and a variety of fungi, indicating that cell-mediated immunity is severely impaired in these patients.[52] The prophylactic measures should be taken for patients with ATL. The mechanism of drug resistance in ATL cells has been studied. One mechanism is that ATL cells show elevated NF-κB activity, which induces antiapoptotic genes such as *bcl-xL* and *inhibitor of apoptosis protein*.[9] To overwhelm the drug resistance mediated by NF-κB, the proteasome inhibitor, PS-341, is a candidate for treatment.[68,69]

Although the frequency of opportunistic infections is much higher in patients with ATL than in those with other hematologic malignancies, the underlying mechanism(s) remained unsolved. Opportunistic malignancies, Kaposi's sarcoma,[70] and Epstein–Barr virus (EBV)–associated lymphoma[71] have also been reported in patients with ATL, which also indicates a state of immunodeficiency in these patients.

α-Interferon (α-IFN) combined with azidothymidine (AZT) was administered to 19 patients with ATL, and major responses (complete plus partial remissions) were achieved in 58% of the patients (11 of 19), including complete remission in 26% (5 of 19).[72] The mechanism of this combination therapy remains unknown since these drugs have no effect in vitro. In primary effusion lymphoma (PEL), α-IFN induced the expression of tumor necrosis factor–related apoptosis-inducing ligand and AZT suppressed NF-κB activity.[73] Both effects are considered to synergistically induce the apoptosis of PEL cells. Humanized monoclonal antibody against IL-2 receptor was also used for patients with ATL,[74] although its effect was limited.

Allogeneic stem cell transplantation (allo-SCT) for patients with ATL has been reported.[75] Median leukemia-free survival after allo-SCT was more than 17.5 months. Since autologous transplantation has been shown to be ineffective for ATL, graft versus leukemia should play an important role in anti-ATL effect. In this regard, it is noteworthy that two patients without graft-versus-host disease relapsed with ATL. The immune response by cytotoxic T lymphocytes against Tax protein has been augmented after BMT, indicating that such anti-Tax cytotoxic T cells exert an antitumor effect on ATL cells.[76]

It is obvious that the reduced transmission of HTLV-I directly leads to prevention of ATL. Since the breast feeding is thought to be major route of vertical transmission, bottle feeding is recommended for seropositive mothers instead of breastfeeding in Japan. About 18% of infants have been seroconverted by breast feeding from seropositive mothers. Refraining from breastfeeding could reduce the seroconversion rate to about 3%.[77] The transmission route of HTLV in seroconverted children in spite of complete bottle feeding remains unknown, although intrapartum transmission is suspected.

For HTLV-I transmission by blood transfusion, all donated blood at blood centers were subjected to HTLV-I antibody testing beginning in November 1986 in Japan. After this, none of the recipients, even patients with hematologic disorders who received multiple transfusions, were seroconverted. In Japan, absolute decline of the carrier rate among the young generation was observed, possibly due to complete achieving of blood donor screening, and success in preventing most maternal transmission by refraining from breastfeeding.

In HIV-1, the prophylactic administration of antiviral drugs to individuals who had accidental exposure to infected blood can reduce the transmission. Since nucleoside reverse transcriptase inhibitors such as azidothymidine can block the replication of HTLV-I,[48] prophylactic administration should be considered after accidental exposure to blood of HTLV-I–infected individuals.

HTLV-I–RELATED DISORDERS

HTLV-I is the causative virus of not only ATL, but also other inflammatory diseases, such as HTLV-I–associated myelopathy/tropical spastic paraparesis (HAM/TSP), chronic lung diseases, infective dermatitis, arthropathy, and uveitis. In patients with HAM/TSP and HTLV-I uveitis, an increased number of HTLV-I–infected cells has been reported, suggesting that inflammatory reactions, which include excessive production of cytokines and increased expression of adhesion molecules in HTLV-I–infected cells, and host immune response against infected cells, play a critical roles in the pathogenesis of these diseases.

References

1. Takatsuki K, Uchiyama T, Sagawa K, et al. Adult T cell leukemia in Japan. In: Seno S, Takaku F and Irino S, eds. Topics in Hematology. The 16th International Congress of Hematology. Amsterdam: Excerpta Medica, 1977:73–7.
2. Poiesz BJ, Ruscetti FW, Gazdar AF, et al. Detection and isolation of type C retrovirus particles from fresh and cultured lymphocytes of a patient with cutaneous T-cell lymphoma. Proc Natl Acad Sci U S A 1980;77:7415–9.
3. Hinuma Y, Nagata K, Hanaoka M, et al. Adult T-cell leukemia: antigen in an ATL cell line and detection of antibodies to the antigen in human sera. Proc Natl Acad Sci U S A 1981; 78:6476–80.
4. Matsuoka M. Human T-cell leukemia virus type I and adult T-cell leukemia. Oncogene 2003;22:5131–40.
5. Seiki M, Hattori S, Hirayama Y, et al. Human adult T-cell leukemia virus: complete nucleotide sequence of the provirus genome integrated in leukemia cell DNA. Proc Natl Acad Sci U S A 1983;80:3618–22.
6. Yoshida M. Multiple viral strategies of htlv-1 for dysregulation of cell growth control. Annu Rev Immunol 2001;19:475–96.
7. Jeang KT. Functional activities of the human T-cell leukemia virus type I Tax oncoprotein: cellular signaling through NF-kappa B. Cytokine Growth Factor Rev 2001;12:207–17.
8. Yamaoka S, Inoue H, Sakurai M, et al. Constitutive activation of NF-kappa B is essential for transformation of rat fibroblasts by the human T-cell leukemia virus type I Tax protein. EMBO J 1996;15:873–87.
9. Tsukahara T, Kannagi M, Ohashi T, et al. Induction of Bcl-x(L) expression by human T-cell leukemia virus type 1 Tax through NF-kappaB in apoptosis-resistant T-cell transfectants with Tax. J Virol 1999;73:7981–7.
10. Nicot C, Mahieux R, Takemoto S, et al. Bcl-X(L) is up-regulated by HTLV-I and HTLV-II in vitro and in ex vivo ATLL samples. Blood 2000;96:275–81.
11. Zhao LJ, Giam CZ. Human T-cell lymphotropic virus type I (HTLV-I) transcriptional activator, Tax, enhances CREB binding to HTLV-I 21-base-pair repeats by protein–protein interaction. Proc Natl Acad Sci U S A 1992;89:7070–4.
12. Kwok RP, Laurance ME, Lundblad JR, et al. Control of cAMP-regulated enhancers by the viral transactivator Tax through CREB and the co-activator CBP. Nature 1996;380:642–6.
13. Suzuki T, Uchida-Toita M, Yoshida M. Tax protein of HTLV-1 inhibits CBP/p300-mediated transcription by interfering with recruitment of CBP/p300 onto DNA element of E-box or p53 binding site. Oncogene 1999;18:4137–43.
14. Suzuki T, Kitao S, Matsushime H, et al. HTLV-1 Tax protein interacts with cyclin-dependent kinase inhibitor p16INK4A and counteracts its inhibitory activity towards CDK4. EMBO J 1996;15:1607–14.
15. Mori N, Morishita M, Tsukazaki T, et al. Human T-cell leukemia virus type I oncoprotein Tax represses Smad-dependent transforming growth factor beta signaling through interaction with CREB-binding protein/p300. Blood 2001;97: 2137–44.
16. Lee DK, Kim BC, Brady JN, et al. Human T-cell lymphotropic virus Type 1 Tax inhibits transforming growth factor-beta signaling by blocking the association of smad proteins with smad-binding element. J Biol Chem 2002;277:33766–75.
17. Jin DY, Spencer F, Jeang KT. Human T cell leukemia virus type 1 oncoprotein Tax targets the human mitotic checkpoint protein MAD1. Cell 1998;93:81–91.
18. Nicot C, Dundr M, Johnson JM, et al. HTLV-1-encoded p30(II) is a post-transcriptional negative regulator of viral replication. Nat Med 2004;10:197–201.
19. Basbous J, Arpin C, Gaudray G, et al. The HBZ factor of human T-cell leukemia virus type I dimerizes with transcription factors JunB and c-Jun and modulates their transcriptional activity. J Biol Chem 2003;278:43620–7.
20. Collins ND, Newbound GC, Albrecht B, et al. Selective ablation of human T-cell lymphotropic virus type 1 p12I reduces viral infectivity in vivo. Blood 1998;91:4701–7.
21. Albrecht B, Collins ND, Burniston MT, et al. Human T-lymphotropic virus type 1 open reading frame I p12(I) is required for efficient viral infectivity in primary lymphocytes. J Virol 2000;74:9828–35.
22. Ding W, Albrecht B, Kelley RE, et al. Human T-cell lymphotropic virus type 1 p12(I) expression increases cytoplasmic calcium to enhance the activation of nuclear factor of activated T cells. J Virol 2002;76:10374–82.
23. Pique C, Ureta-Vidal A, Gessain A, et al. Evidence for the chronic in vivo production of human T cell leukemia virus type I Rof and Tof proteins from cytotoxic T lymphocytes directed against viral peptides. J Exp Med 2000;191: 567–72.
24. D'Agostino DM, Ranzato L, Arrigoni G, et al. Mitochondrial alterations induced by the p13II protein of human T-cell leukemia virus type 1. Critical role of arginine residues. J Biol Chem 2002;277:34424–33.
25. Silic-Benussi M, Cavallari I, Zorzan T, et al. Suppression of tumor growth and cell proliferation by p13II, a mitochondrial protein of human T cell leukemia virus type 1. Proc Natl Acad Sci U S A 2004;101(17):6629–34.
26. Blattner WA, Gallo RC. Epidemiology of HTLV-I and HTLV-II infection. In: Takahashi K, ed. Adult T-Cell Leukemia. New York: Oxford University Press, 1994:45–90.
27. Tajima K, Inoue M, Takezaki T, et al. Ethnoepidemiology of ATL in Japan with special reference to the Mongoloid dispersal. In Takatsuki K, ed. Adult T-Cell Leukemia. New York: Oxford University Press, 1994:91–112.
28. Arisawa K, Soda M, Endo S, et al. Evaluation of adult T-cell leukemia/lymphoma incidence and its impact on non-Hodgkin lymphoma incidence in southwestern Japan. Int J Cancer 2000;85:319–24.
29. Okochi K, Sato H, Hinuma Y. A retrospective study on transmission of adult T cell leukemia virus by blood transfusion: seroconversion in recipients. Vox Sang 1984;46:245–53.
30. Derse D, Hill SA, Lloyd PA, et al. Examining human T-lymphotropic virus type 1 infection and replication by cell-free infection with recombinant virus vectors. J Virol 2001;75: 8461–8.
31. Igakura T, Stinchcombe JC, Goon PK, et al. Spread of HTLV-I between lymphocytes by virus-induced polarization of the cytoskeleton. Science 2003;299:1713–6.

32. Manel N, Kim FJ, Kinet S, et al. The ubiquitous glucose transporter GLUT-1 is a receptor for HTLV. Cell 2003;115:449–59.
33. Yasunaga J, Sakai T, Nosaka K, et al. Impaired production of naive T lymphocytes in human T-cell leukemia virus type I-infected individuals: its implications in the immunodeficient state. Blood 2001;97:3177–83.
34. Akagi T, Ono H, Shimotohno K. Characterization of T cells immortalized by Tax1 of human T-cell leukemia virus type 1. Blood 1995;86:4243–9.
35. Jacobson S, Shida H, McFarlin DE, et al. Circulating CD8+ cytotoxic T lymphocytes specific for HTLV-I pX in patients with HTLV-I associated neurological disease. Nature 1990; 348:245–8.
36. Hanon E, Hall S, Taylor GP, et al. Abundant tax protein expression in CD4+ T cells infected with human T- cell lymphotropic virus type I (HTLV-I) is prevented by cytotoxic T lymphocytes. Blood 2000;95:1386–92.
37. Hisada M, Okayama A, Shioiri S, et al. Risk factors for adult T-cell leukemia among carriers of human T-lymphotropic virus type I. Blood 1998;92:3557–61.
38. Etoh K, Yamaguchi K, Tokudome S, et al. Rapid quantification of HTLV-I provirus load: detection of monoclonal proliferation of HTLV-I-infected cells among blood donors. Int J Cancer 1999;81:859–64.
39. Arisawa K, Katamine S, Kamihira S, et al. A nested case-control study of risk factors for adult T-cell leukemia/lymphoma among human T-cell lymphotropic virus type-I carriers in Japan. Cancer Causes Control 2002;13:657–63.
40. Hanabuchi S, Ohashi T, Koya Y, et al. Regression of human T-cell leukemia virus type I (HTLV-I)-associated lymphomas in a rat model: peptide-induced T-cell immunity. J Natl Cancer Inst 2001;93:1775–83.
41. Hoshida Y, Li T, Dong Z, et al. Lymphoproliferative disorders in renal transplant patients in Japan. Int J Cancer 2001;91: 869–75.
42. Hanon E, Stinchcombe JC, Saito M, et al. Fratricide among CD8(+) T lymphocytes naturally infected with human T cell lymphotropic virus type I. Immunity 2000;13:657–64.
43. Iga M, Okayama A, Stuver S, et al. Genetic evidence of transmission of human T cell lymphotropic virus type 1 between spouses. J Infect Dis 2002;185:691–5.
44. Wodarz D, Hall SE, Usuku K, et al. Cytotoxic T-cell abundance and virus load in human immunodeficiency virus type 1 and human T-cell leukaemia virus type 1. Proc R Soc Lond B Biol Sci 2001;268:1215–21.
45. Seiki M, Eddy R, Shows TB, et al. Nonspecific integration of the HTLV provirus genome into adult T-cell leukaemia cells. Nature 1984;309:640–2.
46. Etoh K, Tamiya S, Yamaguchi K, et al. Persistent clonal proliferation of human T-lymphotropic virus type I–infected cells in vivo. Cancer Res 1997;57:4862–7.
47. Cavrois M, Leclercq I, Gout O, et al. Persistent oligoclonal expansion of human T-cell leukemia virus type 1-infected circulating cells in patients with tropical spastic paraparesis/HTLV-1 associated myelopathy. Oncogene 1998; 17:77–82.
48. Hill SA, Lloyd PA, McDonald S, et al. Susceptibility of human T cell leukemia virus type I to nucleoside reverse transcriptase inhibitors. J Infect Dis 2003;188:424–7.
49. Taylor GP, Hall SE, Navarrete S, et al. Effect of lamivudine on human T-cell leukemia virus type 1 (HTLV-1) DNA copy number, T-cell phenotype, and anti-tax cytotoxic T-cell frequency in patients with HTLV-1–associated myelopathy. J Virol 1999;73:10289–95.
50. Vine AM, Witkover AD, Lloyd AL, et al. Polygenic control of human T lymphotropic virus type I (HTLV-I) provirus load and the risk of HTLV-I-associated myelopathy/tropical spastic paraparesis. J Infect Dis 2002;186:932–9.
51. Tsukasaki K, Miller CW, Kubota T, et al. Tumor necrosis factor alpha polymorphism associated with increased susceptibility to development of adult T-cell leukemia/lymphoma in human T-lymphotropic virus type 1 carriers. Cancer Res 2001;61: 3770–4.
52. Matsuoka M, Takatsuki K. Adult T-cell leukemia. In: Henderson ES, Lister TA, Greaves MF, eds. Leukemia, 7th ed. Philadelphia: Saunders, 2002:705–12.
53. Arai F, Miyamoto T, Ohneda O, et al. Commitment and differentiation of osteoclast precursor cells by the sequential expression of c-Fms and receptor activator of nuclear factor kappaB (RANK) receptors. J Exp Med 1999;190:1741–54.
54. Nosaka K, Miyamoto T, Sakai T, et al. Mechanism of hypercalcemia in adult T-cell leukemia: overexpression of receptor activator of nuclear factor kappaB ligand on adult T-cell leukemia cells. Blood 2002;99:634–40.
55. Yoshie O, Fujisawa R, Nakayama T, et al. Frequent expression of CCR4 in adult T-cell leukemia and human T-cell leukemia virus type 1–transformed T cells. Blood 2002;99: 1505–11.
56. Hasegawa H, Nomura T, Kohno M, et al. Increased chemokine receptor CCR7/EBI1 expression enhances the infiltration of lymphoid organs by adult T-cell leukemia cells. Blood 2000; 95:30–8.
57. Tamiya S, Etoh K, Suzushima H, et al. Mutation of CD95 (Fas/Apo-1) gene in adult T-cell leukemia cells. Blood 1998;91:3935–42.
58. Takeda S, Maeda M, Morikawa S, et al. Genetic and epigenetic inactivation of tax gene in adult T-cell leukemia cells. Int J Cancer 2004;109:559–67.
59. Tamiya S, Matsuoka M, Etoh K, et al. Two types of defective human T-lymphotropic virus type I provirus in adult T-cell leukemia. Blood 1996;88:3065–73.
60. Furukawa Y, Kubota R, Tara M, et al. Existence of escape mutant in HTLV-I tax during the development of adult T-cell leukemia. Blood 2001;97:987–93.
61. Koiwa T, Hamano-Usami A, Ishida T, et al. 5'-long terminal repeat-selective CpG methylation of latent human T-cell leukemia virus type 1 provirus in vitro and in vivo. J Virol 2002;76:9389–97.
62. Kibler KV, Jeang KT. Taxing the cellular capacity for repair: human T-cell leukemia virus type 1, DNA damage, and adult T-cell leukemia. J Natl Cancer Inst 1999;91:903–4.
63. Kamada N, Sakurai M, Miyamoto K, et al. Chromosome abnormalities in adult T-cell leukemia/lymphoma: a karyotype review committee report. Cancer Res 1992;52:1481–93.
64. Tsukasaki K, Krebs J, Nagai K, et al. Comparative genomic hybridization analysis in adult T-cell leukemia/lymphoma: correlation with clinical course. Blood 2001;97:3875–81.
65. Shimoyama M. Diagnostic criteria and classification of clinical subtypes of adult T-cell leukaemia-lymphoma. A report from the Lymphoma Study Group (1984–87). Br J Haematol 1991;79:428–37.
66. Shimoyama M. Chemotherapy of ATL. In: Takatsuki K, ed. Adult T-Cell Leukemia. New York: Oxford University Press, 1994:221–37.
67. Yamada Y, Tomonaga M, Fukuda H, et al. A new G-CSF-supported combination chemotherapy, LSG15, for adult T-cell leukaemia-lymphoma: Japan Clinical Oncology Group Study 9303. Br J Haematol 2001;113:375–82.
68. Mitra-Kaushik S, Harding JC, Hess J, et al. Effects of the proteasome inhibitor PS-341 on tumor growth in HTLV-1 Tax transgenic mice and Tax tumor transplants. Blood 2004; 104(3):802–9.
69. Satou Y, Nosaka K, Koya Y, et al. Proteasome inhibitor, bortezomib, potently inhibits the growth of adult T-cell leukemia cells both in vivo and in vitro. Leukemia 2004;18(8):1357–63.

70. Greenberg SJ, Jaffe ES, Ehrlich GD, et al. Kaposi's sarcoma in human T-cell leukemia virus type I–associated adult T-cell leukemia. Blood 1990;76:971–6.
71. Tobinai K, Ohtsu T, Hayashi M, et al. Epstein–Barr virus (EBV) genome carrying monoclonal B-cell lymphoma in a patient with adult T-cell leukemia-lymphoma. Leuk Res 1991;15:837–46.
72. Gill PS, Harrington W Jr, Kaplan MH, et al. Treatment of adult T-cell leukemia-lymphoma with a combination of interferon alfa and zidovudine. N Engl J Med 1995;332:1744–8.
73. Ghosh SK, Wood C, Boise LH, et al. Potentiation of TRAIL-induced apoptosis in primary effusion lymphoma through azidothymidine-mediated inhibition of NF-kappa B. Blood 2003;101:2321–7.
74. Waldmann TA, White JD, Carrasquillo JA, et al. Radioimmunotherapy of interleukin–2R alpha-expressing adult T-cell leukemia with Yttrium-90–labeled anti-Tac. Blood 1995; 86:4063–75.
75. Utsunomiya A, Miyazaki Y, Takatsuka Y, et al. Improved outcome of adult T cell leukemia/lymphoma with allogeneic hematopoietic stem cell transplantation. Bone Marrow Transplant 2001;27:15–20.
76. Harashima N, Kurihara K, Utsunomiya A, et al. Graft-versus-Tax response in adult T-cell leukemia patients after hematopoietic stem cell transplantation. Cancer Res 2004;64: 391–9.
77. Hino S. Primary prevention of ATL. In Sugamura K, Uchiyama T, Matsuoka M, Kannagi M, eds. Two Decades of Adult T-Cell Leukemia and HTLV-I Research. Tokyo: Japan Scientific Societies Press, 2003:241–51.

30

Hodgkin's Lymphoma: Diagnosis and Treatment

30A Diagnosis

Jonathan W. Friedberg, M.D.

Classical Hodgkin's lymphoma is a lymphoproliferative disorder that is defined histologically by characteristic Reed–Sternberg cells. A hallmark of this neoplasm is a paucity of malignant cells surrounded by abundant "bystander" cells. Age-specific incidence rates suggest a bimodal distribution, with one peak between ages 15 and 34, and a second peak older than age 50. Like non-Hodgkin's lymphomas, the incidence of Hodgkin's lymphoma is increasing, due only in part to association with HIV. There are several patterns of presentation, but the disease generally involves lymph nodes, is unicentric in origin, progresses in a predictable manner, and is fatal without therapy.

The etiology of Hodgkin's lymphoma is unknown; however, epidemiologic studies, including case clustering, familial associations, and relationship to infectious mononucleosis, support a viral pathogenesis.[1–3] Molecular studies have determined that diagnostic Reed–Sternberg cells are clonal populations of transformed germinal-center B cells with disabling V gene mutations. These cells contain Epstein–Barr virus (EBV) DNA in a subset of patients,[4,5] and, when present, have been shown to be monoclonal in origin, suggesting that defective immune control of EBV-infected cells may contribute to Hodgkin's lymphoma in a subset of patients.[6]

Although the majority of patients with Hodgkin's lymphoma are cured, significant limitations to therapy remain.[7] Treatment-related morbidity, including a rising incidence of secondary malignancies, mandates improved staging and minimization of toxic therapy as important future goals for patients with a favorable prognosis. Alternatively, patients with advanced-stage disease, who relapse early after standard therapy, who achieve only a partial initial remission or present with clinically high-risk features, represent a poor prognostic group. Even with aggressive approaches, the long-term cure of these patients is less than 50%.

DISEASE PRESENTATION

The vast majority of patients with classical Hodgkin's lymphoma present with painless enlargement of a superficial lymph node.[8] In about 75% of cases, the first node appreciated is in the neck, more often on the left side than the right side. Axillary nodes are involved approximately 25% of the time, and inguinal and iliac adenopathy occurs approximately 10% of the time, at disease presentation.[9] The enlarged nodes may wax and wane in size over time, and are almost always nontender. Pain in an involved nodal site may occur a few minutes after ingestion of alcohol.[10] Although this symptom is uncommon, alcohol-induced pain in lymph nodes is rarely caused by conditions other than Hodgkin's lymphoma.

Approximately one-third of Hodgkin's lymphoma patients have systemic symptoms (B symptoms: fever, weight loss, night sweats) at time of diagnosis. Fever is present in about 25% of patients at diagnosis, and is most often low grade, occurring in the afternoon and evening. "Pel-Ebstein" fevers, which are pathognomonic of Hodgkin's lymphoma and recur at variable intervals of days to weeks, are not common.[11]

Pruritus is commonly seen in patients with Hodgkin's lymphoma, and may be the initial symptom that patients experience, often predating symptomatic lymphadenopathy by several months.[12] The pruritus is usually diffuse, and refractory to topical therapy and antihistamines. Empiric systemic steroids may transiently improve the condition, often contributing to a delay in the appearance of lymphadenopathy, and definitive diagnosis.

Patients who present without peripheral lymphadenopathy usually have symptomatic mediastinal involvement (cough, fatigue, or dyspnea), or an asymptomatic mass on a chest x-ray examination. Splenomegaly may be present at the time of diagnosis, but is rarely symptomatic and the only site of disease. Unlike the non-Hodgkin's lymphomas, Hodgkin's lymphoma is rarely of extranodal origin and usually does not compress vascular structures or the trachea at initial presentation.

Subdiaphragmatic presentations of Hodgkin's lymphoma are uncommon. In a study of 719 patients with biopsy-proven Hodgkin's lymphoma, 27% had splenic involvement on pathologic staging.[13] Only 14% had upper abdominal nodal involvement, and 11% had lower abdominal nodal involvement. Inguinal and femoral involvement is even less common at presentation. When present, retroperitoneal lymphadenopathy may contribute to back discomfort, abdominal swelling, or even ureteral obstruction.

Again, unlike many of the non-Hodgkin's lymphomas, contiguous spread of disease is commonly seen in Hodgkin's lymphoma, and accounts for many of the localized presentations of early Hodgkin's lymphoma above the diaphragm. Such contiguous spread occurs in a highly predictable manner;[14] for example, the presence of lymphatic channels connecting the lymph nodes of the lower neck with those of the mediastinum explains the frequent simultaneous

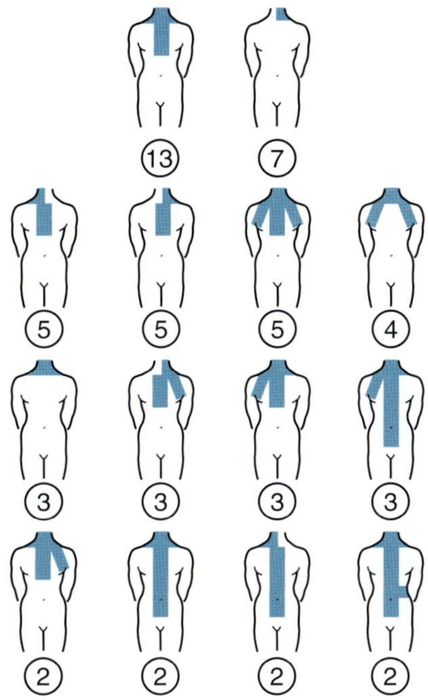

Figure 30–1. Most common anatomic patterns of Hodgkin's disease in 100 consecutive patients who underwent staging laparotomy. The *circled numbers* are the numbers of patients. (From Rosenberg SA and Kaplan HS. Evidence of an orderly progression in the spread of Hodgkin's disease. Cancer Res 1996;26:1255, with permission.)

Table 30–1. Involved Sites of Disease in Pathologically Staged Patients with Hodgkin's Lymphoma

Sites Involved >10% of the Time	% Involved
Cervical	
Left	60–70
Right	50–60
Axilla	
Left	30–35
Right	25–35
Mediastinum	50–60
Hilar nodes	15–35
Spleen	30–35
Para-aortic nodes	30–40
Iliac nodes	15–20
Sites Involved <10% of the Time	
Waldeyer's ring	
Liver	
Mesenteric nodes	
Bone marrow	
Other extranodal sites	

Adapted from Gupta RK, Gospodarowicz MK, and Lister TA. Clinical evaluation and staging of Hodgkin's disease. In: Mauch PM, Armitage JO, Diehl V, et a., eds. Philadelphia: Lippincott Williams and Wilkins, 1999:231, with permission.

occurrence of disease in those two regions. Fig. 30–1 demonstrates the most common anatomic patterns of Hodgkin's lymphoma presentation. The frequency of involved disease sites in untreated pathologically staged patients with Hodgkin's lymphoma is summarized in Table 30–1.

Pulmonary parenchymal involvement also follows the lymphatic pathways of the lung, from the anterior mediastinum, successively to the hilar and bronchopulmonary nodes, then through the lymphatic channels of the bronchovascular bundle into the lung parenchyma and pleural surface. Hematogenous spread of Hodgkin's lymphoma is less common; when this occurs, usually the spleen is the first site, followed by the liver and bone marrow.

Leptomeningeal involvement with Hodgkin's lymphoma at presentation has been reported, but is extremely rare.[15,16] When this occurs, there is often a paraspinal mass arising from an involved lymph node with localized dural infiltration. At recurrence, particularly of chemorefractory disease, both brain parenchymal involvement and leptomeningeal lymphomatosis have been reported.[17]

The clinical features of nonclassical Hodgkin's lymphoma (lymphocyte predominance subtype) differ significantly from classical Hodgkin's lymphoma. This disease is rare (approximately 5% of Hodgkin's lymphoma), and presents most commonly in young males as low-stage disease in the cervical or axillary lymph nodes unaccompanied by systemic symptoms.[18,19] Lymphocyte-predominant Hodgkin's lymphoma may be associated with "progressive transformation of germinal centers" reactive lymphadenopathy.[20] Late recurrences are more common in this subtype in some series, but are usually highly responsive to therapy. For this reason, many consider this disease to be similar to indolent non-Hodgkin's lymphoma. As with other indolent B-cell neoplasms, transformation to diffuse large B-cell lymphoma may occur, although this is uncommon (<5% of patients) and may have a better outcome than other large-cell transformations.[21]

HISTOLOGIC EVALUATION

As with all lymphomas, the diagnosis of Hodgkin's lymphoma requires histologic review of tissue. Although immunophenotyping plays an important confirmatory role, morphologic identification of Reed–Sternberg cells and variants in the appropriate reactive cellular background remains essential for a definitive diagnosis. Even in classical forms of Hodgkin's lymphoma, these cells may frequently be in the minority; therefore, whenever possible, a large, intact, incisional biopsy of a lymph node from the center of the disease process is desirable. Mediastinoscopy specimens and core needle biopsies often do not provide adequate tissue, and patients without palpable lymphadenopathy may require more invasive Chamberlain thoracic procedures in order to fully characterize the malignancy. In addition to benign causes of lymphadenopathy, such as thymoma, T-cell lymphoblastic lymphomas and T-cell–rich B-cell lymphomas and large-cell mediastinal lymphomas with sclerosis may be confused with Hodgkin's lymphoma in the absence of adequate diagnostic material.

Complete discussion of pathologic classification appears in Chapter 1. Malignant Reed–Sternberg cells and variants are the minority of cells in the specimen, which consists of a rich inflammatory infiltrate of lymphocytes, eosinophils, neutrophils, histiocytes and plasma cells. All subtypes of classical Hodgkin's lymphoma have Reed–Sternberg cells with a characteristic immunophenotype: CD15 and CD30 positive, and negative for T-cell markers and CD45. It is critical for specimens to be reviewed by an experienced hematopathologist to confirm the diagnosis.

Nodular sclerosis (NS) is the most common subtype of classical Hodgkin's lymphoma in the United States. Diagnosis requires a nodular growth pattern, bands of fibrosis, and "lacunar" RS cells, with abundant cytoplasm. The disease usually presents in young adults, and anterior mediastinal involvement is very common. The *mixed cellularity* (MC) subtype is associated with diffuse architectural effacement, and classic RS cells with prominent inclusion-like nucleoli. It is more common in men, older people, the immunosuppressed (including HIV-associated Hodgkin's lymphoma), children, and associated with disseminated disease at presentation. *Classical Hodgkin's lymphoma, lymphocyte-rich* is similar in clinical presentation to nodular sclerosis, and must be differentiated from nodular lymphocyte predominance. The immunophenotype is classical Hodgkin's, with CD15 and CD30 generally positive, and about 40% of cases are EBV associated. Most patients with the lymphocyte-rich variant are adult males presenting with asymptomatic axillary or cervical lymphadenopathy, but without mediastinal involvement.

As previously mentioned, *nodular-lymphocyte predominance* Hodgkin's lymphoma differs from classical (NS or MC) Hodgkin's disease (HD) in its immunophenotypic profile and clinical behavior. Classic Reed–Sternberg cells are rare. The neoplastic cells ("popcorn cells"), also known as lymphocytic/histiocytic cells, are CD20-positive and CD15-negative. The disease has an indolent course that is characterized by sensitive relapses, much like indolent B-cell lymphomas. *Lymphocyte depletion* Hodgkin's lymphoma is extremely rare (<1% of Hodgkin's lymphoma), and in most cases actually represents an atypical non-Hodgkin's lymphoma such as T-cell–rich B-cell diffuse large-cell lymphoma. The diagnosis of lymphocyte depletion Hodgkin's lymphoma should always be questioned, and it is essential that this diagnosis be confirmed by an experienced hematopathologist.

HISTORY, PHYSICAL EXAMINATION, AND LABORATORY ASSESSMENT

The recommended diagnostic evaluation for *de novo* Hodgkin's lymphoma is outlined in Table 30–2. Once definitive pathologic diagnosis has been made, a detailed history, including the presence or absence of constitutional "B-symptoms" should be obtained. Risks of infection with human immunodeficiency virus should be assessed, and it is recommended that an HIV test be performed routinely upon diagnosis, as Hodgkin's lymphoma incidence is clearly increased in this population, and such history may have important implications on choice of therapy.[22] Since a subset of Hodgkin's lymphoma may be familial, this history should also be obtained. Finally, a history of exposure to EBV virus (or history of symptomatic mononucleosis) should also be obtained.

On examination, involved lymph nodes are typically nontender, and possess a rubbery consistency on palpation.

Table 30–2. Diagnostic Evaluation of Classical Hodgkin's Lymphoma

1. Adequate diagnostic biopsy sample (excision of node recommended)
   Reviewed by experienced hematopathologist
2. History and physical examination
   Specific attention to "B symptoms" (fevers, weight loss, night sweats)
   Measure all nodal sites
   Evaluate liver size, spleen size
   Complete skin examination
   Determine sites of bone discomfort
3. Laboratory studies
   CBC, differential, platelet count, erythrocyte sedimentation rate
   Liver function testing
   Renal function testing
   Serum calcium
   HIV testing
4. Radiographic studies
   Plain chest radiograph
   CT of chest, abdomen, and pelvis
   Consider FDG-PET
   Bone films or MRI in areas of bone pain
5. Bone marrow biopsy
   Mandatory if advanced stage, B symptoms, relapsed disease, or abnormal CBC
6. Pretreatment evaluation
   Pulmonary function testing, including DLCO
   Radionucleotide ventriculography (preferred) or echocardiogram
   Pregnancy testing (premenopausal female)
   Semen analysis and cryopreservation (males desiring fertility preservation)
   Baseline thyroid function evaluation

A measurement of the largest mass in each lymph node region should be recorded. Waldeyer's ring should always be examined, and may be involved in up to 5% of patients. The size of the liver and spleen on examination should be assessed. It is important to perform a whole body skin examination, as skin lesions that have been associated with Hodgkin's lymphoma include excoriations from severe pruritus, urticaria, hyperpigmentation, and rarely direct skin infiltration with lymphoma.

A complete blood count, and differential and platelet count should be performed on every patient at diagnosis. Routine blood counts are normal in most untreated patients at the time of diagnosis of Hodgkin's lymphoma. Nonetheless, they can provide useful information at the onset of disease, and are frequently abnormal in advanced disease. The latter is manifested as leukocytosis in 25% of patients at diagnosis, usually with neutrophil predominance and along with lymphopenia. This is considered an unfavorable prognostic factor.[23] Eosinophilia is common, and is thought to be a cytokine-mediated phenomenon.[24] An additional 5% of Hodgkin's lymphoma patients present with leukopenia, either on the basis of marrow infiltration or more commonly thought to be cytokine mediated. Anemia and thrombocytopenia are both less commonly seen in patients with newly diagnosed Hodgkin's lymphoma. Usually, cytopenias associated with Hodgkin's lymphoma are not secondary to significant bone marrow infiltration. Anemia is usually normochromic and normocytic, with a "chronic-disease" picture. Coombs-positive autoimmune hemolytic anemia is occasionally seen, most often with far-advanced disease.[25] Thrombocytosis is commonly observed as an acute phase reactant, but immune-mediated thrombocytopenia has also been reported in conjunction with Hodgkin's lymphoma or preceding the diagnosis.[26]

The erythrocyte sedimentation rate (ESR) is a useful but highly nonspecific index of Hodgkin's lymphoma activity.[27,28] It is elevated in about half of newly diagnosed patients, more frequently in those with constitutional symptoms or advanced-stage disease. ESR has been shown to correlate with the extent of disease, and subsequent relapse, and can provide prognostic information, so should be checked at baseline in all patients prior to beginning therapy.

The results of routine liver function testing may influence dosing of chemotherapy and should be performed in all patients. In one series of 421 patients, 1.4% presented with liver function abnormalities consistent with cholestasis, and in three of these patients, the liver was the only diagnostic abnormality observed.[29] Liver function abnormalities, especially elevated alkaline phosphatase, can be cytokine mediated and independent of direct involvement. Tumor in the liver is more common in mixed cellularity subtype, and advanced stages of disease. Low serum albumin is also an unfavorable prognostic factor in advanced-stage disease, but rarely may be secondary to an immunomediated nephrotic syndrome.[30] In this situation, assessing urinary protein excretion is warranted.

Serum calcium may be elevated in advanced disease, or when bone involvement is present, secondary to elevated vitamin D levels, and should be determined on diagnosis.[31] Baseline thyroid studies may be helpful in all patients with planned mantle irradiation therapy, as a significant number of these patients will develop hypothyroidism as a result of treatment.[32]

All patients should be counseled on the use of birth control. Premenopausal females require pregnancy testing. Male patients requiring chemotherapy should undergo semen analysis and discussions regarding sperm cryopreservation, although a significant number of these patients may have limited viable sperm at presentation, usually in symptomatic patients.[33,34]

STAGING

Staging, defined by anatomic location of involved sites and presence or absence of specific symptoms, has an important role in the treatment of all malignancies, but is critically important in Hodgkin's lymphoma. Accurate staging allows optimization of therapy, improving overall survival by decreasing relapse rates. In addition, the unnecessary toxicities of overly aggressive therapy may be avoided with appropriate staging. The risk of secondary malignancies, which exceeds 10% in several series of patients with early-stage Hodgkin's lymphoma, may also be minimized.[35,36] Patient quality of life during and after therapy may be improved with tailored therapy defined by staging.[37] Patients with relapsed disease should be staged in a similar fashion to patients presenting de novo.

Table 30–3. Ann Arbor Staging System

Stage	Criteria
I	Involvement of single lymph node region (I) or of single extralymphatic organ or site (I_E)
II	Involvment of ≥2 lymph node regions on the same side of the diaphragm alone (II) or with involvement of limited, contiguous extralymphatic organ or tissue (II_E)
III	Involvement of lymph node regions on both sides of diaphragm (III), which may include spleen (III_S), or limited, contiguous extralymphatic organ or site (III_E), or both (III_{ES})
IV	Multiple or disseminated foci of involvement of ≥1 extralymphatic organs or tissues, with or without lymphatic involvement

Notes: All cases are subclassified to indicate the absence (A) or presence (B) or the systemic symptoms of significant fever, night sweats, or unexplained weight loss exceeding 10% of normal body weight. The clinical stage (CS) denotes the stage as determined by all diagnostic examinations and a single diagnostic biopsy only. If a second biopsy of any kind has been obtained, whether negative or positive, the term "pathologic stage" (PS) is used.

The four-part Cotswold revision of the Ann Arbor Staging Classification remains in general use as detailed in Table 30–3.[38,39] CT scanning is recommended for the detection of intra-abdominal disease, and the concept of bulky disease comprising more than 10 cm or more than a one-third widening of the mediastinum is now widely considered standard.

Bone Marrow Assessment

There is significant controversy and variation in clinical practice over the role of routine unilateral or bilateral bone marrow biopsy in the staging of de novo Hodgkin's lymphoma, since it rarely affects choice of therapy in an era when most patients receive chemotherapy.[40] Bone marrow dissemination is reported in up to 5% of patients with newly diagnosed Hodgkin's lymphoma. When performed, aspiration is insufficient to diagnose involvement with Hodgkin's lymphoma, so trephine biopsy is required. Spleen involvement almost always accompanies Hodgkin's lymphoma in the marrow, and most patients are ill with constitutional symptoms. In a German study of over 2,000 patients, 32% of Stage IV patients had bone marrow involvement.[41] Marrow involvement had no prognostic relevance with regard to freedom from treatment failure and overall survival, and did not define a special high-risk group in which a different treatment approach was indicated. We continue to perform bone marrow evaluations routinely, particularly for patients with B symptoms, bulky disease, advanced-stage disease, and abnormal peripheral blood counts. Patients with recurrent disease, particularly candidates for autologous stem cell transplantation, require a bone marrow biopsy.

Radiographic Assessment

Conventional chest radiography is typically the initial radiologic examination obtained in patients with suspected Hodgkin's lymphoma.[42] Computed tomography is more sensitive in the assessment of chest disease than is conventional chest radiography, and is considered standard.[43] Historically, bipedal lymphangiography was the procedure of choice for staging abdominal Hodgkin's lymphoma. Although lymphangiography was useful in assessing enlarged retroperitoneal and pelvic lymph nodes, computed tomography has completely supplanted it as the imaging modality of choice for evaluating the abdomen and pelvis. Bone radiographs are obtained in patients who are symptomatic, and typically reveal predominantly osteoblastic or mixed lesions; lytic lesions are much less common. In the spine, an "ivory vertebrae" may be seen, and is often associated with an adjacent soft tissue mass.[44]

Functional Imaging

Nuclear imaging at diagnosis can clarify findings of uncertain significance on conventional radiographic staging. More importantly, baseline imaging allows accurate response assessment, and evaluation of residual masses after therapy. Fluorodeoxyglycose (FDG) positron emission tomography (discussed in detail in Chapter 10) has largely replaced gallium scintigraphy in the evaluation of Hodgkin's lymphoma.[45] FDG-PET appears to accurately assess Hodgkin's lymphoma activity, and several studies have shown at least equal sensitivity and increased specificity of PET when compared to CT or MRI. Moreover, PET, in contrast to gallium scintigraphy (which is of limited value below the diaphragm), may be useful in detecting splenic involvement as well as bone marrow involvement.[46] PET may be helpful in the evaluation of residual masses after therapy, and preliminary data suggests a rapid complete response on PET imaging confers a favorable prognosis. Clinical trials are ongoing incorporating PET response into treatment evaluation. At the present time, however, results from PET imaging are not integrated into the formal staging paradigm, and the authors strongly discourage treatment decisions from being made on the basis of PET imaging alone.

Cardiac and Pulmonary Evaluation

Patients with any history of cardiac disease, symptoms, or above age 40 to 50, should undergo evaluation of cardiac function if therapy is to include chest irradiation or an anthracycline. Patients with abnormal function at baseline require aggressive monitoring to limit the incidence of doxorubicin-associated cardiomyopathy.[47] Complete pulmonary function testing, including DLCO (diffusing capacity of lungs for carbon monoxide) adjusted for volume and hemoglobin, is recommended if the patient is to receive mantle irradiation or bleomycin as part of a chemotherapy regimen. Although significant controversy exists on the relationship between DCLO and development of bleomycin-induced pulmonary toxicity, patients with significant abnormalities at baseline warrant an aggressive monitoring strategy.[48]

Laparotomy and Splenectomy

The growing use of combined modality therapy for patients with early-stage disease, and effective salvage chemotherapy regimens for patients who fail radiation as initial treatment, have limited the value of surgical abdominal staging, and the vast majority of large centers have abandoned the use of staging laparotomy and splenectomy, which historically was a standard diagnostic approach in this histology.[49,50] Laparoscopic staging has been used in some centers, with decreased morbidity; however, the technique has never been prospectively compared with conventional laparotomy in adult patients with Hodgkin's lymphoma.[51]

PROGNOSTIC FEATURES

Clinical

Constitutional complaints, including B symptoms and pruritus, contribute to a poor prognosis in an incremental manner. Additionally, male gender, advanced age (usually defined as over age 40), and advanced stage all contribute to a worse prognosis in several studies. *Mixed cellularity* histology had an independent negative prognostic contribution when radiation therapy also is used.

Several centers have reported that cure with radiation therapy alone is reduced dramatically when the tumor mass exceeds one-third of the maximum chest diameter. The Danish National Hodgkin's Disease Group has extended the study of the relation of tumor bulk to prognosis; total tumor burden (a complex parameter obtained by summation of the tumor bulk of each involved site), not mediastinal mass alone, is the most important factor in predicting disease-free survival of patients in pathologic Stages I and II.[52]

Recently, the data from 5141 patients with advanced-stage Hodgkin's lymphoma were used to develop a parametric model for predicting freedom from disease progression (Table 30–4). Seven factors had similar prognostic effects, that on multivariate analysis were independent: serum albumin of less than 4 g/dL, age under 45, male gender, Stage IV disease, leukocytosis greater than 15,000/mL^3, and lymphopenia less than 600/mL^3 or less

Table 30–4. Advanced-Stage Hodgkin's Lymphoma Clinical Prognostic Factors

Number of Factors[a]	% of Patients	% FFS
0	7	84
1	22	77
2	29	67
3	23	60
4	12	51
≥5	7	42

[a] Factors: serum albumin <4 g/dL, age >45, male gender, Stage IV disease, leukocytosis >15,000/mL^3, lymphopenia <600/mL^3, lymphopenia <8%.

FFS, failure-free survival.

From Hasenclever D and Diehl V. A prognostic score for advanced Hodgkin's disease. International Prognostic Factors Project on Advanced Hodgkin's Disease. N Engl J Med 339:1506–14, 1998 [see comments],[23] with permission.

than 8%.[23] Although only 19% of patients had a score of 4 or higher, these patients had a 47% rate of freedom from disease progression at 5 years. Future clinical trials will incorporate this prognostic information, and it is anticipated that clinical treatment decisions will depend on risk at presentation.[53]

Other

Chemokines appear to be critical in maintaining the microenvironment necessary for the Reed–Sternberg cell.[54] Serum cytokine levels have been shown to correlate with clinical symptoms, stage, and extent of disease.[55] Interleukin-7, interleukin-8, soluble TNF receptor, and p53 protein levels are elevated in the serum of patients with Hodgkin's lymphoma.[56] Interleukin-6 (IL-6) levels are increased in patients with Hodgkin's lymphoma, and are correlated with a poorer response to chemotherapy. Persons with genetically determined lower IL-6 levels may be less susceptible to developing Hodgkin's lymphoma.[57] Other cytokines that may provide prognostic information include IL-9,[58] IL-13,[59] IL-10,[60–62] and TNF.[63] As previously stated, evidence of clonal EBV within Reed–Sternberg cells may provide prognostic information.[64] Tissue eosinophilia, when present, confers a poor prognosis.[65] Similar to non-Hodgkin's lymphoma, unique gene expression profiles have been determined defining Hodgkin's lymphoma.[66,67] Interestingly, there appears to be overlap between expression signatures of Hodgkin's lymphoma and primary mediastinal large B-cell lymphoma, which are significantly different from other forms of large B-cell lymphoma.[68] It is anticipated that novel therapeutic targets for high-risk subsets of Hodgkin's lymphoma will be discovered on the basis of gene expression profiles.

References

1. Thorley-Lawson DA and Gross A. Persistence of the Epstein–Barr virus and the origins of associated lymphomas. N Engl J Med 2004;350:1328–37.
2. Hjalgrim H, Askling J, Rostgaard K, et al. Characteristics of Hodgkin's lymphoma after infectious mononucleosis. N Engl J Med 2003;349:1324–32.
3. Ambinder R. Infection and lymphoma. N Engl J Med 2003;349:1309–11.
4. Kuppers R, Klein U, Hansmann ML, et al. Cellular origin of human B-cell lymphomas. N Engl J Med 1999;341:1520–9.
5. Weiss LM, Movahed LA, Warnke RA, et al. Detection of Epstein–Barr viral genomes in Reed–Sternberg cells of Hodgkin's disease. N Engl J Med 1989;320:502–6.
6. Mueller N, Evans A, Harris NL, et al. Hodgkin's disease and Epstein–Barr virus. Altered antibody pattern before diagnosis. N Engl J Med 1989;320:689–95.
7. DeVita VT Jr. Hodgkin's disease—clinical trials and travails. N Engl J Med 2003;348:2375–6.
8. Kennedy BJ, Loeb V Jr, Peterson VM, et al. National survey of patterns of care for Hodgkin's disease. Cancer 1985; 56:2547–56.
9. Kaplan HS, Dorfman RF, and Nelson TS. Staging laparotomy and splenectomy in Hodgkin's disease: analysis of indications and patterns of involvement in 285 consecutive untreated patients. NCI Monograph. Bethesda, MD: National Cancer Institute, 1973.
10. Atkinson K, Austin DE, McElwain TJ, et al. Alcohol pain in Hodgkin's disease. Cancer 1976;37:895–9.
11. Good GR and DiNubile MJ. Images in clinical medicine. Cyclic fever in Hodgkin's disease (Pel–Ebstein fever). N Engl J Med 1995;332:436.
12. Gobbi PG, Cavalli C, Gendarini A, et al. Reevaluation of prognostic significance of symptoms in Hodgkin's disease. Cancer 1985;56:2874–80.
13. Mauch PM, Kalish LA, Kadin M, et al. Patterns of presentation of Hodgkin disease. Implications for etiology and pathogenesis. Cancer 1993;71:2062–71.
14. Rosenberg SA and Kaplan HS. Evidence for an orderly progression in the spread of Hodgkin's disease. Cancer Res 1966;26:1225–31.
15. Steinherz PG, Walker R, Kroll G, et al. Lymphomatous leptomeningitis as a presenting syndrome of Hodgkin's disease. Ann Intern Med 1983;99:342–3.
16. Anselmo AP, Proia A, Cartoni C, et al. Meningeal localization in a patient with Hodgkin's disease. Description of a case and review of the literature. Ann Oncol 1996;7:1071–5.
17. Chim CS, Shek TW, Ooi GC, et al. Meningeal relapse in Hodgkin's disease. J Clin Oncol 2000;18:1153–5.
18. Aster JC. Lymphocyte-predominant Hodgkin's disease: how little therapy is enough? J Clin Oncol 1999;17:744–6.
19. Diehl V, Sextro M, Franklin J, et al. Clinical presentation, course, and prognostic factors in lymphocyte-predominant Hodgkin's disease and lymphocyte-rich classical Hodgkin's disease: report from the European Task Force on Lymphoma Project on Lymphocyte-Predominant Hodgkin's Disease. J Clin Oncol 1999;17:776–83.
20. Osborne BM, Butler JJ. Clinical implications of progressive transformation of germinal centers. Am J Surg Pathol 1984; 8:725–33.
21. Sundeen JT, Cossman J, and Jaffe ES. Lymphocyte predominant Hodgkin's disease nodular subtype with coexistent "large cell lymphoma." Histological progression or composite malignancy? Am J Surg Pathol 1988;12:599–606.
22. Hartmann P, Rehwald U, Salzberger B, et al. Current treatment strategies for patients with Hodgkin's lymphoma and HIV infection. Expert Rev Anticancer Ther 2004;4:401–10.
23. Hasenclever D and Diehl V. A prognostic score for advanced Hodgkin's disease. International Prognostic Factors Project on Advanced Hodgkin's Disease. N Engl J Med 1998;339: 1506–14.
24. Di Biagio E, Sanchez-Borges M, Desenne JJ, et al. Eosinophilia in Hodgkin's disease: a role for interleukin 5. Int Arch Allergy Immunol 1996;110:244–51.
25. Levine AM, Thornton P, Forman SJ, et al. Positive Coombs test in Hodgkin's disease: significance and implications. Blood 1980;55:607–11.
26. Waddell CC and Cimo PL. Idiopathic thrombocytopenic purpura occurring in Hodgkin disease after splenectomy: report of two cases and review of the literature. Am J Hematol 1979;7:381–7.
27. Henry-Amar M, Friedman S, Hayat M, et al. Erythrocyte sedimentation rate predicts early relapse and survival in early-stage Hodgkin disease. The EORTC Lymphoma Cooperative Group. Ann Intern Med 1991;114:361–5.
28. Friedman S, Henry-Amar M, Cosset JM, et al. Therapeutic implications and sites of relapse predicted by elevated post-therapy erythrocyte sedimentation rate in early stage Hodgkin disease. Am J Hematol 1991;37:253–7.
29. Cervantes F, Briones J, Bruguera M, et al. Hodgkin's disease presenting as a cholestatic febrile illness: incidence and main characteristics in a series of 421 patients. Ann Hematol 1996; 72:357–60.
30. Dabbs DJ, Striker LM, Mignon F, et al. Glomerular lesions in lymphomas and leukemias. Am J Med 1986;80:63–70.
31. Rieke JW, Donaldson SS, and Horning SJ. Hypercalcemia and vitamin D metabolism in Hodgkin's disease. Is there an under-

lying immunoregulatory relationship? Cancer 1989;63: 1700–7.
32. Hancock SL, Cox RS, and McDougall IR. Thyroid diseases after treatment of Hodgkin's disease. N Engl J Med 1991; 325:599–605.
33. Fitoussi, Eghbali H, Tchen N, et al. Semen analysis and cryoconservation before treatment in Hodgkin's disease. Ann Oncol 2000;11:679–84.
34. Shekarriz M, Tolentino MV Jr, Ayzman I, et al. Cryopreservation and semen quality in patients with Hodgkin's disease. Cancer 1995;75:2732–6.
35. Ng AK, Bernardo MP, Weller E, et al. Long-term survival and competing causes of death in patients with early-stage Hodgkin's disease treated at age 50 or younger. J Clin Oncol 2002;20:2101–8.
36. Ng AK, Bernardo MV, Weller E, et al. Second malignancy after Hodgkin disease treated with radiation therapy with or without chemotherapy: long-term risks and risk factors. Blood 2002;100:1989–96.
37. Ng AK, Weeks JC, Mauch PM, et al. Decision analysis on alternative treatment strategies for favorable-prognosis, early-stage Hodgkin's disease. J Clin Oncol 1999;17:3577–85.
38. Carbone PP, Kaplan HS, Musshoff K, et al. Report of the Committee on Hodgkin's Disease Staging Classification. Cancer Res 1971;31:1860–1.
39. Lister TA, Crowther D, Sutcliffe SB, et al. Report of a committee convened to discuss the evaluation and staging of patients with Hodgkin's disease: Cotswolds meeting. J Clin Oncol 1989;7:1630–6, [see comments] [erratum appears in J Clin Oncol 1990;8:1602].
40. Howell SJ, Grey M, Chang J, et al. The value of bone marrow examination in the staging of Hodgkin's lymphoma: a review of 955 cases seen in a regional cancer centre. Br J Haematol 2002;119:408–11.
41. Munker R, Hasenclever D, Brosteanu O, et al. Bone marrow involvement in Hodgkin's disease: an analysis of 135 consecutive cases. German Hodgkin's Lymphoma Study Group. J Clin Oncol 1995;13:403–9, [see comments].
42. Castellino RA, Blank N, Hoppe RT, et al. Hodgkin disease: contributions of chest CT in the initial staging evaluation. Radiology 1986;160:603–5.
43. Hopper KD, Diehl LF, Lesar M, et al. Hodgkin disease: clinical utility of CT in initial staging and treatment. Radiology 1988;169:17–22.
44. Edeiken-Monroe B, Edeiken J, and Kim EE. Radiologic concepts of lymphoma of bone. Radiol Clin North Am 1990; 28:841–64.
45. Friedberg JW and Chengazi V. PET Scans in the staging of lymphoma: current status. Oncologist 2003;8:438–47.
46. Friedberg JW, Fischman A, Neuberg D, et al. FDG-PET is superior to gallium scintigraphy in staging and more sensitive in the follow-up of patients with de novo Hodgkin lymphoma: a blinded comparison. Leuk Lymphoma 2003; 45:85–92.
47. Singal PK and Iliskovic N. Doxorubicin-induced cardiomyopathy. N Engl J Med 1998;339:900–5, [see comments].
48. Comis RL. Bleomycin pulmonary toxicity: current status and future directions. Semin Oncol 1992;19:64–70.
49. Multani PS and Grossbard ML. Staging laparotomy in the management of Hodgkin's disease: is it still necessary? Oncologist 1996;1:41–55.
50. Ng AK, Weeks JC, Mauch PM, et al. Laparotomy versus no laparotomy in the management of early-stage, favorable-prognosis Hodgkin's disease: a decision analysis. J Clin Oncol 1999;17:241–52.
51. Lefor AT, Flowers JL, and Heyman MR. Laparoscopic staging of Hodgkin's disease. Surg Oncol 1993;2:217–20.
52. Specht L, Nordentoft AM, Cold S, et al. Tumor burden as the most important prognostic factor in early stage Hodgkin's disease. Relations to other prognostic factors and implications for choice of treatment. Cancer 1988;61:1719–27.
53. Brice P. Prognostic factors in advanced Hodgkin's disease—can they guide therapeutic decisions? N Engl J Med 1998; 339:1547–9.
54. Teruya-Feldstein J, Tosato G, and Jaffe ES. The role of chemokines in Hodgkin's disease. Leuk Lymphoma 2000; 38:363–71.
55. Gorschluter M, Bohlen H, Hasenclever D, et al. Serum cytokine levels correlate with clinical parameters in Hodgkin's disease. Ann Oncol 1995;6:477–82.
56. Trumper L, Jung W, Dahl G, et al. Interleukin-7, interleukin-8, soluble TNF receptor, and p53 protein levels are elevated in the serum of patients with Hodgkin's disease. Ann Oncol 1994;5 Suppl 1:93–6.
57. Cozen W, Gill PS, Ingles SA, et al. IL-6 levels and genotype are associated with risk of young adult Hodgkin lymphoma. Blood 2004;103:3216–21.
58. Fischer M, Bijman M, Molin D, et al. Increased serum levels of interleukin-9 correlate to negative prognostic factors in Hodgkin's lymphoma. Leukemia 2003;17:2513–6.
59. Fiumara P, Cabanillas F, Younes A. Interleukin-13 levels in serum from patients with Hodgkin disease and healthy volunteers. Blood 2001;98:2877–8.
60. Vassilakopoulos TP, Nadali G, Angelopoulou MK, et al. Serum interleukin-10 levels are an independent prognostic factor for patients with Hodgkin's lymphoma. Haematologica 2001; 86:274–81.
61. Viviani S, Notti P, Bonfante V, et al. Elevated pretreatment serum levels of Il-10 are associated with a poor prognosis in Hodgkin's disease, the milan cancer institute experience. Med Oncol 2000;17:59–63.
62. Sarris AH, Kliche KO, Pethambaram P, et al. Interleukin-10 levels are often elevated in serum of adults with Hodgkin's disease and are associated with inferior failure-free survival. Ann Oncol 1999;10:433–40.
63. Warzocha K, Bienvenu J, Ribeiro P, et al. Plasma levels of tumour necrosis factor and its soluble receptors correlate with clinical features and outcome of Hodgkin's disease patients. Br J Cancer 1998;77:2357–62.
64. Herling M, Rassidakis GZ, Medeiros LJ, et al. Expression of Epstein–Barr virus latent membrane protein-1 in Hodgkin and Reed–Sternberg cells of classical Hodgkin's lymphoma: associations with presenting features, serum interleukin 10 levels, and clinical outcome. Clin Cancer Res 2003;9: 2114–20.
65. von Wasielewski R, Seth S, Franklin J, et al. Tissue eosinophilia correlates strongly with poor prognosis in nodular sclerosing Hodgkin's disease, allowing for known prognostic factors. Blood 2000;95:1207–13.
66. Garcia JF, Camacho FI, Morente M, et al. Hodgkin and Reed–Sternberg cells harbor alterations in the major tumor suppressor pathways and cell-cycle checkpoints: analyses using tissue microarrays. Blood 2003;101:681–9.
67. Kuppers R, Klein U, Schwering I, et al. Identification of Hodgkin and Reed–Sternberg cell-specific genes by gene expression profiling. J Clin Invest 2003;111:529–37.
68. Savage KJ, Monti S, Kutok JL, et al. The molecular signature of mediastinal large B-cell lymphoma differs from that of other diffuse large B-cell lymphomas and shares features with classical Hodgkin lymphoma. Blood 2003;102:3871–9.

30B

Management of Localized Disease

Andrea K. Ng, M.D., M.P.H.

Early-stage Hodgkin's lymphoma comprises about 60% of all cases of Hodgkin's lymphoma. The treatment approach for these patients has evolved over time, and cure rates of 80% to 90% have been achieved in recent years. Because of the excellent survival in this relatively young group of patients, late effects of therapy have been increasingly recognized. The current clinical focus on early-stage Hodgkin's lymphoma is to classify patients into risk groups, and to identify ways to safely modify and reduce treatment within subsets of patients while preserving the high cure rates of the disease.

PROGNOSTIC FACTORS

Classifying patients into prognostic groups allows tailored therapy and exploration of treatment reduction in low-risk patients. Prognostic factors that have been identified for early-stage Hodgkin's lymphoma, based largely on patients treated with radiation therapy alone, include large mediastinal adenopathy, constitutional symptoms, number of involved sites, disease burden, gender, erythrocyte sedimentation rate, and histology.[1–5] These factors were mostly predictive of freedom from recurrence, but seldom of overall survival. The only factor that has been consistently shown to have a negative prognostic impact on survival is older age at diagnosis. Furthermore, most of these factors lose their prognostic significance in the setting of combined modality therapy. Nevertheless, these prognostic factors have been adopted by various groups for patient stratification in the conduction of clinical trials for early-stage Hodgkin's lymphoma. Table 30–5 shows examples of the prognostic classification system used by the European Organization for Research and Treatment of Cancer (EORTC), German Hodgkin's Study Group (GHSG), and the National Cancer Institute of Canada (NCIC) in their trials on early-stage Hodgkin's lymphoma.

RADIATION THERAPY ALONE

Historically, the general strategy in the management of early-stage Hodgkin's lymphoma had been to treat patients with favorable prognosis disease with extended-field radiation therapy alone, and to add chemotherapy in the presence of unfavorable features. Identification of appropriate candidates for radiation therapy alone relies on the performance of staging laparotomy to rule out occult disease below the diaphragm. The main rationale for pathologic staging, developed in the 1960s, was to select patients who can be spared the then-standard chemotherapy for Hodgkin's lymphoma, the mechlorethamine, vincristine, procarbazine, prednisone (MOPP) regimen, with its associated risk of significant myelosuppression, sterility, and leukemogenesis. Subsequently, results from the EORTC H-5 trial randomizing pathologic Stage (PS) I–II patients to mantle versus mantle and para-aortic-splenic pedicle irradiation showed that these patients can be safely treated with mantle irradiation alone.[6] The excellent survival outcome with this approach was confirmed by results from a single institutional prospective study on patients with PS I–II disease treated with mantle radiation therapy alone, in which the 5-year freedom-from-treatment failure (FFTF) and overall survival were 86% and 100%, respectively.[7] Although rarely employed at present, given the high survival rate, this approach remains a reasonable option for patients who wish to avoid extended-field radiation therapy or chemotherapy.

Selection of patients to be treated with radiation therapy alone using staging laparatomy has largely been eliminated in current clinical practice since the introduction of adriamycin, bleomycin, vinblastine, and decarbazine (ABVD), a more effective and less toxic combination chemotherapy regimen than MOPP.[8] In the last 10 to 15 years, there has been a shift to the use of combined modality therapy in early-stage patients. The addition of chemotherapy helps to eradicate occult abdominal disease, obviating the need for pathologic staging. It also allows the use of more limited radiation fields than in patients treated with radiation therapy alone. Furthermore, randomized studies have shown a significantly higher freedom from treatment failure with combined modality therapy than with radiation therapy alone.[9–13]

COMBINED MODALITY THERAPY

There are a number of controversial issues that have recently been or are currently being addressed by clinical trials in the use of combined modality therapy for early-stage Hodgkin's lymphoma. These include alternatives of or modification of the ABVD regimen to limit toxicity in favorable patients or to improve efficacy in unfavorable patients, the optimal number of cycles of chemotherapy, and the optimal radiation field size and dose when used in combination with chemotherapy. The following discussion includes trials that looked at patients with early-stage

Table 30–5. Prognostic Classification Systems for Clinical Stages I–II of Hodgkin's Lymphoma

Institution	Prognostic Classification
EORTC	*Unfavorable Prognosis:* Presence of any one of the following: Age >50 years No B symptoms with ESR ≥50 B symptoms with ESR ≥30 ≥4 Sites of involvement Bulky mediastinal involvement *Favorable Prognosis:* Absence of all factors in unfavorable prognosis group
GHSG	*Unfavorable Prognosis:* Presence of *any* one of the following: Elevated erythrocyte sedimentation rate (≥50 mm without or ≥30 mm with B symptoms) ≥3 Sites of involvement Extranodal involvement Large mediastinal mass *Favorable Prognosis:* Absence of all factors in unfavorable prognosis group
NCIC (excluded patients with bulky disease)	Low risk: Presence of all the following: LP/NS Age <40 ESR <50 <3 Sites of involvement High risk: All other patients

EORTC, European Organization for Research and Treatment of Cancer; ESR, erythrocyte sedimentation rate; GHSG, German Hodgkin's Study Group; LP, lymphocyte predominance; NCIC, National Cancer Institute of Canada; NS, nodular sclerosis.

disease, while trials that consisted of advanced-stage patients and some unfavorable early-stage patients will be discussed in a separate section of the chapter.

WHAT IS THE OPTIMAL SYSTEMIC REGIMEN?

Although ABVD is considered by most as the standard chemotherapy for early-stage Hodgkin's lymphoma, investigators have explored alternative regimens that were felt to be associated with lower toxicity profile, by eliminating or substituting specific drugs, modifying dose and dose schedule, or employing shorter course therapy. Examples include vinblastine, bleomycin and methotrexate (VBM)[14–17]; methotrexate, vinblastine, and prednisone (MVP)[15]; doxorubicin, cyclophosphamide, etoposide, vincristine, bleomycin, and prednisolone (VAPEC-B)[13]; doxorubicin, vinblastine (AV)[10]; mitoxantrone, vincristine, vinblastine, and prednisone (NOVP)[18]; and epirubicin, bleomycin, vinblastine, and prednisone (EBVP II, administered monthly).[12,19] The Stanford V regimen (nitrogen mustard, adriamycin, vincristine, vinblastine, etoposide, bleomycin, and prednisone, followed by radiation therapy to initial nodal involvement in selected cases), a short but intensive 12-week regimen, was originally developed for patients with advanced-stage disease or bulky early-stage disease.[20,21] A modified 8-week regimen is being investigated in nonbulky, Clinical Stage (CS) I–IIA patients, and in the most recent version (Stanford V-C), the nitrogen mustard is substituted by cyclophosphamide, and the radiation dose is reduced from 30 Gy to 20 Gy. Of the regimens listed above, only a limited number have been evaluated in randomized studies.

The Southwest Oncology Group (SWOG) compared three cycles of AV followed by subtotal nodal irradiation with subtotal nodal irradiation in patients with CS I–IIA Hodgkin's lymphoma, and found a significant failure-free survival (FFS) benefit in the combined modality therapy arm, with 3-year FFS of 94% and 81%, respectively ($p<0.001$).[10] In the EORTC H7F trial, patients with early-stage, favorable prognosis Hodgkin's lymphoma were randomized to receive EBVP II and involved-field radiation therapy versus subtotal nodal irradiation.[12] The 6-year relapse-free survival was significantly higher in the combined modality therapy arm (92% vs. 81%, $p = 0.004$). The Medical Research Council compared VAPEC-B and involved-field radiotherapy vs mantle radiotherapy in patients with nonbulky, Stage I–IIA Hodgkin's lymphoma. Significantly higher relapse-free survival (87% vs. 70%, $p = 0.002$) and overall survival (98% vs. 92%, $p = 0.036$) were found, favoring the combined modality therapy arm.[13] In these trials, although the comparison arms were all radiation therapy alone, which is no longer considered standard therapy, excellent results were demonstrated in the arms using the abbreviated chemotherapy regimen. The GHSG 13 trial is a recently opened four-arm study comparing two cycles of ABVD, AVD, ABV, and AV, all followed by 30 Gy of involved-field irradiation in CS I–II patients without risk factors. The results of this trial will shed light on the feasibility of delivering less chemotherapy than the gold standard of ABVD in patients with early-stage, favorable prognosis disease.

In patients with early-stage, unfavorable prognosis disease, attempts to use less intensive regimens have not been as successful. In the EORTC H7U study, comparing unfavorable prognosis CS I–II patients treated with six cycles of EBVP II and involved-field irradiation versus six cycles of MOPP/ABV and involved-field irradiation, the 6-year event-free survival was significantly lower in the EBVP II arm (68% vs. 90%, $p<0.0001$).[12] Three ongoing trials are addressing whether these patients may benefit from the regimen bleomycin, etoposide, doxorubicin, cyclophosphamide, vincristine, procarbazine, and prednisone (BEACOPP), originally developed for patients with advanced-stage disease. Both the EORTC H9U and the GHSG HD11 studies are comparing four to six cycles of ABVD with four cycles of BEACOPP-baseline, followed by involved-field irradiation to 20 to 30 Gy. In the recently opened GHSG HD 14 trial, patients with CS I–II disease with risk factors are randomized to four cycles of ABVD versus two cycles of dose-escalated BEACOPP and two cycles of ABVD, followed by involved-field irradiation to 30 Gy.

In addition to the specific combination chemotherapy included, another question regarding systemic therapy is the duration of therapy. In patients with favorable prognosis disease, this was addressed by the GHSG 10 trial, randomizing CS I–II patients without risk factors to four cycles or two cycles of ABVD, followed by 30-Gy or 20-Gy involved-field irradiation.[22] At a median follow-up of 28 months, the 2-year freedom from treatment failure was 96.6% and the 2-year overall survival was 98.5%, with no significant differences between the four arms. The follow-up time, however, is too short for definitive conclusions at this time. In patients with unfavorable prognosis disease, the optimal number of cycles of chemotherapy was one of the study questions in two successive EORTC trials. In the EORTC-H8U trial, patients were randomized to six cycles of MOPP/ABV followed by involved-field irradiation, four cycles of MOPP/ABV followed by involved-field irradiation, or four cycles of MOPP/ABV followed by extended-field irradiation.[23] At a median follow-up of 39 months, the failure-free survival rates were 89%, 92%, 92%, respectively (p = 0.32), and the overall survival rates were 90%, 94%, and 92%, respectively (p = 0.19). In the EORTC-H9U trial, randomizing patients to six cycles of ABVD, four cycles of ABVD or four cycles of BEACOPP, all followed by involved-field irradiation, the most recent interim analysis showed 4-year event-free survival and overall survival of 90% and 94%, respectively (no arm comparison provided).[24]

WHAT ARE THE APPROPRIATE RADIATION FIELD SIZE AND DOSE?

One key advantage of the combined modality approach in the treatment of early-stage Hodgkin's lymphoma is the opportunity to limit the radiation field size and dose when used in conjunction with effective chemotherapeutic agents. Three randomized trials on patients with early-stage disease confirmed that involved-field irradiation is adequate as part of combined modality therapy. In the GHSG HD8 trial, 1,204 patients with CS I–II Hodgkin's lymphoma with risk factors were randomized to receive two cycles of cyclophosphamide, vincristine, procarbazine, and prednisone (COPP) and ABVD followed by extended-field or involved-field radiotherapy.[25] At a median follow-up time of 54 months, the 5-year FFTF rates of the two arms were 86% and 84%, respectively (p = 0.56), and the 5-year overall survival rates were 91% and 92%, respectively (p = 0.24). The results of this trial also suggested that two cycles of chemotherapy may be effective in eradicating occult disease, although the trial was not specifically designed to answer this question. In an Italian trial, 136 patients with CS I unfavorable and CS IIA favorable and unfavorable Hodgkin's lymphoma received four cycles of ABVD followed by either subtotal nodal irradiation or involved-field radiation therapy.[26] At a median follow-up of 116 months, the 12-year freedom from progression of the two arms were 93% and 94%, respectively, and the 12-year overall survival were 96% and 94%, respectively. Three cases of second malignancies were reported, all of which were in the extended-field radiation therapy arm. As described above, two of the three arms in the EORTC H8U trial compared four cycles of MOPP/ABV followed by either involved-field irradiation or extended-field irradiation, and no significant differences in failure-free or overall survival were detected at a median follow-up of 39 months.[23]

Investigators have also explored the option of lowering the radiation dose as part of combined modality therapy. The previously described GHSG HD10 trial on low-risk, early-stage patients showed no differences between two versus four cycles of ABVD followed by 20 Gy versus 30 Gy of involved-field radiation therapy.[22] However, this was based on only 2-year results, and additional follow-up is needed to establish the safety of 20 Gy of radiation treatment. The EORTC H9F trial is a three-arm trial in which patients receive six cycles of EBVP II.[19] After a complete response, patients were randomized to receive no further treatment, or 36 Gy or 20 Gy of involved-field irradiation. Patients with a partial response all received 36 Gy of involved-field irradiation with or without a 4-Gy boost. In an interim analysis of 771 patients, the chemotherapy-alone arm was closed due to lower than expected event-free survival (discussed below). The 4-year event-free survival of all patients in this trial was 80% and the 4-year overall survival was 98% (no arm comparisons provided).

CHEMOTHERAPY ALONE

Multiple studies have documented late effects of radiotherapy for Hodgkin's lymphoma, based largely on patients treated with radiation therapy alone using larger fields and higher doses of radiation than currently employed, with second malignancies and cardiovascular disease being the leading concerns. This has prompted investigators to explore the option of treating patients with chemotherapy alone.

Can Radiation Therapy Be Safely Eliminated?

Six randomized trials have been performed, examining whether radiation therapy can be safely eliminated, four of which included only early-stage patients and two included patients of all stages (Table 30–6).[19,27–31] The study design, patient population, chemotherapy, and radiation therapy employed varied among the trials. Three trials included a significant proportion of, or exclusively, pediatric patients,[27–29] and two included patients of all stages.[28,29] In three of the trials, randomization to radiation therapy or no radiation therapy occurred only in patients who had achieved a complete response to the chemotherapy.[19,28,29] The chemotherapy alone arm was closed in two of the trials due to high number of relapses.[19,28] The findings and the limitations of each of the trials are discussed below.

Pavlovsky and colleagues from the Grupo Argentino de Tratamiento de la Leucemia Aguda (GATLA) randomized 277 patients with CS I–II Hodgkin's lymphoma to receive six monthly cycles of a MOPP variant, cyclophosphamide, vinblastine, procarbazine, and prednisone (CVPP), followed by involved-field radiation therapy to 30 Gy, versus six cycles of CVPP alone.[27] At 84 months, the disease-free survival (DFS) of the combined modality therapy arm was significantly higher than that of the chemotherapy alone arm (71% vs. 62%, p = 0.01). On subgroup analysis, the difference between the two arms were highly significant among patients with unfavorable features (age >45, more than two sites, or bulky disease), with DFS of 75% in the combined modality therapy arm versus 34% in the

Table 30–6. Randomized Trials Comparing Combined Modality Therapy and Chemotherapy Alone in Early-Stage Hodgkin's Lymphoma

Institution	No.	Patient Population	Treatment Arms	Median F/U	Results: CMT	Results: Chemo Alone
GATLA	277	CS I–II (Included patients with unfavorable factors: age >45, >2 sites or bulky disease) 45% >16 years	CVPP × 6: (1) 30 Gy IFRT, (2) No RT	84 months	DFS: 71% OS: 89% Favorable group: DFS: 77% OS: 92% Unfavorable group: DFS: 75% OS: 84%	62% (p = 0.01) 82% 70% 91% 34% (p = 0.001) 66%
CCG	829	Group 1: CS I–II without adverse factors[a] and without B Sx in CS II Group 2: CS I–II with adverse factors and CS III Group 3: CS IV	Group 1: COPP/ABV × 4 Group 2: COPP/ABV × 6 Group 3: intensive multidrug chemotherapy with GCSF support If CR: (1) 21 Gy IFRT, (2) No RT If PR: (1) 21 Gy IFRT	Not reported	Intent to treat: 3-year EFS: 92% As-treated: 3-year EFS: 93% 3-year OS: 98%	87% (p = 0.057) 85% (p = 0.0024) 99% *Arm closed*
Tata Memorial Hospital	251	CS I–IV (55% CS I–II 46% age < 15 years 71% MC histology 15% bulky disease)	ABVD × 6 If CR: (1) RT[b], (2) No RT	63 months	8-year EFS: 88% 8-year OS: 100%	76% (p = 0.01) 89% (p = 0.002)
MSKCC	152	CS IA–IIB, CS IIIA (bulky disease excluded)	ABVD × 6: (1) RT[c], (2) No RT	60 months	5-year FFP: 86% 5-year OS: 97%	81% (p = 0.61) 90% (p = 0.08)
NCIC/ECOG	399	CS I–IIA (bulky disease excluded) Low risk: LP/NS, age < 40, ESR < 50 and < 3 sites High risk: all other	Low risk: (1) STNI, (2) ABVD × 4–6 STNI: ABVD × 2+ High risk: ABVD × 4–6	4.2 years	(Low risk: STNI; High risk: CMT) 5-year PFS: 93% 5-year EFS: 88% 5-year OS: 94%	87% (p = 0.006) 86% (p = 0.06) 96% (p = 0.42)
EORTC H9F	771	CS I–II, favorable prognosis	EBVP II × 6 If CR: (1) 36 Gy IFRT, (2) 20 Gy IFRT, (3) No RT If PR: 36 Gy IFRT +/–4 Gy	29 months	Not separately reported	<20% cumulative proportion of adverse events *Arm closed*

[a] Adverse factors: hilar disease, >4 sites, larger mediastinal adenopathy (LMA) or bulky disease >10 cm.
[b] IFRT 30 + 10 Gy boost for early stage, and EFRT 25 + 10 Gy boost for advanced stage.
[c] Modified extended-field RT in 83% of patients (91% received 36 Gy).
CCG, Children's Cancer Group; CMT, combined modality therapy; CR, complete response; DFS, disease-free survival; ECOG, Eastern Cooperative Onealogy Group; EFS, event-free survival; EORTC, European Organization for Research and Treatment of Cancer; F/U, follow-up; GATLA, Grupo Argentino de Tratamiento de la Leucemia Aguda; GHSG, German Hodgkin's Study Group; IFRT, involved-field radiation therapy; MC, mixed cellularity; MSKCC, Memorial Sloan Kettering Cancer Center; NCIC, National Cancer Institute of Canada; OS, overall survival; PFS, progression-free survival; PR, partial response; RT, radiotherapy; STNI, subtotal nodal irradiation.

Table 30–7. Standard Alkylating Agent–Containing Regimens: Variants of MOPP

Drug	Dose (mg/m2)	Route	Schedule (days)	Cycle Length (days)
MOPP				28
Mechlorethamine	6	IV	1,8	
Oncovin (vincristine)	1.4	IV	1,8	
Procarbazine	100	PO	1–14	
Prednisone	40	PO	1–14	
ChlVPP				28
Chlorambucil	6 (max10)	PO	1–14	
Vinblastine	6	IV	1,8	
Procarbazine	100	PO	1–14	
Prednisone	40	PO	1–14	
COPP				28
Cyclophosphamide	650	IV	1,8	
Oncovin (vincristine)	1.4	IV	1,8	
Procarbazine	100	PO	1–14	
Prednisone	40	PO	1–14	
MVPP				42
Nitrogen mustard	6	IV	1,8	
Vinblastine	6	IV	1,8	
Procarbazine	100	PO	1–14	
Prednisone	40 total	PO	1–14	
LOPP				28
Chlorambucil (Lerkeran)	10 total	PO	1–10	
Oncovin (vincristine)	1.4	IV	1,8	
Procarbazine	100	PO	1–10	
Prednisone	25	PO	1–14	

Notes: Some studies capped vincristine at 2 mg. Prednisone was given in Cycles 1 and 4 only by some groups. Chlorambucil and vinblastine were capped at 10 mg, and procarbazine was capped at 200 mg in some studies.
IV, intravenous; PO, orally.
From Longo DL. The use of chemotherapy in the treatment of Hodgkin's disease. Semin Oncol 1990;17:716–735,[2] with permission.

tomography (CAT scans) with their greater accuracy and also the higher detection of a "residual" mass. It is anticipated that PET scans (positron emission tomography) will be useful in the assessment of residual disease still present on the CAT scan or routine radiograph (Chapter 10). The current assessment of patients regarding "completeness" of remission includes radionuclide scans, gallium-SPECT or PET, usually 2 to 3 weeks following completion of six or eight cycles of chemotherapy. PET scans following therapy of Hodgkin's lymphoma have shown that a significant fraction of patients will show some faint residual or low-intensity uptake. A significant fraction (~40%) will eventually revert to negative in follow-up and not relapse.[22] It is advisable, in that circumstance, to repeat the PET scan in 4 to 6 weeks as long as there is no clinical progression by clinical or routine radiographic evaluation.

NEWER REGIMENS

The fact that 30% to 35% of patients with advanced disease will relapse or fail to enter complete remission with ABVD has prompted further efforts to intensify the chemotherapy, and thereby hopefully improve the CR rate and ultimately overall survival. The preliminary results of these newer programs are encouraging, and are currently in randomized comparative trials with ABVD.

The first approach, as introduced by the Stanford University group as the Stanford V regimen, was compacting the chemotherapy within 12 weeks with different agents given on a weekly basis to increase the duration of drug exposure.[23] PACEBOM and VAPEC-B, which are similar to the Stanford V regimen, have been studied in the United Kingdom.[24,25] All of the above included radiation therapy to sites of original bulk or "residual" disease. The details are shown on Table 30–9. A randomized trial presented by one of the Italian cooperative groups suggested that Stanford V, as given by them, was not as effective in their hands as ABVD.[26] It should be noted that the Stanford University results with Stanford V were exceptionally good, with freedom from progression at 5 years of 89% and 96% overall survival.[27] If avoidance of radiotherapy is a goal, then all of these regimens need to be compared to a standard with radiation therapy or preferably without radiation to assess their basic cytotoxic impact. There is currently a North American Intergroup trial comparing Stanford V/radiation therapy to ABVD with optional radiation therapy. The pilot trial in the Eastern Cooperative Oncology Group in 47 patients was very positive with estimated freedom from progression of 85% at 5 years.[28] After completion of 12 weeks of chemotherapy, patients receive radiation therapy to sites that were 5 cm or greater. This resulted in a majority having to receive radiation therapy. The degree of immunosup-

Table 30–8. Nonalkylating Combination Chemotherapy Regimens

Regimen (Reference)	Dose (mg/m^2)	Schedule (days)
ABVD (4)		
Doxorubicin	25 IV	1,15
Bleomycin	10 units	1,15
Vinblastine	6	1,15
Dacarbazine	375	1,15
EVA (18)		
Etoposide	100	1,2,3
Vinblastine	6	1
Doxorubicin	50	1 q. 28 days
AV (19)		
Doxorubicin	25	1,15
Vinblastine	6 q. 28 days	1,15
VEEP (20)		
Vincristine	1.4(2.0)	1,8
Epirubicin	50	1 q. 21 days
Etoposide	100	1–4
Prednisolone	100 PO	1–8
NOVP (21)		
Mitoxantrone	10	1
Vincristine	1.4	8 q. 21 days
Vinblastine	6	1
Prednisone	100 PO	1–5

IV, intravenous; q, every; PO, orally.

pression in Stanford V required continuous oral co-trimoxazole and acyclovir. These excellent results entailed about 20% of patients requiring hospitalization. The amount of nitrogen mustard appears to be minimal enough (three injections) to avoid sterilization and secondary myelodysplasia. It is actually unknown whether the Stanford V or PACEBOM could stand alone as a systemic therapy without radiation therapy.

The second approach to increase the CR rate and survival is an intensification of the chemotherapy doses, and this was introduced by the German Hodgkin's Disease Study Group.[29] The BEACOPP regimen has been given as "standard" or escalated regimen[30] (Table 30–10). The BEACOPP regimen showed a statistical superiority to their standard (COPP alternated with four cycles of ABVD) in a large prospective randomized trial with 1,200 patients.[31] The BEACOPP regimen, especially in escalated dosage, also showed superiority in overall survival to COPP/ABVD. The "standard" dose BEACOPP, although more active than COPP/ABVD in failure-free survival at 5 years, did not achieve a superior survival. Myelosuppression was significantly higher with the escalated dosage. In addition, the actuarial risk of secondary myelodysplasia/leukemia was 2.5% at 5 years, analogous to that seen previously with MOPP. This same randomized trial also included radiation therapy to sites of prior disease greater than 5 cm or convincing residual disease. Current trials have modified the program to four cycles of escalated BEACOPP and four cycles of standard dose BEACOPP to attempt to diminish the toxicity. This regimen has been shown to be comparable to eight cycles of escalated BEACOPP, but the analysis

Table 30–9. Hodgkin's Lymphoma Regimens Delivered Weekly, Over 3 Months Only (Radiation Therapy Included)

Regimen (Reference)	Dose (mg/m^2)	Route	Schedule (days)
Stanford V (23)			
Mechlorethamine	6	IV	Weeks 1,5,9
Adriamycin (doxorubicin)	25	IV	Weeks 1,3,5,9,11
Vinblastine	6	IV	Weeks 1,3,5,9,11
Vincristine	1.4	IV	Weeks 2,4,6,8,10,12
Bleomycin	5	IV	Weeks 2,4,6,8,10,12
Etoposide	60 × 2	IV	Weeks 3,7,11
Prednisone	40	PO	Weeks 1–10 q. other day
G-CSF			Dose reduction or delay
PACE-BOM (United Kingdom) (24)			
Doxorubicin	35		Days 1,15,29,43,57,91
Cyclophosphamide	300		Days 1,15,29,43,57,91
Etoposide	150		Days 1,15,29,43,57,91
Bleomycin	10		Days 8,22,36,50,69,78
Vincristine	1.4		Days 8,22,36,50,69,78
Methotrexate	50		Days 8,22,36,50,69,78
Prednisolone	50	PO	Daily for 4 weeks, then alternate days for 8 weeks
VAPEC-B (United Kingdom) (25)			
Doxorubicin	35		Weeks 1,3,5,7,9,11
Cyclophosphamide	350		Weeks 1,5,9
Etoposide	75–100	PO q. day × 5	Weeks 3.7.11
Vincristine	1.4		Weeks 2,4,6,8,10
Bleomycin	10,000 units		Weeks 2,4,6,8,10
Prednisolone	50		PO daily to week 6, then taper over 10 days

IV, intravenous; q, every; PO, orally.

Table 30–10. Intensive and Hybrid Regimens

Drug Regimen (Reference)	Dose (mg/m^2)	Route	Schedule (days)	Cycle Length (days)
ChlVPP/EVA (12)				28
Chlorambucil	10 total	PO	1–7	
Vinblastine	10 total	IV	1	
Procarbazine	150 total	PO	1–7	
Prednisolone	50 total	PO	1–7	
Etoposide	200	IV	8	
Vincristine	2 total	IV	8	
Adriamycin (doxorubicin)	50	IV	8	
BEACOPP (escalated BEACOPP) (30)				28
Bleomycin	10	IV	8	
Etoposide	100 (200)	IV	1–3	
Adriamycin (doxorubicin)	25	IV	1	
Cyclophosphamide	650 (1250)	IV	1	
Oncovin (vincristine)	1.4*	IV	8	
Procarbazine	100	PO	1–7	
Prednisone	40	PO	1–14	
G-CSF	– (+)	SQ	8+	
MOPP/ABV hybrid (Vancouver) (9)				28
Mechlorethamine	6	IV	1	
Oncovin (vincristine)	1.4[a]	IV	1	
Procarbazine	100	PO	1–7	
Prednisone	40	PO	1–14	
Adriamycin (doxorubicin)	35	IV	8	
Bleomycin	10	IV	8	
Vinblastine	6	IV	8	

[a]Vincristine dose capped at 2 mg.
IV, intravenous; PO, orally.

is only at 24 months. Also, the addition of radiation therapy in this GHSG trial (HD12) did not show any early advantage.[32] A certain caution is required with dose escalation, since this trial had a 3.3% mortality rate due to toxicity, and acute myeloid leukemia/myelodysplastic syndrome (AML/MDS) continues to be seen.

Patients presenting with poor prognostic features clearly need a more effective program than ABVD. Fortunately, such patients represent no more than 15%, but with a higher rate of relapse (40% to 60%) with "standard" regimens. Whether a significant improvement can be achieved with regimens like BEACOPP is the subject of the current international prospective trial comparing four/four BEACOPP to ABVD *without* radiation therapy in both arms of the trial.

COMBINED MODALITY THERAPY FOR ADVANCED DISEASE

The value of complementary radiotherapy in advanced Hodgkin's disease (HD) after achieving a CR or CR undetermined (CRu) partial response but with a negative PET scan has been questioned. Randomized trials and an extensive meta-analysis have suggested that overall survival is *not* significantly improved by adding radiation therapy to patients effectively treated with chemotherapy. The meta-analysis featured trials in which radiation was given concurrently or sequentially and in no subgroups was survival improved.[33] Randomized trials that compared the addition of radiation therapy after achieving complete remission to two additional cycles of chemotherapy showed no difference in survival outcome.[34,35] The EORTC (European Organization for Research and Development of Cancer) has completed a trial testing whether radiation therapy to prior sites of disease adds to the survival of patients with advanced disease who achieved a complete response. It did not improve the survival achieved with chemotherapy alone. Patients in partial response were irradiated and did as well as the CR patients.[36] These patients were not assessed with radionuclide scans. It is possible that some "partial response" patients may have been "CR" with a residual CAT scan abnormality that may have been rendered free of tumor. Ten years previously, the Southwest Oncology Group (SWOG) trial of radiation following a CR achieved by MOP-BAP showed no impact on survival by the combined modality arm of the trial.[37]

Up until recently, radiation therapy was routinely given to "bulky" or prior sites of disease after a full course of chemotherapy. After the above mentioned results, it would appear that patients in CR could be spared radiation if a CR or CRu is confirmed with a negative PET scan. The issue is not insignificant since the actuarial risk of radiation-induced secondary solid tumors and serious cardiovascular disease approaches 20% to 30% at 20 to 25 years of follow-up.[38–41] The cardiovascular complications of radiation therapy include vascular, coronary, and myocardial toxicities.[42,43] It is anticipated and hoped that current limitations in doses and fields confined to involved-field radiation will significantly reduce these risks. Parenthetically, almost all trials of chemotherapy followed by a randomization to extended-field or involved-field radiation showed no survival advantage for the combined modality.[44]

BIOLOGIC MARKERS OF RESPONSE TO SYSTEMIC THERAPY

The clinical features which contributed to International Prognostic Scheme (IPS) for advanced HD remain the best determinant of subsequent response and survival. Few biologic features have been studied. One report suggested that interleukin 6 (IL-6) expression by the Reed–Sternberg cells was associated with a higher rate of B symptoms and a lower CR rate, but no difference in survival.[45] Circulating serum-soluble CD30 is known to be correlated with greater burden of disease. A recent series suggested that an IPS greater than 2, and a high serum concentration (>100 IU/mL) of soluble CD30 had a failure-free survival of only 44%.[46] A number of other biologic measurements appear to be associated with a comparatively poorer outcome. They include detectable circulating IL-10 levels[47]; tissue eosinophilia[48]; and mast cell infiltration.[49] Epstein–Barr virus encoded latent membrane protein-1 when present was associated with a small improvement in failure-free survival in two series in long-term follow-up for patients under age 30.[50,51] The differences are small and not placed in a multivariate analysis with the IPS system.

ADVANCED NODULAR LYMPHOCYTE–PREDOMINANT HODGKIN'S LYMPHOMA

NLPHD has an indolent natural history with an impressive (over 90%) 20-year survival despite a relapse rate of about 50% over the same period.[52] The immunophenotype is distinctly different from classic HL and more reflective of a low-grade B-cell lymphoma but with an even better outcome. The very low-grade nature calls into question whether cell-cycle active agents, such as doxorubicin, can achieve the same long-term benefits seen in classic HL. There are virtually no comparative studies of chemotherapy alone for NLPHD, and thus ABVD continues to be used. There is a small series of salvage chemotherapy with ABVD for patients relapsing from radiation, which showed a poor outcome with only 2 or 6 achieving durable responses, as opposed to durable responses in 8 of 12 treated with MOPP or MOPP-like regimens.[53] The role of CD20 positivity in classic HL as to response to ABVD is controversial. A small retrospective series suggested a poorer outcome with ABVD, but no differences with alkylating agent-containing regimens.[54] This could not be supported by a large (300 patients) multiinstitutional review of CD20 positivity and ABVD chemotherapy in classic HD.[55] The CD20 positivity of NLPHD and rarely in classic HL may contribute to the utility of the anti-CD20 antibody rituximab in patients requiring systemic therapy. Two published series showed a very high response rate in previously treated NLPHD patients of 100% and 86%, respectively, including CR in 41% and 57%.[56,57] The responses last a median of 10 to 20 months. Conversion to large-cell lymphoma (LCL) can occur as a result of clonal progression in 3% to 7% of patients.[58] Treatment of this eventuality requires more aggressive chemotherapy tailored to a large-cell lymphoma.[59]

CHEMOTHERAPY IN THE ELDERLY

The overall survival of patients over age 60 treated with standard regimens is consistently poorer than that seen in younger patients.[60] In the assessment of efficacy, the University of Nebraska experience suggests that the inclusion of doxorubicin, however, significantly increases the 5-year survival results to 67% compared to a regimen, ChlVPP, without doxorubicin (30%).[61] A recent modified regimen, VEPEMB (vinblastine, cyclophosphamide, procarbazine, etoposide, mitoxantrone, and bleomycin) was adapted as a less aggressive regimen for the elderly, but the failure-free survival was only 34% in advanced disease.[62] No clear conclusion for the treatment of the elderly can be drawn, except to say that ABVD can be given to many at full doses. There are few data on the use of liposomal encapsulated doxorubicin, which is likely to be more cardioprotective. In all instances, good clinical judgment should prevail on the selection of treatment and its goals.

Summation

The approach to the newly diagnosed patient with advanced HL is likely to change in the future, but the commonly used standard regimen remains ABVD with or without radiation, and this is the standard against which the newer and more intense programs, such as BEACOPP and Stanford V, are being compared. It is uncertain at this time (2004) whether the short-term and long-term toxic risks associated with increased intensity, especially with alkylating agents and etoposide or the extensive application of radiation therapy added to the 3-month weekly regimens, Stanford V or PACE-BOM, will subtract from any disease-free and survival superiority compressed to ABVD. The value of complementary radiotherapy to prior sites of disease of patients in CR or residual areas that are PET-scan negative is questionable, based on both randomized trials and meta-analysis. The long-term risks of radiation to the cardiovascular system and radiation-induced cancer are considerable, especially in patients younger than 30 or 35. It is anticipated that clinical research with radionuclide scans will define patients who may benefit from complementary radiation therapy. Until some of these issues are clarified, clinical judgment based on the current body of experience should prevail.

SALVAGE THERAPY

Failure of initial systemic chemotherapy for advanced disease occurs on average in about 30% of patients, the percentage varying according to presence of the number of negative prognostic factors. A breakdown of the types of failure includes one-third as induction failures, which encompasses true partial remission, and a minority defined as primary progressive disease (5% to 6% of the total); and two-thirds as relapse from CR, the majority will occur within 12 months of CR, leaving about 20% of all relapses as late relapsers in excess of 12 months.[63] The latter dura-

Table 30–11. Selected Salvage Regimens (Published Since 1995)

Drug Regimen (Reference)	Dose, Route	Schedule
DHAP (76)		
Dexamethasone	40 mg/m^2 IV	Days 1–4
Cisplatin	100 mg/m^2 IV continuous infusion	Day 1
Cytarabine	2 g/m^2 IV over 3 hours q. 12 hours	Day 2
G-CSF corticosteroid eye drops	q. 12–17 days	
Mini-BEAM (77)		
BCNU (carmustine)	60 mg/m^2 IV	Day 1
Etoposide	75 mg/m^2 IV q. 12 hours	Days 2–5
Cytarabine	100 mg/m^2 IV q. 12 hours	Days 205
Melphalan	30 mg/m^2 IV × 1; repeated q. 4–6 weeks	Day 6
ICE (72)		
Ifosfamide (equal dose of Mesna)	5.0 g/m^2 continuous infusion 24 hours	Day 2
Carboplatin	AUC 5 IV (maximum 800 mg)	Day 2
Etoposide	100 mg/m^2 IV	Days 1–3
G-CSF	Usual 2 cycles with 2-week interval	Days 5–12
MINE (GELA) (75)		
Mitoguazone	500 mg/m^2	Days 1 and 5
Ifosfamide	1500 mg/m^2	Day 1–5
Vinorelbine	15 mg/m^2	Days 1 and 5
Etoposide	150 mg/m^2, q. 28 Days	Day 1–3
DEXABEAM (German Hodgkin'sStudy Group) (78)		
Dexamethasone	8 mg PO q. 8 hours	Days 1–10
Carmustine	60 mg/m^2 IV	Day 2
Etoposide	250 mg/m^2 IV	Days 4–7
Cytarabine	100 mg/m^2 IV q. 8 hours	Days 4–7
Melphalan	20 mg/m^2 IV, next cycle given when counts recover	Day 3

IV, intravenous; q, every; PO, orally.

tion has been defined in a large number of prognostic series as a favorable circumstance for successful second-line salvage.[64–66] The German Hodgkin's Disease Study Group in a study of 2,422 patients based the outcome of salvage therapy on three risk factors: clinical stage at relapse, time to relapse, and the presence of anemia.[67] In general, freedom from second failure and overall survival at a median of 45 months was 33% and 46%, respectively, for early relapse, and 43% and 71% for late relapse. Primary progressive disease is defined as progression of disease without response, or relapse within 90 days at end of treatment. It has a particularly poor second-line outcome with only 17% freedom from failure and 26% 5-year survival with conventional dose salvage therapy. However, a subgroup that received high-dose therapy with stem cell transplant had 31% freedom from failure and survival of 43% at 5 years.[68] Another series with 75 consecutive patients emphasized the feasibility and success of high-dose chemotherapy (HDCT) for primary progressive HL.[69] The widespread availability of facilities for high-dose chemotherapy (HDCT) and peripheral or bone marrow support has expanded its use in salvage therapy. With the exception for those who relapse *late* (more than 12 months later) in an *isolated* site and are *asymptomatic*, all other patients should be considered for high-dose therapy. It is in this setting that conventional dose salvage chemotherapy appears to have the same survival outcome as HDCT.[65,70] The criteria that predict a favorable outcome following HDCT can also be correlated with the International Prognostic Factors score.[71] In addition, most series add responsiveness to conventional dose second-line chemotherapy prior to HDCT[72,73] as a predictor of outcome.

SALVAGE REGIMENS

There are a number of commonly applied second-line regimens that have not been compared to one another. Long-term assessment is complicated by the fact that many go on to HDCT. A listing of salvage regimens published between 1990 and 1995 are outlined in a prior review.[74] Those regimens published since 1995 are included in Table 30–11.[72,75–77] All are active to the point that 40% to 70% of patients can respond mostly with partial responses, since only two cycles are given in responsive patients before going on to HDCT (see Chapter 9 on transplantation). In addition to the above criteria of chemosensitivity, the more recent experience in relapsed/refractory HL suggests that the outcome is even better when patients are treated with

Table 30–12. High-Dose Therapy with Autologous Peripheral or Bone Marrow Transplant

Relapse/refractory disease, 1993–2004 (26 publications)
3206 patients
Progression-free survival, 25%–62%, median 45%
Follow-up, 3–5 years
Toxic deaths, 7.4%

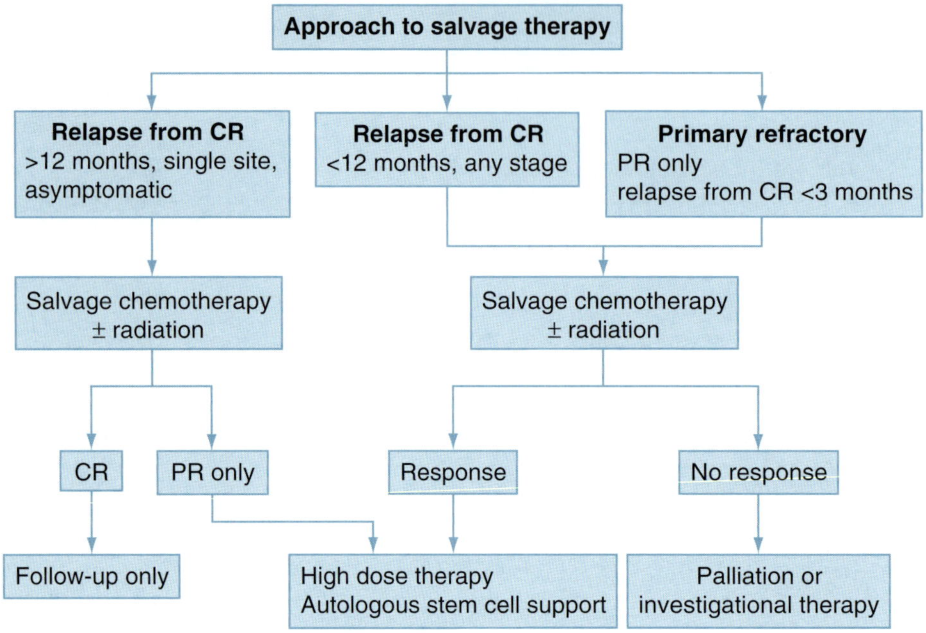

Figure 30–2. Approach to salvage therapy for advanced disease

HDCT while in remission. Table 30–12 summarized the results from 26 series published from 1993 to 2004, including 3,206 patients who showed a median 5-year progression-free survival of 45% (25% to 62%). A trial of comparing aggressive conventional chemotherapy (Dexa-BEAM) versus HDCT limited to chemosensitive patients showed a significant advantage in freedom-from-treatment failure for HDCT, but interestingly *no* overall survival advantage.[78] Most attempts to employ HDCT as part of initial therapy for patients considered at "higher" risk for relapse have been limited to selected Phase II trials. However, a recent prospective Italian Lymphoma Group trial comparing HDCT after four cycles of ABVD versus four more cycles of ABVD showed no difference in rates of CR, relapse-free survival, or overall survival at 5 years.[79] This trial focused on patients with poor prognostic features having at least two of the following: high LDH, inguinal involvement, more than one extranodal site, and bulky mediastinal disease. An algorithm for the approach to salvage therapy is shown in Fig. 30–2.

Relapse following HDCT can be managed with conventional doses of a number of single agents; vinblastine is the most noteworthy.[80] Gemcitabine as a single agent has shown activity, and has been incorporated into salvage regimen with vinorelbine and liposomal encapsulated doxorubicin with good results, especially in patients prior to HDCT.[81,82]

Some patients who fail HDCT may be eligible for allotransplantation, assuming a compatible donor, good performance status, and chemotherapy responsiveness to salvage chemotherapy.[83,84] The same issues pertain to reduced intensity or nonmyeloablative allogeneic transplantation.[85] The approach uses nonmyeloablative techniques for allotransplantation, wherein the HLA compatable donor lymphocytes exert a presumed antitumor effect via a graft-versus-tumor response. Unfortunately, this is not a selective treatment since graft-versus-host (GVH) disease also supervenes. There is experience with this approach that has been associated with some long-term disease control, but the GVH remains a continuing problem. The lower acute mortality rate (20%) is seen with reduced intensity allo-transplantation with a progression-free rate of 35% to 40%. Most chemoresistant patients die within 2 years.

BIOLOGIC AGENTS IN SALVAGE THERAPY

There are no standard biologic treatments for relapsed/refractory HD. The current areas of investigation include monoclonal antibodies rituximab (mentioned above for NLPHD) and perhaps selected CD20-positive classic HD, and more recently, investigational use of humanized anti-CD30, which is only now beginning Phase II trials and is of uncertain benefit. Other antibody infusions have been the subject of investigations with limited numbers of patients. Bispecific antibody preparations consisting of anti-CD30/CD16, the latter to activate natural killer (NK) cells after binding to CD30 on the Reed–Sternberg cells. The preparation was well tolerated with 1 CR and 3 PR out of 16 patients, lasting 3 to 9 months.[86] Similarly, a bispecific molecule consisting of the F(ab) fragments of anti-CD30 and hybridized with antiCD64 has also demonstrated some activity in 4 of 10 responses lasting 3 weeks to 4 months.[87] Experimental cellular immunotherapy has also been approached by ex vivo sensitization of autologous lymphocytes to Epstein–Barr antigens followed by reinfusion of the lymphocytes.[88] Even in clinical relapse, patients can be kept alive for relatively long periods with some of the above mentioned treatments. New agents targeting specific molecular lesions in HL have only recently begun. The constitutively activated proteosome NFκB in Reed–Sternberg cells is the basis for clinical trials of bortezomid.

References

1. DeVita VT, Simon RM, Hubbard SM, et al. Curability of advanced Hodgkin's disease with chemotherapy. Annn Intern Med 1980;92:587–95.

2. Longo DL. The use of chemotherapy in the treatment of Hodgkin's disease. Semin Oncol 1990;17:716–35.
3. Delwail V, Jais J-P, Colonna, et al. Fifteen-year secondary leukaemia risk observed in 761 patients with Hodgkin's disease prospectively treated by MOPP or ABVD chemotherapy plus high-dose irradiation. Br J Haematol 2002;118: 189–94.
4. Bonadonna G, Zucali R, Monfardini S, et al. Combination chemotherapy of Hodgkin's disease with adriamycin, bleomycin, vinblastine, and imidazole carboxamide versus MOPP. Cancer 1975;36:252–9.
5. Bonadonna G, Valagussa P, and Santoro A. Alternating non–cross-resistant combination chemotherapy or MOPP in stage IV Hodgkin's disease. Annn Intern Med 1986;104: 739–46.
6. Canellos GP, Anderson JR, Propert KJ, et al. Chemotherapy of advanced Hodgkin's disease with MOPP, ABVD, or MOPP alternating with ABVD. N Engl J Med 1992;327:1478–84.
7. Canellos GP and Niedzwiecki D. Long-term follow-up of Hodgkin's disease trial. N Engl J Med 2002;346:1417–8.
8. Somers R, Carde P, Henry-Amar M, et al. A randomized study in stage IIIB and IV Hodgkin's disease comparing eight courses of MOPP versus an alternation of MOPP with ABVD: a European Organization for Research and Treatment of Cancer lymphoma cooperative group and Groupe Pierre-et-Marie-Curie controlled clinical trial. J Clin Oncol 1994;12:279–87.
9. Klimo P and Connors JM. MOPP/BV hybrid program: combination chemotherapy based on early introduction of seven effective drugs for advanced Hodgkin's disease. J Clin Oncol 1985;3:1174–82.
10. Glick JH, Young ML, Harrington D, et al. MOPP/ABV hybrid chemotherapy for advanced Hodgkin's disease significantly improves failure-free and overall survival: the 8-year results of the Intergroup trial. J Clin Oncol 198;16:19–26.
11. Duggan DB, Petroni GR, Johnson JL, et al. Randomized comparison of ABVD and MOPP/ABV hybrid for the treatment of advanced Hodgkin's disease: report of an intergroup trial. J Clin Oncol 2003;21:607–14.
12. Radford JA, Crowther D, Rohatiner AZS, et al. Results of a randomized trial comparing MVPP chemotherapy with a hybrid regimen, ChlVPP/EVA, in the initial treatment of Hodgkin's disease. J Clin Oncol 1995;13:2379–85.
13. Viviani S, Bonadonna G, Santoro A, et al. Alternating versus hybrid MOPP and ABVD combinations in advanced Hodgkin's disease: ten-year results. J Clin Oncol 1996;13:1421–30.
14. Connors JM, Klimo P, Adams G, et al. Treatment of advanced Hodgkin's disease with chemotherapy—comparison of MOPP/ABV hybrid regimen with alternating courses of MOPP and ABVD: a report from the National Cancer Institute of Canada Clinical Trials Group. J Clin Oncol 197;15:1638–45.
15. Sieber M, Tesch H, Pfistner B, et al. Treatment of advanced Hodgkin's disease with COPP/ABV/IMEP versus COPP/ABVD and consolidating radiotherapy: final results of the German Hodgkin's Lymphoma Study Group HD6 trial. Ann Oncol 2004;15:276–82.
16. Hirsch A, Els NV, Straus DJ, et al. Effect of ABVD chemotherapy with and without mantle or mediastinal irradiation on pulmonary function and symptoms in early-stage Hodgkin's disease. J Clin Oncol 1996;14:1297–305.
17. Canellos GP, Duggan D, Johnson J, et al. How important is bleomycin in the adriamycin + bleomycin + vinblastine + dacarbazine regimen? J Clin Oncol 2004;22:1532–3.
18. Canellos GP, Gollub J, Neuberg D, et al. Primary systemic treatment of advanced Hodgkin's disease with EVA (etoposide, vinblastine, doxorubicin): 10-year follow-up. Ann Oncol 2003;14:268–72.
19. Press OW, LeBlanc M, Lichter AS, et al. Phase III randomized intergroup trial of subtotal lymphoid irradiation versus doxorubicin, vinblastine, and subtotal lymphoid irradiation for stage IA to IIA Hodgkin's disease. J Clin Oncol 2001;19: 4238–44.
20. Shankar AG, Ashley S, Atra A, et al. A limited role for VEEP (vincristine, etoposide, epirubicin, prednisolone) chemotherapy in childhood Hodgkin's disease. Eur J Cancer 1998;34: 2058–63.
21. Hagemeister FB, Purugganan R, Fuller L, et al. Treatment of early stages of Hodgkin's disease with novantrone, vincristine, vinblastine, prednisone, and radiotherapy. Semin Hematol 1994;31:36–43.
22. de Wit M, Bohuslavizki KH, Buchert R, et al. ^{18}FDG-PET following treatment as valid predictor for disease-free survival in Hodgkin's lymphoma. Ann Oncol 2001;12:29–37.
23. Bartlett NL, Rosenberg SA, Hoppe RT, et al. Brief chemotherapy, Stanford V, and adjuvant radiotherapy for bulky or advanced-stage Hodgkin's disease: a preliminary report. J Clin Oncol 1995;13:1080–8.
24. Simmonds PD, Mead GM, Sweetenham JW, et al. PACE BOM chemotherapy: a 12-week regimen for advanced Hodgkin's disease. Ann Oncol 1997;8:259–66.
25. Radford JA, Rohatiner AZS, Ryder WDJ, et al. ChlVPP/EVA hybrid versus the weekly VAPEC-B regimen for previously untreated Hodgkin's disease. J Clin Oncol 2002;20:2988–94.
26. Federico J, Levis A, Luminari S, et al. ABVD vs. Stanford V (SV) vs. MOPP-EBV-CAD (MEC) in advanced Hodgkin's lymphoma. Final results of the IIL HD9601 randomized trial. Proc Am Soc Clin Oncol 2004;23:557.
27. Horning SJ, Hoppe RT, Breslin S, et al. Stanford V and radiotherapy for locally extensive and advanced Hodgkin's disease: mature results of a prospective clinical trial. J Clin Oncol 2002;20:630–7.
28. Horning SJ, Williams J, Bartlett NL, et al. Assessment of the Stanford V regimen and consolidative radiotherapy for bulky and advanced Hodgkin's disease: Eastern Cooperative Oncology Group Pilot Study E1492. J Clin Oncol 2000;18:972–80.
29. Diehl V, Sieber M, Rüffer U, et al. BEACOPP: an intensified chemotherapy regimen in advanced Hodgkin's disease. Ann Oncol 1997;8:143–8.
30. Diehl V, Franklin J, Hasenclever D, et al. BEACOPP, a new dose-escalated and accelerated regimen, is at least as effective as COPP/ABVD in patients with advanced-stage Hodgkin's lymphoma: interim report from a trial of the German Hodgkin's Lymphoma Study Group. J Clin Oncol 1998;16: 3810–21.
31. Diehl V, Franklin J, Pfreundschuh M, et al. Standard and increased-dose BEACOPP chemotherapy compared with COPP-ABVD for advanced Hodgkin's disease. N Engl J Med 2003;348:2386–95.
32. Diehl V, Schiller P, Engert A, et al. Results of the third interim analysis of the HD-12 trial of the GHSG: 8 courses of BEACOPP with or without additive radiotherapy for advanced stage Hodgkin's lymphoma. Blood 2003;102:27a [abstract].
33. Loeffler M, Brosteanu O, Hasenclever D, et al. Meta-analysis of chemotherapy versus combined modality treatment trials in Hodgkin's disease. J Clin Oncol 1998;16:818–29.
34. Diehl V, Loeffler M, Pfreundschuh M, et al. Further chemotherapy versus lows-dose involved-field radiotherapy as consolidation of complete remission after six cycles of alternating chemotherapy in patients with advanced Hodgkin's disease. Ann Oncol 1995;6:901–10.
35. Ferme C, Sebban C, Hennequin C, et al. Comparison of chemotherapy to radiotherapy as consolidation of complete or good partial response after six cycles of chemotherapy for patients with advanced Hodgkin's disease: results of the Group d'études des Lymphomes de l'Adulte H89 trial. Blood 2000; 95:2246–52.

36. Aleman BMP, Raemaekers JMM, Tirelli U, et al. Involved-field radiotherapy for advanced Hodgkin's lymphoma. N Engl J Med 2003;348:2396–06.
37. Fabian CJ, Mansfield CM, Dahlberg S, et al. Low-dose involved field radiation after chemotherapy in advanced Hodgkin disease. A Southwest Oncology Group randomized study. Ann Intern Med 1994;120:903–12.
38. Aleman BMP, van den Belt-Dusebout AW, Klokman WJ, et al. Long-term cause-specific mortality of patients treated for Hodgkin's disease. J Clin Oncol 2003;21:3431–9.
39. Ng AK, Bernardo MP, Weller E, et al. Long-term survival and competing causes of death in patients with early stage Hodgkin's disease treated at age 50 or younger. J Clin Oncol 2002;20:2101–8.
40. Bhatia S, Yasui Y, Robison LL, et al. High risk of subsequent neoplasms continues with extended follow-up of childhood Hodgkin's disease: report from the Late Effects Study Group. J Clin Oncol 2003;21:4386–94.
41. Dores GM, Metayer C, Curtis RE, et al. Second malignant neoplasms among long-term survivors of Hodgkin's disease: a population-based evaluation over 25 years. J Clin Oncol 2002;20:3483–94.
42. Adams MJ, Hardenberg PH, Constine LS, et al. Radiation-associated cardiovascular disease. Crit Rev Oncol/Hematol 2003; 345:55–75.
43. Adams MJ, Lipsitz SR, Colan SD, et al. Cardiovascular status in long-term survivors of Hodgkin's diease treated with chest radiotherapy. J Clin Oncol 2004;22:3139–48.
44. Eghbali H, Soubeyran P, Tchen N, et al. Current treatment of Hodgkin's disease. Crit Rev Oncol/Hematol 2000;35:49–73.
45. Reynolds GM, Billingham LJ, Gray LJ, et al. Interleukin 6 expression by Hodgkin/Reed–Sternberg cells is associated with the presence of 'B' symptoms and failure to achieve complete remission in patient with advanced Hodgkin's disease. Br J Haematol 2002;118:195–201.
46. Zanotti R, Trolese A, Ambrosetti A, et al. Serum levels of soluble CD30 improve International Prognostic Score in predicting the outcome of advanced Hodgkin's lymphoma. Ann Oncol 2002;13:1908–14.
47. Sarris AH, Kliche K-O, Pethambaram P, et al. Interleukin-10 levels are often elevated in serum of adults with Hodgkin's disease and are associated with inferior failure-free survival. Ann Oncol 1999;19:430–40.
48. von Wasielewski R, Seith S, Franklin J, et al. Tissue eosinophilia correlates strongly with poor prognosis in nodular sclerosing Hodgkin's disease, allowing for known prognostic factors. Blood 2000;95:1207–13.
49. Molin D, Edström A, Glimelius I, et al. Mast cell infiltration correlates with poor prognosis in Hodgkin's lymphoma. Br J Haematol 2002;119:122–4.
50. Montalban C, Abraira V, Morente M, et al. Epstein–Barr virus-latent membrane protein 1 expression has a favorable influence in the outcome of patients with Hodgkin's disease treated with chemotherapy. Leuk Lymphoma 2000;39:563–72.
51. Flavell KJ, Billingham LJ, Biddulph JP, et al. The effect of Epstein–Barr virus status on outcome in age- and sex-defined subgroups of patients with advanced Hodgkin's disease. Ann Oncol 2003;14:282–90.
52. Diehl V, Sextro M, Franklin J, et al. Clinical presentation, course, and prognostic factors in lymphocyte-predominant Hodgkin's disease and lymphocyte-rich classical Hodgkin's disease: report from the European Task Force on Lymphoma Project on Lymphocyte-Predominant Hodgkin's Disease. J Clin Oncol 1999;17:776–83.
53. Bodis S, Kraus MD, Pinkus G, et al. Clinical presentation and outcome in lymphocyte-predominant Hodgkin's disease. J Clin Oncol 1997;15:3060–6.
54. Portlock CS, Donnelly GB, Qin J, et al. Adverse prognostic significance of CD20 positive Reed–Sternberg cells in classical Hodgkin's disease. Br J Haematol 2004;125:701–8.
55. Rassidakis GZ, Jedeiros LJ, Viviani S, et al. CD20 expression in Hodgkin's and Reed–Sternberg cells of classical Hodgkin's disease: associations with presenting features and clinical outcome. J Clin Oncol 2002;20:1278–87.
56. Ekstrand BC, Lucas JB, Horwitz SM, et al. Rituximab in lymphocyte-predominant Hodgkin disease: results of a phase 2 trial. Blood 2003;101:4285–9.
57. Rehwald U, Schulz H, Reiser M, et al. Treatment of relapsed CD20+ Hodgkin lymphoma with the monoclonal antibody rituximab is effective and well tolerated: results of a phase 2 trial of the German Hodgkin Lymphoma Study Group. Blood 2003;101:420–4.
58. Wickert RS, Weisenburger DD, Tierens A, et al. Clonal relationship between lymphocytic predominance Hodgkin's disease and concurrent or subsequent large-cell lymphoma of B lineage. Blood 1995;86:2312–20.
59. Huang JZ, Weisenburger DD, Vose JM, et al. Diffuse large B-cell lymphoma arising in nodular lymphocyte predominant Hodgkin lymphoma: a report of 21 cases from the Nebraska lymphoma Study Group. Leuk Lymphoma 2004;45:1551–7.
60. Stark GL, Wood KM, Jack F, et al. Hodgkin's disease in the elderly: a population-based study. Br J Haematol 2002;119: 432–40.
61. Weekes CD, Vose JM, Lynch JC, et al. Hodgkin's disease in the elderly: improved treatment outcome with a doxorubicin-containing regimen. J Clin Oncol 2002;20:1087–93.
62. Levis A, Anselmo AP, Ambrosetti A, et al. VEPEMB in elderly Hodgkin's lymphoma patients. Report of an Intergruppo Italiano Linfomi (IIL) study. Ann Oncol 2004;15:123–8.
63. Bonfante V, Santoro A, Viviani S, et al. Outcome of patients with Hodgkin's disease failing after primary MOPP-ABVD. J Clin Oncol 1997;15:528–34.
64. Lohri A, Barnett M, Fairey RN, et al. Outcome of treatment of first relapse of Hodgkin's disease after primary chemotherapy: identification of risk factors from the British Columbia experience 1970–1988. Blood 1991;77:2292–8.
65. Brice P, Bastion Y, Divine M, et al. Analysis of prognostic factors after the first relapse of Hodgkin's disease in 187 patients. Cancer 1996;78:1293–9.
66. Garcia-Carbonero R, Paz-Ares L, Arcediano A, et al. Favorable prognosis after late relapse of Hodgkin's disease. Cancer 1998;83:560–5.
67. Josting A, Franklin J, May M, et al. New prognostic score based on treatment outcome of patients with relapsed Hodgkin's lymphoma registered in the database of the German Hodgkin's Lymphoma Study Group. J Clin Oncol 2001;20: 221–30.
68. Josting A, Rueffer U, Franklin J, et al. Prognostic factors and treatment outcome in primary progressive Hodgkin lymphoma: a report from the German Hodgkin Lymphoma Study Group. Blood 2000;96:1280–6.
69. Moskowitz CH, Kewalramani T, Nimer SD, et al. Effectiveness of high dose chemoradiotherapy and autologous stem cell transplantation for patients with biopsy-proven primary refractory Hodgkin's disease. Br J Haematol 2004;124:645–52.
70. Yuen AR, Rosenberg SA, Hoppe RT, et al. Comparison between conventional salvage therapy and high-dose therapy with autografting for recurrent or refractory Hodgkin's disease. Blood 1997;89:814–22.
71. Bierman PJ, Lynch JC, Bociek RG, et al. The International Prognostic Factors Project score for advanced Hodgkin's disease is useful for predicting outcome of autologous hematopoietic stem cell transplantation. Ann Oncol 2002;13: 1370–7.

72. Moskowitz CH, Nimer SD, Zelenetz AD, et al. A 2-step comprehensive high-dose chemoradiotherapy second-line program for relapsed and refractory Hodgkin disease: analysis by intent to treat and development of a prognostic model. Blood 2001;97:616–23.
73. Germe C, Mounier N, Divine M, et al. Intensive salvage therapy with high-dose chemotherapy for patients with advanced Hodgkin's disease in relapse or failure after initial chemotherapy: results of the Group d'Etudes des Lymphomes de l'Adulte H89 trial. J Clin Oncol 2002;20:467–75.
74. Canellos GP. Treatment of relapsed Hodgkin's disease: strategies and prognostic factors. Ann Oncol 1998;9:S91–6.
75. Ferme C, Bastion Y, Lepage E, et al. The MINE regimen as intensive salvage chemotherapy for relapsed and refractory Hodgkin's disease. Ann Oncol 1995;6:543–9.
76. Josting A, Rudolph C, Reiser M, et al. Time-intensified dexamethasone/cisplatin/cytarabine: an effective salvage therapy with low toxicity in patients with relapsed and refractory Hodgkin's disease. Ann Oncol 2002;13:1628–35.
77. Colwill R, Crump M, Couture F, et al. Mini-BEAM as salvage therapy for relapsed or refractory Hodgkin's disease before intensive therapy and autologous bone marrow transplantation. J Clin Oncol 1995;13:396–402.
78. Schmitz N, Pfistner B, Setro M, et al. Aggressive conventional chemotherapy compared with high-dose chemotherapy with autologous haemopoietic stem-cell transplantation for relapsed chemosensitive Hodgkin's disease: a randomised trial. Lancet 2002;359:2065–71.
79. Federico M, Bellei M, Brice P, et al. High-dose therapy and autologous stem cell transplantation versus conventional therapy for patients with advanced Hodgkin's lymphoma responding to front-line therapy. J Clin Oncol 2003;21:2320–5.
80. Little R, Wittes RE, Longo DL, et al. Vinblastine for recurrent Hodgkin's disease following autologous bone marrow transplant. J Clin Oncol 1998;16:584–8.
81. Santoro A, Bredenfeld H, Devizzi L, et al. Gemcitabine in the treatment of refractory Hodgkin's disease: results of a multicenter phase II study. J Clin Oncol 2000;18:2615–9.
82. Bartlett N, Niedzwiecki D, Johnson J, et al. A phase I/II study of gemcitabine, vinorelbine, and liposomal doxorubicin for relapsed Hodgkin's disease: preliminary results of CALGB 59804. Proc Am Soc Clin Oncol 2003;22:141.
83. Akpek G, Ambinder RF, Piantadosi S, et al. Long-term results of blood and marrow transplantation for Hodgkin's disease. J Clin Oncol 2001;19:4314–21.
84. Cooney JP, Stiff PJ, Toor AA, et al. BEAM allogeneic transplantation for patients with Hodgkin's disease who relapse after autologous transplantation is safe and effective. Biol Blood Marrow Transplant 2003;9:177–82.
85. Schmitz N, Sureda A, and Robinson S. Allogeneic transplantation of hematopoietic stem cells after nonmyeloablative conditioning for Hodgkin's disease: indications and results. Semin Oncol 2004;31:27–32.
86. Hartmann F, Renner C, Jung W, et al. Anti-CD16/CD30 Bispecific antibody treatment for Hodgkin's disease: role of infusion schedule and contimulation with cytokines. Clinical Cancer Research 2001;7:1873–81.
87. Borchmann P, Schnell R, Fuss I, et al. Phase 1 trial for the novel bispecific molecule H22xKi-4 in patients with refractory Hodgkin lymphoma. Blood 2002;100:3101–7.
88. Su Z, Peluso MV, Raffegerst SH, et al. The generation of LMP2a-specific cytotoxic T lymphocytes for the treatment of patients with Epstein–Barr virus-positive Hodgkin's disease. Eur J Immunol 2001;31:947–58.

4 Lymphomas in Special Populations

31

Non-Hodgkin's Lymphomas of Childhood

A. Shankar, M.D.
Vaskar Saha, M.D.

Cancer is a rare disease in children, as malignancies among children up to age 14 years account for only 1 of every 200 cancers. Of these, about one-third are acute leukemias, and one-fourth are brain tumors. The lymphomas are the third most common, and comprise about 10% of cancers in this age group. Of these, about 5.5% are non-Hodgkin's lymphomas (NHL) and 4.5% are Hodgkin's disease (HD). In the adolescent age group (15 to 19 years), lymphomas comprise almost a third of malignancies. After that, with increasing age, the incidence of NHL steadily rises.

NHL is a heterogeneous condition, reflecting the diversity and stage of differentiation of the lymphoid cells from which they originate. The histologic spectrum of disease in children is different from that seen in adults. Though low- or intermediate-grade follicular lymphomas do occur in childhood and adolescence, the majority are high-grade diffuse lymphomas. Each type of lymphoma is characterized by a definite immunophenotype and distinctive biological characteristics. All lymphoid malignancies, particularly those that are high grade, may present with diffuse involvement of the bone marrow. This has led to considerable confusion in distinguishing leukemia from lymphoma. An arbitrary criterion of the presence of greater than 25% blast cells in the marrow has been widely used to define those with a diagnosis of "leukemia." It is important to recognize that there is no biological basis for this. Within each lymphoma category, bone marrow involvement is a sign of extensive disease and not a different pathologic process. Although we do not understand the basis for the difference in clinical presentations, acute lymphoblastic leukemia (ALL) and lymphoblastic lymphomas are part of the spectrum of the same disease and should be treated accordingly.

CLASSIFICATION

Prior to the advent of modern immunophenotyping, cytogenetic, and molecular methods of diagnosis, there was considerable confusion in the classification of lymphomas. A plethora of terms existed, and a number of classification schemes compounded this by using the same term for different tumors. The Kiel classification began the process of rectifying this by classifying tumors according to the cell of origin.[1] The revised European–American classification of lymphoid neoplasms (REAL)[2] extended this to include karyotype. The World Health Organization classification further refined this approach and extended it to include all hematopoietic and lymphoid malignancies.[3] As shown in Table 31–1, in children, NHL is mainly classified into one of four categories: (1) lymphoblastic lymphomas (LL); (2) Burkitt's (BL) and Burkitt's-like lymphoma (BLL)/small non-cleaved B-cell lymphoma; (3) diffuse large-cell lymphomas (B, T, or null) (DLBCL); and (4) anaplastic large-cell lymphoma (ALCL). Other types of lymphomas occur rarely in children.

EPIDEMIOLOGY AND ETIOLOGY

While there has been an overall increase in the incidence of NHL in the Western world population over the last two decades,[4–6] this has been primarily in the older population. The incidence of NHL among children younger than 15 years has remained fairly constant over the past 21 years, with a slight increase in incidence for the 15- to 19-year-old population.[7] There is considerable geographic variation in the incidence of disease (Table 31–2). In equatorial Africa, almost 50% of childhood cancers are lymphomas with a preponderance of BL.[8] In the Western world, approximately one-third of childhood lymphomas are LL, one half are BL or BLL, and approximately 15% are large-cell lymphomas (50% DLBCL, and 50% ALCL).[7,9] There is a notable male preponderance, and curiously, in the United States, the incidence is 1.5 times higher in white than in black children.

In 1958, Denis Burkitt described a common jaw tumor primarily affecting children in specific regions of Africa.[10] Burkitt believed that a virus might be responsible for the cancer, given the climatic and geographic distribution of the cases. Epstein–Barr virus (EBV) was first identified in 1964 when Anthony Epstein's group discerned virus-like particles by electron microscopy in a cell line that had been established from a Burkitt's lymphoma biopsy.[11] Later, it was found that sera from patients with the lymphoma that Burkitt had described had much higher antibody titers to EBV than did controls without the lymphoma. The subsequent detection of EBV DNA in BL and the experimental production of lymphomas in cotton-top marmosets and owl monkeys established EBV as the first virus clearly implicated in the development of a human tumor. With infection occurring early in childhood, once infected the individual remains a lifelong carrier of the virus. EBV infects more than 90% of the world's adult population. In central Africa, 95% of BLs carry the EBV genome, while in the Western world, this figure is around 15% to 20%.[12] Two subtypes of EBV, EBV-1 and EBV-2, are known to infect humans,[13] but differ in geographic distribution. While EBV-1 is observed more frequently in most populations; EBV-2 is nearly as prevalent as EBV-1 in New Guinea and in equatorial Africa.[14,15] Immunocompromised patients commonly harbor both subtypes of EBV.[16] Endemic BL and holoendemic malaria are common in equatorial Africa, and it has been shown that almost half of all African BL tumors carry

Table 31–1. Characteristics of Childhood Non-Hodgkin's Lymphomas

WHO Classification/ Updated REAL	Category	Morphology	Immunophenotype	Clinical Presentation	Chromosome Translocations
B-cell neoplasms					
Lymphoblastic	Lymphoblastic convoluted and nonconvoluted	Monomorphic small to medium cells with scanty cytoplasm	Pre-B cell CD19+; CD20+; CD10+	Skin, bone	t(9;22); t(v;11q23); t(1;19)
Mature					
Burkitt's/Burkitt-like (BL)	Small non-cleaved	Medium sized basophilic cytoplasm round nuclei with several nucleoli tingible body macrophages starry sky pattern	Mature B cell CD20+; CD10+; CD79a+ K67+	Jaw (endemic) Abdominal (sporadic)	t(8;14) in 80% t(2;8); t(8;22)
Diffuse large B-cell (DLBCL)	Large cell	Large cells with basophilic cytoplasm. Large nuclei with prominent nucleoli	Mature B cell ± CD30+	Nodal, abdomen, bone, primary CNS mediastinal	Poorly characterized in children, t(8;14) in adults 3q27
T cell neoplasms					
Lymphoblastic	Lymphoblastic convoluted and nonconvoluted	Monomorphic small to medium cells with scanty cytoplasm	T-cell CD3+; CD7+; TdT+	Mediastinal mass Bone marrow	t(1;14); t(11;14);
Mature					
Anaplastic large-cell, systemic	Immunoblastic or large	Large cells with eosinophilic abundant cytoplasm, irregular nuclei (small cell and lymphohistiocytic variant)	CD30+; ALK1+; EMA± NMP± T-cell or null cell	Variable but systemic symptoms predominate	t(2;5)
Anaplastic large-cell, cutaneous	Immunoblastic or large		CD30+; EMA–; TIA+ T-cell	Skin only; single or multiple lesions	Lacks t(2;5)
Others					
Angioimmunoblastic		Small to medium-sized proliferative arborizing venules	CD4+ T-cell markers ±		Clonal TCR rearrangements
Peripheral T cell Mycosis fungoides		Small or large cells with convoluted nucleus (Sezary cell)	CD4+; CD8– T-cell markers VC	Various Cutaneous	Clonal TCR rearrangements Clonal TCR rearrangements
Follicular lymphoma	Intermediate or high grade	Centrocytes or cleaved follicular centre cell [FCC] and centroblasts or non-cleaved FCC	B-cell markers; BCL6+; CD 10+	Nodal disease of head and neck with or without tonsillar involvement or extranodal testicular disease	Poorly characterized in children, t(14;18) in adults

Table 31–2. Geographical Variations in Incidence of Childhood NHL (Incidence per million population)

	Male	Female	Total
Africa			
Uganda	48.5	25.2	36.1
Nigeria	24.1	11.9	18
America			
Colombia	7.7	4.6	6.2
USA (Whites)	4.1	0.7	2.5
USA (Blacks)	0.9	0.3	0.6
Europe			
Spain	8.3	2.5	5.5
UK	0.7	0.2	0.5
Germany	1.7	0.3	1
Netherlands	3.9	0.9	2.4
Asia			
Kuwait	7.2	7.4	7.3
India	0.6	0.3	0.5
Japan	0.7	0.3	0.5
Israel	11.7	5.3	8.6

NHL, non-Hodgkin's lymphoma.

EBV-2. A model for EBV's contribution in the pathogenesis of BL could be that it initiates tumorigenesis where there is a persisting immunosuppressed condition (e.g., HIV or malaria).[17] In endemic BL, it is thought that EBV and malarial infection together stimulate B-cell proliferation and thereby increase the probability of occurrence of the specific chromosomal translocations. Malarial infection is known to cause polyclonal activation of B cells through the production and release of soluble mitogenic antigens, and a general immunosuppression with impairment of the EBV specific cytotoxic T lymphocyte (CTL) response. The immunosuppressive effects are reflected in an observed five-fold increase in the number of EBV-infected B cells in the systemic circulation during acute malaria, after which, during convalescence the EBV-specific CTL response and the number of EBV-infected circulating B cells return to normal values.[18] In regions where BL is endemic, children may suffer several bouts of acute malarial infection each year before the development of lymphoma.

EBV maintains a latent infection in B lymphocytes by either integration of the viral DNA into the host genome or as a multicopy circular episome.[13] The virus is thus able to ensure transmission to cell progeny when B lymphocytes replicate. Although these cells are not oncogenic, if they proceed unchecked or acquire oncogenic mutations they can become neoplastic. While EBV is most closely associated with BL, it has been implicated in a number of other cancers (Table 31–3).

BL is a particularly aggressive tumor, and the hallmark is a chromosomal translocation between chromosome 8 and chromosome 14, 2, or 22. However, it is also true that BLs account for only 30% of lymphomas bearing a *C-MYC* translocation at presentation.[19] Furthermore, the *C-MYC* translocation is not the only genetic lesion found in BL,[20] and *MYC*-transformed cells are usually characterized by the loss of expression of several genes. Cooperating alterations of cell cycle associated genes probably contribute to the pathogenesis of BL,[21] and p53 mutations have been found in 30% to 40% of BL samples.[22] There are subtle phenotypic differences between endemic and nonendemic BL (Table 31–4).

Table 31–3. Malignancies Associated with Epstein–Barr Virus

	Subtype	% EBV Positivity
Hodgkin's disease	Mixed cellularity	70
	Lymphocyte depleted	>95
	Nodular sclerosing	10–40
	Lymphocyte predominant	<5
Non-Hodgkin's Lymphoma		
	BL	
	Endemic	>95
	Nonendemic	15–30
	Nasal T/NK	>90
	Angioimmunoblastic	?
	Anaplastic	>95
Nasopharyngeal carcinoma		
Breast cancer	Medullary carcinoma	0–51
	Adenocarcinoma	
Gastric cancer	Lymphoepithelioma-like	>90
	Adenocarcinoma	5–25
Post-transplant lymphoproliferative disorder		>90
AIDS-associated lymphomas		>95
Leiomyosarcomas in immunosuppressed		?

BL, Burkitt's lymphoma.

The etiology of other NHLs in childhood is not so clear. LL is uncommon in equatorial Africa. Although HTLV-1 is associated with adult T-cell leukemia, this disease is rare in children.[23] As shown in Table 31–5, patients at increased risk of NHL include those with congenital immunodefi-

Table 31–4. Differences Between Endemic and Nonendemic Burkitt's Lymphoma

	Nonendemic BL	Endemic BL
Prevalence	Western Countries	Central Africa
Abdomen	80–90%	50%
Jaw	<5%	50–70%
Orbit	<5%	10%
Bone marrow	15%	5–10%
CNS	15%	20%
EBV	15–30%	>95%
c-MYC breakpoint	5′ or within 1st intron or exon	Outside MYC region

Table 31–5. Immunodeficiency and NHL

Immunodeficiency	AIDS	Burkitt's Burkitt-like Lymphoblastic Diffuse large cell Primary CNS lymphoma (20%)
	Ataxia teleangiectasia Nijmegen breakage syndrome Post-organ transplant	
Viral infections	Epstein Barr	Endemic Burkitt's Immunodeficient patients
	HTLV-1	Adult T-cell NHL

NHL, non-Hodgkin's lymphoma.

ciency syndromes (ataxia telangiectasia [AT], Wiskott–Aldrich syndrome, severe combined immunodeficiency, and the X-linked lymphoproliferative syndrome), acquired immunodeficiency syndrome, and those who receive immunosuppressive therapy.[24] In some of these immunodeficiency states, the genetic instability associated with chromosomal abnormality contributes to the increased risk of lymphoid malignancy. In AT, inherited biallelic mutations of the ATM gene lead to the clinical syndrome,[25] and 10% to 15% present with NHL in childhood or early adulthood.[24] In adult sporadic noninherited pro–T-lymphocytic leukemia, biallelic missense mutations in the ATM gene can be detected in 40% to 60% of cases.[26,27] This suggests that the ATM gene acts as a tumor suppressor gene in the pathogenesis of lymphomas.

There is a link between long-term immunosuppressive therapy in transplant recipients and NHL. Although adults treated with combined modality therapy for Hodgkin's disease have an increased risk for developing secondary NHL, it is not clear if this is so for children.[28] Hydantoin derivatives are known to cause pseudolymphomas that regress with cessation of therapy, and there are isolated reports of NHL in long-term recipients of therapy.[29] Various organic solvents, including dioxins, benzene, herbicide, and hair dyes have been implicated in adult NHL, but there is no evidence to suggest that they represent significant factors in the occurrence of childhood lymphomas.

PATHOLOGY AND DIAGNOSIS

This section provides a brief overview relevant to childhood lymphoma. For a more detailed description of the pathology, see the comprehensive chapter on the classification and histopathology of lymphomas (Chapter 1).

There are a number of pitfalls in the diagnosis of children with NHL. Table 31–1 lists the common diagnostic features, but tumors may vary in the antigens present or absent causing a difficulty in interpretation. Benign lymph node enlargement, particularly in the head and neck region is a relatively common occurrence in children. Often this is due to cutaneous infections such as staphylococcus, head lice, or systemic viral infections such as infectious mononucleosis.[30] Rare benign disorders such as sinus histocytosis with massive lymphadenopathy (Rosai–Dorfman disease),[31] Kikuchi–Fujimoto disease,[32] and other reactive lymphadenopathies,[33] as well as acute myeloid leukemia,[34] may also pose diagnostic dilemmas. Thus, for the pathologist the history and sites of involvement are vital clues to the diagnosis.

While in most cases, a diagnosis can be confidently established on the basis of morphology and immunophenotype alone, a small proportion of diagnostically difficult cases will rely on molecular studies to enable a definitive diagnosis. Analysis of antigen receptor gene rearrangements and chromosomal translocations not only helps with diagnosis, but can also be used for minimal residual disease (MRD) detection and monitoring. Various molecular techniques are available, including Southern blotting (SB), polymerase chain reaction (PCR), fluorescence in situ hybridization (FISH) (including multicolor-FISH/spectral karyotyping), and comparative genomic hybridization (CGH). Currently, flow cytometric analysis of differentiation-linked surface antigens expressed by malignant cells is essential for the accurate diagnosis and optimal therapeutic planning for patients with lymphomas. The latest and perhaps the most powerful tool is gene expression profiling. This enables the analysis of RNA expression by clonal populations of lymphoma cells on a genome-wide scale and has the potential of replacing immunophenotyping.[35–37] Laboratories performing these tests need to have expertise in these areas of testing, and there is a need for greater standardization of molecular tests. It is important to know the sensitivity and specificity of each test as well as its limitations and pitfalls in the interpretation of results. Above all, results of molecular testing should never be considered in isolation, and must always be interpreted in the context of clinical and other laboratory data.[38]

Burkitt's Lymphoma

The BL cell of origin is thought to be the germinal center B cell,[39] although several other studies suggest that its origins may be from the memory B cells.[40] Histologically, BL is composed of intermediately sized monomorphic lymphoblasts with round nuclei, numerous nucleoli, and an abundant vacuolated basophilic cytoplasm typical of the L3 morphology of the French American British (FAB) classification of hematologic malignancies. The presence of the numerous apoptotic tumor cells within the pale benign phagocytic macrophages imparts the "starry sky" appearance, the classic histologic hallmark of BL. Immunophenotypically, the lymphoblasts in BL are relatively mature and express B-cell–specific markers such as CD19, CD20, CD21, and surface immunoglobulins, usually IgM and Ig κ or λ light chains, with absence of terminal deoxynucleotidyl transferase expression (Tdt). Almost all childhood B-cell lymphomas express CD10. Ki-67, a cell-cycle–specific protein and a marker of proliferative activity, is highly expressed in BL. BLL is considered to have larger cells than BL, somewhere intermediate in size between DLBCL and BL. It too has rearranged *C-MYC* and greater than 99% positivity for Ki-67.[2]

Diffuse Large-Cell Lymphoma

DLBCL are a heterogeneous group of lymphomas, and morphologic appearances may vary from being predominantly large non-cleaved cell to large cleaved cells or immunoblastic. Extensive reactive T-cell infiltration is often present.[41,42] The lymph node involvement may be complete, partial, interfollicular, or less commonly, sinusoidal. Immunophenotypically, DLBCLs express a mature B-cell phenotype, that is, CD 79a, CD 19+, CD20+, CD22+, and surface immunoglobulin. An unusual subtype of DLBCL is the T-cell–rich large B-cell lymphoma,[41] which has often been confused with Hodgkin's disease and other reactive lymphadenopathies. This variant of DLBCL mainly occurs in adults and is not well recognized in the pediatric population. The histology is characterized by a predominant population of small mature lymphocytes with a few large lymphoid cells. Immunophenotyping shows that the large lymphoid cells are CD20+, whereas the majority of the small mature lymphocytes will be immunoreactive with CD3 and CD45RO. The extensive T-cell infiltrate has been postulated to be due to either an immune reaction to the malignant B cells and/or the production of cytokines by the neoplastic B cells.[43]

Primary mediastinal large B-cell lymphoma (PMBL) is rare in children.[44] The neoplastic cells are compartmentalized into groups by fine bands of sclerosis. They vary in size and usually have abundant pale cytoplasm. Interspersed among the lymphoma cells are benign lymphocytes and eosinophils, which may raise the suspicion of nodular sclerosing subtype of Hodgkin's lymphoma. However, the malignant cells express CD45, which are typically negative in classic Hodgkin's disease.

Anaplastic Large-Cell Lymphoma

ALCL represents a distinct type of large-cell lymphoma, and is composed of large cells with abundant cytoplasm, pleomorphic indented nuclei, and single or multiple prominent nucleoli. Multinucleated cells are frequently present and may resemble Reed–Sternberg cells. Lymph node involvement by ALCL is characterized by preferentially sinusoidal and usually cohesive growth pattern. Morphologically, they show features that overlap with DLBCL and classic Hodgkin's disease. The malignant cells in ALCL have a diverse and heterogeneous histologic spectrum and are subclassified into three main variant types: common or classic type, small-cell variant, and lymphohistiocytic variant. The common type is composed of sheets of large lymphoid cells with horseshoe-shaped nuclei containing multiple nucleoli. Cells with these cytologic features are called hallmark cells[45] because they are also seen in the other ALCL variants. Multinucleated giant cells resembling Reed–Sternberg cells may also be seen among the malignant cells. The small-cell variant[2] is composed of a mixture of small, medium, and large lymphoid cells. The dominant feature of the lymphohistiocytic variant[46,47] is the presence of a large number of histiocytes frequently obscuring anaplastic tumor cells. Other rare variants include the giant-cell–rich ALCL,[48] Hodgkin's-like ALCL, and rare subforms such as the sarcomatoid variant.[49]

This heterogeneous group of ALCLs are characterized by the cell membrane associated expression of the Ki-1/CD30 antigen, with cytoplasmic CD30 positivity being of uncertain significance. By using conventional T-cell and B-cell markers, three immunophenotypes of ALCLs have been identified: T-cell type; null cell type, and the B-cell type of ALCL. The most frequent is the T-cell phenotype.[50,51] Most if not all null phenotypes of ALCL belong to the T-cell type, as they harbor clonally rearranged TCR γ and β genes and express cytotoxic molecules perforin, granzyme B, and T-cell–restricted intracellular antigen.[52,53] In some ALCLs, the natural killer cell (NK cell) antigen CD56 is also expressed.[54] ALCLs that express B-cell antigens are rare,[55] and are now regarded as a morphologic and immunophenotypic variant of DLBCL.[2] Another frequently expressed antigenic marker is the epithelial membrane antigen (EMA), seen more often in the ALK-positive ALCL.[56]

Lymphoblastic Lymphoma

The lymphoblasts vary from small blasts with scanty cytoplasm, condensed nuclear chromatin, and indistinct nucleoli to larger cells with moderate amounts of light blue to blue-grey cytoplasm, occasionally vacuolated, dispersed nuclear chromatin, and multiple variably prominent nucleoli. Coarse azurophilic granules are present in some lymphoblasts. The morphology of T- and B-cell LL is similar and cannot be used as a distinguishing feature. T-cell LL comprises about 85% to 90% of LL in childhood. In general, the blasts are TdT-positive. T-cell diseases commonly express CD3 and CD7, and variably express CD4, CD5, CD7, and CD8. B-cell disease is characterized by CD10, CD19, CD79a, and HLA-DR positivity. Occasionally, either type may express additional myeloid markers such as CD13 and CD33. Rarely, bi-lineage clones carrying both T- and B-cell markers may be detected.

Angioimmunoblastic T-Cell Lymphoma

Based on the lymph node architecture, there are three patterns of angioimmunoblastic T-cell lymphoma (AITL).[57,58] In pattern I (20%), there is preservation of the lymph node architecture. Hyperplastic B-cell follicles with poorly developed mantle zones and ill-defined borders are seen in the lymph node cortex. These merge into the expanded paracortex containing a polymorphic infiltrate of lymphocytes, transformed lymphoid blasts, occasional multinucleate cells that are reminiscent of Reed–Sternberg cells, plasma cells, macrophages, and eosinophils with a prominent vascular network. Pattern II (30%) is characterized by the loss of normal lymph node architecture, except for the presence of occasional depleted follicles with concentrically arranged follicular dendritic cells. The remainder of the node shows a polymorphic infiltrate with increased numbers of transformed lymphoblasts and vascular proliferation. In Pattern III (50%), the normal architecture is completely effaced and no B-cell follicles are seen.

AITL tumor cells are characterized by CD10+ T cells.[58] However, these cells only contribute to a fraction of the cells seen as there are an intermixed population of CD3+, CD4+, and occasionally CD8+ T cells, as well as B cells and follicular dendritic cells. Although reproducibility of the diagnosis based on the histologic appearances is high,[59] in a small number of patients it can be confused with reactive lymphadenopathies, Castelman's disease, DLBCL, and HD.[58] As for most T-cell malignancies, mono- or oligoclonality can be demonstrated.

Natural Killer–Cell Lymphomas

The NK cell represents a distinctive subset of T lymphocytes that lack CD3 surface expression, but express CD56 (neuronal cell adhesion molecule). Neoplasms of NK cells are rare and more common in Asian, Mexican, and South American populations. There are three categories. The first type, extranodal NK/T-cell lymphoma replaces the old classification of angiocentric. The term "nasal" is appended when the nasal cavity is the primary site of involvement, and "extranasal" when sites other than the nose are involved.[60] The second type is the aggressive NK cell leukemia.[60,61] The third, "blastic NK-cell lymphoma," is rare.[62] Histologically, the lymphomas can show a broad cytologic spectrum, but apoptosis, necrosis, and angioinvasion are common. The most common immunophenotype is CD2(+), surface CD3(−), cytoplasmic CD3(+), and CD56(+) with the NK cell leukemias showing large granular cells. In the blastic NK lymphoma, all cells are EBV-negative and agranular. A diagnosis is primarily based on the characteristic immunophenotypic profile, that is, CD4+, CD56+, CD3−, CD13−, CD33−, and CD19−.[62]

Follicular Lymphoma

Unlike in adults, follicular non-Hodgkin's lymphoma (FNHL) in childhood is exceptionally rare, representing approximately 1% to 2% of all childhood NHL.[63,64] They remain poorly characterized with respect to their biology, cellular origin, and molecular genetics. The morphologic features of childhood FNHL are similar to adult follicular lymphomas, though some reports suggest that the lymph node architecture in childhood FNHL may not be predominantly follicular, but a blend of follicular and diffuse patterns.[63] However, in contrast to adult FNHLs, which are low-grade histology, the majority of childhood FNHLs are either of intermediate- or high-grade histology.[63,65]

Molecular Genetics

All subtypes of BL are characterized by one of three balanced chromosomal translocations, each involving the *C-MYC* gene on chromosome 8 band q24. All involve the juxtaposition of the DNA coding sequence of the *C-MYC* gene with the enhancer/regulatory sequences of the immunoglobulin heavy- or light-chain gene resulting in the formation of an oncogene. In more than 80% of cases of BL, the c-myc proto-oncogene is juxtaposed with the IgH gene on 14q32, leading to the formation of t(8;14) (q24;q32). In the remaining 20%, the variant translocation partner is either the κ immunoglobulin light-chain locus (15%) on chromosome 2 (2p11) or the λ light-chain locus (5%) on chromosome 22 (22q11). As shown in Fig. 31–1, the position of the chromosomal breakpoints relative to the *c-myc*

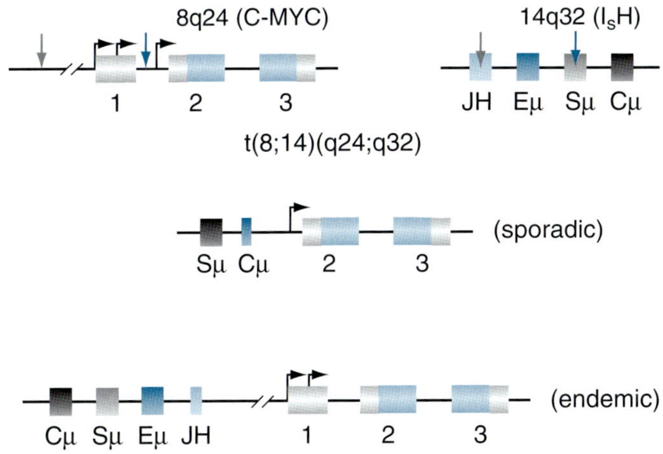

Figure 31–1. Schematic representation of the t(8;14) translocation in Burkitt's lymphoma (BL). The *boxes* represent exons, the *dark shade* shows the coding regions, and the *light shade* shows the noncoding regions. The *line* represents intronic space. *Black arrows* show the promoter regions. The *green* and *red arrows* show breakpoints for sporadic and endemic BL–associated translocations, respectively. On the **top left** is the genomic structure of the C-MYC oncogene, and on the **top right** the IgH locus. In the endemic BL–associated translocation, the IgH locus lies upstream of what appears to be the intact C-MYC gene. In sporadic BL, the breakpoint in C-MYC is within intron 1. As a result of the translocation, the normal promoter region is lost, and a novel transcriptional site is created but the coding region is kept intact.

gene varies according to the type of BL. The breakpoint in endemic BL occurs upstream 5′ of *C-MYC*, whereas in sporadic or AIDS-related BL, it occurs between exons 1 and 2. In the two variant translocations, the breakpoints in chromosome 8 occur in the noncoding sequences 3' to exon 3. Similarly, the breakpoint on chromosome 14 in endemic BL is in the J region, while in sporadic BL or AIDS-related BL, it occurs within the S μ switch region on chromosome 14. In the two variant translocations involving chromosomes 2 and 8, the breakpoints are 5′ of the κ and λ gene constant regions, respectively.

The juxtaposition of the *C-MYC* gene to the regulatory or enhancer sequences of immunoglobulin gene and/or a deletion or mutation of the negative regulatory sequences within *C-MYC* leads to its deregulation and aberrant expression. Exons 2 and 3 of the *C-MYC* gene contain the coding sequences of the *C-MYC* protein, while exon 1 encodes a negative regulatory sequence that blocks transcriptional elongation.[66] It has been postulated that intron 1 of the *C-MYC* gene contains a binding site for the negative transcriptional regulator known as the *C-MYC* intron binding factor. In sporadic BL with t(8;14), the breakpoints are usually in the first intron, which results in the removal of exon 1, as well as the negative regulatory sequences of intron 1. In sporadic BL with variant translocations and in endemic BL, mutations within the *C-MYC* regulatory sequences of exon 1 and intron 1, including the binding site for the negative transcriptional regulator within intron 1 result in abolition of negative regulation.[67,68]

There are no typical cytogenetic abnormalities associated with DLBCL in children and adolescents. Thirty percent of adults with DLBCL have a t(14;18) (q32;q21) as seen in follicular lymphoma.[69] Recent molecular cytogenetic studies suggest that PMBL is a distinct entity in the large B-cell lymphoma group, and that there is a relationship with classic Hodgkin's disease.[70] Gene expression profiling studies further support this relationship. Over one-third of the genes that were more highly expressed in PMBL are also over-expressed in Hodgkin's lymphoma cells.[71]

The majority of pediatric ALCLs carry the t(2;5)(p23;q35) chromosomal translocation that juxtaposes the N-terminal portion of nucleophosphomin (NPM) gene located at 5q35 to fuse with a gene at 2p23 encoding the receptor tyrosine kinase anaplastic lymphoma kinase (ALK)[72] to form the aberrant NPM–ALK hybrid gene. As shown in Fig. 31–2, the resultant NPM–ALK fusion leads to the formation of a 75-kDa hybrid protein that contains the amino-terminal 117 amino acid residues of NPM joined to the entire cytoplasmic portion of the ALK, and exhibits unregulated tyrosine kinase activity. The NPM–ALK protein forms homodimers, cross-linking with other NPM–ALK proteins, or heterodimers, cross-linking with wild-type NPM. NPM–ALK homodimers constitutively activate the catalytic ALK domain in the NPM–ALK fusion protein with consequent aberrant activation of cellular signaling pathways.[73,74] Activated ALK can interact with phospholipase C, inducing mitogenic activity and subsequent neoplastic transformation.[73]

Other variants of the classic t(2;5)(p23;q35) translocation in ALCL include a t(1;2)(q21;p23) and a t(2;3)(p23;q21).[75,76] In both variant translocations, immunohistochemical studies on the tumor cells confirmed positivity for the ALK protein, which suggests that genes other than NPM can also activate the ALK gene by providing alternate fusion partners responsible for activation of ALK. ALK expression correlates with younger age groups and has a good prognosis. The rarer ALK-negative ALCL is similar to the peripheral T-cell lymphoma of unspecified subtype (PTCL-U) and AILT, is seen in older patients, and generally has a poorer prognosis.[77]

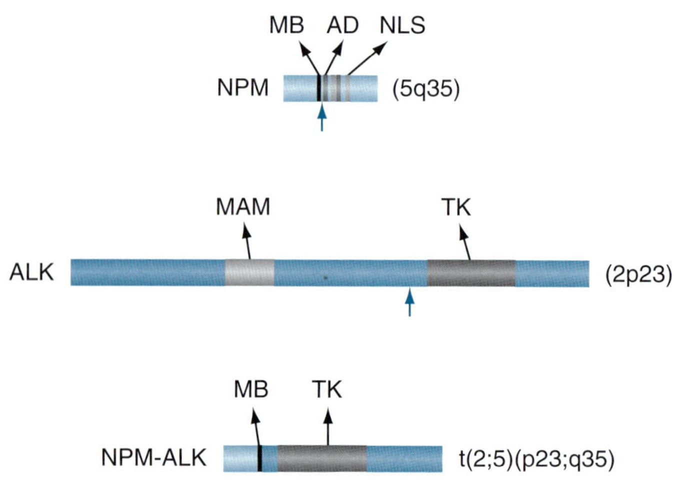

Figure 31–2. Schematic representation of the NPM–ALK fusion as a result of a t(2;5) translocation seen in anaplastic non-Hodgkin's lymphoma. The **top** figure represents the putative protein structure of the nucleophosmin (NPM) gene. This is 294 amino acids in size, and has a metal-binding domain (MB), two acidic domains (AD), and two nuclear localizing signals (NLS). The **middle** figure represents the putative protein structure of the anaplastic lymphoma Kinase-1 (ALK) gene. This is 1620 amino acids in size, and has a conserved MAM (meprin/A5/protein tyrosine phosphatase Mu) and tyrosine kinase domain (TK). The *red arrows* mark the points of fusion. The t(2;5) translocation produces an in-frame fusion of the 5′ end of NPM with the 3′ end of ALK. The figure at the **bottom** shows the putative protein structure of the 680 amino acids fusion product that retains the MB and TK domains.

The lymphoblastic lymphomas are characterized by clonal proliferation of immature T and B cells, and therefore, clonal markers for T-cell receptors and immunoglobulin gene rearrangements are typical. In T-cell lymphomas, gene expression analyses suggest that aberrant expression of *HOX11*, *TAL1*, *LYL1*, *LMO1*, and *LMO2* are critical for lymphomagenesis.[78] There are a number of chromosomal translocations associated with these malignancies, and many of the genes targeted by these events have been identified. These are the subject of recent reviews and will not be discussed further in this chapter.[79,80]

About 90% of AITL patients have cytogenetic abnormalities. Trisomy 3, trisomy 5, and a gain of an X chromosome are the most frequent recurrent abnormalities seen in AITL, as well as in other peripheral T-cell lymphomas.[81,82] Not much is known about the genetic changes in extranodal NK–T-cell lymphoma. Thus far, the commonly observed changes involve del(6)(q21-q25), del(17)(p12-p13), del(13)(q14-q34), and a gain of 1p32-pter.[83,84]

The majority of FNHLs in adults are associated with the characteristic translocation t(14;18)(q23;q21) with the consequent *BCL-2* gene rearrangement and over-expression that protects the malignant cells from apoptotic death.[85,86] In contrast, *BCL-2* expression in childhood FNHLs is uncommon,[64,65,87] which clearly suggests a distinct fundamental difference in their molecular pathogenesis. Most tumors also express *BCL-6* and CD10, which is consistent with the follicular center cell origin of FNHL.[65]

STAGING

Several different staging schemes exist for childhood NHL; none are perfect. The most widely used staging system is that of the St. Jude Children's Research Hospital (also called Murphy's staging), which separates patients with limited disease from those with extensive thoracic or intra-abdominal tumor[88] (Table 31–6). The Murphy staging not only quantifies the tumor burden by separating patients with limited disease from those with extensive disease, but also helps to stratify patients into treatment groups based on prognostic outcome. Patients with extensive bone marrow infiltration or those with central nervous system (CNS) disease have a poorer outcome and are categorized as having advanced-stage disease. A new FAB staging classification based on resectability, CNS, and/or bone marrow involvement better defines the staging of childhood BL (Table 31–6).

Staging Investigations

Appropriate and relevant investigations for accurate staging of lymphomas of childhood are shown in Table 31–7. Modern imaging modalities such as ultrasonography, computed tomography (CT), and magnetic resonance imaging (MRI) are exceptionally good in delineating the extent of disease. Ultrasound examination may be useful as a complementary study to abdominal CT and is particularly

Table 31–6. Staging Systems for Childhood Non-Hodgkin's Lymphoma

Murphy Staging System

Stage I
Single tumor (extranodal) or single anatomic area (nodal) excluding mediastinum or abdomen

Stage II
Single extranodal tumor with regional node involvement
Two or more nodal areas on same side of diaphragm
Two single extranodal tumors with or without regional node involvement on same side of diaphragm
Primary gastrointestinal tract tumor usually in ileocaecal region with or without involvement of associated mesenteric nodes only, grossly completely resected

Stage III
Two single extranodal tumors on opposite sides of diaphragm
Two or more nodal areas above or below diaphragm
All primary intrathoracic tumors (pleural, thymic, mediastinal)
All extensive primary intraabdominal disease, unresectable
All paraspinal or epidural tumors, regardless of other tumor site(s)

Stage IV
Any of above with initial CNS and/or bone marrow involvement (<25%)

FAB Staging for Malignant Small Non–Cleaved Lymphoma

Group A
Completely resected Stage I tumors
Completely resected abdominal Stage II tumors
(Can include lymph node involvement if completely resected)

Group B
Unresected Stage I and II tumors
Resected Stage II tumors other than abdominal completely resected tumors
Stage III disease

Group C
Any CNS involvement and/or bone marrow infiltration ≥25% blasts
CNS involvement includes
1) L3 blasts in cerebrospinal fluid
2) Cranial nerve palsy unexplained by extracranial tumor
3) Clinical spinal cord compression
4) Isolated intracerebral mass
5) Parameningeal extension: cranial and or spinal

CNS, central nervous system.

Table 31–7. Staging Investigations

(1) Clinical examination
(2) Laboratory studies
  a. Full blood count (FBC)
  b. Serum biochemistry including liver function tests (LFTs), electrolytes, creatinine, blood urea nitrogen, uric acid, lactate dehyrogenase (LDH)
(3) Bone marrow examination (bilateral bone marrow aspirates and bone marrow trephine biopsies): morphology, immunophenotyping, molecular cytogenetic studies
(4) Paracentesis or thoracentesis for cytogenetic studies if ascites or pleural effusion is present
(5) Cerebrospinal fluid (CSF) examination
(6) Imaging studies
  a. Chest x-ray
  b. Abdominal ultrasound examination (liver, spleen, kidneys, pelvis)
  c. CT scans of chest and abdomen
  d. MRI scans of chest and abdomen (optional)
  e. CT or MRI scans of head and/or spine if neurological signs and symptoms are present
(7) Radio nuclear imaging
  a. Isotope bone scans for patients with signs or symptoms of bone involvement
  b. PET studies (optional)

useful in assessing for liver or testicular involvement as well as in monitoring response to therapy. MRI is best for examination of the CNS and bone involvement. Positron emission tomography (PET) using fluorine-18-labeled fluorodeoxyglucose (18FDG) is now routinely used for initial staging of aggressive (NHLs) in adults.[89] A recent report of its use in the staging of childhood NHL suggests that FDG PET is very sensitive, showing more lesions than conventional imaging techniques, with a 50% patient upstaging rate. It was also reported to be very accurate for monitoring response to treatment and for characterization of residual masses.[90] Gallium scanning, although very useful in the detection of small volume disease, adds little to the other imaging modalities such as CT and ultrasonography. If a pleural effusion or ascites is present, a cytologic diagnosis is frequently possible using thoracentesis or paracentesis. Bilateral bone marrow aspiration and trephine biopsies are recommended for detecting marrow infiltration because of the unpredictable pattern of marrow disease.[91]

All children with NHL, even those with localized disease, should be considered to have disseminated disease. There are two potentially life-threatening situations seen in NHL. These are the obstruction of the airway by a mediastinal mass (superior mediastinal syndrome), commonly seen in LL; and tumor lysis syndrome, more commonly seen in BL/BLL. Due to the risk of general anesthesia or sedation, a careful clinical evaluation of the patient should be carried out and the least invasive approach chosen to establish a diagnosis. Bone marrow aspirate and biopsy should be performed early. If there is a pleural effusion, a cytologic diagnosis is often made from a thoracocentesis. A lymph node biopsy or a CT-guided core needle should be done where possible to avoid more invasive procedures such as thoracoscopy or thoracotomy. Sometimes, these investigative procedures are best done in an intensive care setting.

CLINICAL PRESENTATIONS

Burkitt's Lymphoma

About 90% of patients with sporadic BL present with abdominal tumors, with or without gross ascites.[8,92] Clinical symptoms include abdominal distension or swelling in the right iliac fossa, abdominal pain, and vomiting, which are due to intestinal obstruction caused either by tumor compression of the bowel lumen or intussusception. The primary site is usually in the ileocacal region, although the appendix or colon may also be involved. About 15% to 20% of patients present with bone pain, pallor, and mucosal bleeding due to bone marrow infiltration. CNS involvement, although uncommon in sporadic BL, usually presents as meningeal infiltration, cranial nerve palsies, or as an epidural mass with spinal cord compression.

The predominant primary site of disease in children with endemic BL is the jaw. This is age dependent and more common in children under age 5 years. Abdominal tumors are also common in endemic BL occurring in approximately 50% of patients. Other primary sites include the orbit, ovary, and spine. CNS involvement is more common in endemic BL than in sporadic BL, whereas bone marrow involvement is distinctly uncommon. Table 31–5 compares the primary sites of disease in endemic and sporadic BL.

Diffuse Large-Cell Lymphoma

Most children and adolescents with DLBCL have advanced-stage disease at diagnosis, and usually present with an intra-abdominal tumor or less often as PMBL. The clinical behavior of primary abdominal tumors is very similar to BL and will not be discussed any further.

Primary Mediastinal Large B-Cell Lymphoma with Sclerosis

Large-cell lymphoma (LCL) arising in the mediastinum is a heterogeneous group of NHL that includes B-cell lymphomas as well as T-cell lymphomas and ALCL. PMBL is now considered as a separate and distinct form of large B-cell lymphoma, which is thought to be derived from mature thymic B cells.[93–95] It generally affects older children or young adults, and patients usually have large anterior mediastinal tumors that often infiltrate adjacent structures including the lungs. Patients may present with clinical symptoms and signs of acute superior vena caval obstruction, as well as respiratory distress with pleural and/or pericardial effusion. Involvement of the bone marrow or CNS at diagnosis is rare.

Lymphoblastic Lymphomas

T-cell LL presents with a mediastinal mass and symptoms of airway compression. Children may have dyspnea, coughing, and swelling of the face, neck, and upper trunk (superior vena cava or superior mediastinum syndrome). Occasionally, a Horner syndrome or hoarseness of the voice may indicate peripheral nerve involvement. Many children will have an associated pleural effusion, and some may have high white cell counts and involvement of the bone marrow.[96] A child with a large mediastinal mass is a medical emergency, as there can be rapidly progressing compromise of the airway leading to respiratory failure. B-cell LL usually presents with bone marrow failure as a consequence of bone marrow involvement. A small number of patients present with primary extramedullary disease with deposits in the skin, bone, gonads, and/or lymph nodes.[97]

Anaplastic Large-Cell Lymphoma

ALCL usually affects the older male child with the median age of diagnosis being between 10 to 11 years. The usual clinical presentation in more than 90% of patients is one of painless generalized lymphadenopathy. More than 50% of patients with ALCL will have B symptoms at diagnosis and, unlike other childhood NHLs, extranodal involvement is seen in more than two thirds of the patients. The usual extranodal sites include skin, bone, lungs, soft tissue, and the gastrointestinal tract. Dissemination to the bone marrow is very uncommon, and CNS involvement is extremely rare. Most patients present with advanced-stage disease.

The Murphy staging system is inappropriate for ALCL, as the majority of patients have advanced-stage disease at diagnosis. The current international collaborative ALCL study groups patients on the basis of known adverse risk factors, which is more appropriate as it allows for stratification of treatment according to risk rather than stage (Table 31–8).

Table 31–8. Prognostic Grouping for Anaplastic Large-Cell Lymphoma

Group A	Completely resected localized disease
Group B (Good risk)	No skin or mediastinal involvement Nonlymphohistiocytic variant
Group C (Poor risk)	Any of the following Biopsy-proven skin lesion (unless fully resected/Group A) Mediastinal and/or lung involvement Lymphohistiocytic variant
Group D	CNS involvement[a]

[a] CNS involvement is defined as presence of cranial nerve paralysis and/or demonstration of an intracerebral lesion and/or presence of malignant cells on a CSF cytospin preparation.

Other Peripheral T-Cell Diseases

AITL is mainly a disease of the elderly and rarely seen in childhood.[98,99] It typically presents with a systemic illness, fever, night sweats, and loss of weight, often mimicking an infectious process. The majority of patients have a hepatosplenomegaly and a pruritic skin rash. NK-cell neoplasms are highly aggressive, and show a strong association with EBV.[100] Extranodal NK/T-cell lymphoma most commonly affects the nasal cavity and other mucosal sites of the upper airway and esophagus. Patients present with nasal obstruction or midfacial destruction.[60,101] Patients with the extranasal form of the lymphoma often present with advanced disease, commonly involving the skin, gastrointestinal tract, testes, and soft tissue, and the prognosis is even worse.[102,103] **Hepatosplenic T-cell lymphoma** is an extranodal and systemic neoplasm derived from cytotoxic T cells usually of $\gamma\delta$ T-cell receptor type. Patients present with marked hepatosplenomegaly but with no peripheral lymphadenopathy. The bone marrow is almost nearly always involved, although neoplastic cells may be difficult to detect.[104–106]

Follicular Lymphoma

FNHL presents with cervical lymphadenopathy without tonsillar involvement[64,65] or as extranodal disease with a predilection for the testes.[87,107,108] In children, the disease tends to be localized and has an indolent clinical course.

TREATMENT

Burkitt's Lymphoma

Prognostic Factors

A number of studies have confirmed that serum LDH is the most reliable pre-treatment prognostic factor in childhood BL.[109–112] Even with intensive regimens such as the Children's Cancer Group (CCG) "Orange Regimen" (B-cell NHL and B-ALL 89 (LMB 89), Berlin-Frankfurt-Münster 90 (BFM 90), it is still predictive of a 5% to 10% difference in event-free survival (EFS). The BFM group currently stratifies patients into risk groups based on tumor resection and serum LDH (Table 31–9). A critically important prognostic determinant of treatment outcome is response to therapy, and the current French Pediatric Oncology Society (SFOP) practice is to intensify therapy early for those who do not respond to treatment. Patients with progressive disease or who do not completely respond have a dismal outcome. CNS disease at presentation is an adverse risk factor, predictive of a higher risk of treatment failure in some studies,[109,111,113] although some recent reports suggest that it is no longer an independent prognostic factor with the use of more intensive treatment regimens.[112,114]

Age may be of prognostic significance,[111,112,114] but this has not been clearly established. Use of more aggressive pediatric chemotherapy regimens in adults with small non-cleaved cell lymphoma (SNCL) has shown improved survival outcome comparable to pediatric studies.[115]

The outstanding successes achieved in the treatment of childhood BL is mainly due to the use of intensive multiagent combination chemotherapy along with the refinements in staging procedures and the management of acute tumor lysis syndrome including metabolic emergencies and improvements in supportive care.

Initial Management

BL has one of the highest rates of cell division.[116] Many patients may actually present with biochemical abnormalities of acute tumor lysis syndrome (TLS), including hyperuricemia, hyperphosphatemia, hyperkalemia, hypocalcemia, and renal failure due to the rapid cell turnover of the malignant cells, as well to a high tumor burden. These occur when the kidneys cannot process and/or excrete the large amounts of intracellular contents released during spontaneous or chemotherapy-induced cell lysis. It is therefore imperative that preventive measures be adopted early. This should be prior to and after commencement of specific therapy to minimize occurrence of this potentially fatal metabolic complication. Ideally, children with BL should be initially managed in a pediatric high-dependency or intensive care setting. Measures to prevent TLS are described below.

Intravenous hyper-hydration with dextrose saline (125 to 250 mL/m^2/h) is used primarily to increase renal perfusion and glomerular filtration, and to ensure adequate renal tubular function. Urine alkalinization is best avoided as calcium phosphate is poorly soluble in alkaline urine and may result in phosphate precipitation within the renal tubules. Urine output should be maintained at above 100 mL/m^2/hour.

Hyperuricemia can potentially lead to acute renal failure secondary to precipitation of uric acid and xanthine within the distal renal tubules. Administration of allopurinol or recombinant urate oxidase (Rasburicase) should be commenced early to prevent this complication. Urate oxidase catalyses the enzymatic oxidation of uric acid into allantoin, which is approximately 10 times more soluble than uric acid in urine. Recent studies have shown that Rasburicase is more effective than allopurinol in reducing serum urate levels and in preventing precipitation of uric acid and xanthine within the renal tubules.[117–119] There is, however, a 5% risk of serious allergic complication with Rasburicase. Allopurinol and urate oxidase must not be used simultaneously, as their actions counteract with one another.[120]

Massive TLS on commencement of specific therapy can cause hyperkalemia, which is a life-threatening emergency, as it can lead to cardiac arrhythmias and arrest. Hydration fluids should contain no potassium, and all patients should have continuous cardiac monitoring as well as frequent serum potassium measurements. As long as high urine output is maintained, life-threatening hyperkalemia is unlikely. A rising serum potassium greater than 6 mmol/L is an ominous sign and may require hemo-filtration or dialysis. Fluid overload, especially third-space sequestration such as ascites or pleural effusion, is another potential complication and may require use of diuretics.

Specific Therapy

For treatment purposes, DLBCL, BL, and BLL are considered as a single group of mature or peripheral B-cell lymphomas. Most investigators categorize patients into prognostic risk groups based on tumor burden and stage of disease (Table 31–9).

Limited-Stage Disease (Stages I and II)

Children who have localized disease have an excellent prognosis with cure rates in excess of 90% (Table 31–10). In view of the very good treatment outcome for this favorable risk group of patients, current treatment regimens are less intensive and of shorter duration than those in advanced-stage disease. The success of this risk-stratified approach is

Table 31–9. **Definition of Risk Groups in Berlin-Frankfurt-Munster Group Non-Hodgkin's Lymphoma Trial 90 (NHL–BFM 90)**

Risk Groups	Site of Disease
R1	Complete resection of disease
R2	Unresected extra abdominal tumor
	Unresected abdominal tumor and LDH <500
R3	Unresected abdominal tumor and LDH >500
	Bone marrow involvement
	CNS disease
	Multifocal bone involvement

Table 31–10. Survival Outcome for Children with Localized Burkitt's Lymphoma/Burkitt's-Like Lymphoma

Study Group	Years	Patient	Treatment Duration	EFS/OS
BFM 86	1986–1990	42	6 weeks	7-year 98%
LMB 89	1989–1996	52	6 weeks	5-year 98%
BFM 90	1990–1995	71	6 weeks	6-year 100%
CCG[a]	1979–1985	104	6 vs.18 months	2-year 98%
UKCCSG	1985–1989	33	27 weeks	3-year 91%
UKCCSG	1990–1996	57	24 weeks	3-year 84%

[a]CCG study included patients from CCG 551 and CCG 501. Of the 211 patients with localized non-Hodgkin's lymphoma, 104 were randomized between 6 and 18 months of COMP therapy.

BFM, Berlin-Frankfurt-Munster Group; CCG, Children's Cancer Group; LMB, B-cell NHL and B-all; UKCCSG, United Kingdom Children Cancer Study Group.

reflected in the results of the BFM, CCG, and the SFOP groups. The Children's Cancer Study Group (CCSG) studies CCG 551 and CCG 501 confirmed that a 6-month course of COMP chemotherapy treatment was as effective as an 18-month course in children with localized disease.[121] A more recent study by the same group showed that a 9-week treatment program was an adequate and effective therapy for children and young adults with early-stage disease.[122]

In the BFM NHL 86 and 90 trials, the total duration of treatment for patients with Stage I and fully resected Stage II disease (II-R), was around 6 weeks. The 6-year EFS in both trials was 100%.[109,123] The SFOP group[111] treated patients with completely resected Stage I and intra-abdominal Stage II disease with two courses of COPAD chemotherapy alone. The 5-year overall survival (OS) and EFS were 100% and 98%, respectively (95% CI, 90%–100%).

The recent United Kingdom Children Cancer Study Group (UKCCSG) results of the outcome of 90 children with localized B-NHL treated on two short intensive regimens are comparable.[124] With a median follow-up of 7.5 years, the 3-year OS for patients treated on regimens NHL 8501 and NHL 9001 were 94% and 89%, respectively, and the 3-year EFS rates were 91% and 84%, respectively. Regimen NHL 8501 was given over 27 weeks and included cyclophosphamide, while the NHL 9001 was a noncyclophosphamide-containing regimen given over 24 weeks. Although the failure rate was nonsignificantly higher in the NHL 9001 regimen, substantial long-term survival was achieved without the use of cyclophosphamide. Thus, short- and reduced-intensity treatment regimens are effective in the treatment of children with localized disease. Although the various chemotherapy regimens seem similarly efficacious, toxicity and possible late effects will ultimately determine the regimen of choice in this favorable group of patients.

Role of Radiotherapy

Radiation is not used as front-line therapy for children with NHL. In the NHL BFM 86 trial, although patients received either local radiotherapy or underwent surgical resection if residual tumor was present after induction chemotherapy, neither of these forms of local therapy improved outcome.[123] This was because most of the patients who had relapsed did so with disseminated disease. The results of the randomized trial by the Pediatric Oncology Group (POG) group,[125] in which patients with localized disease were randomized to receive or not to receive local radiotherapy, confirms that local radiotherapy can be omitted without affecting overall outcome. Similarly successful outcomes have been obtained in other trials in which radiotherapy has not been used.[109,111,126] Local irradiation of the testes is also unwarranted, even in children with testicular involvement as the disease is curable with chemotherapy alone.[127] Radiotherapy has therefore no role in the management of children with localized BL.

CNS Prophylaxis in Patients with Localized Disease

There is little need for intensive CNS prophylaxis in patients with localized BL. In the BFM 90 regimen (R1 and R2), patients received between three and nine intrathecal treatments, while in the LMB 89 regimen, Group A patients received no intrathecal treatment. Table 31–10 shows the treatment outcome for patients with localized disease according to various treatment regimens and national groups, showing little difference in outcome between the BFM 90 and LMB 89 regimen.

Widespread or Extensive Disease

Patients with extensive unresectable primary intra-abdominal or primary mediastinal/intrathoracic tumors as well as those with bone marrow and/or CNS involvement are defined as having extensive disease. Table 31–11 summarizes treatment outcomes.

The SFOP group using the LMB 0281 protocol first confirmed that bone marrow infiltration was not an adverse prognostic factor.[128] Fifty-four percent with Stage IV disease achieved long-term survival, although patients with CNS disease had a poorer outcome (2-year DFS 19%). In subsequent LMB 86 studies, patients with CNS disease had intensified induction with higher dose of methotrexate (8 g/m^2/dose) and consolidation treatment with high-dose cytarabine (HD ARA-C), etoposide, and cranial radiotherapy. The EFS for these patients improved significantly to 75% (±9%).[129] The outcome of children with primary abdominal disease, without either bone marrow and/or CNS involvement, was found to be significantly better than those with disseminated disease.[128,130,131] The SFOP group therefore stratified patients into three risk groups of differing treatment intensity[111] based on tumor burden and initial

Table 31–11. **Treatment Outcome for Children with Extensive BL/BLL**

Study Group	Stage/Risk Group	Number	Duration	EFS/OS
LMB 84	III	167	4–7 months	2-year 80%
	IV	34	4–7 months	2-year 68%
LMB 89	B	386	4–5 months	5-year 92%
	C	123	4–7 months	5-year 84%
	CNS+	67		5-year 79%
BFM 86	B-RG	117	11–13 weeks	7-year 79%
	B-IV/ALL	66	11–13 weeks	7-year 75%
BFM 90	R2	167	13–15 weeks	6-year 96%
	R3	175	20 weeks	6-year 78%
	CNS+	26		6-year 65%
CCG 552	III/IV	52	9 months	4-year 58%
CCG 5911	III/1V	46	6 months	4-year 80%
POG[a]	III	70 (Arm A)	6 months	2-year 64%
		64 (Arm B)	6 months	2 years 79%
UKCCSA 9002[b]	III/IV	112	4–6 months	2-year 84%
HiC-COM	III/IV	20	2 months	2-year 75%

[a] POG study was a randomized study, and patients were randomized to the standard arm (Arm A) or the intensified experimental arm (Arm B).

[b] No central nervous system involvement, and bone marrow infiltration <70%.

BFM, Berlin-Frankfurt-Munster Group; CCG, Children's Cancer Group; HiC-COM, High dose cytarabine, cyclophosphamide, vincristine and high dose methotrexate; LMB, B-cell NHL and B-ALL; UK 9002, United Kingdom Children's Cancer Study Group.

response to treatment. All patients with CNS disease were given 24-Gy cranial irradiation. The strategy employed proved to be successful with a 5-year OS and EFS for Group B of 94% and 92%, respectively, while for Group C they were 85% and 84%, respectively. For patients with CNS disease, the 5-year EFS was 79%.[111]

The BFM group also used a similar risk-adapted treatment strategy. This has shown equally impressive results for patients with advanced disease. In the BFM 86 study, treatment was intensified for Stage IV patients by increasing the dose of intravenous methotrexate to 5 g/m^2 and triple intrathecal therapy. Cranial irradiation (24 Gy) was optional for those with CNS disease, and those without CNS disease were not irradiated. With this strategy, the 7-year EFS was 79% and 75% for Stage III patients and Stage IV patients, respectively.[123] In a more recent report by the same group,[109] using a slightly modified risk-adapted approach (see Table 31–8 for risk stratification) based on tumor resectability, stage, and serum LDH, the reported 6-year EFS rates for patients in risk Groups 2 and 3 were 96% and 78%, respectively. A significant deviation from previously established practice was that patients with CNS disease received additional intrathecal therapy with a higher-dose IV methotrexate but no cranial irradiation. The 6-year EFS for the 26 patients with initial CNS disease was 65%, thus demonstrating that cranial irradiation is not necessary for the control of CNS disease.

The UKCCSG obtained comparable results for patients with advanced-stage disease and without CNS involvement, using the SFOP LMB 84 chemotherapy regimen.[132]

The results of the early North American studies for patients with disseminated disease were uniformly disappointing.[131,133] The most recent report from the CCG suggests that the outcome for children with disseminated disease has significantly improved with the use of a short and intensive B-NHL cell–specific regimen.[112] For four different CCG trials (CCG 551, 503, 552, 5911), the 4-year EFS and OS were 57% and 64%, respectively. Patients treated on the shorter and more intensive CCG 5991 protocol (intensified methotrexate and cytarabine) had an EFS significantly better than those of patients treated on earlier regimens (80% vs. 54%, $p = 0.003$). The POG showed a significant improvement in survival for Stage III BL with the use of a short 6-month intensified treatment regimen, based on fractionated cyclophosphamide with high-dose methotrexate and cytarabine.[134]

With modern intensive chemotherapy regimens there is no need to extend therapy beyond a few months, even in patients with widespread or disseminated disease. The SFOP's randomized trial comparing 4 months of treatment with 7 months of therapy not only showed little difference in EFS between the two arms (89% vs. 87%) but also showed lower treatment morbidity with shorter duration of therapy.[129] The HiC-COM trial, a 2-month intensive chemotherapy regimen for children with advanced-stage disease (Stage III and IV) showed excellent results, with a 2-year EFS of 75%.[135]

Summarizing the results of all published studies from the major pediatric cooperative groups, the current recommendations for the treatment of advanced B-cell lymphoma (BL, BLL, and DLBCL) is that of a short dose-intensive induction phase with high-dose methotrexate, fractionated cyclophosphamide, and doxorubicin over a few days followed by short sequential blocks of high-dose cytarabine and etoposide. Since effective CNS prophylaxis has been achieved without the use of systematic cranial radiotherapy, a combination of aggressive intrathecal therapy with high-dose methotrexate represents optimal treatment.

Management of Relapse

Children who have recurrent disease after completing current intensive treatment regimens tend to have a poor outcome.[136,137] Relapses are early with rapid disease progression. Chemotherapy regimens such as BEAM,[138] CYVE,[139] and ICE[140] have been used to re-induce remission, with some encouraging results. The European Lymphoma Bone Marrow Registry results of autologous bone marrow rescue (ABMT) in 89 children with poor-risk BL (primary refractory disease, recurrent disease, or partial responders) demonstrated that the remission status of the patients both before and after ABMT was a major determinant of long-term survival.[141] Only those who had responsive relapse to salvage chemotherapy benefited from ABMT. Forty-two of the 67 who achieved CR after ABMT remained in continuous CR. In contrast, all patients who failed to achieve CR before ABMT died of progressive disease. The St. Jude's and Spanish Groups have also reported similar results in children with refractory or recurrent nonlymphoblastic NHL. St. Jude's demonstrated that intensive salvage chemotherapy followed by high dose therapy was only of benefit for patients with chemosensitive disease. Of the 22 children in the study, 11 were alive and in remission. Ten of the 11 had nonlymphoblastic NHL, and all 10 had chemosensitive disease at the time of transplantation.[142] In the Spanish study, disease status at ABMT was the only predictive factor for EFS.[143]

Allogeneic BMT is a potentially effective treatment option for patients with relapsed BL. However, the pace of progression of recurrent disease often does not allow search for a matched unrelated donor if a matched sibling donor is unavailable. Only those who survive long enough and remit with second-line salvage chemotherapy will be candidates for allo-BMT. Patients with isolated CNS relapse may be managed with aggressive intrathecal chemotherapy along with intensive systemic re-induction therapy followed by either ABMT or allo BMT. The need for cranial irradiation is largely unsubstantiated though it may be incorporated either as a boost along with TBI in children undergoing allo BMT, or separately for patients undergoing ABMT.

Diffuse Large-Cell Lymphoma

An elevated serum LDH (>500 U/L) at diagnosis is a poor prognostic factor, and is associated with a high risk of treatment failure.[44] This may help identify a subset of high-risk patients who may benefit from dose-intensification chemotherapy. Other predictive factors of poor outcome include performance status, presence of pericardial effusion, and bulky mediastinal disease.[144]

The treatment strategy for DLBCL is identical to BL/BLL, and for treatment purposes it is appropriate to consider them together. The results of the recent POG randomized Phase III study in children with advanced-stage DLBCL showed that the omission of cyclophosphamide from the treatment regimen did not impact adversely on the treatment outcome.[145] Stage III patients with DLBCL were randomized to receive cyclophosphamide-based ACOP or the noncyclophosphamide regimen APO. Radiation was given to patients with bulky disease if there was progression or no response to induction therapy. The 5-year EFS rates were 62% for patients treated with ACOP compared to 72% for those treated with APO ($p = 0.28$). The majority did not receive radiation, confirming that chemotherapy alone is sufficient therapy for children with DLBCL.

Primary Mediastinal Large B-Cell Lymphoma

Most pediatric cooperative groups treat progressive multifocal leucoencephalopathy BL (PMBL) with chemotherapy regimens identical to BL/BLL. The BFM group has recently published its results on the treatment outcome of children with PMBL, all of whom had Stage III disease.[44] Treatment intensity was based on clinical stage, serum LDH values, and response to therapy. Almost all received a combination of dexamethasone, cyclophosphamide, ifosfamide, cytarabine, doxorubicin, intermediate or high-dose methotrexate, etoposide or teniposide with standard triple intrathecal chemotherapy (methotrexate, cytarabine and prednisone), and CNS prophylaxis similar to that used for BL.[109,123] The 5-year EFS for the whole cohort was 70%. The CCG has also reported similar results on the treatment outcome of children with mediastinal large-cell NHL[146] with a 5-year EFS of 75% (±10%). However, they used four different chemotherapy regimens, some patients received mediastinal radiotherapy, and the series included some patients with ALCL.

It is unclear whether patients with PMBL require local mediastinal radiotherapy as part of their overall treatment strategy. Published reports on adults with PMBL suggest that a treatment strategy based on a B-NHL chemotherapy regimen with local radiotherapy is effective in the treatment of this distinct form of large-cell lymphoma.[147–149] While some of the patients in the CCG studies received local irradiation, it is difficult to know whether it was of benefit to them. In the French LMB 89 study, all patients with PMBL were treated with the COPADM-based chemotherapy regimen,[111] and the cure rate for these patients was similar to that obtained for BL/BLL patients treated with the same regimen. In the BFM study, radiotherapy was not part of the treatment strategy, and the presence of a residual mediastinal mass on computed tomography (CT) at the end of chemotherapy did not prejudice outcome. CT may not be the best tool for assessing residual mediastinal disease. Future trials will assess the role of PET scan or Gallium-67 single positron emission computed tomography (^{67}Ga-SPECT) scans in predicting the long-term treatment outcome of patients with a residual mediastinal mass after chemotherapy.[149,150]

Role of Stem Cell Transplantation for Recurrent Disease

Adults with relapsed and/or refractory PMLBL appear to benefit from high-dose chemotherapy when compared with other types of relapsed/refractory BL.[151] Similar encouraging results have also been reported in children with relapsed PMLBL by the BFM group.[44] Caution must be exercised in interpreting these results, as patient numbers are small. Cooperative international trials will be required to ascertain the value of stem cell transplantation for these patients.

Anaplastic Large-Cell Lymphoma

Prognostic Factors

Several prognostic determinants have been identified in childhood ALCL that are known to be associated with poor treatment outcome. Patients with B symptoms, visceral, and/or mediastinal involvement are at a higher risk of treatment failure.[152,153] Other variables that have been reported to have an unfavorable prognostic significance include the small-cell ALCL variant,[154] ALK-negative ALCL,[155] and CD56+ ALCL,[156] although none have been clearly established in large published clinical trials of children and adults. Of the biochemical correlates of prognosis examined thus far, only a serum LDH greater than 800 IU/L appears to be predictive of a higher risk of failure.[157] Recently, both the BFM and SFOP groups have proposed that tumor CD3 expression is a poor prognostic factor with respect to OS, as well as outcome after relapse.

The treatment strategy has been varied, partly due to varying definitions applied to this unusual form of NHL. In Europe, most cooperative study groups have a consensus view on the diagnosis of childhood ALCL. This is the co-expression of CD30 and EMA in large-cell NHL, which has anaplastic morphologic features, with either a T or null immunophenotype. These patients benefit from short intensive chemotherapy regimens as used for BL/BLL. In North America, however, all large-cell NHLs are treated identically, irrespective of histologic subgroup or immunophenotype. This complicates not only interpreting treatment results but also clearly defining prognostic risk factors predictive of outcome.

European Studies

B-Cell–Type Chemotherapy Regimens

In an early BFM study,[158] a short intensive chemotherapy regimen was used, identical to that used to treat peripheral B-cell NHL. Treatment intensity was stratified according to stage (Murphy), and the 9-year EFS for the entire cohort was 81% (5% standard error). A more recent report by the same group showed similar results, with 5-year EFS of 76% (±5%) for the group as a whole and 100% for early-stage disease and 79% (±11%) for advanced-stage disease.[159] The SFOP group obtained similar results with a short intensive treatment protocol, with an OS of 83%, but an EFS of only 66%.[157] The UKCCSG obtained inferior results when compared to either the BFM or the SFOP groups, with a 5-year OS of 65% and EFS of only 59%.[160] All three groups used similar COPADM-based treatment regimens, the BFM using ifosfamide in addition. Staging systems used by all three groups were also identical. Mediastinal involvement rates were, however, higher in both the UK and French studies compared to the BFM patients (40% and 39%, respectively, vs. 31%), and this may have contributed to the poorer outcome in both the UK and French studies.

Acute Lymphoblastic Leukemia–Type Regimens

A few European studies[161,162] have reported favorable treatment outcomes using T-lymphoblastic NHL regimens, but patient numbers were small in these studies.

North American Studies

Acute Lymphoblastic Leukemia–Type Chemotherapy Regimens

The Memorial and Sloan Kettering Cancer Center reported inferior results in children with ALCL treated with ALL-like protocols, when compared to other large-cell lymphomas.[163] On the basis of their results, the study investigators recommended that ALCL patients should be treated with a higher-intensity regimen similar to that used for B-cell lymphomas followed by a prolonged period of maintenance therapy, as used for T-lymphoblastic NHL. It is difficult to justify this conclusion as European studies using short intensive regimens have reported superior results.

B-Cell Chemotherapy Regimens

A recent report from the CCSG described the treatment results of 279 children with diffuse large-cell lymphoma treated over a 20-year period in five consecutive CCSG trials.[164] The chemotherapy regimens used included COMP; COMP with daunorubicin; CHOP-based regimen with etoposide, cytarabine, and methotrexate; or the LMB regimen C. The 5-year EFS was 92% (±3.3%) for patients with localized disease (n = 67) and 50% (±3.5%) for those with disseminated disease (N = 212). Serum LDH >500 IU/L and age below 5 years were predictors of treatment failure. It is difficult to interpret these results, as patients were not subcategorized as ALCL or non-ALCL, and immunophenotyping and molecular genetic studies were not performed on any patient sample. Nevertheless, the EFS rates for patients with disseminated disease are lower than that reported by either the BFM or SFOP groups.

Central Nervous System Prophylaxis

CNS involvement in ALCL is uncommon, whether at presentation or as a site of recurrent disease, and the SFOP and Italian groups have successfully omitted intrathecal treatment from their treatment regimens. This suggests that prophylactic CNS-directed therapy is not required.

Local Radiotherapy

Residual mass at the end of treatment, especially in the mediastinum,[159] is not uncommon in children with ALCL and mostly represents necrotic tissue. Although local recurrence is common in ALCL, most relapses are associated with new sites of disease with or without local recurrence. Local radiotherapy is therefore unlikely to be of benefit in improving outcome.

Treatment of Relapse

On current regimens, 15% to 20% of children will relapse. Of these, 40% will experience several relapses. Almost all relapses occur within 2 years of completion of treatment. Most relapses involve the primary site as well as new sites. Unlike patients with relapsed BL or LL, the majority of ALCL patients with relapsed disease respond well to second-line salvage chemotherapy. Using a combination of lomustine, vinblastine, and cytarabine (CVA) with or without bleomycin (CVAB) for the majority of their relapsed patients, the SFOP group showed that 88% achieved CR2. Remarkably, 8 of 13 patients treated with weekly vinblastine, including six who relapsed after ABMT, achieved long-lasting remission. Likewise in the MSK series, all five patients who were CD30+ and had a late relapse achieved a second CR. In contrast, most of the UK patients who relapsed failed second-line therapy. This may be related either to the use of a Hodgkin's-like salvage therapy and/or due to an inherently aggressive disease, as most of the relapses occurred early (median 5 months) after completion of treatment.

The role of PBSCT in relapsed ALCL is uncertain despite some reports of its efficacy in this setting. In the BFM series of patients, 8 of the 20 patients with relapsed ALCL who underwent PBSCT achieved long-term survival. The SFOP recently published its results of ABMT in children with relapsed ALCL.[165] Their results suggest that prolonged conventional salvage therapy based on vinblastine was as effective as ABMT. The EBMT reported their results of ABMT in patients with ALCL. They have showed that patients who underwent ABMT while in CR maintained durable remission, but those transplanted in PR or with refractory disease had a less successful outcome.[166] Interestingly, the survival outcome of patients less than 20 years of age was significantly superior to older patients, although there was no difference in PFS.

With the use of vinblastine as first-line therapy in the current international ALCL trial, its use as salvage treatment strategy may no longer be feasible. A recent report suggests that oral trofosfamide may be effective in the treatment of relapsed ALCL.[167] Only international collaborative trials based on prognostic factors that prospectively evaluate the role of salvage chemotherapy with peripheral blood stem transplantation will help to increase cure rates for children with relapsed ALCL.

Lymphoblastic Leukemia

As stated earlier, ALL and LL are the same disease. Short-course therapy for aggressive BL and BLL has inferior outcome as compared to standard ALL-type treatment.[133] Within this group, precursor B-cell disease was initially considered to have a better outcome when compared to precursor T-cell disease.[97,168] However, most groups treat high-risk T-cell disease with augmented intensification protocols first pioneered by the BFM,[169] and the outcome for T-cell disease has now considerably improved.[169–171] Treatment of LL consists of a three- or four-drug induction with steroids, L-asparaginase, vincristine, and/or an anthracyclines. Post-induction intensification is carried out twice,[172] and therapy is continued for at least 2 years with thiopurines and methotrexate.[173] CNS-directed therapy even in those without evident CNS disease is required, and frequent intrathecal methotrexate appears to be effective without the requirement of cranial irradiation. Mediastinal irradiation is not necessary in the majority of patients with a mediastinal mass. This should only be considered in the emergency treatment of an airway obstruction or when there is absence of complete radiologic resolution of the mass at the end of induction. Bone marrow transplantation is not advocated in CR1, and is reserved for those who have a delayed response to treatment or those who relapse.

Angioimmunoblastic T-Cell Lymphoma

Single-agent and combination chemotherapy with CHOP,[174] CVP, VAP,[175] steroids with or without cyclophosphamide, high-dose methylprednisolone,[176] COPBLAM, or IMVP-16[177] have been used. Other therapeutic approaches include immunomodulation with interferonα[174] and cyclosporine.[178] In general, while 50% remission rates are achieved with combination chemotherapy and remission duration may be improved with immune modulation, relapse rates remain high.[179] On conventional chemotherapy, therefore, the outcome of AITL remains dismal,[59,174,177] with most patients dying of infections rather than disease, suggesting an underlying immunodeficiency. Given that the tumors are chemosensitive, high-dose therapy followed by autologous rescue or transplantation may offer a cure.[180,181]

Natural Killer Cell

Nasal Natural Killer/T-Cell Lymphoma

This is a rare disease, and all information on therapeutic outcome is based on retrospective analysis of patient series. Radiation appears to be the key,[182] with no convincing benefit of adding chemotherapy.[183] The high rate of resistance to chemotherapy has been attributed to the overexpression of the MDR-1 gene[184] and poor drug delivery due to the prominent tissue necrosis.[60] Attempts to overcome these problems have included the use of anticancer drugs not affected by the MDR pump,[185,186] or high-dose therapy with peripheral stem cell rescue.[185,187] The clinical factors reported to have prognostic significance include stage, performance status, B symptoms, age, and bulk. Advanced-stage disease (Stage III and IV) has been associated with the worst outcome.

Patients with the aggressive NK cell leukemia follow a highly fulminant course. They are usually critically ill with coagulopathy and multiorgan failure.[188] Response to chemotherapy is poor, and the curability of this disease with transplantation is unproven.[189,190]

Follicular Non-Hodgkin's Lymphoma

The rarity of this disease entity combined with the fact that there are few published series on childhood FNHL, makes it difficult to produce strategic guidelines on the treatment of this uncommon NHL. UKCCSG experiences of children with localized FNHL supports a strategy of either a reduced-intensity chemotherapy treatment or a watch-and-wait policy after initial lymph node excision. With a median follow-up of 1.5 years, six of seven patients with FNHL were alive in complete remission, including three who had no chemotherapy after initial lymphadenectomy.[64] Chemotherapy comprised daunorubicin, vincristine, and prednisolone, with intrathecal methotrexate during the induction phase followed by intravenous methotrexate, etoposide, cytarabine, and thioguanine as consolidation/intensification with intermittent IT methotrexate, and the total duration of treatment was around 24 weeks.

An earlier study from the St. Jude's group[63] showed similar survival outcomes; 16 of the 17 patients with FNHL achieved complete remission with a 5-year EFS of 94%. Most were treated with a combination of chemotherapy with or without local radiotherapy. The most common chemotherapy combinations used included a CHOP or a cyclophospamide/vincristine/prednisolone–based induction regimen followed by a methotrexate and 6-mercaptopurine maintenance. The radiation dose ranged from 2.1 Gy to 3.85 Gy. However, children with *BCL-2*-positive FNHL present with disseminated and aggressive disease, and have a poorer outcome.[65]

A significant observation from these studies is that the long-term outcome in children with FNHL is more favorable than in adults, and relatively nonintensive therapy is curative in the majority. These studies suggest that childhood FNHL has a different pathogenesis to FNHL in adults, and future studies based on microarray techniques will throw more light on the etiopathogenesis of childhood FNHL.

Others

EBV-Associated Lymphomas in Immunocompromised Individuals

There are several distinct classes of EBV-associated lymphoproliferative disorders in immunocompromised individuals, sometimes called severe chronic active EBV infection (CAEBV).[191] First, there is a disorder resulting from an inherited immunodeficiency known as X-linked lymphoproliferative disorder. Second, there are lymphomas associated with immunosuppressive drugs given to transplant recipients. Finally, there are AIDS-related lymphoproliferative disorders. For the most part, EBV-associated lymphomas in the immunocompromised host are aggressive and difficult to treat.

X-Linked Lymphoproliferative Disorder

X-linked lymphoproliferative disorder (XLPD) is an inherited immunodeficiency, involving primarily T and NK cells, which in the majority of cases is exacerbated following exposure to EBV. Before EBV infection, most boys with the defective XLP gene appear to be clinically healthy. EBV infection in males with the defective XLP gene leads to three main phenotypes: severe and mostly fatal infectious mononucleosis (58%), lymphoproliferative disorders mostly of B-cell origin (30%), and/or dysgammaglobulinemia (31%).[192] Later in life, dysgammaglobulinemia and malignant lymphoma may also develop in EBV-negative XLP males.[193] This suggests that EBV acts as a potent trigger of the earliest and most serious clinical phenotype of XLP, that is, fatal infectious mononucleosis. The gene responsible for the disease has been cloned and named *SAP* (for SLAM-associated protein) or *SH2D1A*.[194,195] *SAP* encodes a polypeptide of 128 amino acids containing a single SH2 domain. XLPD patients have inactivating mutations in the SH2 domain.[194] Most of the lymphomas are extranodal, usually of the BL type, and often involve the intestine. XLPD has an unfavorable prognosis. Death, which is virtually universal by age 40, is generally because of hepatic necrosis and bone marrow failure secondary to an uncontrolled cytotoxic T-cell response.[196] Successful transplantation of hematopoietic stem cells can cure this immunodeficiency.[197] In the future, gene therapy may eventually become an additional option to prevent XLP.

Post-Transplant Lymphoproliferative Disorders

A variety of post-transplant lymphoproliferative disorders (PTLDs) have been described, and include plasmacytic hyperplasia, polymorphic lymphoproliferative disorder (encompassing polymorphic B-cell hyperplasia and polymorphic B-cell lymphoma), malignant NHL, and multiple myeloma. The incidence of PTLDs ranges from 0.5% to 30%, and varies greatly depending on the organ being transplanted,[198–200] the EBV status of the transplant recipient and donor,[201] and the therapies used to achieve immunosuppression.[202] Most PTLDs are B-cell neoplasms, and arise in the setting of therapeutic immunosuppression after organ transplantation. In decreasing order of frequency, PTLDs occurs after combined liver-kidney, cardiac, liver, lung, and renal transplants. PTLDs arising in bone marrow transplant recipients are generally of donor origin, whereas those in solid organ recipients are usually of recipient origin. EBV seronegativity at the time of transplant and age are predisposing factors. Constitutional factors such as cytokine gene polymorphism, intensity of immunosuppression, receiving T-cell–depleted marrow, and concurrent cytomegalovirus seropositivity may also be important.

Nearly all forms of the disorder harbor EBV, and these lymphomas tend to be aggressive.[203] Their development is probably a multistep process. Iatrogenic immunosuppression leading to primary EBV infection or reactivation of latent EBV infection is followed by polyclonal expansion of B-cell populations with a selective growth advantage. These cells are susceptible to genetic changes, and *BCL-6* may be one of the first such genes altered.[204] Subsequently, other molecular aberrations emerge and drive malignant growth. There appears to be a correlation between PTLDs and EBV viral load measured by quantitative PCR of the peripheral blood.[201] In biopsy tissues, molecular detection of EBER transcripts by in situ hybridization remains the gold standard for proving that the histopathologic lesion is EBV related. EBER hybridization and EBV-LMP-1 immunostains are used routinely to detect latent EBV in tissues affected by PTLD.[203] Molecular testing is therefore increasingly important in the diagnosis and monitoring of patients affected by these diseases.

The most appropriate strategy appears to be the quantitative monitoring of EBV DNA levels and prompt, rather than preemptive, intervention at the onset of clinical symptoms and signs of PTLD.[201] The initial treatment of PTLD is reduction of immunosuppression. Antiviral agents, IFN, monoclonal antibodies such as rituximab,[205,206] cell-based therapy,[207] and chemotherapy have also been used.[208]

AIDS-Related Lymphoproliferative Disorders

AIDS-related lymphoproliferative disorders are a heterogeneous group of diseases that arise in the presence of HIV-associated immunosuppression, a state that permits the unchecked proliferation of EBV-infected lymphocytes.[209] These aggressive disorders include both CNS and systemic lymphomas. Pleural effusion lymphomas also occur and often contain EBV, in addition to human herpesvirus 8.[210] AIDS-related CNS lymphomas are derived from germinal center B cells and almost always contain EBV.[211,212] CNS lymphomas include immunoblastic and large non-cleaved lymphomas. The immunoblastic subtype expresses LMP-1 and BCL-2, but not BCL-6. The large non-cleaved subtype expresses BCL-6, but not LMP-1 or BCL-2.[213]

The AIDS-related systemic lymphomas consist of several subtypes. These include DLBCL, immunoblastic lymphomas, BL, and BLL. EBV positivity for these lymphomas ranges from 30% to more than 90%.[212] The use of highly active anti-retroviral therapy (HAART) has resulted in a decrease in the incidence of HIV-associated NHL.[214] Current evidence suggests that HAART may be safely combined with cytotoxic therapy. Ongoing studies are evaluating the role of rituximab, infusional therapy, and high-dose therapy.[215]

FUTURE CONSIDERATIONS

Despite the greatly improved outcome for children with limited and advanced-stage B-cell lymphomas, approximately 20% will succumb to the disease. But these results have been achieved with intense and toxic chemotherapy regimens, and many survivors will have serious long-term sequelae of treatment, which can include anthracycline-related cardiomyopathy, impaired fertility secondary to alkylating agents, and second malignant neoplasms. There is thus a need to adapt and tailor treatment strategies to reduce the toxicity of therapy, but equally important, to further improve treatment outcome in the highest-risk patients. These strategies will include gene expression profiling, introduction of new chemotherapy agents, and development of novel treatment regimens like targeted immunotherapy and/or gene therapy.

Minimal Residual Disease

The majority of patients with advanced lymphoma achieve a complete clinical remission after initial treatment, but approximately 20% of these patients will relapse from residual tumor cells detectable in clinical remission only by the most sensitive methods. Molecular monitoring of residual lymphoma by quantitative PCR techniques may provide important information about the effectiveness of treatment and the risk of recurrent disease as shown by minimal residual disease (MRD) analysis in patients with childhood lymphoblastic leukemia. A recent study has demonstrated the feasibility of PCR to detect MRD in staging, and follow-up specimens of children with NHL.[216] Quantification of MRD by real-time quantitative PCR techniques will have a major impact in defining prognostic subgroups and possibly permit tailoring treatment strategies and monitoring response to treatment.

Gene Expression Profiling

Microarray gene expression analysis of T-cell leukemia has identified clinically important molecular subtypes predictive of outcome.[78] Recent gene expression profiling of adult PMBL strongly supported a relationship between PMBL and Hodgkin's lymphoma: over one-third of the genes that were more highly expressed in PMBL than in other DLBCLs were also expressed in HL cells. *PDL2*, which encodes a regulator of T-cell activation, was the gene that best discriminated PMBL from other DLBCLs.[71] The same group using DNA microarray techniques also demonstrated three distinct gene expression subtypes of DLBL; germinal-center B-cell–like, activated B-cell–like, and Type-3 diffuse large B-cell lymphoma, that were predictive of overall survival after chemotherapy for DLBLs.[71] It is likely, therefore, that increasingly gene expression analysis will become not only a diagnostic tool but also a prognostic one, allowing stratification for therapeutic intensification.

Pharmacogenomics

An individual's response to a drug is the complex interaction of both genetic and nongenetic factors. Genetic variants in the drug target itself, disease pathway genes, or drug-metabolizing enzymes may all be used as predictors of drug efficacy or toxicity. In oncology, the detection of single-nucleotide polymorphisms has focused on detecting the predisposition for cancer, predicting toxic responses to drugs, and selecting the best individual and combinations of anticancer drugs. Pharmacogenomics involves the application of whole genome technologies (e.g., gene and protein expression data) for the prediction of the sensitivity or resistance of an individual's disease to a single or group of drugs. Genomic microarrays and transcriptional profiling have the ability to generate hundreds of thousands of data points requiring sophisticated and complex information systems necessary for accurate and useful data analysis. This technique has generated a wealth of new information in the fields of leukemia/lymphoma, solid tumor classification and prediction of metastasis, drug and biomarker target discovery, and pharmacogenomic drug efficacy testing. So, ideally in the future, using these high-throughput techniques, it will be possible to not only accurately identify different therapeutic risk groups but also tailor-make therapy to reduce toxicity while maximizing efficacy.

New Agents

A number of monoclonal antibodies are entering clinical use. The most prominent of these is rituximab, a genetically engineered chimeric murine/human monoclonal antibody directed against the CD20 antigen. This was the first monoclonal antibody that was approved for the treatment of low-grade follicular lymphoma.[217] More recently, promising results have been shown with use of rituximab in the treatment of adults with previously untreated aggressive high-grade B-cell lymphomas when used in combination with CHOP (cyclophosphamide, doxorubicin, vincristine, and prednisolone chemotherapy).[218] Recent reports also suggest that the combination of rituximab and chemotherapy (ICE—ifosfamide, carboplatin and etoposide) may be the future treatment strategy to be considered in the treatment of refractory and/or relapsed B-cell lymphomas.[219] The Children's Oncology Group is currently conducting Phase I and II studies that combine rituximab with FAB-type chemotherapy for advanced DLBCL, and results are awaited.

The ubiquitin-proteasome pathway plays a central role in the targeted destruction of cellular proteins, including cell cycle regulatory proteins. Because these pathways are critical for the proliferation and survival of all cells, and in particular cancerous cells, proteasome inhibition is a potentially attractive anticancer therapy. An example of a drug that does this is bortezomib. Phase I and II trials of bortezomib, alone or in combination with other drugs, have shown promise in patients with NHL.[220]

The interleukin-2 (IL-2) receptor is a marker of T-cell differentiation, and is expressed in some T-cell malignancies. Denileukin diftitox (DAB389IL-2 or Ontak) is a fusion molecule of IL-2 to diphtheria toxin, and has been shown to have efficacy in patients with T-cell lymphoma.[221, 222] In addition, antibodies to the IL-2 receptor are also in clinical trials. Histone deacetylase inhibitors are a new class of drugs being evaluated in hematologic malignancies. The drug depsipeptide (FK228) has been shown to be active in some varieties of T-cell lymphoma.[223] Treatment with depsipeptide increases the expression of the IL-2 receptor, and combination therapy with denileukin diftitox in cell lines has been shown to be additive.[224] Thus, many of the new agents hold the promise of inducing molecular targets that will allow the design of molecularly targeted combination chemotherapy.

References

1. Stansfeld AG, Diebold J, Noel H, et al. Updated Kiel classification for lymphomas. Lancet 1988;1:292–3.
2. Harris NL, Jaffe ES, Stein H, et al. A revised European–American classification of lymphoid neoplasms: a proposal from the International Lymphoma Study Group. Blood 1994;84: 1361–92.
3. Harris NL, Jaffe ES, Diebold J, et al. World Health Organization classification of neoplastic diseases of the hematopoietic and lymphoid tissues: report of the Clinical Advisory Committee meeting—Airlie House, Virginia, November 1997. J Clin Oncol 1999;17:3835–49.
4. Chiu BC, Weisenburger DD. An update of the epidemiology of non-Hodgkin's lymphoma. Clin Lymphoma 2003;4: 161–8.
5. Liu S, Semenciw R, Mao Y. Increasing incidence of non-Hodgkin's lymphoma in Canada, 1970–1996: age-period-cohort analysis. Hematol Oncol 2003;21:57–66.
6. Clarke CA, Glaser SL. Changing incidence of non-Hodgkin lymphomas in the United States. Cancer 2002; 94:2015–23.
7. Percy CL, Smith MA, Linet M, et al. Lymphomas and reticuloendothelial neoplasms. In: Ries LAG, Smith MA, Gurney JG, et al., eds. Cancer Incidence and Survival among Children and Adolescents: United States SEER Program 1975–1995. Bethesda, MD: National Cancer Institute, 1999: 35–49.
8. Magrath IT. African Burkitt's lymphoma. History, biology, clinical features, and treatment. Am J Pediatr Hematol Oncol 1991;13:222–46.
9. Birch JM, Alston RD, Quinn M, et al. Incidence of malignant disease by morphological type, in young persons aged 12–24 years in England, 1979–1997. Eur J Cancer 2003;39: 2622–31.
10. Burkitt D. A sarcoma involving the jaws in African children. Br J Surg 1958;46:218–23.
11. Epstein MA, Barr YM, Achong BG. A Second Virus-Carrying Tissue Culture Strain (Eb2) of Lymphoblasts from Burkitt's Lymphoma. Pathol Biol (Paris) 1964;12:1233–4.
12. Levine PH, Kamaraju LS, Connelly RR, et al. The American Burkitt's Lymphoma Registry: eight years' experience. Cancer 1982;49:1016–22.
13. Thompson MP, Kurzrock R. Epstein–Barr virus and cancer. Clin Cancer Res 2004;10:803–21.
14. Sixbey JW, Shirley P, Chesney PJ, et al. Detection of a second widespread strain of Epstein–Barr virus. Lancet 1989;2: 761–5.
15. Young LS, Yao QY, Rooney CM, et al. New type B isolates of Epstein–Barr virus from Burkitt's lymphoma and from normal individuals in endemic areas. J Gen Virol 1987; 68:2853–62.
16. Borisch B, Finke J, Hennig I, et al. Distribution and localization of Epstein–Barr virus subtypes A and B in AIDS-related lymphomas and lymphatic tissue of HIV-positive patients. J Pathol 1992;168:229–36.
17. Buisson M, Morand P, Genoulaz O, et al. Changes in the dominant Epstein–Barr virus type during human immunodeficiency virus infection. J Gen Virol 1994;75:431–7.
18. Lam KM, Syed N, Whittle H, et al. Circulating Epstein–Barr virus-carrying B cells in acute malaria. Lancet 1991;337: 876–8.
19. Bellan C, Lazzi S, De Falco G, et al. Burkitt's lymphoma: new insights into molecular pathogenesis. J Clin Pathol 2003;56:188–92.
20. Magrath I. The pathogenesis of Burkitt's lymphoma. Rec Adv Cancer Res 1990;55:133–270.
21. Hangaishi A, Ogawa S, Imamura N, et al. Inactivation of multiple tumor-suppressor genes involved in negative regulation of the cell cycle, MTS1/p16INK4A/CDKN2, MTS2/p15INK4B, p53, and Rb genes in primary lymphoid malignancies. Blood 1996;87:4949–58.
22. Preudhomme C, Dervite I, Wattel E, et al. Clinical significance of p53 mutations in newly diagnosed Burkitt's lymphoma and acute lymphoblastic leukemia: a report of 48 cases. J Clin Oncol 1995;13:812–20.
23. Pombo-de-Oliveira MS, Dobbin JA, Loureiro P, et al. Genetic mutation and early onset of T-cell leukemia in pediatric patients infected at birth with HTLV-I. Leuk Res 2002;26: 155–61.
24. Taylor AM, Metcalfe JA, Thick J, et al. Leukemia and lymphoma in ataxia telangiectasia. Blood 1996;87:423–38.
25. Shiloh Y. ATM and related protein kinases: safeguarding genome integrity. Nat Rev Cancer 2003;3:155–68.
26. Stoppa-Lyonnet D, Lauge A, Sigaux F, et al. No germline ATM mutation in a series of 16T-cell prolymphocytic leukemias. Blood 2000;96:374–6.
27. Stilgenbauer S, Schaffner C, Litterst A, et al. Biallelic mutations in the ATM gene in T-prolymphocytic leukemia. Nat Med 1997;3:1155–9.
28. Wolden SL, Lamborn KR, Cleary SF, et al. Second cancers following pediatric Hodgkin's disease. J Clin Oncol 1998; 16:536–44.
29. Garcia-Suarez J, Dominguez-Franjo P, Del Campo F, et al. EBV-positive non-Hodgkin's lymphoma developing after phenytoin therapy. Br J Haematol 1996;95:376–9.
30. Tsuruta S, Ohyama S, Arai H, et al. Atypical lymphocytosis resembling non-Hodgkin's lymphoma in peritoneal effusion of infectious mononucleosis: a case report. Pathol Res Pract 2004;200:47–51.
31. Lu D, Estalilla OC, Manning JT Jr, et al. Sinus histiocytosis with massive lymphadenopathy and malignant lymphoma involving the same lymph node: a report of four cases and review of the literature. Mod Pathol 2000;13:414–9.
32. Emir S, Gogus S, Guler E, et al. Kikuchi-Fujimoto disease (histiocytic necrotizing lymphadenitis) confused with lymphoma in a child. Med Pediatr Oncol 2001;37: 546–8.
33. Handa U, Mohan H, Bal A. Role of fine needle aspiration cytology in evaluation of paediatric lymphadenopathy. Cytopathology 2003;14:66–9.
34. Lillington DM, Jaju RJ, Shankar AG, et al. Cytogenetic and molecular evidence of marrow involvement in extramedullary acute myeloid leukaemia. Br J Haematol 2000; 110:547–51.
35. Shipp MA, Ross KN, Tamayo P, et al. Diffuse large B-cell lymphoma outcome prediction by gene-expression profiling and supervised machine learning. Nat Med 2002;8:68–74.
36. Alizadeh A, Eisen M, Davis RE, et al. The lymphochip: a specialized cDNA microarray for the genomic-scale analysis of gene expression in normal and malignant lymphocytes. Cold Spring Harb Symp Quant Biol 1999;64:71–8.

37. Hans CP, Weisenburger DD, Greiner TC, et al. Confirmation of the molecular classification of diffuse large B-cell lymphoma by immunohistochemistry using a tissue microarray. Blood 2004;103:275–82.
38. Spagnolo DV, Ellis DW, Juneja S, et al. The role of molecular studies in lymphoma diagnosis: a review. Pathology 2004;36:19–44.
39. Tamaru J, Hummel M, Marafioti T, et al. Burkitt's lymphomas express VH genes with a moderate number of antigen-selected somatic mutations. Am J Pathol 1995;147: 1398–407.
40. Isobe K, Tamaru J, Nakamura S, et al. VH gene analysis in sporadic Burkitt's lymphoma: somatic mutation and intraclonal diversity with special reference to the tumor cells involving germinal center. Leuk Lymphoma 2002;43: 159–64.
41. Lones MA, Cairo MS, Perkins SL. T-cell–rich large B-cell lymphoma in children and adolescents: a clinicopathologic report of six cases from the Children's Cancer Group Study CCG-5961. Cancer 2000;88:2378–86.
42. Perkins SL, Segal GH, Kjeldsberg CR. Classification of non-Hodgkin's lymphomas in children. Semin Diagn Pathol 1995;12:303–13.
43. Ng CS, Chan JK, Hui PK, et al. Large B-cell lymphomas with a high content of reactive T cells. Hum Pathol 1989;20: 1145–54.
44. Seidemann K, Tiemann M, Lauterbach I, et al. Primary mediastinal large B-cell lymphoma with sclerosis in pediatric and adolescent patients: treatment and results from three therapeutic studies of the Berlin-Frankfurt-Munster Group. J Clin Oncol 2003;21:1782–9.
45. Benharroch D, Meguerian-Bedoyan Z, Lamant L, et al. ALK-positive lymphoma: a single disease with a broad spectrum of morphology. Blood 1998;91:2076–84.
46. Stein H, Mason DY, Gerdes J, et al. The expression of the Hodgkin's disease associated antigen Ki-1 in reactive and neoplastic lymphoid tissue: evidence that Reed–Sternberg cells and histiocytic malignancies are derived from activated lymphoid cells. Blood 1985;66:848–58.
47. Pileri S, Falini B, Delsol G, et al. Lymphohistiocytic T-cell lymphoma (anaplastic large cell lymphoma CD30+/Ki-1 + with a high content of reactive histiocytes). Histopathology 1990;16:383–91.
48. Pileri SA, Piccaluga A, Poggi S, et al. Anaplastic large cell lymphoma: update of findings. Leuk Lymphoma 1995;18–: 17–25.
49. Chan JK, Buchanan R, Fletcher CD. Sarcomatoid variant of anaplastic large-cell Ki-1 lymphoma. Am J Surg Pathol 1990;14:983–8.
50. Penny RJ, Blaustein JC, Longtine JA, et al. Ki-1-positive large cell lymphomas, a heterogenous group of neoplasms. Morphologic, immunophenotypic, genotypic, and clinical features of 24 cases. Cancer 1991;68:362–73.
51. Chan JK, Ng CS, Hui PK, et al. Anaplastic large cell Ki-1 lymphoma. Delineation of two morphological types. Histopathology 1989;15:11–34.
52. Suzuki R, Seto M, Nakamura S, et al. Sarcomatoid variant of anaplastic large cell lymphoma with cytoplasmic ALK and alpha-smooth muscle actin expression: a mimic of inflammatory myofibroblastic tumor. Am J Pathol 2001;159: 383–4.
53. Krenacs L, Wellmann A, Sorbara L, et al. Cytotoxic cell antigen expression in anaplastic large cell lymphomas of T- and null-cell type and Hodgkin's disease: evidence for distinct cellular origin. Blood 1997;89:980–9.
54. Felgar RE, Salhany KE, Macon WR, et al. The expression of TIA-1+ cytolytic-type granules and other cytolytic lymphocyte-associated markers in CD30+ anaplastic large cell lymphomas (ALCL): correlation with morphology, immunophenotype, ultrastructure, and clinical features. Hum Pathol 1999;30:228–36.
55. Nakamura S, Takagi N, Kojima M, et al. Clinicopathologic study of large cell anaplastic lymphoma (Ki-1-positive large cell lymphoma) among the Japanese. Cancer 1991;68: 118–29.
56. ten Berge RL, Snijdewint FG, von Mensdorff-Pouilly S, et al. MUC1 (EMA) is preferentially expressed by ALK positive anaplastic large cell lymphoma, in the normally glycosylated or only partly hypoglycosylated form. J Clin Pathol 2001; 54:933–9.
57. Ree HJ, Kadin ME, Kikuchi M, et al. Bcl-6 expression in reactive follicular hyperplasia, follicular lymphoma, and angioimmunoblastic T-cell lymphoma with hyperplastic germinal centers: heterogeneity of intrafollicular T-cells and their altered distribution in the pathogenesis of angioimmunoblastic T-cell lymphoma. Hum Pathol 1999;30:403–11.
58. Attygalle A, Al-Jehani R, Diss TC, et al. Neoplastic T cells in angioimmunoblastic T-cell lymphoma express CD10. Blood 2002;99:627–33.
59. Rudiger T, Weisenburger DD, Anderson JR, et al. Peripheral T-cell lymphoma (excluding anaplastic large-cell lymphoma): results from the Non-Hodgkin's Lymphoma Classification Project. Ann Oncol 2002;13:140–9.
60. Cheung MM, Chan JK, Wong KF. Natural killer cell neoplasms: a distinctive group of highly aggressive lymphomas/leukemias. Semin Hematol 2003;40:221–32.
61. Lamy T and Loughran TP Jr. Clinical features of large granular lymphocyte leukemia. Semin Hematol 2003;40:185–95.
62. Jacob MC, Chaperot L, Mossuz P, et al. CD4+ CD56+ lineage negative malignancies: a new entity developed from malignant early plasmacytoid dendritic cells. Haematologica 2003;88:941–55.
63. Ribeiro RC, Pui CH, Murphy SB, et al. Childhood malignant non-Hodgkin lymphomas of uncommon histology. Leukemia 1992;6:761–5.
64. Atra A, Meller ST, Stevens RS, et al. Conservative management of follicular non-Hodgkin's lymphoma in childhood. Br J Haematol 1998;103:220–3.
65. Lorsbach RB, Shay-Seymore D, Moore J, et al. Clinicopathologic analysis of follicular lymphoma occurring in children. Blood 2002;99:1959–64.
66. Bentley DL, Groudine M. A block to elongation is largely responsible for decreased transcription of c-myc in differentiated HL60 cells. Nature 1986;321:702–6.
67. Cesarman E, Dalla-Favera R, Bentley D, et al. Mutations in the first exon are associated with altered transcription of c-myc in Burkitt lymphoma. Science 1987;238:1272–5.
68. Zajac-Kaye M, Gelmann EP, Levens D. A point mutation in the c-myc locus of a Burkitt lymphoma abolishes binding of a nuclear protein. Science 1988;240:1776–80.
69. Cigudosa JC, Parsa NZ, Louie DC, et al. Cytogenetic analysis of 363 consecutively ascertained diffuse large B-cell lymphomas. Genes Chromosomes Cancer 1999;25: 123–33.
70. Moller MB, Christensen BE, Pedersen NT. Prognosis of localized diffuse large B-cell lymphoma in younger patients. Cancer 2003;98:516–21.
71. Rosenwald A, Wright G, Leroy K, et al. Molecular diagnosis of primary mediastinal B cell lymphoma identifies a clinically favorable subgroup of diffuse large B cell lymphoma related to Hodgkin lymphoma. J Exp Med 2003;198:851–62.
72. Raetz EA, Perkins SL, Carlson MA, et al. The nucleophosmin-anaplastic lymphoma kinase fusion protein induces c-Myc expression in pediatric anaplastic large cell lymphomas. Am J Pathol 2002;161:875–83.

73. Bischof D, Pulford K, Mason DY, et al. Role of the nucleophosmin (NPM) portion of the non-Hodgkin's lymphoma-associated NPM-anaplastic lymphoma kinase fusion protein in oncogenesis. Mol Cell Biol 1997;17:2312–25.
74. Ladanyi M. The NPM/ALK gene fusion in the pathogenesis of anaplastic large cell lymphoma. Cancer Surv 1997;30: 59–75.
75. Rosenwald A, Ott G, Pulford K, et al. t(1;2)(q21;p23) and t(2;3)(p23;q21): two novel variant translocations of the t(2;5)(p23;q35) in anaplastic large cell lymphoma. Blood 1999;94:362–4.
76. Hernandez L, Pinyol M, Hernandez S, et al. TRK-fused gene (TFG) is a new partner of ALK in anaplastic large cell lymphoma producing two structurally different TFG-ALK translocations. Blood 1999;94:3265–8.
77. ten Berge RL, de Bruin PC, Oudejans JJ, et al. ALK-negative anaplastic large-cell lymphoma demonstrates similar poor prognosis to peripheral T-cell lymphoma, unspecified. Histopathology 2003;43:462–9.
78. Ferrando AA, Neuberg DS, Staunton J, et al. Gene expression signatures define novel oncogenic pathways in T cell acute lymphoblastic leukemia. Cancer Cell 2002;1:75–87.
79. Rabbitts TH. Chromosomal translocations in human cancer. Nature 1994;372:143–9.
80. Look AT. Oncogenic transcription factors in the human acute leukemias. Science 1997;278:1059–64.
81. Schlegelberger B, Himmler A, Bartles H, et al. Recurrent chromosome abnormalities in peripheral T-cell lymphomas. Cancer Genet Cytogenet 1994;78:15–22.
82. Schlegelberger B, Nolle I, Feller AC, et al. Angioimmunoblastic lymphadenopathy with trisomy 3: the cells of the malignant clone are T cells. Hematol Pathol 1990; 4:179–83.
83. Wong KF. Genetic changes in natural killer cell neoplasms. Leuk Res 2002;26:977–8.
84. Siu LL, Chan JK, Kwong YL. Natural killer cell malignancies: clinicopathologic and molecular features. Histol Histopathol 2002;17:539–54.
85. Weisenburger DD, Gascoyne RD, Bierman PJ, et al. Clinical significance of the t(14;18) and BCL2 overexpression in follicular large cell lymphoma. Leuk Lymphoma 2000;36: 513–23.
86. Lambrechts AC, Hupkes PE, Dorssers LC, et al. Translocation (14;18)-positive cells are present in the circulation of the majority of patients with localized (stage I and II) follicular non-Hodgkin's lymphoma. Blood 1993;82:2510–6.
87. Pileri SA, Sabattini E, Rosito P, et al. Primary follicular lymphoma of the testis in childhood: an entity with peculiar clinical and molecular characteristics. J Clin Pathol 2002;55: 684–8.
88. Murphy SB. Classification, staging and end results of treatment of childhood non-Hodgkin's lymphomas: dissimilarities from lymphomas in adults. Semin Oncol 1980;7: 332–9.
89. Kasamon YL, Wahl RL, Swinnen LJ. FDG PET and high-dose therapy for aggressive lymphomas: toward a risk-adapted strategy. Curr Opin Oncol 2004;16:100–5.
90. Montravers F, McNamara D, Landman-Parker J, et al. [(18)F]FDG in childhood lymphoma: clinical utility and impact on management. Eur J Nucl Med Mol Imaging 2002;29:1155–65.
91. Haddy TB, Parker RI, Magrath IT. Bone marrow involvement in young patients with non-Hodgkin's lymphoma: the importance of multiple bone marrow samples for accurate staging. Med Pediatr Oncol 1989;17:418–23.
92. Magrath IT, Sariban E. Clinical features of Burkitt's lymphoma in the USA. IARC Sci Publ 1985:119–27.
93. Addis BJ, Isaacson PG. Large cell lymphoma of the mediastinum: a B-cell tumour of probable thymic origin. Histopathology 1986;10:379–90.
94. Kanavaros P, Gaulard P, Charlotte F, et al. Discordant expression of immunoglobulin and its associated molecule mb-1/CD79a is frequently found in mediastinal large B cell lymphomas. Am J Pathol 1995;146:735–41.
95. Menestrina F, Chilosi M, Bonetti F, et al. Mediastinal large-cell lymphoma of B-type, with sclerosis: histopathological and immunohistochemical study of eight cases. Histopathology 1986;10:589–600.
96. Magrath IT. Malignant non-Hodgkin's lymphomas in children. Hematol Oncol Clin North Am 1987;1:577–602.
97. Neth O, Seidemann K, Jansen P, et al. Precursor B-cell lymphoblastic lymphoma in childhood and adolescence: clinical features, treatment, and results in trials NHL-BFM 86 and 90. Med Pediatr Oncol 2000;35:20–7.
98. Arrowsmith ER, Macon WR, Kinney MC, et al. Peripheral T-cell lymphomas: clinical features and prognostic factors of 92 cases defined by the revised European American lymphoma classification. Leuk Lymphoma 2003;44:241–9.
99. Leake J, Kellie SJ, Pritchard J, et al. Peripheral T-cell lymphoma in childhood. A clinicopathological study of six cases. Histopathology 1989;14:255–68.
100. Peh SC, Quen QW. Nasal and nasal-type natural killer (NK)/T-cell lymphoma: immunophenotype and Epstein– Barr virus (EBV) association. Med J Malaysia 2003;58:196–204.
101. Graham DK, Liang X, Miller KL, et al. Disseminated nasopharyngeal natural killer cell lymphoblastic lymphoma in a child. Med Pediatr Oncol 2003;40:251–3.
102. Child FJ, Mitchell TJ, Whittaker SJ, et al. Blastic natural killer cell and extranodal natural killer cell–like T-cell lymphoma presenting in the skin: report of six cases from the UK. Br J Dermatol 2003;148:507–15.
103. DuBois SG, Etzell JE, Matthay KK, et al. Pediatric acute blastic natural killer cell leukemia. Leuk Lymphoma 2002;43:901–6.
104. Gaulard P, Belhadj K, Reyes F. Gammadelta T-cell lymphomas. Semin Hematol 2003;40:233–43.
105. Belhadj K, Reyes F, Farcet JP, et al. Hepatosplenic gammadelta T-cell lymphoma is a rare clinicopathologic entity with poor outcome: report on a series of 21 patients. Blood 2003; 102:4261–9.
106. Gassas A, Kirby M, Weitzman S, et al. Hepatosplenic gammadelta T-cell lymphoma in a 10-year-old boy successfully treated with hematopoietic stem cell transplantation. Am J Hematol 2004;75:113–4.
107. Lu D, Medeiros LJ, Eskenazi AE, et al. Primary follicular large cell lymphoma of the testis in a child. Arch Pathol Lab Med 2001;125:551–4.
108. Pakzad K, MacLennan GT, Elder JS, et al. Follicular large cell lymphoma localized to the testis in children. J Urol 2002; 168:225–8.
109. Reiter A, Schrappe M, Tiemann M, et al. Improved treatment results in childhood B-cell neoplasms with tailored intensification of therapy: a report of the Berlin-Frankfurt-Munster Group Trial NHL-BFM 90. Blood 1999;94:3294–306.
110. Sandlund JT, Murphy SB, Santana VM, et al. CNS involvement in children with newly diagnosed non-Hodgkin's lymphoma. J Clin Oncol 2000;18:3018–24.
111. Patte C, Auperin A, Michon J, et al. The Societe Francaise d'Oncologie Pediatrique LMB89 protocol: highly effective multiagent chemotherapy tailored to the tumor burden and initial response in 561 unselected children with B-cell lymphomas and L3 leukemia. Blood 2001;97:3370–9.
112. Cairo MS, Sposto R, Perkins SL, et al. Burkitt's and Burkitt-like lymphoma in children and adolescents: a review of the Children's Cancer Group experience. Br J Haematol 2003; 120:660–70.

113. Vannier JP, Patte C, Philip T, et al. [Treatment of extensive B-cell lymphoma in children: studies of the French Pediatric Oncology Society]. Bull Cancer 1988;75:61–8.
114. Gururangan S, Sposto R, Cairo MS, et al. Outcome of CNS disease at diagnosis in disseminated small noncleaved-cell lymphoma and B-cell leukemia: a Children's Cancer Group study. J Clin Oncol 2000;18:2017–25.
115. Soussain C, Patte C, Ostronoff M, et al. Small noncleaved cell lymphoma and leukemia in adults. A retrospective study of 65 adults treated with the LMB pediatric protocols. Blood 1995;85:664–74.
116. Murphy SB, Melvin SL, Mauer AM. Correlation of tumor cell kinetic studies with surface marker results in childhood non-Hodgkin's lymphoma. Cancer Res 1979;39:1534–8.
117. Goldman SC, Holcenberg JS, Finklestein JZ, et al. A randomized comparison between rasburicase and allopurinol in children with lymphoma or leukemia at high risk for tumor lysis. Blood 2001;97:2998–3003.
118. Annemans L, Moeremans K, Lamotte M, et al. Pan-European multicentre economic evaluation of recombinant urate oxidase (rasburicase) in prevention and treatment of hyperuricaemia and tumour lysis syndrome in haematological cancer patients. Support Care Cancer 2003;11:249–57.
119. Patte C, Sakiroglu C, Ansoborlo S, et al. Urate-oxidase in the prevention and treatment of metabolic complications in patients with B-cell lymphoma and leukemia, treated in the Societe Francaise d'Oncologie Pediatrique LMB89 protocol. Ann Oncol 2002;13:789–95.
120. van den Berg H, Reintsema AM. Renal tubular damage in rasburicase: risks of alkalinisation. Ann Oncol 2004; 15:175–6.
121. Meadows AT, Sposto R, Jenkin RD, et al. Similar efficacy of 6 and 18 months of therapy with four drugs (COMP) for localized non-Hodgkin's lymphoma of children: a report from the Children's Cancer Study Group. J Clin Oncol 1989;7:92–9.
122. Link MP, Shuster JJ, Donaldson SS, et al. Treatment of children and young adults with early-stage non-Hodgkin's lymphoma. N Engl J Med 1997;337:1259–66.
123. Reiter A, Schrappe M, Parwaresch R, et al. Non-Hodgkin's lymphomas of childhood and adolescence: results of a treatment stratified for biologic subtypes and stage—a report of the Berlin-Frankfurt-Munster Group. J Clin Oncol 1995; 13:359–72.
124. Amos Burke GA, Imeson J, Hobson R, et al. Localized non-Hodgkin's lymphoma with B-cell histology: cure without cyclophosphamide? A report of the United Kingdom Children's Cancer Study Group on studies NHL 8501 and NHL 9001 (1985–1996). Br J Haematol 2003;121:586–91.
125. Link MP, Donaldson SS, Berard CW, et al. Results of treatment of childhood localized non-Hodgkin's lymphoma with combination chemotherapy with or without radiotherapy. N Engl J Med 1990;322:1169–74.
126. Gasparini M, Rottoli L, Massimino M, et al. Curability of advanced Burkitt's lymphoma in children by intensive short-term chemotherapy. Eur J Cancer 1993;29A:692–698.
127. Dalle JH, Mechinaud F, Michon J, et al. Testicular disease in childhood B-cell non-Hodgkin's lymphoma: the French Society of Pediatric Oncology experience. J Clin Oncol 2001;19:2397–403.
128. Patte C, Philip T, Rodary C, et al. Improved survival rate in children with stage III and IV B cell non-Hodgkin's lymphoma and leukemia using multi-agent chemotherapy: results of a study of 114 children from the French Pediatric Oncology Society. J Clin Oncol 1986;4:1219–26.
129. Patte C, Philip T, Rodary C, et al. High survival rate in advanced-stage B-cell lymphomas and leukemias without CNS involvement with a short intensive polychemotherapy: results from the French Pediatric Oncology Society of a randomized trial of 216 children. J Clin Oncol 1991;9:123–32.
130. Muller-Weihrich S, Henze G, Langermann HJ, et al. [Childhood B-cell lymphomas and leukemias. Improvement of prognosis by a therapy developed for B-neoplasms by the BFM study group]. Onkologie 1984;7:205–8.
131. Murphy SB, Bowman WP, Abromowitch M, et al. Results of treatment of advanced-stage Burkitt's lymphoma and B cell (SIg+) acute lymphoblastic leukemia with high-dose fractionated cyclophosphamide and coordinated high-dose methotrexate and cytarabine. J Clin Oncol 1986;4:1732–9.
132. Atra A, Imeson JD, Hobson R, et al. Improved outcome in children with advanced stage B-cell non-Hodgkin's lymphoma (B-NHL): results of the United Kingdom Children Cancer Study Group (UKCCSG) 9002 protocol. Br J Cancer 2000;82:1396–402.
133. Anderson JR, Wilson JF, Jenkin DT, et al. Childhood non-Hodgkin's lymphoma. The results of a randomized therapeutic trial comparing a 4-drug regimen (COMP) with a 10-drug regimen (LSA2-L2). N Engl J Med 1983;308: 559–65.
134. Brecher ML, Schwenn MR, Coppes MJ, et al. Fractionated cylophosphamide and back to back high dose methotrexate and cytosine arabinoside improves outcome in patients with stage III high grade small non-cleaved cell lymphomas (SNCCL): a randomized trial of the Pediatric Oncology Group. Med Pediatr Oncol 1997;29:526–33.
135. Schwenn MR, Blattner SR, Lynch E, et al. HiC-COM: a 2-month intensive chemotherapy regimen for children with stage III and IV Burkitt's lymphoma and B-cell acute lymphoblastic leukemia. J Clin Oncol 1991;9:133–8.
136. Atra A, Gerrard M, Hobson R, et al. Outcome of relapsed or refractory childhood B-cell acute lymphoblastic leukaemia and B-cell non-Hodgkin's lymphoma treated with the UKCCSG 9003/9002 protocols. Br J Haematol 2001;112: 965–8.
137. Philip T, Hartmann O, Pinkerton R, et al. Curability of relapsed childhood B-cell non-Hodgkin's lymphoma after intensive first line therapy: a report from the Societe Francaise d'Oncologie Pediatrique. Blood 1993;81:2003–6.
138. Colombat P, Biron P, Laporte JP, et al. BEAM protocol and autologous bone marrow transplantation in first chemosensitive relapse of non-Hodgkin's lymphomas. Eur J Cancer 1990;26:858.
139. Gentet JC, Patte C, Quintana E, et al. Phase II study of cytarabine and etoposide in children with refractory or relapsed non-Hodgkin's lymphoma: a study of the French Society of Pediatric Oncology. J Clin Oncol 1990;8:661–5.
140. Kung FH, Harris MB, Krischer JP. Ifosfamide/carboplatin/etoposide (ICE), an effective salvaging therapy for recurrent malignant non-Hodgkin lymphoma of childhood: a Pediatric Oncology Group phase II study. Med Pediatr Oncol 1999;32:225–6.
141. Ladenstein R, Pearce R, Hartmann O, et al. High-dose chemotherapy with autologous bone marrow rescue in children with poor-risk Burkitt's lymphoma: a report from the European Lymphoma Bone Marrow Transplantation Registry. Blood 1997;90:2921–30.
142. Sandlund JT, Bowman L, Heslop HE, et al. Intensive chemotherapy with hematopoietic stem-cell support for children with recurrent or refractory NHL. Cytotherapy 2002; 4:253–8.
143. Bureo E, Ortega JJ, Munoz A, et al. Bone marrow transplantation in 46 pediatric patients with non-Hodgkin's lymphoma. Spanish Working Party for Bone Marrow Transplantation in Children. Bone Marrow Transplant 1995; 15:353–9.

144. Lazzarino M, Orlandi E, Paulli M, et al. Treatment outcome and prognostic factors for primary mediastinal (thymic) B-cell lymphoma: a multicenter study of 106 patients. J Clin Oncol 1997;15:1646–53.
145. Laver JH, Mahmoud H, Pick TE, et al. Results of a randomized phase III trial in children and adolescents with advanced stage diffuse large cell non-Hodgkin's lymphoma: a Pediatric Oncology Group study. Leuk Lymphoma 2002;43:105–9.
146. Lones MA, Perkins SL, Sposto R, et al. Large-cell lymphoma arising in the mediastinum in children and adolescents is associated with an excellent outcome: a Children's Cancer Group report. J Clin Oncol 2000;18:3845–53.
147. Bieri S, Roggero E, Zucca E, et al. Primary mediastinal large B-cell lymphoma (PMLCL): the need for prospective controlled clinical trials. Leuk Lymphoma 1999;35:139–46.
148. Cazals-Hatem D, Lepage E, Brice P, et al. Primary mediastinal large B-cell lymphoma. A clinicopathologic study of 141 cases compared with 916 nonmediastinal large B-cell lymphomas, a GELA ("Groupe d'Etude des Lymphomes de l'Adulte") study. Am J Surg Pathol 1996;20:877–88.
149. Zinzani PL, Martelli M, Magagnoli M, et al. Treatment and clinical management of primary mediastinal large B-cell lymphoma with sclerosis: MACOP-B regimen and mediastinal radiotherapy monitored by (67)Gallium scan in 50 patients. Blood 1999;94:3289–93.
150. Schot B, van Imhoff G, Pruim J, et al. Predictive value of early 18F-fluoro-deoxyglucose positron emission tomography in chemosensitive relapsed lymphoma. Br J Haematol 2003; 123:282–7.
151. Popat U, Przepiork D, Champlin R, et al. High-dose chemotherapy for relapsed and refractory diffuse large B-cell lymphoma: mediastinal localization predicts for a favorable outcome. J Clin Oncol 1998;16:63–9.
152. Sandlund JT, Santana V, Abromowitch M, et al. Large cell non-Hodgkin lymphoma of childhood: clinical characteristics and outcome. Leukemia 1994;8:30–4.
153. de Andrea ML, de Camargo B, Correa Alves A, et al. Factors of prognostic importance in childhood non-Hodgkin's lymphoma treated with two modified LSA2-L2 protocols. A multivariate analysis approach. Cancer 1988;62:240–50.
154. Hodges KB, Collins RD, Greer JP, et al. Transformation of the small cell variant Ki-1+ lymphoma to anaplastic large cell lymphoma: pathologic and clinical features. Am J Surg Pathol 1999;23:49–58.
155. Lin CN, Hou CC, Hwang WS, et al. Anaplastic large cell lymphoma—a rare disorder in southern Taiwan. Leuk Lymphoma 2003;44:1727–31.
156. Suzuki R, Kagami Y, Takeuchi K, et al. Prognostic significance of CD56 expression for ALK-positive and ALK-negative anaplastic large-cell lymphoma of T/null cell phenotype. Blood 2000;96:2993–3000.
157. Brugieres L, Deley MC, Pacquement H, et al. CD30(+) anaplastic large-cell lymphoma in children: analysis of 82 patients enrolled in two consecutive studies of the French Society of Pediatric Oncology. Blood 1998;92:3591–8.
158. Reiter A, Schrappe M, Tiemann M, et al. Successful treatment strategy for Ki-1 anaplastic large-cell lymphoma of childhood: a prospective analysis of 62 patients enrolled in three consecutive Berlin-Frankfurt-Munster group studies. J Clin Oncol 1994;12:899–908.
159. Seidemann K, Tiemann M, Schrappe M, et al. Short-pulse B-non-Hodgkin lymphoma-type chemotherapy is efficacious treatment for pediatric anaplastic large cell lymphoma: a report of the Berlin-Frankfurt-Munster Group Trial NHL-BFM 90. Blood 2001;97:3699–706.
160. Williams DM, Hobson R, Imeson J, et al. Anaplastic large cell lymphoma in childhood: analysis of 72 patients treated on The United Kingdom Children's Cancer Study Group chemotherapy regimens. Br J Haematol 2002;117:812–20.
161. Massimino M, Gasparini M, Giardini R. Ki-1 (CD30) anaplastic large-cell lymphoma in children. Ann Oncol 1995;6:915–20.
162. Vecchi V, Burnelli R, Pileri S, et al. Anaplastic large cell lymphoma (Ki-1+/CD30+) in childhood. Med Pediatr Oncol 1993;21:402–10.
163. Mora J, Filippa DA, Thaler HT, et al. Large cell non-Hodgkin lymphoma of childhood: Analysis of 78 consecutive patients enrolled in 2 consecutive protocols at the Memorial Sloan-Kettering Cancer Center. Cancer 2000;88:186–97.
164. Cairo MS, Sposto R, Hoover-Regan M, et al. Childhood and adolescent large-cell lymphoma (LCL): a review of the Children's Cancer Group experience. Am J Hematol 2003; 72:53–63.
165. Brugieres L, Quartier P, Le Deley MC, et al. Relapses of childhood anaplastic large-cell lymphoma: treatment results in a series of 41 children—a report from the French Society of Pediatric Oncology. Ann Oncol 2000;11:53–8.
166. Fanin R, Ruiz de Elvira MC, Sperotto A, et al. Autologous stem cell transplantation for T and null cell CD30-positive anaplastic large cell lymphoma: analysis of 64 adult and paediatric cases reported to the European Group for Blood and Marrow Transplantation (EBMT). Bone Marrow Transplant 1999;23:437–42.
167. Andersson PO, Braide I, Nilsson-Ehle H. Trofosfamide as salvage therapy for anaplastic large cell lymphoma relapsing after high-dose chemotherapy. Leuk Lymphoma 2002; 43:2351–3.
168. Lin P, Jones D, Dorfman DM, et al. Precursor B-cell lymphoblastic lymphoma: a predominantly extranodal tumor with low propensity for leukemic involvement. Am J Surg Pathol 2000;24:1480–90.
169. Reiter A, Schrappe M, Ludwig WD, et al. Intensive ALL-type therapy without local radiotherapy provides a 90% event-free survival for children with T-cell lymphoblastic lymphoma: a BFM group report. Blood 2000;95:416–21.
170. Goldberg JM, Silverman LB, Levy DE, et al. Childhood T-cell acute lymphoblastic leukemia: the Dana-Farber Cancer Institute acute lymphoblastic leukemia consortium experience. J Clin Oncol 2003;21:3616–22.
171. Grenzebach J, Schrappe M, Ludwig WD, et al. Favorable outcome for children and adolescents with T-cell lymphoblastic lymphoma with an intensive ALL-type therapy without local radiotherapy. Ann Hematol 2001;80(Suppl 3):B73–6.
172. Schrappe M, Reiter A, Zimmermann M, et al. Long-term results of four consecutive trials in childhood ALL performed by the ALL-BFM study group from 1981 to 1995. Berlin-Frankfurt-Munster. Leukemia 2000;14:2205–22.
173. Uckun FM, Reaman G, Steinherez PG, et al. Improved clinical outcome for children with T-lineage acute lymphoblastic leukemia after contemporary chemotherapy: a Children's Cancer Group Study. Leuk Lymphoma 1996;24: 57–70.
174. Pautier P, Devidas A, Delmer A, et al. Angioimmunoblastic-like T-cell non Hodgkin's lymphoma: outcome after chemotherapy in 33 patients and review of the literature. Leuk Lymphoma 1999;32:545–52.
175. Awidi AS, Tarawneh MS, Abu Khalaf MS, et al. Therapeutic effect of vincristine, adriamycin and prednisolone (VAP) in angioimmunoblastic lymphadenopathy (AIL). Cancer Chemother Pharmacol 1983;10:221–2.
176. Colbert N, Andrieu JM, Bernard J. Pulse methylprednisolone therapy in angioimmunoblastic lymphadenopathy. Acta Haematol 1982;68:307–8.

177. Siegert W, Agthe A, Griesser H, et al. Treatment of angioimmunoblastic lymphadenopathy (AILD)-type T-cell lymphoma using prednisone with or without the COPBLAM/IMVP-16 regimen. A multicenter study. Kiel Lymphoma Study Group. Ann Intern Med 1992;117:364–70.
178. Takemori N, Kodaira J, Toyoshima N, et al. Successful treatment of immunoblastic lymphadenopathy-like T-cell lymphoma with cyclosporin A. Leuk Lymphoma 1999;35: 389–95.
179. Dogan A, Attygalle AD, Kyriakou C. Angioimmunoblastic T-cell lymphoma. Br J Haematol 2003;121: 681–91.
180. Jantunen E, D'Amore F. Stem cell transplantation for peripheral T-cell lymphomas. Leuk Lymphoma 2004;45: 441–446.
181. Schetelig J, Fetscher S, Reichle A, et al. Long-term disease-free survival in patients with angioimmunoblastic T-cell lymphoma after high-dose chemotherapy and autologous stem cell transplantation. Haematologica 2003;88:1272–8.
182. Logsdon MD, Ha CS, Kavadi VS, et al. Lymphoma of the nasal cavity and paranasal sinuses: improved outcome and altered prognostic factors with combined modality therapy. Cancer 1997;80:477–88.
183. Li YX, Coucke PA, Li JY, et al. Primary non-Hodgkin's lymphoma of the nasal cavity: prognostic significance of paranasal extension and the role of radiotherapy and chemotherapy. Cancer 1998;83:449–56.
184. Yamaguchi M, Kita K, Miwa H, et al. Frequent expression of P-glycoprotein/MDR1 by nasal T-cell lymphoma cells. Cancer 1995;76:2351–6.
185. Nagafuji K, Fujisaki T, Arima F, et al. L-asparaginase induced durable remission of relapsed nasal NK/T-cell lymphoma after autologous peripheral blood stem cell transplantation. Int J Hematol 2001;74:447–50.
186. Weidmann E, Boehrer S, Chow KU, et al. Treatment of aggressive, or progressing indolent peripheral T- and NK-cell neoplasias by combination of fludarabine, cyclophosphamide and doxorubicine. Onkologie 2001;24:162–4.
187. Liang R, Chen F, Lee CK, et al. Autologous bone marrow transplantation for primary nasal T/NK cell lymphoma. Bone Marrow Transplant 1997;19:91–3.
188. Mori N, Yamashita Y, Tsuzuki T, et al. Lymphomatous features of aggressive NK cell leukaemia/lymphoma with massive necrosis, haemophagocytosis and EB virus infection. Histopathology 2000;37:363–71.
189. Chan JK, Sin VC, Wong KF, et al. Nonnasal lymphoma expressing the natural killer cell marker CD56: a clinicopathologic study of 49 cases of an uncommon aggressive neoplasm. Blood 1997;89:4501–13.
190. Kwong YL, Chan AC, Liang R, et al. CD56+ NK lymphomas: clinicopathological features and prognosis. Br J Haematol 1997;97:821–9.
191. Kanegane H, Nomura K, Miyawaki T, et al. Biological aspects of Epstein–Barr virus (EBV)-infected lymphocytes in chronic active EBV infection and associated malignancies. Crit Rev Oncol Hematol 2002;44:239–49.
192. Gilmour KC, Gaspar HB. Pathogenesis and diagnosis of X-linked lymphoproliferative disease. Expert Rev Mol Diagn 2003;3:549–61.
193. Cohen JI. Benign and malignant Epstein–Barr virus-associated B-cell lymphoproliferative diseases. Semin Hematol 2003;40:116–23.
194. Nichols KE, Harkin DP, Levitz S, et al. Inactivating mutations in an SH2 domain-encoding gene in X-linked lymphoproliferative syndrome. Proc Natl Acad Sci U S A 1998; 95:13765–70.
195. Sayos J, Wu C, Morra M, et al. The X-linked lymphoproliferative-disease gene product SAP regulates signals induced through the co-receptor SLAM. Nature 1998;395:462–9.
196. Nistala K, Gilmour KC, Cranston T, et al. X-linked lymphoproliferative disease: three atypical cases. Clin Exp Immunol 2001;126:126–30.
197. Kawa K, Okamura T, Yasui M, et al. Allogeneic hematopoietic stem cell transplantation for Epstein–Barr virus-associated T/NK-cell lymphoproliferative disease. Crit Rev Oncol Hematol 2002;44:251–7.
198. Atkison PR, Ross BC, Williams S, et al. Long-term results of pediatric liver transplantation in a combined pediatric and adult transplant program. Cmaj 2002;166:1663–71.
199. Juvonen E, Aalto SM, Tarkkanen J, et al. High incidence of PTLD after non-T-cell-depleted allogeneic haematopoietic stem cell transplantation as a consequence of intensive immunosuppressive treatment. Bone Marrow Transplant 2003;32:97–102.
200. Bates WD, Gray DW, Dada MA, et al. Lymphoproliferative disorders in Oxford renal transplant recipients. J Clin Pathol 2003;56:439–46.
201. Wagner HJ, Cheng YC, Huls MH, et al. Prompt versus preemptive intervention for EBV lymphoproliferative disease. Blood 2004;103:3979–81.
202. Birkeland SA, Hamilton-Dutoit S. Is posttransplant lymphoproliferative disorder (PTLD) caused by any specific immunosuppressive drug or by the transplantation per se? Transplantation 2003;76:984–8.
203. Capello D, Cerri M, Muti G, et al. Molecular histogenesis of posttransplantation lymphoproliferative disorders. Blood 2003;102:3775–85.
204. Delecluse HJ, Rouault JP, Jeammot B, et al. Bcl6/Laz3 rearrangements in post-transplant lymphoproliferative disorders. Br J Haematol 1995;91:101–3.
205. Bueno J, Ramil C, Somoza I, et al. Treatment of monomorphic B-cell lymphoma with rituximab after liver transplantation in a child. Pediatr Transplant 2003;7:153–6.
206. Garcia VD, Bonamigo-Filho JS, Neumann J, et al. Rituximab and rapamycin for posttransplant lymphoproliferative disease treatment: report of three cases. Transplant Proc 2002;34:2993–5.
207. Haque T, Taylor C, Wilkie GM, et al. Complete regression of posttransplant lymphoproliferative disease using partially HLA-matched Epstein Barr virus-specific cytotoxic T cells. Transplantation 2001;72:1399–402.
208. Ambinder RF. Posttransplant lymphoproliferative disease: pathogenesis, monitoring, and therapy. Curr Oncol Rep 2003;5:359–63.
209. Sparano JA. Human immunodeficiency virus associated lymphoma. Curr Opin Oncol 2003;15:372–8.
210. Schulz TF. Kaposi's sarcoma-associated herpesvirus (human herpesvirus 8): epidemiology and pathogenesis. J Antimicrob Chemother 2000;45(Suppl T3):15–27.
211. Gates AE, Kaplan LD. Biology and management of AIDS-associated non-Hodgkin's lymphoma. Hematol Oncol Clin North Am 2003;17:821–41.
212. Pollock BH, Jenson HB, Leach CT, et al. Risk factors for pediatric human immunodeficiency virus-related malignancy. JAMA 2003;289:2393–9.
213. Braaten KM, Betensky RA, de Leval L, et al. BCL-6 expression predicts improved survival in patients with primary central nervous system lymphoma. Clin Cancer Res 2003; 9:1063–9.
214. International Collaboration on HIV and Cancer. Highly active antiretroviral therapy and incidence of cancer in human immunodeficiency virus-infected adults. J Natl Cancer Inst 2000;92:1823–30.
215. AIDS Malignancy Consortium. Available at: www.cancer.gov/clinical_trials. Accessed September 24, 2005.
216. Sabesan V, Cairo MS, Lones MA, et al. Assessment of minimal residual disease in childhood non-hodgkin

lymphoma by polymerase chain reaction using patient-specific primers. J Pediatr Hematol Oncol 2003;25:109–13.

217. Grillo-Lopez AJ, White CA, Varns C, et al. Overview of the clinical development of rituximab: first monoclonal antibody approved for the treatment of lymphoma. Semin Oncol 1999;26(Suppl 14):66–73.
218. Vose JM, Link BK, Grossbard ML, et al. Phase II study of rituximab in combination with chop chemotherapy in patients with previously untreated, aggressive non-Hodgkin's lymphoma. J Clin Oncol 2001;19:389–97.
219. Kewalramani T, Zelenetz AD, Nimer SD, et al. Rituximab and ICE as second-line therapy before autologous stem cell transplantation for relapsed or primary refractory diffuse large B-cell lymphoma. Blood 2004;103:3684–8.
220. Adams J. The development of proteasome inhibitors as anticancer drugs. Cancer Cell 2004;5:417–21.
221. Paschal BR. Remission of follicular non-Hodgkin's lymphoma with denileukin diftitox (ONTAK) after progression during rituximab, CHOP and fludarabine therapy. Leuk Lymphoma 2003;44:731–3.
222. Di Venuti G, Nawgiri R, Foss F. Denileukin diftitox and hyper-CVAD in the treatment of human T-cell lymphotropic virus 1-associated acute T-cell leukemia/lymphoma. Clin Lymphoma 2003;4:176–8.
223. Piekarz RL, Robey R, Sandor V, et al. Inhibitor of histone deacetylation, depsipeptide (FR901228), in the treatment of peripheral and cutaneous T-cell lymphoma: a case report. Blood 2001;98:2865–8.
224. Piekarz RL, Robey RW, Zhan Z, et al. T-cell lymphoma as a model for the use of histone deacetylase inhibitors in cancer therapy: impact of depsipeptide on molecular markers, therapeutic targets, and mechanisms of resistance. Blood 2004;103:4636–43.

32

Non-Hodgkin's Lymphoma in the Elderly

Bertrand Coiffier, M.D.

Lymphoma in elderly patients needs special attention because elderly patients represent half of the cases (the median age for all lymphomas is around 60 years), and because elderly patients usually require a different management compared to younger patients. Indeed, these patients usually had one or several other diseases diagnosed before the lymphoma, diseases that may alter the capacity to tolerate lymphoma treatment.[1,2] Moreover, the incidence of lymphoma in elderly patients has increased in recent years, probably more than that of young patients,[3] and although recent results showed a trend to stabilization during the 1990s, this will not occur for the elderly, given that people live longer, and thus the number of elderly patients will increase.[4,5] Very few differences have been described for morphology and clinical presentation between young and elderly patients with lymphoma.[6] However, outcomes in elderly patients with lymphoma are worse, particularly for those with aggressive subtypes, because of the difficulties encountered during treatment, difficulties related to the presence of other diseases, diminished organ functions, and altered drug metabolism.[1,2,7] Recent studies have concluded that the best way to improve the survival of elderly patients with lymphoma is correct intention to treat, that is, an optimal chemotherapy regimen.[5,8,9]

INCREASED INCIDENCE OF LYMPHOMA IN THE ELDERLY

Rising human life expectancy has naturally resulted in an increase in the number of elderly patients: current estimates indicate that the percentage of persons older than 65 years of age will increase from 12% to 20% over the next 25 years.[10] An increase in the incidence of lymphomas has been documented in Europe and the United States, particularly for elderly patients.[4,11–13] For the last 25 years, incidence of lymphoma has increased by more than 50%, even more in patients older than 60 years, and now it is 15 to 16 new cases a year for 100,000 inhabitants in the United States.[14] Half of all newly diagnosed patients with lymphoma are above 60 years of age. All lymphoma subtypes increased among the elderly, but diffuse large B-cell lymphoma registered the greatest increase.[15]

LYMPHOMA SUBTYPES IN ELDERLY

All lymphoma subtypes may be observed in elderly patients, but with small differences compared to those encountered in younger patients.[6,16] Most of the large epidemiologic studies have been done with the Working Formulation for Clinical Usage,[17] and found a higher percentage of patients with aggressive lymphoma in elderly.[4,11,12,14,18] Recent studies used the Revised European–American Lymphoma classification,[19] not greatly different from the World Health Organization classification,[16] allows more precise definition of the subtypes. Only one large study has defined the differences between young and elderly patients, but it was not an epidemiologic study.[6,20] All other cases included in this study were reviewed by five expert pathologists. This study showed that in eight referral centers around the world there were some differences: elderly patients more frequently had lymphocytic/lymphoplasmacytoid lymphoma, diffuse large B-cell lymphoma, and peripheral T-cell lymphoma, and less frequently, anaplastic large cell lymphoma, lymphoblastic lymphoma, and Burkitt's lymphoma (Table 32–1). In all studies, the two most frequent subtypes were diffuse large B-cell lymphoma and follicular lymphoma, accounting for 40% and 20% of all cases, respectively.

No specific chromosomal or genetic abnormalities have been described in elderly patients, but very few studies have examined them. The application of new molecular tools has enormous potential to show any age-related variation.[21,22] However, to date, they have mainly been used to define the level of heterogeneity among subtypes.[23,24]

STAGING IN THE ELDERLY

As in young patients, the Ann Arbor staging system for Hodgkin's lymphoma has proved inappropriate in the elderly, and since 1993, prognosis is better described by the International Prognostic Index than the stage.[25] The International Prognostic Index includes age (less than or more than 60 years); disease stage (localized or disseminated); performance status (good, 0 to 1; poor, >1); lactate dehydrogenase (LDH) levels (normal or above normal); and number of extranodal disease sites (0 to 1 or >1) to classify patients into four risk categories, ranging from low-risk to high-risk categories. For patients older than 60 years, a simplified index, the age-adjusted International Prognostic Index, only uses stage, performance status, and LDH level to estimate the risk of failure or death. Because the International Prognostic Index applies mostly to aggressive lymphomas, a specific index, the FLIPI, has been described for patients with follicular lymphoma.[26] Otherwise, staging is comparable to young patients with clinical examination, CT scan of the body, other examinations as warranted by clinical symptoms, blood counts, bone marrow biopsy, LDH and β2-microglobulin measurements, human immunodeficiency virus, and hepatitis B and C virus serology.

In assessing treatment options for elderly patients, a great deal of attention must be paid to age-related factors.

Table 32–1. Frequency of Lymphomas Reported in REAL Classification in 1283 Patients by Age Group

Lymphoma Subtypes	Number of Patients	Percentage of Patients				
		<35	35–49	50–59	60–69	≥70
Small lymphocytic/lymphoplasmacytoid lymphoma	98	1	14	18	33	34
MALT lymphoma	108	9	14	24	26	27
Marginal zone lymphoma (splenic and nodal)	32	6	22	22	34	16
Follicular lymphoma	317	8	22	22	26	22
Mantle cell lymphoma	72	—	11	31	33	25
Diffuse large B-cell lymphoma	448	16	15	16	21	32
Peripheral T-cell lymphomas	93	11	18	17	26	28
Anaplastic large T/null-cell lymphoma	32	53	19	6	13	9
Burkitt's lymphoma	9	78	—	11	11	—
Lymphoblastic lymphoma	28	68	14	14	4	—
Unclassified	46	6	22	20	22	30
All patients	1283	13	17	19	24	27

Adapted from The Non-Hodgkin's Lymphoma Classification Project. Effect of age on the characteristics and clinical behavior of non-Hodgkin's lymphoma patients. Ann Oncol 1997;8:973–8,[6] with permission.

Presence of other diseases,[27] diminished organ function, and health problems resulting from long-term use or abuse of tobacco, alcohol, and medications are factors that can compromise the ability of elderly patients to tolerate therapy. In one survey, 61% of the patients 70 years or older had at least one comorbid condition compared to 20% of patients younger than 60 years.[28] Furthermore, older patients typically have reduced emotional or physiologic tolerance to invasive and toxic procedures. Elderly patients often have alterations in the absorption, distribution, activation, detoxification, metabolism, and clearance of drugs, which modify the pharmacodynamics of therapeutics.[29,30] Finally, elderly patients take more drugs than younger patients, which places them at increased risk for drug–drug and drug–disease interactions. Decreased glomerular filtration rate and tubular reabsorption delay drug excretion, such that doses may have to be tailored to creatinine clearance.[31] Because of decreased liver function, the metabolism of certain drugs such as cyclophosphamide or anthracyclines may be altered. However, the adjustment to any hepatic function was not associated with a better tolerance.[32] Hematopoietic reserve capacity may be altered as well, and myelotoxicity increased with standard doses.[33] However, decreasing dosage because of putative increased toxicity was proven to be associated with poorer therapeutic results.[34]

In a recently reported study with 577 patients treated in community and academic hospitals, patients older than 65 years had more heart disease and comorbid conditions, and received lower average-dose intensity and fewer cycles than younger patients.[35] Even with this less intensive treatment, they had more hospitalizations for febrile neutropenia (28% compared to 16% in younger patients). None of these patients had received G-CSF, and such a preventive treatment must be considered for elderly patients, particularly those with poor performance status or comorbid conditions. Such an early use was associated with a decrease of repeated hospitalizations and shorter length of stay in hospital in another study.[36]

AGE AS A PROGNOSTIC FACTOR

Several studies described that older age correlated with shorter disease-free and overall survivals. A retrospective analysis of 312 diffuse large B-cell lymphoma patients showed that age of more than 60 years was the only prognostic factor affecting survival.[37] In a study of 307 patients treated with CHOP, disease-free survival rates fell from 65% at 96 months for subjects less than 40 years old to 50% at 36 months for those older than 65 years.[34] Although comparable complete response rates were observed in patients less than 60 years or greater than 60 years of age who were treated with CAP/BOP regimen, the survival rate was much significantly lower for older patients (34% vs. 62%, $p = 0.001$).[38] Likewise, age more than 50 years versus less than 50 years was a major factor predicting outcome in an English study of 459 patients treated with two dissimilar regimens.[39] A Scottish study demonstrated that stage and histology are comparable in patients under and over age 60, although the elderly have a significantly poorer survival.[40] Advancing age has also been associated with increased treatment-related death rates. In patients with advanced-stage diffuse large B-cell lymphoma treated with VAPEC-B, the treatment-related death rate was higher in subjects older than 60 years compared with younger patients.[41] In Peru, patients older than 60 years treated with CHOP plus granulocyte-macrophage colony-stimulating factor had a good response rate and a 50% 4-year disease-free survival, although toxicity was greater in those older than 70 years.[42]

We recently demonstrated that elderly patients usually have more severe disease than young and middle-age patients; complete remission rates decline steadily with age, from 68% in the young to 45% in the elderly.[6] Median event-free and overall survival rates also decline with age (Table 32–2).[6] All published studies show shorter survival in elderly compared with younger patients matched for lymphoma and clinical characteristics.[6,12] This difference persists after correction for non–lymphoma-related deaths. The shorter survival has been ascribed to two main causes: a ten-

Table 32–2. **Response to Treatment and Survival By Age at Diagnosis**

Treatment Outcome	Number of Patients	Percentage of Patients				
		<35	35–49	50–59	60–69	≥70
Response to treatment						
Complete response	686	68	64	64	56	45
Partial response	313	21	18	27	32	30
No response	119	8	12	6	9	13
Not precise	65	3	6	3	3	12
Progression at time of analysis						
Yes	595	38	49	49	51	43
No	688	62	51	51	49	57
Relapse from complete response	253	20	41	40	42	36
Event-free survival						
3-year	—	59	54	55	50	47
5-year	—	59	48	44	43	41
Median	—	NR	4.0	3.9	3.4	2.4
Overall survival						
3-year	—	65	70	0	61	44
5-year	—	61	66	62	51	34
Median	—	NR	NR	7.9	5.5	2.2

Adapted from The Non-Hodgkin's Lymphoma Classification Project. Effect of age on the characteristics and clinical behavior of non-Hodgkin's lymphoma patients. Ann Oncol 1997;8:973–8,[6] with permission.
NR, not reached.

dency by physicians to administer weaker, "better tolerated" (hence less effective) treatment in the elderly[34]; and poor drug tolerance in the elderly, largely due to the presence of concomitant disease.[38] In the absence of concomitant disease, survival is no shorter in those aged over 70 years compared with those aged 70 years or less.[43] As in young patients, therapy in the elderly must be based on the type of lymphoma and the presence/absence of adverse prognostic factors.

Several studies have demonstrated that elderly patients treated with the appropriate therapy and effective management of putative toxicities may have a survival rate comparable to that observed in younger patients.[44–46] Once a complete response has been obtained, disease-free survival in elderly patients may be comparable to that of younger patients even if the initial chemotherapy regimen was less aggressive.[43] However, this did not result in an identical survival rate because the complete response rate was inferior to that observed in younger patients (Fig. 32–1). The major difficulty for physicians treating elderly lymphoma patients is the administration of the chemotherapy required by the lymphoma without adverse toxicities and to reach a high complete remission rate. Using G-CSF from the first cycle may certainly help.[9]

TREATMENT OF DIFFUSE LARGE B-CELL LYMPHOMAS

Given their age and the presence of concomitant disease, the elderly have sometimes been considered ineligible for treatment regimens that are potentially curative in the young. Two approaches have been proposed: the first prioritizes the possibility of cure and uses the same regimens as in the young, provided that there is no severe concomitant disease contraindicating their use; the second prioritizes quality of life, and uses specific treatment regimens tailored to the elderly, which are reputedly less toxic but also less effective.[9] The debate has essentially centered on the treatment of diffuse large B-cell lymphoma, since it is potentially curable with proper treatment, CHOP being the reference therapy.[47] When CHOP is used at lower doses in the elderly, the remission rate declines and survival shortens compared with results in patients aged less than 60 years.[34] The standard CHOP regimen, on the other hand, achieves similar progression-free survival to that in younger patients, but carries a much higher risk of severe toxicity or death: 15% to 30% in different retrospective series. Several recent randomized studies have compared results obtained with the standard CHOP to those obtained using less intensive therapy in elderly patients with diffuse large B-cell lymphoma.[9] Sonneveld showed that CHOP was well tolerated in patients aged over 60 years: toxicity did not differ from that of a reputedly less toxic regimen, CNOP, in which mitoxantrone replaced doxorubicin. The complete remission rate was also higher and survival longer with the CHOP regimen.[48] These results were confirmed in a larger study.[49] In another study, CHOP was compared with "chop," using the same drugs at the same overall doses but in three weekly injections instead of a single injection every 3 weeks, leading to decreased drug toxicity.[50] In this study, survival at 2 years was longer in patients receiving standard CHOP than in those receiving "chop." In a similar study, the Central Lymphoma Group in the United Kingdom reported the failure of CAPOMEt, a weekly regimen based on CHOP drugs plus etoposide, to increase survival over that reached with the CHOP regimen and reported an increase in neurologic toxicity.[51] Finally, CHOP was compared to VMP in an Italian study, and was demonstrated as

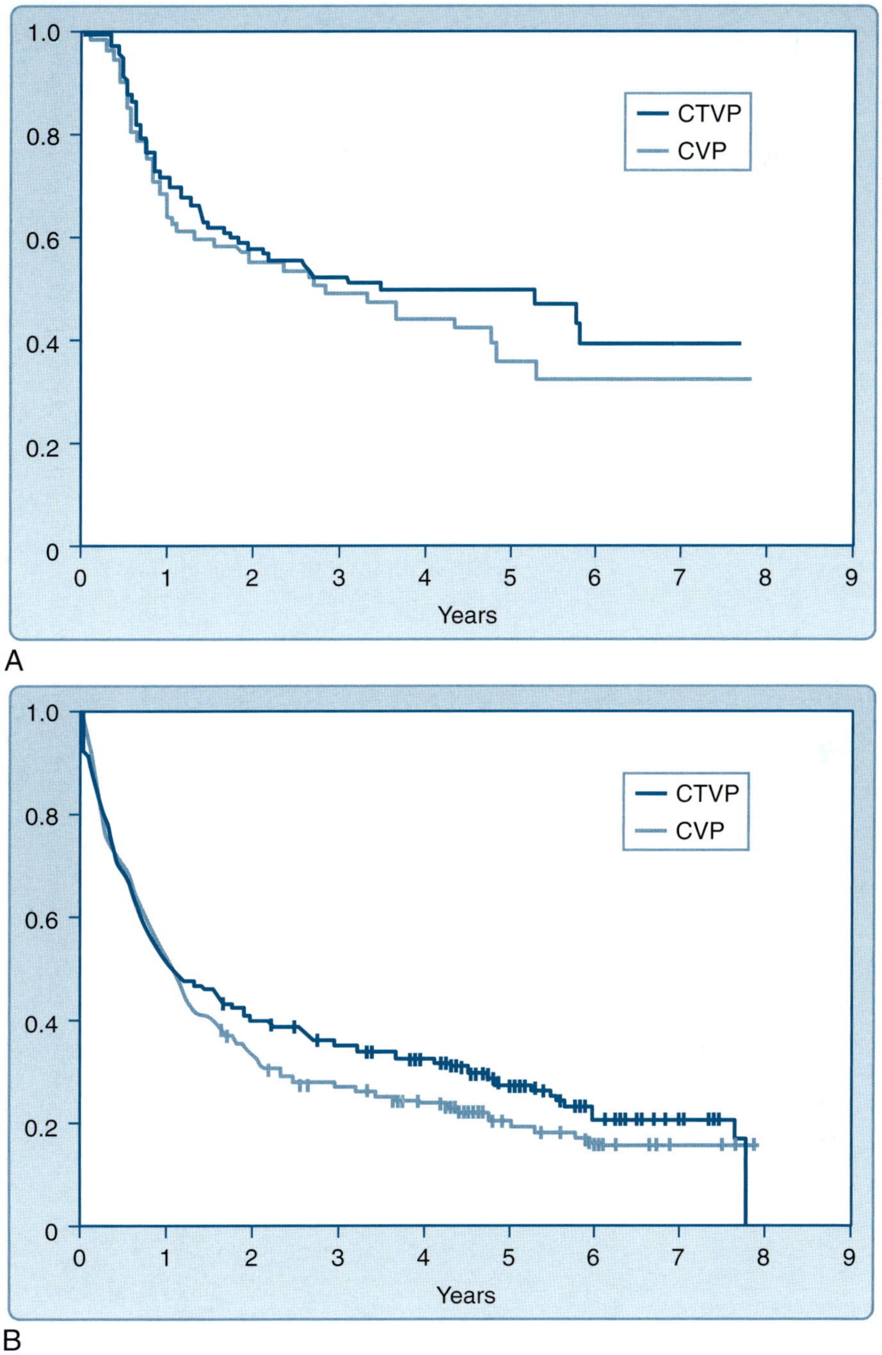

Figure 32–1. Disease-free survival (**A**) and overall survival (**B**) in elderly patients treated with CVP or CHOP-like regimen.[43] Disease-free survival is very good for this group of patients; because there is no difference between the two treatment arms, complete remission must be the first goal of treatment. Overall survival was not good because few of the patients reached complete remission, and all others progressed and died from the disease or toxicity of the treatment.

superior to this previously used regimen in the EORTC group.[52] These data confirmed the similarity of response rates in elderly and younger patients, and also the high correlation between complete response and long survival, irrespective of patient age (Fig. 32–1).[43]

The only comparative study that has shown a regimen to be superior to the anthracyline-base regimen for elderly patients compared PAdriaCEBO to PMitCEBO and used the low dose of doxorubicin (35 mg/m^2) combined with cyclophosphamide (300 mg/m^2), etoposide, vincristine, and bleomycine.[53] In this study, complete remission rates were 60% and 52%, and 4-year survival was 50% and 28% for PMitCEBO and PAdriaCEBO, respectively. This did not signify that PMitCEBO may be superior to CHOP.

A recent German trial showed that therapeutic results may be improved if the dose intensity of the CHOP regimen is increased, that is, CHOP given every 2 weeks (CHOP-14) in spite of the classical 3 weeks (CHOP-21) in patients over 60 years old.[54] In a multivariate analysis, chemotherapy given every 2 weeks was associated with a longer event-free survival rate when etoposide was added; survival was not statistically different. This increase in dose intensity was not associated with an increase of severe complications. However, the median age of the patients included in this

Table 32–3. Randomized Studies in Elderly Patients with Diffuse Large-Cell Lymphoma

Study (first author and reference)	Number of Patients	Chemotherapy Regimens	Lymphoma-Free Survival	P Value	Overall Survival	P Value
Aoki[77]	37	Low-dose CHOP vs. T-COP vs. T-COPE	NS	—	At 2 years 18% vs. 58% vs. 48%	—
Aviles[78]	169	CEOP vs. CIOP	3-Year relapse-free survival 73% vs. 37%	0.01	At 3 years 72% vs. 34%	0.01
Bastion[43]	453	CTVP vs. CVP	5-Year time to treatment failure 24% vs. 14%	<0.05	At 5 years 27% vs. 19%	<0.05
Bayley[51]	381	CHOP-Mtx vs. CAPOMEt	NS	—	Median 31 vs. 24 months At 5 years 43% vs. 37%	NS
Coiffier[55]	399	CHOP vs. R-CHOP	2-Year event-free survival 38% vs. 57%	<0.001	At 2 years 57% vs. 70%	0.007
Cooper[79]	77	CHOP vs. MACOP-B	Failure-free survival 46% vs 45%	—	At 4 years 48% vs. 49%	—
DeLena[80]	24	CHOP-B vs. CEOP-B	NS	—	NS	—
Gordon[81]	167	CHOP vs. m-BACOD	NS	—	NS	—
Jelic[82]	47	BEP vs. MEP	NS	—	At 2 years 30% vs. 50%	>0.2
Mainwaring[53]	516	PAdriaCEBO vs. PMitCEBO	NS	—	At 4 years 28% vs. 50%	0.0001
Meyer[83]	38	CHOP vs. chop	2-year progression -free survival 57% vs. 46%	0.16	At 2 years 74% vs. 51%	0.05
Montserrat[84]	78	CHOP vs. ProMACE-CytaBOM	NS	—	NS	—
Osby[49]	455	CHOP vs. CNOP +/– G-CSF	3-Year failure-free survival 40% vs. 38% vs. 19% vs. 27%	<0.001	At 3 years 61% vs. 51% vs. 33% vs. 33%	<0.001
Pfreundschuh[54]	689	CHOP-21 vs. CHOP-14 vs. CHOEP-21 vs. CHOEP-14	5-Year event-free survival 33% vs. 44% vs. 41% vs. 40%	Not done	At 5 years 51% vs. 53% vs. 46% vs. 50%	NS
Silingardi[85]	71	ProMECE-CytaBOM vs. MACOP-B	NS	—	NS	—
Sonneveld[48]	148	CHOP vs. CNOP	Median disease-free survival 27 vs. 15 m 3-Year survival 17% vs. 13%	0.2 0.12	Median 26 vs. 12 months 3-year survival 42% vs. 26%	0.029 0.034
Tirelli[52]	120	CHOP vs. VMP	Median progression-free survival 26 vs 8 months	0.002	Median 36 vs. 13 months	0.004
Zinzani[86]	306	8-Week vs. 12-week VNCOP-B	5-year relapse-free survival 59% vs. 55%	NS	5-year survival 52% vs. 37%	0.01

CHOP: cyclophosphamide, doxorubicin, vincristine, and prednisone; T-COP; pirarubicin, cyclophosphamide, vincristine, and prednisone; T-COPE: T-COP + etoposide; CEOP: cyclophosphamide, epirubicin, vincristine, and prednisone; CIOP: cyclophosphamide, idarubicin, vincristine, and prednisone; CTVP: cyclophosphamide, pirarubicin, vincristine, and prednisone; CVP: cyclophosphamide, vincristine, and prednisone; CHOP-Mtx: CHOP + methotrexate; CAPOMEt: cyclophosphamide, doxorubicin, prednisone, vincristine, methotrexate, and etoposide; R-CHOP: CHOP + rituximab; MACOP-B: methotrexate, doxorubicin, cyclophosphamide, vincristine, prednisone, and bleomycin; CHOP-B: CHOP + bleomycin; CEOP-B: CEOP + bleomycin; m-BACOD: methotrexate, bleomycin, doxorubicin, cyclophosphamide, vincristine, and dexamethosone; BEP: BCNU, etoposide, and prednisone; MEP: mitoxantrone, etoposide and prednisone; PAdriaCEBO: prednisone, doxorubicin, cyclophosphamide, etoposide, bleomycin, and vincristine; PMitCEBO: prednisone, mitoxantrone, cyclophosphamide, etoposide, bleomycin, and vincristine; chop: low-dose CHOP; ProMACE-CytaBOM: procarbazine, methotrexate, doxorubicin, cyclophosphamide, etoposide and cytarabine, bleomycin, vincristine, mitoxantrone; CNOP: cyclophosphamide, mitoxantrone, vincristine, and prednisone; CHOEP: cyclophosphamide, doxorubicin, vincristine, etoposide, and prednisone; ProMECE-CytaBOM: procarbazine, methotrexate, epirubicin, cyclophosphamide, etoposide and cytarabine, bleomycin, vincristine, mitoxantrone; VMP: vincristine, mitoxantrone, prednisone; VNCOP-B: etoposide, mitoxantrone, cyclophosphamide, vincristine, prednisone, and bleomycin; NS, not significant.

study was only 65 years, and only 20% of the patients were older than 70 years. The conclusion of all these trials is that CHOP can be recommended for the treatment of elderly patients with diffuse large B-cell lymphoma, except for patients with a formal cardiac contraindication to doxorubicin.

Recently, the combination of rituximab plus CHOP (R-CHOP) for eight cycles was demonstrated as being superior to CHOP alone in elderly patients.[55] In this prospective randomized study, patients aged 60 to 80 years with untreated diffuse large B-cell lymphoma were included. The complete response rate was 15% higher in patients treated with the R-CHOP combination. Event-free, disease-free, and overall survivals were significantly longer in a recent update with 4-year median follow-up (Fig. 32–2). Because of the magnitude of the difference between CHOP and R-CHOP and the very good safety ratio, these data have rendered R-CHOP as the new standard for the treatment for previously untreated elderly patients with diffuse large B-cell lymphoma. These results have recently been confirmed in two studies. The Intergroup trial initially randomized elderly patients between CHOP and R-CHOP, and the responding patients were further randomized between no treatment or a maintenance with Rituximab for 2 years.[56] Although the analysis of this study is complicated by double randomization, R-CHOP was better than CHOP and maintenance was associated with a longer time to progression in patients treated with CHOP. A population–case analysis comparing CHOP and R-CHOP also showed longer time to progression and survival in patients treated with R-CHOP.[57]

Questions that remain to be settled follow: How many cycles of CHOP and infusions of rituximab? Is there any indication for a prolonged treatment with rituximab to decrease the relapse rate? Will maintenance with rituximab further improve the results? Will increasing the dose intensity with R-CHOP every 2 weeks increase efficacy without increasing toxicity? Currently, no randomized study has shown that six cycles of CHOP do the same as the classical eight cycles.[58] Moreover, with the use of G-CSF, all studies have shown that full-dose CHOP can be safely administered to elderly patients.[59,60] Decreasing the number of rituximab infusions may decrease the cost of this regimen, but may also decrease efficacy.

PATIENTS WITH CONTRAINDICATION TO ANTHRACYCLINES

Patients with altered cardiac function and a decrease in ventricular ejection rates are not able to tolerate doxorubicin or other anthracyclines, or even mitoxantrone. The use of cisplatin-containing regimen such as DHAP or ESHAP is also frequently contraindicated because of the hydration necessary to avoid renal toxicity, or because of altered renal function associated with the cardiac disease. Protocols with good efficacy but less cardiac toxicity have been designed for these patients; however, they never have been compared to CHOP. Comparison of these trials is impeded by differences in the inclusion criteria (age limits, clinical features at diagnosis), and length of follow-up that may well explain the dissimilarities in their results. Overall survival rates in these Phase II trials, for example, ranged from 34% to 64%.[61,62] None of the reported regimens seems to have a better efficacy. In our center, we often use a combination of rituximab, ifosfamide, and etoposide.[63]

The first question to be asked when considering treatment of an elderly patient is whether there is really any contraindication to use CHOP. A recent study in Netherlands showed that patients not treated with CHOP have a worse survival rate and a much higher death rate from lymphoma (77% compared to 53% for those treated with CHOP).[8,64] The addition of G-CSF allowed more patients to receive the correct chemotherapy regimen without decreasing the results. In conclusion, outcome of elderly patients with diffuse large B-cell lymphoma will be good only if their physicians decide to treat them as younger patients with CHOP chemotherapy.[8]

THERAPEUTIC STRATEGIES FOR OTHER LYMPHOMA SUBTYPES

If therapeutic strategies are beginning to be settled for the treatment of elderly patients with diffuse large B-cell

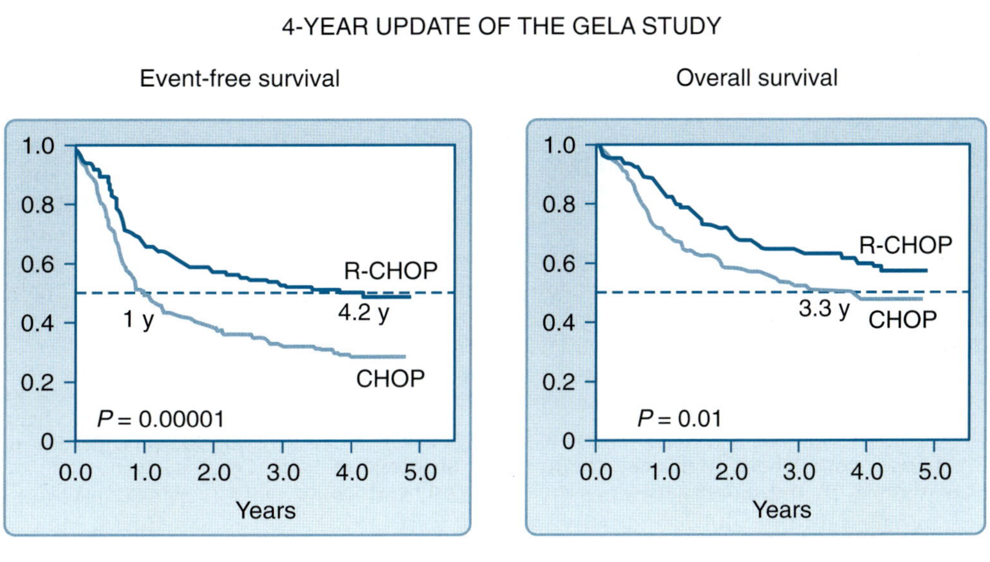

Figure 32–2. Event-free survival and overall survival with a median follow-up of 4 years in patients included in the Groupe d'Etude des Lymphomes de l'Adulte (GELA) trial comparing CHOP and CHOP plus rituximab (R-CHOP) in previously untreated elderly patients with diffuse large B-cell lymphoma.[55]

lymphoma, very few proposals have been made for the treatment of other lymphoma subtypes. Burkitt's lymphoma is a problem because of less positive results obtained with classical CHOP and the near impossibility of increasing dose intensity, except in young elderly patients, that is, between 60 and 65 or 68 years. R-CHOP is recommended and, if outcome is poor, palliative treatment is certainly the best option.

For patients with indolent lymphomas, conclusions drawn for diffuse large B-cell lymphoma may be applied, that is, to treat them in the same way as younger patients. Mantle cell lymphoma and peripheral T-cell lymphoma are the only two problems because no standard has been defined for young patients, and the currently recommended treatments use high-dose therapy with autologous stem cell transplantation.[65] This high-dose therapy should be reserved for a small subgroup of elderly patients, while other patients are treated with standard chemotherapy approaches. The best treatment known for mantle cell lymphoma, even if it only cures a small percentage of patients, is the combination of CHOP plus rituximab.[66] There is no better regimen recommended for patients with peripheral T-cell lymphoma.

Elderly patients with Hodgkin's lymphoma are rare, but it seems that the disease is frequently disseminated with B symptoms and poor performance status.[67,68] No randomized study has been presented in this specific age group, but several studies conclude that doxorubicin-containing regimen do better. ABVD is rarely used because of the vomiting associated with DTIC, but ABV or ABV hybrids are certainly recommended.[68,69] In our center, we used a regimen called ABVPP, that is, the classic ABV regimen plus procarbazine and corticosteroid for 7 days.[70]

AT TIME OF RELAPSE

Very few studies have been dedicated to the treatment of elderly patients who have relapsed. It is usually recognized that the prognosis is very poor with few therapeutic possibilities.[71] Some patients with concomitant diseases or aggressive lymphoma may not be treated at the time of progression because of low performance status. Even if treated, the response rate is around 30%, and median survival is usually less than 6 months. The best therapeutic intervention is palliative chemotherapy with the intention to maintain the best possible quality of life, and preferably at home. In indolent lymphoma, the outcome is better, and rituximab is probably the best solution.

HIGH-DOSE THERAPY WITH AUTOLOGOUS STEM CELL TRANSPLANTATION

High-dose chemotherapy with autologous stem cell transplantation (ASCT) is an established procedure in the treatment of poor-prognosis lymphoma,[72] and advances in supportive care have allowed consideration of its extension to older patients who are otherwise medically fit.[73–75] Gopal et al. presented a series of 53 patients aged 60 to 68 years in relapse treated with high-dose therapy and autologous transplant.[73] Treatment-related mortality was 22%, and 4-year progression-free and overall survival rates were 24% and 33%, respectively. Collection of a sufficient number of CD34+ stem cells does not seem to be an obstacle in these patients. This combination can thus be regarded as a good salvage regimen at the time of relapse for a well-defined and restricted group of patients.

TREATMENT FOR PATIENTS AGED OVER 80 YEARS

Currently, patients older than 80 years are not rare and always pose a difficult problem because of the presence of minor or major dysfunction in practically all organs. However, very few, if any, studies have reported data on these patients. They may have a lymphoma while their performance status is still good, their dependence low, and their intellectual functions near normal. For these patients, except for indolent disease, the solution of no treatment is not considered as satisfactory, at least by the patient. Moreover, clinical status may deteriorate rapidly either because of the lymphoma, other diseases, or hospitalization. A palliative treatment with an appropriate chemotherapy regimen is the best solution.[76] This may be defined as a regimen associated with efficacy, which is disappearance of lymphoma symptoms and low toxicity. In this setting, we use the combination of ifosfamide, 1000 mg/m^2, and etoposide, 300 mg/m^2, plus rituximab for B-cell lymphomas, which are given the same day on an outpatient basis every 2 or 3 weeks. This regimen is nearly devoid of hematologic toxicity, and may decrease tumor volume, which usually gives the patient a few more weeks to arrange her affairs.

CONCLUSION

Age has been described as an adverse prognostic factor for survival of patients with diffuse large B-cell lymphoma, especially when comorbid conditions are present. These poorer results in the elderly may reflect, at least partially, the use of lower doses of chemotherapeutic agents. However, once a complete remission was reached, the disease-free survival of elderly patients does not differ from that of younger patients, emphasizing the importance of achieving complete remission.[11,43] As CHOP plus rituximab is a very well-tolerated regimen, it must be recommended for treatment of these patients, and reducing the dosage in hopes to achieving better tolerance would only decrease the benefits associated with chemotherapy. Treatment with less toxicity must formally be reserved for patients having a contraindication to doxorubicin. Inclusion of growth factors in the therapeutic protocol can offset the risk of neutropenia, neutropenic infection, and a higher treatment-related death rate, and these must certainly be used in the management of elderly patients, particularly for patients with a poor performance status at diagnosis where the risk of treatment-related death is the highest.[58,59]

REFERENCES

1. Armitage JO and Potter JF. Aggressive chemotherapy for diffuse histiocytic lymphoma in the elderly: increased complications with advancing age. J Am Geriatr Soc 1984; 32:269–73.
2. Rao AV, Seo PH, and Cohen HJ. Geriatric assessment and comorbidity. Semin Oncol 2004;31:149–59.

3. Devesa SS, Blot WJ, Stone BJ, et al. Recent cancer trends in the united states. J National Cancer Inst 1995;87:175–82.
4. Howe HL, Wingo PA, Thun MJ, et al. Annual report to the nation on the status of cancer (1973 through 1998), featuring cancers with recent increasing trends. J Natl Cancer Inst 2001;93:824–42.
5. Westin EH and Longo DL. Lymphoma and myeloma in older patients. Semin Oncol 2004;31:198–205.
6. The Non-Hodgkin's Lymphoma Classification Project. Effect of age on the characteristics and clinical behavior of non-Hodgkin's lymphoma patients. Ann Oncol 1997;8:973–8.
7. Balducci L and Ballester OF. Non-Hodgkin's lymphoma in the elderly. Cancer Control 1996;3:5–14.
8. Peters FPJ, Lalisang RI, Fickers MMF, et al. Treatment of elderly patients with intermediate- and high-grade non-Hodgkin's lymphoma: a retrospective population-based study. Ann Hematol 2001;80:155–9.
9. Kouroukis CT, Browman GP, Esmail R, et al. Chemotherapy for older patients with newly diagnosed, advanced-stage, aggressive-histology non-Hodgkin lymphoma: a systematic review. Ann Intern Med 2002;136:144–52.
10. Kennedy BJ. Aging and cancer. J Clin Oncol 1988;6:1903–11.
11. Maartense E, Hermans J, Kluin-Nelemans JC, et al. Elderly patients with non-Hodgkin's lymphoma: population-based results in The Netherlands. Ann Oncol 1998;9:1219–27.
12. d'Amore F, Brincker H, Christensen BE, et al. Non-Hodgkin's lymphoma in the elderly. A study of 602 patients aged 70 or older from a Danish population-based registry. The Danish LYEO-Study Group. Ann Oncol 1992;3:379–86.
13. Carbone A, Tirelli U, Volpe R, et al. Non-Hodgkin's lymphoma in the elderly. A retrospective clinicopathologic study of 50 patients. Cancer 1986;57:2185–9.
14. Greiner TC, Medeiros LJ, and Jaffe ES. Non Hodgkin's lymphoma. Cancer 1995;75:370–80.
15. Groves FD, Linet MS, Travis LB, et al. Cancer surveillance series: non-Hodgkin's lymphoma incidence by histologic subtype in the United States from 1978 through 1995. J Natl Cancer Inst 2000;92:1240–51.
16. Jaffe ES, Harris NL, Stein H, et al., eds. World Health Organization Classification of Tumours. Pathology and Genetics of Tumours of Haematopoietic and Lymphoid Tissues. Lyon: International Agency for Research on Cancer, 2001.
17. The Non-Hodgkin's Lymphoma Pathologic Classification Project. National Cancer Institute sponsored study of classifications of non-Hodgkin's lymphomas. Summary and description of a working formulation for clinical usage. Cancer 1982; 49:2112–35.
18. Carbone A, Volpe R, Gloghini A, et al. Non-Hodgkin's lymphoma in the elderly. I. Pathologic features at presentation. Cancer 1990;66:1991–4.
19. Harris NL, Jaffe ES, Stein H, et al. A revised European–American classification of lymphoid neoplasms. A proposal from the International Lymphoma Study Group. Blood 1994; 84:1361–92.
20. The Non-Hodgkin's Lymphoma Classification Project. A clinical trial of the International Lymphoma Study Group classification of non-Hodgkin's lymphoma. Blood 1997;89: 3909–18.
21. Staudt LM. Molecular diagnosis of the hematologic cancers. N Engl J Med 2003;348:1777–85 [review].
22. Rosenwald A, Wright G, Chan WC, et al. The use of molecular profiling to predict survival after chemotherapy for diffuse large-B-cell lymphoma. N Engl J Med 2002;346:1937–47.
23. Rosenwald A, Wright G, Wiestner A, et al. The proliferation gene expression signature is a quantitative integrator of oncogenic events that predicts survival in mantle cell lymphoma. Cancer Cell 2003;3:185–97.
24. Savage KJ, Monti S, Kutok JL, et al. The molecular signature of mediastinal large B-cell lymphoma differs from that of other diffuse large B-cell lymphomas and shares features with classical Hodgkin lymphoma. Blood 2003;102:3871–9.
25. The International Non-Hodgkin's Lymphoma Prognostic Factors Project. A predictive model for aggressive non-Hodgkin's lymphoma. N Engl J Med 1993;329:987–94.
26. Solal-Celigny P, Roy P, Colombat P, et al. Follicular lymphoma international prognostic index. Blood 2004;104:1258–65.
27. Balducci L. Cancer in the elderly: tailoring treatment. Hosp Pract 2000;35:73–9; discussion 9–80; quiz 135.
28. van Spronsen DJ, Janssen-Heijnen MLG, Breed WPM, et al. Prevalence of co-morbidity and its relationship to treatment among unselected patients with Hodgkin's disease and non-Hodgkin's lymphoma, 1993–1996. Ann Hematol 1999;78: 315–9.
29. Balducci L, Parker M, Sexton W, et al. Pharmacology of antineoplastic agents in the elderly patient. Semin Oncol 1989; 16:76–84.
30. Lichtman SM. Chemotherapy in the elderly. Semin Oncol 2004;31:160–74.
31. Lindeman RD, Tobin J, and Shock NW. Longitudinal studies on the rate of decline in renal function with age. J Am Geriatr Soc 1986;33:278–85.
32. Durnas C, Loi CM, and Cusack BJ. Hepatic drug metabolism and aging. Clin Pharmacokinet 1990;19:359–80.
33. Lipschitz DA. Age-related declines in hematopoietic reserve capacity. Sem Hematol 1995;22(Suppl 1):3–5.
34. Dixon DO, Neilan B, Jones SE, et al. Effect of age on therapeutic outcome in advanced diffuse histiocytic lymphoma: the Southwest Oncology Group experience. J Clin Oncol 1986; 4:295–305.
35. Morrison VA, Picozzi V, Scott S, et al. The impact of age on delivered dose intensity and hospitalizations for febrile neutropenia in patients with intermpediate-grade non-Hodgkin's lymphoma receiving initial CHOP chemotheerapy: a risk factor analysis. Clin Lymph 2001;2:47–56.
36. Chrischilles E, Delgado DJ, Stolshek BS, et al. Impact f age anc colony-stimulating factor use on hospital lenght of stay for febrile neutropenia in CHOP-treated non-Hodgkin's lymphoma. Cancer Control 2002;9:203–11.
37. Simon R, Durrleman S, Hoppe RT, et al. The Non-Hodgkin Lymphoma Pathologic Classification Project. Long-term follow-up of 1153 patients with non-Hodgkin lymphomas. Ann Intern Med 1988;109:939–45.
38. Vose JM, Armitage JO, Weisenburger DD, et al. The importance of age in survival of patients treated with chemotherapy for aggressive non-Hodgkin's lymphoma. J Clin Oncol 1988; 6:1838–44.
39. Linch DC, Hudson BV, Hancock BW, et al. A randomised comparison of a third-generation regimen (PACEBOM) with a standard regimen (CHOP) in patients with histologically aggressive non-Hodgkin's lymphoma: a British National Lymphoma Investigation report. Br J Cancer 1996;74:318–22.
40. Neilly IJ, Ogston M, Bennett B, et al. High grade non-Hodgkin's lymphoma in the elderly:12 year experience in the Grampian Region of Scotland. Hematol Oncol 1995;13: 99–106.
41. Radford JA, Whelan JS, Rohatiner AZS, et al. Weekly VAPEC-B chemotherapy for high grade non-Hodgkin's lymphoma: results of treatment in 184 patients. Ann Oncol 1994;5: 147–51.
42. Gomez H, Mas L, Casanova L, et al. Elderly patients with aggressive non-Hodgkin's lymphoma treated with CHOP chemotherapy plus granulocyte-macrophage colony-stimulating factor: identification of two age subgroups with differing hematologic toxicity. J Clin Oncol 1998;16:2352–8.

43. Bastion Y, Blay JY, Divine M, et al. Elderly patients with aggressive non-Hodgkin's lymphoma: disease presentation, response to treatment, and survival—a Groupe d'Etude des Lymphomes de l'Adulte study on 453 patients older than 69 years. J Clin Oncol 1997;15:2945–53.
44. Zinzani PL, Storti S, Zaccaria A, et al. Elderly aggressive-histology non-Hodgkin's lymphoma: first-line VNCOP-B regimen experience on 350 patients. Blood 1999;94:33–8.
45. Tirelli U, Carbone A, Monfardini S, et al. A 20-year experience on malignant lymphomas in patients aged 70 and older at a single institute. Crit Rev Oncol Hematol 2001; 37:153–8.
46. Miller TP, Dahlberg S, Cassady JR, et al. Chemotherapy alone compared with chemotherapy plus radiotherapy for localized intermediate-and high-grade non-Hodgkin's lymphoma. N Engl J Med 1998;339:21–6.
47. Fisher RI, Gaynor ER, Dahlberg S, et al. Comparison of a standard regimen (CHOP) with three intensive chemotherapy regimens for advanced non-Hodgkin's lymphoma. N Engl J Med 1993;328:1002–6.
48. Sonneveld P, de Ridder M, van der Lelie H, et al. Comparison of doxorubicin and mitoxantrone in the treatment of elderly patients with advanced diffuse non-Hodgkin's lymphoma using CHOP versus CNOP chemotherapy. J Clin Oncol 1995; 13:2530–9.
49. Osby E, Hagberg H, Kvaloy S, et al. CHOP is superior to CNOP in elderly patients with aggressive lymphoma while outcome is unaffected by filgrastim treatment: results of a Nordic Lymphoma Group randomized trial. Blood 2003; 101:3840–8.
50. Meyer RM, Browman GP, Samosh ML, et al. Randomized phase II comparison of standard CHOP with weekly CHOP in elderly patients with non-Hodgkin's lymphoma. J Clin Oncol 1995;13:2386–93.
51. Bailey NP, Stuart NSA, Bessell EM, et al. Five-year follow-up of a prospective randomised multi-centre trial of weekly chemotherapy (Capomet) versus cyclical chemotherapy (Chop-Mtx) in the treatment of aggressive non-Hodgkins-lymphoma. Ann Oncol 1998;9:633–8.
52. Tirelli U, Errante D, Vanglabbeke M, et al. CHOP is the standard regimen in patients greater-than or equal-to 70 years of age with intermediate-grade and high-grade non-Hodgkin's Lymphoma. Results of a randomized study of the European Organization for Research and Treatment of Cancer Lymphoma Cooperative Study Group. J Clin Oncol 1998;16: 27–34.
53. Mainwaring PN, Cunningham D, Gregory W, et al. Mitoxantrone is superior to doxorubicin in a multiagent weekly regimen for patients older than 60 with high-grade lymphoma: results of a BNLI randomized trial of PAdriaCEBO versus PMitCEBO. Blood 2001;97:2991–7.
54. Pfreundschuh M, Truemper L, Kloess M, et al. 2-weekly or 3-weekly CHOP Chemotherapy with or without Etoposide for the Treatment of Elderly Patients with Aggressive Lymphomas: results of the NHL-B2 trial of the DSHNHL. Blood 2004;104:626–41.
55. Coiffier B, Lepage E, Brière J, et al. CHOP chemotherapy plus rituximab compared with CHOP alone in elderly patients with diffuse large B-cell lymphoma. N Engl J Med 2002; 346:235–42.
56. Habermann TM, Weller EA, Morrison VA, et al. Phase III trial of rituximab-CHOP (R-CHOP) vs. CHOP with a second randomization to maintenance rituximab (MR) or observation in patients 60 years of age and older with diffuse large B-cell lymphoma (DLBCL). Blood 2003;102(Suppl 1) (abstract 8).
57. Sehn LH, Donaldson J, Chhanabhai M, et al. Introduction of combined CHOP-rituximab therapy dramatically improved outcome of diffuse large B-cell lymphoma (DLBC) in British Columbia (BC). J Clin Oncol 2005;23:5027–33.
58. Gomez H, Hidalgo M, Casanova L, et al. Risk factors for treatment-related death in elderly patients with aggressive non-Hodgkin's lymphoma: results of a multivariate analysis. J Clin Oncol 1998;16:2065–9.
59. Guerci A, Lederlin P, Reyes F, et al. Effect of granulocyte colony-stimulating factor administration in elderly patients with aggressive non-Hodgkin's lymphoma treated with a pirarubicin-combination chemotherapy regimen. Groupe d'Etudes des Lymphomes de l'Adulte. Ann Oncol 1996;7:966–9.
60. Jacobson JO, Grossbard M, Shulman LN, et al. CHOP chemotherapy with preemptive granulocyte colony-stimulating factor in elderly patients with aggressive non-Hodgkin's lymphoma: a dose-intensity analysis. Clin Lymphoma 2000; 1:211–7;discussion 8.
61. Coiffier B. What treatment for elderly patients with aggressive lymphoma? Ann Oncol 1994;5:873–5.
62. Bertini M, Boccomini C, and Calvi R. The Influence of advanced age on the treatment and prognosis of diffuse large-cell lymphoma (DLCL). Clin Lymphoma 2001;1:278–84.
63. Tigaud JD, Demolombe S, Bastion Y, et al. Ifosfamide continuous infusion plus etoposide in the treatment of elderly patients with aggressive lymphoma. A phase II study. Hematol Oncol 1991;9:225–33.
64. Peters FP, Fickers MM, Erdkamp FL, et al. The effect of optimal treatment on elderly patients with aggressive non-Hodgkin's lymphoma: more patients treated with unaffected response rates. Ann Hematol 2001;80:406–10.
65. Lazzarino M, Arcaini L, Bernasconi P, et al. A sequence of immuno-chemotherapy with Rituximab, mobilization of in vivo purged stem cells, high-dose chemotherapy and autotransplant is an effective and non-toxic treatment for advanced follicular and mantle cell lymphoma. Br J Haematol 2002;116:229–35.
66. Howard OM, Gribben JG, Neuberg DS, et al. Rituximab and CHOP induction therapy for newly diagnosed mantle-cell lymphoma: molecular complete responses are not predictive of progression-free survival. J Clin Oncol 2002;20:1288–94.
67. Stark GL, Wood KM, Jack F, et al. Hodgkin's disease in the elderly: a population-based study. Br J Haematol 2002;119: 432–40.
68. Landgren O, Algernon C, Axdorph U, et al. Hodgkin's lymphoma in the elderly with special reference to type and intensity of chemotherapy in relation to prognosis. Haematologica 2003;88:438–44.
69. Weekes CD, Vose JM, Lynch JC, et al. Hodgkin's disease in the elderly: improved treatment outcome with a doxorubicin-containing regimen. J Clin Oncol 2002;20:1087–93.
70. Ferme C, Sebban C, Hennequin C, et al. Comparison of chemotherapy to radiotherapy as consolidation of complete or good partial response after six cycles of chemotherapy for patients with advanced Hodgkin's disease: results of the Groupe d'etudes des Lymphomes de l'Adulte H89 trial. Blood 2000;95:2246–52.
71. Jabbour E, Chalhoub B, Suzan F, et al. Outcome of elderly patients with aggressive non-Hodgkin's lymphoma refractory to or relapsing after first-line CHOP pr CHOP-like chemotherapy: a low possibility of cure. Leuk Lymph 2004;45:1391–4.
72. Haioun C, Lepage E, Gisselbrecht C, et al. Survival benefit of high-dose therapy in poor-risk aggressive non-Hodgkin's lymphoma: final analysis of the prospective LNH87-2 protocol—A Groupe d'Etude des Lymphomes de l'Adulte Study. J Clin Oncol 2000;18:3025–30.
73. Gopal AK, Gooley TA, Golden JB, et al. Efficacy of high-dose therapy and autologous hematopoietic stem cell transplantation for non-Hodgkin's lymphoma in adults 60 years of age and older. Bone Marrow Transplant 2001;27:593–9.

74. Jantunen E, Mahlamaki E, and Nousiainen T. Feasibility and toxicity of high-dose chemotherapy supported by peripheral blood stem cell transplantation in elderly patients (>= 60 years) with non-Hodgkin's lymphoma: comparison with patients <60 years treated within the same protocol. Bone Marrow Transplant 2000;26:737–41.
75. Zallio F, Cuttica A, Caracciolo D, et al. Feasibility of peripheral blood progenitor cell mobilization and harvest to support chemotherapy intensification in elderly patients with poor prognosis: Non-Hodgkin's lymphoma. Ann Hematol 2002; 81:448–53.
76. Fiorentino MV. Lymphomas in the elderly. Leukemia 1991; 5(Suppl 1):79–85.
77. Aoki S, Tsukada N, Nomoto N, et al. Effect of pirarubicin for elderly patients with malignant lymphoma. J Exp Clin Cancer Res 1998;17:465–70.
78. Aviles A, Nambo MJ, Talavera A, et al. Epirubicin (CEOP-Bleo) versus idaurubicin (CIOP-Bleo) in the treatment of elderly patients with aggressive non-Hodgkin's lymphoma: dose escalation studies. Anti-Cancer Drugs 1997;8:937–42.
79. Cooper IA, Wolf MM, Robertson TI, et al. Randomized comparison of MACOP-B with CHOP in patients with intermediate-grade non-Hodgkin's lymphoma. J Clin Oncol 1994; 12:769–78.
80. De Lena M, Maiello E, Lorusso V, et al. Comparison of CHOP-B vs CEOP-B in 'poor prognosis' non-Hodgkin's lymphomas. A randomized trial. Med Oncol Tumor Pharmacother 1989;6:163–9.
81. Gordon LI, Harrington D, Andersen J, et al. Comparison of a second-generation combination chemotherapeutic regimen (m-BACOD) with a standard regimen (CHOP) for advanced diffuse non-Hodgkin's lymphoma. N Engl J Med 1992; 327:1342–9.
82. Jelic S, Milanovic N, Tomasevic Z, et al. Comparison of two non-anthracycline-containing regimens for elderly patients with diffuse large-cell non Hodgkin's lymphoma—possible pitfalls in results reporting and interpretation. Neoplasma 1999;46:394–9.
83. Meyer RM, Browman GP, Samosh ML, et al. Randomized phase II comparison of standard CHOP with weekly CHOP in elderly patients with non-Hodgkin's lymphoma. J Clin Oncol 1995;13:2386–93.
84. Montserrat E, Garciaconde J, Vinolas H, et al. CHOP vs promace-cytabom in the treatment of aggressive non-Hodgkins lymphomas—long-term results of a multicenter randomized trial. Eur J Hematol 1996;57:377–83.
85. Silingardi V, Federico M, Cavanna L, et al. Promece-cytabom vs macop-b in advanced aggressive non-Hodgkins lymphoma—long term results of a multicenter study of the Italian Lymphoma Study Group (GISL). Leuk Lymph 1995; 17:313–20.
86. Zinzani PL, Gherlinzoni F, Storti S, et al. Randomized trial of 8-week versus 12-week VNCOP-B plus G-CSF regimens as front-line treatment in elderly aggressive non-Hodgkin's lymphoma patients. Ann Oncol 2002;13:1364–9.

33

Lymphoma and Pregnancy

Catherine Traullé, M.D.

Bertrand Coiffier, M.D.

Coincidental lymphoma and pregnancy is a rare event, occurring in about 1 in 1000 deliveries. The number of pregnant women with newly diagnosed Hodgkin's lymphoma (HL) is undoubtedly greater than with non-Hodgkin's lymphoma (NHL). For a long time, it was thought that HL was exacerbated by pregnancy, and that the disease itself affected the course of gestation and delivery, but recent studies showed that this was not the case. If pregnant women with HL usually present with typical manifestations, those with NHL, in contrast, present with unusual manifestations, aggressive subtypes, advanced-stage disease, and poor outcome.

Management of these patients must be individualized, and should involve a multidisciplinary team: hematologist, radiation oncologist, obstetrician, neonatologist, pediatrician, and mental health professional. Indeed it is hard to imagine a more difficult time to receive diagnosis of malignancy than during pregnancy. The choice of staging procedures depends on their efficiency and their lack of toxicity for the fetus. Treatment includes chemotherapy with or without radiotherapy. Both staging and treatment depend on the term of the pregnancy. Major toxicities for the fetus occur during the first trimester of pregnancy, so treatment should be avoided during this period and delayed until the second trimester. If the treatment cannot be delayed until the end of first trimester, often in case of aggressive NHL requiring early chemotherapy, a therapeutic abortion should be proposed. However, most of these women, especially those with HL or DLCL in the second trimester of pregnancy, will be cured, remain fertile, and potentially become pregnant again.

INCIDENCE OF LYMPHOMAS DURING PREGNANCY

HL and NHL are the fourth most frequent malignancies diagnosed among pregnant women, after breast, cervix, and ovarian cancers.[1] The number of women with coincident HL and pregnancy is uncertain, estimated from 1 in 1000 to 1 in 6000 deliveries.[1,2] Among the general population of women, the median age of patients with NHL is older than with HL and the incidence is nearly eight times higher.[3–5] But even if among women of childbearing age the incidence rates are curiously similar, the number of pregnant women with newly diagnosed HL or relapsed disease is clearly superior to what is expected. On the other hand, we know that incidence of HL remains stable, whereas incidence of NHL has been increasing at 3% per year since the 1980s.[5] Consequently, the number of coincidental pregnancy and lymphoma cases is likely to increase.

IMPACT OF PREGNANCY ON LYMPHOMA

Hodgkin's Lymphoma

Most reports in the literature conclude that the characteristics and prognosis of HL in pregnant women do not differ significantly from those seen in nonpregnant women.[6–16] Only three studies note a slightly higher proportion of advanced-stage cases among pregnant women, or a greater than expected incidence of Hodgkin's during the first 6 months postpartum, suggesting a delay in the diagnosis, as the illness's symptoms mimic pregnancy's discomfort.[12,15,17]

Non-Hodgkin's Lymphoma

In 1989, Ward and Weiss reported a series of 42 women with poor outcome.[18] Only 13 patients were alive, among them two with active disease. But they had been obviously undertreated: 6 received a multidrug regimen during the pregnancy and 14 were treated with a single agent—radiotherapy or steroids—or with surgery, while 22 received no treatment at all. Pohlman and Macklis published a retrospective review of 96 pregnant patients.[19] Among the 90 mothers in whom the outcome was known, only 39 were alive and disease-free at a median of 21 months (range 2 to 132) after delivery, 4 were alive with disease, and 47 died at a median of 6 (range <1 to 36) months after delivery. Patients diagnosed during the third trimester and patients with early-stage disease tended to have a better prognosis. Patients with Burkitt's lymphoma had a very poor outcome.

Recent observations tend to demonstrate that if modern treatment modalities are applied early in the course of the illness during the pregnancy, the response to treatment, and failure and progression rates are quite similar to that of nonpregnant women.[20–29]

Nevertheless, most pregnant women have an aggressive histological subtype, uncommon presentation, and advanced-stage disease. Even if predominance of aggressive forms is usual in young patients, their proportion is higher among pregnant women,[18,30–32] with a high rate of Burkitt's lymphoma.[3,19]

A high incidence of breast, uterine, cervical, and ovarian involvement is reported.[3,29,33–50] The predilection for these organs has been attributed to hormonal influence and/or increased blood flow to these organs during pregnancy.[3,38,40,41] In the Dhedin and Coiffier series among 45 women, 13 had breast involvement; the majority had a Burkitt's subtype and a poor outcome. On the other hand, it has been suggested that hormonal and immunologic changes occurring during pregnancy could stabilize the lymphoma's proliferation until delivery.[18,32]

Placenta involvement was only reported in five cases: one case of T-cell immunoblastic lymphoma,[31] two cases of diffuse large B-cell lymphoma,[51,52] one case of anaplastic large-cell lymphoma,[20] and one case of natural-killer-cell lymphoma.[53] Dissemination of the maternal non-Hodgkin's lymphoma to the fetus was described in only one case.[53]

Most of the lymphomas associated with pregnancy are disseminated. In the review of Dhedin and Coiffier,[3] among 73 patients, 67% were Stage IV, 12% Stage III, 5% Stage II, and 16% Stage I. In the Moore and Taslimi series,[54] among 37 patients, 28 presented with extranodal involvement other than bone marrow, and the initial diagnosis was correct in only 16. One likely explanation for this pattern is the frequent delayed diagnosis, as some symptoms of pregnancy mimic symptoms of lymphoma (e.g., asthenia, vomiting with lost of weight, breast enlargement, colicky abdominal pain). Moore and Taslimi reported that the correct diagnosis was delayed for more than 3 weeks in 40% of the 37 patients, and by more than 3 months in 20%.[54]

IMPACT OF LYMPHOMA ON PREGNANCY

Hodgkin's Disease

There is no consensus in the literature concerning consequences of Hodgkin's disease on gestation course, delivery, incidence of spontaneous abortions and prematurity, and fetal outcome. Lishner et al. reported on 22 patients, collected from 1958 to 1984, 12 of whom were diagnosed before conception, treated with radiotherapy (16), chemotherapy (1 in the first trimester), or combined chemotherapy-radiotherapy, with no difference in the stage at diagnosis, maternal outcome, or pregnancy outcome with a similar group of nonpregnant patients.[55]

Ebert et al. identified 24 cases from the literature between 1983 and 1995 who received chemotherapy during pregnancy.[56] Three women had therapeutic abortions, all having received chemotherapy (MOPP, MOP, ABVD or chemotherapy plus radiotherapy in one) in the first trimester, and all three fetuses had multiple anomalies. Two women had spontaneous abortions after chemotherapy (MOPP, vinblastine, and procarbazine) beginning in the first trimester; one fetus had multiple anomalies. Three other infants were born with anomalies and died: two mothers had received chemotherapy during the first trimester and another had received vinblastine, vincristine, and procarbazine beginning in week 25. In contrast, 15 infants were normal and remained healthy for a median of 9 (range 0 to 17) years after delivery; five mothers had received chemotherapy during the first trimester.

Finally, Aviles and Neri reviewed 26 women treated with ABVD, ABD, EBVD, or MOPP, 10 of them during the first trimester, who delivered 26 normal babies.[27]

Non-Hodgkin's Lymphoma

Ortega reported the first successful pregnancy associated with advanced NHL after treatment with a multidrug chemotherapy regimen including cyclophosphamide, vincristine, bleomycin, and prednisone.[57] Zuazu et al. observed no difference within a healthy population in the incidence of spontaneous abortions, prematurity, and malformations among 56 pregnant women with associated hematologic malignancies.[58] Ward and Weiss have suggested interestingly that NHL had adverse effect on pregnancy due primarily to the mother's death.[18]

In the Pohlman et al. series,[2] among 96 pregnancies, 71 babies were reported alive, but the follow-up was short for most of them (<1 month) or unknown.

Aviles and Neri reviewed 29 pregnant women with NHL between 1970 and 1995, who received CHOP or a CHOP-like regimen (17 during the first trimester)[27]; all delivered healthy infants with normal height and weight, and no congenital abnormalities. Aviles et al. had previously reported on 19 pregnant women between 1975 and 1986 who had received doxorubicin-based combination chemotherapy (8 during the first trimester)[21]; three mothers and their fetuses died during induction, with the 16 remaining women delivering healthy infants spontaneously (n = 12) or by caesarean section (n = 4) between 35 and 39 weeks of gestation. Babies had subnormal birth weights, and no apparent congenital abnormalities.

Staging Evaluation

Lymphoma staging is based on history and physical examination, hematologic and biochemical testing, bone marrow testing, eventual lumbar puncture, and radiologic imaging. In pregnant women, ionizing imaging must be avoided, except a chest x-ray that has negligible exposure to the fetus. Thus, CT scan, lymphangiography (now widely excluded from the staging process), isotopic scans, and PET scan are contraindicated. CT scan can be substituted with MRI, which is at least comparable in the detection of lymphadenopathy, but with a lower performance in detecting pathologic mediastinal lymph nodes.[59] Many MR examinations of the chest, abdomen, and pelvis have been performed on pregnant women, with no observable adverse effects on the fetus.[60] However, it is recommended that MRI be used sparingly during the first trimester. Ultrasound and echocardiography can be used without any toxicity. Thus, it is possible to realize a high-quality staging during pregnancy, which dictates the right treatment and prognosis.

CHEMOTHERAPY AGENTS AND PREGNANCY

Pharmacology of Antineoplastic Agents During Pregnancy

Physiologic changes that occur during pregnancy can potentially alter the effectiveness and increase the toxicity of antineoplastic agents, by changing their metabolism or clearance: increasing plasma volume results in dilution; binding of drugs is modified because of a decreased serum albumin concentration; and hepatic function and renal excretion are enhanced.[61–63]

The transplacental crossing of antineoplastic drugs is conditioned by their physicochemical characteristics: passive diffusion increases with decreasing molecular weight, increasing solubility, and decreasing protein-binding capacity. Most antineoplastic drugs have a high placental diffusion.[61,64]

Adverse Effects of Antineoplastic Agents on Fetus

Potential effects of chemotherapy on the fetus depend on several factors: time of exposure, type of drugs, and dose of various drugs. During the first 2 weeks after conception, chemotherapy is likely to result in spontaneous abortion; during the period of organogenesis, from the 2nd to 8th week of gestation, administration of chemotherapy is at high risk of inducing congenital malformations; after the beginning of the 3rd month, chemotherapy may result in growth retardation and low birth weight. If the exact risk of fetal anomalies following exposure of pregnant women to chemotherapy is not known, many case reports describe both normal and abnormal fetal outcome, even if chemotherapy had been administered during the first trimester. It is admitted that antimetabolites and alkylating agents should be avoided during the first trimester because of fetal toxicity.[63,65] Whereas bleomycin, doxorubicin, daunorubicin, vinblastine, and vincristine have not been reported to cause adverse fetal outcome.

In the Aviles and Neri study,[27] among 84 pregnant women with hematologic malignancy, 38 received chemotherapy during the first trimester, including 11 with acute myeloid or lymphoblastic leukemia received standard treatment (cytosine arabinoside and doxorubicin, or cyclophosphamide, vincristine, prednisone, and doxorubicin); 10 with Hodgkin's lymphoma were treated with ABVD, ABD, EBVD or MOPP; and 17 with non-Hodgkin's Lymphoma received CHOP-like regimen. They all delivered normal babies. Germann et al. published recently information concerning 160 pregnant women treated with anthracyclines (71.5% of whom with hematological malignancies, only 21.5% with lymphoma), from a review of literature between 1976 and 2001.[66] Fetal death was frequently related to maternal death (40%), which may account for the significantly higher frequency of unfavorable fetal outcomes in patients with acute leukemia. Abnormalities included malformations (3%), fetal death (9%), spontaneous abortion (3%), fetal complications (8%, cardiac toxicity and bone marrow depletion), and prematurity (6%). The risks associated with chemotherapy are increased by combination with antimetabolites (ara-C) and alkylating agents (cyclophosphamide), which rapidly cross the placenta and have a complete transfer, whereas anthracyclines cross the placenta incompletely. They also depend on the date of administration: in patients with solid tumors, the first trimester is significantly associated with more complications; cardiotoxicity and bone marrow depression are related to late administration, that is, in the second trimester and predelivery. Finally, the risks depend on the dose of treatment, the toxicity being increased 30-fold when the dose of doxorubicin per cycle exceeded 70 mg/m^2. The authors recommend standard dosage in bolus or short infusion from the second trimester, to prevent malformations, until 2 weeks before delivery, to prevent neonatal infection or neutropenia.

RADIATION TREATMENT AND PREGNANCY

The effects of x-rays on fetal development are estimated from extrapolation of experimental animal irradiations, and mainly from the study of Japanese victims of the atomic bomb and unintentional medical exposures. The risks consist of prenatal or neonatal death, congenital malformations, severe mental retardation, and temporary or permanent growth retardation.

The risk of a radiation-induced hereditary disorder is reported to be approximately 1% per gray. Most authors estimate that with appropriate abdominal shielding in place, the fetal dose can be reduced by 50% or more in most cases, and that mantle radiotherapy may be delivered safely to a pregnant patient after the first trimester.[67–71]

Hodgkin's Lymphoma

Several authors, based on their own patients and the review of literature, have published treatment recommendations, which have changed from the 1970s to the present because of more experience and the evolution in treatment. Indeed, in the 1970s, radiotherapy was an essential part of the treatment, as well for limited stages in advanced disease, and the standard chemotherapy was MOPP, known for its fetal toxicity. Currently, for most early-stage diseases, chemotherapy followed by radiotherapy is recommended, which allows delaying radiotherapy until the second trimester, or after delivery. ABVD, less toxic for the fetus after the first trimester, is the standard treatment for advanced-stage disease.

More recent guidelines proposed by Dhedin and Coiffier, and Pohlman and Macklis, are quite similar[3,19]:

During the first trimester, therapeutic abortion may be proposed if a delay in treatment is unacceptable but must usually be avoided. In case of bulky disease, B symptoms, visceral involvement, subdiaphragmatic disease, or rapid disease progression, a treatment must be proposed, but the choice of the drugs is difficult. If continuation of pregnancy is elected because abortion is refused by the patient despite an urgent need for treatment, vinblastine may be used alone, until the second trimester or progression, or ABVD without dacarbazine.

After the first trimester or during the second half of pregnancy, treatment must de delayed as long as possible in case of localized or stable disease. If not possible, ABVD without dacarbazine or CHOP-like regimen is recommended by Dhedin and Coiffier, whereas Pohlman and Macklis propose standard ABVD. Radiotherapy should be postponed until the end of pregnancy, and no more than 9 weeks after last chemotherapy. Occasionally, mantle (or "mini-mantle") radiation therapy may be an acceptable option in some patients, if clinical Stage IA, progression on chemotherapy, or if chemotherapy for some reason is not feasible.

Among women with refractory or relapsed disease, in which ABVD and/or radiotherapy are not indicated, MOPP and MOPP-like regimens have documented efficacy, and limited adverse effect on the fetus if administered after the first trimester.

Non-Hodgkin's Lymphoma

Dhedin and Coiffier and Pohlman and Macklis again propose similar strategies for the treatment of pregnant women. Lymphomas associated with pregnancy usually have an aggressive histology, and maternal outcome is poor without an efficient treatment administered as soon as possible[3,19]:

For Dhedin and Coiffier, during the first trimester patients should be considered for a therapeutic abortion and immediate multidrug regimen. In a small fraction of these women, with Stage I disease, an involved irradiation could be proposed, or a "watch-and-wait" attitude, until the second trimester. Treatment with supradiaphragmatic radiotherapy or single-drug chemotherapy to stabilize a disseminated disease until the second trimester is not a valid option for the mother. However, when the patient and her family refuse therapeutic abortion, a decision regarding treatment must be made, which balances the prognosis of the mother and the hazards to the fetus. Pohlman and Macklis recommend as well a therapeutic abortion during the first trimester.

During the second and third trimesters, all recommend to treat the women with full doses of a multidrug regimen known to have efficacy in these aggressive lymphomas (CHOP). For Pohlman and Macklis concerning women with localized disease who have completed three to eight cycles of CHOP chemotherapy, radiotherapy should be delayed until after delivery, but no more than nine weeks after last cycle of chemotherapy. For the Groupe d'Etudes des Lymphomes de l'Adulte (GELA) group, radiotherapy is not indicated in the treatment of these localized aggressive lymphomas. Patients with Burkitt's lymphoma or lymphoblastic lymphoma may be treated with appropriate high-dose chemotherapy.[19,26]

Only one paper reported the safety and efficacy of a combined rituximab-chemotherapy during pregnancy.[72] This treatment was selected because of the superiority of rituximab plus CHOP over CHOP alone.[73] Rituximab is a humanized immunoglobulin G that passes the placental barrier, and so may affect the fetal B-cell subset. The chemotherapy was a CHOP regimen without cyclophosphamide. The patient (Stage IIA bulky, CD20+ diffuse large B-cell lymphoma) received four full-dose cycles without adverse event, and then, in very good partial remission, delivered a healthy girl via caesarian section. After two more cycles, the mother was in complete remission. The child developed well, and a normal peripheral B-cell population was noted at 4 months. This treatment combining anti-CD20 with chemotherapy seems to be a promising option.

There are no data concerning relapses during pregnancy. For patients in whom a second remission and long-term survival are realistic goals, salvage chemotherapy should not be compromised. Patients who relapse during the first half of pregnancy should have a therapeutic abortion. Those who relapse during the second half of pregnancy could receive salvage treatment, and benefit, if possible, from high-dose therapy with autologous or allogeneic hematopoietic cell transplantation, after delivery.[19]

As of this writing, no case of low-grade nodular lymphoma during pregnancy has been reported, and only two cases of indolent cutaneous lymphomas have been published (two mycosis fungoides, one treated with efficacy and no toxicity by alpha-interferon).[74,75]

OUTCOME FOR CHILDREN

Dienstbier et al. described the data on the course of pregnancy, delivery, and subsequent development of 20 children born from parents with Hodgkin's lymphoma.[76] Thirteen women delivered 16 infants, and three men had three daughters. The parents were treated by radiotherapy alone (1), chemotherapy alone (2), or chemotherapy (COPP/ABVD) plus radiotherapy (13). The parameters of the infants at delivery, and the subsequent physical and mental development were normal. Only one girl (followed up to 10.5 years) was born with malformations of the extremities, not related to the previous treatment of the mother for the geneticist, whose second child was normal.

Aviles and Neri analyzed the 84 children whose mothers had received chemotherapy during pregnancy.[27] The growth, development, educational performance, and behavior of these children were normal. Abnormalities were not observed in hematologic, renal, hepatic, or cardiac function, and cytogenetic studies were normal. With a median follow-up of 18 years (range 6 to 29 years), no cancer or hematologic malignancy was reported. Twelve of these people had normal babies, without congenital abnormalities, but further clinical or laboratory studies were refused by the parents.

CONCLUSION

Hodgkin's and non-Hodgkin's lymphomas occurring during or after a pregnancy are not infrequent diseases in young women. This is mainly considered a coincidence because the two usually occur at the same age. Hodgkin's lymphoma usually has the same characteristics as in nonpregnant woman. Non-Hodgkin's lymphoma is usually of a more aggressive subtype, frequently Burkitt's lymphoma. Therapeutic abortion should be envisaged only during the first weeks of the pregnancy in women who need an urgent therapeutic intervention. During the second and first trimesters, the treatment must not differ from the one proposed for nonpregnant women. Consequences for the fetus are rare, except in cases where treatment is realized during the first trimester or radiation therapy is used. Treatment, as in nonpregnant women, must be curative.

REFERENCES

1. Haas JF. Pregnancy in association with a newly diagnosed cancer: a population-based epidemiologic assessment. Int J Cancer 1984;34:229–35.
2. Pohlman B, Lyons SA, and Macklis RM. Lymphoma in pregnancy. In: Trimble EL, Trimble CL, eds., Cancer Obstetrics and Gynecology. Philadelphia: Lippincott Williams & Wilkins, 1999: 202–38.

3. Dhedin N and Coiffier B. Lymphoma and pregnancy. In: Canellos GP, Lister AT, Young B, eds., The Lymphomas. New York: Elsevier, 1993: 549–56.
4. Landis SH, Murray T, Bolden S, et al. Cancer statistics, 1999. CA Cancer J Clin 1999;49:8–31.
5. Lin AY and Tucker MA. Epidemiology of Hodgkin's disease and non-Hodgkin's lymphoma. In: Canellos GP, Lister TA, Sklar JL, eds. The Lymphomas. Philadelphia: WB Saunders, 1998: 43–61.
6. Barry RM, Diamond HD, and Craver LF. Influence of pregnancy on the course of Hodgkin's disease. Am J Obstet Gynecol 1962;84:445–54.
7. Lishner M, Zemlickis D, Sutcliffe SB, et al. Non-Hodgkin's lymphoma and pregnancy. Leuk Lymphoma 1994;14:411–3.
8. Gelb AB, Vanderijn M, Warnke RA, et al. Pregnancy-associated lymphomas. A clinicopathologic study. Cancer 1996;78:304–10.
9. Aviles A, Diaz-Maqueo JC, Garcia EL, et al. Late lethal events in patients with diffuse large B cell lymphoma: a review of 714 patients treated in a single centre. Leuk Lymph 2001; 42:631–7.
10. Hennessy JP and Rottino A. Hodgkin's disease in pregnancy. Am J Obstet Gynecol 1963;87:851–3.
11. Jacobs C, Donaldson SS, Rosenberg SA, et al. Management of the pregnant patient with Hodgkin's disease. Ann Intern Med 1981;95:669–75.
12. Gobbi PG, Attardo-Parrinello A, Danesino M, et al. Hodgkin's disease and pregnancy. Haematologica 1984;69:336–41.
13. Tawil E, Mercier JP and Dandavino A. Hodgkin's disease complicating pregnancy. J Can Assoc Radiol 1985;36:133–7.
14. Nisce LZ, Tome MA, He S, et al. Management of coexisting Hodgkin's disease and pregnancy. Am J Clin Oncol 1986; 9:146–51.
15. Lambe M and Ekbom A. Cancers coinciding with childbearing: delayed diagnosis during pregnancy? BMJ 1995;311: 1607–8.
16. Anselmo AP, Cavalieri E, Enrici RM, et al. Hodgkin's disease during pregnancy: diagnostic and therapeutic management. Fetal Diagn Ther 1999;14:102–5.
17. Jouet JP, Buchet-Bouverne B, Fenaux P, et al. Influence de la grossess sur le développement de la maladie de Hodgkin. Presse Med 1988;17:423–7.
18. Ward FT and Weiss RB. Lymphoma and pregnancy. Semin Oncol 1989;16:397–409.
19. Pohlman B and Macklis RM. Lymphoma and pregnancy. Semin Oncol 2000;27:657–66.
20. Meguerian-Bedoyan Z, Lamant L, Hopfner C, et al. Anaplastic large cell lymphoma of maternal origin involving the placenta. Case report and literature survey. Am J Surg Pathol 1997;21:1236–41.
21. Aviles A, Diaz-Maqueo JC, Torras V, et al. Non-Hodgkin's lymphomas and pregnancy: presentation of 16 cases. Gynecol Oncol 1990;37:335–7.
22. du Bois A, Meerpohl HG, Gerner K, et al. Effect of pregnancy on the incidence and course of malignant diseases. Geburtshilfe Frauenheilkd 1993;53:619–24.
23. Vicdan K, Alaybeyoglu L, Oguz S, et al. Ultrasonographic appearance of non-Hodgkin's lymphoma in a pregnant woman. Gynecol Obstet Invest 1996;41:284–5.
24. Barnes MN, Barrett JC, Kimberlin DF, et al. Burkitt lymphoma in pregnancy. Obstet Gynecol 1998;92:675–8.
25. Antic N, Colovic M, Cemerikic V, et al. Disseminated Burkitt's-like lymphoma during pregnancy. Med Oncol 2000; 17:233–6.
26. Drevet C, Rosenau L, Francois S, et al. Management of lymphoblastic lymphomas during pregnancy. J Gynecol Obstet Biol Reprod 2000;29:22–7.
27. Aviles A and Neri N. Hematological malignancies and pregnancy: a final report of 84 children who received chemotherapy in utero. Clin Lymphoma 2001;2:173–7.
28. Reimer P, Rudiger T, Muller J, et al. Subcutaneous panniculitis-like T-cell lymphoma during pregnancy with successful autologous stem cell transplantation. Ann Hematol 2003; 82:305–9.
29. Kirkpatrick AW, Bailey DJ, and Weizel HA. Bilateral primary breast lymphoma in pregnancy: a case report and literature review. Can J Surg 1996;39:333–5.
30. Steiner-Salz D, Yahalom J, Samuelov A, et al. Non-Hodgkin's lymphoma associated with pregnancy. A report of six cases, with review of the literature. Cancer 1985;56:2087–91.
31. Kurtin PJ, Gaffey TA, Habermann TM, et al. Peripheral T-cell lymphoma involving the placenta. Cancer 1992;70: 2963–8.
32. Ioachim HL and Moroson H. Lymphoma and pregnancy. Clinical observations and experimental investigations. Leukemia 1994;8:201.
33. Vieaux JW and McGuire DE. Reticulum cell sarcoma of the cervix. Am J Obstet Gynecol 1964;89:134–5.
34. Shepherd JJ and Wright DH. Burkitt's tumour presenting as bilateral swelling of the breast in women of child-bearing age. Br J Surg 1967;54:776–80.
35. Henderson M and Paterson WG. Perforation of jejunum by reticulum cell sarcoma in pregnancy. Am J Surg 1968;115: 385–9.
36. Ludanyi I and Donko A. [Reticulosarcoma in pregnancy]. Zentralbl Gynakol 1969;91:1609–13.
37. Finkle HI and Goldman RL. Burkitt's lymphoma—gynecologic considerations. Obstet Gynecol 1974;43:281–4.
38. Armitage JO, Feagler JR, and Skoog DP. Burkitt lymphoma during pregnancy with bilateral breast involvement. JAMA 1977;237:151.
39. Tunca JC, Reddi PR, Shah SH, et al. Malignant non-Hodgkin's-type lymphoma of the cervix uteri occurring during pregnancy. Gynecol Oncol 1979;7:385–93.
40. Jones DE, d'Avignon MB, Lawrence R, et al. Burkitt's lymphoma: obstetric and gynecologic aspects. Obstet Gynecol 1980;56:533–6.
41. Ioachim HL. Non-Hodgkin's lymphoma in pregnancy. Three cases and review of the literature. Arch Pathol Lab Med 1985;109:803–9.
42. Roumen FJME, de Leeuw JW, van der Linden PJQ, et al. Non-Hodgkin lymphoma of the puerperal uterus. Obstetrics and Gynecology 1990;75:527–9.
43. Azouri J, Afif N, Ghosn M, Nader N, et al. [Primary breast lymphoma. A case report]. J Med Libar 1992;40(4):202–6.
44. Bobrow LG, Richards MA, Happerfield LC, et al. Breast lymphomas. A clinicopathologic review. Hum Pathol 1993; 24:274–8.
45. Arber DA, Simpson JF, Weiss LM, et al. Non-Hodgkin's lymphoma involving the breast. Am J Surg Pathol 1994;18: 288–95.
46. Illes A, Banyai A, Jenei K, et al. Bilateral primary malignant lymphoma of the breast during pregnancy. Haematologia 1996;27(2):99–105.
47. Vicdan K, Alaybeyoglu L, Oguz S, et al. Ultrasonographic appearance of non-Hodgkin's lymphoma in a pregnant woman. Gynecol Obstet Invest 1996;41(4):284–5.
48. Antic N, Colovic M, Cemerikic V, et al. Disseminated Burkitt's-like lymphoma during pregnancy. Med Oncol 2000;17:233–6.
49. Wang PH, Chao KC, Lin G, et al. Primary malignant lymphoma of the cervix in pregnancy. A case report. J Reprod Med 1999;44:630–2.
50. Durodola JI. Administration of cyclophosphamide during late pregnancy and early lactation: a case report. J Natl Med Assoc 1979;71:165–6.

51. Tsujimura T, Matsumoto K, and Aozasa K. Placental involvement by maternal non-Hodgkin's lymphoma. Arch Pathol Lab Med 1993;117:325–7.
52. Pollack RN, Sklarin NT, Rao S, et al. Metastatic placental lymphoma associated with maternal human immunodeficiency virus infection. Obstet Gynecol 1993;81:856–7.
53. Catlin EA, Roberts JD, Erana R, et al. Transplacental transmission of natural-killer-cell lymphoma. N Engl J Med 1999; 341:85–91.
54. Moore DT and Taslimi MM. Non-Hodgkin's lymphoma in pregnancy: a diagnostic dilemma. Case report and review of the literature. J Tenn Med Assoc 1992;85:467–9.
55. Lishner M, Zemlickis D, Degendorfer P, et al. Maternal and foetal outcome following Hodgkin's disease in pregnancy. Br J Cancer 1992;65:114–7.
56. Ebert U, Loffler H, and Kirch W. Cytotoxic therapy and pregnancy. Pharmacol Ther 1997;74:207–20.
57. Ortega J. Multiple agent chemotherapy including bleomycin of non-Hodgkin's lymphoma during pregnancy. Cancer 1977;40:2829–35.
58. Zuazu J, Julia A, Sierra J, et al. Pregnancy outcome in hematologic malignancies. Cancer 1991;67:703–9.
59. Nicklas AH and Baker ME. Imaging strategies in the pregnant cancer patient. Semin Oncol 2000;27:623–32.
60. Levine D, Barnes PD, and Edelman RR. Obstetric MR imaging. Radiology 1999;211:609–17.
61. Redmond GP. Physiological changes during pregnancy and their implications for pharmacological treatment. Clin Invest Med 1985;8:317–22.
62. Powis G. Anticancer drug pharmacodynamics. Cancer Chemother Pharmacol 1985;14:177–83.
63. Doll DC, Ringenberg QS, and Yarbro JW. Antineoplastic agents and pregnancy. Semin Oncol 1989;16:337–46.
64. Delmer A, Bauduer F, Ajchenbaum-Cymbalista F, et al. Grossesse et hémopathies malignes: approche thérapeutique. Bull Cancer 1994;81:277–86.
65. Glantz JC. Reproductive toxicology of alkylating agents. Obstet Gynecol Surv 1994;49:709–15.
66. Germann N, Goffinet F, and Goldwasser F. Anthracyclines during pregnancy: embryo-fetal outcome in 160 patients. Ann Oncol 2004;15:146–50.
67. Woo SY, Fuller LM, Cundiff JH, et al. Radiotherapy during pregnancy for clinical stages IA-IIA Hodgkin's disease. Int J Radiat Oncol Biol Phys 1992;23:407–12.
68. Friedman E and Jones GW. Fetal outcome after maternal radiation treatment of supradiaphragmatic Hodgkins disease. CMAJ 1993;149:1281–3.
69. Cygler J, Ding GX, Kendal W, et al. Fetal dose for a patient undergoing mantle field irradiation for Hodgkin's disease. Med Dosim 1997;22:135–7.
70. Fenig E, Mishaeli M, Kalish Y, et al. Pregnancy and radiation. Cancer Treat Rev 2001;27:1–7.
71. Nuyttens JJ, Prado KL, Jenrette JM, et al. Fetal dose during radiotherapy: clinical implementation and review of the literature. Cancer Radiother 2002;6:352–7.
72. Herold M, Schnohr S, and Bittrich H. Efficacy and safety of a combined rituximab chemotherapy during pregnancy. J Clin Oncol 2001;19:3439.
73. Coiffier B, Lepage E, Briere J, et al. CHOP chemotherapy plus rituximab compared with CHOP alone in elderly patients with diffuse large-B-cell lymphoma. N Engl J Med 2002;346: 235–42.
74. Castelo-Branco C, Torne A, et al. Mycosis fungoides and pregnancy. Oncol Rep 2001;8:197–9.
75. Echols KT, Gilles JM, and Diro M. Mycosis fungoides in pregnancy: remission after treatment with alpha-interferon in a case refractory to conventional therapy: a case report. J Matern Fetal Med 2001;10:68–70.
76. Dienstbier Z, Hermanska Z, Zamecnik J, et al. Children of parents treated for Hodgkin's disease using irradiation and chemotherapy. Vnitr Lek 1994;40:163–6.

34

Lymphoma in the Immunosuppressed

34A

Lymphoma in the Setting of HIV Infection

Alexandra M. Levine, M.D.

Lymphoma is known to occur in patients with underlying immunodeficiency, dysregulation, or both, and its incidence is statistically increased in these settings. Thus, patients with congenital immunodeficiency diseases, such as Wiskott–Aldrich syndrome,[1] ataxia telangiectasia,[2] and X-linked lymphoproliferative disorder[3], are at increased risk for lymphoma. Patients with autoimmune disorders such as Sjögren's syndrome[4,5] and Hashimoto's thyroiditis[6] are diagnosed with lymphoma more frequently than expected; the lymphomas that ensue may occur at the specific sites of prior autoimmune disease.[7]

Monoclonal B-cell lymphomas or polyclonal lymphoproliferative disorders are also seen with increased frequency in patients who have undergone organ transplantation[8] occurring 25 to 50 times more commonly than expected in the general population, with a latent period of approximately 33 months from transplantation. The association between profound immunodeficiency and the subsequent development of transplant-related lymphoma may be also surmised by the data from Swinnen and colleagues, who demonstrated that the use of more intensive regimens of immunosuppression, such as monoclonal antibody-induced T-cell depletion, was associated with a greater likelihood of subsequent lymphoma, occurring at shorter latent periods.[9] Patients who have undergone cardiac transplantation appear most at risk. This may be related to the fact that episodes of incipient cardiac rejection are more likely to be treated with increasing immunosuppressive regimens in an attempt to preserve the transplant, in contrast with renal allografts, which can more easily be removed, with return to long-term dialysis.

In 1982, approximately 1 year after the first descriptions of *Pneumocystis carinii* pneumonia (PCP) and Kaposi's sarcoma, the Centers for Disease Control and Prevention (CDC) first reported a small group of homosexual men with Burkitt's-like (diffuse undifferentiated) lymphomas.[10] Lymphoma primary to the brain, occurring in patients younger than 60 years of age, was included as an acquired immunodeficiency syndrome (AIDS)-defining diagnosis in the same year,[11] and systemic lymphoma, high-grade or intermediate-grade large-cell type occurring in human immunodeficiency virus (HIV)-seropositive patients, became AIDS-defining in 1985.[12] Although lymphoma occurred in only 2% of patients diagnosed with AIDS in the United States between 1981 and 1989,[13] recent data suggest that lymphoma has now become much more common. Thus, with the widespread use of highly active antiviral therapy (HAART), the occurrence of AIDS-defining opportunistic infections has declined remarkably, such that lymphoma has now become one of the most common of the initial AIDS-defining illnesses.[14–16]

The known relationship between underlying immune dysfunction and the subsequent development of lymphoma would be fully consistent with the occurrence of lymphomas in the setting of HIV-induced immune dysregulation. Indeed, certain similarities exist among all these immunodeficiency-related lymphomas, including the B-lymphoid origin of the disease; the development of aggressive pathologic types; the frequent presence of extranodal disease at initial presentation; and short survival times, despite therapy.[17]

EPIDEMIOLOGY

Incidence

The incidence of lymphoma doubled in the United States between 1940 and 1980[18] for reasons that are not well understood. The AIDS epidemic has had an additional impact, associated with a risk of lymphoma between 60 and 100 times that expected in the general population.[13,19,20] Lymphoma is a late manifestation of HIV infection, more likely to occur in the setting of significant immune suppression,[21] with CD4 cells below 200/mm^3, and prior history of an AIDS-defining illness. Following an earlier diagnosis of AIDS, the relative risk of immunoblastic lymphoma is increased approximately 627-fold, while that of diffuse large-cell lymphoma is 145-fold higher than that expected in the general population.[22,23] Of interest, when linking cancer and AIDS registries, even low-grade lymphoma was found to be increased 14-fold,[22,23] while the incidence of T-cell lymphoma is also increased among patients with AIDS.[24]

Lymphoma is the second most common malignancy occurring in patients with AIDS, serving as the initial AIDS-defining diagnosis in approximately 16% of HIV-infected persons in the United States and Europe.[16] Data regarding the true incidence of AIDS-related lymphoma in the United States are problematic, however, since the CDC collects inclusive information only on initial AIDS-defining conditions.[13] Thus, lymphoma developing in a person initially diagnosed with PCP will remain unknown to the CDC in statistical terms, in the absence of linkage analyses between AIDS and cancer registries.

Population Groups at Risk for AIDS-Lymphoma

In sharp distinction to Kaposi's sarcoma, which occurs primarily in homosexual or bisexual men, lymphoma appears to occur with relatively equal frequency in persons from all categories of risk for the acquisition of HIV infection. Thus, as shown in data on 53,042 AIDS cases in 21 European countries,[25] the frequency of lymphoma ranged from 1.1 in children infected perinatally to 2.6 in injection drug users, 2.6 in heterosex, 3.2 in blood transfusion recipients, 3.4 in homosexual men, and 3.9 in hemophiliacs. After controlling for the effects of age, gender, and year of AIDS diagnosis, an excess of borderline statistical significance was found among homosexual or bisexual men (odds ratio 1.2; 95% confidence interval 1.0–1.3).[25] Similarly, although the incidence of lymphoma among homosexual or bisexual men in the United States is identical to that described in Europe, the incidence in injection drug users also appears somewhat less.[13]

The demographic features of patients with AIDS-related lymphoma may differ among HIV risk groups. Thus, as described by Monfardini and colleagues in a study of 150 cases from the Italian Cooperative Group,[26] the median age of homosexual men diagnosed with AIDS-related lymphoma was 38 years, whereas that of injection drug users was 26 years. No differences were seen in pathologic type or sites of lymphomatous disease. Likewise, median survival after diagnosis of lymphoma was similar in both groups.[26]

In a prospective study of 1295 HIV-infected men with hemophilia, 5.5 developed lymphoma, at a median interval of 59 months from the initial HIV infection.[27] The relative risk of lymphoma was 36.5 times higher than that observed in a group of HIV-negative hemophiliacs, followed prospectively in the same study, and 29 times higher than expected in the general population. The mean CD4 cell count at diagnosis of AIDS-related lymphoma was 64×10^9/L. All pathologic and clinical characteristics of lymphomatous disease appeared similar to those described in patients with history of homosexuality or injection drug use.

Demographic Factors

The usual age of patients with AIDS-related lymphoma seems to vary in a bimodal distribution pattern.[13] Thus, the first peak of disease appears in adolescence (10 to 19 years of age), with the second peak in middle age (50 to 59 years). In data from the United States, where the relationship between age and pathologic type has also been studied, younger patients were shown to be more likely to present with Burkitt's lymphoma, whereas immunoblastic lymphoma was seen in older patients.[13] In the United States, AIDS-related lymphoma is more common in men than in women and is diagnosed in whites more often than in African Americans.[13] These data are fully consistent with the demographic pattern of "de novo" lymphoma in the United States, occurring in patients without underlying HIV infection.[20]

Epidemiologic Changes in the Era of Highly Active Antiretroviral Therapy (HAART)

Highly active antiretroviral therapy (HAART) has resulted in a significant decline in mortality due to AIDS, as well as a remarkable decrease in the development of new opportunistic infections, Kaposi's sarcoma, and/or primary central nervous system lymphoma among patients with AIDS.[14–16] While significant decreases in the incidence of systemic AIDS related lymphoma have also occurred in the era of HAART, the decline is not as profound as that seen in other AIDS-defining conditions,[15,16] and lymphoma has now become one of the more common of the initial AIDS-defining illnesses.[16,28]

Genetic Epidemiology

AIDS-related lymphoma, similar to lymphoma occurring in immunocompetent hosts, is more common in men than in women.[29] Although major environmental factors have not been associated with an increased risk for AIDS-lymphoma,[30] genetic factors in the host may be operative. Heterozytes for the Δ32 deletion of the CCR5 co-receptor gene are statistically less likely to develop lymphoma,[31] while those with SDF-1 mutations (3′A) are statistically more likely to develop lymphoma.[32]

ETIOLOGY AND PATHOGENESIS

The development of lymphoma in patients with underlying HIV infection represents the accumulation of multiple factors occurring over a relatively short period in a given person. Full understanding does not yet exist of factors that are necessary and sufficient for the development of lymphoma. However, multiple insights have been made, allowing an understanding of those factors that may lead to the development of lymphoma in persons infected by HIV.

Underlying Immunodeficiency

Immunodeficient states per se may be associated with the development of lymphoma, as evidenced by its increased incidence in patients with congenital immunodeficiency diseases,[1,3] in those with acquired autoimmune disorders,[4–6] and in the setting of organ transplantation with iatrogenic immunosuppression.[8,9]

The significance of immunosuppression in the development of AIDS-lymphoma may be surmised by the fact that lymphoma is most likely to occur in patients with more profound degrees of CD4 lymphocytopenia, as demonstrated by Besson[33] and colleagues from France. Thus, among a cohort of HIV infected individuals, the risk of AIDS-lymphoma increased progressively as the CD4 count fell. Studies by Grulich and colleagues from Australia have also confirmed the importance of falling CD4 cells, as well as ongoing B-cell stimulation, as risk factors for development of AIDS-lymphoma.[21]

Ongoing B-Cell Stimulation and Proliferation

Aside from the myriad of qualitative and quantitative abnormalities of T lymphocytes in HIV-infected persons,[34] B-lymphocytic function is also deranged, with polyclonal activation induced by HIV, as well as by other antigens, mitogens, and additional infecting organisms.[35] This polyclonal expansion results in the florid follicular hyperplasia seen in enlarged reactive lymph nodes ("persistent generalized lymphadenopathy"), and in the polyclonal hypergammaglobulinemia that often accompanies HIV infection.[34,35] The description of an HIV-infected patient with multiple myeloma, in whom the abnormal paraprotein was found to have activity against the p24 antigen of HIV, lends further credence to the concept that HIV per se may lead to ongoing B-cell expansion, with eventual clonal selection.[36] Although associated with polyclonal expansion of B lymphocytes, HIV infection may also be associated with an intrinsic impairment in B-cell maturation, as described by Berberian and colleagues.[37] The ongoing B-cell expansion in HIV infection, with subsequent intrinsic impairment in B-cell maturation, may mimic the usual setting in lymphoproliferative malignancies, characterized by clonal expansion of cells that have been arrested at a specific stage of maturation or activation.[38]

Cytokine Networks

Ongoing production of various inflammatory cytokines may also contribute to the chronic B-cell proliferation that characterizes HIV infection. Numerous cytokines are responsible for B-cell proliferation and differentiation, including interleukin-1 (IL-1), IL-2, IL-4, IL-6, IL-7, and IL-10.[39–44] B cells from HIV-infected patients with polyclonal hypergammaglobulinemia constitutively express TNF-a and IL-6.[45]

IL-6 may play a critical role in the development of AIDS-related lymphoma, as is the case in other lymphoproliferative malignancies. Thus, IL-6 functions as an autocrine growth factor in multiple myeloma[46] and is constitutively expressed in chronic lymphocytic leukemia[47] and in Castleman's disease.[48] High levels of IL-6 expression have been demonstrated in both HIV-positive and HIV-negative cases of B-cell large-cell lymphoma, independent of Epstein–Barr virus (EBV) status, but dependent on the presence of immunoblasts within the lymphoma tissue.[49] Thus, although not unique to AIDS-lymphoma, IL-6 may play an important role in the pathogenesis of diverse types of B-cell neoplasia, in which terminally differentiated cells predominate. Elevated levels of serum IL-6 levels at study entry, with subsequent further elevations in time, were documented before the development of large-cell lymphoma in a group of patients with symptomatic HIV infection followed by Pluda and associates from the National Cancer Institute[50]; elevated serum IL-6 levels and depressed CD4 cells were the only predictors of lymphoma in this cohort.

IL-10 may also play an important role in the development of AIDS-related lymphoma. Human IL-10 shares significant homology with the EBV-associated protein BCRF-1.[51] IL-10 and BCRF-1 specifically impair the ability of the activated Th-1 subset of CD4 cells to synthesize interferon-gamma and IL-2, serving to suppress T-helper cell antiviral and anti-tumor surveillance activities.[52] These functions alone could have an impact in terms of lymphomagenesis. In addition, however, constitutive expression of IL-10 has been demonstrated in EBV-positive B-cell lines derived from patients with AIDS-related lymphoma.[53] Further, human IL-10 has been shown to function as an autocrine growth factor in similar cell lines.[54]

It is thus apparent that several cytokines may be operative in the full pathogenesis of AIDS-related lymphoma. HIV itself may induce the production of a cascade of such cytokines from infected monocytes, T cells, and bone marrow stromal cells, serving to up-regulate HIV. These cytokines may also affect the proliferation, differentiation, and expression of both B cells and cytotoxic T cells, creating the milieu in which polyclonal B-cell expansion may occur, with eventual clonal selection and continued paracrine- and autocrine-induced B-cell growth.

The Multi-Center AIDS Cohort Study (MACS) recently evaluated the cytokine profile in serum of homosexual/bisexual men who went on to develop lymphoma within the next 6-month period.[55] Markers of activation, including soluble CD27, CD30, and CD44 were elevated when compared with HIV positive controls who did not develop lymphoma. In addition, markers of isotype switching, including soluble CD23 and IgE, were elevated, as was serum IL10. Serum levels of IgM and IgG were decreased when compared with controls. In multivariate analysis, serum CD23, CD27, IgM, IgG, IgE, and IL10 were independently associated with lymphoma. While it is highly likely that lymphoma had already developed in these patients, who were formally diagnosed within 1 to 6 months after serum collection, it is of interest that a particular pattern of markers, related to B-cell activation, stimulation and isotype switching were consistently expressed. These markers may provide the ability to predict which HIV-infected patients are at increased risk for development of B-cell lymphoma.[55]

Epstein–Barr Virus

In addition to cytokine pathways, EBV may be implicated in the pathogenesis of HIV-associated lymphoma, perhaps related to the impaired immunosurveillance of EBV-infected cells in patients with AIDS. EBV has consistently been implicated in the etiology of Burkitt's lymphoma in Africa, in which the EBV genome is uniformly present within tumor cells,[56,57] and EBV infection has been shown to precede the development of lymphoma.[58] Additional relationships between EBV infection and subsequent lymphoma may be seen in the model of X-linked lymphoproliferative disorder, in which affected boys may develop high-grade B-cell lymphomas after primary infection with EBV.[59] Theoretically, EBV could lead to malignant transformation via multiple diverse mechanisms. First, activation of various EBV latent genes, encoding Epstein–Barr nuclear antigens (EBNAs), and latent membrane proteins (LMPs), may prolong the survival of EBV-infected host cells by blocking apoptosis.[60] LMP-1 has also been shown to have direct transforming and oncogenic properties in the rodent model.[61] Expression of the EBNA2 gene has been shown to induce the expression of CD21 and CD23 B-cell surface antigens, which in turn induce B-cell proliferation. In this regard, CD21 is a receptor for EBV, possibly allowing EBV-induced autostimulation.[62] In addition, EBV could lead to a malignant phenotype by its down regulation of lymphocyte function-associated antigens (LFA-1 and LFA-3), leading to a "nonadhesive" phenotype that could then allow cells to escape immune surveillance by cytotoxic T cells.[63] Another mechanism whereby EBV could cause malignant transformation relates to its ability to form complexes with the p53 protein so as to inactivate the protein's tumor suppressor function.[64] Furthermore, EBV could lead to ongoing B-cell activation and polyclonal expansion by means of its BCRF1 protein, which is similar in its functional and structural characteristics to human IL-10.[51] BCRF-1 leads to a decrease in interferon-gamma and IL-2 production from T cells, resulting in decreased T-cell-induced antiviral activity, enhanced viral survival, and resultant ongoing B-cell activation and expansion.[63] This ongoing B-cell proliferation may generate increased numbers of B cells that are susceptible to genetic errors, such as chromosome breaks and translocations.

Although EBV may thus induce malignant transformation through multiple pathways, its precise relationship to the etiology of AIDS-lymphomas still remains somewhat controversial. Shibata and associates[65] studied the reactive lymphadenopathy tissues from 35 HIV-infected patients, employing polymerase chain reaction (PCR) and in situ hybridization. EBV DNA was detected in 13 (35%) patients; the presence of detectable amounts of EBV DNA in these 13 reactive biopsies was associated with an increased incidence of concurrent lymphoma at another site, or development of lymphoma over time.

Primary CNS AIDS-related lymphoma has been uniformly associated with the presence of EBV DNA within tumor cells, with identification of the EBV early region (EBER) protein in all 21 cases described by MacMahon and colleagues,[66] with expression of LMP-1 in 45%. These PCNSLs were all of large-cell or immunoblastic pathologic subtype.

Although AIDS-related PCNSLs are thus associated with EBV, the relationship between EBV and systemic HIV-associated lymphoma is less clear. Thus, MacMahon and colleagues[66] detected EBV genome in only 3 of 7 (43%) such cases, whereas Subar and associates[67] found EBV sequences or protein in only 6 of 16 (36%) systemic lymphoma cases. The differences in EBV expression may be a function of the site of disease or may be related to differing histologic types. Thus, Hamilton-Dutoit and associates detected the EBV genome by in situ hybridization in 11 of 17 (65%) cases of systemic immunoblastic lymphoma, versus only 1 of 5 cases of Burkitt's lymphoma, similar to the findings of others.[68] In a subsequent study of 101 cases of systemic AIDS-related lymphoma, Hamilton-Dutoit et al.[69] demonstrated EBER1 expression in 46 of 60 (77%) immunoblast-rich, large-cell lymphomas, but in only 12 of 35 (34%) small non-cleaved cases, and in 1 of 6 (17%) cases of diffuse large-cell lymphoma. In contrast, employing Southern blot analysis, PCR, and in situ hybridization in 59 cases of systemic AIDS-lymphoma, Shibata et al.[70] have demonstrated the presence of EBV in the majority of cases, including 85% of immunoblastic, 55% of large-cell, and 57% of small non-cleaved lymphomas. These discrepancies may be related to differing assessments of histologic type, differing geographic patterns of disease, or other unidentified factors. However, clonal EBV infection has been demonstrated in all systemic EBV-positive cases yet reported, thus indicating that EBV integration occurred before clonal B-cell expansion and lymphomagenesis.[70,71] Although not proving that EBV caused these lymphomas, the finding of clonal EBV would be consistent with the hypothesis that this virus was critically involved in the process of lymphomagenesis.

B-Lymphoid Genomic Mutations

As discussed previously, ongoing B-cell expansion and activation is expected during the long asymptomatic course of HIV infection, induced by HIV itself, by multiple cytokines, and potentially by EBV as well. This continual B-cell proliferation may allow the milieu in which genetic "errors" may occur, simply because of the increased numbers of cells that may be susceptible to chromosome translocations and abnormal rearrangements. Thus, as hypothesized by Ames and Gold,[72] high proliferative activity alone may predispose cells to genomic mutations, leading eventually to neoplastic transformation. In the adult, lymphocytes normally undergo DNA rearrangement during B-cell differentiation. These normal DNA rearrangements may provide vulnerable, abnormal recombination-prone sites, leading to chromosome translocations involving the immunoglobulin heavy-chain or light-chain genes. These recombinase errors could lead to the specific chromosome translocations that have been described in AIDS-lymphoma, as well as in Burkitt's lymphoma, including t(8;14), t(8;22), and t(8;2).[73–78] Consistent with this hypothesis, Pelicci and colleagues[79] described the presence of one or more faint or low-intensity immunoglobulin gene rearrangement bands within reactive persistent generalized lymphadenopathy tissues in 4 of 11 HIV-infected persons. The rearrangement bands were occasionally accompanied by a hybridization smear, suggesting the presence of additional oligoclonal B-cell expansions. These B-cell clones did not carry c-myc rearrangements, suggesting that they were immortalized but not fully transformed. These results suggest that within reactive lymphoid tissues, there may be one or several occult clonal B-cell populations that are not identifiable by morphologic or immunophenotypic analysis alone. The subsequent selection and growth advantage of one such clone, perhaps by abnormal activation of c-myc or other oncogenes, could explain the eventual development of monoclonal B-cell malignancy from an ongoing polyclonal B-cell response. The oligoclonal B-cell expansions would thus represent a premalignant condition, from which true lymphoma could develop. In this regard, chromosome abnormalities have been described in such reactive lymph nodes.[78] Furthermore, the development of lymphoma in patients with persistent generalized lymphadenopathy has been shown to occur 850 times more frequently than expected in the usual population.[80]

c-myc Dysregulation

One mechanism that may lead to malignant transformation of B lymphocytes is the translocation of a normal growth-promoting gene (proto-oncogene) to one of the immunoglobulin genes of the B cell in question. The juxtaposition of this proto-oncogene with the transcriptionally active enhancer sequences of the immunoglobulin molecule would result in over-expression of the translocated gene, now functioning as a true oncogene. The classic example of such a translocation is the t(8;14) rearrangement, which occurs uniformly in Burkitt's lymphoma.[73] This translocation leads to abnormal activation of the c-myc oncogene on chromosome 8 (8q24), which is now juxtaposed to the immunoglobulin gene heavy-chain locus on chromosome 14 (q32). In this setting, transcriptional activation of c-myc can occur from direct juxtaposition to the immunoglobulin gene enhancer sequences or from the action of long-range enhancers on chromosome 14, without the need for proximity to c-myc. Although c-myc dysregulation has been well documented in many cases of AIDS-related lymphoma, this abnormality has not uniformly been observed. Thus, activation of c-myc has been detected in approximately 60% to 80% of AIDS- associated systemic lymphomas.[67,79,81,82] Differences in c-myc dysregulation have been observed in different pathologic types of lymphoma. Thus, as shown by at least two groups of investigators, the AIDS-related small non-cleaved lymphomas (Burkitt's or Burkitt's-like) are uniformly associated with c-myc dysregulation, whereas only one-third or fewer of the immunoblastic or large-cell lymphomas demonstrate this abnormality.[81,82] The molecular mechanisms leading to c-myc dysregulation may also differ in the AIDS-related lymphomas. Thus, c-myc translocation, similar at the molecular level to sporadic Burkitt's lymphoma, has been observed in several series.[68,83] In contrast, point mutations within c-myc, similar to that seen in endemic Burkitt's lymphoma, have been documented in another well-studied patient.[84] Dysregulation of c-myc has been associated with transformation of human B cells in vitro and may cause B-cell lymphoma in transgenic animals carrying immunoglobulin-myc chimeric constructs.[85,86] The relationship between c-myc dysregulation and underlying HIV infection may also be seen from the work of Laurence and Astrin,[87] who demonstrated that HIV Type I infection of immortalized B-cell lines can itself result in up-regulation of c-myc transcripts. Pauza and associates[88] have also demonstrated that HIV may directly affect cellular c-myc gene expression. In summary, myc protein is a potent regulator of cell proliferation. Its abnormal expression may provide an important mechanism for the development of lymphoma in the setting of HIV infection. However, it is also clear that c-myc dysregulation is not present in all cases of AIDS-related lymphoma, indicating that alternative mechanisms of lymphomagenesis must also be operative.

Role of *bcl-6*

A new proto-oncogene was recently described on chromosome 3, consistent with chromosome breakpoints that have been documented in cases of diffuse large-cell lymphoma at chromosome 3q27. This proto-oncogene has been termed *bcl-6*. Rearrangements of the *bcl-6* gene have been found in 30% to 40% of de novo diffuse large-cell lymphoma.[89,90] Gaidano and colleagues[91] studied 24 cases of AIDS-associated diffuse large-cell lymphoma, demonstrating rearrangements of *bcl-6* in 20%, including 2 of 8 cases of large non-cleaved lymphoma, and 3 of 16 cases of immunoblastic lymphoma. Rearrangement of *bcl-6* was found in none of the 13 cases of small non-cleaved lymphoma that were evaluated. These rearrangements were found in both the presence and the absence of EBV infection of the tumor clone. The discovery of *bcl-6* mutations or rearrangements exclusive to diffuse large-cell lymphoma serves to broaden the understanding of the multiple molecular pathways that are operative in the eventual development of AIDS-related lymphoma.

Role of Tumor Suppressor Genes

Tumor suppressor genes such as the p53 or retinoblastoma (Rb) genes are believed to play a significant role in the development and progression of various human malignancies when their loss or dysregulation removes the normal negative regulatory signals from affected cells. In this regard, p53 gene mutations have been described in de novo lymphomas, specifically of the small non-cleaved type, or its leukemic counterpart, French-American-British L3 acute lymphoblastic leukemia.[92] In addition, p53 gene mutations have been demonstrated in approximately 37% of AIDS-related lymphomas.[81] The presence of p53 abnormalities was shown to vary between pathologic subtypes of disease, with approximately 60% of small non-cleaved lymphomas demonstrating p53 abnormalities, whereas no case of immunoblastic or large-cell lymphoma did so. A relationship was seen between the occurrence of p53 suppressor gene inactivation and c-myc proto-oncogene dysregulation in the same tumor in vivo,[81] suggesting that cells carrying the over-expressed c-myc are under additional pressure to delete a p53 pathway. Aside from the tumor suppressor p53 abnormalities in AIDS-related small non-cleaved lymphoma, there is no current evidence to indicate inactivation of other such suppressor genes. Thus, abnormalities of the Rb gene have not been demonstrated in AIDS-related lymphoma thus far reported.[81,93]

PATHOLOGIC CHARACTERISTICS

The AIDS-associated lymphomas are classically of B-lymphoid derivation and high-grade pathologic type, described in approximately 70% to 90% of reported cases.[94–99] The more common subtypes of disease include B-immunoblastic or small non-cleaved lymphomas,[100] the latter of which may be further subclassified into Burkitt's or Burkitt-like types. Intermediate-grade, diffuse large-cell lymphomas have also been included in the expanded case definition of AIDS published in 1987[101]; these diffuse large B-cell lymphomas constitute approximately 30% of all AIDS lymphomas. Although unusual, HIV-infected patients with low-grade, B-cell lymphomas have also been described, including persons diagnosed with plasmacytomas, chronic lymphocytic leukemia, and multiple myeloma.[102–106] Of interest, when combining data from national AIDS and cancer registries in the USA, the risk of low grade lymphoma was found to be increased 14-fold over expected in HIV-infected patients.[22,23] Such patients appear to fare reasonably well with standard approaches to management, similar to the expected course of disease in patients with de novo low-grade lymphoma.[107,108]

T-Cell Lymphomas in HIV Setting

Although HIV-infected patients with various T-cell lymphomas have been reported, these cases are unusual and such conditions are not considered among the criteria for the diagnosis of AIDS. Nonetheless, when combining data from AIDS and cancer registries in the United States, a statistically increased incidence of T-cell lymphoma among AIDS patients was identified.[24] A whole range of T-cell lymphomas has been described among HIV-infected individuals, including T-lymphoblastic lymphomas[109,110]; cutaneous T-cell lymphomas[111–113]; and peripheral T-cell lymphomas.[114] Of interest, human T-cell lymphotropic virus, Type I (HTLV-I)–associated lymphoma/leukemia has also been diagnosed in several patients who were dually infected with HIV and HTLV I.[115–117]

Several small series of anaplastic large-cell lymphoma, occurring in HIV-infected patients have also been described.[118,119] The clinical, pathologic, and molecular characteristics of anaplastic large-cell lymphoma appear identical in patients with or without underlying HIV infection. It is possible that these cases simply represent the chance occurrence of two unrelated events.

PROGNOSTIC FACTORS

The factors associated with shorter survival in patients with AIDS-lymphoma include CD4 cells less than 100/mm^3, Stage III or IV disease, age greater than 35 years, history of injection drug use, and elevated LDH.[120] The International Prognostic Index (IPI) for aggressive lymphoma has also been validated in patients with AIDS-lymphoma.[121]

THERAPY OF PATIENTS WITH SYSTEMIC AIDS-LYMPHOMA

Standard Versus Low-Dose Chemotherapy

Prior to the development of HAART, Phase II and III clinical trials demonstrated that low-dose chemotherapeutic regimens, such as m-BACOD, were as efficacious as standard-dose regimens, but had the advantage of statistically decreased rates of hematologic and other toxicity.[122,123] With the addition of HAART to chemotherapy, standard-dose therapy has become feasible and advantageous, and a nihilistic approach is no longer tenable for a substantial population of patients.

Safety and Pharmacokinetics of Concomitant HAART Plus Chemotherapy

The use of HAART, along with dose-reduced and standard-dose CHOP was evaluated by the National Cancer Institute (NCI)–sponsored AIDS Malignancy Consortium in a group of 65 patients with newly diagnosed AIDS-lymphoma.[124] HAART therapy consisted of indinavir, stavudine and lamivudine, the former of which is a protease inhibitor, while the latter two are nucleoside reverse transciptase inhibitors. Grade 3 or 4 neutropenia was more common among patients receiving full-dose CHOP (25% vs. 12%), but there were similar numbers of patients with other toxicities. Doxorubicin clearance and indinavir concentration curves were similar in patients on this study when compared to historical controls. Cyclophosphamide clearance was decreased 1.5 fold when compared to controls, although there was no apparent clinical consequence of this change. The authors concluded that HAART could be administered safely with concomitant low dose or standard dose CHOP chemotherapy.[124] Caution should be used, however, when using chemotherapy together with zidovudine, since this antiretroviral agent may cause significant bone marrow compromise in itself.[125]

Efficacy of HAART Plus Chemotherapy

The vast majority of both retrospective and prospective clinical studies has shown a highly significant advantage, in terms of overall survival, when HAART therapy is combined with multiagent chemotherapy in patients with systemic AIDS-lymphoma.[33,126–128] The efficacy of HAART in prolonging survival in patients with AIDS-lymphoma would be consistent with the ability of effective antiretroviral therapy to prolong survival in patients with other AIDS-related conditions, such as opportunistic infections, in whom the death rate declined by approximately 75% after the widespread use of HAART in the United States.[14] The efficacy of HAART in reducing the HIV-1 viral load has also been associated statistically with attainment of complete remission after chemotherapy in a retrospective study of patients with systemic AIDS-lymphoma.[126]

Infusional Cyclophosphamide, Doxorubicin, and Etoposide

The 96-hour continuous infusion of cyclophosphamide, doxorubicin, and etoposide (CDE) regimen[129,130] has been tested in a large, multi-institutional ECOG trial of 107 patients, including 48 who were also given antiretroviral therapy with didanosine (ddI), and 59 who received HAART regimens.[129,130] For the group as a whole, the rate of complete remission was 44%, similar in patients who received either HAART or single agent didanosine. However, as has been described in the setting of other AIDS conditions, the median overall survival was significantly longer in AIDS-lymphoma patients who received combination antiretroviral therapy. Thus, response rates to infusional CDE appear similar to those achieved with either low-dose or standard-dose m-BACOD, although survival is certainly superior in those patients who receive concomitant HAART.

Infusional, Risk-Adjusted EPOCH Regimen

Wilson and his group at the NCI developed the dose-adjusted EPOCH regimen (Table 34–1), consisting of a 4-day infusion of etoposide, vincristine, and doxorubicin, with risk-adjusted bolus dosing of cyclophosphamide on day 5, and prednisone given orally on days 1 through 5 of

Table 34–1. EPOCH Regimen of Infusional Chemotherapy

Etoposide 50 mg/m^2/day × 4 days
Vincristine 0.4 mg/m^2/day × 4 days
Doxorubicin 10 mg/m^2/day × 4 days
Cyclophosphamide 187 mg/m^2 IV on day 5 for CD4+ <100 cells/mm^3 or 375 mg/m^2 IV on day 5 for CD4+ ≥100 cells/mm^3
Prednisone 60 mg/m^2 orally, days 1 to 5
G-CSF: start on day 6
Repeat on day 22 times 6 cycles

each 22-day cycle.[131] G-CSF was used uniformly, beginning at day 6, and intrathecal methotrexate was given at a dose of 12 mg on days 1 and 5 of cycles 3 through 6. Of interest, all antiretroviral therapy was withheld until day 6 of the last dose and last cycle of chemotherapy. A total of 39 patients were accrued, including 41% with CD4 cells less than 100/mm^3, and 59% who had IPI scores of 2 or 3, indicating high-risk disease. A complete remission rate of 74% was achieved, including 56% in those with CD4 lymphocyte counts less than 100/mm^3 and 87% among patients with CD4 lymphocyte counts greater than 100/mm^3. With a median follow-up of 56 months, there have been only two relapses, and the disease free survival is 92%. Overall survival at 56 months is 60%, while the overall survival of patients with CD4 cells greater than 100/mm^3 at entry is 87%. One controversial aspect of this regimen is the discontinuation of antiretroviral therapy until completion of all chemotherapy. In this regard, the median HIV viral load rose by 0.83 log over the first month of chemotherapy, but fell promptly to pre-EPOCH levels very quickly after re-institution of HAART. Likewise, although CD4 lymphocyte counts fell by a median of 189 cells/mm^3 by the completion of cycle 6, the CD4s had returned to baseline levels by 12 to 18 months following completion of EPOCH. No new opportunistic infections (OI) occurred during chemotherapy, although three patients developed OIs within the first 3 months of completion of EPOCH. During EPOCH, neutropenia (<500 cells/mm^3) was evident in 30% of cycles, febrile neutropenia was seen in 13% of cycles, and 21% of cycles were associated with a platelet count of less than 50,000/mm^3.

Several biologic markers associated with prognosis in lymphoma were studied as part of this trial, and their impact upon prognosis was assessed. High MIB-1 activity (>80%), associated with greater proliferative rate and poor prognosis in HIV-negative patients was present in 85% of these HIV positive individuals, but did not correlate with response or survival after EPOCH. Similarly, p53 expression, associated with poor prognosis in HIV-negative cases, was of no significance in terms of predicting survival in these EPOCH-treated patients. Bcl 2 expression, however, was predictive of shorter survival.

Most recent studies have demonstrated the advantage of combination antiretroviral and chemotherapy for AIDS-lymphoma, and there is no question that HAART has been associated with a remarkable prolongation in survival of these patients.[33,126–128] Thus, Antinori and colleagues demonstrated that virologic response to HAART was the only factor associated with improved rates of complete remission to CHOP or CHOP-like chemotherapy.[126] These data are in contrast to the NCI's results with EPOCH, in which outstanding rates of complete remission and long-term, disease-free survival were achieved, while purposely omitting HAART during chemotherapy.[131] The immediate re-institution of HAART at the completion of chemotherapy is clearly an important aspect of this approach.

Value of Rituximab When Combined with CHOP Chemotherapy in AIDS-Lymphoma

The addition of rituximab to the CHOP regimen has been associated with statistically significant improvements in response and survival among elderly patients with de novo diffuse large B-cell lymphoma.[132] With these facts in mind, the NCI-sponsored AIDS-Malignancy Consortium (NCI/AMC) conducted a Phase III randomized trial of the standard CHOP regimen versus CHOP plus rituximab, in a group of 151 patients with newly diagnosed AIDS-lymphoma.[133]

The regimens employed included cyclophosphamide (750 mg/m^2, IV on day 1); doxorubicin (50 mg/m^2, IV on day 1), vincristine (1.4 mg/m^2 IV on day 1, capped at 2.0 mg total), and prednisone, 100 mg orally from days 1 through 5. In patients randomized to R-CHOP, rituximab was given at a dose of 375 mg/m^2 on day 1 of each cycle, while the same doses of CHOP were begun on day 3 of each 21-day cycle. After completion of 6 cycles of R-CHOP chemotherapy, the R-CHOP patients also received three monthly doses of the antibody. All patients were treated until achievement of complete remission, plus two additional cycles, or a minimum of 6 cycles of therapy. Antiretroviral therapy, filgrastim, and prophylaxis for *Pneumocystis* pneumonia were mandated. Meningeal prophylaxis was not routinely given.

The median CD4 cell count in the R-CHOP group was 128/mm^3, versus 154/mm^3 in the CHOP patients. Approximately half of the patients on each arm had received prior antiretroviral therapy including a protease inhibitor. Diffuse large B-cell lymphoma was present in 82% of the R-CHOP, and 74% of the CHOP-treated patients. Approximately 80% of both groups had Stage III or IV disease.

Complete remission rates (including CR unconfirmed) were statistically similar, achieved in 58% of the R-CHOP patients, and in 47% of those who received CHOP alone. Death due to lymphoma occurred in 14% of R-CHOP and 29% of CHOP patients.

In terms of toxicity, absolute neutrophil counts less than 500/mm^3 occurred in 62% of R-CHOP versus 48% of CHOP patients ($p = 0.11$), and in 21% of R-CHOP cycles versus 17% of CHOP cycles ($p = 0.19$). Rates of febrile neutropenia were also similar, occurring in 31% of R-CHOP cycles and 24% of CHOP cycles ($p = 0.35$). Nonetheless, there was a significant increase in death due to infection in the R-CHOP group, occurring in 14% of R-CHOP patients versus 2% of the CHOP group ($p = 0.035$). Thus, 14 of the 15 patients who died of infection had been randomized to R-CHOP. Of note, the CD4 cell count was available on 13 of these individuals, and 8 (61%) had CD4 cells less than

50/mm^3. Forty percent (6/15) of the fatal infections occurred during the maintenance phase of rituximab, after completion of all chemotherapy. In contrast, death due to lymphoma occurred in 10% of the R-CHOP group versus 19.5% of CHOP-treated patients.

The results of this study are somewhat difficult to interpret, especially in terms of the reported increase in infectious deaths in the patients treated with R-CHOP. The fact that over 60% of these deaths occurred in patients with CD4 cells of less than 50/mm^3 would suggest the possibility that this fatal complication was more related to the severe underlying immune deficiency[134] than to the use of rituximab per se. The fact that there was no statistically significant difference in the incidence of infection, or in the occurrence of neutropenic sepsis, would also mandate a consideration of the myriad of factors that may predict whether a neutropenic patient with sepsis actually dies.

The finding that R-CHOP was no more efficacious than CHOP alone in the AMC/NCI trial is also noteworthy. The R+CHOP-treated patients tended to have a higher CR rate than those treated with CHOP alone. Further, 29% of CHOP-treated patients died of progressive lymphoma, versus 14% of those who received CHOP with rituximab. A recent Phase II French study of R-CHOP in patients with AIDS-lymphoma[135] reported a higher complete remission rate (77%) than that reported by the AMC/NCI (59%). Nonetheless, the majority (54%) of the French patients had low-risk IPI scores (0 or 1), and the study was therefore "driven" by the inclusion of these individuals. Further, the median CD4 cell count was relatively high (180/mm^3), and the median HIV viral load was relatively low (9236 copies/cc) in the French study. It is possible that the excellent results in the French R+CHOP trial were due to the addition of rituximab to CHOP. Alternatively, these results may also be due to the fact that a relatively low-risk group of patients was enrolled. The French study was also smaller than that of the NCI/AMC, and was not randomized.[135]

It is clearly possible that rituximab does *not* improve the response rate of patients with AIDS-lymphoma, when added to the standard CHOP regimen. In this regard, *Bcl 2* has been associated with poor prognosis in patients with aggressive B-cell lymphoma.[136] *Bcl 2* expression is also important in determining response to R-CHOP in elderly HIV-negative patients, with *Bcl-2*–positive cases more likely to benefit from addition of rituximab.[137] It is certainly possible that AIDS-related aggressive lymphomas may be less likely to express *Bcl-2*, and thus less likely to benefit from the addition of rituximab. In this regard, Little and colleagues from the NCI have compared *Bcl-2* expression in 25 HIV-infected and 33 HIV-negative patients with diffuse large B-cell lymphoma.[131] *Bcl 2* was expressed in 16% of the AIDS-related cases, and 41% of the de novo lymphomas. If these data hold true in larger series, one might expect that addition of rituximab would be less beneficial in the setting of AIDS-lymphoma, since *Bcl-2* is less frequently expressed in these cases.

A full understanding of the results of the current AMC/NCI trial will require further elucidation of *Bcl-2* status of these patients, and further detailed analysis of the factors associated with infectious death among the R-CHOP-treated patients.

Therapy of Patients with Relapsed or Primary Resistant AIDS-Lymphoma

Treatment options for patients with relapsed or refractory AIDS-lymphoma are limited. The infusional CDE regimen has been associated with a complete remission rate of 4% in a group of 24 patients with relapsed/refractory disease, and a median survival of 2 months.[138] A regimen consisting of etoposide, prednimustine, and mitoxantrone resulted in complete response in 8 of 21 patients (38%), but a median survival of only 2 months.[139] While associated with uniform Grade 4 neutropenia, the infusional etoposide, solo-medrol, high-dose cytosine cis-platia (ESHAP) regimen, when given to 13 patients with relapsed or refractory AIDS-lymphoma led to complete remission in 31%, overall response in 54%, and median survival of 7.1 months from the time of ESHAP.[140] High-dose chemotherapy, followed by autologous stem cell rescue has been efficacious in patients with relapsed/refractory AIDS-lymphoma, with complete remission rates and toxicity profiles similar to that seen in HIV-negative patients, provided that effective antiretroviral therapy is also employed.[141] Primary central nervous system lymphoma, occurring in the HIV setting, carries a very poor prognosis but is fortunately declining in frequency since the introduction of HAART. (See Chapter 16C.) The optimal management of patients with AIDS related primary CNS lymphoma has yet to be defined.

PRIMARY EFFUSION LYMPHOMA

Primary effusion lymphoma (PEL) is an aggressive B-cell lymphoma, usually confined to body cavities, which occurs primarily, but not exclusively, in HIV-infected patients.[142,143] Patients with HIV associated PEL tend to be homosexual/bisexual males, with severe immunosuppression. PEL is caused by a gamma 2 herpes virus termed Kaposi sarcoma–associated herpes virus (KSHV), also known as human herpes virus Type 8 (HHV-8).[142,143] HHV-8 is also the cause of Kaposi sarcoma (KS), from which it was first isolated.[144]

The malignant cells in PEL are large and pleomorphic, and may resemble Reed–Sternberg cells, although they are CD15 negative. Phenotypically, the cells stain for leukocyte common antigen CD45 and various activation antigens (HLA-DR, EMA, CD30, CD38, CD77), but are usually negative for other B- and T-cell markers including CD20 and CD19. The B-cell nature can be demonstrated by the presence of immunoglobulin gene rearrangements by Southern blot or PCR. The malignant cells in PEL are derived from postfollicular B cells, which harbor somatic hypermutations of the immunoglobulin genes. The pathogenesis of PEL is of interest, since HHV 8 carries a number of oncogenic sequences including a *bcl-2* like sequence, a G-protein coupled receptor, and a Type D cyclin similar to PRAD1.[145] The virus also produces cytokines such as viral IL-6, capable of contributing to angiogenesis and tumor cell growth.[146]

Patients with PEL classically present with symptoms and signs of an effusion (pleural, pericardial, or ascitic) in the absence of a tumor mass. Extension to adjacent structures such as the chest wall, pleura, or peritoneum may also occur. Rarely, PEL may be diagnosed in the absence of an effusion, either at diagnosis or during the course of disease. With standard CHOP chemotherapy, median survival has been in the range of only 60 days.[142] Several case reports have documented the successful use of HAART, either with[147] or without[148] antiherpetic therapy. While the PEL cells do not classically express CD20, a case of pathologically confirmed complete remission of PEL after HAART and rituximab has also been described.[149]

CASTLEMAN'S DISEASE

Multicentric Castleman's disease (MCD) is a polyclonal lymphoproliferative disorder characterized by recurrent fevers, lymphadenopathy, hepatosplenomegaly, and autoimmune phenomena, which often progresses to malignant lymphoma. The plasma cell variant of MCD has been described in the setting of underlying HIV infection, and appears to be associated with HHV-8 infection, with a high degree of HHV-8 lytic gene activity and high-titer viremia.[150] While cidofovir and ganciclovir have been effective against HHV-8 in vitro, cidofovir was shown to be ineffective when used in patients with AIDS-KS.[151] Nonetheless, AIDS patients receiving ganciclovir for cytomegalovirus retinitis had a 40% reduction in the risk of developing KS over time, suggesting that antiherpetic therapy may be of some clinical value in HHV-8-related diseases.[152] The optimal therapy of HIV-associated MCD is unknown. Recently, Casper and colleagues demonstrated the efficacy of ganciclovir (5 mg/kg twice daily for 1 week, and then once daily) given to three HIV-infected patients with MCD.[153] Rituximab has also shown activity in this setting, with complete remission attained in four of six such patients.[154] Of interest, splenectomy has also been efficacious in HIV-infected patients with MCD, associated with resolution of fevers, and improvement in anemia.[155] Long-lasting remission was described in 8 of 10 such patients, after receipt of both splenectomy and HAART.[155]

HODGKIN'S DISEASE IN SETTING OF HIV INFECTION

While not considered an AIDS-defining illness, the incidence of Hodgkin's disease is clearly increased among HIV-infected individuals.[156] Unusual clinical and pathologic characteristics of HD have been described in this setting. Thus, systemic "B" symptoms are almost always present, mixed cellularity HD is the predominant pathologic subtype of disease, and advanced, extranodal disease is expected in the majority.[156] Bone marrow involvement has been documented in 40% to 60% of patients at initial diagnosis, and patients often undergo the initial diagnostic bone marrow examination for the evaluation of fever of unknown origin in the setting of HIV infection and pancytopenia. While standard multiagent chemotherapy may be curative in most HIV-negative patients with Stage III or IV HD, the median survival for HIV-infected patients has been in the range of 1 to 2 years.[156] Standard-dose ABVD with hematopoietic growth factor support was evaluated in a multi-institutional trial of 21 HIV-infected patients.[157] Antiretroviral therapy was not used. Neutropenia (<500 cells/dL) developed in almost 50%, and median survival for the group was only 18 months. It is possible that results would have improved with concomitant use of highly active antiretroviral therapy (HAART), as was demonstrated with the Stanford V regimen, employed in 59 HIV-infected patients from Italy.[158] In this study, complete remission was attained in 81%, and 56% of these (i.e., 45% of all patients treated) were estimated to remain disease-free at a median follow-up interval of 33 months.[158] Grade 3 or 4 neutropenia occurred in 78%, despite use of G-CSF. Further work will be required to define the optimal therapy for such patients.

References

1. Frizzera C, Rosai J, Dehner LP, et al. Lymphoreticular disorders in primary immunodeficiency: New findings based on an updated histologic classification of 35 cases. Cancer 1950;46:692.
2. Penn I. Tumors of the immunocoinpromised patient. Annu Rev Med 1988;39:63–73.
3. Purtilo DT. Opportunistic non-Hodgkin's lymphoma in X-linked recessive immunodeficiency and lymphoproliferative syndromes. Semin Oncol 1977;4:335–43.
4. Zulman J, Jaffe R, and Talal N. Evidence that the malignant lymphoma of Sjogren's syndrome is a monoclonal D cell neoplasm. N Engl J Med 1978;299:1215–20.
5. Anderson LG and Talal N. The spectrum of benign to malignant lymphoproliferation in Sjogren's syndrome. Clin Exp Immunol 1972;10:199–201.
6. Burke JS, Butler J, and Fuller LM. Malignant lymphomas of the thyroid;A clinical-pathologic study of 35 patients including ultrastructural observations. Cancer 1977;39: 1587–602.
7. Levine AM, Taylor CR, Schneider DR, et al. Immunoblastic sarcoma of T cell versus B cell origin. I. Clinical features. Blood 1981;58:52–61.
8. Penn I. Cancers complicating organ transplantation. N Engl J Med 1990;323:1767–9.
9. Swinnen LJ, Costanzo-Nordin MR, Fisher SG, et al. Increased incidence of lymphoproliferative disorder after immunosuppression with the monoclonal antibody OKT3 in cardiac transplant recipients. N Engl J Med 1990;323: 1723–8.
10. Centers for Disease Control and Prevention. Diffuse, undifferentiated non-Hodgkin's lymphoma among homosexual males—United States. MMWR Morb Mortal Wkly Rep 1982;31:277–9.
11. Centers for Disease Control and Prevention. Update on acquired immune deficiency syndrome (AIDS)–United States. MMWR Morb Mortal Wkly Rep 1982;31:507–8.
12. Centers for Disease Control and Prevention. Revision of the case definition of acquired immunodeficiency syndrome for national reporting-United States. Ann Intern Med 1985; 103:373–5.
13. Beral V, Peterman T, Berkelman R, et al. AIDS-associated non-Hodgkin's lymphoma. Lancet 1991;337:805–9.
14. Palella FJ Jr, Delaney KM, Moorman AC, et al. Declining morbidity and mortality among patients with advanced human immunodeficiency virus infection. N Engl J Med 1998;338:853–60.
15. Ledergerber B, Telenti A, and Effer M. Risk of HIV related Kaposi's sarcoma and non-Hodgkin's lymphoma with potent antiretroviral therapy: prospective cohort study. BMJ 1999; 319:23–4.
16. Mocroft A, Katama C, Johnson AM, et al. AIDS across Europe, 1994–1998: the EuroSIDA study. Lancet 2000;356: 291–6.
17. Levine AM. Lymphoma complicating immunodeficiency disorders. Ann Oncol 1994;4(Suppl 2):S29–35.

18. DeVesa SS and Fears T. Non-Hodgkin's lymphoma time trends: U.S. and international data. Cancer Res 1992;52: 5432–40.
19. Rabkin CS, Biggar RJ, and Horm JW. Increasing incidence of cancers associated with the human immunodeficiency virus epidemic. Int J Cancer 1991;47:692–6.
20. Biggar RJ and Rabkin CS. The epidemiology of acquired immunodeficiency syndrome-related lymphomas. Curr Opin Oncol 1992;4:883.
21. Grulich AE, Wan X, Law MG, et al. B cell stimulation and prolonged immune deficiency are risk factors for non-Hodgkin's lymphoma in people with AIDS. AIDS 2000;14: 144–0.
22. Cote TR, Biggar RF, Rosenberg PS, et al. Non-Hodgkin's lymphoma among people with AIDS. Incidence, presentation and public health burden. Int J Cancer 1997;73:645–50.
23. Biggar RJ, Rosenberg PS, and Cote T. Kaposi's sarcoma and non-Hodgkin's lymphoma following the diagnosis of AIDS. Int J Cancer 1996;68:754–8.
24. Biggar RJ, Engels EA, Frisch M, et al. Risk of T cell lymphomas in persons with AIDS. J AIDS 2001;26:371–6.
25. Serraino D, Salamina C, Franceschi S, et al. The epidemiology of AIDS-associated non-Hodgkin's lymphoma in the World Health Organization European Region. Br J Cancer 1992;66:912–6.
26. Monfardini S, Vaccher E, and Tirelli U. AIDS associated non-Hodgkin's lymphoma in Italy: Intravenous drug users versus homosexual men. Ann Oncol 1990;1:203–11.
27. Ragni MV, Belle SH, Jaffe RA, et al. Acquired immunodeficiency syndrome-associated non-Hodgldn's lymphomas and other malignancies in patients with hemophilia. Blood 1993;81:1889–97.
28. Peters BS, Beck E, Coleman DG, et al. Changing disease patterns in patients with AIDS in a referral center in the United Kingdom: the changing face of AIDS. BMJ 1991;302:203–7.
29. Nelson RA, Levine AM, and Bernstein L. Reproductive factors and risk of intermediate or high grade B cell non-Hodgkin's lymphoma in women. J Clin Oncol 2001;19: 1381–7.
30. Holly EA, Lele C, and Bracci P. Non-Hodgkin's lymphoma in homosexual men in the San Francisco Bay area: Occupational, chemical and environmental exposures. J AIDS 1997; 15:223–31.
31. Dean M, Jacobson LP, McFarlane G, et al. Reduced risk of AIDS lymphoma in individuals heterozygous for the CCR5-Δ32 mutation. Cancer Res 1999;59:3561–4.
32. Rabkin CS, Yang Q, Goedert JJ, et al. Chemokine and chemokine receptor gene variants and risk of non-Hodgkin's lymphoma in human immunodeficiency virus–1 infected individuals. Blood 1999;93:1838–42.
33. Besson C, Goubar A, Gabarre J, et al. Changes in AIDS related lymphoma since the era of highly active antiretroviral therapy. Blood 2001;98:2339–44.
34. Pantaleo G, Craziosi C, and Fauci AS. Mechanisms of disease: the immunopathogenesis of human immunodeficiency virus infection. N Engl J Med 1993;328:327–35.
35. Schnittman SM, Lane HC, Higgins SE, et al. Direct polyclonal activation of human B lymphocytes by the AIDS virus. Science 1986 233:1084–6.
36. Konrad RJ, Kricka LJ, Goodman DBF, et al. Myeloma-associated paraprotein directed against the H1V-1 p24 antigen in an HIV-1 seropositive patient. N Engl J Med 1993;328:1817–9.
37. Berberian L, Valles-Ayoub Y, SunN, et al. A Vh clonal deficit in human HIV immunodeficiency virus-positive individuals reflects a B-cell maturational arrest. Blood 1991;78:175–9.
38. Karp J. Overview of AIDS-related lymphomas: a paradigm of A IDS malignancies. In: Broder S, Merigan TC Jr, Bolognesi D, eds., Textbook of AIDS Medicine. Baltimore, Williams & Wilkins, 1994:415–29.
39. Paul WE. Interleukin 4/B cell stimulatory factor 1: one lymphokine, many functions. FASEB J 1987;1:456–61.
40. Jelinek DF and Lipsky PE. Enhancement of human B cell proliferation and differentiation by tumor necrosis factor-alpha and interleukin 1. J Immunol 1987;139:2970–6.
41. Jelinek DF, Splawski JB, and Lipsky PE. The roles of interleukin-2 and interferon-gamma in human B cell activation, growth, and differentiation. Eur J Immunol 1986;16:925–32.
42. Hirano T, Yasukawa K, Harada H, et al. Complementary DNA for a novel human interleukin (BSF-2) that induces B lymphocytes to produce immunoglobulin. Nature 1986; 324:73–6.
43. Saeland S. Duvert V, Pandrau D, et al. Interleukin-7 induces the proliferation of normal human B cell precursors. Blood 1991;78:2229–38.
44. Zlotnik A and Morre KW. Interleukin 10. Cytokine 1991; 3:366.
45. Fauci A, Schnittman SM, Poli G, et al. Immunopathogenetic mechanisms in human immunodeficiency virus (HIV) infection. Ann Intern Med 1991;114:678–93.
46. Kawano M, Hirano T, Matsuda T, et al. Autocrine generation and requirement of BSF-2/IL-6 for human multiple myelomas. Nature 1988;332:83–5.
47. Biondi A, Rossi V, Bassan R, et al. Constitutive expression of IL-6 gene in chronic lymphocytic leukemia. Blood 1989; 73:1279–84.
48. Yoshizald K, Matsuda T, Nishimoto N, et al. Pathogenic significance of IL-6 (IL-6/BSF-2) in Castleman's disease. Blood 1989;74:1360–7.
49. Emilie D, Coumbaras J, Raphael M, et al. Interleukin-6 production in high-grade B lymphomas: correlation with the presence of malignant immunoblasts in acquired immunodeficiency syndrome and in human immunodeficiency virus-seronegative patients. Blood 1992;80:498–504.
50. Pluda JM, Venzon DJ, Tosato G, et al. Parameters affecting the development of non-Hodgkin's lymphoma in patients with severe human immunodeficiency virus infection receiving antiretroviral therapy. J Clin Oncol 1993;11:1099–107.
51. Moore KW, Vieria P, Fiorentino DF, et al. Homology of cytokine synthesis inhibitory factor (IL-10) to the Epstein–Barr virus gene (BCHF). Science 1990;248:1230–4.
52. Fiorentino DF, Bond MW, and Mossmann TR. Two types of mouse helper T cells: IV. Th2 clones secrete a factor that inhibits cytokine production by Th-1 clones. J Exp Med 1989;170:2081–2095.
53. Benjamin D, Knobloch TJ, and Dayton MA. Human B cell interleuldn-10: B cell lines derived from patients with acquired immunodeficiency syndrome and Burkitt's lymphoma constitutively secrete large quantities of interleukin-10. Blood 1992;80:1289–98.
54. Masood R, Zhang Y, Bond MW, et al. Interleukin 10 is an autocrine growth factor for acquired immunodeficiency syndrome related B cell lymphoma. Blood 1995;85:3423–30.
55. Breen EC, Boscardin WJ, Epeldegui M, et al. Multifactorial analyses of serum markers of B cell activation prior to the development of AIDS associated non-Hodgkin's B cell lymphoma. Paper presented at 7th International Conference on Malignancies in AIDS and Other Immunodeficiencies, Bethesda, MD, April 28–29, 2003 [abstract 8].
56. Birx DI, Redfield RR, and Tosato G. Defective regulation of Epstein–Barr virus infection in patients with acquired immunodeficiency syndrome (AIDS) or AIDS-related disorders. N Engl J Med 1986;314:874–9.
57. Undahl T, Klein G, Reedman BM, et al. Relationship between Epstein–Barr virus DNA and the EBV determines nuclear antigen (EBNA) in Burkitt lymphoma biopsies and other

lymphoproliferative malignancies. Int J Cancer 1974; 13:764.

58. Ceser A, DeThe G, Lcnoir G, et al. Final case reporting from the Uganda prospective study of the relationship between EBV and lymphoma. Int J Cancer 1982;29:397.
59. Purtilo DT. Opportunistic non-Hodgkin's lymphoma in X-linked recessive immunodeficiency and lymphoproliferative syndromes. Semin Oncol 1977;4:335.
60. Gregory CD, Dive C, Henderson S, et al. Activation of Epstein–Barr virus latent genes protects human B cells from death by apoptosis Nature 1991;349:612–4.
61. Wang D, Tjebowjtz D, and Kief TE. An EBV membrane protein expressed in immortalized lymphocytes transforms established rodent cells. Cell 1985;43:831–40.
62. Calender A, Cordier M, Billaud M, et al. Modulation of cellular gene expression in B lymphoma cells following in vitro infection by Epstein–Barr virus (EBV), Int J Cancer 1990; 46:658–63.
63. Gregory CD, Murray RJ, Edwards CF, et al. Downregulation of cell adhesion molecules LFA-3 and ICAM-1 in Epstein–Barr virus–positive Burkitt's lymphoma underlies tumor cell escape from virus-specific T cell surveillance. J Exp Med 1988;167:1811–24.
64. Luka J, Jornvall H, and Klein G. Purification and biochemical characterization of the Epstein–Barr virus–determined nuclear antigen and an associated protein with a 53,000-dalton subunit. J Virol 1980;35:592–602.
65. Shibata D, Weiss LM, Nathwani BN, et al. Epstein–Barr virus in benign lymph node biopsies from individuals infected with the human immunodeficiency virus is associated with concurrent or subsequent development of non-Hodgkin's lymphoma. Blood 1991;77:1527–33.
66. MacMahon EME, Class D, Hayward SD, et al. Epstein–Barr virus in AIDS-related primary central nervous system lymphoma Lancet 1991:338:969–73.
67. Subar M, Neri A, Inghirami G, et al. Frequent c-myc oncogene activation and infrequent presence of Epstein–Barr virus genome in AIDS-associated lymphoma. Blood 1988; 72:667–71.
68. Hamilton-Dutoit SJ, Pallesen C, Franzmann MB, et al. AIDS-related lymphoma;Histopathology, immunophenotype, and association with Epstein–Barr virus as demonstrated by in situ nucleic acid hybridization. Am J Pathol 1991;138: 149–63.
69. Hamilton-Dutoit SJ, Raphael M, Audouin J, et al. In situ demonstration of Epstein–Barr virus Early Regional (EBER 1) in acquired immunodeficiency syndrome-related lymphomas: Correlation with tumor morphology and primary site. Blood 1993;82:619–24.
70. Shibata D, Weiss LM, Hemandez AM, et al. Epstein–Barr virus-associated non-Hodgkin's lymphoma in patients infected with the human immunodeficiency virus. Blood 1993;81:2102–9.
71. Neri A, Barriga F, Inghirami G, et al. Epstein–Barr virus infection precedes clonal expansion in Burkitt's and acquired immuno-deficiency-associated lymphoma. Blood 1991; 77:1092–5.
72. Ames BN and Gold LS. Too many rodent carcinogens: mitogenesis increases mutagenesis. Science 1990;249:970–1.
73. Zech I, Haglund U, Nilsson K, et al Characteristic chromosomal abnormalities in biopsies and lymphoid cell lines from patients with Burkitt and non-Burkitt lymphomas. Int J Cancer 1976;17:47.
74. Berger R, Bernheim A, Bertrand S, et al. Variant chromosomal t(8;22) translocation in four French cases with Burkitt lymphoma-leukemia. Nouv Rev Fr Hematol 1981;23:39.
75. Chaganti RSK, Jhanwar SC, Koziner B, et al. Specific translocations characterize Burkitt's-like lymphoma of homosexual men with the acquired immunodeficiency syndrome. Blood 1983;61:1269–74.
76. Peterson JM, Tubbs RR, Savage RA, et al. Small noncleaved B cell Burkitt-like lymphoma with chromosome t(8;14) translocation and Epstein Barr–virus nuclear associated antigen in a homosexual man with acquired immunodeficiency syndrome. Am J Med 1985;78:141.
77. Groopman JE, Sullivan L, Mulder C, et al. Pathogenesis of B-cell lymphoma in a patient with AIDS. Blood 1986; 67:612–5.
78. Alonso ML, Richardson ME, Metroka CE, et al. Chromosome abnormalities in AIDS-associated lymphadenopathy. Blood 1987;69:855–8.
79. Pelicci PG, Knowles DM II, Arlin ZA, et al. Multiple monoclonal B cell expansions and c-myc oncogene rearrangements in acquired immune deficiency syndrome-related lymphoproliferative disorders: implications for lymphomagenesis. J Exp Med 1986;164:2049–60.
80. Levine AM. Gill PS, Krailo M, et al. Natural history of persistent generalized lymphadenopathy (PGL) in gay men: risk of lymphoma and factors associated with development of lymphoma. Blood 1986;68:130a.
81. Ballerini P, Caidano G, Gong JZ, et al. Multiple genetic lesions in AIDS-related non-Hodgkin's lymphoma. Blood 1993;81:166–76.
82. Delecluse HJ, Raphael M, Magaud JP, et al. Variable morphology of human immunodeficiency virus-associated lymphomas with c-myc rearrangements. Blood 1993;82:552–63.
83. Ballerini P, Caidano C, Gong JZ, et al. Molecular pathogenesis of HIV-associated lymphomas. AIDS Res Hum Retroviruses 1992;8:731–5.
84. Haluska FG, Russo G, Kant J, et al. Molecular resemblance of an AIDS-associated lymphoma and endemic Burkitt lymphomas: implications for their pathogenesis. Proc Natl Acad Sci U S A 1989;86:8907–11.
85. Lombardi L, Newcomb EW, and Dalla-Favera R. Pathogenesis of Burkitt lymphoma: expression of an activated c-myc oncogene causes the tumorigenic conversion of EBV infected human B lymphoblasts. Cell 1987;46:161.
86. Adams JM, Harris AW, Pinkert CA, et al. The c-myc oncogene driven by immunoglobulin enhancers induces lymphoid malignancy in transgcnic mice. Nature 1985;318: 553.
87. Laurence J and Astrin SM. Human immunodeficiency virus induction of malignant transformation in human B lymphocytes. Proc Natl Acad Sci U S A 1991;88:7635–9.
88. Pauza CD, Galindo J, and Richman DD. Human immunodeficiency virus infection of monoblastoid cells;Cellular differentiation determines the pattern of vinis replication. J Virol 1988;62:3558.
89. Ye BH, Lista F, Lo Coco F, Knowles DM, et al. Alterations of a zinc finger-encoding gene, BCL-6, in diffuse large cell lymphoma. Science 1993;262:747–50.
90. Gaidano G, Lo Coco F,Ye BH, et al. Rearrangements of the BCL-6 gene in acquired immunodeficiency syndrome associated non-Hodgkin's lymphoma: association with diffuse large cell subtype. Blood 1994:84:397–402.
91. Gaidano G, Carbone A, Pastore C, et al. Frequent mutation of the 5' noncoding region of the BCL 6 gene in acquired immunodeficiency syndrome related non-Hodgkin's lymphomas. Blood 1997;89;3755–62.
92. Gaidano G, Ballerini P, Gong JZ, et al. p53 mutations in human lymphoid malignancies: Association with Burkitt lymphoma and chronic lymphocytic leukemia. Proc Natl Acad Sci U S A 1991;88:5413–7.
93. Dryja TP, Rapaport JM, Joyce JM, et al. Molecular detection of deletions involving band ql4 of chromosome 13 in retinoblastoma. Proc Natl Acad Sci U S A 1986;83:7391–4.

94. NCI Non-Hodgkin's Lymphoma Classification Project Writing Committee. Classification of non-Hodgkin's lymphomas: reproducibility of major classification systems. Cancer 1985;55:91.
95. Levine AM, Gill PS, Meyer PR, et al. Retrovirus and malignant lymphoma in homosexual men. JAMA 1985;254: 1921–5.
96. Knowles DM, Chamulak GA, Subar M, et al. Lymphoid neoplasia associated with the acquired immunodeficiency syndrome (AIDS): the New York University experience. Ann Intern Med 1988;108:744–53.
97. Lowenthal DA, Straus DJ, Campbell SW, et al. AIDS-related lymphoid neoplasia: the Memorial Hospital experience. Cancer 1988;61:2325–37.
98. Kaplan LD, Abrams DI, Feigal E, et al. AIDS-associated non-Hodgkin's lymphoma in San Francisco. JAMA 1989;261: 719–24.
99. Ziegler JL, Beckstead JA, Volberding PA, et al. Non-Hodgkin's lymphoma in 90 homosexual men: relation to generalized lymphadenopathy and the acquired immunodeficiency syndrome. N Engl J Med 1984;311:565–70.
100. Lukes RJ, Parker JW, Taylor CR, et al. Immunologic approach to non-Hodgkin's lymphomas and related leukemias: analysis of the results of multiparameter studies of 425 cases. Semin Hematol 1978;15:322–51.
101. Centers for Disease Control and Prevention. Revision of the CDC surveillance case definition for acquired immunodeficiency syndrome. MMWR Morb Mortal Wkly Rep 1987;36(Suppl):1S.
102. Raphael J, Centihomme O, Tulliez M, et al. Histolopathologic features of high-grade non-Hodgkin's lymphomas in acquired immunodeficiency syndrome. Arch Pathol Lab Med 1991;115:15–20.
103. Carbone A, Tirelli U, Vaccher E, et al. A clinicopathologic study of lymphoid neoplasms associated with human immunodeficiency virus infection in Italy. Cancer 1991; 68:842–52.
104. Ioachim HL, Dorsett B, Cronin W, et al. Acquired immunodeficiency syndrome-associated lymphomas: Clinical, pathological, immunologic and viral characteristics of 111 cases. Hum Pathol 1991;22:659–73.
105. Levine AM, Burkes RL, Walker M, et al. Development of B cell lymphoma in two monogamous homosexual men. Arch Intern Med 1985;145:479–81.
106. Levine AM. Acquired immunodeficiency syndrome-related lymphoma. Blood 1992;80:8–20 [review].
107. Levine AM, Sadeghi S, Espina B, et al. characteristics of indolent non-Hodgkin's lymphoma in patients with type 1 human immunodeficiency virus infection. Cancer 2002;94: 1500–6.
108. Horning SJ and Rosenberg SA. The natural history of initially untreated low-grade non-Hodgkin's lymphomas. N Engl J Med 1984;311:1471–5.
109. Ciobanu N, Andreef M, Safai B, et al. Lymphoblastic neoplasia in a homosexual patient with Kaposi's sarcoma. Ann Intern Med 1983;98:151.
110. Presant CA, Gala K, Wiseman C, et al. Human immunodeficiency virus-associated T-cell lymphoblastic lymphoma in AIDS. Cancer 1987;60:1459–61.
111. Janier M, Katlama C, Flageui B, et al. The pseudo-Sezary syndrome with CD8 phenotype in a patient with the acquired immunodeficiency syndrome (AIDS). Ann Intern Med 1989;110:738–40.
112. Goldstein J, Becker N, DelRowe J, et al. Cutaneous T-cell lymphoma in a patient infected with HIV, type 1. Cancer 1990;66:1130.
113. Crane GA, Variakojis D, Rosen ST, et al. Cutaneous T-cell lymphoma in patients with human immunodeficiency virus infection. Arch Dermatol 1991;127:989–94.
114. Sternlieb J, Mintzer D, Kwa D, et al. Peripheral T-cell lymphoma in a patient with the acquired immunodeficiency syndrome. Am J Med 1988;85:445.
115. Baurmann H, Miclea M, Ferchal F, et al. Adult T-cell leukemia associated with HTLV-I and simultaneous infection by HIV type 2 and human herpes virus 6 in an African woman: a clinical, virofogic, and familial serologic study. Am J Med 1988;85:853–7.
116. Shibata D, Brynes R, Rabinowitz A, et al. HTLV-I associated adult T cell leukemia lymphoma in a patient infected with HIV-1. Ann Intern Med 1989;111:871–5.
117. Gill PS, Harrington W, Kaplan MH, et al. Treatment of adult T cell leukemia-lymphoma with a combination of interferon alpha and zidovudine. N Engl J Med 1995;332:1744–8.
118. Gonzalez-Clemente JM, Ribera JM, Campo E, et al. Ki-1 positive anaplastic large cell lymphoma of T cell origin in an HIV-infected patient. AIDS 1991;5:751–5.
119. Chadburn A, Cesarman E, Jagirdar J, et al. CD30 (Ki-1) positive anaplastic large cell lymphomas in individuals infected with the HIV. Cancer 1993;72:3078–90.
120. Straus DJ, Juang J, Testa MA, et al. Prognostic factors in the treatment of HIV associated non-Hodgkin's lymphoma. Analysis of AIDS Clinical Trials Group protocol 142: Low dose versus standard dose m-BACOD plus GM-CSF. J Clin Oncol 1998;16:3601–6.
121. Rossi G, Donisi A, Casari S, et al. The International Prognostic Index can be used as a guide to treatment decisions regarding patients with HIV related systemic non-Hodgkin's lymphoma. Cancer 1999;86:2391–7.
122. Levine AM, Wernz JC, Kaplan L, et al. Low dose chemotherapy with central nervous system prophylaxis and zidovudine maintenance in AIDS-related lymphoma: a prospective multi-institutional trial. JAMA 1991;266:84–8.
123. Kaplan LD, Straus DJ, Testa MA, et al. Randomized trial of standard-dose versus low dose m-BACOD chemotherapy for HIV-associated non-Hodgkin's lymphoma. N Engl J Med 1997;336:1641–8.
124. Ratner L, Lee J, Tang S, et al. Chemotherapy for HIV associated non-Hodgkin's lymphoma in combination with highly active anti-retroviral therapy. J Clin Oncol 2001;19:2171–8.
125. Gill PS, Rarick MU, Brynes RL, et al. Azidothymidine and bone marrow failure in AIDS. Ann Intern Med 1987; 107:502–5.
126. Antinori A, Cingolani A, Alba L, et al. Better response to chemotherapy and prolonged survival in AIDS related lymphomas responding to highly active antiretroviral therapy. AIDS 2001;15:1483–91.
127. Vaccher E, Spina M, de Gennaro G, et al. concomitant cyclophosphamide, doxorubicin, vincristine, and prednisone chemotherapy plus highly active antiretroviral therapy in patients with human immunodeficiency virus–related non-Hodgkin's lymphoma. Cancer 2001;91:155–63.
128. Hoffmann C, Wolf E, Fatkenheuer G, et al. Response to highly active antiretroviral therapy strongly predicts outcome in patients with AIDS related lymphoma. AIDS 2003; 17:1521–9.
129. Sparano JA, Wiernik PH, Hu X, et al. Pilot trial of infusional cyclophosphamide, doxorubicin and etoposide plus didanosine and filgrastim in patients with HIV associated non-Hodgkin's lymphoma. J Clin Oncol 1996;14:3026–35.
130. Sparano JA, Lee S, Henry DH, et al. Infusional cyclophosphamide, doxorubicin and etoposide in HIV associated non-Hodgkin's lymphoma: a review of the Einstein, Aviano, and ECOG experience in 182 patients. Abstracts of the 4th International AIDS Malignancy Conference, May 16–18, 2000, Bethesda, MD. J AIDS 2000;23:A11 [abstract S15].

131. Little RF, Pittaluga S, Grant N, et al. Highly effective treatment of acquired immunodeficiency syndrome related lymphoma with dose adjusted EPOCH. Impact of antiretroviral therapy suspension and tumor biology. Blood 2003;101: 4653–9.
132. Coiffier B, Lepage E, Briere J, et al. CHOP chemotherapy plus rituximab compared with CHOP alone in elderly patients with diffuse large B cell lymphoma. N Engl J Med 2002; 346:235–42.
133. Kaplan LD, Lee JY, Ambinder RF, et al: Rituximab does not improve clinical outcome in a randomized phase III trial of CHOP with or without rituximab in patients with HIV associated non-Hodgkin's lymphoma: AIDS Malignancies Consortium Trial 010. Blood 2005;106:1538–43.
134. Meynard J-L, Guiguet M, Fonquernie L, et al. Impact of highly active antiretroviral therapy on the occurrence of bacteraemia in HIV infected patients and their epidemiologic characteristics. HIV Med 2003;4:127–32.
135. Boue F, Gabarre J, Gisselbrecht C, et al. CHOP chemotherapy plus rituximab in HIV patients with high grade lymphoma-results of an ANRS trial. Blood 2002;100:470a [abstract 1824].
136. Gascoyne RD, Adomat SA, Krajewski S, et al. Prognostic Significance of Bcl-2 protein expression and Bcl-2 gene rearrangement in diffuse aggressive non-Hodgkin's lymphoma. Blood 1997;90:244–51.
137. Mounier N, Briere J, Gisselbrecht C, et al. Rituximab plus CHOP (R-CHOP) overcomes bcl–2 associated resistance to chemotherapy in elderly patients with diffuse large B cell lymphoma (DLBCL). Blood 2003:101:4279–84.
138. Errante D, Santarossa S, Antinori A, et al. Second line chemotherapy with CDE in patients with resistant HIV related non-Hodgkin's lymphoma. Proc ASCO 1998;17:57a.
139. Tirelli U, Errante D, Spina M, et al. Second line chemotherapy in HIV related non-Hodgkin's lymphoma. Cancer 1996; 77:2127–31.
140. Bi J, Espina BM, Tulpule A, et al. High dose cytosine arabinoside and cisplatin regimens as salvage therapy for refractory or relapsed AIDS related non-Hodgkin's lymphoma. J AIDS 2001;28:416–21.
141. Krishnan A, Zaia J, and Forman SJ. Should HIV positive patients with lymphoma be offered stem cell transplants? Bone Marrow Transplant 2003:32:741–8.
142. Nador RG, Cesarman E, Chadburn A, et al. Primary effusion lymphoma: a distinct clinicopathologic entity associated with the Kaposi's sarcoma-associated herpes virus. Blood 1996;88:645–56.
143. Nador RG, Cesarman E, Knowles DM, et al. Herpes-like DNA sequences in a body-cavity-based lymphoma in an HIV-negative patient. N Engl J Med 1995;333:943.
144. Chang Y, Cesarman E, Pessin MS, et al. Identification of herpes virus-like DNA sequences in AIDS-associated Kaposi's sarcoma. Science 1994;266:1865–9.
145. Cesarman E, Mesri EA, and Gershengorn MC. Viral G protein-coupled receptor and Kaposi's sarcoma: a model of paracrine neoplasia? J Exp Med 2000;191:417–22.
146. Aoki Y, Jaffe ES, Chang Y, et al. Angiogenesis and hematopoiesis induced by Kaposi's sarcoma–associated herpes virus–encoded interleukin-6. Blood 1999;93: 4034–43.
147. Hocqueloux L, Agbalika F, Oksenhender E, et al. Long-term remission of AIDS-related primary effusion lymphoma. AIDS 2001;15;280–2.
148. Oksenhendler E, Clauvel JP, Jouveshomme S, et al. Complete remission of primary effusion lymphoma with antiretroviral therapy. Am J Hematol 1998;57:266.
149. Rubin N, Said J, and Levine AM. Successful therapy of relapsed HIV related primary effusion lymphoma with HAART and rituxan. Paper presented at 7th International Conference on Malignancies in AIDS and Other Immunodeficiencies. Bethesda, MD, April 28–29, 2003 [abstract 91].
150. Dupin N, Diss TL, Kellam P, et al. HHV-8 is associated with a plasmablastic variant of Castleman disease that is linked to HHV-8-positive plasmablastic lymphoma. Blood 2000;95: 1406–12.
151. Little RF, Merced-Galindez F, Humphrey R, et al. A clinical trial of cidofovir in patients with Kaposi's sarcoma. Paper presented at 5th International AIDS Malignancy Conference, Bethesda, MD, April 23–25, 2001 [abstract 52].
152. Martin DF, Juppermann BD, Wolitz RA, et al. Oral ganciclovir for patients with cytomegalovirus retinitis treated with a ganciclovir implant N Engl J Med 1999:340;1063–70.
153. Casper C, Nichols WG, Huang M-L, et al. Remission of HHV-8 and HIV-associated multicentric Castleman's Diseaes with Ganciclovir treatment. Blood 2004;103:1632–4.
154. Marcelin AG, Aaron L, Mateus C, et al. Rituximab for HIV associated Castleman's disease. Paper presented at 7th International Conference on Malignancies in AIDS and Other Immunodeficiencies, Bethesda, MD, April 28–29, 2003 [abstract 10].
155. Coty P, Astrow A, Gallinson D, et al. Splenectomy is an effective treatment for HIV associated Castleman's Disease. Paper presented at 7th International Conference on Malignancies in AIDS and Other Immunodeficiencies. Bethesda, MD, April 28–29, 2003 [abstract 11].
156. Levine AM. Hodgkin's disease in the setting of human immunodeficiency virus infection. J Natl Cancer Inst 1998; 23:37–42.
157. Levine AM, Li P, Cheung T, et al. Chemotherapy consisting of DTIC with G-CSF in HIV infected patients with newly diagnosed Hodgkin's Disease: a prospective multi-institutional AIDS Clinical Trials Group Study (ACTG 149). J AIDS 2000;24:444–50.
158. Spina M, Gabarre J, Rossi G, et al. Stanford V regimen and concomitant HAART in 59 patients with Hodgkin's disease and HIV infection. Blood 2002;100:1984–8.

34B

Post-Transplant Lymphoproliferative Disease

Jonathan W. Friedberg, M.D.
Lode J. Swinnen, M.D.

Post-transplant lymphoproliferative disease (PTLD) is a heterogeneous clinical entity manifested by an abnormal expansion of lymphoid cells in patients following solid organ or hematopoietin stem cell transplantation. Clinically, the disease ranges from benign polyclonal lymphocyte expansions to aggressive, often fatal, monoclonal non-Hodgkin's lymphoma. The clinical, pathologic, and molecular features of PTLD differ significantly from those of non-Hodgkin's lymphomas encountered in immunocompetent individuals. Despite the curability of a proportion of patients, both morbidity and mortality from the disease has typically been high, and the disease is responsible for a significant proportion of deaths more than 1 year after solid organ transplantation; in several series the most common invasive malignancy that occurs in this group of patients.[1,2] Several studies suggest a rising prevalence of PTLD over the past decade, including patients surviving more than 10 years following transplant. The outcome of PTLD, particularly monoclonal disease, remains poor. However, several novel treatment approaches are under investigation, and new approaches toward prevention will hopefully decrease morbidity from PTLD in the future.

EPIDEMIOLOGY

Penn has reported 562 neoplasms that occurred in 548 heart and combined heart–lung allograft recipients.[1] Forty-two percent of these malignancies were lymphomas, and in the 33 pediatric patients with malignancy after transplantation, lymphomas were seen in 82% of these patients. The incidence of PTLD was significantly higher after cardiac transplant than in renal transplant recipients. Similarly, Lanza et al. found a twofold greater incidence in neoplasms, particularly PTLD, after cardiac transplantation compared with after renal transplantation.[3] In a French series of 701 cardiac recipients, 13 developed PTLD, for a frequency of 1.8%.[4]

A multicenter, collaborative project quantified the risk of PTLD after kidney or heart transplantation in over 50,000 patients.[5] The risk of PTLD was higher in heart transplant patients compared with renal transplant patients. During the first post-transplant year, 1.2% of heart transplant patients developed NHL. The incidence of NHL was lower in subsequent years, with a risk of 0.3%/year in cardiac transplant recipients. With longer patient follow-up, the incidence of PTLD after solid organ transplantation is rising.[6] Recent series of thoracic organ transplant recipients with long-term follow-up have reported cumulative risk of development of PTLPD that exceeds 5%.[7] While PTLD occurs most commonly in the early post-transplant period, there is a second wave later in follow-up. Children are at considerably higher risk than adults.

Risk Factors

In the multicenter collaborative project, three factors were found to increase the risk of PTLD after transplantation using multivariate analysis.[5] PTLD was significantly increased in the United States as compared with Europe, possibly secondary to more aggressive immunosuppression regimens used in the United States during the early 1990s. Patients given either ATG or OKT3 as prophylaxis showed a higher incidence of NHL. Finally, the incidence of PTLD was increased if immunosuppression included the combination of cyclosporine and azathiaprine as compared with cyclosporine with or without steroids.

Significant increases in PTLD incidence have repeatedly been linked with specific immunosuppressive drugs or regimens. Agents specifically targeting or depleting T cells result in the highest levels of risk, and the effect is at least partially dependent on the intensity and duration of T-cell suppression. The immunosuppressive antibody OKT3, a potent anti T-cell agent, resulted in a nine fold higher incidence of PTLD in cardiac transplant recipients receiving induction immunotherapy, with an incidence of 35.7% in patients who had received two courses of the drug.[8] In a recent analysis of the United Network for Organ Sharing (UNOS) registry data for 2713 renal transplant recipients, the use of various immunotherapy induction agents was compared with no induction therapy. The use of monoclonal antilymphocyte antibodies resulted in a 72% increase in risk, from an incidence of 0.51% to an incidence of 0.85%. The use of polyclonal antilymphocyte antibodies, or of anti- IL-2 receptor antibody, resulted in nonsignificant increases of 29% and 14%, respectively.[9] Many other observations are consistent with the view that the intensity of immunosuppression and particularly the use of selective anti–T-cell agents, correlates well with the risk for PTLD.[10]

Pre-transplant EBV seronegativity is perhaps the single greatest risk factor for PTLD. Seronegative recipients will almost all seroconvert within 1 year of transplantation. The majority of seronegative patients are children, with the likelihood of seronegativity being determined by age and by social and geographic factors. The incidence of PTLD in the pediatric age group is not as well defined as among adults, but is clearly appreciably higher, with up to 15% incidence after heart transplantation; a series from the University of Pittsburgh identified a four times higher risk of PTLD for pediatric than for adult transplant recipients.[11] In a series of 381 nonrenal transplant patients from the Mayo Clinic, including 43 heart transplant recipients, 14 cases of PTLD were identified.[12] EBV seronegative recipients had a 24-fold higher risk of PTLD compared with EBV seropositive recipients. OKT3 therapy and CMV seromismatch further increased this risk. PTLD in EBV seronegative patients also had a worse prognosis in this series.[12] EBV primary infection after cardiac transplantation in seronegative pediatric recipients resulted in PTLD in 12 of 19 patients in a report from Columbia University.[13]

Specific risk factors for the development of PTLD after allogeneic stem cell transplantation are well established, and include HLA mismatching, T-cell depletion, and the use of antilymphocyte antibodies as conditioning or treatment of graft-versus-host disease (similar to the solid organ experience).[14]

In the setting of immunosuppression, DNA polymorphisms have been shown to confer a risk of the development of non-Hodgkin's lymphoma.[15,16] A polymorphism associated with low expression of the interferon-γ (IFN-γ) has been reported to be a risk factor for PTLD[17]; specifically, the A allele at a T/A polymorphism in intron 1 is associated with low expression, and also with increased risk of PTLD.[18,19] In one study, 6 or 9 (67%) PTLD patients were homozygous for the low producer IFN-γ gene compared with 37 of 143 (37%) kidney transplant patients without PTLD.[19] Studies are ongoing to clarify this and other potential risk groups.

Therefore, the two major risk factors for the development of PTLD after transplantation are pre-transplant–negative recipient EBV serology, and the degree of post-transplant immunosuppression (Table 34–2).[20] Prophylactic approaches under investigation include elimination, when possible, of these risk factors.[20]

ETIOLOGY AND PATHOPHYSIOLOGY: ROLE OF EPSTEIN–BARR VIRUS

The majority of cases of PTLD are EBV associated, suggesting that the virus plays a central role in the pathogenesis of this disease. One of the earliest observations was that clinical or serologic indications of a primary or reactivated EBV infection were frequent around the time of clinical appearance of the disorder. Tumor tissue was subsequently found to often contain EBV-DNA in much larger quantities than normal tissue, and to actively express viral proteins.[21] Suppression of T-cell function or numbers to prevent graft rejection is believed to result in uncontrolled EBV-driven proliferation of B cells. Continued proliferation would then result in clones with a growth advantage, giving rise to one or more clonal populations. In fact, tumor-associated EBV is clonal, further supporting an etiologic role for the virus, rather than incidental subsequent infection of an already expanded neoplastic B-cell proliferation.

The virus is usually of Type A (Type 1).[22] In addition, lesions consisting of polyclonal B-cell proliferations contain multiple EBV clones, while monoclonal proliferations show evidence of a single infectious event.[23,24] A preclinical phase for PTLD is also suggested by observations that viral load, as determined in peripheral blood mononuclear cells, increases prior to the appearance of clinically detected disease (discussed in detail below).[25,26] It is not clear whether such rises in EBV load necessarily indicate EBV-driven neoplasia, or are reflective of severe immunodeficiency at that point in time. The clinical observations of increased PTLD risk following primary EBV infection, and in association with progressively more potent anti–T-cell drugs, are very consistent with a disease model based on insufficient or inadequate T-cell surveillance of EBV-driven lymphoproliferation. This model is less informative in cases of PTLD that occur late after transplantation, and in cases of T-cell or EBV-negative PTLD.

EBV infection of resting B cells in vitro results in immortalized lymphoblastoid cell lines that express the full range of latent viral cycle proteins (six nuclear antigens: EBNA-1, EBNA-2, EBNA-3A, -3B, -3C, EBNA-LP, and three membrane proteins: LMP-1, LMP-2A, LMP-2B), the so-called latency III pattern. It is often stated that expression of viral latency proteins in PTLD is essentially that seen in lymphoblastoid cell lines, consistent with severely diminished EBV-specific T-cell function. Restoration of T-cell surveillance by withdrawal or reduction in immunosuppressive therapy can in fact result in permanent regression of PTLD, particularly those presenting early after transplantation. In the setting of allogeneic stem cell transplantation, donor lymphocyte infusion often results in eradication of PTLD.[14] However, in many instances PTLD will not regress with such measures, despite expression of immunodominant EBNAs in the tumor. Varying degrees of restriction of antigenic expression have been identified in tumor tissue, possibly reflecting varying degrees of immune control, or evolution over time to proliferations with structural genetic alterations.[27,28]

Table 34–2. Populations at High Risk for Post-Transplant Lymphoproliferative Disease

Pre-transplant Epstein–Barr virus seronegative/pediatric age group
Thoracic organ transplant recipient
Monoclonal anti-CD3 antibodies as immunosuppression
Mismatched bone marrow transplant or T-cell depleted bone marrow transplant
Low expression interferon-γ (DNA polymorphism)

PATHOLOGY

Marked variability is characteristic of the pathology and the molecular features of PTLD. Nonetheless, a spectrum appears to exist, with polymorphic, polyclonal proliferations at one end, and monomorphic, predominantly monoclonal tumors closely resembling aggressive non-Hodgkin's lymphomas at the other. Whether transition along this spectrum occurs in vivo, or whether the different entities are reflective of an individual pathogenesis in each case, remains an open question. Unlike the situation following allogeneic stem cell transplantation, PTLD following solid organ transplantation is most often of recipient origin.[29,30]

Like NHL in the non-immunocompromised setting, adequate histology is necessary for diagnosis of PTLD. Excisional biopsy should be performed whenever possible, as needle biopsy and cytologic evaluations are often inadequate or not representative of the tumor. Microscopic examination should be performed by a pathologist experienced in lymphoproliferative diseases. In addition to standard histologic evaluation, the clonality of B and T cells should be determined. Immunoperoxidase studies, in particular CD20, may provide important therapeutic information.[20] Several pathologic classifications have been used, the most recent being that of the World Health Organization (Table 34–3).[17,31,32] However, polymorphic post-transplant lymphoproliferative disorder, with EBNA-2 expression, does not occur in normal individuals, and therefore is a separate classification. Rare cases of indolent B-cell malignancies and Hodgkin's disease have been reported posttransplant.[33,34] These are not considered as PTLDs at the present time, and should be approached as disease in the nonimmunosuppressed host.

EBV status of the malignancy should be determined using in situ assays or immunostaining (Fig. 34–1). Paraffin sections of diagnostic biopsy specimens may be stained for EBV latent membrane protein-1 (LMP-1) using a commercially available antibody, or for EBV small nuclear RNAs (EBERs) using a commercially available nucleic acid probe. Quantitative EBV PCR is an emerging technology that may allow early, more reliable diagnosis; however, additional study is required before routine clinical use, as detailed below.[25,26]

Histologically, PTLD occurring early after transplantation appears polymorphic and classified as plasmacytic hyperplasia and infectious mononucleosis-like PTLD (IM-PTLD). The proliferations are typically polyclonal or show only small clonal components. IM-PTLD closely resembles infectious mononucleosis, and may simply be infectious mononucleosis in an immunocompromised host. Whether this represents a true PTLD, with the same potential for morbidity, is controversial. With the exception of bcl-6 mutations, seen in somewhat less than half the cases, additional genotypic abnormalities are not expected. The vast majority of PTLD presenting early after transplantation are EBV associated.

Table 34–3. Categories of Post-Transplant Lymphoproliferative Disease

1. Early lesions
   Reactive plasmacytic hyperplasia
   Infectious mononucleosis-like
2. Polymorphic PTLD
3. Monomorphic PTLD
   B-cell:
      Diffuse large-cell lymphoma-like
      Burkitt-like
      Plasmacytoma-like
      Myeloma-like
   T-cell neoplasms
4. Hodgkin's lymphoma and Hodgkin's lymphoma–like PTLD

Adapted from Harris NL, Swerdlow SH, Frizzera G, et al. Post transplant lymphoproliferative disorders. In: Jaffe ES, Harris NL, Stein H, et al., eds. World Health Organization Classification of Tumours. Pathology and Genetics of Haematopoietic and Lymphoid Tissues. Lyon: International Agency for Research on Cancer Press, 2001: 264–9,32 with permission.
PTLD, post-transplant lymphoproliferative disease.

This spectrum of EBV-driven proliferation has been difficult to categorize beyond simple clonality studies. The transition from polyclonal to monoclonal proliferation, recognized for 25 years,[35] continues to be poorly understood, and is likely multifactorial.[36] In a series of 28 PTLDs, Knowles et al. identified three categories exhibiting distinctive morphologic and molecular genetic characteristics.[37] Plasmacytic hyperplasia lesions were polyclonal, EBV positive, usually were found in the oropharynx or lymph nodes, and may represent the earliest lymphoid proliferations post-transplant. Polymorphic B-cell hyperplasia/lymphomas were observed in both lymph nodes and extranodal sites. These lesions were almost always monoclonal. Finally, malignant lymphomas were clonal lymphoproliferations with p53, ras, or c-myc mutations. These designations were found to be clinically relevant in a subsequent analysis. Plasmacytic hyperplasia and polymorphic lesions were likely to respond to a reduction in immunosuppression or surgery alone, whereas malignant lymphomas were likely to be resistant even to aggressive clinical interventions.[38]

PTLD occurring early after transplantation characteristically contains admixture of reactive T cells. Polymorphic PTLD especially can have more than 50% T cells with some monomorphic PTLD also reported to be T-cell rich.[39,40] The nature of these T cells is variable and has not been extensively studied, with some cases showing a predominance of CD8+ cells and others predominantly CD4+ cells.[41]

With longer follow-up, increasing numbers of patients with PTLD not associated with EBV have been reported. These usually occur late after solid organ transplantation. In a French series that included 15 patients with PTLD after cardiac transplantation, 11 of 35 lymphomas failed to express EBV. Among 13 lymphomas diagnosed after more than 2 years post-transplant, only 5 were associated with EBV.[42] Similarly, in a series of 15 patients who developed PTLD a median of 79 months after organ transplant, only 44% of samples demonstrated the presence of EBV.[43] These lymphomas demonstrated a histologic and clinical presentation similar to immunocompetent subjects; however, clinical outcome was poor, with a median survival of only 7 months. There is considerable heterogeneity in immunophenotype, with some cases having a phenotype-like follicular center cells (CD10+, bcl-6+, CD138–) and others being clearly post-follicular (CD10–, bcl-6–, CD138+). Lesions are predominantly clonal, and most will have Bcl-6 mutations; various genotypic abnormalities have been described, including c-myc rearrangements and p53 mutations.[37,44,45]

T-cell NHL, unrelated to EBV or HHV-8, also appears to be increased late after solid organ transplantation. Six patients described by Hanson et al. had a particularly

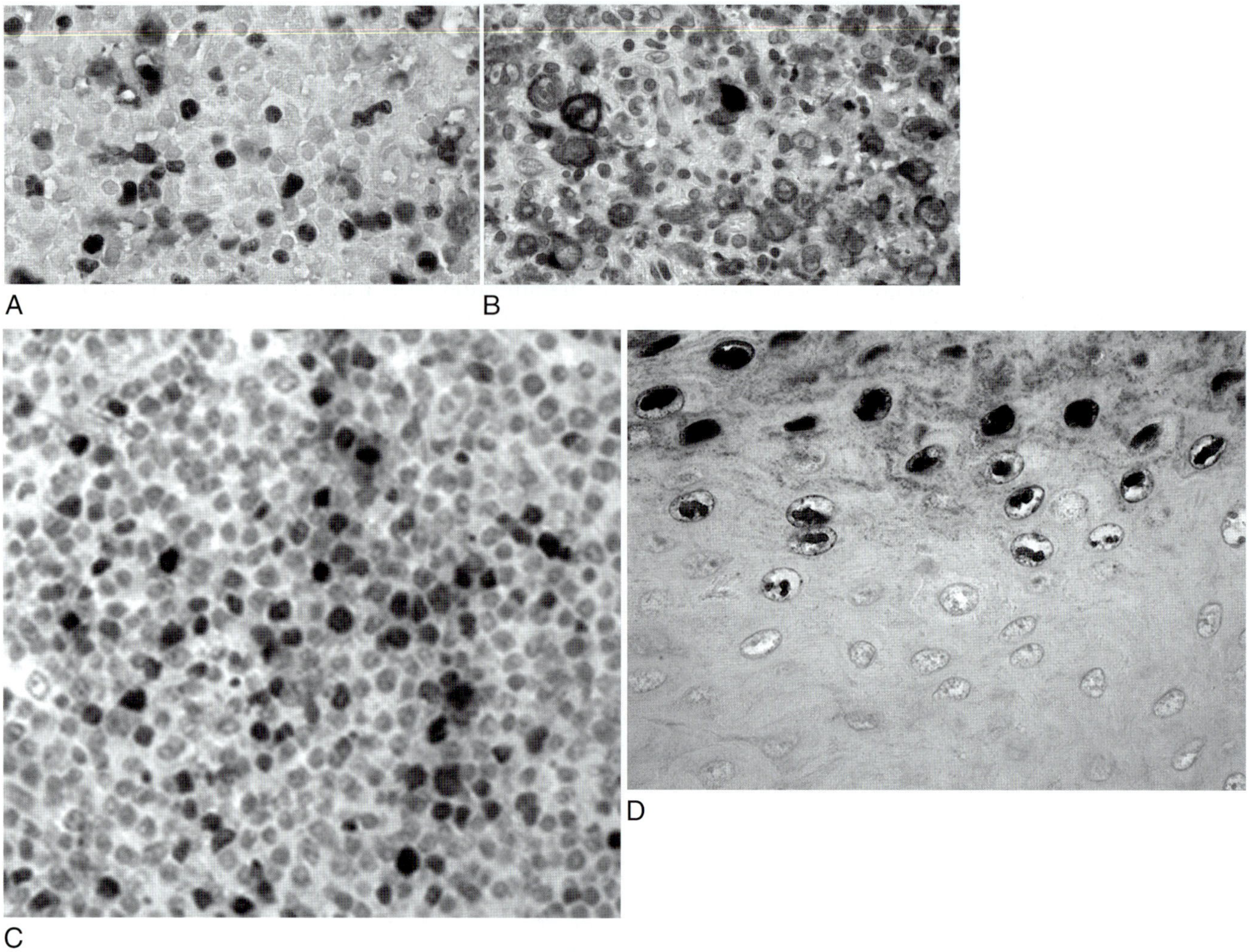

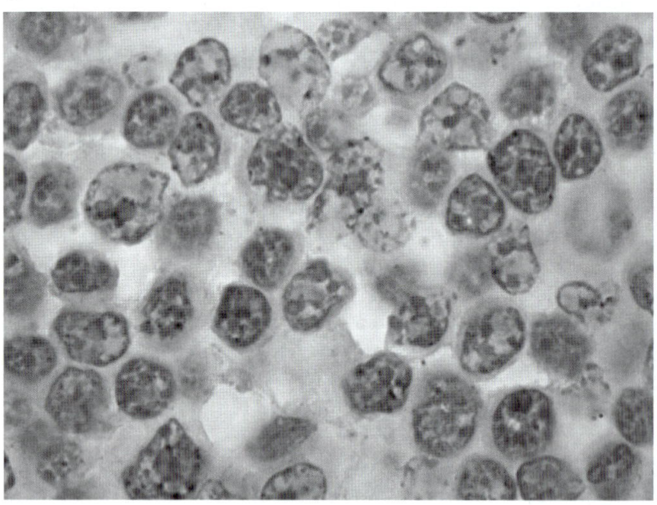

E

Figure 34–1. Examples of detection of EBV and related herpes viruses in situ. **A:** Chromogenic in situ hybridization for small nuclear RNAs (EBERs). **B:** Immunostaining for LMP-1. **C:** Immunostaining for EBNA2. **D:** Chromogenic in situ hybridization for the rhesus EBV-like lymphocryptovirus. **E:** Chromogenic in situ hybridization for the human EBV genomes. **A**, **B**, **C**, and **E** represent stains performed on tissue sections prepared from human PTLDs that are latently infected with EBV. **D** is an example of chromogenic in situ hybridization for the LCV genome performed on sections taken from an epithelial lesion wherein cells are lytically infected. In each instance, staining is developed with a horseradish peroxidase-based method that produces a brown color. Individual EBV genomes in (**E**) are seen as small nuclear dots. (See color insert.)

aggressive course, with a median survival of 5 weeks.[46] A single case of EBV-negative primary effusion lymphoma related to HHV8 has been reported in a cardiac transplant recipient with a history of Kaposi's sarcoma.[47]

CLINICAL PRESENTATION AND OUTCOME

PTLD after solid organ transplantation has several unique features, which differentiate it from non-Hodgkin's lymphoma (NHL) in the immunocompetent host. Most patients present with lymphadenopathy or a mass; however, extranodal involvement, a poor prognostic indicator in aggressive non-Hodgkin's lymphoma,[48] is often present. In many series, isolated extranodal disease is the most common presentation of PTLD, and in a minority of patients, disease is confined to the lymphatic system. CNS involvement occurred in 22% of PTLDs in a registry experience of over 1000 patients.[49] Other common extranodal sites include the lung and gastrointestinal tract, which may be associated with a better prognosis.[50] The allograft may be involved; 22% of the time in a study evaluating heart, lung, and liver transplants.[1] Particularly in patients following lung and liver transplantation, this phenomenon has been confused with rejection, emphasizing the importance of experienced hematopathologists in evaluating questionable biopsies. Diagnosis is made by autopsy in a minority of cases, often when concomitant infection or rejection is present.

The prognosis for PTLD is again highly variable, determined in part by clinical variables in the individual patient, and by response to the treatment modality used. Attempts at identifying factors predictive of outcome have been made; one large retrospective series of 61 patients identified EBV negativity in the tumor or T-cell phenotype as negative tumor-related prognostic factors. The International Prognostic Index for aggressive lymphoma in immunocompetent patients[48] was less predictive in PTLD than was a specific index using two risk factors: performance status 0 or 1 versus more than 2, and number of involved sites (1 vs. >1).[51] A similar retrospective review of 54 cases with analysis for prognostic variables found advanced-stage involvement of the allograft, poor performance status, and CD20 negativity, to be statistically significant negative prognostic factors.[52] In view of the therapeutic value of the anti-CD20 antibody rituximab (see below), it is important accurately assess CD20 positivity, as many of the cells in a PTLD may be infiltrating benign T cells.[53]

CLINICAL EVALUATION

Evaluation of patients with PTLD should follow guidelines for aggressive lymphomas outside the setting of immunodeficiency, including a careful history for "B" symptoms (fever, night sweats, weight loss), and complete physical examination. Standard radiographic evaluation includes CT scan of the chest, abdomen, and pelvis. An MRI of brain with gadolinium enhancement should be performed for any neurologic symptoms. The role of nuclear imaging with FDG-PET[54] has yet to be defined in this histology, but may be helpful in differentiating between a residual mass after therapy, and persistent involvement with lymphoma. Laboratory evaluation should include complete blood count, differential, and platelet count, chemistry panel for liver and renal function, uric acid, calcium, and LDH. All patients with advanced-stage disease or an abnormal complete blood count should undergo bone marrow biopsy and aspiration. A lumbar puncture for cytology is recommended for patients with advanced-stage disease, or with neurologic symptoms. Patients who present with fever must have a careful microbiologic assessment to exclude concurrent opportunistic infections that may complicate therapy, given the immunosuppressed nature of this patient population.

THERAPY

Withdrawal of Immunosuppression

Reduction or discontinuance of immunosuppression is the initial therapeutic intervention for PTLD, and may result in complete regression of early-stage disease, often without subsequent rejection of the graft.[55] The optimal approach to the reduction in immunosuppression remains to be defined and varies depending on the transplanted organ. In general, much more caution is indicated in the thoracic organ recipient than in the abdominal organ recipient. In addition, the individual patient's rejection history will strongly influence the approach to reduction of immunosuppression. At the present time, most research studies support the complete elimination of azathiaprine and mycophenolate mofetil, and a reduction of calcineurin inhibitors. Polyclonal disease, and PTLD occurring early after transplantation, has a much higher rate of response to immunosuppression modulation.[13]

Antiviral Therapy

Acyclovir inhibits viral DNA polymerase, and in clinical studies has been shown to decrease oropharyngeal shedding of EBV. Many early treatment algorithms for PTLD included antiviral therapy in an attempt to control EBV infection. Polyclonal disease, in particular, has shown responses to ganciclovir in anecdotal reports.[56] Plasmacytic hyperplasia, and mononucleosis-type syndromes after transplant may respond to antiviral therapy. Foscarnet has been shown in case reports to have activity against PTLD.[57] In vitro studies also suggest that rapamycin can inhibit the IL-10 signal transduction pathway, and growth of EBV related PTLD,[58] however anecdotal evidence is conflicting regarding in vivo activity.[59,60] The recent availability of oral valganciclovir[61] suggests another treatment option that warrants clinical evaluation.

Other Approaches to Localized Disease

Interferon-alpha is a cytokine that has been shown to decrease EBV-induced B-cell outgrowth. Anecdotal cases suggest a benefit in the treatment of PTLD. However, particularly in renal allograft patients, the use of interferon post transplant has been associated with rejection.[62] Since this drug is also associated with significant morbidity, including severe depression,[63,64] this is generally not used as standard treatment. Complete surgical resection followed by radiation therapy has been recommended for the rare case of localized, accessible PTLD, in conjunction with other treatments such as reduction in immunosuppression, however there are no controlled studies to support this approach. Cranial XRT, with or without additional therapy, is the most effective treatment of PTLD of the central nervous system (CNS).[49]

Cytotoxic Chemotherapy

Many published reports indicate a high mortality and failure rate for combination cytotoxic chemotherapy in PTLD, as compared with nonimmunosuppressed patients.[4,6] The majority of these reports are anecdotal, with short follow-up. Small series of patients treated in uncontrolled studies suggest that responses may be seen in anthracycline-based chemotherapy regimens, such as CHOP (cyclophosphamide, doxorubicin, vincristine, and prednisone), the current standard therapy for diffuse large B-cell NHL and ProMACE-CytaBOM.[65,66] In a prospective multicenter trial conducted prior to the advent of rituximab in patients refractory to reduced immunosuppression, the ProMACE-CytaBOM regimen resulted in a complete response rate of 67%, and 57% durable complete response at more than 2 years follow-up.[67] Less aggressive alkylating agent-based chemotherapy regimens have also provided responses, particularly in pediatric organ transplant recipients.[68] However, in general, chemotherapy is poorly tolerated in the PTLD patient population, and novel, less toxic strategies are needed for the majority of patients.

Cellular Immunotherapy

In a disease model where PTLD is the result of inadequate T-cell control over EBV-driven lymphoproliferation, infusion of EBV-specific T cells would be expected to cause regression or resolution of the proliferation. Adoptive transfer of EBV-specific T-cell immunity in solid organ recipients is constrained by the MHC-restricted nature of the T-cell response, and the fact that the majority of PTLDs arise from recipient rather than donor lymphocytes in the organ transplant setting.[69] Although encouraging preliminary data using autologous EBV-specific T cells expanded in vitro have been reported,[70,71] this technique is cumbersome, and with present technology, is difficult to apply to large numbers of patients in multiple institutions. Further research is ongoing in this area.

In the setting of PTLD following bone marrow or stem cell transplantation, the efficacy of unselected donor leukocytes (DLI) in reconstituting the recipient's immune system has been well described, and this approach has been frequently utilized to both prevent and treat PTLD.[14,72] Unfortunately, unselected DLI also significantly increases the risk of GVHD. Small studies suggest that EBV-specific donor T cells are effective both prophylactically and as primary therapy for PTLD after allogeneic bone marrow transplantation.[73] This has lead to interest in expanding populations of autologous cytotoxic T lymphocytes against EBV antigen or lymphokine-activated killer cells in vitro as a therapeutic modality for malignant EBV-driven lymphoproliferation after solid organ transplantation.[74] Ongoing efforts to refine either autologous or HLA-matched allogeneic EBV-specific lymphocyte processing and administration may provide effective treatment or prevention of PTLD in both the solid-organ transplant population, and allogeneic stem cell population.

Antibody Therapy

Anti-B-cell serotherapy has been successfully employed in the treatment of PTLD. A cohort of transplanted patients who developed severe PTLD were treated with murine monoclonal anti-B-cell antibodies to CD21 and CD24, with a 1-year remission rate of 69%, and overall survival at 1 year of 61%.[75] Multivariate analysis identified multivisceral disease, CNS involvement and late onset of PTLD as poor prognostic factors. Therapy was well tolerated, with only minimal infusional toxicity, and a minority of patients developing antimouse antibodies. The antibodies to CD21 and CD24 are not commercially available in the United States.

Initial reports of rituximab therapy (Rituxan®; Biogen Idec, Cambridge, MA; and Genentech Inc., South San Francisco, CA[76]) for CD20+ PTLD are promising.[77–80] A retrospective analysis of 26 patients in Europe treated with rituximab for PTLD after solid organ transplantation revealed an overall response rate of 65%.[81] The agent is clearly safe, as contrasted with cytotoxic chemotherapy, without reports of significant toxicity or damage to the allograft. Preliminary results from a larger, more recent, retrospective study of 44 patients with PTLD who did not respond to taper of immunosuppression suggest a response rate of 45% following treatment with single agent rituximab, with 15 patients achieving CR. Elevated EBV viral load appeared to predict response in these patients.[82] Finally, a multicenter study of 25 patients with PTLD treated with rituximab demonstrated a 52% CR rate, with a mean duration of response of 25 months.[83] Adverse events were rare in both of these studies. Clearly, rituximab is an active agent for PTLD, and is evolving to be a standard first-line therapy (after immunosuppressive withdrawal) for these patients.[84,85] Current ongoing investigations include the evaluation of rituximab in combination with cytotoxic chemotherapy for PTLD.[86]

Radioimmunotherapy

Because antibody-dependent cellular cytotoxicity (ADCC) may be an important component of rituximab therapy, inadequate effector cell responses may limit efficacy of this therapy, particularly in the case of PTLD, where effector cell function is frequently impaired by concomitant immunosuppressive therapy.[87] Radioimmunoconjugates—for example, murine monoclonal antibodies with an attached radioisotope—may overcome these resistance mechanisms.[88] Due to the inherent radiosensitivity of PTLD, radioimmunoconjugates have the ability to provide direct cytotoxicity in the absence of host effector mechanisms, and in the presence of impaired ADCC. Further, the bystander or "crossfire effect," which delivers radiation to neighboring cells inaccessible to antibody or with insufficient antigen expression, can result in cytotoxicity even in the absence of antibody binding to a particular target cell.[89] Ongoing clinical trials are evaluating radioimmunotherapy in the setting of PTLD, which has progressed following treatment with rituximab.

Gene Therapy

Franken et al. have described a provocative animal model suggesting a role for gene therapy techniques in the treatment of PTLD.[90] In a murine system, an EBNA2-responsive EBV promoter selectively targeted EBV-related lymphoma cells by virus-regulated expression of a suicide gene. Sensitivity to ganciclovir was selectively enhanced in cells expressing EBNA2, and moreover, there was complete macroscopic regression of established B-cell lymphomas in SCID mice treated with a single course of ganciclovir.

Summary: Sequential Approach to Therapy

Most centers currently utilize a sequential approach to therapy of EBV-associated PTLD, particularly in the solid organ transplant recipient (Table 34–4).[20,67] If immunosuppression withdrawal, with or without antiviral therapy, immunoglobulin, or interferon, does not induce a remission within 14 to 21 days, then chemotherapy is considered. Although data are limited, the promising results and low toxicity associated with monoclonal antibody therapy suggest an early role for this evolving modality. Studies in the immunocompetent host setting have suggested a role for combining immunotherapy with chemotherapy in the setting of aggressive lymphoma,[91,92] although this approach has not been prospectively evaluated in the treatment of PTLD, and has been shown to have increased toxicity in the setting of HIV-associated lymphoma.[93] The treatment of EBV-negative PTLD is less defined, but the general principle of sequential therapy is valid.[42] In the allogeneic transplant recipient, it is imperative to consider possible DLI early in the course of the disease. When possible, all patients with PTLD should be offered participation in an ongoing clinical trial. A treatment algorithm is summarized in Fig. 34–4.

Table 34–4. Sequential Therapy of Post-Transplant Lymphoproliferative Disease

All patients:
Immunosuppression taper (see below).
Consider IVIg, interferon, antiviral therapy.

Localized, accessible disease:
Consider surgery and/or localized radiation therapy.

Diffuse disease, or if no response in 14 to 21 days:
Monoclonal antibody therapy, if CD20+ (rituximab).
Combination chemotherapy, with or without rituximab.
Donor lymphocyte infusion (for stem cell transplant patients).
Novel approaches in the context of a clinical trial are always recommended.
A standard immunosuppressive taper schedule is outlined below. This should be attempted in all patients unless there is evidence of ongoing allograft rejection.
Eliminate azathiaprine and Mycophenolate Mofetil (MMF).
Reduce calcineurin inhibitor (cyclosporine or tacrolimus) by 50%.
Taper prednisone by 50% or as tolerated.

PREVENTION: SCREENING AND MONITORING

EBV Viral Load

PTLD can be subtle and is frequently misdiagnosed as infection or rejection. A definitive diagnostic test for clinically evident disease would clearly be desirable, in view of the poor prognosis attached to extensive disease or to declining performance status. Of even greater value would be a reliable test for subclinical lymphoproliferation, which should permit early preemptive treatment for PTLD. There are extensive data supporting the existence of a detectable subclinical phase to the disease. Analysis of prior liver biopsy specimens in liver transplant recipients has shown that the presence of EBV, as determined by PCR or by in situ immunohistochemical staining for EBER expressing cells, could be detected in 70% of cases who subsequently developed PTLD. Only 10% of cases who did not go on to develop PTLD had such findings.[21] More accessible indications of a preclinical phase of the disease are evident from observations that circulating viral load, as determined in peripheral blood mononuclear cells or in serum, increases prior to the appearance of clinically detected disease, which resolve following eradication of the PTLD. Some transplant centers already perform routine EBV viral load determinations, and attempt to integrate that information into the clinical management of patients. However, many uncertainties exist.[94] It is not clear when such increases in EBV load are indicative of EBV-driven neoplasia, and when they might only reflect the degree of immunodeficiency at the time. Pediatric cases are particularly challenging, as viral load may be chronically high in patients who underwent a post-transplant primary EBV infection.[95] Existing data are generally from small series with, at times, conflicting results.[25,26,96–102]

Multiple questions still need to be resolved before an effective test for routine post-transplant screening can be defined, including determination of the best compartment (peripheral blood mononuclear cells, serum, or whole blood) to sample,[99] the most suitable probes and methodologies for detection, and the establishment of stringent parameters of sensitivity and specificity in specific patient populations.[103] Also, whether quantitative measurement of EBV DNA is best used to enable prompt versus preemptive treatment of PTLD remains controversial.[104] Moreover, the role of viral load testing in the era of rituximab therapy has not been defined. At the present time, viral load testing remains investigational, and it is difficult to make definitive treatment recommendations based on results of viral load testing.

Interleukin 10

Interleukin 10 (IL-10) is an anti-inflammatory cytokine that also has activity as a growth regulator for B lymphocytes.[105] Increases in peripheral blood IL-10 have been seen in association with, and even preceding, the diagnosis of PTLD.[106,107] The EBV gene BCRF1 is a homolog of human IL-10 and its protein product has IL-10–like biological activity.[108] Although BCRF1 is usually not expressed in EBV latency III—which is associated with lymphoma in immunodeficiency states—PTLD is usually accompanied by active EBV infection and this may contribute to increasing the level of IL-10.[17] Furthermore, there is some evidence that the promoter genotype for IL-10 has an impact on primary EBV infection.[109,110] Using peripheral blood IL-10 as a screening strategy is currently under investigation.

EBV Vaccines

The lower incidence of PTLD in EBV-seropositive organ recipients in comparison with seronegative recipients provides evidence for the protective nature of an established immune response prior to transplantation and accompanying immune suppression.[11] Similarly, it may provide a rationale for boosting the existing immune response in seropositive recipients. EBV vaccines have been tested for the prevention of infectious mononucleosis and of EBV-associated malignancies. One major focus of investigation has been the major envelope glycoprotein, gp340, the principal target of the virus-neutralizing antibody response.[111] In a tamarin vaccination model, subunit antigen formulations or recombinant viral vectors expressing gp340 are protective against the development of EBV-induced B-cell lymphoma.[112,113] Whether efficacy in this model is a function of humoral or cellular immunity, or both, is unclear. Other approaches to vaccines have used defined epitopes. Moss et al. are studying "polytopes" that combine immunodominant epitopes that are recognized by the natural virus-induced CTL response.[114] Although promising, concerns remain that targeting single antigens or epitopes may engender an immune response inadequate to control virus-induced proliferation.

Cell-based therapeutic tumor vaccines have been studied in both animal models and patient trials. In contrast to peptide-based vaccines, a tumor vaccine may generate immune responses to a spectrum of antigens. For the prevention of tumors, an autologous "tumor vaccine" is not possible; however, EBV-immortalized autologous lymphocytes are readily generated in the laboratory, and express the full panel of viral latency antigens expressed in PTLD. EBV-immortalized lymphoblastoid cell lines (LCLs) are potent stimulators of the cytotoxic T-cell response in vitro, and adoptively transferred cells expanded with irradiated LCL stimulators mediate tumor regression or prevent tumor development in many instances.[115–117] Ongoing studies are addressing EBV vaccination strategies to prevent PTLD in patients at high clinical risk.

CONCLUSIONS

Although rare, PTLD warrants intensive future studies, given the increasing indications for both allogeneic stem cell transplants and solid organ transplants, and the high mortality of this disease. PTLD is a biologically fascinating disorder that greatly illuminates the roles of the immune system and viral infection in the development of lymphoma, and has implications in the understanding of other infection-driven lymphomas. Therapy of PTLD provides a prime and exciting example of successful immunotherapy of lymphoma, and novel approaches should decrease the morbidity of this disorder in the future.

Acknowledgment

Dr. Friedberg is supported in part by a career development award from the National Cancer Institute (CA 102216-01).

References

1. Penn I. Incidence and treatment of neoplasia after transplantation. J Heart Lung Transplant 1993;12:S328–36.
2. Fridell JA, Jain A, Reyes J, et al. Causes of mortality beyond 1 year after primary pediatric liver transplant under tacrolimus. Transplantation 2002;74:1721–4.
3. Lanza RP, Cooper DK, Cassidy MJ, et al. Malignant neoplasms occurring after cardiac transplantation. JAMA 1983; 249:1746–8.
4. Leblond V, Sutton L, Dorent R, et al. Lymphoproliferative disorders after organ transplantation: a report of 24 cases observed in a single center. J Clin Oncol 1995;13:961–8.
5. Opelz G and Henderson R. Incidence of non-Hodgkin lymphoma in kidney and heart transplant recipients. Lancet 1993;342:1514–6 [see comments].
6. Armitage J, Kormos R, Stuart R, et al. Posttransplant lymphoproliferative disease in thoracid organ transplant patients: ten years of cyclosporine-based immunosuppression. J Heart Lung Transplant 1991;10:877–87.
7. Gao SZ, Chaparro SV, Perlroth M, et al. Post-transplantation lymphoproliferative disease in heart and heart-lung transplant recipients:30-year experience at Stanford University. J Heart Lung Transplant 2003;22:505–14.
8. Swinnen LJ, Costanzo-Nordin MR, Fisher SG, et al. Increased incidence of lymphoproliferative disorder after immunosuppression with the monoclonal antibody OKT3 in cardiac- transplant recipients. N Engl J Med 1990;323: 1723–8 [see comments].
9. Cherikh WS, Kauffman HM, McBride MA, et al. Association of the type of induction immunosuppression with posttransplant lymphoproliferative disorder, graft survival, and patient survival after primary kidney transplantation. Transplantation 2003;76:1289–93.
10. Penn I. The changing pattern of posttransplant malignancies. Transplant Proc 1991;23:1101–3.
11. Ho M, Jaffe R, Miller G, et al. The frequency of Epstein–Barr virus infection and associated lymphoproliferative syndrome after transplantation and its manifestations in children. Transplantation 1988;45:719–27.
12. Walker R, Paya C, Marshall W, et al. Pretransplantation seronegative Epstein–Barr virus status is the primary risk factor for posttransplantation lymphoproliferative disorder in adult heart, lung, and other solid organ transplantations. J Heart Lung Transplant 1995;14:214–21.
13. Zangwill SD, Hsu DT, Kichuk MR, et al. Incidence and outcome of primary Epstein–Barr virus infection and lymphoproliferative disease in pediatric heart transplant recipients. J Heart Lung Transplant 1998;17:1161–6.
14. Loren AW, Porter DL, Stadtmauer EA, et al. Post-transplant lymphoproliferative disorder: a review. Bone Marrow Transplant 2003;31:145–55.
15. Breen EC, Boscardin WJ, Detels R, et al. Non-Hodgkin's B cell lymphoma in persons with acquired immunodeficiency syndrome is associated with increased serum levels of IL10, or the IL10 promoter—592 C/C genotype. Clin Immunol 2003;109:119–29.
16. Lin MT, Storer B, Martin PJ, et al. Relation of an interleukin-10 promoter polymorphism to graft-versus-host disease and survival after hematopoietic-cell transplantation. N Engl J Med 2003;349:2201–10.
17. Nalesnik MA. Clinicopathologic characteristics of post-transplant lymphoproliferative disorders. Recent Results Cancer Res 2002;159:9–18.

18. Pravica V, Perrey C, Stevens A, et al. A single nucleotide polymorphism in the first intron of the human IFN-gamma gene: absolute correlation with a polymorphic CA microsatellite marker of high IFN-gamma production. Hum Immunol 2000;61:863–6.
19. VanBuskirk AM, Malik V, Xia D, et al. A gene polymorphism associated with posttransplant lymphoproliferative disorder. Transplant Proc 2001;33:1834.
20. Paya CV, Fung JJ, Nalesnik MA, et al. Epstein–Barr virus-induced posttransplant lymphoproliferative disorders. ASTS/ASTP EBV-PTLD Task Force and The Mayo Clinic Organized International Consensus Development Meeting. Transplantation 1999;68:1517–25.
21. Randhawa PS, Jaffe R, Demetris AJ, et al. Expression of Epstein–Barr virus-encoded small RNA (by the EBER-1 gene) in liver specimens from transplant recipients with post-transplantation lymphoproliferative disease. N Engl J Med 1992;327:1710–4.
22. Frank D, Cesarman E, Liu YF, et al. Posttransplantation lymphoproliferative disorders frequently contain type A and not type B Epstein–Barr virus. Blood 1995;85:1396–403.
23. Cleary ML, Nalesnik MA, Shearer WT, et al. Clonal analysis of transplant-associated lymphoproliferations based on the structure of the genomic termini of the Epstein–Barr virus. Blood 1988;72:349–52.
24. Kaplan MA, Ferry JA, Harris NL, et al. Clonal analysis of posttransplant lymphoproliferative disorders, using both episomal Epstein–Barr virus and immunoglobulin genes as markers. Am J Clin Pathol 1994;101:590–6.
25. Riddler SA, Breinig MC, and McKnight JL. Increased levels of circulating Epstein–Barr virus (EBV)-infected lymphocytes and decreased EBV nuclear antigen antibody responses are associated with the development of posttransplant lymphoproliferative disease in solid-organ transplant recipients. Blood 1994;84:972–84.
26. Rooney CM, Loftin SK, Holladay MS, et al. Early identification of Epstein–Barr virus-associated post-transplantation lymphoproliferative disease. Br J Haematol 1995;89:98–103.
27. Cen H, Williams PA, McWilliams HP, et al. Evidence for restricted Epstein–Barr virus latent gene expression and anti-EBNA antibody response in solid organ transplant recipients with posttransplant lymphoproliferative disorders. Blood 1993;81:1393–403.
28. Delecluse HJ, Kremmer E, Rouault JP, et al. The expression of Epstein–Barr virus latent proteins is related to the pathological features of post-transplant lymphoproliferative disorders. Am J Pathol 1995;146:1113–20.
29. Larson RS, Scott MA, McCurley TL, et al. Microsatellite analysis of posttransplant lymphoproliferative disorders: determination of donor/recipient origin and identification of putative lymphomagenic mechanism. Cancer Res 1996;56:4378–81.
30. Chadburn A, Suciu-Foca N, Cesarman E, et al. Post-transplantation lymphoproliferative disorders arising in solid organ transplant recipients are usually of recipient origin. Am J Pathol 1995;147:1862–70.
31. Harris NL, Jaffe ES, Diebold J, et al. World Health Organization classification of neoplastic diseases of the hematopoietic and lymphoid tissues: report of the Clinical Advisory Committee meeting—Airlie House, Virginia, November 1997. J Clin Oncol 199;17:3835–49.
32. Harris NL, Swerdlow SH, Frizzera G, et al. Post transplant lymphoproliferative disorders. In: Jaffe ES, Harris NL, Stein H, et al., eds. World Health Organization Classification of Tumours. Pathology and Genetics of Haematopoietic and Lymphoid Tissues. Lyon: International Agency for Research on Cancer Press, 2001:264–9.
33. Hood IM, Mahendra P, McNeil K, et al. Hodgkin's disease after cardiac transplant: a report of two cases. Clin Lab Haematol 1996;18:115–6.
34. Hsi ED, Singleton TP, Swinnen L, et al. Mucosa-associated lymphoid tissue-type lymphomas occurring in post- transplantation patients. Am J Surg Pathol 2000;24:100–6.
35. Hanto DW, Frizzera G, Gajl-Peczalska KJ, et al. Epstein–Barr virus-induced B-cell lymphoma after renal transplantation: acyclovir therapy and transition from polyclonal to monoclonal B-cell proliferation. N Engl J Med 1982;306:913–8.
36. Yarbro JW. The Epstein–Barr virus and the distinction between benign and malignant lymphoproliferative processes. Semin Oncol 1993;20:658–61 [editorial].
37. Knowles DM, Cesarman E, Chadburn A, et al. Correlative morphologic and molecular genetic analysis demonstrates three distinct categories of posttransplantation lymphoproliferative disorders. Blood 1995;85:552–65.
38. Chadburn A, Chen JM, Hsu DT, et al. The morphologic and molecular genetic categories of posttransplantation lymphoproliferative disorders are clinically relevant. Cancer 1998; 82:1978–87.
39. Minervini MI, Swerdlow SH, and Nalesnik MA. Polymorphism and T-cell infiltration in posttransplant lymphoproliferative disorders. Transplant Proc 1999;31:1270.
40. Kowal-Vern A, Swinnen L, Pyle J, et al. Characterization of postcardiac transplant lymphomas. Histology, immunophenotyping, immunohistochemistry, and gene rearrangement. Arch Pathol Lab Med 1996;120:41–8.
41. Perera SM, Thomas JA, Burke M, et al. Analysis of the T-cell micro-environment in Epstein–Barr virus-related post-transplantation B lymphoproliferative disease. J Pathol 1998;184:177–84.
42. Leblond V, Davi F, Charlotte F, et al. Posttransplant lymphoproliferative disorders not associated with Epstein–Barr virus: a distinct entity? J Clin Oncol 1998;16:2052–9.
43. Dotti G, Fiocchi R, Motta T, et al. Epstein–Barr virus–negative lymphoproliferate disorders in long-term survivors after heart, kidney, and liver transplant. Transplantation 2000;69:827–33 [see comments].
44. Cesarman E, Chadburn A, Liu YF, et al. BCL-6 gene mutations in posttransplantation lymphoproliferative disorders predict response to therapy and clinical outcome. Blood 1998;92:2294–302.
45. Locker J and Nalesnik M. Molecular genetic analysis of lymphoid tumors arising after organ transplantation. Am J Pathol 1989;135:977–87.
46. Hanson MN, Morrison VA, Peterson BA, et al. Posttransplant T-cell lymphoproliferative disorders—an aggressive, late complication of solid-organ transplantation. Blood 1996; 88:3626–33 [see comments].
47. Jones D, Ballestas ME, Kaye KM, et al. Primary-effusion lymphoma and Kaposi's sarcoma in a cardiac-transplant recipient. N Engl J Med 1998;339:444–9 [see comments].
48. The International Non-Hodgkin's Lymphoma Prognostic Factors Project. A predictive model for aggressive non-Hodgkin's lymphoma. N Engl J Med 1993;329:987–94.
49. Penn I and Porat G. Central nervous system lymphomas in organ allograft recipients. Transplantation 1995;59: 240–4.
50. Chen JM, Barr ML, Chadburn A, et al. Management of lymphoproliferative disorders after cardiac transplantation. Ann Thorac Surg 1993;56:527–38.
51. Leblond V, Dhedin N, Mamzer Bruneel MF, et al. Identification of prognostic factors in 61 patients with posttransplantation lymphoproliferative disorders. J Clin Oncol 2001;19: 772–8.
52. Ghobrial IM, Habermann TM, Maurer MJ, et al. Proposed prognostic model for survival in solid organ transplant recip-

ients with post transplant lymphoproliferative disorders. Blood 2003;102:392a.
53. Gulley ML, Swinnen LJ, Plaisance KT Jr, et al. Tumor origin and CD20 expression in posttransplant lymphoproliferative disorder occurring in solid organ transplant recipients: implications for immune-based therapy. Transplantation 2003;76:959–64.
54. Friedberg JW and Chengazi V. PET scans in the staging of lymphoma: current status. Oncologist 2003;8:438–47.
55. Starzl TE, Nalesnik MA, Porter KA, et al. Reversibility of lymphomas and lymphoproliferative lesions developing under cyclosporin-steroid therapy. Lancet 1984;1:583–7.
56. Pirsch JD, Stratta RJ, Sollinger HW, et al. Treatment of severe Epstein–Barr virus-induced lymphoproliferative syndrome with ganciclovir: two cases after solid organ transplantation. Am J Med 1989;86:241–4.
57. Oertel SH, Ruhnke MS, Anagnostopoulos I, et al. Treatment of Epstein–Barr virus-induced posttransplantation lymphoproliferative disorder with foscarnet alone in an adult after simultaneous heart and renal transplantation. Transplantation 1999;67:765–7.
58. Nepomuceno RR, Balatoni CE, Natkunam Y, et al. Rapamycin inhibits the interleukin 10 signal transduction pathway and the growth of Epstein Barr virus B-cell lymphomas. Cancer Res 2003;63:4472–80.
59. Sindhi R. Sirolimus in pediatric transplant recipients. Transplant Proc 2003;35:113S–114S.
60. Dominguez J, Mahalati K, Kiberd B, et al. Conversion to rapamycin immunosuppression in renal transplant recipients: report of an initial experience. Transplantation 2000; 70:1244–7.
61. Reusser P. Oral valganciclovir: a new option for treatment of cytomegalovirus infection and disease in immunocompromised hosts. Expert Opin Invest Drugs 2001;10: 1745–53.
62. Magnone M, Holley JL, Shapiro R, et al. Interferon-alpha-induced acute renal allograft rejection. Transplantation 1995;59:1068–70.
63. Musselman DL, Lawson DH, Gumnick JF, et al. Paroxetine for the prevention of depression induced by high-dose interferon alfa. N Engl J Med 2001;344:961–6.
64. Malik UR, Makower DF, and Wadler S. Interferon-mediated fatigue. Cancer 2001;92:1664–8.
65. Garrett TJ, Chadburn A, Barr ML, et al. Posttransplantation lymphoproliferative disorders treated with cyclophosphamide-doxorubicin-vincristine-prednisone chemotherapy. Cancer 1993;72:2782–5.
66. Swinnen LJ. Durable remission after aggressive chemotherapy for post-cardiac transplant lymphoproliferation. Leuk Lymphoma 1997;28:89–101.
67. Swinnen LJ, LeBlanc M, Kasamon Y, et al. Phase II study of seqential reduction in immunosuppression, interferon alpha-2b, and ProMACE-CytaBOM chemotherapy for post-transplant lymphoproliferative disorder (SWOG/ECOG S9239). Blood 2003;102:403a.
68. Gross TG, Park J, Bucuvalas J, et al. Low-dose chemotherapy for refractory EBV associated post transplant lymphoproliferative disease following solid organ transplantation. Blood 2002;100:159a.
69. Liu Z, Savoldo B, Huls H, et al. Epstein–Barr virus (EBV)-specific cytotoxic T lymphocytes for the prevention and treatment of EBV-associated post-transplant lymphomas. Recent Results Cancer Res 2002;159:123–33.
70. Khanna R, Bell S, Sherritt M, et al. Activation and adoptive transfer of Epstein–Barr virus-specific cytotoxic T cells in solid organ transplant patients with posttransplant lymphoproliferative disease. Proc Natl Acad Sci U S A 1999; 96:10391–6.
71. Comoli P, Labirio M, Basso S, et al. Infusion of autologous Epstein–Barr virus (EBV)–specific cytotoxic T cells for prevention of EBV-related lymphoproliferative disorder in solid organ transplant recipients with evidence of active virus replication. Blood 2002;99:2592–8.
72. Bollard CM, Savoldo B, Rooney CM, et al. Adoptive T-cell therapy for EBV-associated post-transplant lymphoproliferative disease. Acta Haematol 2003;110:139–48.
73. Rooney CM, Smith CA, Ng CY, et al. Infusion of cytotoxic T cells for the prevention and treatment of Epstein–Barr virus-induced lymphoma in allogeneic transplant recipients. Blood 1998;92:1549–55.
74. Nalesnik MA, Rao AS, Furukawa H, et al. Autologous lymphokine-activated killer cell therapy of Epstein–Barr virus-positive and -negative lymphoproliferative disorders arising in organ transplant recipients. Transplantation 1997; 63:1200–5.
75. Fischer A, Blanche S, Le Bidois J, et al. Anti-B-cell monoclonal antibodies in the treatment of severe B-cell lymphoproliferative syndrome following bone marrow and organ transplantation. N Engl J Med 1991;324:1451–6.
76. Rastetter W, Molina A, and White CA. Rituximab: expanding role in therapy for lymphomas and autoimmune diseases. Annu Rev Med 2004;55:477–503.
77. Cook RC, Connors JM, Gascoyne RD, et al. Treatment of post-transplant lymphoproliferative disease with rituximab monoclonal antibody after lung transplantation. Lancet 1999;354:1698–9.
78. O'Dwyer ME, Launder T, Rabkin JM, et al. Successful treatment of aggressive post transplant lymphoproliferative disorder using rituximab. Leuk Lymphoma 2000;39:411–9.
79. Zilz ND, Olson LJ, and McGregor CG. Treatment of post-transplant lymphoproliferative disorder with monoclonal CD20 antibody (rituximab) after heart transplantation. J Heart Lung Transplant 2001;20:770–2.
80. Ganne V, Siddiqi N, Kamaplath B, et al. Humanized anti-CD20 monoclonal antibody (Rituximab) treatment for post-transplant lymphoproliferative disorder. Clin Transplant 2003;17:417–22.
81. Milpied N, Vasseur B, Parquet N, et al. Humanized anti-CD20 monoclonal antibody (Rituximab) in post transplant B-lymphoproliferative disorder: a retrospective analysis on 32 patients. Ann Oncol 2000;11(Suppl 1):113–6.
82. Choquet S, Herbrecht R, Soucie G, et al. Efficacy and safety of rituximab in B-cell post transplantation lymphoproliferative disorders: preliminary results of a multicenter, open label, phase II trial. Blood 2002;100:467a.
83. Oertel S, Zeidler K, Grefer J, et al. Monotherapy with the anti-CD20 antibody rituximab in patients with post transplant lymphoproliferative disease: results of a multicentre phase II study. Blood 2002;100:573a.
84. European best practice guidelines for renal transplantation. Section IV: Long-term management of the transplant recipient. IV.6.1. Cancer risk after renal transplantation. Post-transplant lymphoproliferative disease (PTLD): prevention and treatment. Nephrol Dial Transplant 2002;17(Suppl 4):31–3, 35–6.
85. Garnier JL, Stevenson G, Blanc-Brunat N, et al. Treatment of post-transplant lymphomas with anti-B-cell monoclonal antibodies. Recent Results Cancer Res 2002;59:113–22.
86. Orjuela M, Gross TG, Cheung YK, et al. A pilot study of chemoimmunotherapy (cyclophosphamide, prednisone, and rituximab) in patients with post-transplant lymphoproliferative disorder following solid organ transplantation. Clin Cancer Res 2003;9:3945S–52S.
87. Multani PS and Grossbard ML. Monoclonal antibody-based therapies for hematologic malignancies. J Clin Oncol 1998; 16:3691–710.

88. Cheson BD. Radioimmunotherapy of non-Hodgkin lymphomas. Blood 2003;101:391–8.
89. Friedberg JW and Fisher RI. Iodine-131 tositumomab (Bexxar(R)): radioimmunoconjugate therapy for indolent and transformed B-cell non-Hodgkin's lymphoma. Expert Rev Anticancer Ther 2004;4:18–26.
90. Franken M, Estabrooks A, Cavacini L, et al. Epstein–Barr virus-driven gene therapy for EBV-related lymphomas. Nat Med 1996;2:1379–82.
91. Haberman TM, Weller EA, Morrison VA, et al. Phase III trial of rituximab-CHOP vs. CHOP with a second randomization to maintenance rituximab or observation in patients 60 years of age and older with diffuse large B cell lymphoma. Blood 2003;102:6a.
92. Coiffier B, Lepage E, Briere J, et al. CHOP chemotherapy plus rituximab compared with CHOP alone in elderly patients with diffuse large-B-cell lymphoma. N Engl J Med 2002; 346:235–42.
93. Kaplan LD and Scadden DT. No benefit from rituximab in a randomized phase III trial of CHOP with or without rituximab for patients with HIV-associated non-Hdogkin's lymphoma: AIDS malignancies consortium study 010. Proc ASCO 2003;2:564a.
94. Stevens SJ, Verschuuren EA, Verkuujlen SA, et al. Role of Epstein–Barr virus DNA load monitoring in prevention and early detection of post-transplant lymphoproliferative disease. Leuk Lymphoma 2002;43:831–40.
95. Boyle GJ, Michaels MG, Webber SA, et al. Posttransplantation lymphoproliferative disorders in pediatric thoracic organ recipients. J Pediatr 1997;131:309–13.
96. Lucas KG, Burton RL, Zimmerman SE, et al. Semiquantitative Epstein–Barr virus (EBV) polymerase chain reaction for the determination of patients at risk for EBV-induced lymphoproliferative disease after stem cell transplantation. Blood 1998;91:3654–61.
97. Rose C, Green M, Webber S, et al. Detection of Epstein–Barr virus genomes in peripheral blood B cells from solid-organ transplant recipients by fluorescence in situ hybridization. J Clin Microbiol 2002;40:2533–44.
98. Rowe DT, Qu L, Reyes J, et al. Use of quantitative competitive PCR to measure Epstein–Barr virus genome load in the peripheral blood of pediatric transplant patients with lymphoproliferative disorders. J Clin Microbiol 1997;35: 1612–5.
99. Wagner HJ, Wessel M, Jabs W, et al. Patients at risk for development of posttransplant lymphoproliferative disorder: plasma versus peripheral blood mononuclear cells as material for quantification of Epstein–Barr viral load by using real-time quantitative polymerase chain reaction. Transplantation 2001;72:1012–9.
100. Smets F, Latinne D, Bazin H, et al. Ratio between Epstein–Barr viral load and anti-Epstein–Barr virus specific T-cell response as a predictive marker of posttransplant lymphoproliferative disease. Transplantation 2002;73:1603–10.
101. Tsai DE, Hardy CL, Tomaszewski JE, et al. Reduction in immunosuppression as initial therapy for posttransplant lymphoproliferative disorder: analysis of prognostic variables and long-term follow-up of 42 adult patients. Transplantation 2001;71:1076–88.
102. Swinnen LJ, Gulley ML, Hamilton E, et al. EBV DNA quantitation in serum is highly correlated with the development and regression of post-transplant lymphoproliferative disorder in solid organ transplant recipients. Blood 1998; 98:314–15.
103. Gartner BC, Fischinger J, Schafer H, et al. Epstein–Barr viral load as a tool to diagnose and monitor post-transplant lymphoproliferative disease. Recent Results Cancer Res 2002;159:49–54.
104. Wagner HJ, Cheng YC, Huls MH, et al. Prompt versus preemptive intervention for EBV-lymphoproliferative disease. Blood 2004;103:3979–81.
105. Moore KW, de Waal Malefyt R, Coffman RL, et al. Interleukin-10 and the interleukin-10 receptor. Annu Rev Immunol 2001;19:683–765.
106. Birkeland SA, Bendtzen K, Moller B, et al. Interleukin-10 and posttransplant lymphoproliferative disorder after kidney transplantation. Transplantation 1999;67:876–81.
107. Muti G, Klersy C, Baldanti F, et al. Epstein–Barr virus (EBV) load and interleukin-10 in EBV-positive and EBV-negative post-transplant lymphoproliferative disorders. Br J Haematol 2003;122:927–33.
108. Thompson MP and Kurzrock R. Epstein–Barr virus and cancer. Clin Cancer Res 2004;10:803–21.
109. Helminen M, Lahdenpohja N, and Hurme M. Polymorphism of the interleukin-10 gene is associated with susceptibility to Epstein–Barr virus infection. J Infect Dis 1999;180:496–9.
110. Helminen ME, Kilpinen S, Virta M, et al. Susceptibility to primary Epstein–Barr virus infection is associated with interleukin-10 gene promoter polymorphism. J Infect Dis 2001;184:777–80.
111. Hoffman GJ, Lazarowitz SG, and Hayward SD. Monoclonal antibody against a 250,000-dalton glycoprotein of Epstein–Barr virus identifies a membrane antigen and a neutralizing antigen. Proc Natl Acad Sci U S A 1980;77:2979–83.
112. Wilson AD, Lovgren-Bengtsson K, Villacres-Ericsson M, et al. The major Epstein–Barr virus (EBV) envelope glycoprotein gp340 when incorporated into Iscoms primes cytotoxic T-cell responses directed against EBV lymphoblastoid cell lines. Vaccine 1999;17:1282–90.
113. Wilson AD, Shooshstari M, Finerty S, et al. Virus-specific cytotoxic T cell responses are associated with immunity of the cottontop tamarin to Epstein–Barr virus (EBV). Clin Exp Immunol 1996;103:199–205.
114. Moss DJ, Khanna R, Sherritt M, et al. Developing immunotherapeutic strategies for the control of Epstein–Barr virus-associated malignancies. J AIDS 1999;21(Suppl 1): S80–3.
115. Savoldo B, Goss J, Liu Z, et al. Generation of autologous Epstein–Barr virus-specific cytotoxic T cells for adoptive immunotherapy in solid organ transplant recipients. Transplantation 2001;72:1078–86.
116. Orentas RJ, Lemas MV, Mullin MJ, et al. Feasibility of cellular adoptive immunotherapy for Epstein–Barr virus-associated lymphomas using haploidentical donors. J Hematother 1998;7:257–61.
117. Wagner HJ, Rooney CM, and Heslop HE. Diagnosis and treatment of posttransplantation lymphoproliferative disease after hematopoietic stem cell transplantation. Biol Blood Marrow Transplant 2002;8:1–8.

Index